# Coronary Care

# Coronary Care

*Editor*

## Joel S. Karliner, M.D.

*Associate Professor of Medicine*
*University of California, San Diego*
*Director, Clinical Cardiology Section*
*University of California Medical Center*
*San Diego, California*

*Associate Editor*

## Gabriel Gregoratos, M.D.

*Professor of Medicine*
*University of California, San Diego*
*Director, Coronary Care Unit*
*University of California Medical Center*
*San Diego, California*

## Churchill Livingstone

*New York, Edinburgh, London, and Melbourne 1981*

© Churchill Livingstone Inc. 1981

Distributed in the United Kingdom by Churchill Livingstone,
Robert Stevenson House, 1–3 Baxter's Place, Leith Walk,
Edinburgh EH1 3AF and by associated companies, branches
and representatives throughout the world.

First published 1981
Printed in U.S.A.

ISBN 0–443–08061–5
7 6 5 4 3 2 1

**Library of Congress Cataloging in Publication Data**

Main entry under title:

Coronary care.

    Includes bibliographies and index.
    1. Heart—Infarction.  2. Coronary care units.
I. Karliner, Joel S., 1936–    II. Gregoratos,
Gabriel. [DNLM: 1. Coronary diseases—Diagnosis.
2. Coronary disease—Therapy.  3. Coronary care
units.  WG300 C8213]
RC685.I6C68     616.1′23706     80–19651
ISBN 0–443–08061–5

Manufactured in the United States of America

*To Adela and Eva*

# *Preface*

Despite an encouraging reduction in mortality from cardiovascular disease over the past decade, this group of disorders continues to be the prime cause of death in the United States today. Among the various forms of cardiovascular disease, coronary heart disease claims the largest number of lives, often among individuals in their most productive years. It is estimated that over one million patients suffer an acute myocardial infarction in the United States each year and that the vast majority of such individuals are treated in a Coronary Care Unit or an Intensive Care Unit. Thus, in terms of both morbidity and mortality, coronary heart disease remains our most pressing medical problem. It was with these considerations in mind that we set out to create a text that would deal with this major health problem in the most comprehensive fashion possible. We hope that this book will fill the void that currently exists by providing a detailed treatment of the vast array of newer concepts and techniques that make up contemporary coronary care.

The current volume is divided into seven sections which deal with the fundamental aspects of acute myocardial infarction, the historical and organizational aspects of the Coronary Care Unit, the approach to the patient with acute myocardial infarction, the diagnosis of acute myocardial infarction, complications of acute myocardial infarction and their treatment, additional monitoring and diagnostic methods, and, finally, a section comprising further aspects of therapy in the patient with acute ischemic heart disease. These sections are further divided into a total of 43 chapters, many of which contain new and important information not previously available in one volume. Wherever appropriate, fundamental material from the basic sciences has been incorporated into a number of the chapters, with emphasis on clinical application. Contributions of contemporary electrophysiology, pharmacology, enzymology, nuclear methods, echocardiography, pathophysiology, and surgery have been included in this book.

The editors are authors or coauthors of six of the chapters, and one of us (JSK) has personally edited the entire volume, both in manuscript and galley form. A careful attempt has been made to avoid overlap, and, where such overlap exists, it is intentional—as, for example, in the chapters on complications of acute myocardial infarction and surgical treatment. Revisions have been made to incorporate the most recent available evidence, and many chapters contain references ranging from the last half of 1979 through the middle of 1980.

In this volume, we have also recognized that the Coronary Care Unit has assumed an increasing role in the care of patients who may have other manifestations of ischemic heart disease, such as arrhythmias, and in the treatment of individuals who have critical cardiac dysfunction of other etiology and who require intensive care and monitoring. Thus, the techniques of pacemaker implantation, hemodynamic monitoring, and vasodilator therapy described in this book can be easily applied to these patients as well.

We would like to extend our grateful thanks to all our contributors, whose efforts have enhanced the quality of this volume beyond measure. We would also like to acknowledge the consistent encouragement and help we have received from our publisher, Mr. Lewis Reines, and from the staff at Churchill Livingstone, especially Ms. Brooke Dramer and Ms. Carole Baker. Our grateful thanks also go to our secretarial staff—Ms. Billie Adair, Ms. Linda Long, Ms. Rosemary Montoya, and Ms. Barbara Wilson. We also wish to acknowledge the artistic and photographic efforts of Ms. Sue Adornato and Mr. Don Luczak and their associates in the Office of Learning Resources at the University of California, San Diego. We hope that the efforts of all these individuals have resulted in a volume that in this and future editions will provide an important resource to those engaged in the care of patients with acute and chronic ischemic heart disease.

Joel S. Karliner, M.D.
Gabriel Gregoratos, M.D.

# Contributors

Joseph S. Alpert, M.D.
Professor of Medicine
University of Massachusetts
Director, Division of Cardiology
University of Massachusetts Medical
  Center
Worcester, Massachusetts

William Ashburn, M.D.
Professor of Radiology
University of California, San Diego
Head, Division of Nuclear Medicine
University of California Medical Center
San Diego, California

Alexander Battler, M.D.
Staff Cardiologist
Heart Institute, The Chaim Sheba Medical
  Center
Tel Hashomer, Israel

Jonathan L. Benumof, M.D.
Associate Professor of Anesthesia
University of California, San Diego
School of Medicine
San Diego, California

Colin M. Bloor, M.D.
Professor of Pathology
University of California, San Diego
School of Medicine
La Jolla, California

Ned H. Cassem, M.D.
Associate Professor of Psychiatry
Harvard Medical School
Director, Psychiatric Consultation-Liaison
  Service
Massachusetts General Hospital
Boston, Massachusetts

Dennis L. Costello, M.D.
Assistant Professor of Medicine

University of California, San Diego
Director, Cardiac Catheterization
  Laboratory
Veterans Administration Medical Center
La Jolla, California

James W. Covell, M.D.
Professor of Medicine and Bioengineering
University of California, San Diego
School of Medicine
La Jolla, California

Michael H. Crawford, M.D.
Associate Professor of Medicine
University of Texas, San Antonio
Director, Cardiac Non-invasive Diagnostic
  Laboratories
The University of Texas Health Science
  Center at San Antonio
San Antonio, Texas

Guy P. Curtis, M.D., Ph.D.
Assistant Professor of Medicine,
University of California, San Diego
School of Medicine
San Diego, California

Roy V. Ditchey, M.D.
Assistant Professor of Medicine
University of Colorado School of Medicine
Denver, Colorado

Robert L. Engler, M.D.
Assistant Professor of Medicine
University of California, San Diego
Director, Coronary Care Unit
Veterans Administration Medical Center
La Jolla, California

Victor F. Froelicher, M.D.
Associate Professor of Medicine,
University of California, San Diego

Director, Cardiac Rehabilitation and Exercise Testing
University of California Medical Center
San Diego, California

Leslie A. Geddes, M.E., Ph.D
Showalter Distinguished Professor
Director, Biomedical Engineering Center
Purdue University
Lafayette, Indiana

Elizabeth A. Gilpin, M.S.
Senior Programmer
Ischemic Heart Disease Specialized Center of Research
University of California Medical Center
San Diego, California

Evelyn Gleeson, R.N.
Patient Care Coordinator
Coronary Care Unit
University of California Medical Center
San Diego, California

Herman K. Gold, M.D.
Associate Professor of Medicine
Harvard Medical School
Cardiac Unit
Massachusetts General Hospital
Boston, Massachusetts

Ary Goldberger, M.D.
Assistant Professor of Medicine
University of California, San Diego
Director, Electrocardiography
Veterans Administration Medical Center
La Jolla, California

Nora Goldschlager, M.D.
Associate Clinical Professor of Medicine
University of California, San Francisco
Director, Coronary Care Unit
San Francisco General Hospital Medical Center
San Francisco, California

Gabriel Gregoratos, M.D.
Professor of Medicine
University of California, San Diego
Director, Coronary Care Unit
University of California Medical Center
San Diego, California

Richard W. Gross, M.D.
Research Fellow
Cardiovascular Division, Department of Medicine
Washington University School of Medicine
St. Louis, Missouri

Charles Higgins, M.D.
Professor of Radiology
University of California, San Diego
School of Medicine
San Diego, California

David S. Janowsky, M.D.
Professor of Psychiatry
University of California, San Diego
School of Medicine
San Diego, California

Allen D. Johnson, M.D.
Director of Critical Care Services
Scripps Clinic, La Jolla, California
Associate Clinical Professor of Medicine
University of California, San Diego
School of Medicine
San Diego, California

Joel S. Karliner, M.D.
Associate Professor of Medicine
University of California, San Diego
Director, Clinical Cardiology Section
University of California Medical Center
San Diego, California

Robert Leinbach, M.D.
Associate Professor of Medicine
Harvard Medical School
Cardiac Unit
Massachusetts General Hospital
Boston, Massachusetts

Martin M. LeWinter, M.D.
Associate Professor of Medicine
University of California, San Diego
Director, Cardiac Graphic Methods
Veterans Administration Medical Center
La Jolla, California

Peter E. Maroko, M.D.
Director, Cardiovascular Research
Deborah Heart and Lung Center
Browns Mills, New Jersey

M. D. McKirnan, Ph.D
Staff Research Associate
University of California, San Diego
Co-Director, Cardiac Rehabilitation
University of California Medical Center
San Diego, California

James A. Meyer, M.D.
Professor of Anesthesiology
Loma Linda University School of Medicine
Chief of Anesthesiology
Veterans Administration Hospital
Loma Linda, California

Kenneth M. Moser, M.D.
Professor of Medicine
University of California, San Diego
Chief, Pulmonary Division
University of California Medical Center
San Diego, California

William P. Nelson, M.D.
Professor of Medicine
University of Kansas School of Medicine
Section of Cardiovascular Diseases, Department of Medicine
University of Kansas Medical Center
Kansas City, Kansas

Robert L. North, M.D.
Professor of Medicine
University of Texas Southwestern Medical School
Chief, Department of Internal Medicine
Presbyterian Hospital of Dallas
Dallas, Texas

Robert A. O'Rourke, M.D.
Professor of Medicine
University of Texas, San Antonio
Chief, Division of Cardiology
Department of Medicine
University of Texas Health Science Center at San Antonio
San Antonio, Texas

Robert W. Peters, M.D.
Assistant Professor of Medicine
University of California, San Francisco
School of Medicine
San Francisco, California

Kirk L. Peterson, M.D.
Associate Professor of Medicine
University of California, San Diego
Director, Cardiac Catheterization Laboratory
University of California Medical Center
San Diego, California

Douglas R. Reynolds, J.D.
Attorney-at-Law
Ault, Midlam and Reynolds
San Diego, California

S. Craig Risch, M.D.
Staff Psychiatrist
Clinical Neuropharmacology Branch
NIMH, NIH Clinical Center
Bethesda, Maryland

Robert Roberts, M.D.
Associate Professor of Medicine
Washington University School of Medicine
Director, Cardiac Care Unit
Barnes Hospital
St. Louis, Missouri

John Ross, Jr., M.D.
Professor of Medicine
University of California, San Diego
Head, Division of Cardiology
University of California, San Diego
School of Medicine
La Jolla, California

Melvin Scheinman, M.D.
Professor of Medicine
University of California, San Francisco
Chief, Electrocardiography and Clinical Cardiac Electrophysiology Section
Moffitt Hospital
San Francisco, California

Ralph Shabetai, M.D.
Professor of Medicine
University of California, San Diego
Chief, Cardiology Section
Veterans Administration Medical Center
La Jolla, California

Burton E. Sobel, M.D.
Professor of Medicine
Washington University School of Medicine
Director, Cardiovascular Division

Barnes Hospital
St. Louis, Missouri

Roger G. Spragg, M.D.
Assistant Professor of Medicine
University of California, San Diego
Director, Medical Intensive Care Unit
University of California Medical Center
San Diego, California

Joe R. Utley, M.D.
Professor of Surgery
University of California, San Diego
Head, Division of Cardiothoracic Surgery
University of California Medical Center
San Diego, California

Richard A. Walsh, M.D.
Assistant Professor of Medicine
University of Texas, San Antonio
Co-Director, Cardiac Catheterization Lab-
    oratories
University of Texas Health Science Center
    at San Antonio
San Antonio, Texas

John Watkins, M.B.
Visiting Research Cardiologist and Hark-
    ness Fellow
Division of Cardiology
Department of Medicine
University of California, San Diego
School of Medicine
San Diego, California

Robert T. Weibert, Pharm. D.
Associate Clinical Professor
University of California School of Phar-
    macy, San Francisco
UCSD/UCSF—San Diego Program
University of California Medical Center
San Diego, California

Kathryn F. Witztum, M.D.
Assistant Research Radiologist
University of California, San Diego
School of Medicine
San Diego, California

# Contents

# Section 1
# FUNDAMENTAL ASPECTS OF ACUTE MYOCARDIAL INFARCTION

# 1 | Pathogenesis and Pathology of Acute Myocardial Infarction

*Colin M. Bloor, M.D.*

Acute myocardial infarction is the most dramatic and lethal clinical presentation of coronary heart disease. It represents the single most frequent cause of death in the United States and other economically affluent countries. In most cases atherosclerotic involvement of the coronary arteries is severe. Presumably, coronary atherosclerosis is the basic lesion, although occlusive lesions are not always present in individual cases.

In this chapter the pathogenesis of atherosclerosis and associated risk factors are briefly discussed, with special emphasis on the coronary circulation. Then the pathology of acute myocardial infarction including ultrastructural features is presented. The pathology of significant complications of myocardial infarction and postoperative changes in coronary bypass vein grafts are discussed next. The concluding section addresses the nonatherosclerotic causes of acute myocardial infarction.

## DEFINITION OF ATHEROSCLEROSIS

Atherosclerosis is an arterial disease that has for many years been recognized as a principal cause of myocardial infarction and thrombosis. Nevertheless, the cause and pathogenesis of atherosclerosis remain unsolved, mainly because the disease can develop insidiously for many years before symptoms appear. This makes it difficult to follow the early stages of atherosclerosis in individual patients and to causally relate any of its several types of lesions to the stages observed. However, the key features of atherosclerotic lesions are well recognized.

Atherosclerosis is characterized by arterial intimal lesions resulting from the deposition of lipid material, particularly cholesterol, and the formation of fibrous tissue. The lipid deposits and complicated lesions (atheroma) may be either primary or secondary to sclerotic changes. In early stages, the atheroma may be reversible if they are limited to the intima; but, in the more advanced lesions, the media and adventitia are also affected, resulting in irreversible lesions.

## DEVELOPMENT OF THE ATHEROSCLEROTIC PLAQUE

There are few topics in pathology that have elicited more heated or prolonged controversy than atherosclerosis and its pathogenesis. The essential nature of the disease process is still unknown. However recent reviews of the topic—e.g., papers by McCullagh [1] and Ross and Glomset[2,3]—are recommended for detailed discussion of current concepts of pathogenesis. This section briefly presents the major current hypotheses of the pathogenesis of atherosclerosis and the features of the lesions.

3

## Lesions

Three types of atherosclerotic lesions are classically recognized: the fatty streak, the fibrous plaque or proliferative lesion, and the atheroma or complicated lesion.

The *fatty streak* comprises focal accumulations of small numbers of intimal smooth mus-

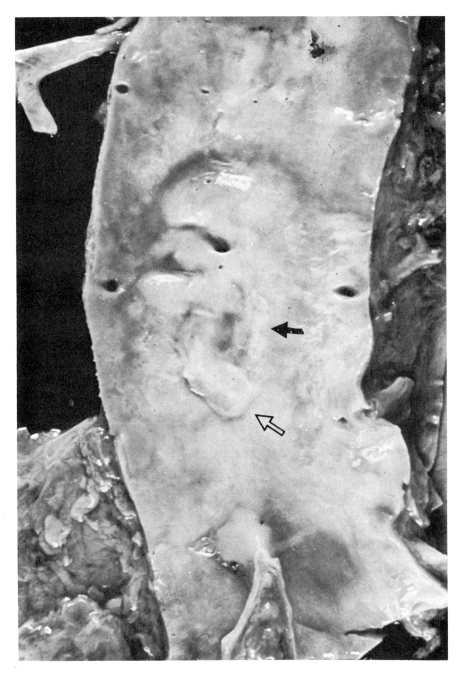

Fig. 1.1 Atherosclerosis. This view of the opened aorta shows the early lesions of atherosclerosis. Fatty streaks (solid arrow) are bright yellow linear streaks along the intimal surface. The proliferative lesion (open arrow) is in a more advanced stage in which the intima is elevated and is opaque and pale white. (Bloor CM: Cardiac Pathology, p. 185, Philadelphia, J. B. Lippincott, 1978.)

cle cells containing lipid deposits. Grossly, bright yellow streaks are evident on the intimal surface of the involved vessels (Fig. 1.1). Microscopically, lipid deposits are easily identified with appropriate lipid stains (Fig. 1.2). Fatty streaks appear at different stages and different regions of the arterial bed, but they occur in the aortas of everyone by the age of 10 years, regardless of race, sex, or geographic location.[4,5] Up to the age of 25 years, the extent of aortic intimal surface covered by fatty streaks increases from about 10 percent to 30 to 50 percent.[4,5,6] Most of the lipids in fatty streaks are in the form of cholesterol and cholesterol esters. Most of the cholesterol found within fatty streaks probably results from imbibition from plasma, but it is also likely that plasma lipids are hydrolyzed and reesterified once they have been taken up by the cells.[2,3,7] Fatty streaks are considered to be reversible lesions;

they show evidence of regression when plasma cholesterol levels are reduced.

The *fibrous plaque* or proliferative lesion is the most characteristic lesion of atherosclerosis. Grossly, it is gray-white in appearance, is elevated above the intimal surface, and protrudes into the lumen of the involved vessel (Fig. 1.1). The fibrous plaque comprises an intimal accumulation of lipid-laden smooth muscle cells, with the lipids being in the form of cholesterol and cholesterol esters (Fig. 1.3). These lipid-laden smooth muscle cells are surrounded by additional lipids, collagen, elastic fibers, and proteoglycans. These cells and the extracellular matrix components combine to form a fibrous cap that covers a large, deep deposit of free extracellular lipids intermixed with cell debris.

Earlier studies suggested that the fatty streak was a precursor of the fibrous plaque or proliferative lesion. Population studies showed that

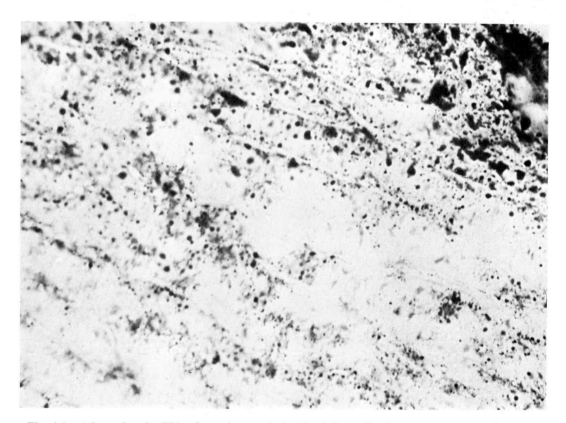

Fig. 1.2  Atherosclerosis. This photomicrograph (×40) of the wall of a coronary artery shows the early lesions of atherosclerosis. Darkly stained lipid droplets are diffusely scattered throughout the coronary artery wall. Near the intimal surface (upper right) the lipid droplets are densely accumulated. Oil red O stain. (Bloor CM: Cardiac Pathology, p. 187, Philadelphia, J. B. Lippincott, 1978.)

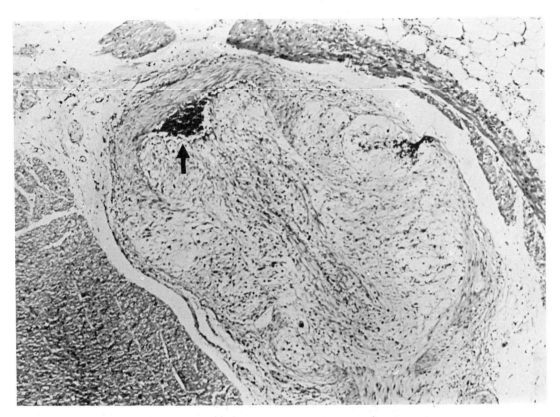

Fig. 1.3  Atherosclerosis. Photomicrograph (×40) of a large coronary artery shows extensive intimal proliferation. The intimal cells are swollen and laden with fat and have a foamy appearance. The intimal proliferation is sufficiently extensive to encroach upon the vessel lumen (arrow), which is about 10 percent of its normal size. (Bloor CM: Cardiac Pathology, p. 187, Philadelphia, J. B. Lippincott, 1978.)

fatty streaks occurred earlier than fibrous plaques, and, in some cases, in the same anatomic position, particularly in the coronary and cerebral arteries. However, in the aorta, the anatomic sites where fatty streaks occur are different from those where fibrous plaques appear.[8,9] The reasons for these differences are not apparent; thus, the current view is that fibrous plaques and fatty streaks are unrelated lesions of atherosclerosis.

The *atheroma* or complicated lesion (Figs. 1.4 and 1.5) is a fibrous plaque which has been altered by hemorrhage, calcification, cell necrosis, and mural thrombosis. Calcification is the distinguishing feature of this lesion. Atheroma usually progresses to significant occlusive disease, particularly when thrombosis complicates the lesion.

The focal lesions of atherosclerosis are characterized by three fundamental phenomena: (1) proliferation of smooth muscle cells; (2) deposition of intracellular and extracellular lipids, and (3) accumulation of extracellular matrix components including collagen, elastic fibers, and proteoglycans. Any hypothesis concerning the pathogenesis of atherosclerosis must account for all three phenomena and ultimately explain the effect of risk factors on the incidence and clinical sequelae of the disease.

Current Hypotheses

The current hypotheses concerning pathogenesis of atherosclerosis are: (1) the reaction-to-injury hypothesis, (2) the monoclonal hypothesis, and (3) differences in growth control.

The reaction-to-injury hypothesis is based largely on Virchow's theory with later modifications by Ross and associates and by other investigators.[10-13] Basically, this hypothesis states that the lesions of atherosclerosis result from the response of arterial endothelium to some form of injury (Fig. 1.6). Focal injury to arterial endothelium results in increased permeability to plasma constituents (e.g., lipoproteins) and allows platelets to adhere to the subendothelial connective tissue, to aggregate, and to release the contents of their granules. As platelets and plasma components build up, smooth muscle cells from the arterial media migrate into subintimal and intimal locations and then proliferate. Simultaneously, large amounts of connective tissue matrix are formed and lipid accumulates. If injury is a single event, then endothelial regeneration will occur, the endothelial barrier will be restored, and the lesion will regress. However, more often, repeated or chronic injury occurs which results finally in the development of an atheromatous plaque.

Platelets and other components of thrombosis also have a role in the reaction-to-injury hypothesis. After endothelial injury, platelets adhere to such sites and may become incorporated along with other thrombotic material within the atheromatous plaque. Platelets may play a more critical role: Ross and his associates have shown the platelet-derived growth factor directly stimulates proliferation of smooth muscle cells.[12] The activity of this factor in vivo is suggested by the protective effect that occurs after thrombocytopenia is experimentally induced, or when inhibitors of platelet aggregation are given in some models of experimental atherosclerosis.[12] However, smooth muscle proliferation may occur without the participation of platelet adherence or aggregation.[14] Stimuli for smooth muscle proliferation include not only platelet derived factors but also plasma or cell components which may leak into the vessel wall. Thus, certain components of low-

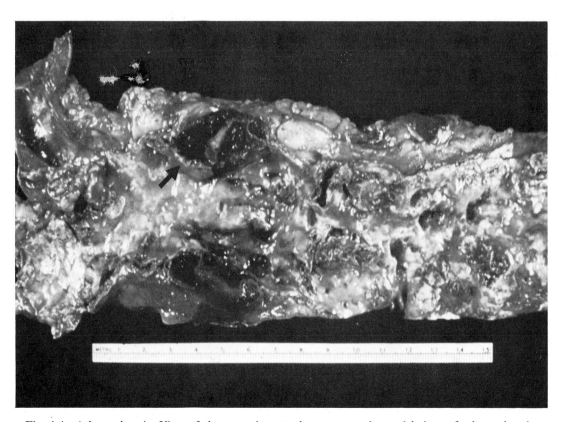

Fig. 1.4 Atherosclerosis. View of the opened aorta shows more advanced lesions of atherosclerosis. Ulcerated plaques are now extensively scattered over the intimal surface. A mural thrombus is formed (arrow) at a site of saccular aneurysm formation of the aortic wall. (Bloor CM: Cardiac Pathology, p. 185, Philadelphia, J. B. Lippincott, 1978.)

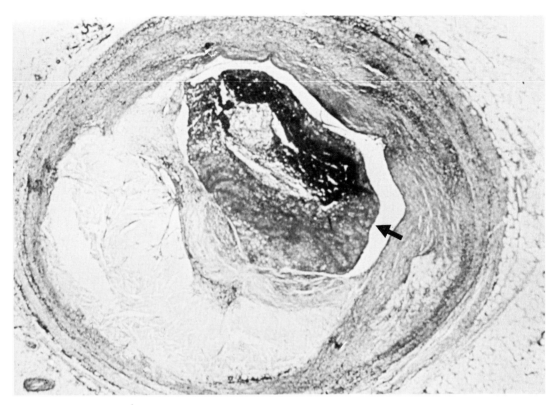

Fig. 1.5   Atherosclerosis. This photomicrograph (×10) of a coronary artery shows the advanced stage of atheromatous lesions. In addition to intimal proliferation, a fibrous plaque has formed. Numerous cholesterol clefts or slits are present within the fibrous plaque. A surface of this plaque has also ulcerated, with resulting thrombus formation (arrow) that completely occludes the vessel lumen. (Bloor CM: Cardiac Pathology, p. 188, Philadelphia, J. B. Lippincott, 1978.)

density lipoprotein (LDL), or other circulating hormones, or factors from macrophages may also supply the growth-stimulating effect. In turn, the smooth muscle cells produce the extracellular components of the atheromatous plaque—namely, collagen, elastic tissue, and proteoglycans. While doing this, the smooth muscle cells accumulate large amounts of cholesterol and cholesterol esters, which are derived largely from plasma lipoproteins. Thus, the majority of extracellular lipids in the atheromatous plaque is also plasma derived. Intracellular lipid accumulation may be caused by a regulatory defect of cholesterol metabolism in the smooth muscle cells and is perhaps initiated by the hyperlipidemic serum.

The reaction-to-injury hypothesis is attractive in that it provides for the important role of lipids in atherogenesis. However, certain questions are left unanswered. For example, if

endothelial injury occurs early, why do some fatty streaks regress and others apparently progress to more severe lesions? Second, although endothelial injury alone may cause smooth muscle proliferation, why is hypercholesterolemia necessary for the atheroma or complicated lesion to occur? Third, what are the determinants of the anatomic location of the lesions? Often these sites are unrelated to hemodynamic factors. The major objection to the reaction-to-injury hypothesis is that, although endothelial injury is the initial event, the development of the atheromatous plaque and complicated lesion could be explained if smooth muscle cell migration and proliferation were the initial events. It is possible that lipids or lipid components that normally reach the smooth muscle layer in hypercholesterolemic individuals may stimulate smooth muscle cells to migrate and proliferate. Alternatively, genetic or acquired defects of smooth muscle cells may induce the initial proliferative response. Thus, two other hypotheses have been proposed to explain the pathogenesis of atherosclerosis. These are briefly discussed below.

The monoclonal hypothesis advanced by Benditt and Benditt [15,16] proposes that each lesion of atherosclerosis is derived from a single smooth muscle cell that serves as progenitor for the remaining proliferative cells. A- or B-isoenzyme of X-linked glucose 6-phosphate dehydrogenase (G-6-PD) was used as a cellular marker in atheromatous plaques.[15,16] Normal tissues in heterozygotes consist of a mosaic of cells having both A- and B-isoenzymes. In contrast, the finding of one or the other of these isoenzymes in the tissue would indicate proliferation of a single cell, or clone.[15,16] Fibrous atheromatous plaques contained either A- or B-isoenzymes and only seldom contained both. This monotypic nature of the smooth muscle cells in the plaque was interpreted as evidence that the plaques are equivalent to benign monoclonal neoplasms (e.g., leiomyomas) and are

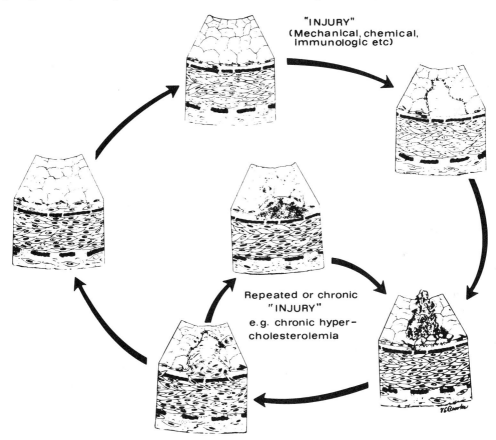

Fig. 1.6   Two possible different cycles of events in the response-to-injury hypothesis. The large cycle may represent what occurs in all persons at varying times. Endothelial injury may lead to desquamation, platelet adherence, aggregation, and release, followed by smooth muscle proliferation and connective-tissue formation. If the injury is a single event, the lesions may go on to heal and regress, leaving a slightly thickened intima. The smaller, inner cycle demonstrates the possible consequences of repeated or chronic injury to the endothelium in which lipid deposition may occur and smooth-muscle proliferation may continue after a sequence of proliferation, regression, proliferation and regression, leading to a complicated lesion containing newly formed connective tissue and lipids which may eventually calcify. This sequence of events could lead to a complicated lesion that goes on to produce clinical sequelae, such as thrombosis and infarction. (Reprinted, by permission, from The New England Journal of Medicine. Ross and Glomset: Pathogenesis of atherosclerosis. N Engl J Med 295:420, 1976.)

initiated by mutation. The mutagenic effect may be induced by transforming agents, such as viruses or chemicals.[16] Pearson and associates [20] have shown a higher proportion of fatty streaks to be monoclonal, which lends further support to this hypothesis. These studies clearly represent a new departure in the study of atherosclerosis and suggest interesting possibilities that deserve to be tested.

The other hypothesis accounting for smooth muscle proliferation in the pathogenesis of atherosclerosis implicated disturbances in growth control, possibly related to senescence in the cells of the media.[17-20] There is evidence supporting the role for growth inhibitors in growth regulation of the arterial wall. In fact, factors inhibiting cell growth in culture have been isolated from aortic walls.[19] Presumably, focal loss of such inhibitors could lead to smooth muscle cell proliferation. However, these concepts are still largely speculative.

The current hypothesis that is most comprehensive is the reaction-to-injury hypothesis. However, no single proposal corresponds to all the accumulated evidence. Clinically significant atherosclerosis appears to be a disease of multiple origins and the cumulative effect of many factors. Thus, investigation continues on the role that serum lipids, other risk factors, and their manipulation have on prevention and treatment of complicated lesions.

Clinically, the presentation of atherosclerosis is as varied as the vessels affected and the extent of the atheromatous change. The lesions cause clinical disease by (1) narrowing vascular lumens resulting in ischemia; (2) sudden occlusion of vessels by thrombotic complications resulting in infarction; (3) providing a site for thrombosis and embolism, or (4) weakening the involved vessel wall resulting in aneurysm formation or rupture. In this chapter, we are concerned with events occurring when the involved vessels are the coronary arteries in which progression of atherosclerosis results in myocardial ischemia or infarction.

## RISK FACTORS

A number of factors are thought to predispose an individual to atherosclerosis. These include race, age, sex heredity, body-build and body weight, occupation, serum cholesterol concentration, hypertension, cardiac hypertrophy, cigarette smoking, diabetes mellitus, hypothyroidism, uric acid concentration, hematocrit and hemoglobin levels, and other factors. Of these various predisposing factors, four are considered to be of prime importance: (1) hypertension, (2) hyperlipidemia, (3) cigarette smoking, and (4) diabetes. A brief discussion of the primary risk factors follows with some comments on the others.

### Hypertension

In individuals with high blood pressure, there is a greater incidence of atherosclerosis and ischemic heart disease. In the Framingham study, the incidence of ischemic heart disease in men 45 to 62 years of age with hypertension was five times that observed in normotensive men of similar age.[21,22] After the age of 45 years, hypertension may be a greater risk factor than hypercholesterolemia. Since hypertension increases the risk of all forms of coronary heart disease, it is probably related to the atherosclerotic process rather than to any effects on thrombotic complications.

### Hyperlipidemia

There is overwhelming evidence that hyperlipidemia is associated with an increased incidence of atherosclerosis and premature heart disease. Although hypercholesterolemia, hypertriglyceridemia, and hyperlipidemia have all been correlated with the severity of atherosclerosis and the incidence of ischemic heart disease, hypercholesterolemia has been studied most extensively.[21,22] Populations having relatively high levels of cholesterol and low-density lipoproteins (LDL) have higher mortality from ischemic heart disease. The Framingham studies have shown that men and women of ages 35 to 44 years, with serum cholesterol levels of 265 mg percent or more, have 5 times higher risk of developing ischemic heart disease than those individuals with cholesterol levels below 220 mg percent. When total serum cholesterol was further analyzed to evaluate the contribution of low-density lipoprotein (LDL), very low-density lipoprotein (VLDL), and high-density lipoprotein (HDL) separately, LDL was independently related to risk for both men and women, while HDL was inversely related to risk.[23] It has also been shown that dietary modification can reduce serum cholesterol levels and, in turn, reduce the risk of developing coronary atherosclerosis and ischemic heart disease.

## Cigarette Smoking

According to some epidemiologic studies, cigarette smoking increases the risk of developing certain forms of coronary atherosclerosis and ischemic heart disease, particularly myocardial infarction or sudden death.[21,24-32] In men who smoke one or more packs of cigarettes per day, the death rate from ischemic heart disease is 70 to 200 percent higher than that for nonsmokers, and the risk is particularly significant in younger men. Autopsy studies have also shown that the degree of aortic and coronary atherosclerosis is greater in smokers than in nonsmokers.[33] However, the incidence of angina pectoris is not increased in cigarette smokers, which suggests that the effect is not on the atherosclerotic process but on coagulation changes—particularly on platelet function, which can increase the incidence of ventricular arrhythmias. The incidence of these forms of the disease is reduced when cigarette smoking ceases. It is also of interest that pipe smokers and cigar smokers do not have an increased risk of developing coronary heart disease.

## Diabetes

The incidence of atherosclerosis is increased in diabetic patients. For example, in diabetic patients over the age of 40, its incidence in women is equal to, or greater than, that in men.[34-38] The incidence of myocardial infarction is greater among diabetic patients. It appears that diabetes mellitus contributes to atherogenesis as a result of abnormal lipid metabolism and associated hypertension, obesity, and aging.[39]

## Other Predisposing Factors

A host of other factors which increase the extent and severity of atherosclerosis has been identified, but their data are more equivocal than those for the major risk factors described above. For example, although obesity correlates with an increased risk of morbidity and mortality from the clinical complications of atherosclerosis, the relationship may be indirect because obese individuals have an increased incidence of hyperlipidemia, hypertension, and diabetes mellitus.

The role of physical activity in the development of atherosclerosis is unclear. The Framingham data showed that the most sedentary of the men who participated in the study had three times the risk of developing significant coronary atherosclerosis or fatal ischemic heart disease as the 15 percent of participants who were classified as most physically active.[22] This does not indicate whether physical activity had a direct effect on the development of atherosclerosis, since those individuals engaging in physical activity frequently alter their lifestyles in many ways. Thus, reduction in serum lipids, body weight, or blood pressure may occur and be the primary factors affecting the development of atherosclerosis. The role of stress and behavior patterns is still controversial.

Most individuals think that stressful life events are related to the risk of coronary heart disease, but statistical studies are by no means conclusive. One study showed that men with aggressive, "type A" behavior patterns had twice the rate of heart disease as men having less competitive, "type B" behavior patterns.[40,41] However, twin studies suggest that the behavior pattern may not be the primary determinant, but rather that the individual's degree of self-esteem and view of success in achieving life goals are more influential.[42]

Finally, it should be noted that, although the major risk factors contribute individually to the development of clinically significant atherosclerosis, when multiple factors occur simultaneously their effect is greater than that of simple addition. The Framingham data indicate that when three risk factors were present—namely, hyperlipidemia, hypertension, and cigarette smoking—the rate of myocardial infarction was 7 times greater than when there were no risk factors. When two risk factors were present, the risk was increased four-fold, and with one risk factor the increase was two-fold. However, since some cardiac patients do not have elevated serum lipids, elevated systemic blood pressure, or diabetes, the etiology and pathogenesis of atherosclerosis remain controversial and subject to continuing speculation.

## PATHOLOGY OF ACUTE MYOCARDIAL INFARCTION

The sequence of events in a developing myocardial infarct has been well-defined in gross and conventional light microscopic terms for many years.[34,43-45] As discussed in the section on atherosclerosis, the disease process starts in the coronary vessels, where lipids are deposited in the subendothelium, resulting in a fatty streak. Later, reaction-to-injury occurs with a proliferative response at that site, with deposition of collagen and elevation of the overlying intima. The proliferative lesion progresses to an atheroma or complicated lesion in which cholesterol esters precipitate and form clefts. A fibrous cap is formed over the lesion, and various degrees of intimal proliferation occur. If the intimal endothelial surface is disrupted by this process, exposing the underlying collagen, then platelets will aggregate and small thrombi will form. This compounds the atheromatous lesion, resulting in severe narrowing or occlusion of major coronary vessels. When such occlusion occurs, the myocardium distal to the lesions is rendered ischemic, and cell death follows. The changes associated with myocardial cell death have been well-defined by gross observation and conventional light microscopy. More recent investigations have shown the sequence of ultrastructural changes that occur in the early stages of an evolving myocardial infarct and have provided additional clues about the pathogenesis of ischemic myocardial injury that results in the clinical event of acute myocardial infarction. In this section, the conventional gross and light microscopic observations will be summarized and then more recent observa-

tions on the sequence of ultrastructual events in ischemic myocardial cell injury will be shown. In discussing the new approaches for defining irreversible injury in ischemic myocardium, the response of myocardial vessels to ischemic injury as well as ultrastructual alterations in ischemic myocardial cells will be presented.

### Gross Changes

Gross morphologic evidence of myocardial infarcts in man does not appear until 6 to 12 hours after the onset of the process.[45] A slight pallor may be present during the first three days of an evolving myocardial infarct. The involved myocardium will have a pale, dry appearance, and there may be focal red-purple areas of hemorrhage and congestion within these zones. Since oxidative enzymes are depleted in the ischemic regions, histochemical stains may be used to demonstrate the region of infarct on gross specimens. Frequently, the nitro-blue tetrazolium (NBT) stain is used to show the absence of dehydrogenase enzymes in the infarct region. About the fourth day after the onset of myocardial infarction, the necrotic zone becomes more sharply defined with a hyperemic border. The fine yellow line at the peripheral margin of the infarct results from leukocytic infiltration of the tissue and engulfment of lipid material released from the necrotic myocardium. This zone becomes broader and may change to a yellow-green color. As the fatty change progresses, the yellow zone extends throughout the infarct, giving it a mottled appearance. Between 6 to 8 days, the central necrotic zone is soft and contains hemorrhagic regions (Fig. 1.7). The marginal zones are intensely red in color and highly vascularized. At 8 to 10 days, removal, by catalysis, of debris of necrotic myocardial fibers and the beginning replacement of the necrotic muscle by the ingrowth of fibrous, vascularized scar tissue results in reduced thickness of the myocardium in the zone of infarction. The infarct surface is yellow in color and surrounded by a red-purple depressed band of granulation tissue. The process of organization continues, and at 3 to 4 weeks the red-purple granulation tissue

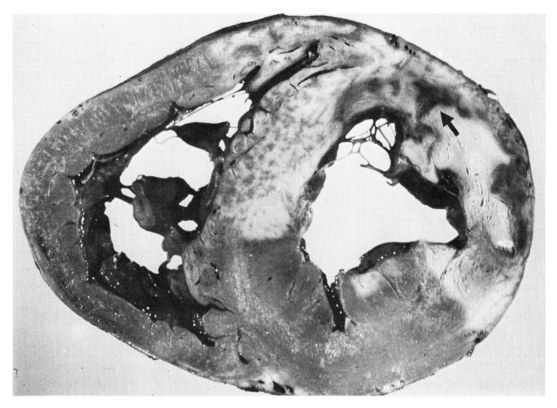

Fig. 1.7   Acute myocardial infarct. Cross-section of the heart shows a myocardial infarct about 1 week old, involving the posterior half of the interventricular septum and posterior-lateral left ventricular walls. This infarct is secondary to occlusion of the left circumflex coronary artery. The myocardium has a mottled appearance and the margins of the infarct are well demarcated. In the central portion of the infarct involving the posterior papillary muscle, there is evidence of hemorrhage (arrow). (Bloor CM: Cardiac Pathology, p. 195, Philadelphia, J. B. Lippincott, 1978.)

extends throughout the infarct. About 2 to 3 months later, the infarct acquires a gelatinous gray appearance until it is transformed into a shrunken-firm scar (Fig. 1.8). After 3 months, the gray scar becomes more white and firmer in consistency.

In the early stages of an evolving myocardial infarct, the morphologic changes present may represent several different time periods. This is because the initial infarct may extend, and, thus, regions of infarct of various ages are present. This mixed appearance is more likely to occur in larger infarcts.

## Microscopic Changes

Light microscopic changes in myocardial infarcts pursue a more or less orderly progression.[34,43] The major microscopic features include: (1) necrosis of muscle, connective tissue, and small blood vessels; (2) hemorrhage; (3) deposition of fatty material; (4) infiltration by polymorphonuclear leukocytes; (5) ingrowth of blood vessels and connective tissue; (6) removal of necrotic muscle and infiltration by pigmented macrophages; (7) appearance of lymphocytes and plasma cells; (8) fibroblastic proliferation with collagen production, and (9) formation of mature scars.

Using routine histologic stains—e.g., hematoxylin and eosin—light microscopic evidence of necrosis does not appear until 5 or 6 hours after the onset of an infarct. Before then, some more subtle changes may be observed. A wavy appearance of myocardial fibers at the margin of an infarct may occur within one hour after

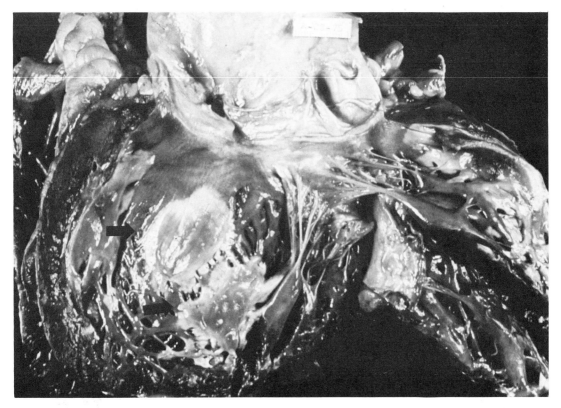

Fig. 1.8  Old myocardial infarct. The left ventricular chamber is opened. Two large infarcts (arrow) can be seen along the endocardial surface of the left ventricular outflow tract. These are located in the interventricular septum and are well-circumscribed, gray scars. (Bloor CM: Cardiac Pathology, p. 196, Philadelphia, J. B. Lippincott, 1978.)

the onset of ischemia (Fig. 1.9). These changes are thought to result from loss of normal contractility of ischemically injured myocardial cells with stretching of those fibers interposed between the surrounding, normal contracting myocardium and the noncontractile zone within the center of the infarct. Contraction bands may also appear in fibers at the border zone of the evolving infarct (Fig. 1.10). Glycogen depletion of ischemic myocardial fibers can occur within 60 minutes, and such change may be readily demonstrated by periodic acid-Schiff stain. However, these special techniques of demonstrating early ischemic injury by light microscopy are only valid in fresh or specially preserved specimens. The usual early evidence of coagulative necrosis is the hyaline appearance of the myocardial fibers, which stain more eosinophilic than normal, and disappearance of their cross striations (Fig. 1.11). The myocar-

dial fibers then become swollen and contain eosinophilic granules and irregular cross-bands. Their nuclei either disappear or become pyknotic. The subendocardial zone of muscle is usually intact, since adequate perfusion of this layer can be maintained by direct diffusion from the ventricular cavity. Focal hemorrhage is usually present throughout the infarct, and venules and capillaries are often severely congested. When red blood cells hemolyze, hemosiderin deposits are present in the evolving infarct and are later ingested by macrophages. Lipid droplets may appear early within the ischemically injured myocardial fibers (Fig. 1.12).

During the first 24 hours, polymorphonuclear leukocytes start to infiltrate the edges of the infarct and spread centrally. They first appear in the interstitial tissue in perivascular locations and gradually extend into necrotic tissue (Fig. 1.13). At 48 hours the leukocytic infiltrate starts to subside, and some polymorphonuclear leukocytes show evidence of degeneration. During subsequent days, the dead fibers become more distinctly coagulated and their nuclei become pyknotic or disappear. Removal of the necrotic debris occurs both by catalysis initiated by release of lysosomal enzymes and phagocytosis caused by infiltrating macrophages. At 4 days a dense leukocytic infiltrate is present along the margin of the infarct, and a day later many of them are necrotic. Thereafter, they gradually disappear and are usually absent by 12 to 14 days. After the fourth day, some eosinophils are present in the infarct. At 4 days, capillaries appear at the margin of the infarct and are accompanied by fibroblasts. They proceed to grow into the infarct. The ingrowth of such granulation tissue is usually greater on the epicardial side of the infarct than on the endocardial side. If the infarct is large, vascular-

ization may not reach the center, and fibrin is strikingly absent. Central islands of persistently necrotic muscle may be present even months after the acute event. When capillary and fibroblastic ingrowth occur, macrophages invade the necrotic tissue and phagocytize the debris. Occasionally, giant cells may be observed during this stage. Eventually, the necrotic myocardial fibers dissolve and disappear (Fig. 1.14). Their lipofuscin pigment remains within the macrophages, which may also contain hemosiderin. Pigment-laden macrophages may persist through 1 to 2 years after the onset of the infarct. Myocardial fibers in the zone adjacent to the infarct are often hypertrophic and have hyperchromatic nuclei. Other evidence of muscle regeneration may be present. As soon as absorption of necrotic myocardial fibers starts, lymphocytes and plasma cells appear. They are particularly prominent during the third week

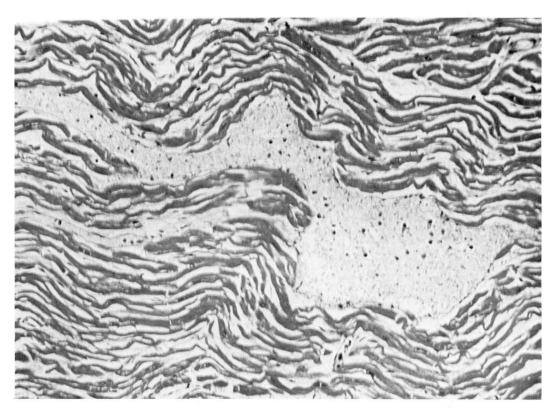

Fig. 1.9  Acute myocardial infarct. This low-power photomicrograph (×40) shows a wavy arrangement of myocardial fibers, which differs from the normal parallel longitudinal array. This change may occur at the margin of the ischemic zone due to asynchronous contraction of the viable and nonviable fibers. (Bloor CM: Cardiac Pathology, p. 200, Philadelphia, J. B. Lippincott, 1978.)

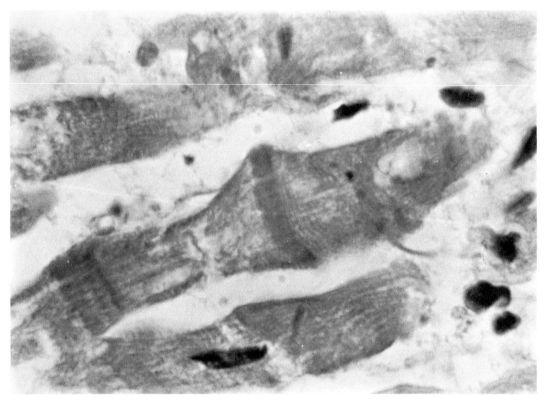

Fig. 1.10  Acute myocardial infarct. Myocardial fibers are disrupted in the region of the intercalated disc and in portions of the fibers lying between the intercalated discs. The individual fibers are also separated from each other by some intracellular edema. Also, the cytoplasm has condensed, forming a dense contraction band (arrow) ($\times$400). (Bloor CM: Cardiac Pathology, p. 198, Philadelphia, J. B. Lippincott, 1978.)

of the evolving myocardial infarct and disappear about the same time as the pigmented macrophages.

About two weeks after the onset of an infarct, fibroblasts show evidence of producing collagen. This is very conspicuous after three weeks and reaches maximum amount at 2 to 3 months. The quantity of collagen present may indicate the age of an infarct. The mature scar of an old infarct contains highly vascular foci, which, on gross inspection, appear red and simulate a recent infarct.

The age of an infarct, during the first 3 weeks, may be judged reasonably accurately on the basis of microscopic changes. In general, they are as follows: During the first 5 to 6 hours of an infarct, the predominant changes include swollen cytoplasm of the involved myocardial fibers with intense acidophilic staining and loss of cross-striations. There is also the appearance of focal hyalinization, eosinophilic granules, and irregular cross-bands in the involved myocardial fibers. The nuclei of these fibers are pyknotic or completely disappear at this stage. During the first 3 days of infarction, capillaries and venules are severely congested and appear hyperemic. There is some edema of the interstitial tissue. Red blood cells may extravasate on occasions, but hemorrhage at this time is rare. A few polymorphonuclear leukocytes may be seen. At 4 days, there is a zone of dense neutrophilic exudate present at the margin of the infarct. At 8 days, the necrotic muscle fibers are dissolved and polymorphonuclear leukocytes are in abundance. The infiltrate extends into the central portion of the infarct. At 8 to 10 days, there is a decrease in the number of polymorphonuclear leukocytes, with the appearance now of lymphocytes and plasma cells. Necrosis of the myocardial fibers is advanced, and a narrow zone of granulation tissue appears at the margin of the infarct. At 12 days, collagen produced by proliferating fibroblasts makes its first appearance. At 3 to 4 weeks, granulation tissue is less cellular and less vascular than in the earlier stages, and newly formed collagen is abundant. At 3 months, a fibrous scar is fully developed.

## Ultrastructural Changes

Jennings and coworkers [46,47] have conducted numerous investigations on myocardial cell injury caused by ischema. Initially after coronary occlusion, arterial flow to the myocardium decreases, leading to a hypoxic environment in which various degrees of anaerobic metabolism occur. Since myocardial cells are completely dependent upon mitochondria for their energy requirements, mitochondrial alterations, which include swelling, a decreased matrix density and the formation of amorphous, dense precipitates in the matrix, are thought to be associated with irreversible cell injury. Transmission electron microscopy permits identification of very early changes in myocardial cells after the onset of ischemia. In a normal myocardial cell (Fig. 1.15), the chromatin material is evenly dispersed within the nucleus. The mitochondria are oval or elongated and lie between myofibrils. Glycogen is abundantly present and the sarcomeres are regularly arranged. After 15 minutes of ischemia, following coronary artery occlusion, there is some depletion of glycogen and slight swelling of mitochondria (Fig. 1.16). However, the sarcomeres are still in regular arrangement. If flow is reestablished at this time, the changes are reversible and the myocardial

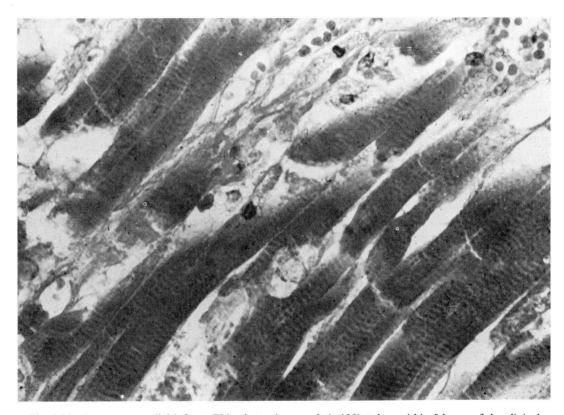

Fig. 1.11 Acute myocardial infarct. This photomicrograph (×100), taken within 5 hours of the clinical onset of acute myocardial infarction, shows increased eosinophilic staining of the myocardial fibers and loss of some cross-striations. The nuclei have disappeared. (Bloor CM: Cardiac Pathology, p. 198, Philadelphia, J. B. Lippincott, 1978.)

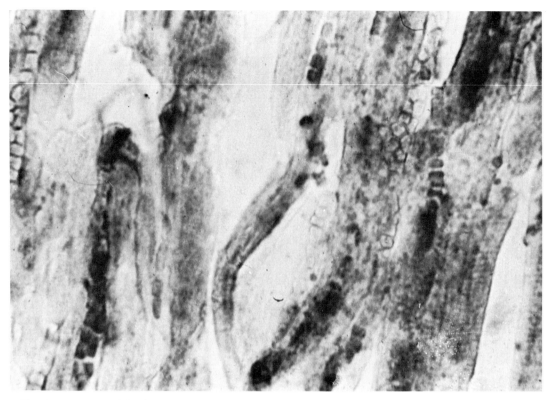

Fig. 1.12  Myocardial infarct. Photomicrograph (×100) in the early stages of acute myocardial infarct shows many darkly stained fat droplets within myocardial fibers. These may represent the earliest light microscopic change. (Bloor CM: Cardiac Pathology, p. 199, Philadelphia, J. B. Lippincott, 1978.)

cell will resume its normal function. With continuing ischemia, glycogen granules are further depleted and clumping of nuclear chromatin occurs at the margins of the nucleus (Fig. 1.17). Mitochondrial swelling becomes more severe, and the depletion of glycogen and loss of nuclear chromatin are apparent. If ischemia persists for 40 to 60 minutes, small, dense bodies are observed in many of the swollen mitochrondria (Fig. 1.18). These dense bodies take a variety of shapes, and their presence correlates well with loss of mitochondrial function. Several investigators have recently studied the nature of these granules.[48-50] When special techniques—for example, x-ray microanalysis—are applied to the study of these granules, calcium and phosphorus peaks have been identified, indicating that the granules are calcium-phosphate precipitates (Fig. 1.19). If reflow to the ischemic zone is now established after 40 to 60 minutes of occlusion, the development of

these granules in the mitochondria is accelerated.[47] Later, as the ischemia persists in the myocardium, calcium further accumulates within the cytoplasm of the injured myocardial cells and extremely contracted sarcomeres are seen in the form of contraction bands which can also be identified by the light microscope (Fig. 1.10).

Transmission electron microscopy of myocardial cells during early ischemia usually shows intact plasma cell membranes, even though other alterations associated with irreversible injury are present within the cell. The changes described earlier indicate that the regulation of calcium levels in the ischemic myocardial cell changes, increasing amounts of calcium phosphate precipitate in the mitochrondria, thus interfering with their function. Such changes in calcium levels in the ischemic cells suggest possible permeability changes within the plasma cell membrane. Thus, other techniques have been used to demonstrate changes in cell membrane permeability during early ischemia. Lanthanum studies after 45 minutes of ischemia show alterations in the plasma cell membranes (Fig. 1.20).[51] Freeze-fracture studies also show changes in the membrane at this time, confirming alterations in cell membrane permeability.[52] As ischemia progresses, breaks appear in the myocardial cell membrane and intramembranous particles aggregate (Fig. 1.21), suggesting that cell permeability has changed.[51]

During persisting myocardial ischemia, changes are not solely confined to the myocardial cell. Scanning electron microscopy studies [51,53] have shown that alterations occur in small coronary vessels throughout the ischemic myocardium. After 45 minutes of ischemia, the endothelial cell nuclei swell and then later bulge into the lumina of the coronary vessels. Cytoplasmic projections may extend from these cells and cross the lumina to form poten-

tial sites for small microthrombi. About 4 hours after occlusion, the luminal surface of the coronary artery is well covered with fibrin in the ischemic region, and red blood cells and leukocytes attach to its surface. Migration of red cells through the intimal surface into a subendothelial position has been observed. Transmission electron microscopy shows similar changes in these vessels. Obliteration of the lumina due to swollen endothelial cells may occur in small intramural vessels. If many vessels develop such lesions after occlusion and the onset of ischemia, then significant functional changes may occur in the coronary vascular bed, affecting its capacity and flow distribution throughout the ischemic myocardium.

## COMPLICATIONS OF ACUTE MYOCARDIAL INFARCTION

There are many complications associated with myocardial infarction. The most important

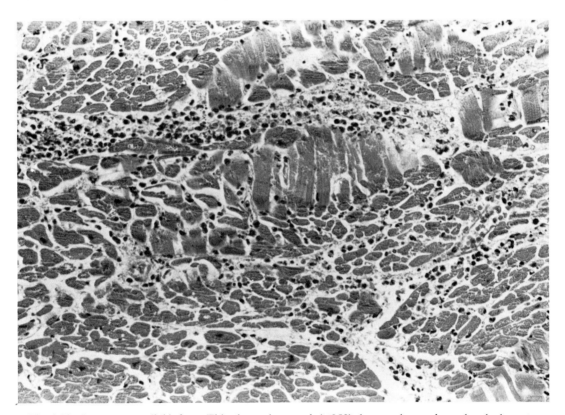

Fig. 1.13  Acute myocardial infarct. This photomicrograph (×250) shows polymorphonuclear leukocyctes infiltrating the interstitial tissue adjacent to the necrotic myocardial fibers.

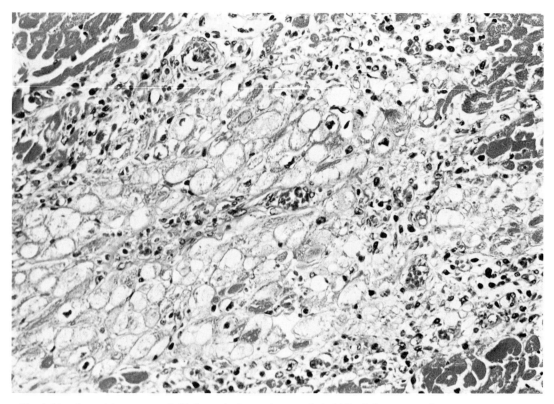

Fig. 1.14   Organizing myocardial infarct. A photomicrograph (×100) of a later stage shows granulomatous response in the necrotic myocardium. Macrophages are now present in the margin of the lesion. In the central portion many myocardial fibers have dissolved and membrane fragments remain. Fibroblasts have grown into the zone of necrotic tissue, and small vessels are starting to appear. (Bloor CM: Cardiac Pathology, p. 201, Philadelphia, J. B. Lippincott, 1978.)

ones to be described here include pericarditis, mural thrombosis, cardiac rupture, papillary muscle rupture, and ventricular aneurysm. Other complications are of striking clinical significance—e.g., arrhythmias, cardiogenic shock, and congestive heart failure—but have few unique morphological aspects. They will be presented in other chapters.

## Pericarditis

Pericarditis occurs about the second or third day after the onset of an infarct and is present in approximately 30 percent of cases.[34,54] It is usually associated with some degree of pericardial effusion and results from extension of the infarct to the epicardial surface. With organization and healing of the infarct, the pericarditis usually resolves, but occasionally it may organize to produce permanent fibrous adhesions.

## Mural Thrombosis

When an infarct extends into the ventricular endocardium, dense fibrous thickening results, which may initiate mural thrombus formation (Fig. 1.22). The incidence of mural thrombosis has been significantly reduced with the widespread use of anticoagulant therapy for patients with acute myocardial infarction.[55] When mural thrombosis occurs, it is most often associated with myocardial infarcts of the left ventricle, less often with atrial infarcts, and least frequently in infarcts involving the right ventricle. About one-third of patients with mural thrombi in the left ventricle have the occurrence of systemic emboli. This is especially frequent when the mural thrombus is attached to the interventricular septum.[34] Embolism from mural thrombi may also result in emboli lodging in coronary arteries, which in turn can cause extension or recurrence of myocardial infarction.

## Cardiac Rupture

About 10 percent of patients coming to autopsy with acute myocardial infarcts and 5 percent of patients observed clinically who die with acute myocardial infarcts have rupture of the ventricular wall at the site of the infarct (Fig. 1.23).[56-58] The most frequent site of rupture is the lower third of the ventral wall of the left ventricle, just above the apex. Cardiac rupture occurs more often in men than in women and most often in individuals over 60 years of age.[34,58] When cardiac rupture occurs, it is usually within the first week of the onset of an acute myocardial infarct. Considering the stages of evolution and organization of myocardial infarction described earlier, this is the time at which maximum necrosis of myocardial fibers has occurred and the structural integrity of the myocardial wall is at its weakest. If rupture occurs in the interventricular septum, then a left-to-right shunt will develop acutely. These patients will have the sudden appearance of a thrill and a loud, harsh, systolic murmur along the lower left sternal border combined with the sudden onset of right heart failure.

Predisposing factors to cardiac rupture in-

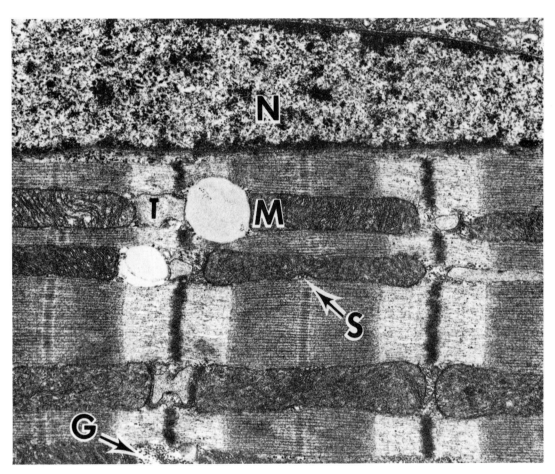

Fig. 1.15 Ischemic myocardial injury. Transmission electron micrograph (×22,500) of control, nonischemic myocardium. Chromatin material is evenly dispersed in a nucleus (N). Mitochondria (M) are elongated and lie between the myofibrils. G-glycogen particles; T-transverse tubule; S-sarcoplasmic reticulum. (Bloor CM, Ashraf M: Pathogenesis of acute myocardial infarction. Advances in Cardiology 23:1, 1978).

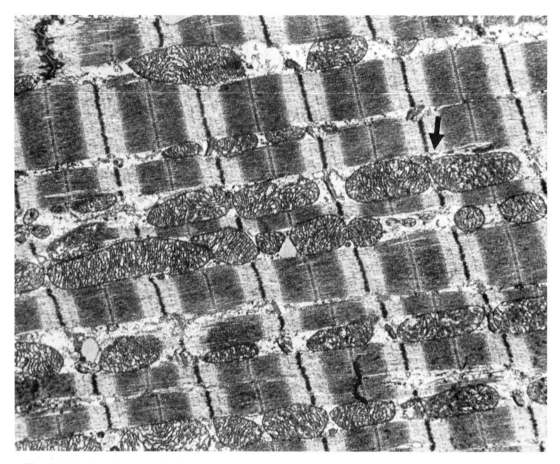

Fig. 1.16   Ischemic myocardial injury. Transmission electron micrograph (×6,200) of ischemic myocardium 15 minutes after the onset of ischemia. Glycogen granules are depleted and mitochondria (arrow) are slightly swollen. These changes are reversible if blood flow is restored at this time. (Bloor CM: Cardiac Pathology, p. 204, Philadelphia, J. B. Lippincott, 1978.)

clude absence of old myocardial scars, presence of a heavy polymorphonuclear leukocytic infiltrate, hemorrhage and an increase in subepicardial fat in the region of the infarct, and the persistence of hypertension after the onset of an acute myocardial infarct. The heavy infiltration of polymorphonuclear leukocytes and the resulting disintegration of the leukocytes in the infarct liberate proteolytic enzymes which digest the necrotic muscle. This contributes to the softening of the ventricular wall, making it more likely to rupture. In patients with previous myocardial infarcts, the presence of old myocardial scars with increased collateral circulation and greater resistance of the fibrous connective tissue to ischemia reduces the likelihood of rupture.

Most cardiac ruptures lead to massive pericardial hemorrhage (hemopericardium) and cardiac tamponade. This is frequently fatal, although the amount of blood present in the pericardial cavity may be relatively small—in most cases ranging from 200 to 250 ml.

## Papillary Muscle Rupture

When rupture occurs in the papillary muscle, it almost always involves papillary muscles of the left ventricle. The posterior papillary muscle is involved twice as frequently as the anterior papillary muscle (Fig. 1.24). When rupture of both heads of the papillary muscle occurs, most patients die suddenly, almost immediately.

However, a rupture involving a single head of a papillary muscle is compatible with longer survival.[50],[60] Such patients develop changes in the character and intensity of murmurs that have been present before the onset of the acute myocardial infarct, or a new murmur may develop over the mitral region which is systolic and is loud and harsh. Rupture of mitral chordae tendineae may also occur, which is compatible with longer survival.

The greater frequency of involvement of the posterior papillary muscle is thought to be related to its remoteness from its source of blood supply and to a poor collateral blood supply to the superficial bulbospiral muscle that forms the papillary muscle. In contrast, the left anterior papillary muscle derives its blood supply only from the left coronary artery. It lies at the greatest distance from the ostium of the artery, and is a favorite site of scarring with increased collateralization.

## Ventricular Aneurysm

With large myocardial infarcts, the resulting fibrous scar may undergo progressive ballooning in the course of months to years, eventually resulting in a ventricular aneurysm. This comprises a persistent localized bulging of a weakened wall of a chamber in response to the high intraluminal pressure. Ventricular aneurysms occur in about 4 percent of the patients dying with myocardial infarcts.[61] They most often involve the left ventricle, rarely the right ventricle, and almost never the atria. The larger cardiac aneurysms are usually located in the anterior apical or anterior septal portions of the left ventricular wall. Posterior basal aneurysms are smaller.

Ventricular aneurysms usually develop during the first two weeks after the onset of a myocardial infarct,[55],[62] although they may occur at a later time. At this time, myocardial necrosis

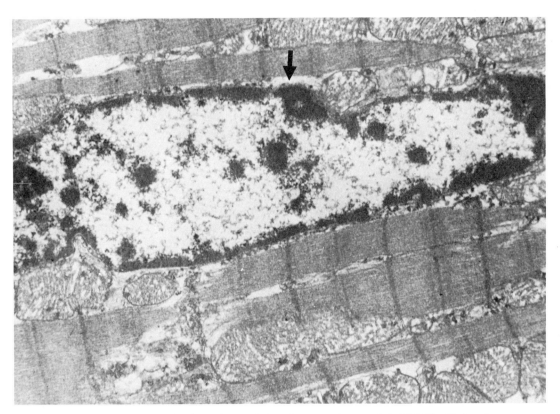

Fig. 1.17 Ischemic myocardial injury. Transmission electron micrograph (×22,550) of ischemic myocardium 2 hours after the onset of ischemia. Nuclear chromatin (arrow) is now clumped at the nuclear membrane. (Bloor CM: Cardiac Pathology, p. 205, Philadelphia, J. B. Lippincott, 1978.)

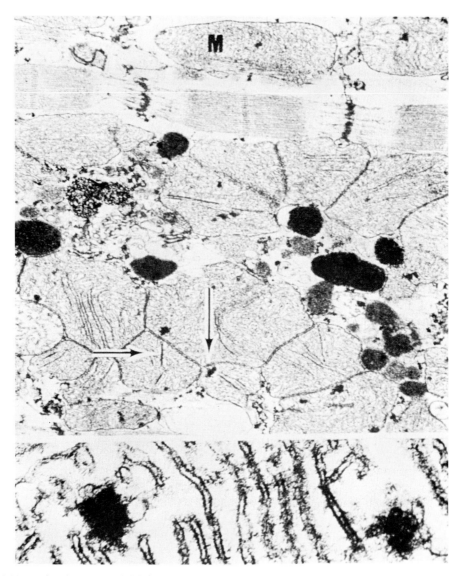

Fig. 1.18  Ischemic myocardial injury. Transmission electron micrograph of ischemic myocardium 2 hours after the onset of ischemia. Upper panel shows swollen mitochondria, which contain dense granules (arrow). Lower panel shows the dense granules at higher magnification. The cristae of the mitochondria are swollen and separated. (Bloor CM: Cardiac Pathology, p. 205, Philadelphia, J. B. Lippincott, 1978.)

is at its maximum development and some collagen is beginning to layer on the surface to aid in maintaining integrity of the wall and preventing cardiac rupture. Grossly, ventricular aneurysms may be saccular, but most frequently they are not sharply demarcated from the ventricular cavity. Mural thrombosis occurs on the endocardial surface and may wall-off the entry site into the aneurysmal chamber (Fig. 1.25). The wall of the aneurysm is thinner than that of the ventricle. Adhesions between the epicardium and pericardium in the region of the thin-walled aneurysm may prevent rupture with cardiac tamponade from occurring. On microscopic examination, the myocardial fibers in the aneurysmal wall are decreased in size and number. There are various degrees of necrosis, fibrosis, hyalinization, and calcium deposits.

When a ventricular aneurysm is present for a long time, calcification may occur in its wall,

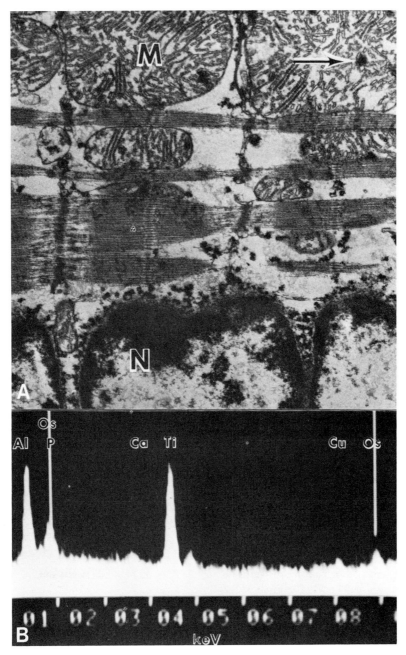

Fig. 1.19   Ischemic myocardial injury. *(A)* Transmission electron micrograph (×22,500) after 2 hours of coronary occlusion. The mitochrondria (M) are swollen and contain electron-dense deposits (arrow). Chromatin material is clumped along the margins of the nucleus (N). *(B)* Energy dispersion spectrum of a mitochondrial deposit (as marked in A) showing calcium (Ca) and phosphorus (P) peaks. The phosphrous (K$\alpha$) peak shows interference from the osmium peak at approximately the level of 2 keV. The other peak originated from the grid and its holder. (Bloor CM, Ashraf M: Pathogenesis of acute myocardial infarction, Adv Cardiol 23:1, 1978.)

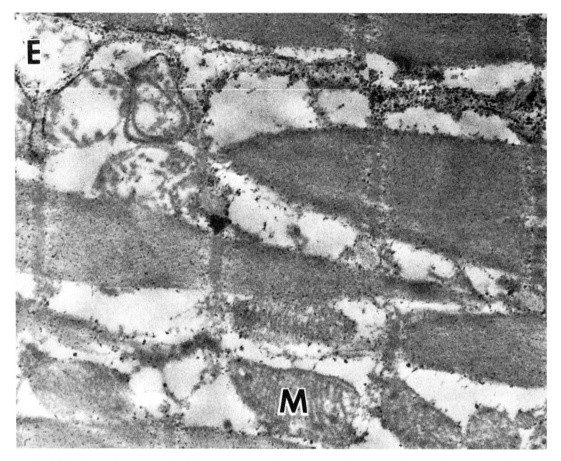

Fig. 1.20 Ischemic myocardial injury. Transmission electron micrograph (×22,500) after 45 minutes of coronary occlusion. The tissue is treated with lanthanum, which is used as an extracellular tracer. Mitochondria (M) are swollen and contain electron-dense deposits. Lanthanum has leaked into the extracellular space (E), indicating an increase in cell membrane permeability. (Bloor CM, Ashraf M: Pathogenesis of myocardial infarction. Adv Cardiol 23:1, 1978.)

resulting in plaque-like zones which appear on a radiograph. Spontaneous rupture of ventricular aneurysm is rare.[55] The usual course of terminal events in the patient with a ventricular aneurysm is the development of progressive congestive heart failure.

## PATHOLOGY OF CORONARY BYPASS VEIN GRAFTS

Coronary artery bypass graft surgery using saphenous vein grafts has been widely and successfully used for the treatment of ischemic

Fig. 1.21 Ischemic myocardial injury. (A) Transmission electron micrograph (×137,000) of a freeze-fractured normal myocardial cell membrane, showing E fracture face. The intramembranous particles are sparse. T-opening of transverse tubule; V-pinocytotic vesicle. (B) P fracture face of a cell membrane, containing numerous particles. V-pinocytotic vesicle (×137,000). (C) P fracture face of the cell membrane from myocardium ischemic for 2 hours showing nicks or breaks (arrows) in the lipid bilayer and various aggregations of intramembrane particles (×65,000). (Bloor CM, Ashraf M: Pathogenesis of acute myocardial infarction. Adv Cardiol 23:1, 1978.)

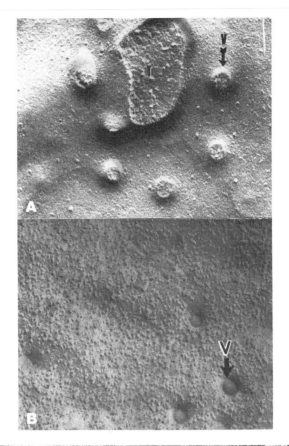

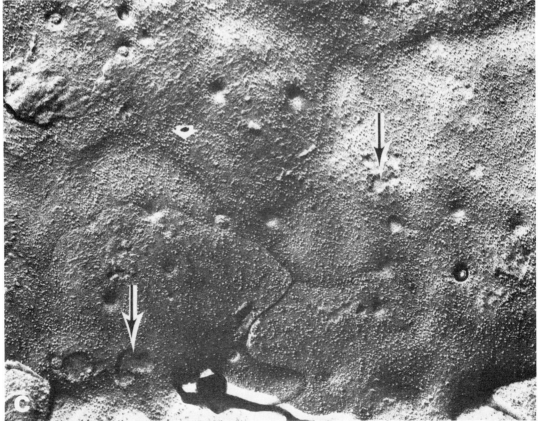

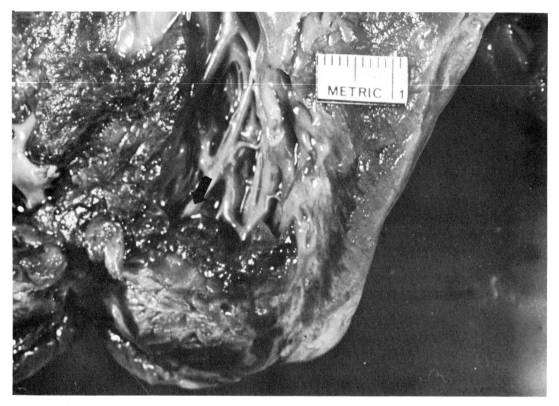

Fig. 1.22  Mural thrombus. In this heart with an acute myocardial infarct involving the apex of the left ventricle, a small mural thrombus (arrow) is present on the endocardial surface, lying over the region of the infarct. (Bloor CM: Cardiac Pathology, p. 196, Philadelphia, J. B. Lippincott, 1978.)

heart disease. Morphological studies of hearts with coronary artery bypass grafts have focused on the internal changes occurring within the graft [63] and on the changes related to the surgical procedure that involve the anastomoses, the coronary arteries, and the myocardium.[64] A brief review of these changes is presented here.

Vlodaver and Edwards [63] studied the segments of saphenous veins used as grafts to the coronary arteries. Except for an occasional thrombotic occlusion of a graft, no lesions were observed in grafts which had been in place for less than 1 month. In grafts present for 3 months or longer, fibrous thickening of the intima was consistently present. This lesion progressed to fibrous intimal proliferation, resulting in near or complete occlusion of the lumen in some patients. This fibrous intimal proliferation appeared to be a response to arterial pressure within the vein graft.

Bulklcy and Hutchins [64] described similar in-

timal changes in vein grafts. However, most occlusions occurred at the site of the anastomosis of the coronary artery bypass graft. Compression of the vascular lumen and thrombosis and dissection of the coronary artery were the most frequent mechanisms of occlusion. In Bulkley and Hutchins' study, the myocardium was also at risk for changes resulting from the bypass operation. Contraction band or reperfusion necrosis was the change most frequently seen. This occurred most often in the distribution of patent grafts.

## NONATHEROSCLEROTIC CAUSES OF ACUTE MYOCARDIAL INFARCTION

In some patients, acute myocardial infarction will occur in the virtual or near absence of significant coronary atherosclerosis. Such cases remind us that myocardial infarction is a dynamic phenomenon in which a number of factors interact with one another. It is a balance among these factors that eventually determines whether infarction will occur and develop. Basically, the balance is between oxygen supply to the myocardium and the oxygen needs of the myocardium. This balance is constantly changing because of a variety of factors. When the balance is disturbed—i.e., the supply is not meeting the metabolic demands of the tissue—then ischemic injury will develop and eventually proceed to cell death, necrosis, and the state called myocardial infarction.

Several investigators have reported the actual incidence of myocardial infarction in the absence of significant coronary occlusion. According to Roberts and Buja,[65] the incidence ranges somewhere between 5 and 10 percent of all autopsy patients presenting with acute myocardial

infarcts. Another study, involving a review of some 5,000 autopsies since 1968 from University and Veterans Administration Hospitals, UCSD School of Medicine, showed that 4 percent of our patients who had documented acute myocardial infarcts at autopsy had coronary artery disease involving the three major vessels, with less than 70 percent occlusion of each. Some narrowing of the vessels was present, but several patients had less than 50 percent narrowing in all three of their major coronary arterial branches. Thus, about 4 to 10 percent of patients who have acute myocardial infarction at autopsy do not have significant narrowing of the coronary arterial bed by atherosclerotic disease. It is true that an autopsy population has certain bias;[66] these patients have more severe clinical disease at the time of initial presentation than surviving patients. Other factors to be accounted for include: (1) different popula-

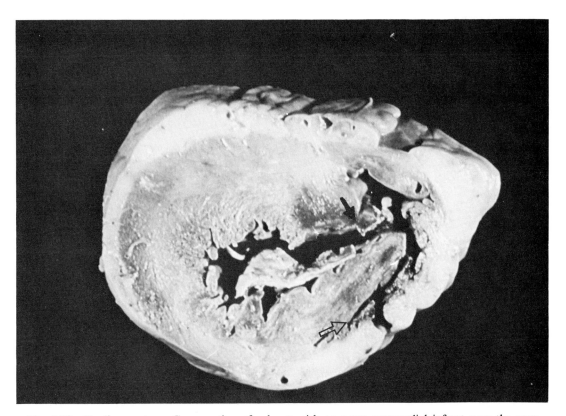

Fig. 1.23 Cardiac rupture. Cross-section of a heart with an acute myocardial infarct near the apex shows rupture of the intraventricular septum (solid arrow) and the anterior left ventricular wall (open arrow). This resulted in hemopericardium and sudden death. (Bloor CM: Cardiac Pathology, p. 209, Philadelphia, J. B. Lippincott, 1978.)

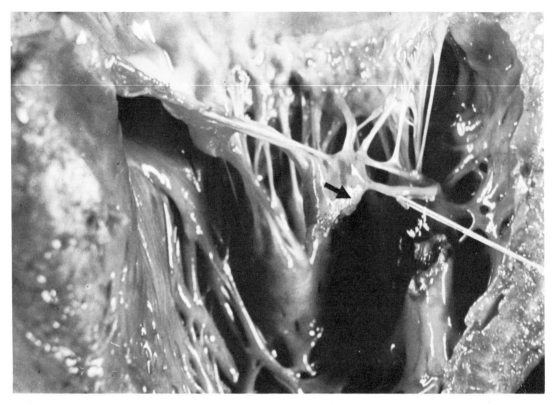

Fig. 1.24  Papillary muscle rupture. This specimen shows papillary muscle rupture in a heart with an acute myocardial infarct involving the posterior left ventricular wall and the posterior papillary muscle. The posterior papillary muscle belly is ruptured (arrow). This resulted in acute mitral regurgitation, rapid onset of left-sided heart failure, and death within 24 hours. (Bloor CM: Cardiac Pathology, p. 211, Philadelphia, J. B. Lippincott, 1978.)

tions from different autopsy services, and (2) the time after death in which the hearts were examined—for example, the longer the time, the greater the chance that thrombi may lyse postmortem. Thus, even with the most careful inspection—including microscopic examination—there may not be any evidence that an occlusive thrombus was present at the time the clinical event occurred. However, in these studies of autopsy patients, coronary atherosclerotic disease was still less than observed in other patients.

Likoff [67] has summarized the pathogenesis of myocardial infarction occurring without significant coronary artery disease and coronary occlusion. The etiologies include limitations of coronary arteriography, functional coronary constriction, small vessel disease, platelet aggre-

gation, abnormal hemoglobin, and redistribution of coronary blood flow. Let us consider these factors individually. First, there may be limitations of arteriography or angiography in demonstrating the presence of significant coronary arterial disease. Techniques today have better resolution than was true a number of years ago, and it is now uncommon to find that occlusion was not documented clinically by angiography when postmortem evidence was available. The second possibility—namely, functional coronary constriction or vasospasm—definitely occurs but its incidence is uncertain (see Ch. 25). It is unlikely that this factor is responsible for the number of cases seen because vasospasm would have to persist for a long time to cause irreversible myocardial cell injury. The next factor, small vessel disease, is a possibility; however, even in large autopsy series the incidence of small vessel disease without significant large vessel disease is very low. Platelet aggregation may induce coronary flow reduction, resulting in myocardial infarction; however, when one sees platelet aggregation at autopsy, it is present in small vessels in the mid-wall and endocardial portions of the myocardium. One would expect these individuals to have subendocardial infarcts, but usually they have transmural infarcts. Platelet aggregation seems an unlikely explanation. Abnormal hemoglobin-oxygen affinity has been demonstrated in patients with acute myocardial infarcts, but this as the sole cause of acute myocardial infarction in the absence of significant coronary disease is, again, a rare occurrence. The last possibility may be redistribution of coronary blood flow. There is experimental evidence for this in animals with partial constriction of a coronary artery. Physiologic stress can redistribute coronary blood flow away from the subendocardium, making it more vulnerable to ischemic change.[68] If individuals with subclinical coronary artery disease are stressed to levels where the metabolic demands of the tissue become so high that actual flow cannot meet them, there may be significant flow diverted away from the subendocardial zones. This makes them more susceptible to ischemic injury, which can progress to myocardial infarction. Thus, current investigations support the view that myocardial infarction can occur without significant coronary atherosclerotic disease

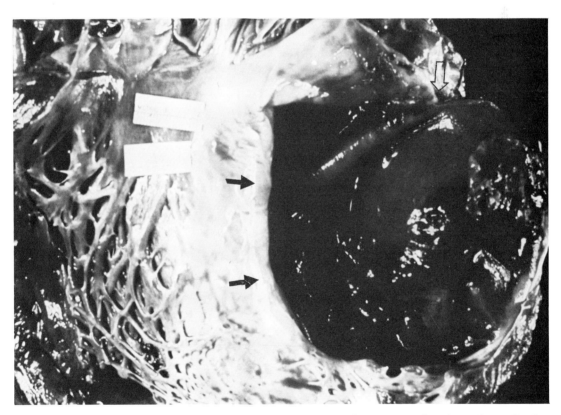

Fig. 1.25  Ventricular aneurysm. This specimen shows a ventricular aneurysm in a heart that suffered acute myocardial infarction 6 months earlier. A massive aneurysm has developed in the posterior portion of the interventricular septum and the posterior left ventricular wall (dark arrow). A large mural thrombus is adherent to the wall of the aneurysm (white arrow). The endocardial surface adjacent to the margin of the aneurysm is thickened secondary to the old infarct beneath. (Bloor CM: Cardiac Pathology, p. 12, Philadelphia, J. B. Lippincott, 1978.)

and coronary occlusion. The actual number of patients in which this does occur, however, remains in the neighborhood of 5 to 10 percent.

## ROLE OF THROMBOSIS IN ACUTE MYOCARDIAL INFARCTION

Acute myocardial infarction is usually considered to be the result of thrombotic occlusion of a major coronary artery. Autopsy studies have reported the frequency of such thrombosis to range from 21 to 91 percent.[65,69-73] Differing techniques of examining coronary arteries at autopsy and differing definitions of what constitutes thrombosis may contribute to the varied incidences of thrombosis reported in acute myocardial infarction. However, the detailed anatomic study of the coronary arterial beds of patients dying of acute myocardial infarction by Roberts and Buja[65] shows that coronary arterial thrombi are present in 54 percent of patients having transmural necrosis, in none having only subendocardial necrosis, and in 8 percent of those dying suddenly. The virtual absence of thrombi in patients dying suddenly and the presence of thrombi in only half of those having myocardial necrosis suggests that coronary arterial thrombi are consequences rather than causes of acute myocardial infarction. The findings of Spain and Bradess[72,73] that the incidence of coronary arterial thrombi increases with longer intervals between the onset of symptoms of myocardial ischemia and death also supports this view. However, although thrombosis may be less important as a precipitating cause of acute myocardial infarction, it still plays a major role in inducing the underlying coronary atherosclerosis. Indeed, there is little doubt that organization of thrombi contributes to the development of the complicated atherosclerotic plaque which significantly narrows the coronary artery.[65]

## REFERENCES

1. McCullagh KG: Revised concepts of atherogenesis. A review. Cleveland Clinic Quart 43:249–266, 1976.
2. Ross R, Glomset JA: The pathogenesis of atherosclerosis. Part 1. N Engl J Med 295:369–377, 1976.
3. Ross R, Glomset JA: The pathogenesis of atherosclerosis. Part 2. N Engl J Med 295:420–425, 1976.
4. Geer JC, McGill HC Jr, Strong JP: The fine structure of human atherosclerotic lesions. Am J Path 33:263, 1968.
5. McGill HC Jr (Ed.): The geographic pathology of atherosclerosis. Lab Invest 18:463, 1968.
6. McGill HC Jr, Geer JC, Strong JP: Natural history of human atherosclerotic lesions. In Sandler M. and Bourne GH, (Eds.): Atherosclerosis and its origin. New York, Academic Press, 1963, pp. 39–65.
7. Hollander W, Kramsch DM, Inove A: The metabolism of cholesterol, lipoproteins, and acid mucopolysaccharides in normal and atherosclerotic vessels. Prog Biochem Pharmacol 4:270, 1968.
8. French JE: Atherosclerosis in relation to the structure and function of arterial intima with special reference to the endothelium. Int. Rev. Pathol. 5:253, 1966.
9. Mitchell JRA, Schwartz CJ: Arterial disease. Oxford, Blackwell Scientific Publications, 1965.
10. Mustard JF, Packham MA: The role of blood and platelets in atherosclerosis and the complications of atherosclerosis. Thromb Diath Haemorrh 33:444, 1975.
11. Ross R, Glomset J, Harker L: Response to injury and atherogenesis. Am J Path 86:675, 1977.
12. Ross R, Vogel A: The platelet-derived growth factor. Cell. 14:203, 1978.
13. Thomas W, Jones R, Scott RF, Morrison E, Goodale F, Imai H: Production of early atherosclerotic lesions in rats characterized by proliferation of modified smooth muscle cells. Exp Mol Pathol 2 (Suppl. I): 40, 1963.
14. Guyton JR, Karnovsky MJ: Smooth muscle proliferation in the occluded rat cartoid artery. Lack of requirement for luminal platelets. Am J Path 94:585, 1979.
15. Benditt EP: Evidence for a monoclonal origin of human atherosclerosis plaques and some implications. Circulation 50:650–652, 1974.
16. Benditt EP, Benditt JM: Evidence for monoclonal origin of human atherosclerotic plaque. Proc Natl Acad Sci 70:1753, 1973.
17. Martin GM: Cellular aging. Am J Path 89:484, 1977.
18. Martin GM, Ogburn C, Sprague C: Senescence and vascular disease. In: Cristofalo VJ (Eds.):

Explorations in aging. New York, Plenum Press, 1976, pp. 163–194.

19. Nam K, Florentin RA, Janakidevi K, Lee KT, Reiner JM, Thomas WA: Population dynamics of arterial smooth muscle cells. III. Inhibition by aortic tissue extracts of proliferative response to intimal injury in hypercholesterolemic swine. Exp Mol Pathol 21:259, 1974.

20. Pearson TA, Dillman JM, Solez K, Heptinstall RH: Clonal markers in the study of the origin and growth of human atherosclerotic lesions. Circulation Res 43:10, 1978.

21. Dawber TR: Coronary heart disease. Morbidity in the Framingham study and analysis of factors of risk. Bibl Cardiol 13:9–24, 1963.

22. Kannel, WB: Serum lipid precursors of coronary heart disease. Human Pathol 2:109, 1971.

23. Castelli WP, Doyle JT, Gordon T, et al: HDL, cholesterol and other lipids in coronary heart disease: The cooperative lipoprotein phenotyping study. Circulation 55:767, 1977.

24. Doll R, Hill AB: Mortality and smoking. Brit Med J I:1399, 1964.

25. Doyle JT, Dawber, TR, Kannel, WB, Heslin AS, Kahn HA: Cigarette smoking and coronary heart disease. Combined experience of the Albany and Framingham studies. Engl J Med 266:796–801, 1962.

26. Hammond EC: In Richardson, RG: (Ed.), Proceedings of the Second World Conference on Smoking and Health. London, Pitman, 1972.

27. Kannel WB, McGee D, Gordon T: A general cardiovascular risk profile: The Framingham study. Am J Cardiol 38:46, 1976.

28. Kannel WB, Dawber TR, Friedman GD, Glennon WE, McNamara PM: Risk factors in coronary heart disease. An evaluation of several serum lipids as predictors of coronary heart disease; the Framingham study. Ann Intern Med 61:888–899, 1964.

29. Kuller, WH: Epidemiology of cardiovascular diseases: Current perspectives. Am J Epidemiol 104:425, 1976.

30. Russek HI, Zohman BL: Relative significance of heredity, diet and occupational stress in coronary heart disease of young adults. Amer J Med Sci 235:266–275, 1958.

31. Stamler J: Life-styles, major risk factors, proof and public policy. Circulation 58:3, 1978.

32. Wilhelmsson C, Vedin, JA, Elmfeldt, D, Tibblin G, Wilhemson L: Smoking and myocardial infarction. Lancel I:415–419, 1975.

33. Strong JP, Richards ML, McGill HC Jr, Egger DA, McMurray MT: On the associations of ciga-

rette smoking with coronary and aortic atherosclerosis. J. Atheroscler. Res. 10:303, 1969.

34. Bloor CM: Cardiac Pathology. Philadelphia, J.B. Lippincott, 1978, pp. 176–221.

35. Epstein FH, Ostrander LD, Johnson BC, Payne MW, Hayner NS, Keller JB, Francis T: Epidemiological studies of cardiovascular disease in total community, Tecumseh, Michigan. Ann Intern Med 62:170, 1965.

36. Keen H, Rose GA, Pyke DA, Boyns DR, Chlouverakis C, Mistry S: Blood sugar and arterial disease. Lancet II: 505, 1965.

37. Ostrander LD, Francis T, Hayner NS, Khelsberg MO, Epstein FH: The relationship of cardiovascular disease to hyperglycaemia. Ann Intern Med 62:1188, 1965.

38. Stearns S, Schlesinger MJ, Rudy A: Incidence and clinical significance of coronary artery disease in diabetes mellitus. Arch Intern Med 80:463–474, 1947.

39. Woolfe N: Atherosclerosis. In Pomerance, A. and Davies, M.J.: The Pathology of the Heart. Oxford, Blackwell, 1975.

40. Morris JN, Gardner MJ: Epidemiology of ischemic heart disease. Am J Med 46:674, 1969.

41. Rosenman RH, Brand RJ, Jenkins CD, Friedman M, Straus R, Wurm, M: Coronary heart disease in the Western Collaborative Group Study: Final follow-up experience of 8½ years. JAMA 233:872, 1975.

42. Liljefois I, Rahe RH: An identical twin study of psychosocial factors in coronary heart disease in Sweden. Psychosom Med 32:523, 1970.

43. Fishbein MC, MacLean D, Maroko PR: The histopathologic evolution of myocardial infarction. Chest 73:843, 1978.

44. Lodge-Patch I: The aging of cardiac infarcts and its influence on cardiac rupture. Brit Heart J 13:37, 1951.

45. Mallory GK, White PD, Salcedo-Salgar J: The speed of healing of myocardial infarction. A study of the pathologic anatomy in seventy-two cases. Amer Heart J 18:647–671, 1939.

46. Jennings RB, Baum JH, Herdson PB: Fine structural changes in myocardial ischemic injury. Arch Path 79:135–143, 1965.

47. Jennings RB, Ganote CE, Reimers KA: Ischemic tissue injury. Am J Path 81:179–198, 1975.

48. Asraf M, Bloor CM: X-ray microanalysis of mitochondrial deposits in ischemic myocardium. Virchows Arch. B. Zellpath, 22:287–297, 1976.

49. Ashraf M, Sybers HD, Bloor CM: X-ray microanalysis of ischemic myocardium. Exp Mol Pathol 24:435, 1976.

50. Shen AC, Jennings RB: Myocardial calcium and magnesium in acute ischemic injury. Am J Path 67:417–440, 1972.

51. Bloor CM, Ashraf M: Pathogenesis of acute myocardial infarction. Advances in Cardiology, 23:19–24, 1977.

52. Ashraf M, Halverson C: Structural changes in the freeze-fractured sarcolemma of ischemic myocardium. Am J Path 88:583–594, 1977.

53. Ashraf M, Livingston L, Bloor CM: Ultrastructural alterations in myocardial vessels after coronary artery occlusion. Scanning Electron Microscopy, Vol. 2, ITT Research Institute, 502–506, Chicago, 1977.

54. Davies MJ, Robertson WB: Diseases of the coronary arteries. In: Pomerance A, and Davies MJ: The Pathology of the Heart. Oxford, Blackwell, 1975.

55. Titus JL: Pathology of coronary heart disease. Cardiovasc. Clinics I:9, 1969.

56. Lewis AJ, Burchell HB, Titus JL: Clinical and pathological features of post infarction cardiac rupture. Amer J Cardiol 23:43, 1969.

57. Naeim F, Maza LM, Robbins SL: Cardiac rupture during myocardial infarction. A review of 44 cases. Circulation 45:1231, 1972.

58. Van Tassel RA, Edwards JE: Rupture of heart complicating myocardial infarction. Chest 61: 104, 1972.

59. Braunwald E: Mitral regurgitation. Physiologic, clinical and surgical considerations. N Engl J Med 281:425, 1969.

60. Cerderqvist L, Soderstrom J: Papillary muscle rupture in myocardial infarction—a study based on autopsy material. Acta Med Scand 176:287, 1964.

61. Dubnow M, Burchell HB, Titus JL: Clinical and pathological features of post infarction ventricular aneurysm. A study of 80 cases. Amer Heart J 70:753, 1965.

62. Davis RW, Ebert PA: Ventricular aneurysm—a clinical pathologic correlation. Amer J Cardiol 29:I, 1972.

63. Voldaver Z, Edwards JE: Pathologic changes in aortic-coronary arterial saphenous vein grafts. Circulation 44:719, 1971.

64. Bulkley BH, Hutchins AM: Pathology of coronary artery bypass graft surgery. Arch Pathol Lab Med 102:273, 1978.

65. Roberts WC, Buja LM: The frequency and significance of coronary arterial thrombi and other observations in fatal acute myocardial infarction: A study of 107 necropsy patients. Amer J Med 52:425, 1972.

66. Bloor CM, Roeske WR, O'Rourke RA: Clinical pathologic correlates in acute myocardial infarction. Adv. Cardiol. 23:14, 1978.

67. Likoff W: Myocardial infarction in subjects with normal coronary arteriograms. Am J Cardiol 28:742, 1971.

68. Bloor CM: An overview of myocardial blood flow. In: Manning GW, Haust DM, eds: Atherosclerosis: Metabolic, Morphologic and Clinical Aspects. Plenum Press, New York, 1977, pp. 668–673.

69. Barnes AR, Ball RG: The incidence and situation of myocardial infarction in one thousand consecutive postmortem examinations. Am J Med Sci 183:215, 1932.

70. Baroldi G: Acute coronary occlusion as a cause of myocardial infarct and sudden coronary heart death. Am J Cardiol 16:589, 1965.

71. Miller RD, Burchell HB, Edwards JE: Myocardial infarction with and without acute coronary occlusion. A pathologic study. Arch Intern Med 88:597, 1951.

72. Spain DM, Bradess VA: The relationship of coronary thrombosis to coronary atherosclerosis and ischemic heart disease. Am J Med Sci 240:701, 1960.

73. Spain DM, Bradess VA: Sudden death from coronary heart disease. Survival time, frequency of thrombi and cigarette smoking. Chest 58:107, 1970.

# 2 | Biochemical and Metabolic Aspects of Ischemia

*Richard W. Gross, M.D.*
*Burton E. Sobel, M.D.*

Knowledge of metabolic derangements resulting in cell death has become increasingly pertinent to the clinical cardiologist concerned with protection of ischemic myocardium and therapy of coronary artery disease. Detailed consideration of the numerous processes involved in myocardial biochemistry is beyond the scope of this brief review. Accordingly, we shall focus on those processes and derangements of particular relevance to the understanding of the function of normal and diseased myocardium and to the management and diagnosis of ischemic heart disease. Emphasis will be placed on those biochemical abnormalities which have been exploited diagnostically and those which are amenable to manipulation for potential therapeutic progress.

In contrast to anoxia per se, ischemia (i.e., inadequate perfusion), which is of course generally accompanied by anoxia, entails accumulation of potentially noxious metabolites within jeopardized myocardium, some of which have been implicated as mediators of malignant ventricular dysrhythmia and contributors to irreversible injury. Accordingly, the rationale for protecting ischemic myocardium has been broadened to include not only considerations based on the need for improving the balance between myocardial oxygen requirements and supply but also for precluding accumulation of deleterious metabolites and facilitating their removal.

The function of the heart as a pump depends on effective transduction of chemical energy derived ultimately from catabolism of substrates. As in other tissues, the "currency" of transduction of chemical to physical energy is adenosine-triphosphate (ATP). When myocardial oxygen supply is limited by the diminished perfusion caused by coronary artery spasm, atherosclerosis, or small vessel disease, the delivery of substrate (primarily glucose and fatty acid) as well as oxygen is compromised. Production of ATP under physiological conditions depends on a close coupling between electron transport from the chemical substrate being utilized to the terminal electron acceptor—oxygen—in a process called oxidative phosphorylation, which is localized to the mitochondria. However, ischemic tissue suffers from double jeopardy: (1) lack of availability of both substrate and the terminal electron acceptor limits electron transport and therefore the genesis of ATP, and (2) anaerobic glycolytic metabolism, which produces some ATP in the absence of oxygen, can only proceed to a limited extent because of the inhibitory effects of metabolites such as hydrogen ion and lactate on critical components of the glycolytic pathway. This double jeopardy helps to explain the resistance to irreversible injury manifested by myocardium rendered anoxic but not ischemic (for example, in isolated hearts perfused with nitrogenated rather than aerated media). Ischemic tissue also suffers from accumulation of other metabolites such as fatty acid esters and catabolites of membrane constituents which may exert deleterious electrophysiological effects on the tissue and contribute to necrosis.

## BIOCHEMICAL AND STRUCTURAL ORGANIZATION WITHIN MYOCARDIUM

Transduction of chemical to mechanical energy in myocardium results primarily from oxidation of organic substrates through the citric acid cycle (Fig. 2.1) and via fatty acid beta oxidation. Enzymes involved in both pathways are located in the mitochondria. Sugars, such as

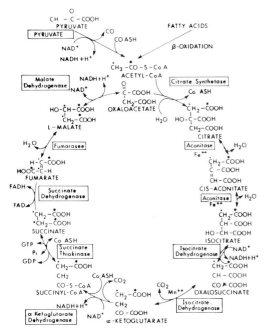

Fig. 2.1 A diagrammatic representation of the tricarboxylic, aerobic pathway of metabolism. Substrate enters the cycle in the form of fatty acids or pyruvate, a catabolic product of carbohydrates. Through a series of enzymatic reactions mediated by enzymes (designated in the rectangular boxes), substrate is oxidized to $CO_2$ and water. Energy liberated during the process of oxidation is conserved in the form of nucleotides including primarily ATP, although some energy conservation occurs with the synthesis of GTP as well. ATP is synthesized via coupling reactions involving conversion of reduced flavine nucleotides (FADH) and reduced pyridine nucleotides (NADH) and concomitant electron transfer in mitochondria (not depicted in the diagram).

glucose, are first partially metabolized via glycolysis in the cytosol and then broken down to two-carbon constituents that can enter the citric acid cycle. Reducing equivalents (reduced pyridine nucleotides and flavoproteins) generated as a byproduct of substrate oxidation donate their electrons to the terminal electron acceptor, oxygen, via a series of electrochemical reactions utilizing the electron transport chain in mitochondria with concomitant production of ATP and formation of water. Myocardial energy requirements are extensive. Thus, it is not surprising that mitochondria comprise between 25 and 50 percent of myocardial mass and that they are dispersed extensively through the tissue in juxtaposition to myofibrils. ATP production per mole of glucose catabolized is 16-fold greater with aerobic compared to anaerobic metabolism. Thus, although brief intervals of anoxia or ischemia may be tolerated during which anaerobic glycolytic metabolism can supply some ATP, more prolonged intervals cannot be tolerated because of the inability of anaerobic intermediary metabolism to produce ATP fast enough to sustain the energy supply required for myocardial viability.[1]

Under conditions in which substrate availability may be limited, but oxygen supply is adequate (e.g., with profound hypoglycemia), myocardial metabolism becomes dependent on utilization of endogenous substrate stored in the form of glycogen, triglycerides, and other moieties serving as depot sources for substrate. Sarcoplasmic storage granules of glycogen comprise approximately 0.4 to 0.6 percent of myocardial wet weight, but depletion of glycogen begins within 30 seconds after the induction of ischemia, and glycogen stores can satisfy substrate requirements for only approximately four minutes in the absence of exogenous fatty acid or carbohydrate. Endogenous triglycerides can supply fatty acid for catabolism when substrate availability is limited. However, fatty acid metabolism requires oxidation. Since the most common cause of substrate limitation is ischemia, and since the limited availability of substrate is accompanied by impaired oxidative capacity, fatty acids released from the endogenous triglycerides accumulate in the cytosol as acyl esters with potentially noxious effects on myo-

cardial membranes. Because of the net limitation of utilization of fatty acids released from
endogenous pools during ischemia, repetitively
insulted tissue is characterized by accumulation
of neutral fat. This reflects deposition of fatty
acids delivered to the cell from the blood under
conditions in which oxidation is repetitively
precluded.[2-4]

## The Contractile Proteins

Myocardium contains contractile elements
called sarcomeres that consist of contractile
proteins (actin and myosin) with regulatory
protein constituents (troponin and tropomyosin) arranged in a highly organized lattice (Fig.
2.2). Thick myosin filaments are interspersed

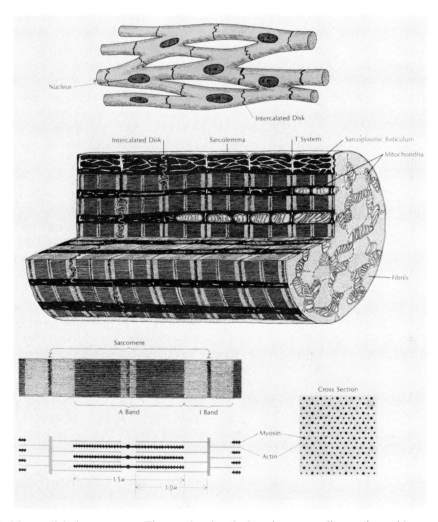

Fig. 2.2 Myocardial ultrastructure. The top drawing depicts the myocardium as it would appear under
the light microscope. Ultrastructural schematization (center drawing) illustrates the division of the fiber
longitudinally into rodlike fibrils, in turn composed of sarcomeres, the basic contractile units. Within
the sarcomeres, thick filaments of myosin, confined to the central dark A band, alternate with thin
filaments of actin which extend from the Z lines (delimiting the sarcomere) through the I band and
into the A band where they overlap with myosin filaments. Also depicted is the T system that mediates
ion transport into the cells and the sarcoplasmic reticulum that releases calcium to activate the contractile
machinery. (Adapted from figure by B. Tagawa from Sonnenblick, E. H., "Myocardial ultrastructure
in the normal and failing heart," *Hospital Practice,* Vol. 5, No. 4 and from "The Myocardium: Failure
and Infarction," E. Braunwald, Editor, HP Publishing Co., Inc., New York, 1974.)

in parallel with thin actin filaments, facilitating chemical interactions between these two contractile proteins. The regulatory proteins are interspersed periodically along the thin actin filaments and serve to modulate the chemical interactions that occur between actin and myosin and account for contraction of the muscle. Although contractile and regulatory proteins had been thought to be composed of a single polypeptide chain in each case until recently, it has been found that they contain aggregates of several different polypeptide subunits. For example, troponin is composed of at least three subunits, each with a specific biological function. One aggregate (41,000 daltons) serves to bind the troponin complex to tropomyosin, an aggregate of 17,000 daltons that binds calcium. Another aggregate (28,000 daltons) inhibits the actin-ATP-myosin interaction.[5]

## Excitation-Contraction Coupling

Electrical depolarization is accompanied by the release of calcium from the sarcoplasmic reticulum to the cytosol, where it gains access to the contractile and regulatory proteins. Myocardial cell contraction is initiated when the calcium that is released binds to the calcium-binding subunit of troponin and displaces the inhibitory subunit in such a way that interaction between myosin and actin is facilitated. Other factors, in particular the myosin light chains, play a role in conferring calcium sensitivity to the contractile apparatus as well.

The most distinctive feature of the cytoplasm of cardiac muscle cells is a regular array of transverse bands recognizable by light microscopy. One band is strongly birefringent (that is, anisotropic) and is therefore called the A-band. The other is only weakly birefringent (isotropic) and is called the I-band. Each I-band is bisected by a dense line called the Z-line, and the sarcomere is defined as a region between two successive Z-lines. The thick myosin filaments are the characteristic structural components comprising the A-bands. On the other hand, the thin actin filaments originate at the Z-line and penetrate into the A-band, where

they interdigitate with myosin. One region of the A-band, in which the thick filaments are not overlapped by actin, is called the H-zone. During contraction, the length of individual thin and thick filaments changes negligibly. However, changes in sarcomere length occur as a result of a change in the extent of overlap of thick and thin filaments. In essence, then, contraction is the result of sliding of thin and thick filaments over each other, mediated by molecular rearrangements in response to binding of calcium by selected portions of contractile and regulatory proteins. Although it is not entirely clear just what the exact chemical nature of the interaction between actin and myosin is that accounts for the change in overlap underlying contraction, it is clear that hydrolysis of ATP is the source of energy transduced into physical work.

Relaxation of cardiac muscle occurs when calcium is taken up again by the sarcoplasmic reticulum, leading to molecular rearrangements that temporarily inhibit the actin-myosin interactions responsible for contraction.

Obviously, effective contraction of the entire ventricle requires coordinated sequential alterations in calcium flux during each cardiac cycle. This is accomplished by coupling of electrical activity to function of the sarcoplasmic reticulum, a syncytium of anastomosing intracellular tubules. As the wavefront of electrical activity reaches the sarcoplasmic reticulum, calcium is released from binding sites. Subsequent relaxation during diastole is mediated by re-uptake of free calcium by the electrically quiescent sarcoplasmic reticulum.

In ischemic myocardium, contractility is impaired virtually instantaneously, despite the relatively slower deterioration of myocardial intermediary metabolism and the comparably slow decline of high-energy phosphate stores. Changes in intracellular pH occur promptly, and it has been suggested that the increased concentration of hydrogen ions accounts for the prompt diminution of contractile function by virtue of interference with function of the regulatory proteins, sarcoplasmic reticulum, or both.[5,6]

Clinical corollaries to these observations include the following: (1) localized regions of dyskinesis are commonly seen during episodes of transitory ischemia when suitably sensitive techniques are employed for studies in vivo. These appear to reflect transient impairment of contractility in cells subjected to ischemia but not irreversibly injured, and (2) prolonged ischemia, leading to irreversible dysfunction of myocardial membranes including the sarcolemma, the sarcoplasmic reticulum, and mitochondrial membranes, impairs intracellular calcium metabolism profoundly by flooding the cytosol and contractile proteins with free calcium, which may be manifest in its extreme form by contracture of myofilaments and production of the so-called stone heart. Excessive accumulation of free calcium leads to binding of radioactive tracers such as $^{99m}$Tc-pyrophosphate. Tissue subjected to irreversible injury of this nature can therefore be visualized by myocardial infarct scintigraphy. Accumulation of tracer in this setting has been correlated with intracellular deposition of calcium detected morphologically. Experiments with doubly labeled $^{99m}$Tc-pyrophosphate demonstrate concordant binding of labeled pyrophosphate and labeled technetium,[6] suggesting that clinically detectable accumulation of tracer is attributable to complexing with calcium. Although some of the tracer accumulates in mitochondria—compatible with independent observations of dense bodies in mitochondria from ischemic heart muscle containing calcium and phosphate—images reflect uptake of tracer and binding to calcium in numerous other subcellular loci as well, since only 29 percent of the tracer is found in the mitochondrial fraction.[7,8]

Regulation of intracellular calcium flux under physiological conditions and derangements in calcium metabolism under pathophysiological conditions are readily understandable when one recognizes the marked concentration gradients for calcium that exist across cell and organelle membranes. Since the concentration of calcium in interstitial fluid is of the order of $5 \times 10^{-3}$ M and the concentration of calcium within the cytosol is precisely regulated within a range of $10^{-7}$ and $10^{-8}$ M throughout the cardiac cycle, it is not surprising that impair-

ment of membrane function results in a flooding of the intracellular environment with exogenous calcium.[9]

## Ultrastructural Manifestations of Myocardial Ischemia

Prolonged ischemia results in mitochondrial swelling with a decrease in mitochondrial matrix density and the appearance of amorphous granules thought to contain lipids. In mitochondria from regions subjected to ischemia for 15 minutes or less, the changes may be reversible. However, when ischemia persists for 20 to 60 minutes, progressive morphological alterations occur that appear to persist even if perfusion is subsequently restored. Swelling is a reversible feature, but deposition of granules in the matrix is among the earliest morphological criteria of irreversible injury. Other granular densities containing calcium and phosphate appear in the intramitochondrial space when ischemia sufficiently prolonged to produce irreversible injury is followed by reperfusion, presumably because of the increased delivery of calcium to regions of myocardium in which exclusion of the free calcium by functionally intact membranes is compromised.[10,11]

Respiratory function of mitochondria is impaired in organelles isolated from tissue subjected to ischemia persisting for 20 to 60 minutes. Thus, despite the persistence of some electron transport function, oxidation of pyruvate, coupling of respiration to synthesis of ATP, and suppression of latent mitochondrial ATPase are markedly impaired.[12]

Severe and prolonged ischemia results in alterations of ultrastructure of other organelles as well. Thus, in contrast to the central location of a nucleus with evenly distributed chromatin in normal myocardium, nuclei from ischemic regions become eccentrically located and aggregate chromatin peripherally. Ischemic cells become swollen, and their sarcolemma exhibits rents and exvaginations. After several hours of ischemia, ultrastructural alterations in contractile proteins become apparent with disruption and thickening of thin filaments accompanied by dense packing of thick filaments and loss of the regular lattice seen under physiological conditions.[13]

## Substrate Utilization

Within the context of the overall biochemical and ultrastructural characteristics described above, myocardium obtains energy from substrate catabolism and transduces it to mechanical energy utilized in contraction, thereby fulfilling the functional requirements of the heart as a pump. Depending on availability of specific substrates and prevailing intracellular biochemical conditions, the tissue may utilize, individually or in combinations, numerous metabolic substrates including free fatty acids, glucose, pyruvate, lactate, ketone bodies, and amino acids. The extraction fraction of a particular substrate is dependent on myocardial energy requirements, availability of alternative substrates, binding of the substrate to circulating moieties such as albumin, prevailing hormonal influences, and interactions between related metabolic pathways.

Under physiological conditions, metabolism of free fatty acid fulfills 60 to 90 percent of myocardial energy requirements. Thus, production of ATP under aerobic conditions is dominated by free fatty acid oxidation. Several factors account for this preponderance: [14]

(1) The extensive activity of enzymes within myocardium involved in fatty acid oxidation.[15]

(2) High activity of enzymes that esterify fatty acids reaching the intracellular space, thereby trapping them within myocardium and precluding their loss through the extracellular fluid in a bidirectional flux.[16]

(3) Extensive deployment of enzymes that facilitate transport of activated fatty acids into the mitochondria via a series of reactions involving interconversion of fatty acid to fatty acid-carnitine and fatty acid-thioester derivatives, resulting in preferential transport of fatty acids to the sites for oxidation under physiological conditions.[17]

(4) High activity of enzymes involved in transporting cofactors utilized in fatty acid catabolism (such as carnitine) from the mitochondria to the cytosol in the form of short chain-carnitine derivatives, facilitating the conversion of cytosolic fatty acid thiolesters to fatty acid-carnitine derivatives which can readily ingress into mitochondria.[18]

Under physiological conditions, uptake of exogenous fatty acid occurs by diffusion of a small amount of free fatty acid in equilibrium with albumin-bound fatty acid, facilitated by incompletely characterized fatty acid-binding proteins in the heart muscle. It is not entirely clear whether or not albumin-bound fatty acid (present in interstitial fluid as well as in plasma) can be taken up directly, bypassing fatty acid in the aqueous phase in equilibrium with albumin-bound fatty acid. The importance of the molar ratio of fatty acid to albumin is underscored by the exquisite dependence of extraction fraction on this ratio. Fatty acid that is taken up into the cell is trapped in the form of acyl (fatty-acid)-Coenzyme A (CoA), in a process called thioesterification. Under conditions in which the cytosolic content of CoA is depleted, trapping of fatty acid will be impaired and the outward flux will therefore increase markedly. Such circumstances prevail in ischemic myocardium because the limited amount of cytosolic CoA normally present is complexed to acetyl groups whose oxidation is precluded. This phenomenon—namely, the reduction in net accumulation of fatty acid by ischemic myocardium due to outward flux increasing and offsetting the persistent inward flux—has been exploited diagnostically in studies with [11]C-labeled palmitate detected by positron emission transaxial tomography to localize regions of myocardium whose metabolism has been altered by ischemia. Diminished uptake in irreversibly injured cells reflects a different underlying phenomenon—namely, the loss of viable myocardium capable of accumulating or oxidizing fatty acid under any circumstances.[19-21]

Under physiological conditions, extraction of free fatty acids is increased when myocardial oxygen requirements are increased. If exogenous fatty acid is not available in quantities sufficient to meet the needs, hydrolysis of intracellular triglycerides ensues, providing the myocardium with preferred fuel even in the absence of an adequate exogenous supply. The teleological advantages of fatty acid as the preferred fuel for myocardium are evident, based on the amount of ATP that can be synthesized from one mole of a long-chain fatty acid (i.e., approximately 140 moles of ATP).

Under physiological conditions, fatty acids extracted by myocardium are metabolized primarily by beta oxidation within the mitochondria. However, during brief intervals of ischemia, uptake continues but oxidation is inhibited; the result is accumulation of cytosolic fatty acids, some of which are deposited in triglycerides. Thus, it is not surprising that increased triglyceride stores, detectable histochemically or by ultrastructural analysis of the tissue, are a hallmark of myocardium subjected to repetitive, brief episodes of ischemia.[4,15]

## Carbohydrate Metabolism

Myocardium can subsist for many hours with glucose as the sole substrate. Some carbohydrate metabolism is essential under all conditions—even when the primary energy supply comes from oxidation of fatty acids, since terminal oxidation of the 2-carbon fragments resulting from catabolism of fatty acids or carbohydrates requires oxidation through the citric acid cycle. However, in contrast to beta oxidation of fatty acids which occurs in the mitochondria, the initial metabolism of carbohydrates occurs in the cytosol.

Transport of glucose into the myocardial cell is both stereospecific and carrier-mediated. It is increased by specific hormones such as insulin, growth hormone, and catecholamines. Transport of glucose, like uptake of fatty acids, is augmented under conditions in which myocardial energy requirements are increased. Extensive availability of exogenous fatty acids inhibits uptake of glucose through mechanisms which are not entirely understood but appear to be dependent on direct effects of fatty acids on the cell membrane.[22]

Once glucose reaches the intracellular environment, it is trapped [23] by phosphorylation in a reaction mediated by hexokinase. Since the product, glucose-6-phosphate, cannot permeate the cellular membrane, outward flux is precluded. In the absence of insulin, transport of glucose across the cell membrane is rate-limiting for glucose utilization. However, when insulin is present, the rate-limiting step is hexokinase activity. Glucose-6-phosphate can undergo one of three major metabolic fates: (1) glycolysis via the Emden-Meyerhof (glycolytic) pathway; (2) deposition in the storage form—glycogen, or (3) oxidation via the hexose monophosphate shunt. Metabolism via the Emden-Meyerhof pathway is involved in both anaerobic glycolysis and aerobic metabolism of glucose. In the case of anaerobiasis, glucose can be broken down only to the 3-carbon level, with lactate as an end product and accumulation of reducing equivalents in the cytosol as a concomitant. During aerobic metabolism, the 3-carbon compound, pyruvate, can undergo further degradation after conversion to acetyl CoA via the pyruvate dehydrogenase reaction. Subsequent complete oxidation of acetyl CoA via the citric acid cycle in mitochondria results in formation of water and carbon dioxide. Relative fluxes through the three major metabolic pathways available to glucose are determined by activities of enzymes at branch points in individual pathways. Under physiological conditions, glycolysis is allosterically restrained at the level of phosphofructokinase. Thus, intracellular concentrations of glucose-6-phosphate are high, formation of glucose-1-phosphate via phosphoglucomutase is facilitated, and glycogenesis is favored since the glucose-1-phosphate can react with a uridyl group permitting subsequent condensation with intracellular glycogen by the action of glycogen synthase.[22-24]

Glycogenesis is regulated primarily at the glycogen synthase step, and is under the influence at this site of both covalent and noncovalent mechanisms.[25] The synthase enzyme is a multiple phosphorylated, single polypeptide chain. Its active (A) form can be converted to an inactive (B) form by phosphorylation of serine in a reaction catalyzed by synthase kinase. The synthase is also influenced by noncovalent modulators which impart a finely graded influence on its activity.[26]

Under conditions of exogenous glucose deprivation, and particularly when exogenous fatty acid is also limited, intracellular glucose can be derived from endogenous myocardial glycogen stores by glycogenolysis. Glycogenolysis is initiated by an enzyme called phosphorylase, which exists in two different forms. The *b* form (inactive under physiological conditions) can be phosphorylated to the active, *a* form by a protein kinase. Under conditions of ischemia, the *b* form may have biological importance because of the release of inhibition of its activity by the declining glucose-6-phosphate concentrations as well as stimulation of its activity by inorganic phosphate and AMP. One important activator of the protein kinase responsible for converting phosphorylase *b* to phosphorylase *a* is cyclic AMP. Thus, it is not surprising that exposure of myocardium to catecholamines which give rise to cyclic AMP results in marked augmentation of glycogenolysis. However, the potential importance of many other possible activators (including calcium), as well as specific sites of covalent modification and substrate specificity of protein kinases remain to be elucidated.[24]

It is important to emphasize that, under conditions in which phosphorylation of many enzymes may occur concomitantly, the covalent modifications of enzymes involved in synthesis of glycogen and degradation of glycogen would be complimentary. In other words, enzyme modification would result in enhanced activity of glycogenolysis (through the phosphorylase *a* reaction) and decreased activity of glycogenesis (due to conversion of the synthase to the inactive B form).

## Minor Contributors to Energy Supply

Ketone bodies, pyruvate, lactate, and amino acids are readily extractable by myocardium. However, under physiological conditions their catabolism contributes little to overall energy requirements of the heart. Beta-hydroxybutyrate and acetoacetate are oxidized and cleaved to form acetyl CoA, which can enter the citric acid cycle. Under conditions of starvation or diabetic ketoacidosis, ketone bodies compete with conventionally utilized substrates and are oxidized preferentially with relative inhibition of glycolysis and fatty acid beta oxidation. Pyruvate formed may enter the citric acid cycle via the pyruvate dehydrogenase reaction.[27]

Amino acids can be metabolized by transamination or deamination (in some cases), giving rise to compounds that can enter directly into carbohydrate-oxidative metabolic pathways.

## Glycolysis

As mentioned previously, the Emden-Meyerhof pathway is important, not only because it provides the initial set of reactions involved in aerobic metabolism of carbohydrates, but also because it can subserve energy requirements to some extent during transitory anaerobiasis. Under anaerobic conditions, ATP is produced by substrate level phosphorylations. As can be seen in Figure 2.3, in the Emden-Meyerhof pathway 1 mole of glucose is phosphorylated, split to form two 3-carbon fragments, and metabolized to form 2 moles of NADH and 2 moles of ATP (net) via substrate phosphorylations. Under aerobic conditions, the 2 moles of NADH give rise to 6 moles of ATP by interaction with the electron transport chain after incorporation of reducing equivalents into mitochondria is facilitated by shuttle reactions. However, when oxygen availability is limited, anaerobic glycolysis results in formation of only 2 moles of ATP per mole of glucose metabolized. Under aerobic conditions, in addition to the 8 moles of ATP formed from catabolism of glucose to the 3-carbon level, a substantial additional amount of ATP is formed when pyruvate is converted to acetyl CoA and incorporated in the citric acid cycle, with subsequent complete oxidation of constituents originally present in glucose.

Rates of glycolytic flux are modulated by several mechanisms affecting the activity of rate-limiting enzymes. Three are particularly important and will be considered separately.

**Phosphofructokinase (PFK).** Under many conditions, phosphofructokinase determines the rate of glycolytic flux. Its activity is under allosteric control, with modulation by at least 10 identified noncovalent effectors.[28] PFK is inhibited by ATP, creatine phosphate, citrate, and low pH. In contrast, its activity is stimulated by fructose-1,6-disphosphate, cyclic AMP, ADP, and inorganic phosphate. The interaction of these effectors is complex, but briefly, the presence of fructose-1,6-disphosphate and inorganic phosphate precludes allosteric inhibition by binding of ATP. On the other hand, cyclic

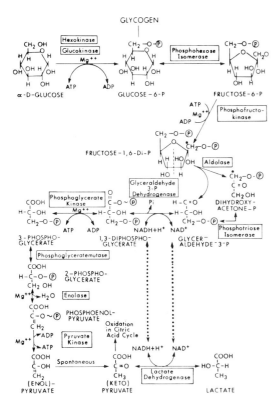

Fig. 2.3 A diagrammatic depiction of glycolysis, a series of reactions by which glucose (either free or derived from glycogen) is converted to pyruvate under aerobic conditions and consequently catabolized via the tricarboxylic acid cycle (see Figure 1) or to lactate under anaerobic conditions. Molecular oxygen is not required for this cycle. Enzymes mediating individual steps of the metabolic pathway are depicted within rectangular boxes. Synthesis of ATP occurs in the form of substrate phosphorylations under anaerobic and aerobic conditions, but additional ATP can be synthesized under aerobic conditions permitting oxidation of NADH by the mitochondrial electron transport chain and the coupled synthesis of ATP.

AMP prevents allosteric inhibition by precluding binding of citrate.[29] When PFK activity is low, fructose-6-phosphate and glucose-6-phosphate accumulate, inhibiting net extraction of glucose from the extracellular space because of a strong product inhibition of hexokinase by glucose-6-phosphate and consequent impairment of trapping. In addition, glycogen synthesis is stimulated by the high concentrations of glucose-6-phosphate. Thus, PFK acts as an intracellular microprocessor, responding to

concentrations of critical intermediates in metabolism and influencing the extraction and biochemical fate of glucose. Under physiological conditions, glycolysis is restrained at the level of the PFK reaction by end-products of free fatty acid metabolism (particularly citrate, ATP, and creatine phosphate formed from the synthesized ATP). Under conditions of hypoxia or ischemia, PFK becomes activated because of the declining concentrations of citrate, ATP, and creatine phosphate. In addition, the increased concentrations of cyclic AMP, ADP, and inorganic phosphate augment its activity. Activation of PFK is amplified because of positive feedback provided by the product of the reaction it catalyzes, 1,6-fructose diphosphate. When PFK is activated under conditions such as these, the rate-limiting step in glycolytic flux shifts. Thus, under conditions of anoxia or ischemia, glycolytic flux is controlled by activity of glyceraldehyde-3-phosphodehydrogenase.

**Glyceraldehyde-3-Phosphate Dehydrogenase (GPDH).** With ischemia, dihydroxyacetone phosphate and glyceraldehyde-3-phosphate accumulate, suggesting that the rate-limiting step in glycolytic flux under these conditions is activity of GPDH. GPDH is transformed from an apoenzyme (protein without cofactor) to a holoenzyme (active enzyme complex with cofactor) by the addition of pyridine nucleotides which appear to influence isomerization. Thus, the enzyme is regulated by allosteric mechanisms. Its critical regulatory role is dependent also on its low affinity for substrates and sensitivity to hydrogen ion accumulating during ischemia with consequent depression of activity.[30,31]

**Pyruvate Dehydrogenase.** Under aerobic conditions, glycolytic flux is coupled to pyruvate oxidation. Thus, pyruvate and lactate do not accumulate within the myocardium. Under conditions of ischemia or hypoxia, however, pyruvate oxidation is precluded or limited. The negative redox potential in the cell leads to conversion of pyruvate to lactate, which first accumulates in myocardium and promptly appears as well in effluents from ischemic regions. Oxidation of pyruvate requires: (1) decarboxylation and formation of an active species (acetyl CoA) by a complex of enzymes collectively referred to as pyruvate dehydrogenase, and (2) oxidative phosphorylation permitting net oxidation of cytosolic NADH produced as a result of the generation of pyruvate. Pyruvate dehydrogenase activity is regulated by both covalent and noncovalent mechanisms. Covalent modification is modulated by activation of pyruvate dehydrogenase kinase, which phosphorylates the enzyme and inhibits enzymatic activity. Pyruvate, ADP, and inorganic phosphate inhibit the kinase and thereby increase activity of pyruvate dehydrogenase. In addition, pyruvate dehydrogenase activity is product-inhibited by acetyl CoA and NADH. Although activity of pyruvate dehydrogenase may control the rate of entry of pyruvate into the citric acid cycle, it is possible that alternative pathways such as the mitochondrial pyruvate transport system may provide another locus of modulation of overall citric acid cycle flux.[32,33]

## Citric Acid Cycle

The citric acid cycle refers to a series of reactions that sequentially oxidize 2-carbon units (acetyl CoA) derived from glycolysis or fatty acid oxidation. The cycle is responsible for generating most of the ATP derived from substrate metabolism. Under physiologic aerobic conditions, one turn of the cycle results in production of 12 moles of ATP and liberation of 2 moles of carbon dioxide per mole of acetyl CoA catabolized. Flux in the cycle is coupled closely to mitochondrial redox potential, maintaining a balance between the generation of reducing equivalents, the energy requirements of myocardium, and the rate of oxidative phosphorylation. The cycle also provides a metabolic link between cytosolic glycolytic flux and mitochondrial metabolism, which must be regulated precisely to provide efficient utilization of substrate.

Citric acid cycle flux is determined principally by the mitochondrial redox potential which operates by influencing citrate synthase, isocitric dehydrogenase, and $\alpha$-ketogluterate dehydrogenase. In isolated mitochondria, citrate synthase activity is regulated by the concentration of oxaloacelate, in turn modulated by the intramitochondrial ratio of NAD/

NADH. This ratio also serves to modulate the activity of the dehydrogenase reactions and thereby links the citric acid cycle flux to the rate of oxidative phosphorylation. Reduced pyridine nucleotides (such as NADH) are unable to penetrate the inner mitochondrial membrane. Accordingly, reducing equivalents formed in the cytosol from glycolytic reactions must be transported into the mitochondrial matrix via one of several shuttle reactions, of which the most important example is the malate-aspartate shuttle. This shuttle provides a communication not only between cytosolic and mitochondrial metabolism, but also between different component reactions of the citric acid cycle. For example, fluxes through the citrate synthase and $\alpha$-ketogluterate dehydrogenase portions of the cycle during the first several minutes after the addition of glucose are markedly disparate. This so-called "unspanning" of the citric acid cycle occurs because of differential rates of entry and exit of intermediates in the cycle utilized in the malate-aspartate shuttle. Thus, the shuttle modulates activity of the citric acid cycle in response to altered conditions of respiratory function in mitochondria such as those occurring at the time of onset of ischemia. When the funtional integrity of the malate-aspartate shuttle is compromised, such as during conditions of prolonged ischemia, cytosolic NADH accumulates. Accumulation of reducing equivalents in the cytosol inhibits glycolytic flux, thereby further compromising the ability of the anoxic and ischemic myocardium to generate ATP, even through the backup mechanism of substrate phosphorylation.[34-37]

To recapitulate, under physiological conditions the mitochondrial ratio of NADH/NAD is relatively high; hence, the citric acid cycle flux is restrained by the relatively low concentrations of oxaloacetate and the low activity of isocitrate dehydrogenase and $\alpha$-ketogluterate dehydrogenase. Under conditions in which myocardial oxygen requirements are high and oxidative phosphorylation is increased, the NADH/NAD ratio declines. This leads to a relative increase in the concentration of oxaloacetate augmenting flux through citrate synthase. Furthermore, the relatively low NADH/NAD ratio augments flux through the dehydrogenase reactions. The overall increase in citric acid cycle flux permits augmented production of reducing equivalents from substrate and, hence, increased synthesis of ATP via oxidative phosphorylation utilizing the mitochondrial electron transport chain. In contrast, under conditions of hypoxia or ischemia, oxidative phosphorylation is precluded. The result is an increase in the NADH/NAD ratio with a consequent decrease of flux through the citric acid cycle. ATP production becomes dependent on substrate level phosphorylation. However, even when anaerobic glycolysis is proceeding at a maximal rate, the rate of synthesis of ATP via this mechanism is insufficient to maintain energy stores required for myocardial viability. Furthermore, persistence of ischemia leads to accumulation of catabolites that preclude maintenance of anaerobic glycolytic flux at a rate similar to that seen during the early burst initiated by anoxia.[38]

## Fatty Acid Metabolism

Intracellular free fatty acids are initially bound to cytosolic proteins and subsequently activated by formation of thioesters in a reaction utilizing ATP. In extracts of myocardium, acyl CoA synthetase activity exceeds the maximum rate of free fatty acid beta oxidation observed in vivo.[39] Thus, acyl CoA synthetase activity does not appear to be rate-limiting for fatty acid utilization. Even though AMP and adenosine inhibit the activity of acyl CoA synthetase and increase the amount of myocardium rendered ischemic, the acyl CoA synthetase step does not appear to become rate-limiting since acyl CoA accumulates in ischemic and hypoxic myocardium.

Acyl CoA may undergo one of two metabolic fates: (1) conversion to acyl carnitine via several specific carnitine–acyl CoA transferases, or (2) incorporation into polar or nonpolar lipids after initial reaction with glycerophosphate mediated via glycerophosphate acyl transferase. The relative preponderance of one of these metabolic pathways depends on the relative activity of glycerophosphate acyl transferase and acyl carnitine transferase under specific prevailing physiological or pathophysiological conditions.

Acyl CoA carnitine transferase activity is high, facilitating utilization of fatty acids by myocardium for production of ATP under physiological conditions. Since long-chain acyl CoA cannot permeate mitochondrial membranes, oxidation of the acyl groups requires transfer of the activated form into the mitochondrial matrix after conversion to carnitine derivatives mediated by carnitine acyl CoA transferase I and II (located on or near the outer and inner mitochondrial membranes respectively). Intramitochondrial acyl carnitine is converted to acyl CoA, the substrate required for the first step of actual oxidation. Reducing equivalents generated from oxidation of fatty acid derivatives are utilized to form ATP in a fashion analogous to that involved in carbohydrate oxidation. Rates of beta oxidation of fatty acids are modulated by intramitochondrial redox potentials as well as the mitochondrial concentration of acyl CoA. Thus, the flux of fatty acid beta oxidation is coupled tightly to citric acid cycle activity, oxidative phosphorylation, and overall myocardial energy balance.

## Synthesis of Polar and Nonpolar Lipids

Myocardial lipids are in dynamic equilibrium. Absolute concentrations of individual species are determined by relative rates of synthesis and degradation. Complex myocardial lipids are synthesized by sequential acylation of glycerophosphate, hydrolysis of phosphatidic acid, and condensation of 1,2-diacyl glycerol with acyl CoA to form triglycerides or with a cytidine diphosphate (CDP)-base to form phospholipids. Thus, 1,2-diacyl glycerol represents a branch point in lipid synthesis with the relative rates of polar compared to nonpolar lipid determined by the flux of 1,2-diacyl glycerol to neutral lipids (mediated by acyl transferase) or to phospholipids (mediated by phosphocholine or phosphoethanolamine cytidyl transferase).

The rate-limiting step for nonpolar lipid synthesis is esterification of glycerol phosphate which is dependent upon the concentrations of both acyl CoA and glycerol phosphate. Under conditions in which fatty acid oxidation is limited by the availability of oxygen as a terminal electron acceptor acyl CoA accumulating in the cytosol is preferentially shunted into the synthesis of triglycerides which appear in increased concentrations as storage forms.[40] Subsequently, when oxygen availability is reestablished, liberation of fatty acids from triglycerides provides endogenous substrate for beta oxidation. This phenomenon—the hydrolysis of nonpolar lipids—is catalyzed by triglyceride lipase activity. In some tissues triglyceride lipase is remarkably sensitive to activation by cyclic AMP and, hence, to activation by catecholamines which augment the rate of synthesis of this secondary messenger. In other tissues (such as adipose tissue) the lipase is stimulated by heparin. Modulation of myocardial triglyceride lipase activity has not been completely elucidated. Nevertheless, it is apparent that triglyceride lipase activity is inhibited by high concentrations of fatty acids within the cell, thus linking triglyceride hydrolysis with the need for endogenous supply of fatty acids to the myocardium.[41]

The rate-limiting step for myocardial polar lipid synthesis is the phosphocholine cytidyl transferase reaction.[42] Polar lipids comprise major structural components of all myocardial membranes including sarcolemma, mitochondrial membranes, and the sarcoplasmic reticulum, and the rates of turnover of individual moieties appear to be finely regulated. Hydrolysis of these membrane constituents proceeds by the action of ubiquitous phospholipases and lysophospholipases, some of which appear to be intimately bound to the membranous structures in which the phospholipids are found. Regulation of activity of these phospholipases is only poorly understood, although it appears likely that, in general, phospholipase activity requires calcium and that hydrolysis of membrane constituents may be accelerated when local concentrations of calcium become excessively high.

## Lysophosphatides

Lysophosphatides are asymmetrical, wedge-shaped phospholipids that have potent, detergent-like effects on membranes in many systems. Although these compounds comprise only a small fraction of the total lipid constituents in membranes, at least two lysophosphatides, lysophosphatidyl choline and lysophosphatidyl ethanolamine, have been found to accumulate in ischemic myocardium.[43,44] Increased concentrations of these moieties have been detected in venous effluents from ischemic zones of myocardium in situ and may contribute to arrhythmogenic properties of such effluents.[45]

The membrane-active effects on cardiac muscle and Purkinje fibers have been demonstrated in several systems. Superfusion of normoxic Purkinje fibers from canine hearts with media containing lysophosphatidyl choline in concentrations less than those seen in extracts of myocardium rendered ischemic in vivo leads to profound alterations in transmembrane action potentials with changes resembling those seen in action potentials recorded from ischemic myocardium in vivo.[46] Furthermore, perfusion of isolated rabbit hearts with media containing lysophosphatidyl choline bound to albumin results in the rapid onset of ventricular dysrhythmia and impairment of diastolic relaxation as well as concomitant coronary vasoconstriction presumably reflecting direct effects of the lysophosphatides on coronary smooth muscle as well as myocardium (unpublished observations). Theoretically, the asymmetry and relatively large volume occupied by the polar head groups of lysophosphoglycerides endows these compounds with properties impairing packing of other phospholipids in the myocardial membranes. Thus, incorporation of even small quantities of these potentially deleterious metabolites may contribute to functional and structural instability manifested by ventricular dysrhythmia and ventricular dysfunction accompanying ischemia. Accumulation of lysophosphatides in ischemic myocardium is compatible with several observations, including:

(1) Identification of phospholipase activity in subcellular constituents of myocardium including the sarcolemma.[47]

(2) Documentation of activity of such phospholipases at physiological pH.

(3) Recognition of prostaglandin release from hearts rendered ischemic,[48] since the rate-limiting step for prostaglandin synthesis and release appears to be phospholipolysis with liberation of arachidonic acid and formation of

prostaglandin endoperoxides mediated by cyclo-oxygenase.

(4) Activation of phospholipolysis in other organs rendered ischemic including the liver with remarkably rapid loss of phospholipid constituents.[49]

(5) Detection of increased quantities of lysophosphatides in extracts of ischemic myocardium and effluents from ischemic zones in situ.[44] Accumulation of these compounds may be mediated not only by activation of phospholipases but also by diminished washout from ischemic zones. Some evidence suggests de novo synthesis of lysophosphatides from glycolytic intermediates which accumulate during ischemia.[50]

One clinical implication of the potentially deleterious effects of membrane-active constituents accumulating in myocardium rendered ischemic or delivered to the ischemic tissue via the circulation is the potential benefit derived from administration of solutions containing glucose, insulin, and potassium. Such infusions reduce circulating levels of free fatty acid and diminish ventricular dysrhythmia accompanying myocardial ischemia in man.[51] The protective effect of the regimen may be dependent upon limitation of ingress of fatty acids into the ischemic heart muscle, reduction of formation and accumulation of moieties such as acyl CoA and acyl carnitine, both of which may exert detergent-like effects on the sarcolemma, and reduction of synthesis of other amphiphilic compounds such as lysophosphatides because of the diminished availability of acyl CoA.

## Protein and Amino Acid Metabolism

Protein synthesis and degradation in the heart are modulated by numerous factors, prominent among which are availability of amino acids and influences of hormones. Influx of amino acids is potentiated by prolonged, sequential, passive stretch and relaxation of myocardium in vitro, suggesting that ingress of amino acids may increase when cardiac work increases in vivo, in part as a direct response to the increased mechanical activity. Under physiological conditions, protein degradation is diminished by insulin and protein synthesis is augmented by it. However, it is not clear to what extent, if any, cardiac dysfunction occurring in patients with diabetes mellitus is a direct reflection of the lack of an insulin effect on myocardium. Ischemia elicits characteristic changes in myocardial amino acid metabolism. The concentrations of alanine and branch-chain amino acids increase; the former because of increased de novo synthesis from transamination of pyruvate accumulating as a result of impaired aerobic metabolism and the latter because of decreased oxidation. Protein synthesis is diminished, not only because of possible effects of the diminished concentrations of selected amino acids but also because of decreased peptide chain initiation and elongation. Deleterious effects of decreased protein synthesis on net protein content may be blunted somewhat, since protein degradation appears to be an energy-dependent process which would, of course, be somewhat limited by the decreased high-energy phosphate stores typical of ischemic tissue. Effects of hypoxia on protein synthesis are partially modified by administration of insulin, at least in isolated perfused heart preparations. Insulin stimulates peptide chain initiation in this setting, but chain elongation remains inhibited. Thus, net protein synthesis does not increase.[52-54]

## INTEGRATED CHANGES IN METABOLISM IN ISCHEMIC MYOCARDIUM—A RECAPITULATION

Under physiologic aerobic conditions, metabolites of the predominant pathway of intermediary metabolism utilized in energy production—i.e., fatty acid beta oxidation—restrain glycolytic activity by inhibiting uptake of glucose and decreasing activity of phosphofructokinase and pyruvate dehydrogenase. When ischemia ensues, the abrupt decline of the intracellular phosphate potential (ATP/ADP + inorganic phosphate) leads to augmentation of glycolytic activity mediated via release of allosteric inhibition of phosphofructokinase due to the decreased concentration of ATP and the diminished concentration of citrate reflecting decreased citric acid cycle flux and facilitated also by the increased concentrations of inorganic phosphate and cyclic AMP. Decreased delivery of substrate from the blood is offset in part by increased glycogenolysis and hydrolysis of triglycerides, both of which may be triggered by the augmentaiton of cyclic AMP content typical of ischemic myocardium and mediated to some extent by local release of catecholamines. The early burst of glycolytic flux persists only briefly, since accumulation of lactate and hydrogen ion limits glycolytic activity by inhibiting glyceraldehyde-3-phosphate dehydrogenase. Because of the lack of oxygen availability, reducing equivalents accumulate in the cytosol in the form of NADH, leading to an alteration in the NADH/NAD ratio which restrains both citric acid cycle flux and fatty acid beta oxidation. This accumulation of reducing equivalents is initially attenuated by increased conversion of pyruvate to lactate as well as by de novo fatty acid biosynthesis. However, as lactate concentrations rise and as intracellular high-energy stores decline, these compensatory mechanisms fail because mass action precludes conversion of pyruvate to lactate and the lack of ATP limits biosynthesis of fatty acids.

Accumulation of noxious metabolites appears to contribute to the accelerating impairment of myocardial metabolism and ultrastructural integrity. Fatty acyl CoA esters inhibit activity of adenine nucleotide translocase, an enzyme involved in the transport of ATP from mitochondria to cytosol.[55] Increased concentrations of acyl CoA, coupled with the increased concentrations of glycerol phosphate, promote synthesis of triglycerides by virtue of the mass action effect.[56] Accumulation of neutral fat is therefore observed in myocardium subjected to repeated ischemia. The acyl esters themselves, and possibly other metabolites such as lysophosphatides, accumulate in the ischemic tissue and may contribute to loss of membrane integrity.

## PROMISING APPROACHES TO ELUCIDATION OF MYOCARDIAL METABOLISM IN VIVO

Most of the information acquired during the past several decades delineating metabolic se-

quelae of ischemia has been obtained by conventional analyses of myocardial constituents and arterial-venous differences for selected metabolites. Recently, implementation of nuclear magnetic resonance to permit quantitative determination of concentrations of selected metabolites in isolated perfused hearts under conditions in which dynamic changes can be detected after the induction of ischemia has proven particularly promising in defining factors influencing energy metabolism. With the use of Fourier transform techniques, Hollis and others have characterized the temporal sequence of changes in concentrations of intracellular ATP, ADP, inorganic phosphate, and pH as a function of ischemia in isolated perfused hearts.[57] Early deviation of pH and its implications regarding regulation of intermediary metabolism and impairment of contractile function have been corroborated. Another promising approach for delineating temporal changes in myocardial metabolism in intact hearts entails the use of positron emission tomography, a technique permitting quantitative delineation of uptake and utilization of radionuclides labeled with positron-emitting tracers such as [11]C-palmitate.[58-62] Positron annihilation results in simultaneous emission of two photons, approximately 180° apart. Thus, algorithms can be employed to correct for attenuation of radiation within the tissue and to quantify the distribution of the source precisely in 3-dimensional space. The regional distribution of myocardium rendered ischemic transiently and myocardium subjected to irreversible injury has been quantified with this technique in experimental animals subjected to coronary occlusion and in patients with coronary artery disease. Interpretation of results has been facilitated, based on information obtained in experiments with isolated perfused hearts. In these experiments, the influence of concentration of substrate, binding to albumin, tissue lipid pool size, hormonal and metabolic environment, and myocardial oxygen requirements on extraction of the labeled substrate, retention in myocardium, and rates of catabolism have been quantified under rigorously controlled conditions. Both techniques—nuclear magnetic resonance and positron emission tomography—offer considerable promise for delineation of intermediary metabolism in myocardium exhibiting a variety of pathogenic phenomena in addition to sequelae of ischemia. With judicious use of these approaches in experimental animal preparations and in clinical research, and with appropriate selection of tracer substances to be employed, it should be possible to identify pathways involved in cryptogenic cardiomyopathies, the response of the myocardium undergoing hypertrophy to increased afterload, and hearts of patients with familial dysrhythmias, to name but a few examples.

## PROTECTION OF ISCHEMIC MYOCARDIUM BIOCHEMICALLY—AN EXAMPLE

To illustrate the therapeutic implications of these and related considerations regarding myocardial metabolism, it may be helpful to briefly review experience gained with administration of glucose-insulin-and-potassium (GIK). The initial interest in this approach was articulated by Sodi-Pallares, who felt that the regimen might protect ischemic myocardium by virtue of its potential to "hyperpolarize" cells subjected to electrophysiological dysfunction. When factors influencing the fate of ischemic myocardium first underwent rigorous experimental evaluation, it became clear that one promising approach entailed favorable modification in the balance between intracellular high-energy phosphate stores and energy requirements associated with cardiac work. Although initial approaches focused largely on reduction of myocardial oxygen requirements achieved by diminishing the energy demands associated with ventricular performance, maintenance of rates of synthesis of intracellular high-energy phosphate stores was actively pursued as well. The most obvious approach to the latter involves facilitation of coronary perfusion, since the increased availability of oxygen will of course potentiate aerobic synthesis of ATP. On the other hand, under conditions in which this is not possible, augmentation of substrate phosphorylation facilitated by increased availability of glucose might retard or diminish the overall depletion of high-energy phosphate stores that would be encountered in the absence of such an intervention. This rationale has been em-

ployed in studies of the potentially protective effects of GIK administered intravenously to experimental animals and patients with myocardial ischemia.[51,63-65]

The provision of GIK appeared attractive because, even though perfusion might be limited in ischemic regions, availability of unusually high concentrations of glucose available for diffusion into the ischemic myocardial cells was thought to be potentially useful in facilitating generation of ATP anaerobically via substrate phosphorylations. Inclusion of potassium in the infusions was felt to counteract the characteristic loss of intracellular potassium accompanying impaired sarcolemmal function early after the onset of ischemia when concentration gradients of intra- to extracellular potassium lead to rapid efflux of potassium from cells. In canine preparations, vulnerability to ventricular fibrillation is reduced by administration of GIK,[65] in keeping with the demonstration of arrhythmogenic effects induced by elevated arterial concentrations of free fatty acids (FFA).[66] Because the administration of GIK diminishes circulating FFA concentrations, the concept that "glucose is good and FFA is bad" for ischemic myocardium gained credence. This orientation was intensified by studies in experimental animals demonstrating that metabolites of FFA (such as acyl carnitine and acyl CoA) exert deleterious effects on myocardial metabolism and/or function, and that selected metabolites such as acyl CoA can inhibit adenine nucleotide translocase, impairing efficient transfer of intramitochondrial ATP to cytosolic high-energy phosphate stores.

The inclusion of insulin in such infusions was predicated on the need to optimize the delivery of glucose to the ischemic myocardium and on known ancillary biochemical effects of the hormone such as its ability to diminish circulating levels of FFA via an antipolytic effect in adipose tissue. Insulin facilitates intracellular glycolysis in myocardium by potentiating uptake of glucose; increases intracellular concentrations of potassium by augmenting ingress of this ion concomitantly with glucose; increases glycogen stores by accelerating glycogenesis and diminishing the need for glycogenolysis, and increases availability of intracellular glycerol phosphate—potentially capable of trapping excess fatty acids in the form of triglycerides and thereby reducing their propensity to exert detergent-like effects on membrane constituents. Nevertheless, potential enthusiasm for GIK must be tempered by several observations, including those by Opie and Owen,[67] who found that, even in ischemic zones of myocardium in situ, the overwhelming majority of ATP is produced via residual oxidative metabolism rather than anaerobic glycolysis, and those by Liedtke et al,[68] who demonstrated that infusion of GIK does not augment glycolytic flux because of persistent inhibition at the glyceraldehyde-3-dehydrogenase step by metabolic alterations occurring in the ischemic tissue. Furthermore, despite the initial view that hyperpolarization might be induced by GIK, ratios of intracellular potassium to sodium did not change in central zones of infarction, even under conditions in which increases in the concentration of glycogen were achieved by administration of GIK.[67]

On the other hand, in experimental animal preparations, augmentation of intracellular glycogen stores prior to imposition of anoxia protects the tissue against the insult.[69] Moreover, the increased plasma osmolality induced by infusion of GIK may facilitate continued perfusion and diminution of the "no-reflow" phenomenon induced by ischemia and the cell swelling it initiates. Although GIK infusion does diminish ST segment elevation after coronary occlusion in canine preparations, definitive documentation of efficacy of hyperosmotic infusions mediated via diminution of "no-reflow" has not been observed with angiographic techniques.[70]

In isolated perfused hearts subjected to prolonged ischemia, administration of GIK diminishes the rate of evolution of criteria of irreversible myocardial injury, such as release of creatine kinase into the effluent.[64] Protective effects appear to be at least partly independent of osmolality, since nonmetabolized sugars such as sorbitol in equiosmolar concentrations failed to exert a comparable protective effect. Based on ultrastructural studies of ischemic tissue, it has been postulated, but not proven, that GIK infusions exert a "membrane-stabilizing effect" that attenuates release of lytic enzymes from

myocardial lysosomes. However, definitive support for this hypothesis is lacking.

In clinical studies—including a prospective, randomized trial of the effect of GIK infusions in 50 consecutive patients treated beginning within 12 hours after the onset of symptoms indicative of acute myocardial infarction—GIK lowered circulating free fatty acid concentrations substantially, diminished ventricular dysrhythmia, and improved ventricular performance.[51]

On the other hand, analyses of plasma enzyme time-activity curves and of mortality have not yet provided conclusive evidence that GIK preserves jeopardized ischemic myocardium or diminishes mortality associated with acute myocardial infarction.

## DIAGNOSTIC IMPLICATIONS OF BIOCHEMICAL CHANGES DELINEATED IN NORMAL AND DISEASED MYOCARDIUM

Increased understanding of myocardial biochemistry has led to several diagnostic applications. Of particular importance are changes observed accompanying ischemia and infarction.

### Myocardial Ischemia

Under physiological conditions, myocardium extracts approximately 20 percent of the lactate presented to it in the arterial blood. Lactate can be converted to pyruvate, with subsequent entry into the citric acid cycle and complete oxidation. However, when myocardial ischemia supervenes, intracellular lactate accumulates because of several factors. First of all, glycolytic flux is markedly accelerated, increasing the rate of production of pyruvate. Concomitantly, the intracellular concentrations of NADH increase because of the lack of a terminal electron acceptor. Augmentation of concentrations of NADH preclude utilization of pyruvate in the citric acid cycle and favor the production of lactate from pyruvate via the lactic dehydrogenase reaction. In contrast to the case of normally oxygenated myocardium, the ischemic tissue produces lactate rather than utilizing exogenous lactate for oxidation. Because the cell membrane is permeable to lactate, ischemic myocardium not only accumulates this moiety in the intracellular space, but liberates it into the venous effluent, where it can be readily detected. Release of lactate and net lactate production rather than net extraction are concomitants of early, reversible, myocardial ischemia. Unfortunately, however, the concentration of lactate in the coronary sinus is influenced by many factors besides the presence or absence of ischemia, including: acid-base balance of the tissue and blood; the presence or absence of adrenergic stimulation to the myocardium, which of course can augment glycogenolysis and production of lactate; the relative preponderance of carbohydrate in contrast to fatty acid as substrate; potential changes in permeability of myocardial cell membranes; the presence or absence of diabetes mellitus, and the prevailing concentrations of arterial free fatty acids. For these reasons, diagnostic sensitivity and specificity of lactate production as a criterion of myocardial ischemia are somewhat limited.

Similar constraints pertain to interpretation of release of other moieties of low molecular weight into the effluents from ischemic zones. For example, it is well recognized that substances such as inorganic phosphate diffuse out of the ischemic myocardium into the effluent; but again the diagnostic sensitivity and specificity of phosphate release is influenced by other factors besides the absolute magnitude and duration of the ischemic insult. One of the earliest consequences of myocardial ischemia is impairment of sarcolemmal function maintaining the physiologically high ratio of intra- to extracellular potassium. Accordingly, the electrochemical gradient for potassium leads to efflux of this ion from the cell with an elevation of concentration of potassium first in the interstitial fluid and promptly thereafter in venous effluents. Again, however, factors influencing the sodium-potassium ATPase pump, prevailing intra- and extracellular pH, availability of macromolecules for binding potassium, and the influence of numerous factors affecting myocardial cell membranes may alter the temporal course and proportionality between release of potassium

and the severity and persistence of ischemia.

Myocardial ischemia is accompanied by a prompt decline in intracellular concentrations of creatine phosphate, due in part to the markedly decreased flux of high-energy phosphate available for phosphorylating creatine in the cytoplasm. The decline in intracellular concentrations of ATP is slower but follows soon after the decline of creatine phosphate and continues during prolonged ischemia. The temporal course of these changes has recently been delineated with the use of nuclear magnetic resonance spectra obtained from isolated perfused hearts.[57] In contrast to other tissues, myocardium has only limited enzymatic machinery necessary for the "salvage pathways" of purine metabolism. Accordingly, as ATP concentrations decline, metabolic products such as adenosine, hypoxanthine, and inosine accumulate and are released into the venous effluents from the ischemic zones.[71-73] Increases as large as 20 fold have been observed for hypoxanthine in coronary sinus blood after myocardial oxygen requirements have been increased in patients with coronary artery disease by acceleration of ventricular rate. Although these catabolic products of purine metabolism are reflections of the deranged intermediary metabolism in ischemic myocardium, the same sorts of constraints that apply to the diagnostic implications of other small molecules apply to these moieties as well. Furthermore, from a diagnostic point of view it appears that production of lactate can be detected even before augmentation of hypoxanthine production.[71]

## Macromolecular Markers of Acute Myocardial Infarction

The diagnosis of acute myocardial infarction is generally suspected on the basis of clinical history and findings. Electrocardiographic criteria of the initiation and progress of irreversible injury continue to be valuable despite their simplicity. Nevertheless, the sine qua non of acute myocardial infarction has become documentation of release of macromolecular markers—particularly enzymes—from the irreversibly injured tissue. Technical progress facilitating precise, prompt, and sensitive assay of some of these markers has increased the diagnostic utility of this approach.[74-84]

The alterations in sarcolemmal integrity accompanying myocardial ischemia lead initially to efflux of small molecules such as potassium, inorganic phosphate, lactate, hypoxanthine, inosine, and other constituents. As the injury to the cell membrane becomes more extensive, macromolecular markers efflux as well. Enzymes such as transaminase (involved in the shuttle reactions facilitating transfer of reducing equivalents from cytoplasm to mitochondria and involved in catabolism of amino acids), lactate dehydrogenase (a glycolytic, cytoplasmic enzyme), and creatine kinase (CK) (catalyzing phosphorylation of creatine from ATP and energy transduction from mitochondrial ATP to myofibrillar ATP) have been particularly useful. Based on extensive clinical and experimental studies, release of these macromolecules into the circulation appears to be tantamount to cell death. Thus, depletion of myocardial CK activity in hearts from experimental animals is directly proportional to the extent of infarction assessed by independent morphometric techniques.[85] Furthermore, in dogs subjected to coronary occlusions for graded intervals with subsequent reperfusion for intervals sufficiently long to permit appearance of macromolecules in the coronary venous effluent, insults sufficient to lead to macromolecule release are sufficient also to produce infarction detected morphometrically. On the other hand, those insults that do not lead to release of macromolecules into the coronary venous effluent also fail to lead to morphometric criteria of necrosis.[86] In patients, enzymatic estimation of infarct size—based on analysis of serial changes in plasma creatine kinase time-activity curves and, more recently, on time-activity curves of the MB ("myocardial") isoenzyme—correlate with independent criteria of the severity of infarction. These criteria include: (1) the frequency of premature ventricular complexes within the first 10 hours after admission;[87] (2) the extent of impairment of ventricular function detected by radionuclide angiocardiography and by contrast medium angiography;[88] (3) early mortality;[89] (4) prognosis late after myocardial infarction (particularly among patients whose

index infarction is the initial infarction);[90] and (5) the persistence and severity of ventricular dysrhythmia late after myocardial infarction.[90]

Although enzymatic indices have been used for many years to document the presence of acute myocardial infarction, diagnostic specificity has been limited in part because of the ubiquitous distribution of such enzymes throughout many organs. Accordingly, interest regarding particular isoenzymes has intensified. Creatine kinase is a useful example for consideration. Cytosolic enzyme exists in three well recognized isoenzyme forms (molecularly distinct species with the same enzymatic catalytic activity), each consisting of a dimer composed of M or B monomers in all possible combinations. The MB isoenzyme contributes 14 percent of total enzymatic activity of the CK type in myocardium in man. This particular species is found virtually exclusively in myocardium in human beings, in contrast to the case in numerous other animal species. Accordingly, in normal human subjects, MB activity in plasma is very low (< 5 mIU/ml), and activity fails to rise after trauma to tissues such as skeletal muscle, abdominal viscera, and virtually any organ besides the heart. On the other hand, when myocardial infarction occurs, MB CK is released from the irreversibly injured myocardium and the activity of MB CK in blood represents approximately 14 percent of total plasma CK activity, which is, of course, elevated. Other phenomena resulting in myocardial injury—such as cardiac surgery, pericarditis with myocardial involvement, or electrical cardioversion with injury to myocardial cells—will, of course, give rise to elevations of plasma MB CK activity. Furthermore, in unusual circumstances (such as those occurring in patients with muscular dystrophy) the isoenzyme profiles of tissues other than the heart may be abnormal, and it is possible that MB CK can be represented in tissues besides the heart. However, for all practical purposes among patients hospitalized with suspected myocardial infarction in whom another major cardiac insult can be excluded, serial changes in plasma MB CK activity provide a highly specific and sensitive diagnostic criterion of the presence of myocardial infarction and permit estimation of infarct size even when CK release from tissues besides the heart may be involved, such as is the case in patients with intramuscular injections or marked hypoperfusion of peripheral tissues.[91-97]

Analysis of plasma MB CK time-activity curves indicates that MB activity peaks slightly earlier than total CK activity after myocardial infarction and that the MB enzyme activity is cleared somewhat more rapidly from blood than activity associated with other CK isoenzymes. Although the fractional disappearance rate of CK and of MB CK varies among individuals, the rates in the same patient appear to remain remarkably constant despite hemodynamic perturbations or exposure to pharmacological agents. Experimental verification of this impression has been gained in studies with conscious dogs in which marked perturbation of hemodynamic parameters such as increments in heart rate, virtual complete elimination of renal blood flow, profound diminution of cardiac output, and gross alteration of hepatic perfusion have been implemented. Under these conditions, the disappearance rates of enzymes appear to vary by less than 10 percent. However, some physiological and pathophysiological factors can profoundly influence enzyme disappearance rates, including those that affect the reticuloendothelial system (RES). Treatment of dogs with zymosan (an inhibitor of the RES) diminishes disappearance rate markedly.[98] This observation is compatible with the view that reticuloendothelial system activity is important in the clearance of enzyme activity from the blood. It is important to recognize also that, despite the fact that plasma enzyme time-activity curves are directly related to loss of enzyme activity from the injured organ, local degradation of enzyme also occurs, perhaps mediated in part by activation of lysosomal hydrolases in ischemic tissue. Furthermore, transport of enzyme into the lymph, with potential inactivation of those enzymes that are labile in response to constituents in circulating lymph, plays a major role in the removal of enzyme from damaged myocardium. Parameters affecting transport in extravascular compartments as well as parameters influencing exchange between the vascular and extravascular pools will therefore be important determinants of the character of

plasma enzyme time-activity curves and their relationship to the absolute magnitude and time course of depletion of enzyme time-activity from the injured heart.[99,100]

Comparison of enzymatic estimates of infarct size among groups of patients treated with interventions potentially useful in preserving ischemic myocardium have been useful in pilot studies designed to determine whether jeopardized tissue can be protected and whether such protection provides a prognostic advantage to the patient. Other approaches, such as those using curve-fitting techniques, have demonstrated that the rate of evolution of infarction and its ultimate extent can be modified in experimental animals in which the implementation of an intervention can be achieved promptly. Based on analogous observations,[101] one subset of patients—namely, those with marked hypertension at the time of onset of acute myocardial infarction—appears to benefit from therapeutic interventions designed to reduce myocardial oxygen requirements.

The nature of this selective review is such that detailed consideration of the many other useful and well characterized macromolecular markers of irreversible injury cannot be undertaken. Nevertheless, on the basis of the observations noted and the availability of extensive, related information from several centers acquiring data over many decades, it is clear that quantitative evaluation of the time course of release of macromolecular markers from ischemic myocardium provides insight into the nature, evolution, and extent of irreversible ischemic injury in man, and that improved understanding of biochemical derangements accompanying myocardial ischemia has facilitated diagnosis and characterization of this entity in the clinical as well as in the experimental setting.

## ACKNOWLEDGMENTS

Research from the authors' laboratory was supported in part by the NHLBI HL17646 (Ischemic Heart Disease SCOR). We thank Ms. Jo Ann Zaccarello for preparation of the typescript.

# REFERENCES

1. Bing RJ: Carciac metabolism. Physiol Rev 45:171, 1965.
2. Soskin S, Levin R: Carbohydrate in Metabolism: Correlation of Physiological, Biochemical and Clinical Aspects. The University of Chicago Press, Chicago, Illinois, p. 305, 1946.
3. Olson. RE: Physiology of cardiac muscle. Handbook of Physiology, Section 2, Circulation 1:199 American Physiological Society, Washington, 1962.
4. Sobel BE: Salient biochemical features in ischemic myocardium. Circ Res 35 (Suppl. III):III–173, 1974.
5. Katz AM: Contractile proteins in normal and failing myocardium. Braunwald, E., Ed. The Myocardium: Failure and Infarction. HP Publishing Co., Inc., New York, p. 15, 1974.
6. Buja LM, Parkey RW, Dees JH, Stokely EM, Harris RA Jr, Bonte FJ, Willerson JT: Morphologic correlates of technetium-99m stannous pyrophosphate imaging of acute myocardial infarcts in dogs. Circulation 52:596, 1975.
7. Coleman RE, Klein MS, Ahmed SA, Weiss ES, Buchholz WM, Sobel BE: Mechanisms contributing to myocardial accumulation of technetium-99m stannous pyrophosphate after coronary arterial occlusion. Am J Cardiol 39:55, 1977.
8. Shen AC, Jennings RB: Kinetics of calcium accumulation in acute myocardial ischemic injury. Am J Pathol 67:441, 1972.
9. Reuter H: Exchange of calcium ions in the mammalian myocardium: Mechanisms and physiological significance. Circ Res 34:599, 1974.
10. Jennings RB, Ganote, CE: Ultrastructural changes in acute myocardial ischemia. Oliver MF, Julian DG, Donald KW, Eds. Effect of Acute Ischemia on Myocardial Function. Churchill Livingstone, Edinburgh, pp. 50–74, 1972.
11. Jennings RB, Ganote CE: Structural changes in myocardium during acute ischemia. Circ Res 34 & 35 (Suppl. III):III–156, 1974.
12. Trump BF, Mergner WJ, Kahng MW, Saladino AJ: Studies on the subcellular pathophysiology of ischemia. Circulation 53 (Suppl. I):I–17, 1974.
13. Sobel BE: Biochemical and morphologic changes in infarcting myocardium. Braunwald E, Ed. The Myocardium: Failure and Infarction. HP Publishing Co., Inc., New York, 1974.
14. Neely JR, Morgan HE: Relationship between carbohydrate and lipid metabolism and the energy balance of heart muscle. Ann. Rev. Physiol. 36:413, 1974.
15. Braunwald E, Sobel BE: Myocardial ischemia. Biochemical and functional considerations. Braunwald E, Ed. Heart Disease. W.B. Saunders Company, Philadelphia 1980.
16. Borrebaek B, Christiansen R, Christophersen BO, Bremer J: The role of acyltransferases in fatty acid utilization. Circ Res 38 (Suppl. I):I-16, 1976.
17. Pande SV: A mitochondrial carnitine acylcarnitine translocase system. Proc Nat Acad Sci USA 72:883, 1975.
18. Oram JF, Wenger JI, Neely JR: Regulation of long chain fatty acid activation in heart muscle. J Biol Chem 250:73, 1975.
19. Evans JR: Cellular transport of long chain fatty acids. Can J Biochem 42:955, 1964.
20. Klein MS, Goldstein RA, Welch MJ, Sobel BE: External assessment of myocardial metabolism with $^{11}$C-palmitate in rabbit hearts. Am J Physiol.: Heart Circ. Physiol. 237(1):H51, 1979.
21. Goldstein RA, Klein MS, Sobel BE: Distribution of exogenous labeled palmitate in ischemic myocardium: Implications for positron emission transaxial tomography. Vogel, JHK, Ed. Advances in Cardiology. S Karger, Basel, Switzerland (in press).
22. Morgan HE, Neely JR: Insulin and membrane transport. Steiner, DF and Freinkel, N, Ed. Handbook of Physiology. American Physiological Society, Washington, pp. 323–331, 1972.
23. Ross J Jr, Sobel BE: Regulation of cardiac contraction. Ann Rev Physiol 34:47, 1972.
24. Sobel BE, Mayer SE: Cyclic adenosine monophosphate and cardiac contractility Circ Res 32:407, 1973.
25. Larner J: Mechanisms of regulation of glycogen synthesis and degradation. I. Regulation of intermediary metabolism. Circ Res 38 (Suppl. I): I-2, 1976.
26. Larner J, Villar-Palasi C: Glycogen synthase and its control. Curr Top Cell Regul 3:195, 1971.
27. Garland PB, Newsholme A, Randle PJ: Effects of free fatty acids, ketone bodies, diabetes, starvation on pyruvate metabolism in rat heart and diaphragm muscle. Nature 195:381, 1962.
28. Mansour TE: Phosphofructokinase. Curr Top Cell Regul 5:1, 1972.
29. Lorenson MY, Mansour TE: Studies on heart phosphofructokinase: Binding properties of na-

30. Neely JR, Rovetto MJ, Whitmer JT: Rate-limiting steps of carbohydrate and fatty acid metabolism in ischemic hearts. Acta Med Scand Suppl 587:9, 1976.
31. Kirschner K: Kinetic analysis of allosteric enzymes. Curr Top Cell Regul 4:167, 1971.
32. Linn TC, Pettet FH, Reed LJ: Regulation of the activity of the pyruvate dehydrogenase complex from beef kidney mitochondria by phosphorylation and dephosphorylation. Proc Nat Acad Sci USA 62:234, 1969.
33. Randle PJ: Regulation of glycolysis and pyruvate oxidation in cardiac muscle. Circ Res 38 (Suppl. I):I–8, 1976.
34. LaNoue KF, Williamson, JR: Interrelationships between malateaspartate shuttle and citric acid cycle in rat heart mitochondria. Metabolism 20:119, 1971.
35. Williamson JR, Ford C, Illingworth J, Safer B: Coordination of citric acid cycle activity with electron transport flux. Circ Res 38 (Suppl. I):I–39, 1976.
36. Purvis JL, Lowenstein JM: The relationship between intra- and extra-mitochondrial pyridine nucleotide. J Biol Chem 236:2794, 1961.
37. LaNoue K, Nicklas WJ, Williamson JR: Control of citric acid activity in rat heart mitochondria. J Biol Chem 245:102, 1970.
38. Kobayashi K, Neely JR: Control of maximum rates of glycolysis in rat cardiac muscle. Circ Res 44:166, 1979.
39. Bremer J, Wojtczak AB: Factors controlling the rate of fatty acid β-oxidation in rat liver mitochondria. Biochim Biophys Acta 280:515, 1972.
40. Evans JR: Importance of fatty acid in myocardial metabolism. Circ Res 14 & 15 (Suppl. II): II–96, 1964.
41. Crass MF III: Exogenous substrate effects on endogenous lipid metabolism in the working rat heart. Biochim Biophys Acta 280:71, 1979.
42. Gross RW: Unpublished observations, 1972.
43. Sobel BE, Corr PB: Biochemical mechanisms potentially responsible for lethal arrhythmias induced by ischemia: The lysolipid hypothesis, 1979. Vogel JHK, Ed. Advances in Cardiology, Vol. 26, S. Karger, Basel Switzerland.
44. Sobel BE, Corr PB, Robison AK, Goldstein RA, Witkowski FX, Klein MS: Accumulation of lysophosphoglycerides with arrhythmogenic properties in ischemic myocardium. J Clin Invest 62:546, 1978.
45. Corr PB, Sobel BE: The importance of metabolites in the genesis of ventricular dysrhythmia induced by ischemia. Mod Concepts Cardiovasc Dis 48:43 and 49, 1979.
46. Corr PB, Cain, ME, Witkowski FX, Price, DA, Sobel BE: Potential arrhythmogenic electrophysiological derangements in canine Purkinje fibers induced by lysophosphoglycerides. Circ Res 44:822, 1979.
47. Weglicki WB, Waite M, Sisson P, Shohet SB: Myocardial phospholipase A of microsomal and mitochondrial fractions. Biochem Biophys Acta 231:512, 1971.
48. Needleman P, Marshall GR, Sobel BE: Hormone interactions in the isolated rabbit heart. Synthesis and coronary vasomotor effects of prostaglandins, angiotensin, and bradykinin. Circ Res 37:802, 1975.
49. Chien KR, Abrams J, Serroni A, Martin, JT, Farber, JL: Accelerated phospholipid degradation and associated membrane dysfunction in irreversible, ischemic liver cell injury. J Biol Chem 253:4809, 1978.
50. Gross RW, Sobel BE: Mechanisms independent of phospholipase activation augmenting synthesis of lysophosphoglycerides in ischemic myocardium. Clin Res 27:172A, 1979.
51. Rogers WJ, Segall PH, McDaniel HG, Mantle JA, Russell RO Jr, Rackley CE: Prospective randomized trial of glucose-insulin-potassium in acute myocardial infarction. Am J Cardiol 43:801, 1979.
52. Morgan HE, Rannels DE, Kao RL: Factors controlling protein turnover in heart muscle. Circ Res 34 & 35 (Suppl. III):III–22, 1974.
53. Kao R, Rannels DE, Morgan HE: Effects of anoxia and ischemia on protein synthesis in perfused rat hearts. Circ Res 38 (Suppl. I):I–124, 1976.
54. Rannels DE, Kao R, Morgan HE: Effect of cardiac ischemia on protein degradation. Circulation 53:I–30, 1976.
55. Shug AL Shrago E, Bittar N, Folts JD, Koke JR: Acyl-CoA inhibition of adenine nucleotide translocation in ischemic myocardium. Am J Physiol 228:689, 1975.
56. Brachfield N, Ohtaka Y, Klein I, Kawade M: Substrate preference and metabolic activity of the aerobic and hypoxic turtle heart. Circ Res 31:453, 1972.
57. Hollis DP, Nunnally RL, Taylor GJ, Weisfeld ML, Jacobus WE: Phosphorus nuclear magnetic resonance studies of heart physiology. Magnetic Resonance 29:319, 1978.

58. Weiss ES, Hoffman EJ, Phelps ME, Welch MJ, Henry PD, Ter-Pogossian MM, Sobel BE: External detection and visualization of myocardial ischemia with ${}^{11}$C-substrates in vitro and in vivo. Circ Res 39:24, 1976.

59. Ter-Pogossian MM, Hoffman EJ, Weiss ES, Coleman RE, Phelps ME, Welch MJ, Sobel BE: Positron emission reconstruction tomography for the assessment of regional myocardial metabolism by the administration of substrates labeled with cyclotron produced radionuclides. Harrison DC, Sandler H, Miller HA, Eds. Proceedings from the Conference on Cardiovascular Imaging and Image Processing Theory and Practice. Vol. 72. Society of Photo-Optical Instrumentation Engineers, Palos Verdes Estates, 1975.

60. Weiss ES, Ahmed SA, Welch MJ, Williamson, JR, Ter-Pogossian MM, Sobel BE: Quantification of infarction in cross sections of canine myocardium in vivo with positron emission transaxial tomography and ${}^{11}$C-palmitate. Circulation 55:66, 1977.

61. Sobel BE, Weiss, ES, Welch MJ, Siegel BA, Ter-Pogossian, MM: Detection of remote myocardial infarction in patients with positron emission transaxial tomography and intravenous ${}^{11}$C-palmitate. Circulation 55:853, 1977.

62. Sobel BE: External quantification of myocardial ischemia and infarction with positron-emitting radionuclides. Vogel, JHK Ed. Advances in Cardiology. Vol. 22. S. Karger, Basel, Switzerland, 1978.

63. Maroko PR, Libby P, Sobel BE, Bloor CM, Sybers HD, Shell WE, Covell JE, Braunwald E: Effect of glucose-insulin-potassium infusion on myocardial infarction following experimental coronary artery occlusion. Circulation 45:1160, 1972.

64. Henry PD, Sobel BE, Braunwald E: Protection of hypoxic guinea pig hearts with glucose and insulin. Am J Physiol 226:309, 1974.

65. Obeid AI, Verrier RL, Lown B: Influence of glucose, insulin, and potassium on vulnerability to ventricular fibrillation in the canine heart. Circ Res 43:601, 1978.

66. Oliver MF, Rowe MJ, Luxton MR, Miller NE, Neilson JM: Effect of reducing circulating free fatty acids on ventricular arrhythmias during myocardial infarction and on ST-segment depression during exercise-induced ischemia. Circulation 53 (Suppl. I):I–210, 1976.

67. Opie LH, Owen P. Effect of glucose-insulin-potassium infusions on arteriovenous differences of glucose and of free fatty acids and on tissue metabolic changes in dogs with developing myocardial infarction. Am J Cardiol 38:310, 1976.

68. Liedtke AJ, Hughes HC, Neely JR: Effects of excess glucose and insulin on glycolytic metabolism during experimental myocardial ischemia. Am J Cardiol 38:17, 1976.

69. Scheuer J, Stezoski SW: Protective role of increased myocardial glycogen stores in cardiac anoxia in the rat. Circ Res 27:835, 1970.

70. Ahmed SS, Lee CH, Oldewurtel HA, Regan, TJ: Sustained effect of glucose-insulin-potassium on myocardial performance during regional ischemia. J Clin Invest 61:1123, 1978.

71. deJong JW, Verdouw PD, Remme WJ: Myocardial nucleotide and carbohydrate metabolism and hemodynamics during partial occlusion and reperfusion of pig coronary artery. J Mol Cell Cardiol 9:297, 1977.

72. Maguire MH, Lukas MC, Rettie JF: Adenine nucleotide salvage synthesis in the rat heart; pathways of adenosine salvage. Biochem Biophys Acta 262:108, 1972.

73. Remme WJ, deJong JW, Verdouw, PD: The effects of pacing-induced ischemia on hypoxanthine release from the human heart. Am J Cardiol 40:55, 1977.

74. Sobel BE, Shell WE: Serum enzyme determinations in the diagnosis and assessment of myocardial infarction. Circulation 45:471, 1972.

75. Roberts R, and Sobel BE: Isoenzymes of creatine phosphokinase and diagnosis of myocardial infarction. Ann Intern Med 79:741, 1973.

76. Roberts R, Gowda KS, Ludbrook PA, Sobel BE: Specificity of elevated serum MB creatine phosphokinase activity in the diagnosis of acute myocardial infarction. Am J Cardiol 36:433, 1975.

77. Sobel BE: Quantification of myocardial ischemic injury. Vogel JHK, Ed. Advances in Cardiology. Vol. 15. S. Karger, Basel, Switzerland, 1975.

78. Sobel BE, Shell WE: Diagnostic and prognostic value of serum enzyme changes in patients with acute myocardial infarction. Yu PN, Goodwin JF, Eds. Progress in Cardiology 4. Lea & Febiger, Philadelphia, 1975.

79. Ahumada G, Roberts R, Sobel BE: Evaluation of myocardial infarction with enzymatic indices. Prog Cardiovasc Dis 18:405, 1976.

80. Sobel BE, Roberts R, Larson, KB: Considerations in the use of biochemical markers of ischemic injury. Circ Res 38 (Suppl I):I–99, 1976.

81. Sobel BE, Markham J, Roberts R: Factors influencing enzymatic estimates of infarct size. Am J Cardiol 39:130, 1977.

82. Roberts R, Sobel BE: Creatine kinase isoenzymes in the assessment of heart disease. Am Heart J 95:521, 1978.

83. Roberts R, Sobel BE, Parker, CW: Radioimmunoassay for creatine kinase isoenzymes. Science 194:855, 1976.

84. Roberts R, Parker CW, Sobel BE: Detection of acute myocardial infarction by radioimmunoassay for creatine kinase MB. Lancet 2:319, 1977.

85. Roberts R, Ahumada G, Sobel BE: Estimation of infarct size: With emphasis on enzymatic techniques. Scope Monograph. The Upjohn Company. Kalamazoo, 1975.

86. Ahmed SA, Williamson JR, Roberts R, Clark RE, Sobel BE: The association of increased plasma MB CPK activity and irreversible ischemic myocardial injury in the dog. Circulation 54:187, 1976.

87. Cox JR Jr, Roberts R, Ambos HD, Oliver GC, Sobel, BE: Relations between enzymatically estimated myocardial infarct size and early ventricular dysrhythmia. Circulation 53 (Suppl. I): I-150, 1976.

88. Kostuk WJ, Ehsani AA, Karliner JS, Ashburn WL, Peterson KL, Ross, J Jr, Sobel BE: Left ventricular performance after myocardial infarction assessed by radioisotope angiocardiography. Circulation 47:242, 1973.

89. Sobel BE, Bresnahan GF, Shell WE, Yoder RD: Estimation of infarct size in man and its relation to prognosis. Circulation 46:640, 1972.

90. Geltman EM, Ehsani AA, Campbell MK, Schechtman K, Roberts R, Sobel BE: The influence of location and extent of myocardial infarction on long-term ventricular dysrhythmia and mortality. Circulation, 60:805, 1979.

91. Roberts R, Henry PD, Witteveen SAGJ, Sobel BE: Quantification of serum creatine phospho-kinase isoenzyme activity. Am J Cardiol. 33:650, 1974.

92. Roberts R, Sobel BE: CPK isoenzymes in evaluation of myocardial ischemic injury. Hosp. Prac. 11:55, 1976.

93. Roberts R, Henry PD, Sobel BE: An improved basis for enzymatic estimation of infarct size. Circulation 52:743, 1975.

94. Roberts R, Ludbrook PA, Weiss ES, Sobel BE: Serum CPK isoenzymes after cardiac catheterization. Br Heart J 37:1144, 1975.

95. Sobel BE, Roberts R, Larson KB: Estimation of infarct size from serum MB creatine phosphokinase activity: Applications and limitations. Am J Cardiol 37:474, 1976.

96. Sobel BE, Kjekshus JK, Roberts R: The quantification of infarct size. Hearse DJ, and DeLeiris J, Ed. Enzymes in Cardiology: Diagnosis and Research. John Wiley and Sons Limited, Chichester, in press.

97. Klein MS, Shell WE, Sobel BE: Serum creatine phosphokinase (CPK) isoenzymes after intramuscular injections, surgery, and myocardial infarction. Experimental and clinical studies. Cardiovasc Res 7:412, 1973.

98. Roberts R, Sobel BE: Effect of selected drugs and myocardial infarction on the disappearance of creatine kinase from the circulation in conscious dogs. Cardiovasc Res 11:103, 1977.

99. Clark GL, Robison AK, Gnepp DR, Roberts R, Sobel BE: Effects of lymphatic transport of enzyme on plasma creatine kinase time-activity curves after myocardial infarction in dogs. Circ Res 43:162, 1978.

100. Sobel BE, Markham J, Karlsberg RP, Roberts R: The nature of disappearance of creatine kinase from the circulation and its influence on enzymatic estimation of infarct size. Circ Res 41:836, 1977.

101. Shell WE, Sobel BE: Protection of jeopardized ischemic myocardium by reduction of ventricular afterload. N Engl J Med 291:481, 1974.

# 3 | Coronary and Left Ventricular Angiography in Coronary Heart Disease

## Kirk L. Peterson, M.D.

Over the last two decades selective coronary and left ventricular angiography have emerged as highly sophisticated and precise methods for defining, in vivo, the pathological anatomy and pathophysiology of coronary atherosclerosis.[1-3] Prior to the development of these methods, physicians were dependent upon indirect methods—e.g., clinical symptoms and/or physical signs, or rest-and-exercise electrocardiography—to assess the presence or absence of significant atherosclerotic obstruction of the coronary arterial tree. Consequently, a large body of knowledge has emerged which relates coronary pathologic anatomy to patient symptoms and physical signs, natural history or survival, electrocardiographic abnormalities, regional and global dysfunction of the left ventricle, myocardial perfusion deficits, and candidacy for surgical revascularization.

The intent of this chapter is to review the historical and technical aspects of coronary and left ventricular angiography and to present the normal, anomalous, and pathologic angiographic anatomy of the coronary arterial tree and left ventricle. Emphasis will be placed upon the typical patterns of atherosclerotic lesions within the coronary arterial tree and their relation to natural history, anatomical and electrocardiographic sites of myocardial ischemia and infarction, and global as well as regional dysfunction of the left ventricle. Finally, the conventional indications for performance of coronary angiography and left ventriculography in

the clinical care of the patient with coronary heart disease will be considered.

## HISTORICAL ASPECTS OF CORONARY ANGIOGRAPHY

The earliest attempts to visualize the coronary arterial tree in the living subject involved nonselective injection of large amounts of contrast agent through a large bore catheter into the ascending aorta. Various associated maneuvers to maximize delivery of dye into the coronary vessels were attempted—including selective injection during diastole, transient cardiac arrest during acetylcholine administration, temporary reduction of cardiac output with balloon catheters in either the caval vessels or ascending aorta, and use of specially designed catheters which directed the contrast stream toward the periphery of the aorta. However, all were found to be suboptimal for adequate resolution of the distal portions of the major coronary vessels.

Sones [1] was the first to recognize the feasibility of selectively catheterizing and injecting contrast agents directly into the coronary orifices, thereby improving the opacification and detailed anatomy of the coronary arterial tree without compromising patient safety. His observations led him to develop flexible catheters which are inserted via a surgically exposed brachial artery and manipulated into either the right or left coronary orifices under fluoroscopic

visualization.[2] In subsequent years, other investigators designed preformed catheters which
can be inserted percutaneously (via the Seldinger technique [4]) into the femoral artery and
which readily engage the orifices of the coronary arteries, provided their anatomical position is not distorted or anomalous.[5-7] Both approaches continue to be used throughout the
world and carry a minimal and acceptable
risk—considering the vital structures which are
visualized, the complexity of the techniques,
and the invasive nature of the procedure.

## TECHNICAL ASPECTS OF CORONARY ANGIOGRAPHY AND LEFT VENTRICULOGRAPHY

### Sones or Retrograde Brachial Approach

Under local anesthesia and through a small
median antecubital incision, the brachial artery
is isolated by blunt dissection and opened by
a transverse arteriotomy. In order to provide
anticoagulation of the patient's blood, heparin
(4000 to 5000 units) is administered, either directly into the distal brachial artery or through
an intravenous line. A 7 to 8F diameter catheter
(80 to 125 cm in length and with a tip which
tapers to approximately 5.5F) is inserted under
direct vision and manipulated under fluoroscopy through the axillary, subclavian, and innominate vessels into the ascending aorta. The
more flexible, tapered tip of the Sones catheter
is then directed toward the left coronary sinus,
looped against the left aortic valve cusp, and
manipulated directly into the left coronary orifice (Fig. 3.1a). Subsequently, the catheter is
rotated clockwise so that the tip traverses the
anterior portion of the proximal aorta and
swings directly into the right coronary orifice.
Alternatively, the tip can be repositioned in the
right coronary sinus, looped upon the right coronary cusp, and then pushed directly into the
right coronary orifice (Fig. 3.1b). Considerable
technical skill, including rapid eye-hand coordination, is requisite in order to rapidly and easily
engage the coronary orifices by the Sones technique. Once mastered, nevertheless, the technique is highly reproducible and relatively

A

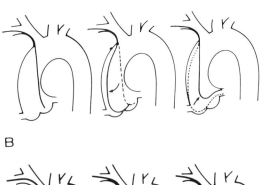

B

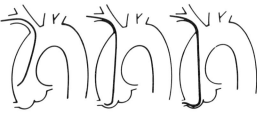

Fig. 3.1  *(A)* Demonstration of route by which a
Sones catheter is passed into the ascending aorta.
Selective engagement of the left coronary orifice is
accomplished by looping the catheter in the left sinus
of Valsalva or upon the aortic leaflets and simultaneously advancing the catheter. Thereafter, the catheter is withdrawn slightly, which lifts it and directs
its tip into the left main coronary artery. *(B)* Engagement of the right coronary artery is accomplished
by rotating the catheter into the right sinus of Valsalva and then looping the tip of the catheter off
the right coronary cusp until the tip engages the
right coronary orifice. (Figure reproduced with permission of the American Heart Association from
Conti CR: Coronary arteriography. Circulation
55:227, 1977.)

atraumatic to the coronary vessels. Since Sones
catheters have superior torque control, modifications of the standard engagement maneuvers
can be made in order to enter coronary arteries
which are congenitally displaced or pushed out
of their normal position by disease of the ascending aorta (e.g., aneurysmal dilatation of the
ascending aorta). Other advantages of the Sones
technique include: (1) the catheters are reusable,
thereby reducing cost; (2) a single catheter can
be used for catheterization of both coronary
arteries and the left ventricle (although some
angiographers prefer to use a catheter with a
lower resistance to injection for left ventriculography); (3) entrance into the ascending aorta

is seldom precluded by disease in the pathway of catheter insertion (as contrasted to the femoral approach, where local disease in the descending aorta or iliac vessels frequently complicates catheter passage), and (4) sideholes and an end-hole in the catheter provide a passageway for distal coronary artery perfusion, even though the tip may significantly occlude the coronary orifice. Some disadvantages of the technique, however, are: (1) a long and rigorous period of training is necessary before successful engagement of both coronary arteries can be accomplished in the full spectrum of patients needing study; (2) a relatively distal insertion of the innominate artery into the aorta can preclude ready entrance into the ascending aorta from either brachial artery; (3) significant tortuosity of the subclavian or innominate arteries makes manipulation of the tip difficult; (4) a clot may form in one of the holes near or at the end of the catheter and embolize into the coronary arterial tree or another systemic artery; and (5) intimal damage to the brachial artery at the point of catheter insertion may lead to thrombotic occlusion of the vessel with symptoms of ischemia in the hand, necessitating surgical repair of the vessel. Rarely, traumatic damage to the median nerve can occur.

## Percutaneous or Retrograde Femoral Approach

Under local anesthesia, an 18 gauge, thin-wall needle is introduced into the lumen of the femoral artery. When backflow is clearly obtained, a guidewire is threaded into and passed retrogradely into the abdominal aorta. The needle is then removed, and a dilating sheath is passed over the guidewire into the artery. Next, the dilator is removed and the preformed catheter is passed over the guidewire and up into the abdominal or thoracic aorta. The guidewire is then removed, and the catheter is carefully aspirated and flushed. Anticoagulation with 4000 to 5000 units of heparin is accomplished at this juncture, as with the Sones technique. The catheter can then be advanced under fluoroscopic control into the ascending aorta. For engagement of the coronary orifices, several types of catheters can be utilized; these are commonly referred to as Judkins,[5] Amplatz,[6] or Schoonmaker (multipurpose)[7] catheters. With the Judkins technique, three different catheters must be utilized in order to opacify both the left and right coronary arteries and the left ventricle. The coronary artery catheters are again 7 or 8F in diameter and 100 cm in length, and they taper at the ends to a 5F tip; however, in contrast to the Sones catheter, there is only one end-hole for purposes of contrast injection and pressure monitoring. As shown in Figure 3.2A, the left coronary artery Judkins catheter has a secondary curve which lies against the right lateral wall of the ascending aorta, and the primary curve directs the tip of the catheter

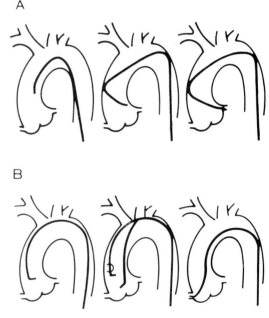

A

B

Fig. 3.2 *(A)* Demonstration of passage of a Judkins preshaped left coronary catheter into the ascending aorta and left coronary orifice. The secondary curve of the catheter sits along the right anterolateral margin of the aorta and serves to direct the tip into the left coronary orifice. *(B)* Engagement of the right coronary artery orifice using a Judkins preshaped right coronary artery catheter. Note that, after pointing the tip towards the left coronary artery orifice, rotation causes the tip to descend and sweep across the anterior portion of the ascending aorta until the right coronary artery orifice is engaged. (Figure reproduced with permission of the American Heart Association from Conti CR: Coronary arteriography. Circulation 55:227, 1977.)

into the left coronary orifice. Depending upon the size of the aortic root, a variable distance between the primary and secondary curves of approximately 4 to 6 cm is necessary in order to reach the left coronary orifice. Simple advancement of the Judkins left coronary artery catheter will usually lead to prompt engagement of the orifice; in fact, the catheter's major danger lies in its high predisposition to seek out the left coronary orifice once it lies in the ascending aorta. Constant surveillance of end-hole pressure and position is mandatory in order to avoid inadvertent obstruction of the left coronary orifice. As shown in Figure 3.2B, the right coronary artery Judkins catheter has two curves, a primary and secondary, and the catheter is preshaped so that the tip points toward the left anterior wall of the aorta when it is first advanced into the ascending aorta. With clockwise rotation, the catheter then descends into and sweeps across the anterior wall of the aorta and engages the orifice of the right coronary artery. Careful attention must be paid to avoid inadvertent obstruction of the right coronary artery, which can produce myocardial ischemia or infarction.

The major advantages of the Judkins technique include: (1) its simplicity requires less manual dexterity on the part of the operator; (2) the unidirectional flow of contrast material as it is injected into the coronary orifices provides superior opacification of the distal coronary arteries, as opposed to the Sones technique; (3) immediate detection of obstruction at the tip of the catheter is possible because of the presence of only one hole for injection and pressure measurement, and (4) tortuosity and/or obstruction of the subclavian or innominate vessels do not interfere with successful entrance into the ascending aorta. Disadvantages of the technique include: (1) dependence upon three catheter exchanges in order to sequentially perform left coronary artery opacification, right coronary artery opacification, and left ventriculography (using a so-called "pigtail" catheter); (2) entrance into the left ventricle for monitoring of left ventricular systolic or end-diastolic pressure is difficult with either the left or right Judkins coronary catheters; (3) multiple catheter exchanges enhance the risk of thrombus

remaining in the catheter and subsequently embolizing into the systemic arterial tree, and (4) anatomical anomalies or distortion of the coronary orifices can preclude successful engagement of the vessels.

With the Amplatz technique, a preshaped catheter is inserted into the ascending aorta and looped on or near the aortic valve; the tip is then advanced upward toward the left coronary orifice. Again, catheters with varying size curvatures are available in order to compensate for abnormal dilatation of the ascending aorta. In contrast to Sones catheters, Amplatz catheters are shaped to seek out the coronary orifices; however, the left coronary orifice may still be difficult to engage with this technique. One must also deal with the potential for increased risk of multiple catheter exchanges.

A single catheter for coronary angiography and left ventriculography has been developed by Schoonmaker and King.[7] It is 8F in diameter, 100 cm in length, and curved to 45° at the tip. After percutaneous insertion of the catheter into the ascending aorta, it is looped against the aortic valve (similar to the manipulations of a Sones catheter from the arm) and directed upward toward the left coronary orifice. Thereafter, because of its superior torque characteristics, it can be rotated clockwise into the right coronary orifice. Also, because it has side holes as well as an end-hole, it can be positioned in the mid left ventricle and used for the left ventricular angiogram. In our experience, its major disadvantages are: (1) frequent stimulation of ventricular premature beats during the left ventricular angiogram despite a slow injection rate of contrast material and careful positioning of the catheter tip, and (2) catheter movement is not as readily controlled as with a Sones catheter from the arm, and, thus, there is a somewhat greater danger of arterial injury (e.g., dissection of the right coronary artery).

## NORMAL ANGIOGRAPHIC ANATOMY OF THE CORONARY ARTERIAL TREE

The normal anatomy of the coronary arterial tree in man must be visualized and conceptualized in several projections in order to appreciate its complex structure and 3-dimensional nature. As shown in Figure 3.3, a coronary angiogram is customarily filmed in multiple projections— including the antero-posterior, the left lateral, the right anterior oblique (RAO), and the left anterior oblique (LAO) projections. In approximately 90 percent of humans, most of the diaphragmatic surface of the left ventricle and the free wall of the right ventricle are supplied by the right coronary artery. This vessel originates from the ascending aorta at an angle of approximately 40° to the right of the anterior sagittal plane, passes beneath the right atrial appendage, and courses caudally in the atrioventricular groove which separates the right atrium and ventricle. After giving off a conus branch which runs anteriorly across the right ventricular outlow tract, and muscular branches which course anteriorly and supply the right ventricular myo-

cardium, the right coronary artery gives off the posterior descending artery at the intersection of the atrioventricular and interventricular sulci posteriorly (the so-called "crus" of the heart). The posterior descending branch of the right coronary artery supplies blood to the inferior surface of the right and left ventricles, as well as septal branches to the interventricular septum. In 55 percent of humans, the sinus node artery arises from the proximal portion of the right coronary artery and courses between the atrial appendage and the aorta to penetrate the sinus node and encircle the ostium of the superior vena cava. Alternatively, it may originate from the proximal portion of the circumflex branch of the left coronary artery. Since in 90 percent of humans the right coronary artery provides the dominant amount of blood to the posterior-diaphragmatic surface of the heart,

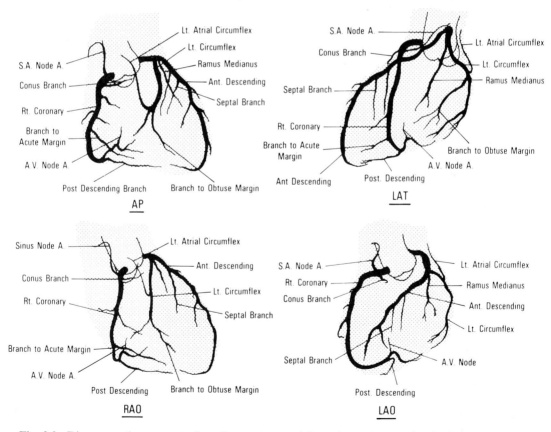

Fig. 3.3  Diagrammatic representation of coronary arterial tree in anteroposterior (AP), lateral (LAT), right anterior oblique (RAO), and left anterior oblique (LAO) projections. See text for details of individual vessels. (Figure modified from Abrams, HL, Adams, DF: The coronary arteriogram. N Engl J Med 281:1277, 1969.)

the arterial supply to the atrioventricular node arises from the right coronary artery with an equivalent incidence.

The left coronary artery and its tributaries supply the anterior, apical, lateral, and portions of the inferior surfaces of the left ventricle. The left main coronary artery varies in length from an immediate postostial bifurcation to a trunk as long as 2 to 4 cm. The vessel then divides into the circumflex and anterior descending arteries. However, there may be other vessels which take off at this point of bifurcation and course over the anterior and lateral surfaces of the left ventricle (labeled as ramus medianus in Figure 3.3). The circumflex vessel arises in a nearly perpendicular fashion from the left main coronary artery and courses down the left atrioventricular sulcus for a variable distance; in only 10 percent of humans, however, does it reach the crus of the heart to give off the posterior descending artery and the atrioventricular nodal artery. In the majority of humans, the circumflex branch of the left coronary artery terminates just beyond the obtuse margin of the heart. The circumflex system may give rise to numerous atrial branches, including the left atrial circumflex artery and, as noted above, the sinus node artery. The anterior descending branch of the left coronary artery courses along the interventricular groove and manifests a variable length, terminating short of (or, alternatively, passing around) the apex of the heart to perfuse the inferior apical surface of the left ventricle. Along its course, the left anterior descending artery gives off a variable number of diagonal branches which course laterally over the anterior surface of the left ventricle (not shown in Fig. 3.3). In addition, the anterior descending artery gives off an array of septal branches, beginning with the first septal branch, which can itself have a characteristic bifurcation in the mid septum. All septal branches are intramyocardial rather than epicardial in location, and thus they are not amenable to revascularization surgery. Occasionally, the left anterior descending artery itself may lie within the myocardium for nearly its entire length, or it may have only segments which lie buried within muscle.

A common anatomical variation of the left anterior descending artery is for it to bifurcate in its final branching. Thus, it can readily be mistaken on a cine angiogram for the large first septal branch, or it may be misinterpreted as a diagonal branch in the setting of total occlusion of the anterior descending branch. Irrespective of its anatomy, accurate recognition of the anterior descending artery is vital, since it usually provides 60 to 70 percent of the total coronary blood flow to the heart.

The normal patterns of coronary artery perfusion to the specialized conduction system of the heart are of considerable importance in understanding rhythm disturbances in patients with coronary heart disease. The atrioventricular node is supplied virtually exclusively by the atrioventricular nodal artery. However, the His bundle has been found to have a dual primary blood supply in 90 percent of human hearts and a single supply via the atrioventricular nodal artery in 10 percent.[8] The blood supply to the proximal right bundle has been found to be from dual sources in 50 percent, from the septal branch alone in 40 percent, and from the atrioventricular nodal artery alone in 10 percent of patients. The posterior fasicle of the left bundle branch system has been found to have a dual blood supply in 40 percent, a sole source via the septal branch in 10 percent, and a sole source via the atrioventricular nodal artery in 50 percent. Using this information and recalling that the atrioventricular nodal artery arborizes from the right coronary artery in 90 percent of patients, various conduction disturbances in acute myocardial infarction can be more readily explained.

Infero-posterior infarction with loss of the atrioventricular nodal artery would be expected to retard atrioventricular nodal conduction with only Mobitz type I block and no Mobitz type II block unless the patient was the one out of ten in whom the atrioventricular nodal artery alone supplied the His bundle, or there was a preceding occlusion of the proximal anterior descending coronary artery. Moreover, such an occlusion alone would not be expected to progress to complete heart block unless the patient was the one out of ten in whom both bundle branches were solely supplied by the first septal artery, or where there was preceding disease impairing flow in the atrioventricular nodal artery.[9] Loss of the anterior septal artery blood supply alone would most often be expected to involve the right bundle and the anterior portions of the left bundle system, leading to right bundle branch block and variable degrees of left ventricular conduction delay.[10]

## DEVELOPMENTAL ANOMALIES OF THE CORONARY ARTERIAL TREE

Developmental anomalies of the coronary arteries can be categorized into: (1) anomalous origin of the left or right coronary artery or their branches from the pulmonary artery; (2) normal origin of both right and left coronary arteries from the aorta, but with a fistulous branch of one or more of these vessels which communicates directly with a cardiac chamber (usually the right ventricle), the pulmonary trunk, the coronary sinus, the superior vena cava, or a pulmonary vein, and (3) displaced origin of either the left or right coronary artery from the aorta. All three categories of developmental anomalies have been implicated in the production of myocardial ischemia and/or infarction and, thus, deserve consideration in any comprehensive discussion of the pathoanatomy of coronary heart disease.

The most important developmental anomaly in the neonatal and childhood periods occurs when the left coronary artery arises from the pulmonary trunk.[11,12] The aberrant artery is usually relatively small and thin-walled, while the portion of the left ventricle supplied by the artery is scarred, dilated, and possibly aneurysmal and calcified. The angiographic pattern on injection of both coronary arteries is characterized by normal antegrade flow in both right and left coronary arteries in the immediate neonatal period (related to a perfusion gradient between the pulmonary artery and the myocardial capillary bed immediately after birth), subsequent decrease in antegrade flow through the left coronary artery as the pulmonary artery pressure declines (with no intercoronary anastamoses), and, later in childhood, the demonstration of retrograde flow through the left coronary artery originating from intercoronary channels

connecting the right with the left coronary arteries. This latter pathophysiologic state may be associated with significant myocardial ischemia or infarction related to a "steal" or "run-off" of coronary blood flow away from the capillary bed of the myocardium. However, myocardial ischemia and/or infarction can also be associated with the stage of decreased antegrade perfusion of the anomalous left coronary artery, potentiated, undoubtedly, by oxygen desaturation of blood coming from the pulmonary artery.

A congenital coronary arterial fistula of large size and with substantial amounts of flow through it can likewise give rise to myocardial ischemia or infarction.[13] On angiography, the lumen of the fistulous coronary artery is generally smaller at its drainage site than at its origin; therefore, the dimensions of the fistulous vessel are believed to increase with the passage of time, sometimes becoming extremely large, thinwalled, and tortuous. Drainage into the coronary sinus can result in significant aneurysmal dilatation of that channel as well. Coronary "steal" of blood from the capillaries of the myocardium can again serve to divert blood from other coronary arteries into the fistulous channel. This mechanism appears to be more important when the steal arises from the left coronary artery, as opposed to its originating from the right coronary artery.

The incidence and types of anomalous aortic origin of the coronary arteries have only become fully appreciated since the use of coronary angiography in clinical practice.[14] As shown in Figure 3.4, the left coronary artery can arise from the right sinus of Valsalva or the right coronary artery itself. The left main coronary artery may course either behind the aorta or between the aorta and the pulmonary artery on its way to the left ventricle. Alternatively, the circumflex and anterior descending branches may arise separately from the right coronary artery and take separate paths around the great vessels. While the circumflex vessel assumes a retroaortic course, the anterior descending artery may pass either behind or in front of the pulmonary artery. Rarely, only the diagonal branch of the lcft anterior descending artery arises from the left sinus of Valsalva. In other patients, the ante-

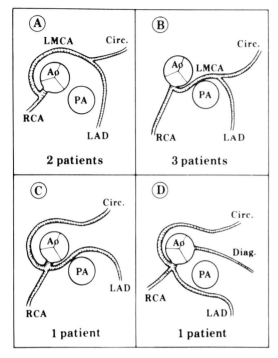

Fig. 3.4 Demonstration of types of aberrant origin of the left coronary artery (LCA) from either the right coronary artery (RCA) or the right sinus of Valsalva. *(A)* Origin of the left coronary artery from the proximal RCA with passage of the vessel posterior to the aorta (Ao). *(B)* Common origin of the left and right coronary arteries from the right sinus of Valsalva with passage of the left main coronary artery (LMCA) between the Ao and pulmonary artery (PA). *(C)* Separate origins of circumflex (Circ.) and left anterior descending (LAD) branches of the LCA with passage of the Circ. behind Ao and of the LAD between Ao and PA. *(D)* Same anomaly as (C) except the diagonal (Diag.) branch of LAD arises separately from left sinus of Valsalva. (Figures 3.4 and 3.5 reproduced with permission of the American Heart Association from Chaitman B et. al.: Clinical, angiographic, and hemodynamic findings in patients with anomalous origin of the coronary arteries. Circulation 53:122, 1976.)

rior descending branch of the left coronary artery arises from the left sinus of Valsalva, but the circumflex branch comes off the right coronary artery and traverses a pathway behind the aorta (Fig. 3.5). Similarly, the right coronary artery can arise from the left coronary artery or as a separate orifice coming off the left sinus of Valsalva; it can then take either a retro- or

anteaortic course to reach the right atrioventricular groove (Fig. 3.5B, C).

Over the last decade, two groups of patients have been identified in whom an anomalous left main coronary artery or anterior descending branch passes between the aorta and the pulmonary artery or right ventricular infundibulum, and in whom myocardial perfusion can be compromised.[15] One subgroup, composed of individuals who are relatively young (under 20 years of age), appears to be prone to sudden death after exertion. At postmortem examination, these individuals are found to have focal proximal obstructions at the origin of the anomalous vessel or in the area where the vessel

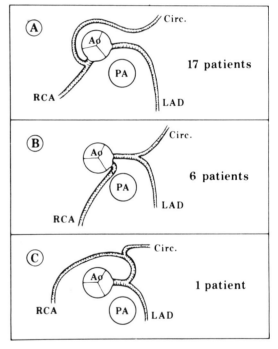

Fig. 3.5 *(A)* Anomalous origin of circumflex (Circ.) artery from the proximal right coronary artery (RCA) and passage of Circ. artery behind the aorta (Ao). Left anterior descending (LAD) arises from left sinus of Valsalva. *(B)* Anomalous origin of right coronary artery (RCA) from left sinus of Valsalva with passage of vessel between aorta (Ao) and pulmonary artery (PA). *(C)* Origin of both the right and left coronary arteries from a common trunk arising from the left sinus of Valsalva. Note that the right coronary artery (RCA) gives off the circumflex (Circ.) and travels behind the Ao to reach the right atrioventricular groove.

passes between the aorta and the right ventricular infundibulum. A second subgroup is comprised of individuals who demonstrate the same point of origin and pathway of the aberrant artery but who exhibit a normal life span and develop symptoms of myocardial ischemia as a consequence of atherosclerosis distal to the congenital abnormality. Interestingly, patients with an anomalous origin of the right coronary artery with passage between the aorta and the pulmonary artery have not been noted to be prone to sudden death.

## ATHEROSCLEROTIC LESIONS OF THE CORONARY ARTERIAL TREE

Coronary atherosclerosis can lead to a wide spectrum of anatomic alterations in the coronary arterial tree, ranging from diffuse narrowing and stiffening of the vessels to discrete narrowing and/or dilatation of segmental areas. Most commonly, however, the atheromatous plaque tends to aggregate in a small section of the artery and extends inward at the expense of the lumen (Fig. 3.6, bottom). Using coronary

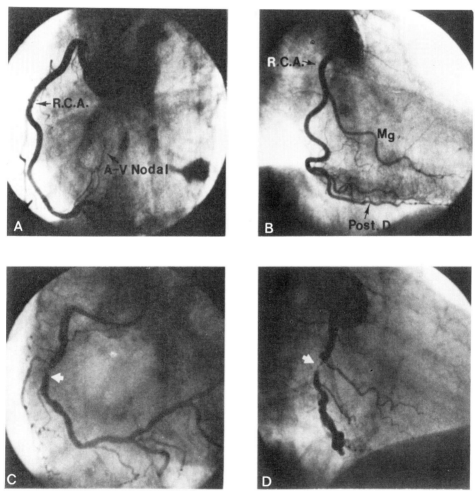

Fig. 3.6  Right coronary arteriogram: *(A)* left anterior and *(B)* right anterior oblique projections of a normal subject. *(C)* left anterior and *(D)* right anterior oblique projections of a patient with a high-grade stenosis (arrows) in the mid portion of the right coronary artery (RCA). Note that the atrioventricular (A-V) nodal artery arises from the distal RCA. The acute marginal (Mg.) branch arises in the mid RCA and supplies the anterior wall of the right ventricle. The psoterior descending (Post. D.) branch of the RCA runs along the interventricular sulcus on the inferior surface of the heart.

angiography, these segmental changes of coronary atherosclerosis have now been confirmed to occur at certain sites of predilection. Hydraulic factors are postulated to influence the specific loci where lesions will have the greatest tendency to develop; points of bifurcation of the major branches of the left coronary artery are noted to be particularly susceptible.[16] For example, since the first septal perforating branch of the anterior descending branch dips in a perpendicular direction into the myocardium, it is postulated that unusually high shear forces occur at this point and predispose the vessel to intimal damage or tear and, ultimately, plaque formation. On the other hand, some investigators have hypothesized that areas of low shear, exemplified by the inside of long, curved vessels such as the right coronary or circumflex arteries, may cause sequestration of platelets and provide a nidus for lipid deposition.[17] Irrespective of the underlying physical factors which might contribute to plaque formation, it is noted empirically that atherosclerotic obstructions tend to occur at bifurcation points in the anterior descending branch (at the first septal perforating branch, at the takeoff of the first diagonal branch), at the bifurcation of the circumflex artery into the first obtuse marginal branch, and in the proximal third of the right coronary artery. These general predilections, however, are less commonly noted in patients who have underlying metabolic disorders (e.g., diabetes mellitus or congenital hyperlipoproteinemias) which predispose to a more diffuse pattern of atheroma development—not only in the coronary arteries but also in other regions of the systemic arterial tree.

On a coronary angiogram, the hemodynamically significant lesion can appear as a long, segmental obstruction with a relatively smooth lumen, reducing the caliber in severe lesions to the size of a pinhole. Or, the lesion may be very short in length and show up with ragged edges as if the intimal surface were violated and ulcerated. In some patients, a thrombus forms either at the time of acute myocardial infarction or subsequent to infarction as part of a low cardiac output state. This thrombus can be recognized by the layering of contrast agent in and around the site of obstruction.

Alternatively, a thrombus may recanalize and appear as a very narrow passageway indistinguishable from that caused by a long, segmental plaque.

Major emphasis in the recognition of lesions of hemodynamic significance is placed upon the extent to which the atheromatous plaque compromises cross-sectional area, as compared to a closely contiguous segment of the same vessel. However, it is widely recognized that both the *length* and the *cross-sectional extent* of the lesion contribute to increased resistance to blood flow.[18] Moreover, diffuse narrowing or dilatation of a vessel can lead to significant errors in the assessment of cross-sectional compromise of a vessel, since the true hemodynamic effect of narrowing is determined by the absolute (not relative) diameter. Finally, the conventional approach of looking for cross-sectional compromise of lumen size is weakened further by the fact that most atherosclerotic lesions are eccentric, rather than concentric, to the center of the vessel. Because two perpendicular views of any given lesion are necessary to determine the true cross-sectional severity of a particular lesion, obtaining even the highest quality angiographic demonstration of coronary stenoses in multiple projections leaves significant intra- and interobserver variability in the interpretation of their hemodynamic severity. It is standard practice in most institutions, therefore, to have both the angiographer (usually a cardiologist) and a nonbiased physician (usually a cardiac radiologist) review the films before final prognostic or therapeutic decisions are rendered to the patient. In recent years, the use of radiographic systems which allow angulation of image intensifier and x-ray tube in multiple projections has greatly facilitated normal (perpendicular) views of all lesions, particularly those occurring in the proximal portion of the anterior descending branch of the left coronary artery.[19,20]

In the setting of subtotal or total obstruction proximally, the distal portion of a coronary artery often fills by collateral sources (Fig. 3.7, bottom). Common pathways for collateral filling of the distal anterior descending artery include channels via (1) the conus branch off the right coronary artery, (2) the posterior descend-

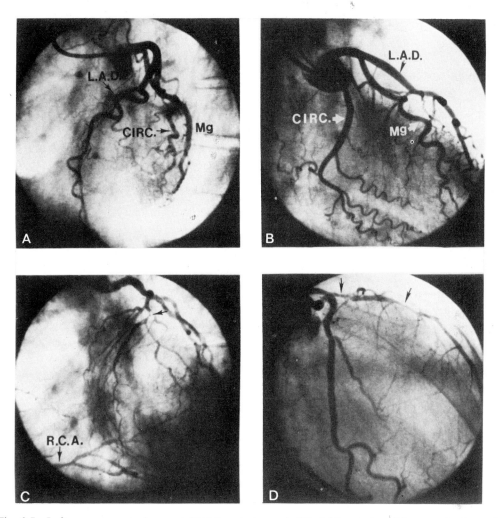

Fig. 3.7  Left coronary arteriogram: *(A)* left anterior and *(B)* right anterior oblique projections of a normal subject. *(C)* left anterior and *(D)* right anterior oblique projections of a patient with several long segmental stenoses of the left anterior descending *(arrows)*. Note that the left coronary artery is comprised of three major tributaries: left anterior descending (LAD), circumflex (CIRC.), and obtuse marginal (Mg.).

ing coronary artery around the apex of the left ventricle, or (3) smaller septal branches originating from the posterior descending artery. Occasionally, an arcade will form between the obtuse marginal branches coming off the circumflex vessel and the distal portion of the anterior descending artery. Some patients survive a complete occlusion of the left main coronary artery, and all of the coronary arterial tree then fills via the right coronary artery. However, with this constellation, a proximal lesion in the right coronary artery can then jeopardize flow to all segments of the myocardium. Collateral

filling of the distal right and posterior descending arteries is often seen via the distal radicals of the anterior descending or circumflex branches of the left coronary artery. It is felt that coronary collaterals are not capable of providing normal coronary blood flow during the stress of exercise and may not even provide adequate levels of flow at rest. Therefore, delivery of contrast material to the area of a vessel beyond a high-grade obstruction is inadequate in most instances to fully assess the size and dimensions of the distal lumen. Also, the distal portions of a vessel may fill by dual sources—

one through the normal antegrade pathway and the other via a collateral source. In this circumstance, selective injection of the collateral source with contrast material will often demonstrate oscillation or layering of contrast at the point where the nonopacified and opacified blood mix. This dynamic phenomenon as witnessed on a cine coronary angiogram has also been referred to as "reciprocating flow."

The underlying stimulus for collateral vessel formation is not fully understood and varies from species to species. In man, collateral channels are felt to represent dilatation of preexistent vessels which, in response to the development of a positive pressure gradient between their ends, begin to convey blood and thicken their walls.[21] Why some patients develop collateral vessels and others do not remains unsettled. There is further uncertainty as to whether the presence of collateral vessels favorably affects left ventricular function. Helfant, et al., have reported that a direct correlation exists between the number of collateral vessels and the severity of ventricular asynergy (wall motion disorders); however, no relationship was found between the presence of collateral vessels and the level of left ventricular end-diastolic pressure or cardiac output.[22] Also it is uncertain whether the development of collateral vessels has any predictable influence on survival or on the subsequent incidence of acute myocardial infarction. Finally, there does not appear to be a significant correlation between the presence of collateral vessels and the presence or absence or severity of clinical manifestations of myocardial ischemia, including angina pectoris. In fact, patients who exhibit collateral vessels demonstrate an ischemic postexercise electrocardiogram and myocardial lactate production more frequently than control patients without collateral vessel formation.[23]

## ANGIOGRAPHIC PATTERNS OF CORONARY ATHEROSCLEROSIS AND THE NATURAL HISTORY OF CORONARY HEART DISEASE

Beginning with the retrospective followup of patients who underwent coronary angiography at the Cleveland Clinic in the 1960s, it became apparent that actuarial survival in coronary heart disease was closely related to the extent of involvement of coronary atherosclerosis in the coronary arterial tree.[24-26] It is now generally agreed that patients with left main coronary artery stenosis of greater than 70 percent have the least favorable natural history, with a 1-year mortality rate of 20 to 32 percent and a cumulative 5-year mortality rate of 60 to 70 percent.[27-29] Patients with single vessel involvement of either the right, anterior descending, or circumflex coronary arteries have an annual mortality rate ranging from 0.7 to 3.6 percent, those with double vessel involvement a mortality rate of 6.6 to 13 percent, and those with triple vessel involvement a rate of 9.0 to 15 percent.[24-26, 30-34] The ranges cited in the above studies are likely related to differences in the definition and interpretation of significant obstructive lesions as well as to some heterogeneity of the population groups reported.

Although the natural history of coronary heart disease appears best predicted by the pathoanatomy found on coronary angiography, there are limitations and weaknesses in most of the previously published studies where followup of medically treated patients is presented. In some studies, patients in the cohorts for left main, single, double, and triple vessel disease were withdrawn for internal mammary artery implantation surgery, a procedure which was performed prior to the advent of saphenous vein bypass graft surgery. Secondly, radiographic resolution of coronary artery lesions was suboptimal in the 1960s and early 1970s, compared to that produced today by the cesium iodide intensifier mounted on an angulating device. Thirdly, propranolol and long-acting nitrates, which have a synergistic action in reducing myocardial oxygen demand, were not commonly utilized together in many of the subjects in these reports. The improved survival rate of patients treated medically in the Veterans Administrative Cooperative Study, as well as that from the University of Oregon, suggests that use of these drugs has significantly improved survival in patients with coronary heart disease.[35,36] Finally, an improved public awareness of the risk factors for coronary artery disease may be responsible for a notable decline in the incidence of deaths due to coronary artery disease over the past decade. Some caution should be exercised, therefore, in accepting the natural history of the disease in the 1960s and 1970s as being applicable to comparable subsets of patients today.

## ANGIOGRAPHIC PATTERNS OF CORONARY ATHEROSCLEROSIS AND THE CLINICAL SYNDROMES OF ANGINA PECTORIS AND MYOCARDIAL INFARCTION

Numerous investigators have attempted to correlate the pattern and extent of coronary artery disease (as viewed by coronary angiography) with the clinical syndromes of angina pectoris and acute myocardial infarction. It is apparent, however, that there are no tidy, irrefutable correlations to be found here. For example, angina pectoris can be experienced as readily by the patient with a single lesion in the right coronary artery as by one with lesions in all three major vessels. Or, conversely, some patients with extensive involvement of all vessels of the coronary arterial tree may exhibit no pain referable to myocardial ischemia. Similarly, a patient with an acute myocardial infarct may manifest no evidence of large vessel obstruction in the corresponding coronary artery, while another individual with an infarct in the same anatomical locale can show severe subtotal occlusion of the vessel serving that area of myocardium. There are dynamic factors relating to regional oxygen supply-and-demand relationships, to transitory spasm of some vessels of the coronary arterial tree, and possibly to coronary arterial embolism or small vessel involvement (beyond the resolution of the coronary anteriogram) which might explain some of the discrepancies noted between clinical syndromes and coronary angiographic pathoanatomy.

Despite the limitations posed above, certain broad correlations can be stated. Patients with a long history of angina pectoris, nocturnal angina, or postprandial angina are more likely to demonstrate multivessel involvement on the coronary arteriogram.[37] Moreover, certain electrocardiographic and hemodynamic findings at the time of stress testing on an exercise treadmill have been noted to correlate with high-risk subsets of coronary pathoanatomy.[38] Triple vessel or significant left main coronary artery involvement are likely to be present when the following electrocardiographic, workload, or hemodynamic responses are noted: (1) ischemic ST-segment changes during the first three minutes of exercise (any of the standard exercise protocols); (2) depressed J point with downsloping (as opposed to horizontal or upsloping) ST segments; (3) persistence of ST segment changes for greater than 8 minutes during recovery; (4) marked depth (2 to 3 mm) of ST segment depression; (5) hypotension or abnormal systolic blood pressure response during progressive exercise; (6) exercise-induced arrhythmias; and (7) reduced and symptom-limited exercise workload or heart rate (inability to complete Bruce protocol Stage II or equivalent, maximal heart rate less than 80 percent of predicted maximal in absence of angina, or heart rate less than 130/minute or less than 70 percent of predicted maximal rate before onset of angina). In general, the association of these treadmill responses with high-risk complexes of lesions in the coronary arterial tree has been made on patients who were symptomatic; thus, their applicability to an asymptomatic population is currently unknown.

Although coronary arteriography has not been performed routinely in most institutions within several months after myocardial infarction, a preliminary study from the University of Alabama reported that, in patients with more than one previous myocardial infarct, there was an 80 percent incidence of significant triple vessel disease and a 20 percent incidence of double vessel disease. In patients with one previous infarct, only approximately 40 percent were found to have significant triple vessel disease, 30 percent to have double vessel disease, 30 percent to have single vessel disease, and 10 percent to have left main coronary artery disease.[39] Thus, depending on the presence or absence of more than one antecedent infarct, between 70 and 100 percent of subjects in this limited study exhibited coronary artery pathologic anatomy characteristic of high-risk subsets and reduced survival. In a further study, Miller, et al. reported on the prospective, routine performance of coronary arteriography in 84 patients with previous uncomplicated isolated inferior myocardial infarction in order to identify those subjects at high risk for early death. Of the 84 subjects, 45 percent had significant stenosis of all three major coronary vessels, 35 percent had stenosis of two, and only 20 percent had stenosis of only one coronary vessel. Sixty-three percent of the patients with disease in the left anterior descending coronary artery had either total or subtotal occlusion of this major vessel.[40]

## LEFT VENTRICULOGRAPHY: TECHNIQUE, INTERPRETATION, AND QUANTITATION

Left ventriculography is routinely performed with coronary angiography and as a part of the same diagnostic procedure. In most cardiac catherization laboratories, cinefilming is utilized in order to fully demonstrate the dynamic aspects of wall motion and to uncover global and regional mechanical dysfunction brought about by coronary arterial lesions. Rapid large-film techniques (4 to 12 frames per second) have also been utilized and provide the advantage of superior anatomic resolution. However, rapid large-film techniques have the following disadvantages: (1) recognition of arrhythmias which might have occurred during the course of filming is difficult unless an electrocardiogram is recorded simultaneously; (2) ventriculographic images cannot be stored on videotape for instant replay, and (3) the ventriculogram cannot be viewed on a television monitor simultaneously with the injection of the contrast agent. Optimal definition of the left ventricular cavity-endocardial interface is obtained with either technique by injecting the contrast agent directly into the left ventricle. In order to avoid catheter recoil and the stimulation of premature ventricular contractions, most operators inject 30 to 60 ml of the contrast agent over 3 to 4 seconds, using a multihole cathether with relatively low resistance to injection. In our own experience, place-

ment of the catheter in the inflow portion of the left ventricular chamber, directly in front of the mitral valve, most consistently provides a contrast injection without ventricular extrasystoles.

Single-plane angiography, most frequently performed in the RAO projection, allows visualization of the anterior, apical, and inferior surfaces of the ventricular chamber but fails to demonstrate septal and posterolateral wall motion. In more sophisticated laboratories, biplane angiography is performed either in the anterior and lateral projections or in the RAO and LAO projections. Several radiographic equipment vendors have now designed and begun testing equipment which provides angulation capability of both the anterior and lateral imaging systems and which allows visualization of the left ventricular chamber directly perpendicular to the long axis of the chamber in both projections. Such design improvements avoid foreshortening and distortion of some elements of the ventricular wall and will undoubtedly improve the detection of regional wall motion abnormalities.

Cine left ventriculography allows both qualitative and quantitative assessment of global and regional function of the left ventricle. As such, the technique allows a more direct assessment of left ventricular function than that provided by the classical hemodynamic measurements of left ventricular end-diastolic pressure, stroke work, or stroke volume. By reviewing the cinefilm in real-time speed (usually 60 frames/sec) a trained observer can identify aberrant areas of segmental wall motion, form a mental integration of the average percent shortening of the chamber, and detect mitral regurgitation, a common consequence of papillary muscle ischemia or infarction. A more objective assessment of the mechanics of shortening is provided by outlining the margins of the chamber and computing either mean or instantaneous indices of shortening for the whole ventricle as well as for specific regions or segments of its wall.

The ejection fraction, or the stroke volume as a fraction of the end-diastolic volume, provides a quantitative index of the percent shortening for the whole chamber. To calculate ventricular volume, the ventriculogram is calibrated to life-size dimensions by means of a cross-hatched grid which corrects for magnification error as well as pincushion distortion of the image; using this grid, a calibration factor (CF) is derived. The left ventricular chamber is then modeled as an ellipse of revolution, and the volume is calculated as:

$$V = \frac{L_m \times D_f \times D_{lat}}{6}$$

where $D_f$ equals the diameter of the chamber in the frontal plane, $D_{lat}$ equals the diameter of the chamber in the lateral plane, and $L_m$ equals the longest length measured in either the frontal or lateral planes (Fig. 3.8). As shown in the same figure, the diameter of each projection is calculated from measurement of the area and the longest length of the ventricular image. Thus,

$$V_m(cc) = \frac{\pi \, D_F \cdot D_{Lat} \cdot L_M}{6}$$

where

$$D_F = \left(\frac{4 \, A_F}{\pi \, L_{M_F}}\right) \cdot CF_F$$

$$D_{Lat} = \left(\frac{4 \, A_{Lat}}{\pi \, L_{M_{Lat}}}\right) \cdot CF_{Lat}$$

In order to correct for errors which arise from inclusion of papillary muscles within the boundaries of the chamber, a linear regression equation, based on the studies of Dodge and coworkers, is utilized.[41] The equation, which relates the true volume ($V_t$) to the measured volume ($V_m$), is as follows:

$$V_t(cc) = 0.928 \, V_m - 3.8$$

In patients with coronary heart disease, the accuracy of left ventricular volume measurement is superior at end-diastole, as opposed to end-systole, due to geometric distortion of the end-systolic frame (nonconformity with ellipsoid reference figure) caused by regional wall motion abnormalities.

Dodge and coworkers have reported that the

minor axes ($D_f$ and $D_{lat}$) do not differ significantly in most patients, permitting calculation of left ventricular volume from a single-plane (usually right anterior oblique) image.[41] However, in the presence of significant regional disturbance of wall motion, the equivalency of the minor axes is less assured; thus, for optimal quantitative analysis of left ventricular function biplane angiography is advisable.

The effects of a regional disturbance of wall motion on the ejection fraction of the left ventri-

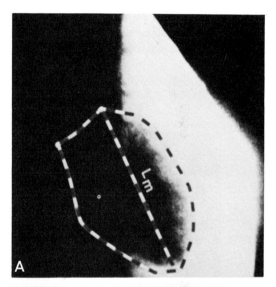

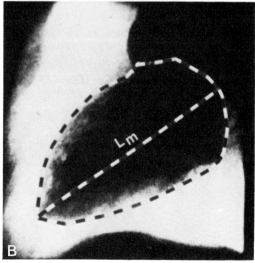

Fig. 3.8  Area-length method for calculation of left ventricular volume from a biplane left ventriculogram showing frontal *(A)* and lateral *(B)* projections of the ventricular image. See text.

cle can be appreciated by viewing Figure 3.9. In a normal patient (top panel) there is symmetrical shortening of the ventricle between the end-diastolic and end-systolic frames, providing an ejection fraction of 0.69—within the normal range of 0.67 ± 0.08 (SD). By contrast, in a patient with a previous antero-apical infarct secondary to a high-grade stenosis of the anterior descending branch of the left coronary artery, there is no movement of the anterior wall between the end-diastolic and end-systolic frames, and the stroke volume is generated almost entirely by contraction of the inferior segment of the left ventricular chamber. Accordingly, the ejection fraction is significantly reduced to 0.41.

Meticulous, frame-by-frame analysis of cine ventriculograms has shown that there are four

types of wall motion abnormalities (asynergy) which occur with coronary heart disease. These are: (1) hypokinesis, where a segment of the ventricular wall exhibits reduced extent of shortening but with normal inward movement during systole; (2) akinesis, where inward movement of the wall is completely absent during systole; (3) dyskinesis, where the wall moves paradoxically (outward) during systole and inward during diastole; and (4) asynchrony, a more subtle form, where each segment of the ventricular wall exhibits a normal extent of shortening, but ischemic segments contract late and are out of phase with normally perfused areas (Fig. 3.10).

The cine left ventriculogram has also been utilized to assess regional wall motion before and after a physiologic or pharmacologic inter-

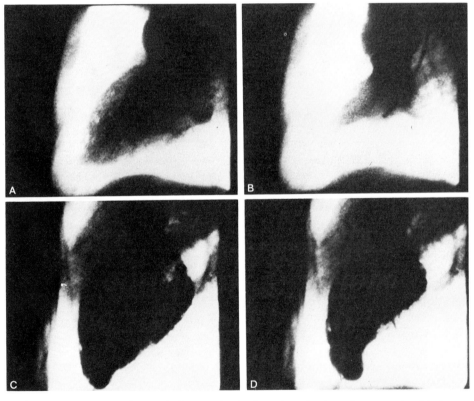

Fig. 3.9 Comparison of the left ventriculogram in the lateral projection of a normal subject at end-diastole *(A)* and at end-systole *(B)* with the left ventriculogram at end-diastole *(C)* and at end-systole *(D)* of a patient who had a previous anteroseptal myocardial infarction. In the normal patient, the ejection fraction (EF) was 0.69, and in the abnormal patient it was 0.41. Note that the abnormal patient demonstrates no systolic movement of the anterior and apical segments of the left ventricular wall.

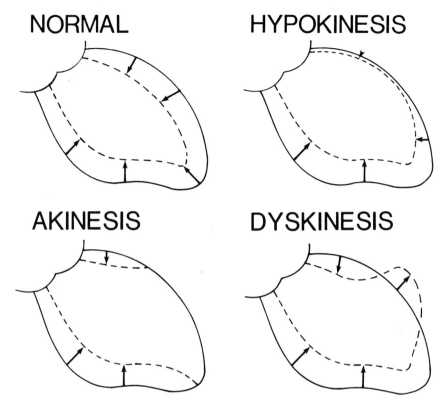

Fig. 3.10   Diagrammatic representation of various types of regional wall motion disorders (asynergy). See text.

vention in order to unmask latent myocardial ischemia or, conversely, to determine contractile reserve. As shown in Figure 3.11, chordal analysis can be performed whereby the long axis is divided into six equal segments, and chords are then drawn perpendicular to their junction to reach the anterior and inferior walls. To assess apical function, the apical end of the long axis is measured frame-by-frame throughout systole in a similar fashion. On a postventricular premature contraction (post-VPC), all segments are shown to exhibit potentiation of contraction, indicating some residual contractile reserve in each area. However, the patient was then paced to a heart rate of 150 beats/ min, until ST-segment depression in leads II, III, and AVF was noted and the patient experienced anginal pain—at which time pacing was stopped abruptly and a second ventriculogram was performed, with filming beginning on the third beat postpacing. By comparison with the control ventriculogram filmed under identical conditions of heart rate and projection, it can

be appreciated that pacing led to ischemia along the inferior wall (chordal segments 9, 10, and 11), which could be recognized by deterioration of wall motion in these segmental areas.

A pharmacologic agent which has been used in conjunction with ventriculography to assess latent ischemia is l-epinephrine, which increases myocardial oxygen demand and induces regional imbalances of myocardial oxygen supply and demand in areas of coronary arterial stenosis.[43] Nitroglycerin has also been used to unload the heart during ventriculography, at which time akinetic areas may exhibit shortening potential which was not apparent in the control state.[44]

## CLINICAL INDICATIONS FOR CORONARY ANGIOGRAPHY AND LEFT VENTRICULOGRAPHY

The spectrum of indications for coronary arteriography has widened in the last decade as

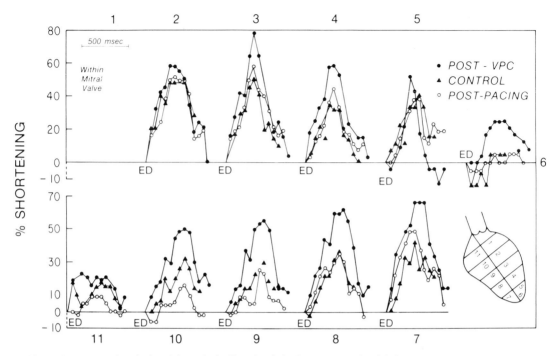

Fig. 3.11  Example of chordal analysis (key in right lower corner) of left ventricular wall motion in control state (closed triangles), postventricular premature contraction (VPC) (closed circles), and immediately after cessation of rapid pacing while the myocardium was still ischemic (open circles). Note the potentiation of shortening of all chords on the post-VPC beat and the deterioration of wall motion in the inferoposterior area (chords 9, 10, 11) with postpacing state.

the safety of the procedure has increased and the value of the information obtained has assumed greater clarity. In broad, general terms the procedure is indicated in any patient in whom there is uncertainty about the presence or absence of coronary arterial disease or in whom the information is considered essential for management. On the one hand, the procedure may be performed in an individual case because of its predictive value for survival. On the other hand, performance of the procedure may be essential in a patient in whom surgical revascularization is being contemplated.

In more specific terms, coronary arteriography is now recommended for individuals who fall into the following categories:

(1) Patients with a characteristic clinical syndrome which points to the presence of underlying coronary heart disease. In this category, the procedure is performed in those who have a chronic, stable anginal syndrome but in whom

pharmacologic and other conservative measures have not sufficiently alleviated symptoms to render both life-style and occupational status satisfactory and tolerable. Such patients are considered candidates for aortocoronary bypass graft surgery and must undergo angiography to assess whether their individual patho-anatomy is amenable to the procedure. Coronary angiography is also indicated in patients with unstable or "preinfarctional" angina in whom knowledge of specific coronary pathoanatomy is necessary for prognostication as well as therapeutic decisions; the feasibility of revascularization surgery is then known, but it is only undertaken if the patient remains refractory to intensive medical therapy while in the hospital. Finally, coronary angiography is advised in any patient who is suspected on the basis of clinical history or exercise testing of harboring a left mainstem lesion. In this subgroup, coronary angiography is indicated because of the well-recognizable, favorable effect of aortocoronary by-pass graft surgery, rather than medical therapy only, in relieving symptoms and prolonging life.[29]

(2) Patients with suspected coronary heart disease but without a definite or characteristic anginal syndrome. A cardiologist encounters some patients who are disabled because they think they have heart disease, although they are frequently proven to have a normal coronary arteriogram. The confirmation of the absence of significant disease can often allay patient anxiety, reduce the cost of future medical attention, and turn physician and patient attention appropriately toward other possible causes of the chest pain syndrome. Another subgroup of patients in this category have cardiac disease for which open heart surgery is being planned and where knowledge of occult coronary artery obstruction may influence operative results and mode of procedure. A third subgroup are individuals who have been resuscitated successfully from ventricular fibrillation, but in whom the underlying cause remains uncertain. Such patients commonly are found to have severe coronary heart disease and are at significant risk for sudden death. As noted earlier, some patients exhibit a markedly positive exercise stress test even though they may not admit to significant or typical symptoms. Patients in this subgroup are now being subjected more frequently to coronary arteriography because of its prognostic value and the insight it gives into the appropriateness of coronary artery bypass graft surgery.

(3) Patients who have complications of either myocardial infarction (e.g., ruptured papillary muscle or ventricular septum) or aortocoronary bypass graft surgery where operation or reoperation is being considered. Although the risk of coronary angiography is greater in some of these patients than in elective candidates, the information provided by the procedure is vital for a sound decision to intervene surgically.

Parenthetically, it should be stated that certain clinical subsets of patients with coronary heart disease are not referred for angiographic visualization of the coronary arteries. These include: (1) older individuals (over 70 years of age) with stable, controlled angina, (2) patients with old or recent myocardial infarcts who are asymptomatic or have mild, readily controlled angina, and (3) patients with a positive exercise test and a high work level without significant anginal pain.

## ACKNOWLEDGMENTS

Supported in part by Roche Foundation for Medical Research during author's sabbatical leave at Centre de Cardiologie, University of Geneva, Geneva, Switzerland.

## REFERENCES

1. Sones FM Jr: Acquired heart disease. Symposium on present and future cineangiocardiography. Am J Cardiol 3:710, 1959.
2. Sones FM Jr, Shirey FK: Cine coronary arteriography. Modern Concepts Cardiovasc Dis 31:735, 1962.
3. Rickets HJ, Abrams HL: Percutaneous selective coronary cine arteriography. JAMA 181:620, 1962.
4. Seldinger SI: Catheter replacement of the needle in percutaneous arteriography. Acta Radiol 39:368, 1953.
5. Judkins MP: Selective coronary arteriography: 1. A percutaneous transfemoral technique. Radiology 89:815, 1967.
6. Amplatz K, Formanek G, Stanger P, Wilson W: Mechanics of selective coronary artery catheterization via femoral approach. Radiology 89:1040, 1967.
7. Schoonmaker FW, King SB: Coronary arteriography by the single catheter percutaneous femoral technique. Experience in 6800 cases. Circulation 50:735, 1974.
8. Frink RJ, James TN: Normal blood supply to the human His bundle and proximal bundle branches. Circulation 47:8, 1973.
9. James TN: The coronary circulation and conduction system in acute myocardial infarction. Progr Cardiov Dis 10:410, 1968.
10. Scheinman M, Brennan B: Clinical and anatomic implications of intraventricular conduction blocks in acute myocardial infarction. Circulation 46:753, 1972.

11. Bland EF, White PD, Garland J: Congenital anomalies of coronary arteries: Report of unusual case associated with cardiac hypertrophy. Am Heart J 8:787, 1933.

12. Gasul BM, Loeffler E: Anomalous origin of the left coronary artery from the pulmonary artery. (Bland-White-Garland syndrome). Pediatrics 4:498, 1949.

13. Edis AJ, Schattenberg TT, Feldt RH, Danielson GK: Congenital coronary artery fistula. Mayo Clinic Proc. 47:567, 1972.

14. Chaitman B, Lesperance J, Saltiel J, Bourassa MG: Clinical, angiographic, and hemodynamic findings in patients with anomalous origin of the coronary arteries. Circulation 53:122, 1976.

15. Liberthson RR, Dinsmore RE, Fallon JT: Aberrant coronary artery origin from the aorta. Report of 18 patients, review of literature and delineation of natural history and management. Circulation 59:748, 1979.

16. Fry DL: Response of the arterial wall to certain physical factors. Atherogenesis: Initiating Factors, Ciba Foundation Symposium 12. Amsterdam, N.Y., Associated Scientific Publishers, 1973, pg. 121.

17. Caro CG: Transport of material between blood and wall in arteries. Atherogenesis: Initiating Factors. Ciba Foundation Symposium 12. Amsterdam, N.Y., Associated Scientific Publishers, 1973, pg. 127.

19. Bunnell IL, Greene DG, Tandon RN, Arani DT: The half-axial projection: A new look at the proximal left coronary artery. Circulation 48:1151, 1973.

20. Arani DT, Bunnell IL, Greene DG: Lordotic right posterior oblique projection of the left coronary artery: A special view for special anatomy. Circulation 52:504, 1975.

21. Schaper J, Borgers M, Schaper W: Ultrastructure of ischemia-induced changes in the precapillary anastamotic network of the heart. Am J Cardiol 29:851, 1972.

22. Helfant RH, Kemp HG, Gorlin R: Coronary atherosclerosis, coronary collaterals, and their relation to cardiac function. Ann Intern Med 73:189, 1970.

23. Helfant RH, Vókonas PS, Gorlin R: Functional importance of the human coronary collateral circulation. N Engl J Med 284:1277, 1971.

24. Moberg CH, Webster JS, Sones FM: Natural history of severe proximal coronary disease as defined by cineangiography. Am J Cardiol. 29:282, 1972.

25. Bruschke AVG, Proudfit WL, Sones FM Jr: Progress study of 590 consecutive nonsurgical cases of coronary disease followed 5–9 years. II. Ventriculographic and other correlations. Circulation 47:1154, 1973.

26. Webster JS, Moberg C, Rincon G: Natural history of severe proximal coronary disease as documented by coronary cineangiography. Am J Cardiol 33:195, 1974.

27. Cohen MV, Cohn PF, Herman MV, et al: Diagnosis and prognosis of left coronary artery obstruction. Circulation 45,46: Suppl. I:I–57, 1972.

28. Lim JS, Proudfit WL, Sones FM, Jr: Left main coronary arterial obstruction: Long-term follow-up of 141 non-surgical cases. Am J Cardiol 36:131, 1975.

29. Takaro T, Hultgren HN, Lipton MJ, et al: The VA Cooperative randomized study of surgery for coronary arterial occlusive disease. II. Subgroup with significant left main lesions. Circulation 54, Suppl. III:III–107, 1976.

30. Brymer JF, Buter TH, Walton JA Jr, Willis PW III: A natural history study of the prognostic role of coronary arteriography. Am Heart J 88:139, 1974.

31. Friesinger GC, Page EE, Ross RS: Prognostic significance of coronary arteriography. Trans Assoc Am Physicians 83:78, 1970.

32. Oberman A, Jones WB, Riley CP, Reeves TJ, Sheffield LT, Turner ME: Natural history of coronary artery disease. Bull NY Acad Med 48:1109, 1972.

33. Reeves TJ, Oberman A, Jones WB, Sheffield T: Natural history of angina pectoris. Am J Cardiol 33:423, 1975.

34. McNeer JF, Starmer CF, Bartel AG, et al: The nature of treatment selection in coronary artery disease: experience with medical and surgical treatment of a chronic disease. Circulation 49:606, 1974.

35. Murphy ML, Hultgren HN, Detre K, Thomsen J, Takaro T: Participants of Veterans Administration Cooperative Study: Treatment of chronic stable angina. A preliminary report on survival data of the Randomized Veterans Administration Cooperative Study. N Engl J Med 297:621, 1977.

36. Kloster FE, Kremkau EL, Ritzmann LW, Rahimtoola SH, Rosch J, Kanarek, PH: Coronary bypass for stable angina: A prospective randomized study. N Engl J Med 300:149, 1979.

37. Cohen LS, Elliott WC, Klein MD, Gorlin R: Coronary heart disease. Clinical cinearteriographic and metabolic correlations. Am J Cardiol 17:153, 1966.

38. Sheffield T, Reeves TJ, Blackburn H, Ellestad MH, Froelicher VF, Roitman DR, Kansal S: The exercise test in perspective. Circulation 55:681, 1977.
39. Russell RO, Rogers WJ, Mantle JA, Kouchoukos NT, Rackley CE: Coronary arteriography within two months of acute myocardial infarction. Cardiovascular Medicine, July, 1977, pg. 769.
40. Miller RR, DeMaria AN, Vismara LA, Salel AF, Maxwell KS, Amsterdam EA, Mason DT: Chronic stable inferior myocardial infarction: unsuspected harbinger of high-risk proximal left coronary arterial obstruction amenable to surgical revascularization. Am J Cardiol 39:954, 1977.
41. Dodge HT, Sandler H, Baxley WA, Hawley RR: Usefulness and limitations of radiographic methods for determining left ventricular volume. Am J Cardiol 18:10, 1966.
42. Herman MV, Heinle RA, Klein, MD, Gorlin R: Localized disorders in myocardial contraction. N Engl J Med 277:222, 1967.
43. Horn H, Teichholz LE, Cohn PF, Herman MV, Gorlin R: Augmentation of left ventricular contraction pattern in coronary artery disease by an inotropic catecholamine: the epinephrine ventriculogram. Circulation 49:1063, 1974.
44. Helfant, RH, Pine R, Meister SG, Feldman MS, Trout RG, Banta VS: Nitroglycerin to unmask reversible asynergy: Correlation with post coronary bypass ventriculography. Circulation 50: 108, 1974.

*Section 2*
# HISTORICAL AND ORGANIZATIONAL ASPECTS OF THE CORONARY CARE UNIT

# 4 | *History of the Coronary Care Unit and Its Contribution to Mortality Reduction*

## *Joel S. Karliner, M.D.*

## HISTORY OF THE CCU

From an historical standpoint, the acceptance of coronary care as an integral part of the medical management of patients with acute myocardial infarction was an exceedingly rapid event, beginning with the establishment of the first Coronary Care Units in 1962 in Kansas City, Toronto, and Philadelphia.[1] By the late 1960s or early 1970s, virtually all large hospitals and many smaller and intermediate hospitals had some kind of intensive care unit that was devoted, in part or in whole, to patients with coronary artery disease. The initial impetus for the establishment of such units came about from the recognition that many patients with acute myocardial infarction died suddenly. It was therefore hoped that resuscitative efforts could reverse this remarkable mortality trend.

It is worthwhile to trace the gestation of the Coronary Care Unit, the conception of which represented the fusion of two separate but parallel lines of investigation. One concerned cardiac resuscitation and the other the mechanism of death in acute myocardial infarction. In 1933, Hooker et al. used animal experiments to propose a specific method of cardiac resuscitation which involved rhythmic manual massage of the heart through a thoracotomy followed by electrical defibrillation.[2] However, attempts in man failed because of the inability of the myocardium to resume normal beating and because there was a critical period of only several min-

utes in which a resuscitation attempt could be made, beyond which death of viable myocardial tissue as well as brain death were irreversible. A milestone event occurred in 1947 when Claude Beck and his colleagues successfully applied Hooker's technique to a 14-year-old boy who had developed ventricular fibrillation just as an operation for funnel chest deformity was being completed.[3] The chest wound was reopened, the heart massaged, and defibrillation performed by delivering 110 volts of AC current through two large electrodes applied directly to the heart. The patient survived and was well thereafter. Subsequent to this report, many hospitals equipped their operating rooms with defibrillators and surgeons were trained in resuscitative techniques. Nine years later, Beck et al. were able to use this method for the first time outside the operating room in a patient with acute myocardial infarction.[3] The patient was a 65-year-old physician who developed ventricular fibrillation. He was rushed to the operating room where thoracotomy was performed only minutes after circulatory collapse. The patient underwent open chest cardiac massage and defibrillation and recovered fully except for minor memory deficit. To quote Beck et al:[4] "This one experience indicates that resuscitation from a fatal heart attack is not impossible and might be applied to those who die in the hospital and perhaps to those who die outside the hospital." About the same time, Reagan et al. also resuscitated a patient with ventricular fibrillation sec-

83

ondary to acute myocardial infarction.[5] As is often the case in science as well as in clinical medicine, the well-prepared investigator was able to seize the opportunity: The patient was having an electrocardiogram recorded in the emergency room when he developed the potentially fatal dysrhythmia; open chest defibrillation was performed without delay, and the patient survived.

Unfortunately, however, these reports did not lead to an increase in the overall survival of patients with acute myocardial infarction because of the obvious requirements that a physician had to be present to rush the patient to the operating room, where an open thoracotomy had to be performed. By 1956, however, it became apparent that one of the major obstacles to routine resuscitation could be avoided when Zoll and his colleagues reported that ventricular fibrillation could be terminated by delivering an electric shock through the intact chest wall.[6] In this original report, four patients were described in whom ventricular fibrillation was abolished on 11 occasions by externally applied countershock. This exceedingly important contribution awaited solution of the second problem of circulatory maintenance until countershock could be applied. The beginnings of cardiopulmonary resuscitation (CPR: see Chapters 17 and 31) as we know it today began when Kouwenhoven et al. demonstrated in 1960 that the heart could be effectively massaged without thoracotomy by rhythmic external compression of the chest wall.[7] Combined with mouth-to-mouth respiration, this maneuver was capable of supporting the circulation until external defibrillation could be performed.

Based on these concepts, Dr. Hughes Day, in Kansas City, Missouri, began attempts to resuscitate patients suffering from cardiac arrest.[1] A mobile crash cart was constructed with a defibrillator and a trained team who responded immediately to a code signal whenever a cardiac arrest was recognized anywhere in the hospital. This attempt yielded disappointing results, primarily because of the delay in reaching the patient after an arrest was recognized. The difficulty identified by Day and his colleagues continues to be an important problem in hospital rooms and wards, where cardiac ar-

rest may be recognized too late. Subsequently, Day and others recognized that, if such resuscitation were to be effective, it would require a unit where constant surveillance was possible. With the financial support of a private foundation (no government support at this time!), Day and his colleagues designed and built an intensive care facility at his institution. Constant physiologic monitoring was introduced from the beginning, as well as constant cardiac monitoring to a central nursing station. Such monitoring equipment had only recently become available for general use and, as indicated above, similar units opened at about the same time in both Philadelphia and Toronto. Thus, the goal of Day's unit was to provide resuscitative capabilities in an intensive care setting. The complementary initial goal of the unit in Philadelphia, begun by Meltzer and Kitchell, was to provide immediate therapy for cardiac arrhythmias which they assumed were the cause of sudden death in patients with acute myocardial infarction.[8] This hypothesis arose out of a previous study of anticoagulation in such patients. Thus, Meltzer and Kitchell realized that the therapeutic aim of anticoagulation, which was to prevent thromboembolism, was an erroneous one. Effective early treatment of dysrhythmias was also proposed by the group in Toronto. Hence, the convergence of a number of lines of research—i.e., electrical defibrillation, cardiopulmonary resuscitation, and the recognition of the probable importance of dysrhythmias—gave birth to the first Coronary Care Units as we know them today. Thus began the organized efforts to save hearts which, in Beck's phrase, were "too young to die." From these early efforts also emerged the routinely accepted designation "Code Blue" because, as Day has pointed out, most of the resuscitated patients were initially cyanotic.[1]

With the advent of routine rhythm surveillance in these early units, it soon became apparent that the vast majority of patients with acute myocardial infarction exhibited ventricular dysrhythmias, thereby confirming earlier studies. Prior to that time, the significance of arrhythmias during acute myocardial infarction had not been recognized. Although the concept of "warning arrhythmias"—i.e., ventricular dysrhythmias that heralded ventricular fibrillation [9]—received considerable support, the significance and treatment of such dysrhythmias nevertheless remains an important and controversal issue [10] (see Chapter 16). Thus, the evolution from the initial goal of resuscitation of patients with cardiac arrest to the establishment of an organized and specialized environment for segregating patients with acute myocardial infarction that permits constant surveillance of cardiac rhythm as well as gauging hemodynamic status, took only several years, and its uncritical acceptance still remains a matter of some controversy, as will be explained later in this section.

Another "mini-revolution" brought about in part by the development of the Coronary Care Unit was the responsibility that was now given to nurses. It became apparent that a physician could not be in constant attendance for 24 hours to provide monitoring. Therefore, it became necessary to have other individuals undertake these responsibilities, and this naturally fell to nurses who staffed the Unit. It should be appreciated that this represented an important change of attitude on the part of the medical profession. Although it is now commonplace for nurses, and even paramedical personnel, to introduce intravenous solutions, interpret electrocardiograms, begin therapy (intravenous lidocaine, defibrillation), perform routine hemodynamic monitoring and obtain arterial blood specimens for determination of oxygen and carbon dioxide tensions, the general acceptance that these procedures could be performed by nurses was in part brought about by the advent of CCUs. Indeed, this alteration in nursing responsibility required changes both in medical and legal practice in most areas of the country. In the early 1960s, Meltzer and Kitchell trained their nurses in defibrillation procedures, and this must be credited as a pioneering effort in the concept of the highly trained coronary care nurse.[1]

As indicated above, the nurse remains the cornerstone of care in the prevention and treatment of dysrhythmias. Even when 'round-the-clock medical coverage is present (and this is often not the case in intermediate-sized and smaller institutions), the CCU nurse must be skilled in cardiac resuscitation and recognition of potentially dangerous dysrhythmias. In this context, the importance of an ongoing training program cannot be overemphasized. The nurse's contribution to the diagnosis of dysrhythmias goes beyond the simple observation of the oscilloscope. He or she must exercise judgment as to the nature of the problem and act upon that decision. The nurse must be alert to early signs of circulatory failure and must be able to assess a patient's hemodynamic status by checking for restlessness, sweating, and pulmonary rales; where such facilities are available, the nurse must be skilled in monitoring intracardiac pressures. It is often routine procedure for nurses to institute resuscitative measures and make critical decisions regarding the nature and treatment of dysrhythmias for prolonged periods, often on the basis of optional standing orders which are implemented at their discretion. Such obligations may create some medical-legal problems, which are discussed in Chapter 41.

## EFFECTIVENESS IN REDUCING MORTALITY RATE

How effective have Coronary Care Units been? It has been estimated that each year some 700,000 persons in the United States die of acute myocardial infarction. Approximately half of these individuals succumb before reaching the hospital so that the existence of an in-hospital CCU has no direct bearing on their mortality, and this observation has led to the notion of precoronary care (see Chapter 36). Before the advent of CCUs the significance of ventricular dysrhythmias went virtually unrecognized except for a few reports (and resuscitative efforts were usually unsuccessful because of the delay in reaching the patient after a cardiac arrest had been recognized). Subsequent to the development of such units, uncontrolled, nonrandomized, retrospective studies purported to demonstrate a 50 percent reduction in mortality from ventricular fibrillation compared with the years preceding the institution of the Unit. However, mortality from "pump failure" and cardiogenic shock remained essentially unaffected, and this observation remains substantially true today.

The Coronary Care Unit and, indeed, other types of intensive care units such as the Respiratory Intensive Care Unit, have gained relatively uncritical acceptance by the medical profession. In this sense, the best analogy is to a surgical procedure which is initially accepted and subsequently undergoes a critical review with a controlled trial. By contrast, the establishment of such units is unlike the acceptance of a new drug which must undergo a critical evaluation in controlled trials prior to general use. Since the introduction of CCUs, there have been only a few appropriately designed and randomized studies that have considered the effects of CCU treatment on short- and long-term patient mortality. In a report published in 1971, Mather and colleagues showed that it was better for some patients to be kept at home.[11] Unfortunately, only 28 percent of all cases were randomized, and most of these came under care after the period of highest mortality had passed. More recently, the same group reappraised the goal of hospital admission in a randomized study of home versus hospital in Bristol in the southwest of England. Again, only 24 percent of their patients with suspected myocardial infarction could be allocated randomly to the two treatment groups, the remainder being electively admitted to the hospital or retained at home.[12] This study has been criticized in the United Kingdom by a joint working party of the Royal College of Physicians and the British Cardiac Society, who found the results to be unacceptable because of defects in design: many patients were seen late after the onset of symptoms, and only a small, ill-defined minority of patients were randomized.[13]

A more recent study by Hill, Hampton, and Mitchell in the Nottingham area of England compared home and hospital management of patients with suspected myocardial infarction in a randomized prospective study.[14] A hospital-based team was responsible for calls from general practitioners, and 349 patients out of 500 were suspected of having myocardial infarction. Of these, 24 percent were excluded from the trial on predetermined medical and social grounds. The medical reasons included dys-

rhythmias such as atrial fibrillation, supraventricular tachycardia, heart block and multiple ventricular ectopic beats, heart failure, cardiac arrest (seven patients), persistent chest pain, urinary retention, cerebral embolus, or cardiogenic shock. Social grounds included a lack of family support, refusal by the patient to care for himself or a relative's refusal to care for him, unsuitable housing, the patient's not living at his own home, or equipment failure. For the remaining patients, there was no significant difference in the 6-week mortality between the home group (13 percent) and the hospital group (11 percent). The authors concluded that, for the majority of patients to whom a general practitioner is called because of suspected infarction, hospital admission confers no clear advantage. Subsequently, this study was subjected to a number of criticisms. Thus, Oliver pointed out that there were eight deaths during the first day among those randomized for home care and only one among those sent to the hospital, implying that hospital care is desirable at this very early stage.[15] He suggested that efficient antidysrhythmic units, in which patients are treated very soon after the onset of symptoms, preferably within six hours, can decrease the mortality significantly and return such patients to active lives. He did not find it surprising that home care was as satisfactory as hospital care for patients once they had passed the time when primary lethal dysrhythmias are most common. Barritt and his colleagues emphasized that the circumstances of the trial were not those in which a usual practitioner is called to see a patient with suspected myocardial infarction.[16] They pointed out that the hospital-based team had technical help from monitoring oscilloscopes, a defibrillator, and considerable experience in their use. The 14 percent of patients who were selected for hospital admission for medical reasons included seven with cardiac arrest, 16 with rhythm disturbances, and eight with cardiac failure. Barritt et. al. reported that of 171 patients admitted to the Coronary Care Unit at Bristol over a 3-year period with proven myocardial infarction, 10 percent had an episode of ventricular fibrillation during their hospital stay.[16] Of the 102 patients with ventricular fibrillation, 62 left the hospital, and previous studies have shown that their fate is not different from patients leaving the hospital who did not have such an attack. They concluded that 6 percent of all patients seem to gain a real advantage from hospital admission, unless it can be shown that admission to the hospital by itself produces ventricular fibrillation. This is an area where further research is clearly called for.

In addressing the study of Hill et. al.,[14] Norris made the case for precoronary care by pointing out that, during the time between the patient's call for help and the arrival of the team, 14 had died and a further seven had a cardiac arrest during the period of domiciliary coronary care.[17] Based on epidemiological studies, Norris thought it likely that at least 20 more deaths occurred before a patient could call for help. Most of those deaths would have been caused by primary ventricular fibrillation which can be effectively treated by highly trained and mobile paramedical units, particularly if cardiopulmonary resuscitation can be initiated by bystanders or relatives before the paramedics arrive (see Chapters 17 and 31).

Where CCUs have been assessed in relation to general hospital ward care, early studies indicated that specialized units conferred a definite advantage. Thus, Hofvendahl in Sweden studied 248 patients with 271 myocardial infarctions.[18] Patients were randomized, according to bed availability, either to the CCU or to the general medical ward. Hospital mortality in the CCU group was 17 percent, which was significantly lower than the 35 percent of the control group. The difference in mortality derived primarily from a lower first-day mortality in the CCU group. Compared with the control group, there was a reduction of deaths due to cardiac dysrhythmias in the CCU group, which was achieved chiefly by preventing primary dysrhythmias. The majority of late hospital deaths were unexpected, and were presumably due to reinfarction and/or ventricular dysrhythmias, thereby justifying the need for postcoronary care (see Chapter 37). After discharge, the patients in the two groups were followed for between two and three years; long-term survival was similar between the two groups. Similar results were reported by Christianson, Iverson, and Scooby in Denmark, who concluded that ". . . the better results obtained in the Coronary Care Unit seem to be due to a selective individualized prophylaxis based on intensive observation, early detection and treatment of arrhythmias, and a schedule for slow reduction of drug therapy under close observation to detect the slightest signs of relapse." [19]

By contrast, Hill, Holdstock, and Hampton could not demonstrate a lower mortality among patients receiving intensive care.[20] In this study, 2,047 patients suspected of having an acute myocardial infarction were seen in a period of 32 months. Of 1,480 patients with definite or probable infarction, 483 were admitted to an ordinary medical ward because of a shortage of CCU beds. There was a higher proportion of successful resuscitations in the CCU, but there was no significant difference in mortality in either group between patients admitted to the CCU or to a ward. As the authors themselves point out, the study was not randomized, and a higher proportion of patients who later proved to have either a definite or a probable infarction were admitted to the CCU. Thus, in some hospitals in the United Kingdom, hospitalization on a ward for uncomplicated myocardial infarction represents an acceptable standard of medical care. Further, in many rural and some urban areas of Great Britain, home care is an acceptable medical alternative for patients who appear to have an uncomplicated course, especially if their symptoms are disappearing or are gone by the time the general practitioner makes the home visit (an event which is less common in the United States).

In a statewide retrospective study of 1,156 patients with acute myocardial infarction who were discharged from Maryland hospitals during a one-year period, Gordis et al. found that, of all patients treated in coronary care units, 30.1 percent died in-hospital compared with 17.8 percent of those not treated in CCUs (P < .0001).[21] This difference persisted when race, sex, age, anticoagulant use, and clinical severity were considered. When the combined effects of differences in prognostic factors between CCU and non-CCU patients were assessed using a multiple regression model, the adjusted mortality rates in CCU patients were almost twice as high as in patients not treated in such units.

In reviewing the literature on the effectiveness of CCUs, Gordis et al. concluded that the studies in which such units were found to be beneficial were generally significantly flawed in design and methodology.[21] Although these authors acknowledged that all the studies thus far published have limitations of differing sorts, they stated that ". . . the literature can be fairly summarized by saying that the better the study the less the benefit that has been shown from coronary care units."[21]

In further examining this issue, Gordis and colleagues suggested that the real question is not whether CCUs are better than no CCUs, but: if CCUs are better, what are the specific components of care provided in such units which produce the benefit?[21] They argue that, in view of a combination of limited resources and increasing expense of medical care, this question is a critical one to answer. In their view, it would therefore be reasonable to design a randomized study in which a CCU provides different arrays of services to different patients. By comparing the outcome, they suggest it would then be possible to conclude whether any of the services provided are of benefit and, if so, which service or services are most beneficial.[21]

In this connection, Peterson has written that "It is discouraging that these expensive services and their increasing application have taken place without regard to efficacy, much less to their cost . . . is it too late to conduct a randomized trial comparing a quiet, less expensive hospital room with intensive care? After all, many cardiologists feel that the atmosphere of the CCU is responsible for the induction of the arrhythmias that Coronary Care personnel have become so adept at treating."[22] Such a statement represents a challenge to cardiologists in this era of rising costs to demonstrate conclusively that the CCU is indeed an efficacious and "cost-effective" method of treating patients. Further, any such studies must take into account the caveat of the anonymous *Lancet* editorialist who cautioned that ". . . the apparent mortality rate of patients admitted to a CCU can be altered drastically by minor variations in the age-structure, infarct-timing, and general health of patients. Claims for a major alteration in mortality cannot therefore be accepted without an assurance that like is being compared with like. Finally . . . we should obey Pasteur's injunction to 'keep your enthusiasm but let strict verification be its constant companion.' "[10]

In considering both cost and efficacy, it should be recognized that the concept of the CCU has expanded with time to include the treatment of many more patients other than those with acute myocardial infarction. Indeed, an argument could be made for changing the name of such units to an Intensive Cardiac Care Unit rather than a Coronary Care Unit, and this, indeed, has occurred in many institutions. Thus, the Coronary or Cardiac Care Unit provides a setting for the treatment of patients having a variety of cardiac disorders with a well-trained staff schooled in resuscitative, hemodynamic, and monitoring techniques. In many such units, the percentage of admitted patients in whom the diagnosis of acute myocardial infarction is subsequently established varies between 35 and 60 percent. The other patients are those with suspected or proved acute or chronic ischemic heart disease in whom an acute myocardial infarction is excluded by appropriate studies, but who are nevertheless monitored because of the possibility of infarction. These individuals may be susceptible to sudden death because of ventricular dysrhythmias without overt infarction and hence are suitable candidates for monitoring. Other patients frequently admitted to Cardiac Care Units for intensive monitoring are those with a history of syncope who may have rapid supraventricular dysrhythmias or who have developed heart block. Under these circumstances, the Cardiac Intensive Care Unit may also be used for the insertion of a temporary or permanent pacemaker, after which patients are usually monitored for one or more days. Other types of patients with cardiac disease who may be admitted to the Unit include those with unstable angina pectoris who are also susceptible to sudden death due to ventricular dysrhythmias. These patients require therapy in an intensive care setting and frequently undergo coronary angiography as part of their diagnostic assessment, after which they may be returned to the Unit and a decision may be made regarding the suitability of coronary artery bypass surgery. Patients undergoing "routine" diagnostic cardiac catheterization and coronary angiography, who may be in an unstable hemodynamic state subsequent to these procedures, are also suitable candidates for monitoring in the intensive care setting.

A more recent addition to the types of patients who may be admitted to the Cardiac Care Unit are those individuals with advanced congestive cardiac failure, whether or not it is due to acute or chronic ischemic heart disease, who require hemodynamic monitoring in association with vasodilator therapy (see Chapter 22). In some institutions, the Coronary Care Unit is also the setting for patients undergoing intraaortic balloon counterpulsation (see Ch. 21). Another potentially beneficial aspect of acute coronary care is the effect on the subsequent extent of myocardial infarction or "infarct size" produced by conventional techniques such as the routine therapy of ventricular dysrhythmias. Current studies in this area may shed some light on the efficacy of Coronary Care Units in this regard (see Ch. 23). Should specific therapy to reduce "infarct size" become established,[23] the Coronary Care Unit will be its natural home.

Finally, both the proponents and opponents of routine coronary care must take into account the prognostic stratification of patients entering the Coronary Care Unit (see Ch. 43). If, after the first 48 hours, low-risk patients could be separated from high-risk patients, the former group could be transferred more rapidly from the Coronary Care Unit to an intermediate monitoring unit or even to a ward bed, possibly equipped with remote telemetry. Such rapid screening and effective prognostic identification would effect considerable savings in CCU costs and, thereby, justify the continued use of such units. Administrators will eventually have to make decisions concerning the allocation of fiscal priorities. However, until such stratifications are tested prognostically and in a controlled fashion, no specific conclusions can be drawn

from the types of information currently available in the medical literature.

## ADMISSION CRITERIA FOR THE CCU

Below are listed the criteria for admission to the Coronary Care Unit, University Hospital, University of California Medical Center, San Diego, California. It is recognized that such criteria may differ from hospital to hospital and that varying criteria will be necessary depending on hospital location and degree of staffing. Nevertheless, the guidelines below provide some "ground rules" which can be adopted by different institutions according to their needs.

Admission Policy

I. Admissions to the Coronary Care Unit may be direct or by transfer, as long as beds are available.

II. Final decision regarding any admission to the Coronary Care Unit will normally rest with the CCU Resident (or covering resident) in accordance with the admission criteria outlined below.

  A. If a difference of opinion develops between the admitting physician and the CCU Resident regarding the appropriateness of a particular admission, the matter will be referred to the next level of authority—i.e., the Cardiology Fellow supervising the Coronary Care Unit, and, if necessary, the Coronary Care attending physician.

III. The Coronary Care Unit will be closed to admissions only when all beds are occupied by priority one patients (see paragraph V).

IV. Admission Criteria

  A. Documented or suspected acute myocardial infarction with symptoms less than 48 hours in duration.

  B. Unstable angina.

  C. Documented or suspected myocardial infarction of any duration currently complicated by:

    1. Significant dysrhythmia
    2. Acute disturbance in CNS function
    3. Hypotension/shock

4. Thromboembolism
5. Persistent or recurrent chest pain/dyspnea
6. Other serious management problems with high therapeutic potential

D. Patients without documented or suspected myocardial infarction, but with serious dysrhythmias, such as:
   1. Ventricular tachycardia or ventricular fibrillation
   2. High-grade atrioventricular block or Stokes-Adams episodes
   3. Tachyarrhythmias of any type associated with hypotension
   4. Any dysrhythmia producing significant symptoms

E. Documented or suspected cardiovascular catastrophies, other than acute myocardial infarction, such as:
   1. Acute pulmonary embolism
   2. Acute pulmonary edema
   3. Acute hypertensive crisis
   4. Dissecting aortic aneurysm
   5. Cardiac tamponade
   6. Overdose of tricyclic antidepressant drugs or other drugs with a high potential for development of serious cardiac dysrhythmias

F. Other cases which the CCU Resident believes can be appropriately treated in this Unit, with the concurrence of the CCU Cardiology Fellow.

V. Admission Priorities
A. PRIORITY I
   1. Suspected or proven ischemic heart disease with:
      a. Symptoms of myocardial infarction or unstable angina 48 hours in duration or less, regardless of complications
      b. Symptoms present more than 48 hours, but one or more complications present (see paragraph IV-C)
   2. No recent symptoms of ischemic heart disease present, but serious dysrhythmias due to any cause exist

B. PRIORITY II
   1. Acutely complicated, nonischemic heart disease (see paragraphs IV-B and IV-E)

   2. Suspected or proven ischemic heart disease without complications, symptoms one week or less, but more than 48 hours duration

Admission to the Coronary Care Unit may have further justification in terms of overall hospitalization. Thus, if the patient follows an uncomplicated course in the CCU, not only earlier mobilization but also earlier discharge from the hospital may be justified. For example, McNeer and his colleagues reported that patients who were uncomplicated through day four had a subsequent hospital mortality rate of zero and an incidence of late serious complications of zero.[24] Earlier studies had also suggested that the duration of bed rest and the timing of early ambulation as well as total hospitalization may be progressively decreased.[25-31] These observations, pioneered by Levine and Lown,[32] represent a major change in thinking over the past 20 to 30 years. Prior to this time, prolonged bed rest and convalescence from acute myocardial infarction were urged; although at least one contemporary report still takes this stance,[33] most practitioners currently feel that early mobilization and discharge are justified, especially when no complications have arisen. These issues are discussed in detail in Chapter 7.

In recent years, the concept of coronary care or cardiac care has been extended to include the treatment of premonitory symptoms as well as subsequent intermediate cardiac care (Chapters 36 and 37). Because in a number of cities in the United States and Europe, approximately half of patients with acute myocardial infarction die suddenly out of hospital, a system of "precoronary care" has been developed with trained paramedics and ambulance teams able to respond to emergencies within short periods of time. Considerable information has been learned from these efforts, and it has become apparent that resuscitation, if it is begun early enough, may lead to considerably enhanced patient survival.[34] Radiotelemetric devices for physician monitoring of dysrhythmias have been developed, and there appears to be an especially great reduction in mortality in patients under the age of 70 who are treated by either mobile or fixed life-support stations for acute myocardial infarction. These represent encouraging statistics and establish the validity of the concept that electrical instability, when treated early, may be less of a life-threatening event.

The role of the intermediate-care unit has also been recognized in the past few years. After the establishment of Intensive Coronary Care Units, it became apparent that a certain number of patients with acute myocardial infarction still exhibited electrical instability following discharge from the Coronary Care Unit and among these patients were a considerable number of presumably preventable deaths. Among the goals of intermediate coronary care, as outlined by Frieden and Cooper,[35] are the following: (1) a decrease in the frequency of cardiac arrest in patients leaving the CCU by early detection and prophylactic therapy of potentially dangerous dysrhythmias; (2) improvement of the success rate of cardiac resuscitation by immediate recognition of ventricular fibrillation and cardiac standstill, (3) a decrease in the total length of hospitalization by monitoring an earlier increase in activity levels, (4) reduction in hospital cost by utilization of a convalescent center rather than a regular hospital floor for patients having an uncomplicated course in the Coronary Care Unit, and (5) an increase in the availability of Coronary Care Unit beds by allowing earlier transfer from the CCU. Indeed, in their study the total duration of the hospital stay of patients with acute myocardial infarction was shortened by three days and the success rate of cardiac resuscitation was improved, although this was an uncontrolled observation.

High-risk profiles for treatment in an intermediate Coronary Care Unit have been developed. Recently, Lie et. al. reported that, among 47 consecutive CCU survivors with anteroseptal infarction complicated by right or left bundle branch block kept in a monitoring area for six weeks after infarction, 17 (36 percent) sustained late in-hospital ventricular fibrillation.[36] Of 884 patients not kept in the monitoring area, only eight (0.9 percent) sustained late ventricular fibrillation, and four others died suddenly in the hospital. They concluded that CCU survivors with anteroseptal infarction complicated by right or left bundle branch block should be kept in the monitoring area for longer periods of time, up to six weeks. Based on such information, it may be possible to identify patients who are at higher risk for late episodes of ventricular fibrillation and justify the use of intermediate Coronary Care Units even further.

In summary, Coronary Care Units have had a relatively short history but an important impact on the practice and approach to the treatment of patients with acute myocardial infarction. The treatment of arrhythmias, both by drugs and by electrical means, has been refined, but new agents are continually on the horizon for the treatment of refractory patients. The problem of pump failure has been attacked with considerable vigor but so far without notable success. The Coronary Care Unit has provided a setting where right heart catheterization of acutely ill patients can be safely performed, a possibility undreamed of before the 1970s. It has helped to revolutionize the role of the nurse and paramedical professional in the treatment of acute cardiac emergencies and has expanded the notion of coronary care to that of cardiac care, thereby encompassing patients with complications of heart disease other than those due to acute myocardial infarction. In addition, it has spawned its own progeny in the form of fixed and mobile life support stations (precoronary care and the postcoronary care telemetry unit). While the Coronary Care Unit is an accepted part of the medical landscape, its impact on medical ecology has been questioned. In an era of rising costs and further limitation of resources, the issue of who should be admitted to the Coronary Care Unit and for how long must be raised. Further, the efficacy of such Units in reducing mortality has been questioned in a number of studies, and this issue can be resolved only by performing well-designed, prospective controlled studies. Such investigations are difficult to mount, not only because of their inherent complexity, but also because of the usual questions of ethics that are always raised when accepted medical procedure is challenged. Sophisticated prognostic schemes may be of use in this regard but in the current context will not eliminate the need for virtually all patients to be hospitalized, at least initially, in the Coronary or Cardiac

Care Unit. Thus, whatever objections to intensive cardiac care in its current state are raised, it will likely be with us for the indefinite future; therefore, it is up to the medical, nursing, and paramedical professions, as well as to all concerned with patient care, to provide the most efficient medical care of the highest standards in the context of the Coronary Care Unit, and it is to this end that the current volume is dedicated.

# REFERENCES

1. Day HW: History of coronary care units. Am J Cardiol 30:405, 1972.
2. Hooker DR, Kouwenhoven WB, Langworthy AR: Effects of alternating electrical currents on the heart. Am J Physiol 103:444, 1933.
3. Beck CF, Veckesser EC, Barry FM: Fatal heart attack and successful defibrillation. JAMA 161:434, 1956.
4. Beck CF, Pritchard WH, Feil HS: Ventricular fibrillation of long duration abolished by electric shock. JAMA 135:985, 1947.
5. Reagan LB, Young KR, Nicholson JW: Ventricular defibrillation in a patient with probable acute coronary occlusion. Surgery 39:482, 1956.
6. Zoll PM, Linenthal AJ, Gibson W, Paul MH, Norman LR: Termination of ventricular fibrillation in man by externally applied electric countershock. N Engl J Med 254:727, 1956.
7. Kouwenhoven WB, Jude JR, Knickerbocker GG: Closed-chest cardiac massage. JAMA 178:1064, 1960.
8. Meltzer LE, Kitchell JR: The development and status of coronary care. In: Textbook of Coronary Care. Meltzer LE and Dunning AJ, editors Charles Press, Philadelphia, 1972.
9. Lown B, Kosowky BD, Klein MD: Pathogenesis, prevention and treatment of arrhythmias in myocardial infarction. Circulation 40 (suppl IV): 261, 1969.
10. Editorial: Antidysrhythmic treatment in acute myocardial infarction. The Lancet 1:193, 1979.
11. Mather HG, Pearson NG, Read KLQ, Shaw DB, Steed GR, Thorne MG, Jones S, Guerrier CJ, Erant CD, McHugh PM, Chowdhury NR, JaFury MH, Wallace TJ: Acute myocardial infarction: home and hospital treatment. Br Med J 3:334, 1971.
12. Mather HG, Morgan DC, Pearson NG, Read KLQ, Shaw DB, Steed GR, Thorne MG, Lawrence CJ, Riley IS: Myocardial infarction: a comparison between home and hospital care for patients. Br Med J 1:925, 1976.
13. Joint working party of the Royal College of Physicians and the British Cardiac Society. J R Coll Physicians Lond 10:5, 1975
14. Hill JD, Hampton JR, Mitchell JRA: A randomized trial of home-versus-hospital management for patients with suspected myocardial infarction. The Lancet 1:837, 1978.
15. Oliver MF: Letter to the editor. The Lancet 1:1089, 1978.
16. Barritt DW, Jordan SC, Marshall AJ, Bennett JEA: Letter to the editor. The Lancet 1:1090, 1978.
17. Norris RM: Letter to the editor. The Lancet 1:1090, 1978
18. Hofvendahl S: Influence of treatment in a CCU on prognosis in acute myocardial infarction. Acta Medica Scandinavica (Suppl) 519:1–78, 1971.
19. Christiansen I, Iverson K, Skooby AP: Benefits obtained by the introduction of a coronary-care unit. A comparative study. Acta Medica Scandinavica 189:285, 1971.
20. Hill JD, Holdstock G, Hampton JR: Comparison of mortality of patients with heart attacks admitted to a coronary care unit and an ordinary medical ward. Br Med J 2:81, 1977.
21. Gordis L, Naggan L, Tonascia J: Pitfalls in evaluating the impact of coronary care units on mortality from myocardial infarction. Johns Hopkins Medical J 141:287, 1977.
22. Petersen OL: Myocardial infarction: unit care or home care? Ann Intern Med 88:259, 1978.
23. Norris RM, Clarke ED, Sammel NL, Smith WM, Williams B: Protective effect of propranolol in threatened myocardial infarction. The Lancet 2:907, 1978.
24. McNeer JF, Wallace AG, Wagner GS, Sturmer CF, Rosati RA: The course of acute myocardial infarction. Feasibility of early discharge of the uncomplicated patient. Circulation 51:410, 1975
25. Harpur JE, Conner WT, Hamilton M, Kellet RJ, Galbraith H-JB, Murray JJ, Swallow JH, Rose GA: Controlled trial of early mobilisation and discharge from hospital in uncomplicated myocardial infarction. The Lancet 2:1331, 1971.
26. Rose G: Early mobilization and discharge after myocardial infarction. Mod Concepts Cardiovas Dis 41:59, 1972.
27. Boyle JA, Lorman AR: Early mobilisation after uncomplicated myocardial infarction. Prospective study of 538 patients. The Lancet 2:346, 1973.

28. Hutter AM, Sobel VW, Shine KI, DeSanctis RW: Early hospital discharge after myocardial infarction. N Engl J Med 288:1141, 1973

29. Tucker HH, Carson PHM, Bass NM, Sharratt GP, Stock JPP: Results of early mobilization and discharge after myocardial infarction. Br Med J 1:10, 1973.

30. Bloch A, Maeder J-P, Haissly J-C, Felix J, Blackburn H: Early mobilization after myocardial infarction. A controlled study. Am J Cardiol 34:152, 1974.

31. Abraham AS, Sever Y, Weinstein M, Dollberg M, Menczel J: Value of early ambulation in patient with and without complications after acute myocardial infarction. N Engl J Med 292:719, 1975.

32. Levine SA, Lown B: "Armchair" treatment of acute coronary thrombus. JAMA 148:1365, 1952.

33. Scherf D, Cohen J: To each according to his desert. Am Heart J 95:536, 1978.

34. Wallace WA, Yu PN: Sudden death and the prehospital phase of acute myocardial infarction. Annu Rev Med 26:1, 1975.

35. Frieden J, Cooper JA: The role of the intermediate cardiac care unit. JAMA 235:816, 1976.

36. Lie KI, Liem KL, Schuilenburg RM, David GK, Durrer D: Early identification of patients developing late in-hospital ventricular fibrillation after discharge from the coronary care unit. A 5½ year retrospective and prospective study of 1,897 patients. Am J Cardiol 41:679, 1978.

# 5 | Organization of a Coronary Care Unit

*Robert L. North, M.D.*

In the 1980s, planning, organization, and other management functions for a CCU must be in accordance with certain general principles, which we will attempt to outline briefly in this introductory note. Chapter 4 discussed the history of the development and implementation of the CCU concept. As we ponder this historical record and attempt to define current trends, several of these principles emerge.

The CCU is often envisioned, and usually discussed, as a self-contained special care unit within a hospital. The unit is geographically distinct, specially equipped, and, at any particular time, has more or less well-defined functions and objectives in patient care. It should be staffed and directed by professional personnel, medical and nursing, with specialized training and competence, and with very broad authority to initiate therapeutic procedures for any patient in the unit. The CCU should have priority in demand for ancillary, supporting, and consultative services within the institution and its medical staff. These essentials distinguish the CCU as unique, and define its importance in in-patient care. If the medical staff and administration of the hospital are not prepared to guarantee these essentials, it is deceitful to employ the label "CCU" while abridging the concept upon which effects are predicated.

Despite these (and other) features unique to the CCU, it is also worthy of emphasis that a CCU is but one segment of a much larger and increasingly complex system for care of cardiac patients. This, too, is implicit in the concept of progressive patient care, which in its simplest form is a plan for matching access to services with anticipated needs within groups of patients. The plan and organization of any particular CCU must also conform to the constraints or characteristics of this larger system. At the very least, weight must be given to community need and the organization of emergency services in the community and within the hospital itself. The character and availability of intermediate care and rehabilitative services in the hospital will also modify the mission of the CCU. In the broadest possible sense, the CCU must be viewed in the perspective of chronic disease with major impact on public health.

These "system" aspects, dependent as they are upon a complex amalgam of geography, people, machines, and natural forces, significantly complicate the organization of services in any CCU. It is the system as a whole which yields some outcome in patient care. Important variables in these outcomes are subject to little or no control, and certainly not by the CCU manager. Changes in one part of the system (e.g., delay time between onset of symptoms and entry) may profoundly affect other parts, sometimes in unanticipated ways. While all CCUs may share the rationale of progressive patient care, there must be substantial and ineluctable differences between individual CCUs in policies, objectives, and performance.

These patient care systems, of which the

CCU is an integral part, historically have been highly dynamic. While changes have characteristically been incremental and rooted in some previous base of skills, knowledge, and technology, the effects over the life span of a particular unit have led to spectacular changes in missions and expectations. The progression from cardiopulmonary resuscitation to aggressive management of pump dysfunction to preservation of jeopardized myocardium in less than 20 years encapsulates not only a very worthy record of success, but the continuing frustration of the strategic battle against a vicious disease. The plan and organization of a CCU must countenance changes of similar magnitude, if uncertain direction, in the future.

Critics of the CCU have been forced to utilize data which is as "soft" and unreliable as the earlier studies interpreted as supporting the concept and implementation of such units.[1] In general, the arguments against the CCU are economic in nature, and it is beyond the scope of this presentation to explore them in detail. Nevertheless, these are not trivial questions, nor will they be easily resolved. The most obvious economic issue is cost—particularly the operational costs due to assigned personnel, but also those due to increased utilization of diagnostic and therapeutic services supporting the CCU. A second major economic problem is that of access. Exactly what levels of care are provided in a particular unit? To which groups of patients are these services provided? Is there some promise implied to the community by the CCU designation which cannot, in fact, be realized in a given unit? Finally, we must recognize the possibility of formal, regulatory rationing of services in the future, as public policies are developed for control of cost and access problems.

## GEOGRAPHIC DESIGN FACTORS

Most CCUs will receive patients in transfer from other patient care areas in the hospital—usually from other medical nursing units, but occasionally from any location in which patients (or visitors) may be. An orderly plan for communication and transport from these areas must be devised. The volume of direct admissions to a particular unit will vary greatly with local practices, but there will always be at least a few patients in this category for whom very prompt access and safe transportation must be arranged, as well as appropriate administrative procedures. In most hospitals, the Emergency Department will be the location from which the majority of patients will be received.

An attempt should be made to minimize the time spent in transportation of patients to the Unit. Current standards require that these patients be transported with an intravenous portal securely established, with portable electrocardiographic monitoring and a defibrillator, and at least two CPR-skilled attendants with lidocaine and atropine prepared for immediate use. However, some patients will have to be transported with endotracheal intubation, continuous oxygen therapy (with an Ambu bag, e.g.), perhaps several intravenous infusions, and multiple attendants. It must be possible to preempt critical portions of the route to the CCU (e.g., elevators), and each portion of the route must have sufficient physical dimension to accommodate this traveling road show. Each member of the transport team must know his job and be familiar with the route, and someone has to be in charge. How much "stabilization" of the patient is accomplished prior to transportation, and the use of routine lidocaine prophylaxis[2] are matters to be established by local policy and availability of services.

Patients will leave the CCU with destinations as diverse as those from which they are received. While the urgency and risks in this exit phase are generally less than on admission and subject to some scheduling, there are at times even more equipment and people involved in the trip. The majority of patients will be moving to an intermediate care unit of some sort (and as many as 5 to 10 percent of these may require a return trip to the CCU before discharge), so this unit should be as close to the CCU as is geographically feasible. Some patients will be transported to and from the catheterization laboratory and to the operating room in hospitals so equipped; and, of course, some must be transported to the morgue.

The nuclear medicine facility plays an increasingly important role even very early in the course of the CCU patient. In some hospitals, it will be necessary to transport patients routinely to and from the central nuclear medicine department. This must be accomplished with the same precautions as on the initial admission of the patient. In other cases, portable scanning equipment may be brought to the bedside or CCU procedure room for many of the more routine nuclear medicine procedures.

These patient flow characteristics are a major determinant of CCU location, second in priority only to availability of adequate space and utilities.

## INTERIOR TRAFFIC

Careful consideration of interior traffic patterns is also essential in CCU design. Of course, all passageways and entry to rooms or other patient treatment spaces should be sufficient in dimension to accommodate the attendants and permit maneuvering of a hospital bed. Generally, other large items of equipment will be accommodated satisfactorily in passageways large enough for the bed. One must remember that the operational plan of the unit may require stationing of crash carts and defibrillators at strategic points near patient rooms. Without care in planning, these necessary devices may impede other traffic in the unit.

There is also heavy traffic between the central monitoring/nursing station, drug storage/preparation areas, equipment and supply storage areas, and each patient room. These routes should also be free of nonessential impediments. Finally, a nurses' lounge should be located within the unit, to obviate the need for assigned staff to be absent from the unit during a tour of duty. In the event of emergency, there must be ready access from the lounge to patient treatment and monitoring areas.

These service access routes take priority in design. However, one must also accommodate visitor traffic between the visitors' waiting area and patient rooms. There must be convenient access for physicians to patient treatment areas, medical records, and the central monitoring area. It is highly desirable that the unit have a means of ingress and egress for staff which

is not subject to direct scrutiny from the visitors' waiting area. A physician's lounge and sleeping room within the unit should also be located in such fashion that access is concealed from visitors. There should, however, be a private consultation room in which physicians or other staff may meet with family members; this may be located in a visitors' waiting area convenient to but outside the unit itself.

## PATIENTS' ROOMS

The duration of patient stay in the CCU probably still averages three to five days, may occasionally be substantially longer, and is rarely less than 48 hours. Unless there are serious complications, the patient is likely to be fully conscious, alert, and free of major physical distress within 12 to 24 hours. Psychic and emotional stimuli can aggravate the tendency to dysrhythmia in susceptible patients. Mental rest and an environment as free of disturbing distractions as possible are important therapeutically for these patients, who, as a group, are wide awake but quite anxious. The environmental requirements are thus much more stringent than for some other forms of intensive care. These patients should be treated in private rooms, protected from disturbing noise, light, and traffic in the unit.

Soundproofing the unit requires particular attention. Audible alarms and public address systems in the nurses' station should be muted to the minimum level essential for function, but it may still be necessary to provide additional soundproofing in the patient rooms. It should be possible to turn audible alarms off from the bedside as well as in the central monitoring station. The false alarm is part of the way of life in most CCUs, as one expects in a "fail safe" system; but the alarms, false or real, should not be disturbing to all patients in the unit.

In direct conflict with the patient's need for peace and privacy is the equally important requirement for visual surveillance of all patients by the nursing staff. Depending upon the size of the unit, whether it is newly constructed or a modification, and similar constraints, this conflict may require the exercise of considerable architectural ingenuity. Surveillance of patients by closed-circuit television is far less satisfactory to patients and staff, and a very inferior means for detecting changes in the physical status of patients or unauthorized activity in the room. Television monitors are also too easily ignored for long periods of time in the press of numerous other duties assigned to the nursing staff, and human factors thus diminish their utility. An experienced hospital architect should be consulted in design of even a small unit, and will have access to a voluminous literature concerning the problem of privacy vs. surveillance.

Additional important design factors in the CCU patient rooms include exterior windows in each room. This is not merely a comfort factor, but an important aid in maintaining patient orientation with respect to time and place. The routines of nursing care and hospital procedure are disruptive enough for most patients without the additional confusion induced by lying for days in a sterile, monastic, artificially lighted cubicle without external reference. By the same token, a clock visible to the patient helps maintain orientation. During emergencies, however, such a device on the wall may be more threatening than reassuring to the patient. My preference for timing events and maintaining a log of medications during resuscitation or other emergencies is a stop watch with an elapsed time indicator on the crash cart rather than a wall clock in the room for the same purposes.

Finally, the individual patient rooms must be spacious. It should be possible to take a 6-foot portable chest x-ray in each room with the patient in bed. In an emergency, it should be possible for five or six staff members who are likely to assemble on either side or end of the bed to have essential contact with the patient while maintaining a corridor of access to the room. In addition to people, the defibrillator, and the crash cart, one must anticipate space requirements for intravenous infusion pumps, hemodynamic monitoring equipment, an electrocardiograph, and a respirator at any bedside in the unit. These considerations lead to a recommendation for minimum room size with about 13 m² of open floor with no dimen-

sion less than about 3.5 m. For patients requiring circulatory assist devices such as an intra-aortic balloon, even this amount of uncluttered floor space is not truly adequate, and it is desirable to dimension one or two rooms more generously to accommodate the additional equipment. (This problem will be touched upon again in a subsequent section of this chapter.) Rooms should be as attractive in appearance and lighting as is consistent with function, and surfaces should be free of glare.

## EQUIPPING PATIENT ROOMS

In new construction, standard equipment and utilities should be built in so as to maintain a maximum of uncluttered floor space. This includes a lavatory and small adjacent shelf space for preparation and temporary storage of medications, intravenous solutions, etc. Built-in cabinets for frequently used small medical supply items are essential, and an area for storage of clean linen and personal care items is highly desirable in each room. Finally, a closet or other built-in storage area for the patient's personal property is necessary. CCU admission policies and operational plans usually allow admission of cardiac patients in whom acute myocardial infarction is not suspected, or who, for other reasons, may be permitted limited bathroom privileges during their CCU stay. Where possible, a toilet, perhaps shared by adjacent rooms, can be justified both for patient comfort and staff efficiency.

Each room should have built-in lines for oxygen, compressed air, and suction. Patient reading lamps, general room illumination, a night light, and an overhead examining light source should be standard, and there should be ceiling-mounted IV solution holders at each side of the bed. Each room should have a wall mounted sphygmomanometer, and a small shelf or clipboard at the head of the bed to hold an airway, a lidocaine syringe, suction tubing, and other small items of frequent or emergency use.

Potential electrical power requirements in patient rooms seem to increase yearly. Provision for 3 kW per room is standard. Power supplies should be dedicated for standard equipment in each room, such as bedside monitors, electric beds, or television. In addition, there should be a minimum of six undedicated duplex receptacles, wall mounted but dispersed conveniently near the head of the bed. Each receptacle should be on a separate circuit rated for 30 amperes, and all should have an emergency power supply automatically provided within 10 seconds of failure of main power systems. (Grounding and other safety requirements are the subject of Chapter 6.)

Bedside monitoring equipment is preferably placed upon a secure, wall mounted, adjustable shelf just above eye level, with all controls within reach of a short adult. This kind of placement facilitates maintenance, replacement, or expansion of the bedside equipment and flexibility in its use. As more physiologic data are collected at the bedside, the number of connections with the central station increases and the conduit should be at least 1¼ inches in diameter, and routed to simplify pulling of new conductors, even if a few "spares" are made available at the time of initial installation.

While it is not customary to provide patients with unrestricted access to telephones, a telephone line with phone plug in each room is desirable, and may be essential if the hospital makes use of centralized data processsing employing this means of communication.

Television receivers, also preferably wall mounted at sufficient height so as not to interfere with personnel or with other equipment in the room, may be regarded as essential to the care of bedridden but otherwise alert patients in most communities. If used, there should, of course, be a bedside speaker and set of controls. The hospital TV system may also be employed as a part of the patient education program in some institutions. The justification for television and radio in patient rooms is not education however, but to provide distraction, maintain orientation, and counter the pernicious effects of boredom. Television and radio are so much a part of the normal life-style and habits of many patients that deprivation can be a very disruptive and unpleasant experience. Even the non-addicted may turn to television to combat the inevitable boredom and monot-

ony of the highly restricted and regimented existence of a cardiac in-patient.

There are occasional patients whose emotional reaction to specific program material may be anticipated as potentially deleterious, as when the patient or family is the subject of public comment. For the most part, however, television viewing cannot be considered as a harmful or disturbing activity for CCU patients.

The final items of room furnishing include a comfortable chair, suitable for patients or visitors but easily moved in emergencies, and the bed itself. Electrically powered beds, controllable by patient or staff, offer numerous advantages in comfort and convenience. These beds may be made sufficiently safe electrically by design, manufacture, and routine maintenance to be preferred as routine furniture for patient rooms. They should be of standard size and design, subject to safety requirements, and interchangeable with similar beds in other units. Headboards should be immediately removable in case of emergency.

Temperature and humidity should be controlled in the CCU, following current standards for hospital construction and equipment. It is highly desirable that temperature controls in each patient room permit easy adjustment for patient comfort over a range of about 16 to 27°C. Ventilation rates and fresh air admixture should also follow current recommended standards, and the air exchange system should be designed to minimize drafts and noise in patient treatment areas.

## CENTRAL WORK AREAS

Space allocation for work and storage of equipment and supplies within the unit must also be generous, while permitting direct and easy access to each patient treatment site. Work space layout should be functional.

One functional grouping is the central monitor and recording site. The monitoring console should be comfortable to view from either a seated or standing position. Oscilloscopes should be grouped closely together to permit monitoring of all patients by one or two people, and controls should be conveniently located with respect to the monitors. Ambient lighting and glare problems have already been mentioned. Strip chart recording apparatus and rate meters may be located adjacent to the central oscilloscope bank. Ample, desk-height work space should be provided at the monitor station, since much of the abundant record-keeping each patient generates will be performed here. Medical record storage should be near the monitoring station, but separate record-keeping work space for physicians visiting the unit should be provided to one side of the monitoring console. It should be possible to view each patient being monitored from a location at which the monitor is also visible.

A secretarial and communications center area is another functional space allocation. Blank forms are stored here, with telephone, computer terminals, paging systems, and other communications devices concentrated at this location. Telephone extensions should also be provided in the monitoring areas and in the physician's work space.

These functional areas should be within earshot and each should be readily accessible from the other. Some physical separation permits cooperation without interference. It should be possible to leave the inner work areas readily to gain immediate access to crash carts and patient rooms in an emergency. Usually, several exitways are provided, none more than a few steps from personnel stations. There is also need within the central work area for a centrally located general purpose cleanup and preparation area, including lavatory and waste disposal facilities. This may or may not be combined with the unit's drug and intravenous solution storage and preparation area, unless necessary cabinets and shelving obstruct traffic, viewing, or communication channels.

There should be a generously proportioned equipment and bulk supply room within or immediately adjacent to the unit; even small units are likely to need the capability for at least temporary storage for bulky items of medical equipment as well as linen and supply items of regular and frequent use. This equipment absolutely must not be parked, even temporarily, in traffic passage-ways to patient rooms. A nurses'

lounge and toilet should be located in the unit itself, and included in the audible alarm system. There should be a small utility room with bedpan washing facilities, if patient room toilets lack this capability or are not provided. Storage and disposal of dirty linen, trash, and disposable items should be in accordance with current standards and hospital routines and may or may not require provision of separate holding and handling space within the unit. The unit should provide space for a refrigerator for patient nourishments and snacks. For larger units, a small office for the head nurse and for maintenance of personnel and unit logs and records is highly desirable.

An integral "procedure room" is probably necessary for all but the smallest and most elementary of CCUs. This room, of at least 55 m² and preferably 70 or 75 m², will be used for invasive procedures in CCU patients. It should be equipped with outlets for oxygen, air, and suction, electrical outlets, an ECG monitor, and a sphygmomanometer, similar to the patient rooms. There should be a bank of wall mounted x-ray view boxes. The procedure room should have an adjustable, ceiling mounted, medium-size operating room lamp. General room lighting should be variable in intensity, but in addition an on/off foot switch for use by the physician is very strongly advised. There should be ample shelf and cabinet storage for sterile supplies and trays, suture materials, Swan-Ganz catheters, pacing wires, etc., all arranged in an orderly fashion, labeled, and readily accessible.

The procedure room should be equipped with image-intensified fluoroscopic equipment with a television monitor. Portable intensifiers are generally satisfactory, and, if the gurney used to transport the patient to the room has a firm radiolucent top and adjustable height, procedures may be readily performed without having to transfer the patient again. Fabric sling transporters are somewhat easier to position patients upon for the move from bed to procedure room, and are also radiolucent. However, the patient in one of these slings generally crumples into a position that renders cutdowns and other procedures considerably more difficult. A procedure room equipped as described offers great advantages in space, organization, speed, and safety of invasive procedures. Its utilization will be sporadic and unpredictable.

Construction and equipment costs will be amortized over at least several years, while additional operating expense is low. Even so, alternatives may be considered. One alternative to consider is the use of the cardiac catheterization laboratory, if there is one nearby. It is sometimes necessary to transport heavily instrumented patients from the CCU to the catheterization laboratory in any event; the closer these two units are, geographically, the better. It is good to remember in this context that invasive procedures for CCU patients are almost always done on an emergency or highly urgent, unscheduled basis. The catheterization laboratory is likely to operate with a full and busy routine schedule. Planning to use the catheterization laboratory for all CCU emergencies may significantly impair the smooth functioning of both units.

Of course, pacemaking wires, Swan-Ganz catheters, and arterial cannulae may be inserted at the bedside, and without fluoroscopic control. This is more cramped, cumbersome, and time-consuming, and does not provide the reassurance of immediate radiologic verification of catheter or wire position. For more elaborate procedures such as intra-aortic balloon placement, a well-equipped and organized procedure room provides convenience, space for assistants and aides, fluoroscopic verification of balloon position, and probably enhances safety as well.

Another alternative is to expand the utilization of the CCU procedure room by making it available on a scheduled and second priority basis for certain other procedures, such as fiberoptic bronchoscopy and biopsy, which must be performed with fluoroscopic control.

There are two final space considerations in CCU design. One is physician sleeping room, bathroom, and office space. Hospitals with house staff are very likely to assign physicians to coverage of the unit, necessitating appropriate space allocation within the unit. Without house staff, there are still likely to be occasions upon which physicians will prefer to spend the night in the hospital to be immediately available to a critically ill patient.

The final major function in all CCUs is education. At minimum, there must be a continuing education program for all staff assigned to the unit, and often these classes will include intermediate care unit staff. Educational sessions are often scheduled at times of shift changes in the unit, and this, along with mandatory requirements, guarantees large attendance. Meanwhile, essential patient care services cannot be ignored. Classroom space within the CCU complex is thus highly desirable, although it need not be dedicated solely to CCU training. Teaching hospitals with additional medical and nursing education programs will have an even greater need for classroom space in patient care areas, and the CCU deserves strong consideration as a desirable location.

The importance of provision of adequate and even seemingly generous floor space for the CCU, functionally laid out, with all necessary utilities, cannot be overemphasized. In time, equipment and staffing may well be subject to modification or expansion, if needed. Inadequate space allocation will be an enduring curse in operation and performance of the unit, never adequately offset by other procedural modifications. Fixed operating costs do obviously increase in proportion to floor space provided in any hospital unit. Accounting procedures may also allocate indirect expense and overhead to a treatment unit in proportion to space occupied. Such considerations should not lead planners into major compromise in space allocation.

## PATIENT VOLUME

While certain general concepts and principles govern location, design, equipment, and procedure employed in any CCU, more specific planning must be developed from estimates of patient volume and the levels of care projected for these patients. Such planning must incorporate long-range projections of the role of the hospital and its medical staff in meeting community and regional needs as well as historical data and trends. Philosophically, each CCU should be regarded as unique, but planners can derive much benefit from consulting planning guides and manuals.[3] Site visits to functioning units are highly recommended as an excellent means for bringing to consideration practical flaws and problems, some of which may be avoidable in new construction.

Criteria employed in planning will necessarily vary greatly from one unit to another, since, as we have emphasized previously, the CCU is but one segment of a larger system of care including extramural as well as intramural elements. It has been customary to initiate planning for CCU services by definition of a need or set of needs for improvement in patient care. These needs, as perceived by the medical staff and the hospital administration, will depend upon the population served as well as whether other services such as cardiac surgery are provided. Historically, these rational and a priori determinations of need have been greatly modified in practice, due to a constantly increasing demand to extend specialized care to broader categories of patients, and to the emergence of new knowledge and technology.

It seems probable at the time of this writing that both the public and the medical profession will accept some restraint in this expansion of demand, if groups of patients at low risk or with little prospect for benefit can be defined, and explicit criteria for assessment of marginal benefits of new technology are enforced. Nevertheless, the modern CCU must be envisioned as a specialized unit for cardiac care, not just coronary care. The often quoted planning guideline is that 50 percent of CCU admissions will have acute myocardial infarction documented during the CCU stay. This will not be realized in many units unless very stringent admission criteria, rigidly enforced, are accepted by the medical staff of the hospital. It is not an uncommon experience to find that as many as half the admissions to a CCU are not clinically suspected of acute myocardial infarction or unstable angina at the time of admission, even when virtually all display acute manifestations of serious cardiac disease. This leads to reported rates of documented infarction in some CCUs as low as 25 or 30 percent.[4] This changed patient mix tends to reduce average duration of patient stay in the unit somewhat, although this variable is also strongly influenced by availability and quality of intermediate care services.

Having established admission policies accept-able to the medical staff and defined in terms of categories of patients to be served, it should be possible to estimate the annual volume and mix of admissions expected for a given CCU. A set of disposition policies and expectations should then be defined for each category of patient. From these considerations, the total annual bed days and mean duration of patient stay can be derived. Dividing the total anticipated bed days by 365 yields a number representing the requirement for CCU beds, assuming 100 percent occupancy and absolutely stable admission and disposition rates.

Unfortunately, planners must then make allowance for the observed fact that fluctuation in demand for CCU beds is not only substantial and significant, but it will not necessarily parallel the more predictable weekly or seasonal variations in hospital utilization in general. The demand for CCU beds may be assumed to follow a random distribution unless there is a sound empirical historical data base revealing another pattern. Two conflicting economic considerations must then be addressed in planning. The first is that of providing timely access to services for the groups of patients recognized as having need. The second is the fixed operating costs of the unit which are ultimately shared in some way by the community and more directly by the patients using the unit. Lower utilization rates in general imply higher fixed operating costs per patient treated. Higher utilization rates in general imply a lower probability that all patients needing services can be accepted without undesirable delay.

To further complicate this problem, there are likely to be other urgent requirements within the institution for capital investment or new and improved patient services, at the time when development or expansion of CCU services is contemplated. Lavish allocation of resources to the CCU may be unwise if it proves detrimental to other essential services.

The CCU plan should establish a target rate or probability that a bed will be available when patients present for admission. Disposition policies should permit some flexibility in judgment for movement of individual patients out of the unit sooner than originally planned in order to make room for high-risk patients. Major urban full-service hospitals, located near principal traffic arteries and in communities with well-coordinated emergency services, will be expected to meet different performance standards than the smaller hospital in areas having low population density or lacking community wide planning. It may be necessary for the former to plan for a 90 or 95 percent probability of bed access because of a key role in caring for high-risk patients. In the second case, 80 percent probability of bed availability may be acceptable, with little discernible effect on statistical measures of outcome within the institution.

Computer simulation or modeling based upon expected volume, distribution, mix, and duration of stay in a given unit is technically feasible but heavily dependent upon the assumptions which must be made. This sort of data can be quite useful in defining boundaries for access and utilization rates for a particular unit, displaying the effects of the several variables involved.

In practice, these estimates of probability of bed availability are still rather crude. An information reporting system should be established to determine patient waiting times or outright refusals for CCU beds. Policies and facilities may require modification based upon actual experience. Even so, if the average utilization or occupancy rate of a cardiac care unit exceeds 70 or 75 percent, lack of bed availability at demand peaks will become increasingly evident and troublesome. Care in planning and organization must be exercised to minimize the impact of overcrowding upon quality in patient care. Because of this, the number of beds required in a given unit will be at least 30 percent greater than the number projected assuming 100 percent utilization.

## LEVELS OF CARE

Another important determinant of planning and organization for a CCU is the levels of care projected. These range from elementary services, including electrocardiographic monitoring, dysrhythmia prevention, and cardiopulmonary resuscitation, to elaborate and innovative research requirements.

## ELEMENTARY CARE

CCU patients will be entirely or almost entirely confined to bed for the greater part of their stay in the unit. In addition to constant physical surveillance by a skilled nursing staff, patients require prompt assistance with all personal care and bodily functions, including in many cases, assistance with meals. The unit staff must also minister to the psychological and emotional needs of the patients and establish an atmosphere which inspires confidence. These aims are more readily attained if the nursing staff establishes personalized relationships with patients. Nursing assignments should therefore be to patients rather than to tasks within the unit. This policy need not preclude some diversification in positions established by task and skill level analysis, particularly in larger units. The ratio of highly trained professional nurses to patients must be sufficient to meet emergency needs in any event, and it is not realistic to staff units in anticipation of less than about 12 hours of skilled nursing coverage per patient per day.

Continuous electrocardiographic monitoring for all patients is, of course, an essential and elementary service provided in the CCU. The choice of equipment for this purpose depends not only on functional specifications but upon availability of service and maintenance, repair capability, and reliable sources of consumable supplies and replacement parts. Time spent in thorough review of locally available equipment and service prior to purchase is essential. Even if the hospital down the street professes satisfaction with brand X, or one's own past experience with a particular manufacturer has been satisfactory, there is an advantage to resurveying the current situation with respect to equipment suitability.

At minimum, the ECG signal must be clearly displayed at both bedside and in a central monitoring station in the unit. The intensity and contrast of the oscilloscopic display in both locations, and the size of the deflections, should be such as to permit recognition of QRS morphology changes or prematurity from a distance of 3 or 4 meters under the most adverse lighting conditions. The "sweep speed" should not be less than 25 mm/sec, though the capability of increasing this to 50 mm/sec is occasionally useful. So-called "nonfading" display of ECG signals significantly enhances dysrhythmia recognition by visual monitoring, and ought to be considered standard in the elementary CCU. These considerations also dictate a minimum oscilloscope diameter or width of 17 or 18 cm.

In addition to the ECG waveform, at minimum there should be some reliable indication of mean heart rate, both at the bedside and in the central station. It should be possible to initiate hardcopy records of ECG data on a strip-chart recorder, identified by bed (and preferably by time), from either bedside or central staion. Signal amplitude and position upon the bedside oscilloscope screen should be capable of modification independently of similar controls at the central monitoring and recording station.

The major weakness in ECG monitoring systems is signal acquisition. If there is hair on the chest, it must be shaved thoroughly and over a large enough area to leave a generous margin at the perimeter of the electrode. The skin should be cleansed thoroughly and vigorously, and then scraped or abraded lightly at the point of electrode contact. After drying the area of electrode attachment completely, the recommended amount of conductive paste or gel must be properly applied, and the electrode firmly cemented to the skin. There are any number of commercially available paste-on electrodes capable of giving satisfactory performance; but, unless these are meticulously applied, the signal will be noisy and even interrupted when the electrode is displaced or pulled off by patient movement. Unless care is taken in application of each electrode, variations in interelectrode resistance may cause the oscilloscope trace to wander madly. Finally, there must be good electrical contact between the shielded lead wires and the electrode itself. Snap-on or clip-on lead lines offer some conveniences in monitoring but must be carefully maintained to provide good electrical contact.

The CCU policy manual should establish standards for electrode positions on the chest and leads to be routinely monitored. It is highly recommended that an extra electrode be applied routinely to each patient so that, whatever the routine lead arrangements, a second lead is readily available to aid in analysis of questionable QRS morphologies. The MCL-1 and MCL-5 leads are standard in many CCUs and generally quite satisfactory.[5] Care should be exercised, however, that electrode positions chosen do not unnecessarily interfere with examination of the patient or the application of defibrillator electrodes.

The elementary monitoring system should include low and high heart rate alarms, triggered within a few seconds, when preset limits are exceeded. In patients with functioning electrical pacemakers, the pacemaker stimulus signal itself must be rejected by the alarm circuitry or through selection of monitor lead positioning to ensure that the QRS complex, not the stimulus artifact, is being monitored. The central station alarms should be both audible and visible but there should be no audible bedside alarms. The monitoring system should also give a "signal loss" alarm in the central station which is distinctive and independent of the rate alarms. The visual indicator of this condition at the bedside should also be separate from the rate alarm indication. Once their purpose has been served, it should be possible to promptly disable audible alarms from either bedside or central station. Finally, the bedside monitor should have a switch which temporarily bypasses alarms but permits continued display of ECG and rate data, for use while the patient is being bathed, for example, or during electrode change.

The central station monitor displays and controls should be grouped for convenience in monitoring, but it should be possible to see both the patient and the monitor from the same location. An ECG strip chart recorder should be an integral part of the central station. The recorder should permit the option of recording rhythm strips of predetermined duration (10 to 16 sec) triggered automatically by the rate alarms or manually from either bedside or central station. Bed number should always be positively identified on these strips. Automatic indication of time of recording is also quite useful but not absolutely essential in smaller units. Finally, it should be possible to operate the recorder continuously from the central station by a manual on/off switch.

There should be an electronic delay line or "memory" preserving at least several seconds of ECG data for recording. At minimum, whatever is still visible on the oscilloscope face should be capable of permanent recording. Occasionally, linking or "cascading" two channels of display is useful and provides in some installations more "remembered" data for recording or review. Electronic delays are far superior to continuous magnetic tape recordings for recall and recording of evanescent events in routine monitoring applications, and much more reliable in operation. Tape recording should be reserved for more specific research or specialized services rather than routine applications.

If the electrode system is the major source of noise and false alarms in the Unit, the second major weak point is in reliable surveillance of the ECG display in the central station. Not only is the continued visual surveillance of a bank of monitors a monotonous and mesmerizing task for the human viewer, but there are numerous other distractions leading to momentary inattention, even when the duty schedule of the observer supposedly permits undivided attention to the displays. There is some practical limit to the number of tracings (8 to 12) that a single individual can be expected to monitor, even with nonfading displays closely grouped. Not only must the monitor watcher recognize departures in rate and rhythm and distinguish these from artifacts, but often a judgment must be made as to the importance of a given event, which requires additional knowledge about the patient. The primary purposes in monitoring ECG data are: (1) detection of harbingers of cardiac arrest so that prophylactic treatment may be instituted, and (2) the assessment of the effects of therapy already administered. The extent to which human oversight may foil these goals is not known, but occasional oversight will almost certainly occur.[6]

For this and other reasons, computerized CCU electrocardiographic monitoring has been the subject of considerable interest and developmental work almost from the time these units were first established. In the past, this approach called for the employment of a dedicated mini-

computer to process data on line from several beds. The more elaborate systems also permit direct acquisition of other physiologic data at the bedside and manual entry of a wide range of patient information. Once the unit is acquired and processed according to the preference of the system designer, a virtually endless variety of terminal output displays or hardcopy reports is possible. The major virtues of minicomputer systems are the versatility in input and output and capability for expanded storage of information. Major drawbacks include expense and the problems associated with downtime for repair or maintenance, which temporarily disable monitoring for several beds simultaneously and require maintenance of a conventional and complete backup monitoring system. Software problems in dysrhythmia recognition and noise rejection have posed major practical drawbacks in these installations as well. Perhaps the most overwhelming difficulty in routine application, however, lies in the interaction between the machine and personnel, especially nurses, charged with patient care responsibility.

In actual practice, the computerized system is likely to be regarded as a nuisance that imposes increased, largely technical, work load demands on the nurse without realization of the expected benefits to the patient. Only when there is very strong and continuing medical and administrative emphasis and participation—which may include hiring of additional employees to serve the machine—are some of the theoretical advantages likely to be attained.

This disappointing situation is, however, at least on the threshold of promising change. The reason for this change is the development of microprocessor technology appropriate to monitoring tasks. The microprocessor "computer on a chip" is outgrowing its earlier role as a rigidly programmed, inflexible, switching and process control device. The hardware itself has become ubiquitous and inexpensive, with satisfactory processing speed, and with relatively sophisticated memory, peripheral, and programming capability. Microprocessor-controlled central stations are cost-effective in medium to large sized units. For arrhythmia monitoring an individual microprocessor module may be dedicated to each bed at total costs approaching those of the older central systems. There is also a tendency to simplify the dysrhythmia recognition algorithms and programs. Finally, the interface with users is being simplified.

At present, several major equipment manufacturers are developing and marketing microprocessor-based systems. These still appear to be undergoing very rapid change and modification, and, except in unusual situations, purchase decisions might profitably be delayed for at least several months. There does appear to be definite potential for some improvement in monitoring reliability. It is doubtful that an absolute reduction in staffing can be achieved; but, in larger installations, it may well be possible to substitute monitoring assistants or technical personnel for nurses, which would both lower costs and improve patient care. These concepts may apply with equal or greater force to intermediate care units in which the number of monitored patients may exceed that in the CCU, while staffing ratios are lower. There is some light at the end of the computer tunnel.

In the elementary level CCU, recognized ventricular ectopic activity which meets or exceeds guidelines specifically defined in the policy manual should automatically empower the nurse to institute prophylactic or therapeutic routines. Generally, in patients suspected of acute myocardial infarction, any ventricular ectopic activity more frequent than 5 or 6 per minute, or any complex ventricular ectopy such as multiform, repetitive, or early beats, have been accepted as an indication for prophylactic therapy. Ventricular fibrillation or ventricular tachycardia of a sustained type with evidence of hemodynamic impairment are indications for nurse-initiated defibrillation and resuscitation. Criteria based upon frequency of ventricular ectopic beats are admittedly arbitrary, and as many as 25 percent of patients with infarction may develop ventricular fibrillation without recognized premonitory dysrhythmia. The tendency in recent years has been to be increasingly liberal in dysrhythmia prophylaxis employing lidocaine, an agent with an excellent reputation for safety and efficacy.[2]

Unfortunately, there is much less data bearing upon the significance of ventricular ectopic activity in patients with nonischemic heart disease. The ventricular ectopic beat per se is a poor marker of risk, commonly documented in otherwise normal individuals. Sudden death, presumably due to dysrhythmia, has been well documented in studies by medical examiners in individuals with virtually any form of heart disease.[7] In most CCUs, complex or frequent ventricular ectopic beats will be treated according to a standard protocol, regardless of etiologic considerations, despite the greater uncertainty concerning risks and benefits in patients with other than ischemic heart disease. In units admitting large numbers of noncoronary suspects, the clinical circumstances permitting routine lidocaine prophylaxis in patients without documented ventricular ectopic beats must be defined with great care.

The medical director of the CCU will find it wise to review all cases daily and not merely those for whom prophylactic therapy was instituted. Nursing or house staff will occasionally label a dysrhythima as "benign" which should have been treated. Aberrant conduction of supraventricular beats may stump the best of us, but those newly introduced to this phenomenon have a tendency to overdiagnose it. Ventricular ectopic beats may be called junctional simply because in a given lead they may not appear as wide as one expects.

Lidocaine, delivered as an intravenous bolus with or without subsequent constant infusion, has earned such respect in dysrhythmia prophylaxis that there is often an unconscious tendency to regard the drug as perfect. This, of course, is not the case. Standard treatment policies in the unit must not only establish clear indications for use, but standardized dosing protocols, and definite end points for therapy as well. If the drug at reasonable dosage does not achieve the targets established for reduction or elimination of ectopic activity, or if toxicity develops, CCU policy should establish secondary antiarrhythmic drug protocols. Chapter 16 provides further discussion of arrhythmia management schemes.

While the ECG monitoring system, dysrhythmia recognition, and standardized drug prophylaxis routines may be considered elementary services in any CCU, they are not trivial.

Personnel should be thoroughly trained in these essentials before assignment as a part of the regular staff of the unit. The protocols devised to cover these routines should be quite specific, defining responsibilities and authority by position, record-keeping requirements, and other communication procedures for each unit. While "standing" orders or treatment protocols may authorize nursing staff to initiate prophylactic and other treatment for defined indications, physicians responsible for the care of the patient must be kept fully informed. Protocols should define the manner and timing of these communications between nursing and physician staff.

For the same reasons, ECG monitoring and treatment routines will constitute the major segment of the continuing education program in the unit. Commercially available teaching systems may form the basis for this aspect of the educational program, but must be amplified and modified to include locally defined procedure.

## CARDIOPULMONARY RESUSCITATION

Cardiopulmonary resuscitation is a second elementary level service in the CCU. All professional personnel working in the unit should be certified annually in Basic Life Support techniques according to American Heart Association standards. There should be at least one individual in the unit at all times certified for Advanced Life Support actions such as use of a defibrillator and intravenous drug therapy. Each hospital should have its own procedures, which may include designated "teams" to respond to cardiac arrest emergencies in any location. The CCU should not depend upon some hospital-wide team for initiation of cardiopulmonary resuscitation, nor should CCU personnel be called away from the unit routinely to function as members of such teams.

In addition to well-drilled and well-trained personnel, the CCU plan should assure that equipment and supplies customarily employed in resuscitation are either present or can be rapidly assembled in an orderly fashion at any bedside. If mobile carts are employed for this pur-

pose, care should be taken to assure a high degree of maneuverability (e.g., large wheels) and a low center of gravity. It is disconcerting in the midst of emergency to see a defibrillator dumped on the floor from an unstable or poorly designed cart. If hand-carried portable defibrillators are used, a stable platform should be available at the bedside for the device to sit upon. Defibrillators and "crash carts" should be strategically located within the unit so as to be accessible without major detours to staff enroute to the location of an emergency; yet, they should not obstruct normal traffic patterns in the unit.

Cardiopulmonary resuscitation is a team effort, and unit protocol should specify in detail the responsibilities of a leader as well as for each individual member of the team. A communication and paging protocol should be established to bring additional personnel to the scene promptly. These may be medical and nursing staff members, electrocardiographic, blood gas, or respiratory therapy technologists, or other essential skilled personnel as dictated by the organization of hospital services, geography, and other considerations. The team leader may release unneeded personnel or change assignments as indicated; but, once an alarm is given, it should not be necessary to continue to search for individuals with needed skills.

The "crash cart" is usually employed to bring to the scene a supply of drugs, fluids, supplies, and equipment most frequently employed in cardiopulmonary resuscitation attempts. Unit protocol should specify not only the quantities and sizes of these various items, but also their location in the various drawers, shelves or cabinets of the cart. Each member of the staff assigned to the unit should be familiar with the organization of the cart, but legible labels listing contents of each section of the cart should also be affixed. It may prove useful to locate duplicate supplies of some items such as syringes, needles, and venous catheters in several locations in the cart, adjacent to other supplies or drugs with which their use is necessarily associated. Other materials should be grouped logically according to use: pacemaker, wires, stylets, etc. in one location; endotracheal tubes, laryngoscope, etc. in another. Do not forget a supply of fresh batteries in the various sizes that may be required, or screwdrivers and wrenches that may be needed for battery charges, electrical connections, or the like. The crash cart should contain a scratch pad, gummed labels, flow sheets, nursing notes, and other stationery supplies necessary for accurate chronological records of the resuscitation attempt, and a stopwatch and elapsed time indicator (unless unit protocol specifies a wall clock in the room for maintenance of chronologic records). A simple, four-function calculator on the cart will be a great aid in calculating drug concentrations or infusion rates and quantities.

Crash carts always seem to lack at least one item that may be needed, particularly during a prolonged or difficult resuscitation attempt. Conversely, the more elaborately stocked carts require more complicated indexing, consume more time and effort in periodic inspection, checking expiration dates, restocking and other maintenance chores. An overly large and bulky cart may hinder access to the patient or need to be located inconveniently far from the scene. Crash carts designed and stocked for use throughout the hospital may contain items which are not always immediately available in general nursing units but are stocked routinely in a CCU or other intensive care unit. Supplies of sterile gauze bandages, suction catheters, armboards, intravenous infusion sets, oral airways, padded tongue blades and similar items may be stocked in the patient rooms in a CCU, permitting use of a smaller and more mobile cart.

The CCU cart should contain an ample "immediate use" supply of standard drugs and electrolyte solutions, which may be replenished in use from other stocks maintained in the unit. These include lidocaine both for local anesthesia and intravenous administration (such as the 100 mg Bristojet syringes), epinephrine in 1:1000 and 1:10,000 concentrations, atropine, propranolol, procaine amide, calcium chloride, potassium chloride, sterile saline for injection, and, of course, an ample supply of sodium bicarbonate. The protocol for the unit should specify who, and under what circumstances, may order administration of these agents, how frequently, and in what dosage. A flow sheet should be developed for documentation of time, rate, and

routine of administration for each agent in the standard repertoire. An ample supply of stopcocks, extension tubing, alcohol and Betadine swabs, and adhesive tape will save many unnecessary steps.

Narcotics, sedatives, most inotropic agents, anticonvulsants, and similar agents should be stocked in the unit, but need not be maintained on the cart, provided the unit has sufficient trained staff members to promptly prepare and transport these agents as required to the scene of the emergency. The CCU protocol and procedure manual should specify initial concentrations, vehicles, and administration rates for all drugs administered by intravenous injection or infusion. These standards may subsequently be modified as dictated by medical judgment in the individual case; but, in the heat of the moment, standardized initial concentrations and infusion rates, familiar to all, simplify decision making.

For some units, equipment and supplies for mechanical respiratory support (endotracheal tubes in a wide range of sizes, stylets, laryngoscope with spare batteries and bulbs, AMBU or similar bag with mask and necessary connectors, and tubing for oxygen supply) will be stocked on the crash cart. Similarly, a pacemaker on the cart, with supplies and equipment for institution of both transvenous and transthoracic pacing, will save the time otherwise required for those items to be brought from the procedure room or other storage site.

A bed board to aid in providing a firm surface for closed chest compression may be kept in each room or may be fitted to the crash cart. Mechanical or pneumatic devices for chest compression, if employed at all, are not, in my estimation, "first use" equipment to be a part of the CCU crash cart.

It must be emphasized that there is no "standard" crash cart recommended for universal use. Any cart should contain a basic complement of drugs and electrolyte solutions most commonly required in resuscitation, and a selection of small items such as syringes and needles which are often consumed copiously. Many patients do not require intubation or pacing, and secondary trays or kits readily accessible within the unit may be used to meet these needs as they emerge. Smaller units with fewer personnel available may find it useful to include an expanded list of supplies on the cart.

Whatever its constitution, the crash cart must be completely restocked and replenished immediately after use. It must be inventoried periodically, and outdated materials must be replaced. The CCU protocol should designate specific individuals with these responsibilities. The cart should, obviously, not be "robbed" of any supplies simply to meet routine needs in the unit. Breakaway locks or other devices are sometimes used to provide a visible indication that the cart has been violated and may not be complete.

## HEART FAILURE

Beyond the elementary CCU functions in basic patient care and dysrhythmia monitoring and treatment, the next level of organization for services is treatment of congestive heart failure. The presence of congestive failure (pulmonary edema) in the patient with acute myocardial infarction, especially if associated with any clinical evidence of compromised cardiac output, has long been recognized as a poor short-term prognostic factor (see Chap. 43). At least half the in-patient mortality from infarction may be due to heart failure with or without shock, and acute pulmonary edema due to any cause remains a grave illness with high mortality risk. As we have seen, very early in the history of CCU implementation, the management objectives expanded rapidly to include heart failure, which remains a major problem. Early treatment of heart failure and the prevention of flagrant pulmonary edema are among the major objectives in CCU care.

One key service indispensable to the diagnosis and management of congestive failure is the provision of standardized chest x-rays. It should not be necessary to transport patients to the X-ray Department to obtain satisfactory chest films, as good portable x-ray machines are available through several manufacturers. It is extremely important, however, that all films be highly standardized for accuracy in interpretation and comparison. For this reason, all CCU films should be obtained by use of a single, portable x-ray machine, or at least by machines of identical design and performance. At the time

of this writing, there are at least four different designs for x-ray equipment in use.

The oldest of these is very conventional in circuitry and manufacture. In order to obtain satisfactory power output and relatively short exposure times, this equipment may be extremely bulky and may require 220 volts of service. This kind of equipment is, in my opinion, unsatisfactory for use in the CCU, even though some hospitals may still have such equipment in service.

Capacitor discharge and battery-powered portable x-ray machines are both capable of obtaining chest films of good quality with reasonably brief exposure times—a prime essential. The design of capacitor discharge equipment is such that the total milliampere-seconds (mAs) required to give satisfactory film density is held constant at a given kvp, but tube current and therefore exposure time will vary considerably with tube voltage changes. In practice, this factor is more likely to produce variations in film quality between patients rather than in the same patient at different times, and this is inevitable in any event. Nevertheless, this is one good reason not to switch indiscriminately between machines for CCU films. The direct current machines (battery powered) will ordinarily yield comparable exposure times for chest films within the customary range of kpv values used. Both types of equipment are generally sturdy and reliable and pose no major power supply problems.

A given piece of equipment may present advantages in size or maneuverability which will be important in a particular unit. This will be particularly noticeable if there is a long distance to be covered in transportation of the machine to the unit, in which case a "high-speed" travel motor control is useful. Low speeds, on the other hand, are more helpful in performing small positioning maneuvers in the patient rooms.

More recently, portable field emission ("high kv") equipment has become available. Since high kv technique routine chest films are standard in many hospitals, one may suppose high kv portable chest films would thus be more comparable in technique to the hospital's routine chest films. The high kv films are sufficiently distinctive in technique to require some modification in criteria, especially for bone density and interstitial disease. One does not expect to rely upon portable films for refined judgments about parenchymal, intracardiac, or lesser degrees of vascular calcification in any event, but the high kv technique is an especially poor choice for revealing parenchymal calcification, and most cardiologists will prefer conventional chest film technique. The author has no personal experience with high kv portable films. The requirements for cassette intensifying screens, film emulsions and development are also different, which could present some problems if more conventional techniques are also employed for portable films in the hospital.

It is possible to purchase portable x-ray equipment with fairly sophisticated film and tube positioning controls and even phototiming devices. These add so substantially to costs that the need must be carefully assessed. Generally, any equipment providing good chest films will perform satisfactorily for the occasional abdominal and bone films obtained in the CCU.

If equipment standardization is important, the question arises as to whether the CCU should be equipped with its "own" x-ray machine. The largest volume of portable chest film requests, particularly on an urgent or "stat" basis, is likely to come from specialized and intensive care units such as the CCU. Substantial amounts of technician time can be absorbed simply in moving these heavy machines from site to site. Stationing portable machines near locations of predominant usage may be highly cost-effective. Ordinarily, however, responsibility for repair, maintenance, supplies, and technician availability and training should remain with the Radiology Department. The clinician will want to review all films, perhaps with the radiologist; but these should be retained with the other film files in Radiology, and the "official" written interpretation should be the responsibility of the Radiology Department in most instances.

In addition to equipment standardization and maintenance, x-ray technique must be highly standardized for comparability in sequential films. Tube-film distances should be measured, not estimated, the standard being either 72 in or 2m in most units. The patient should be

positioned upright if any meaningful judgment is to be made concerning upper lobe vascularity, either by adjusting the head of the bed or by seating the patient on the edge of the bed.

Whether the film is taken in postero-anterior or antero-posterior projection is of less consequence than that all be taken in the same projection. Kilovoltage and mAs settings should be standard, based upon chest dimension or some other objective criterion, and an exposure table should be posted permanently on the machine for guidance of all technicians. The technical data, including patient position, tube-film distance, kv and mAs, should be recorded along with the name, identifying number, date, and time of the film. If not directly recorded on the film, a gummed sticker on the film may be used to provide this necessary information.

If all these precautions are routinely taken, CCU chest films provide useful data in judging degrees of pulmonary congestion, both at the time of admission and during the course of illness (see Ch. 26). A baseline examination should be routinely performed as soon after admission as circumstances permit. The films are also helpful in differential diagnosis, as for aortic dissection or pulmonary embolic disease.

Arterial blood gas determinations are frequently required in CCU patients, especially in management of arrest, failure, and shock, but also in diagnosis of pulmonary embolism and other pulmonary disease. The manner in which this service is provided varies widely in different institutions. If a blood gas machine is located in the CCU in order to provide convenience and speed in reporting, a rigid quality control program will also be necessary for maintenance and standardization of the equipment and technique.

Means for accurately weighing CCU patients must be provided, along with meticulous attention to fluid intake and output records. A chair scale will be adequate for most patients, and the ironing board type of scale will suffice for many who cannot be weighed in a chair. However, a bed scale will be necessary for a small percentage of patients.

A few of these patients will also require endotracheal intubation and mechanical ventilation. (See Ch. 32.)

## HEMODYNAMIC MONITORING

Hemodynamic monitoring of patients is an integral part of more sophisticated programs for management of congestive failure and cardiogenic shock. Of course, the medical staff of the hospital must provide the necessary skills, knowledge, training, and experience to make appropriate use of these techniques. Central venous pressure monitoring alone is of no value in these patients. The manual skill required for passage of a Swan-Ganz catheter is such that it is virtually at the "see-one-do-one" level, although it is occasionally a memorable experience. Data acquisition and display systems have become progressively simpler and more trouble-free in operation. Even so, the appropriate utilization of hemodynamic monitoring in patient care remains the province of experts only. This expertise extends to the nursing staff involved, who must be thoroughly and broadly trained, not only in every aspect of the process itself, but in the wide range of therapeutic alternatives that will be employed in these patients. The subject of hemodynamic monitoring is covered more extensively in Chapter 27. For our present purposes we will merely emphasize some important facets in planning.

Firstly, it should be possible to institute hemodynamic monitoring at any bedside in the unit. My preference has been to use portable monitoring modules rather than fully equipping each bedside for this purpose, since this provides flexibility in use, lower initial expense, and convenience in replacing defective modules, all at little additional cost in floor space. Repeating pressure or flow data displays in the central monitoring station will rarely offer substantial practical benefit in my estimation, and need not be considered essential. However, it is essential that each pressure being monitored have an oscilloscopic waveform display at the bedside in addition to a digital display for accuracy in measurement. The waveform provides diagnostic information as well as an early warning system when the integrity of the data acquisition chain is threatened, as by kinks, bubbles, or clots. The nursing staff must be made expert in waveform recognition. The display will require at least a two-channel oscilloscope, since many patients will have both pulmonary and systemic pressure monitors. A calibrated multipurpose strip-chart recorder, preferably having at least two channels, will also be quite useful for permanent records of pressure or flow data, though a single recorder will usually suffice for the entire CCU. Similarly, a single thermodilution cardiac output "computer" will meet all requirements in most units. The routines established should include a closed, pressurized system for periodic flushing of tubing with a heparinized solution. All the necessary paraphernalia should be maintained in readiness in the procedure room, and expendables should be replaced promptly as used.

## HYPOTENSION AND CARDIOGENIC SHOCK

Hypotension in the patient with an acute myocardial infarct is usually defined somewhat arbitrarily by CCU policy, such as systolic blood pressure persistently less than 90 mm Hg; however, some individuals will display no evidence of underperfusion in this range of indirect (cuff) pressure. The more aggressive and widespread use of vasodilators and beta blockers in cardiac patients also increases the number with relatively low blood pressure but satisfactory perfusion. Shock is clinically defined by evidence of poor organ perfusion, whatever the blood pressure might be. When shock is due to severely impaired cardiac pumping function, it is an exceedingly lethal complication, discussed at length in subsequent chapters in this book.

The treatment of patients with cardiogenic shock may require much more equipment, more personnel at the bedside, and much more traffic in and out of the room than any other activity in the CCU. In some cases, it will be necessary to move the patient and several devices to the catheterization laboratory and to the operating room. At the very least a more generously proportioned room, with additional power supply, is needed to do this job well. A separate shock unit or subunit in the CCU is beyond the scope of this chapter.

Before leaving the subject of cardiogenic

shock, it is probably worthy of emphasis here, for those planning smaller units, that many hypotensive patients will not necessarily progress to irreversible shock. Some of these patients will respond well to volume expansion, which while more confidently accomplished with hemodynamic monitoring, can nonetheless be employed provided there is not radiographic or clinical evidence of pulmonary edema. A transient form of "warm shock" due to a vagal reflex is sometimes encountered, especially with inferior myocardial infarction. These patients usually have bradycardia and may complain of nausea, but have warm, well-perfused skin. They may respond simply to elevation of the legs or small doses of atropine. Patients with milder degrees of cardiogenic shock may sometimes be salvaged with catecholamine infusions alone, as will be discussed in Chapter 20.

## MYOCARDIAL SALVAGE

The patient in severe cardiogenic shock has an extremely poor outlook. Even with the most aggressive management, in-hospital salvage is small, and long-term prognosis is quite poor. Traditionally, these patients have been considered nontransportable, as to larger regional hospitals with specialized shock facilities and programs. There is little reason at present to change this view, since the great majority of these patients have suffered irreversible loss of myocardial mass as the proximate cause of shock. The few with potentially surgically correctible lesions are very high-risk surgical cases. Current thinking is directed more toward preservation of viable myocardium and limitation or reduction of infarct size rather than toward expansion of therapy for severe shock. Myocardial salvage seems a more promising means for improvement of both short- and long-term prognosis. Planning for future services in the CCU should countenance the likelihood that some procedures currently considered experimental or very highly specialized will gradually become generally accepted.

At present, there is no practical program which may be recommended for large-scale, routine use with the objective of reducing in-farct size, although this is a field of intense research activity. Should an efficacious routine emerge, it will probably emphasize pharmacological rather than mechanical procedures, although hemodynamic monitoring of patients undergoing such treatment is likely to be essential.

At this writing, outside of research-oriented units, aggressive treatment intended to preserve jeopardized myocardium is usually reserved for patients who display an unstable course or progressive deterioration early during hospitalization. This may involve mechanical assistance, such as intra-aortic balloon pumping, as well as vasoactive and cardioactive drug therapy. These are practical options in hospitals which offer a broad range of specialized services such as cardiac catheterization and cardiac surgery. In such institutions, the CCU plan should include rooms of larger floor space and power supply, additional staffing to provide virtually constant nursing attention, and an expanded curriculum for the staff educational programs.

## REFERENCES

1. Gordis L, Naggan L, Tonascia J: Pitfalls in evaluating the impact of Coronary Care Units on mortality from myocardial infarction. Johns Hopkins Medical Journal 141:287–295, 1977.
2. Harrison DC: Should lidocaine be administered routinely to all patients after acute myocardial infarction? Circulation 58:581–584, 1978.
3. Clipson CW, Wehrer JJ: Planning for cardiac care. A guide to the planning and design of cardiac care facilities. The Health Administration Press, Ann Arbor Michigan, 1973.
4. Stross JK, Willis PW, Reynolds EW, et al: Effectiveness of coronary care in small community hospitals. Ann Intern Med 85:709–713, 1976.
5. Marriott HJL, Fogg E: Constant monitoring for cardiac dysrhythmias and blocks. Mod Concepts Cardiovasc Dis 39:103–108, 1970.
6. Rombilt DW, Bloomfield SS, Chou TC, Fowler NO: Unreliability of conventional electrocardiographic monitoring for arrhythmia detection in coronary care units. Am J Cardiol 31:457–461, 1973.
7. Kuller L, Lilianfield A, Fisher R: Sudden and unexpected death in young adults. JAMA 198:248, 1966.

# 6 | Electrical Hazards in the Coronary Care Unit and Principles of Equipment Maintenance

*James A. Meyer, M.D.*

The Coronary Care Unit is one part of the hospital where one might be considered to be in a very safe environment. However, in the area of electrical safety this may not always be the case. Electrical safety is of great importance in all walks of life, but it requires special attention in the Coronary Care Unit. It is in such a location that patients and personnel come into contact with electric devices in ways that are not encountered at work or in the home. With recent advances in medicine have come many complex electric devices, some of which in normal use are "hard-wired" to the patient, making him a part of the circuit. The use of invasive conductive paths to the heart renders the patient unusually susceptible to the sudden onset of dysrhythmias which may be fatal if not immediately recognized and treated. These dysrhythmias may be induced by extremely small electric currents. This chapter will present the magnitude of the problem, describe the mechanisms of electric shock, and outline those principles which, when properly applied, will provide safety for the patient and the attending medical personnel.

## BACKGROUND AND "EPIDEMIOLOGY"

Any discussion of electrical hazards in hospitals should be preceded by an appraisal of the degree of actual risk and a review of the peculiar history of the subject. In years past, a physician worked mainly with the patient's history and the use of his own five senses. Now he is greatly assisted by a wide variety of electric devices which diagnose, monitor, and provide therapy for the patient. Unfortunately, electricity—the wonderful, unseen, silent servant—sometimes follows an unusual path that results in injury or death. Several observers noted during the past two decades that patients undergoing diagnosis, monitoring, and treatment with electrical devices could receive electric shocks resulting in ventricular fibrillation and death.[1-15] As physicians and others with an interest in health care problems became aware of this hazard, speculation arose that there were far more cases of accidental electrocution in hospitals than were actually proven. Dr. C. Walter, speaking at the 71st Annual Meeting of the American Hospital Association held in Chicago in 1960, estimated that each year as many as 1,200 deaths might be attributed to electrical accidents in U.S. hospitals.[16] It was in 1970 that Ralph Nader suggested that the number was probably more like 5,000. He credited this new figure to "conversations with doctors and technicians at recent meetings." [17] In 1971, Nader's article in a lay publication indicated that there might be as many as 12,000 such deaths per year.[18] Remarkably, there is still little known about the true incidence of fatal electrical accidents in hospitals. There has been confusion concerning the mechanism in some cases of ventricular fibrillation (VF) where it was seemingly unrelated to any electrical contact. Passage of conductive catheters or a catheter with a metal stylet in place into the heart may allow stray electric current to cause VF. The picture is further clouded when it is reported that mechanical stimulation during passage of a Swan-Ganz catheter can cause VF.[19] Ventricular fibrillation by mechanical stimulation is occasionally seen during cardiac catheterization procedures, although electrocution is not usually considered a factor in these cases.

Since widespread alarm was raised over these frightening numbers of deaths, very few rational studies have been performed to determine more accurately the true incidence of injury and death by electric shock in hospitals.[15] Information that is available seems to indicate that the incidence is probably very low—on the order of from 0.1 to 1.0 percent of the figures so widely quoted. It is probable that some cases go unrecognized where a unique combination of faults occurred and that some cases might go unreported where fear of litigation limits reporting of the facts.

During the past decade, it became clear that better design was needed both in medical instrumentation and in the hospital electric system. Manufacturers responded by improving the design of instruments with regard to better grounding, lower "leakage" currents, and isolation of patient leads. There are still areas of disagreement on appropriate methods for a safer electric system. The inevitable clashes between proponents of one system over another continue into the 1980s. The estimated costs of redundant safeguards have escalated into the tens of millions of dollars where uninformed inspectors misapply standards and require expensive retrofitting of electrical system devices. Efforts at a rational and orderly approach are often disregarded by those who want equipment such as isolated power systems or ground-fault circuit interrupters to substitute for operator education and regular maintenance of well-designed medical devices. If the true incidence of accidental electrocution is very low, as careful studies indicate, it is perhaps partly the result of the following: (1) improved design of equipment; (2) widespread use of third-wire

ground; (3) better grounding of the electric system and receptacles; (4) improved maintenance of both portable equipment and electric systems; and (5) an increasing awareness of electrical safety by having it regularly included as a subject for in-service training programs.

## BASIC CONCEPTS IN ELECTRICITY

To better understand the mechanism of electric shock, it is necessary first to review some basic concepts of electricity and the manner in which electric current can flow through human tissue. Electric current can be thought of as a flow of electric charges which, though invisible, represent energy that is available to perform work. This energy can produce light, heat, or motion—the latter, for example, by inducing magnetic fields in the coils of wire within a motor. It can also produce stimulation of nervous tissue, muscles, and the heart. Electric current flows when a power source such as a flashlight cell is attached to a resistive load such as a light bulb with two lengths of wire. The amount of current that flows in this simple circuit is directly proportional to the "electric pressure" or voltage of the power source and inversely proportional to the resistance of the light bulb and the wires. Electric current flows through any pathway that is made up of "conductive" materials. Those materials (usually nonmetals) that do not conduct electricity are known as nonconductors or insulators. A good analogy to help visualize the relationship among voltage, resistance, and current is that of water flowing from a reservoir through a pipe. The height of the reservoir above the pipe outlet determines the pressure and may be compared with voltage. The diameter and length of the pipe represent the resistance to flow. The flow of water obtained represents the electric current flow and is expressed as quantity per unit time. As the water level in the reservoir is raised, the pressure (voltage) is increased and a greater flow (electric current) is obtained through the same diameter and length (resistance) of pipe. Without raising the height of the water, a greater flow may be obtained by making the delivery pipe shorter or wider in diameter (lower resistance). The analogy must end soon, as the reservoir will be emptied and there is no way for the water to return to the reservoir. In an electric system, energy will only flow when there is a complete or circular path for the electric current to return to the power source—hence the term "circuit." Electrical safety requires that we do not allow the patient or attending personnel to become part of a complete electric circuit. The relationship between voltage and resistance in producing current flow is stated in Ohm's law that voltage (E) is equal to current (I) times resistance (R). (E stands for electromotive force and, although an old symbol, is still seen in electrical diagrams representing voltage.) Voltage is expressed in volts (V) or millivolts (mV) (thousandths of a volt); current is expressed in amperes (A) or milliamperes (mA) (thousandths of an ampere) or microamperes ($\mu$A) (millionths of an ampere); and resistance is expressed in ohms ($\Omega$). In the case of direct current (DC), which flows in only one direction, such as in a flashlight cell, Ohm's law may be applied quite precisely. The power used in hospital electrical systems is alternating current (AC), and this behaves in a somewhat different manner. In alternating current, the direction of energy flow is reversed 120 times per second, resulting in 60 complete cycles each second. The cycle is now referred to as Hertz (Hz). This alternating current is much more economical to transmit over utility lines without loss as heat, and the voltage can easily be changed to different values as needed with a transformer. Alternating current has the added dimension of frequency. The usual frequency of the line current in the United States is 60 Hz.

This frequency may be increased to very high values in such medical equipment as the electrosurgical device that applies electric current at more than 500,000 Hz, or in medical diathermy where the frequency is around 13.56 and 27.12 megahertz (million cycles). In alternating current, there is a constantly changing buildup and collapse of a magnetic field around each conductor as the current flow increases from zero to a maximum value, then reverses passing through zero to a negative maximum value and again returns to zero (Fig. 6.1). As the voltage

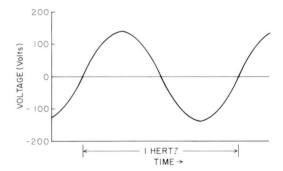

Fig. 6.1 The line voltage in an alternating current system is best visualized by observing the sine wave produced on an oscilloscope. The display shown indicates voltage change plotted against time.

increases from zero to its maximum value, the current increases in phase with the voltage to its maximum value (Fig. 6.2). When two plates of conductive material are in close proximity, an electric charge on one induces an opposite charge on the other. If the applied electric current is removed, there is a brief storage effect as the charges then attempt to equalize. This is known as the capacitor effect. When an alternating current is applied to a capacitor, it is easily passed while direct current is blocked. There is, however, a phase shift with the alternating current due to the capacitor making the current rise lead the voltage rise by 90° (Fig. 6.3).

Another component in electric circuits is the inductor or coil. This is a device that resists the buildup of current flow as the voltage rises from zero to a maximum value, then also resists the fall of current when the voltage decreases from a maximum back through zero. This results in the voltage leading the current by 90°

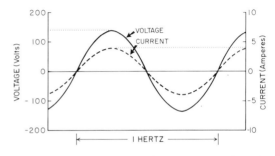

Fig. 6.2 The relationship of current and voltage is shown where the current is in phase with the applied voltage.

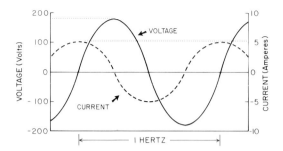

Fig. 6.3   Where AC voltage is applied through a capacitor, the current leads the voltage by 90°.

(Fig. 6.4) The combination of the effects of resistance, capacitance, and inductance is known as impedance. Ohm's law may be applied to AC circuits where the load is entirely resistive, as is the case with direct current. However, there may be some change in values obtained when capacitators and inductors are placed in the circuit. For general purposes in calculating current flows through humans, we may use Ohm's law even though current paths through the body represent an impedance differing somewhat from simple DC resistance.

## THE PHYSIOLOGIC RESPONSE TO ELECTRIC CURRENT

Electric current is often intentionally applied to the body when using various therapeutic instruments such as a nerve stimulator, a pacemaker, a defibrillator, or the electrosurgical apparatus. With these devices, the type of current and the current path are controlled to prevent injury. Accidental electric shock is the uncon-

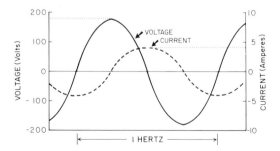

Fig. 6.4   Where AC voltage flows through an inductor the voltage leads the current by 90°. The effects of capacitance and inductance make it difficult to predict the effects of AC currents through the body.

trolled, unintentional application of electric current to the body. It may result in pain, burns, muscle spasm with resultant mechanical injury, paralysis of the respiratory center; or, most important, it may cause ventricular fibrillation, a fatal dysrhythmia when it is not immediately recognized and treated.

Unfortunately, one of the most dangerous frequencies that can be applied to the heart is the 60 Hz supplied by the standard system. The 50-Hz system used in many countries outside of the United States is essentially the same as the 60-Hz with respect to the danger of electric shock. The power distribution systems in many countries distribute 220 to 240 volts rather than the 110 to 120 volts commonly used in the United States. In a given electric shock situation, this higher voltage might result in double the current flow through the human body. The high frequencies utilized in electrosurgery and medical diathermy pass easily through human tissue and, although they produce a heating effect, they do not stimulate nervous, muscular, or cardiac tissue as does 60 Hz. Unless there is a 60-Hz fault, these devices do not represent an electric shock hazard with regard to VF, other than being a source of ground (see below).

The human body represents a resistance (impedance, in the case of AC) to electric current that varies greatly depending on several factors. If the voltage is large, the current will be higher. If the area of contact is large, the resistance will be lower—hence, the current will be higher. Skin moisture also greatly reduces resistance, resulting in larger current flow. Contact with thick, dry skin may result in a resistance as high as 100,000 ohms, while contact with wet hands may lower resistance to less than 1,000 ohms. The amount of current and the degree of injury may be roughly estimated by application of Ohm's law. In the case of contact with dry hands, 100,000 ohms body resistance, and a line voltage of 120 volts, the current would be about 1.2 mA. The threshold of perception is about 1 mA (1,000 $\mu$A). Hence, one might hardly feel a tingle in the latter case. In the case of wet hands and a resistance of 1000 ohms, the current would be 120 mA, a shock that may stop breathing and cause VF.

## MACROSHOCK VS. MICROSHOCK

The effects of electric current on the human body as noted in Table 6.1 are dependent on the part of the body involved. A large current from a foot to the thigh would cause great stimulation of nerves and muscles but would perhaps have little effect on the heart. A smaller current passing through the chest from one arm to a foot or from one arm to the other might readily cause VF (Fig. 6.5). These large currents passing through the intact skin are referred to as *macroshock*. The current required to cause VF in these cases is from 100 to 3000 mA, and the value depends on how moist the skin is and the size and location of the areas of contact with the body. The use of invasive techniques, such as the introduction of pacing leads or catheters which provide a low-impedance conductive pathway to the heart, make patients become extremely vulnerable to very small alternating currents. These small currents which may cause VF are referred to as *microshock* and range from 20 μA up to several mA (Fig. 6.6).

The very low-impedance conductors to the heart (catheters and pacing wires) are often in contact with the endocardium, and the area of the point of contact is so small that the current density is relatively high even with a very small

Table 6.1   Physical Effects of Electrical Shock at 60 Hz Electrical Current on Humans *

| Current Value | Physiologic Effects |
|---|---|
| *Microshock* (internal contact through low-impedance conductor to the heart) | |
| 10 μA | Considered safe for normal heart |
| 20 to 500 μA | Ventricular fibrillation threshold |
| *Macroshock* (external contact through skin or internal without direct contact with the heart) | |
| 0 to 500 μA | No sensation |
| 500 μA (0.5 mA) to 2000 μA (2 mA) | Threshold of sensation, tingle |
| 2 mA to 10 mA | Pain, muscle contraction |
| 15 to 20 mA | Pain and mechanical injury, heart and respiration continue, may be impossible to let go of source as flexors are stronger than extensors |
| 25 to 100 mA | Respiratory paralysis |
| 100 to 3000 mA | Ventricular fibrillation, death without immediate resuscitation including defibrillation |
| over 3000 mA | Cardiac standstill in systole, respiratory paralysis, burns. Heart may return to sinus rhythm with effective pumping if source of current is quickly removed. |

* Compilation from many sources including references 9–12, 20–22, and 27.

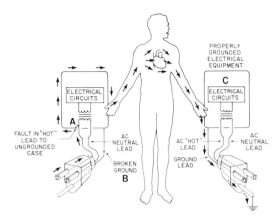

Fig. 6.5 Example of a mechanism for macroshock electrocution. A fault "A" in the instrument case on the left in combination with the broken ground lead "B" allows a large current to flow through the patient who is in contact with the properly grounded instrument "C" on the right.

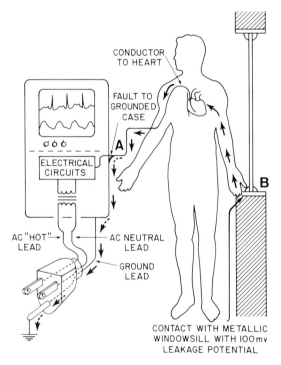

Fig. 6.6 Example of a mechanism for microshock electrocution. Accidental grounding of an intracardiac conductor through a fault in the insulation at "A" allows current flow directly through the heart when patient contacts source of leakage current such as improperly grounded conductive building part "B."

current. The highest risk is when the electrode is actually in contact with the inside of the ventricle rather than when it is floating free or in contact with the atrium. The minimum current value found to produce VF in human hearts varies with investigators. Generally accepted values range between 80 and 180 $\mu$A.[20,21] Values as low as 20 $\mu$A can cause VF in dogs.[9] This 20 $\mu$A value was determined before the research showing that the value was somewhat higher for humans was performed; therefore, it was decided at that earlier time that leakage currents must be kept to 10 $\mu$A or less. Electrical safety standards are still partly based on this low value.[22] In cases where a low-impedance conductive path to the heart is in place, the current required to cause VF is less than one mA (1000 $\mu$A), which is the approximate threshold for feeling current through the skin. This means that the physician or nurse could become a conductive pathway for a leakage current great enough to cause VF without feeling the current himself. Since AC flows in both directions, it is very important that an intracardiac conductor not contact a grounded object, even through the hands of an attendant, while the patient is in contact with a source of AC leakage current.

## LEAKAGE CURRENT

Leakage current is a current that flows from any conductive surface, such as an instrument case, to another conductive surface which is at a lower potential or ground. It is an unintentional current and is usually the result of poor design or a "fault" within an electric device or system. Where two grounded conductors are not at the same potential, a leakage current will flow between them when they are connected by a conductive path. Where metallic instruments, windowsills, or sink tops are present in a CCU, it is very important that they be at the same potential.

## GROUNDING

It is very important to insure that conductive surfaces in the patient area do not become sources of leakage current and to see that they are all maintained at the same ground potential. This is best accomplished by having each conductive surface connected to a high-quality-zero-potential ground. This is referred to as "earth" in European countries. Since ground wires have resistance, it is often difficult to maintain all equipment grounds at the same potential. The use of only high-quality line cords with a third-wire ground is the most effective way to maintain zero or very low-potential grounding in instruments. To prevent faults in equipment from causing unwanted currents to flow in ground conductors within the electrical system, it is important that all patient equipment be plugged in at one location. This will minimize differences in potential occurring on grounded conductive surfaces due to resistance in ground circuits within the electric system. The use of patient circuits for housekeeping or maintenance tools must not be allowed, for such devices may cause ground currents and affect patient safety. The use of "hospital-grade" or equivalent receptacles with proper testing and maintenance will help to assure safe grounding. All humans are susceptible to electric shock and must be protected. The terms "electrically susceptible patient" (ESP) and "electrically susceptible patient location" (ESPL) were coined in the late 1960s to describe those patients and locations within hospitals where patients had invasive monitoring lines to the heart which placed them at increased risk for electric shock. The term ESP is no longer used, but the term ESPL is still in use. The preferred term is now "critical care area," as currently used in the National Electrical Code.[23]

Some of the factors that increase the risk of electric shock are summarized as follows:

1. The presence of low-impedance conductors to the heart which result in a higher current density being applied at a most sensitive location is the primary factor leading to the microshock hazard.

2. The patient may be comatose or have his senses obtunded by medications rendering him unable to call for help or move from the source of the shock.

3. The patient may have wet dressings or lie in a wet bed where solutions with a high electrolyte content greatly reduce the resistance to electrical current flow.

4. The use of two or more line-powered devices increases the opportunity for leakage current to find paths through the patient.

5. Old buildings with inadequate wiring may negate some safety features found in new equipment.

6. The electrical safety provided by new equipment and a well-designed electrical system are soon defeated by the lack of regular periodic testing and preventive maintenance.

7. Lack of experienced personnel who are given regular in-service training and serve on all shifts is a major factor in increasing patient risk.

## ELECTRICAL SAFETY: WHO IS INVOLVED?

Electrical safety in the CCU requires a multifaceted approach. It involves an understanding by all personnel of the several mechanisms of electric shock. These personnel include: physicians, nurses, aides, and technicians as well as members of the housekeeping and engineering staff. This can only be accomplished by holding regular in-service training at all levels. It also means establishing strict rules of electrical safety for all to observe.

## SELECTION OF EQUIPMENT

The equipment used in the CCU should be of up-to-date design. For example, external temporary pacemaker pulse generators should have no exposed conductive surfaces, and pressure transducers should isolate electrically the fluid column within the transducer dome and intravascular catheter. All equipment should meet standards for current leakage limits and, where possible, have "isolated" patient input sections. There should always be a three-wire grounded line cord with adequate strain relief provision where it enters the instrument case. The manufacturer should be conversant with the electrical safety features of his equipment. It is best not to purchase instruments that do not have adequate written instructions and specifications. Beware of equipment that has not been approved by recognized testing organizations. The specifications should give data on leakage limits. The conditions of the warranty should be clearly stated and include what local maintenance is both expected and allowed. A good sales representative should know specific differences between his equipment and what the competition has to offer. Where the features and specifications are approximately equal, it is best to purchase equipment from a manufacturer who has a good local service capability with ability to respond promptly to night and weekend calls. In some locations equipment with modular construction may serve best, since less sophisticated hospital maintenance personnel can exchange plug-in modules or circuit boards and quickly return the instrument to service. The modules or circuit boards may then be returned to the vendor for definitive repair by qualified personnel.

## EQUIPMENT MAINTENANCE

A preventive maintenance program is the key to good electrical safety. Each electrically operated device should be checked for electrical leakage periodically and a record should be carefully maintained. A system of tags placed on the instrument listing the latest maintenance date is very desirable. The line cord and cap account for the majority of instrument failures, especially where equipment is moved about on wheeled stands. The combination of hospital-grade plug caps and receptables gives excellent, very low-resistance ground contact. Unfortunately, when personnel carelessly move wheeled equipment without removing the plug, the tension on the blades of the plug is so great that the cord and its conductors may be damaged. This may result in hidden damage with a breach in the electrical safety normally provided by the third-wire ground. Where hospital maintenance personnel are in short supply, lacking in specialized education, or unable to attend manufacturers' maintenance instruction courses, it may be better for the hospital to purchase maintenance contracts. Unless the

hospital is located in a metropolitan area, the delay in service may be excessive with the latter arrangement. The ideal is to have at least one person who is a certified clinical engineer and an adequate medical equipment repair staff. The exact number of such staff necessary will depend on the number of beds, operating rooms, Intensive/Coronary Care Units, and specialized services that are offered. A hospital with cardiac surgery and renal dialysis programs, for instance, will require extra support. The number of technicians should be such that 24-hour coverage is always available even during times of illness or vacation.

## ELECTRIC SYSTEM CONSIDERATIONS

The electric system serving the CCU should comply with the National Electrical Code, which specifies details of construction designed to provide an electrically safe environment.[23] Some of the special requirements for critical care areas include:

(1) Each patient location shall have at least six single or three duplex receptacles all grounded to the reference ground. It is important that all line-powered devices be plugged in at one location to minimize potential differences in the ground pin of the plugs. When a potential difference exists between two grounds, a current may flow through a patient if both devices are either attached to or even in casual contact with the patient.

(2) All exposed conductive surfaces shall not exceed 100 mV potential difference in the patient vicinity. This is to assure that the patient or someone touching the patient and a conductive surface—e.g., a metal windowsill—will not become the means for passage of leakage currents.

(3) Each patient should be provided with at least two branch circuits. This is so that there will be power available at each bed in case one circuit breaker opens due to a short circuit or overload.

(4) Though not required, isolated power systems shall be permitted in critical care areas. The use of isolated power offers some additional

features though it is not required in CCUs. It provides continuity of power where one line-to-ground fault occurs. This would keep a ventilator in operation while warning of a short-to-ground in another device plugged into the same duplex receptacle. The system includes a line isolation monitor that gives off an alarm when the first line-to-ground fault occurs, giving the operator time to detach the faulty equipment. The line isolation monitor unfortunately provides a high-impedance path to ground which will allow up to two mA to flow to ground before the alarm is sounded. This partly negates the value of this sytem for microshock protection. It does not warn personnel of a line-to-line fault. However, in such a case the circuit-breaker should function by turning off the power.

The receptacles, which should all be mounted at one location to minimize the possibility of unequal ground potentials, play a key role in maintaining electrical safety. Only hospital-grade receptacles should be used, and these should be periodically tested for blade tension and integrity of the ground. Where isolated power systems are installed, the line isolation monitor should be tested periodically.

## THE GROUND FAULT CIRCUIT INTERRUPTER

One method of limiting electric shock hazards is by the use of the Ground Fault Circuit Interrupter (GFCI). This device detects the current flow to ground by comparing the current flow in the hot side of the line with the current flow in the neutral. If the flows are not the same, indicating a line-to-ground fault, the GFCI shuts off the power. This occurs very quickly—in a few msec. This prevents a fault current from flowing long enough to cause VF in macroshock situations. The GFCI is usually set to allow 5 mA but to open the circuit at 6 mA. The GFCI would be of some help in detecting faulty instruments; however, it would not protect against microshock in most cases. In a CCU, the use of a GFCI-protected duplex electric receptacle would be dangerous where an electrically powered ventilator or other item

of life-support equipment depends on continuity of power. A faulty device plugged into the same GFCI duplex receptacle as a ventilator would shut off power to the ventilator. Current electric codes require a GFCI in bathrooms of domestic residential construction in the United States.[24] It is hoped that this move will prevent the growing number of electrocutions of persons dropping hair dryers and such line-operated appliances into sinks and bathtubs. If the GFCI is to be used in the CCU, it should control only single receptacles rather than duplex receptacles, and all life-support equipment should be equipped with power failure alarms and/or self-activating emergency power supplied within the equipment.

## PRACTICAL CONSIDERATIONS IN THE PREVENTION OF ELECTRIC SHOCK

The role of physicians, nurses, and other attendants in the prevention of electric shock is especially important, since it is a matter of continuing education and review rather than a one-time design consideration. The electrical safety provided by low-leakage equipment and a well-designed electric system will be quickly defeated by personnel not instructed in basic electrical safety practices. The following recommendations will help to prevent unintentional electric shocks:

1. The physician or nurse must learn to avoid any situation where he becomes a conductor of electric energy. This is for his own safety as well as that of the patient, since he may inadvertently cause VF in a patient with externalized pacing leads.

2. When touching a line-operated electric device or lighting fixture, use only one hand and keep the other hand away from other electric equipment or conductive surfaces that might be electrically "alive" or grounded. This includes conductive parts of a bed, plumbing fixtures, and metallic building parts such as windowsills.

3. Avoid touching all electric equipment and metallic surfaces that might be "alive" or grounded when the hands are wet. Any mois-

ture greatly reduces the protective resistance provided by dry skin (as much as a hundredfold) and increases the chance of a dangerous electrical shock.

4. When caring for a patient with a low-impedance path to the heart such as an externalized intracardiac electrode, it is best to wear rubber gloves when handling the lead connections or a metal stylet from a central catheter.

In general, it is best to carefully ground all line-operated equipment and as far as possible avoid grounding the patient. Conductive objects not likely to become energized, such as metal tables, should not be grounded. There is no reason to provide extra grounding opportunities for the patient to contact.

Electrically operated beds represent a special hazard unless they are very carefully designed. They may provide additional opportunities for the patient to contact ground if conductive surfaces are exposed. There have been accidents where the line cord is partly severed in the scissor-like mechanism of the bed. This resulted in electrifying the entire bed frame with 120 volts AC. The use of an isolation transformer on the bed is of marginal help in preventing this problem, since it is the line cord that becomes entangled in the mechanism. There is capacitative and inductive coupling leakage from some motors, which makes it difficult to avoid excessive leakage currents from electric beds of the older design. In another case, an electric bed was raised, pushing the attached intravenous pole through a ceiling light fixture and therefore electrifying the bed frame. Some hospitals have removed all electrically operated beds from their critical care areas as a precaution.

fire or explosion from falling television sets, interference with pacemakers, and electric shock from dropping shavers and hair dryers into sinks and bathtubs. The battery-operated radio is safe until an AC adaptor is added. These are not supplied with a grounded plug, and the isolation inherent in battery operation is defeated. The Joint Commission on Accreditation of Hospitals (JCAH) standard now states in Standard 2 of the "Functional Safety and Sanitation" section of its manual that patient-owned equipment, if permitted in the hospital, must be approved as safe. The Accrediation Manual for Hospitals makes it clear in the interpretation of Standard 2 that "Written policies shall be established for prohibition of the use of personal electrical equipment by patients and staff, unless such equipment has been approved as safe in writing by the appropriate hospital personnel prior to its use. Exceptions regarding specific items or categories of items or restricted areas of use may be designated by the safety committee." [25] The term "approved as safe" is intended to give flexibility to the hospital administration in its inspection and control policy.

The hospital may ban all patient-owned devices, ban some and inspect others, or maintain a list of exempted items such as electric toothbrushes and shavers that are battery operated. The latter policy should require that all chargers be kept at the nursing station. Some patients might feel lost without some of their own items for personal care, so each situation may need individual consideration. Overall safety is ultimately in the hands of a well-informed nursing staff who are in a position to observe the patient and vistors and carry out the policy determined by the hospital administration.

## CONTROL OF PATIENT-OWNED APPLIANCES

The use of patient-owned appliances in a CCU introduces some hazards, though there are essentially none reported in the medical literature. Hospitals are in an unclear position with regard to liability for injury caused by the patient-owned appliance. Possible problems include fires from faulty battery charger units,

## EQUIPMENT CONTROL PROGRAM

A good example of an equipment control program protocol has recently been published.[26] This protocol covers such subjects as acquisition, technical support, education and information, monitoring and evaluation, and documentation. It also suggests criteria for retiring obsolete equipment.

## ELECTRIC PLUGS AND LINE CORDS

By far the most common equipment failure is associated with the line cord and plug. Production defects have mandated the removal of molded plugs from use on hospital equipment. The use of three-conductor, U-ground plugs and three-conductor line cords is now standard for medical equipment. Plugs and line cords should be inspected regularly. A high resistance in the ground lead indicates a loose screw connection or possibly a broken wire. Another common problem occurs when the line cord is sheared at the strain relief by improper tightening of "crimp" type cord grips. The "chuck" type cord grip may loosen, allowing the cord to slip out with the strain then taken up by the screw connections. Line cord and plug assemblies on portable equipment mounted on wheeled tables are especially prone to damage when the equipment is carelessly moved without removing the plug. Special care must be exercised by maintenance personnel when repairing these cords, since it is very easy to reverse the hot and neutral leads. Any use of two-prong plugs, "cheater" adaptors, and extension cords in critical care areas should be abolished.

## THE ROLE OF STANDARDS IN ELECTRICAL SAFETY

Since 1964, there have been efforts to write electrical safety standards by several organizations. In 1976, the consensus standard for safe current limits developed by the Association for the Advancement of Medical Instrumentation (AAMI) was revised; in 1978, it received American National Standards Institute (ANSI) approval. ANSI is officially recognized by the U.S. Government, and documents carrying ANSI approval are considered American National Standards. The AAMI document requires that leakage from medical devices be limited to levels that will provide adequate protection for patients in contact with electric devices. The most stringent requirement is for patient connections that are limited to 10 $\mu$A of leakage current. The case of cord-connected equipment must not exceed 100 $\mu$A. Equipment not in patient areas is limited to 500 $\mu$A.

Despite the difficulties in achieving agreement on a standard for safe leakage values, medical equipment manufacturers have greatly improved the electrical safety in their engineering and design of medical equipment during the last 15 years. In general, the equipment currently available meets the AAMI standard and is usually very good. Various techniques, including isolated input sections, isolated power supplies, careful grounding, and double insulation have all contributed to instruments which are far safer than those offered prior to this upsurge in electrical safety. It is undoubtedly these improvements that have reduced the incidence of electric shock.

## ADMINISTRATIVE RESPONSIBILITIES

The hospital administration is responsible for establishing a comprehensive electrical safety program. The administration should:

1. Establish a hospital electrical safety committee.

2. Designate areas of the hospital as critical care areas (NEC). They were formerly called electrically susceptible patient locations (ESPL) by the NFPA 76B-T (tentative) standard, which has been revised to eliminate that designation but still has not become approved as a standard.

3. Establish medical equipment selection and procurement policies that will insure that only safe and well-designed equipment is purchased.

4. Establish policies that require periodic inspection of the electric system, including receptacles and all portable electric equipment with testing and documentation where indicated.

5. Insure that all equipment is equipped with adequate grounding systems. A three-conductor line cord with U-ground polarized plug is necessary on all but those items designated as "doubly insulated." All three-to-two-prong adaptors (cheater adaptors) must be prohibited. Extension cords should also be prohibited.

6. Provide training programs on medical electrical safety for all personnel who work in the hospital, with appropriate emphasis for

those involved in patient care and especially those working in critical care areas.

# REFERENCES

1. Medicine and the Law: Fatal shock from a cardiac monitor. Commentary, Lancet 1:872, 1960.
2. Zoll PM, Linenthal AJ: Long-term electrical pacemakers for Stokes-Adams disease, Circulation 22:341, 1960.
3. Furman S, Schwedel JB, Robinson G, Hurwitt ES: Use of an intracardiac pacemaker in the control of heart block. Surgery 49:98, 1961
4. Noordijk JA, Oey FTI, Tebra W: Myocardial electrodes and the danger of ventricular fibrillation. Lancet 1:975, 1961.
5. Pengelly LD, Klassen GA: Myocardial electrodes and the danger of ventricular fibrillation. Lancet 1:1234, 1961.
6. Bousvaros GA, Conway D, Hopps JA: An electrical hazard of selective angiocardiography. Can Med Assoc J 87:286, 1962.
7. Weinberg DI, Artley JL, Whalen RE, McIntosh HD: Electric shock hazards in cardiac catheterization. Circ Res 11:1004, 1962.
8. Lee WR: The nature and management of electric shock. Br J Anaesth 36:572, 1964.
9. Whalen RE, Starmer CF, McIntosh HD: Electrical hazards associated with cardiac pacemaking. Ann NY Acad Sci III:922 1964.
10. Starmer CF, Whalen RE, McIntosh Hd: Hazards of electric shock in cardiology. Am J Cardiol 14:537, 1964.
11. Whalen RE, Starmer CF, McIntosh HD: Electric shock hazards in clinical cardiology. Mod Conc Cardiovasc Dis 36:2, 1967.
12. Bruner JMR: Hazards of electrical apparatus. Anesthesiology 28:396, 1967.
13. Lee WR: The hazards of electricution during patient monitoring. Potgrad Med 46:355, 1970.
14. Kugelberg J: Accidental ventricular fibrillation of the human heart. Scand J Thorac Cardiovasc Surg 9:133, 1975.
15. Bruner JMR, Aronow S, Cavicchi RV: Electrical incidents in a large hospital: a 42-month register. JAAMI 6:222, 1972.
16. Too many shocks. Time magazine 98(No 16, April 18):63, 1969.
17. Friedlander GD: Electricity in hospitals: elimination of lethal hazards. IEEE Spectrum 8:40, 1971.
18. Nader, R: Ralph Nader's most shocking expose. Ladies Home Journal 88:98, 1971.
19. Cairns JA, Holder DA: Ventricular fibrillation due to the passage of a Swan-Ganz catheter. Am J Cardiol 35:589, 1975.
20. Raferty EB, Green H, Gregory I: Electrical safety: Fibrillation thresholds with 50 Hz leakage currents in man and animals. Br Heart J 35:864, 1973.
21. Starmer CF, Whalen RE: Current density and electrically induced ventricular fibrillation. Med Instrum 7:158, 1973.
22. AAMI Safety standard for electromedical apparatus: Safe current limits. Assoc for the Advanc of Med Instrument April 1964.
23. National Electrical Code, NFPA 70, Article 517, 1978.
24. National Electrical Code, NFPA 70, Article 210, 1978.
25. Joint Commission on Accreditation of Hospitals, Accreditation Manual for Hospitals, 1979 ed. Chicago: JCAH, 1979.
26. Equipment Control Program Protocol. Health Devices 8 (10–11): 225, 1979. Published by the Emergency Care Research Institute, 5200 Butler Pike, Plymouth Meeting, Pa. 19462.
27. Kantrowski P: Electrical safety in hospitals. Instrum Tech 19 (No 8): 35, 1972.

## SUGGESTED READINGS

Bruner JMR: Hazards of electrical apparatus. Anesthesiology 28:396, 1967.

Meyer JA: Electrical hazards in medical instrumentation. Clin. Anesthesia 2:53 (chapter 6) FA Davis 1967.

Meyer JA: Safety in the use of monitoring equipment. Clinical Anesthesia 9:48 (chapter 3) FA Davis 1973.

Roth HH, Telischer ES, Kane IM: Electrical safety in health care facilities Clin. Engineering Series. Academic Press, 1975.

# Section 3

# APPROACH TO THE PATIENT WITH ACUTE MYOCARDIAL INFARCTION

# 7 | Initial Therapy of Acute Myocardial Infarction

## Gabriel Gregoratos, M.D.
## Evelyn Gleeson, R.N.

The importance of appropriate initial therapy for the patient with acute myocardial infarction cannot be overemphasized. It has been repeatedly demonstrated that the risk of ventricular fibrillation and sudden death is highest during the first few hours following the onset of acute myocardial infarction.[1] Of equal importance is the need to recognize that the first few hours following the onset of acute myocardial infarction represent a period of intense psychologic trauma for most patients, as they make the transition from well human beings to patients being rushed through the alien and regimented environments of ambulance, emergency ward, and, finally coronary care unit.[2] As we discuss further the complex and detailed issues facing the coronary care team when a new patient is admitted, it is good to remember the patient's continuing needs for reassurance and explanation of the proceedings.

Although questions have been raised recently concerning the efficacy and cost effectiveness of coronary care units,[3] it is our firm conviction that all patients with documented or suspected acute myocardial infarction must be admitted to a CCU for intensive cardiac rhythm monitoring and/or treatment, as appropriate.[4,5,6] In order to provide the patient with safe and comprehensive care, it is customary to establish guidelines for treatment and standing orders which provide the nursing staff of the CCU with the appropriate framework for monitoring and treatment of the patient with acute myocardial infarction. The standard CCU admission orders utilized at the University of California Medical Center are reproduced in Fig. 7.1. Standard orders are reviewed by the CCU Committee annually and updated as treatment modalities change. The admitting house officer has the prerogative and responsibility of individualizing the routine orders according to the specific needs of the patient. In order to preclude arbitrary deviations from the standard orders, the reason for such deviations must be clearly documented in the patient's record and explained to the unit director.

## RHYTHM MONITORING

Electronic monitoring systems providing continuous surveillance of a patient's rhythm were the initial impetus which led to the establishment of intensive CCUs in the 1960s. Continuous cardiac rhythm surveillance remains today the most valuable and important function of the CCU. Rhythm monitoring provides the capability of detecting early warning signs which may forecast the occurrence of potentially lethal dysrhythmias. The opportunity thereby exists to treat the altered cardiac electrical status prophylactically in the hope of preventing a primary dysrhythmic cardiac death in the presence of an otherwise viable heart.

127

**UNIVERSITY HOSPITAL**
University of California
Medical Center, San Diego

MYOCARDIAL INFARCTION
PHYSICIAN'S ORDERS
STANDARD ORDERS
Source | Date | Patient Identification

PHYSICIAN: Use ball point pen. Cross-off and initial nonapplicable orders. To reinstate or add additional orders after signing and dating this set, use a blank 151.031, Physician's Orders. EVERY page must be signed and dated.
NURSE: Remove Nursing and Pharmacy copies. Retain Nursing copy. Check drugs needed, then forward Pharmacy copy, whether or not medications are ordered or appear on that page.

ANOTHER GENERICALLY EQUIVALENT BRAND IDENTICAL IN DOSAGE AND CONTENTS OF ACTIVE
INGREDIENT(S) MAY BE DISPENSED AND ADMINISTERED UNLESS A DRUG IS SPECIFIED BY CIRCLING.

A. ADMITTING DIAGNOSIS/ADMISSION DATE
1. Diagnosis:
2. Admit to CCU or SCOR bed (Circle one)
3. Comments:

B. ALLERGIES/BLOOD & Rh TYPE
Comments:

C. VITAL SIGNS/I & O/WEIGHT
1. Vital signs (pulse, BP, resp.) q 1 hr x 4, then if stable q 4 hr. Repeat this sequence if patient becomes unstable. Temperature q 8 hrs.
2. Daily weights - use bed scale until patient has chair privileges.
3. I and O q 8 hrs.
4. Comments:

D. EXAMINATIONS/MONITORING
1. Constant cardiac monitoring with modified $V_1$ lead, if possible; set alarm for 40-140 range.
2. Keep a record of examples of arrhythmias; document when leads are switched and place an example of patient's rhythm in chart at least once a shift.
3. Maintain Heparin Lock with 18 Angiocath. - flush with 2 cc Heparin solution (19 cc NS with 1 cc of 1000 U Heparin) q 4 hr.
4. Comments:

E. LABORATORY TESTS REQUIRED
1. ECGs are to be taken and mounted q AM for use in CCU. Copies of admission tracing, day 1, day 2, and discharge from CCU to be sent to Heart Station. Copies of admission, days 1, 2, 3 & discharge from CCU xerox and place in patient's chart. Mark lead positions on chest.
2. CK, SGOT, and LDH sent on admission, then CK q 6 hours x 4 or until CK peaks and AM days 2 & 3.
3. CK isoenzymes on first elevated total CK specimen.
4. CBC on admission.
5. Urinalysis on admission.
6. Creatinine, BUN, electrolytes and glucose on admission.
7. Drug levels; check if required: ___ Digoxin ___ Procainamide ___ Quinidine ___ Dilantin
8. Comments:

B 089 (1-78) SIC 600
Physician's Signature | Date & Time

---

**UNIVERSITY HOSPITAL**
University of California
Medical Center, San Diego

MYOCARDIAL INFARCTION
PHYSICIAN'S ORDERS
STANDARD ORDERS
Source | Date | Patient Identification

PHYSICIAN: Use ball point pen. Cross-off and initial nonapplicable orders. To reinstate or add additional orders after signing and dating this set, use a blank 151.031, Physician's Orders. EVERY page must be signed and dated.
NURSE: Remove Nursing and Pharmacy copies. Retain Nursing copy. Check drugs needed, then forward Pharmacy copy, whether or not medications are ordered or appear on that page.

ANOTHER GENERICALLY EQUIVALENT BRAND IDENTICAL IN DOSAGE AND CONTENTS OF ACTIVE
INGREDIENT(S) MAY BE DISPENSED AND ADMINISTERED UNLESS A DRUG IS SPECIFIED BY CIRCLING.

K. ACTIVITY/AMBULATION/STIMULATION (continued)
e. Day 5: ___ (1) Up in chair as tolerated.
             ___ (2) Up in chair tid.
f. Impending MI or CHF same as Day 1 until otherwise ordered.
2. Stimulation:
a. Day 1: No TV, radio or reading. Visitors: Immediate family only, one at a time for 15 minutes x 4 in 24 hours. No smoking EVER.
b. Day 2 & 3: May read or listen to radio. Visitors: Immediate family qid for 15 minutes each visit.
c. Day 4 & on: at patient's and nurses' discretion.
3. Foot board exercise and deep breathing, cough exercise qid.
4. Passive movement of extremities bid.
5. Bathe patient first 3 days then assist patient.
6. Patients are not allowed to comb their own hair or shave their own faces with a razor (electric shaver OK unless pacemaker patient).
7. Comments:

L. REMINDER OF OTHER FORMS/APPOINTMENTS
Comments:

M. OTHER STATEMENTS REQUIRED BY THE PROCEDURE
1. Arrhythmia Treatment:
a. Ventricular fibrillation: counter shock immediately with 400 watt/sec, repeat if necessary; then give 100 mg of Lidocaine IV push (50 mg if patient on Lidocaine) and follow with IV drip of 4 mg/min; if ventricular fibrillation persists 45 seconds, begin CPR; then call House Officer.
b. Ventricular tachycardia with rate greater than 120: deliver a hard blow over the precordium and give Lidocaine as directed above; if it persists, counter shock with 400 watts/sec. and call House Officer.
c. "Slow" ventricular tachycardia with rate less than 120: call House Officer.
d. Ventricular premature beats greater than 6/min, multifocal, R on T of preceding beat or coupled: give Lidocaine as directed above and call House Officer.
e. Ventricular premature beats less than 6/ min: call House Officer.
f. Asystole: Begin cardiopulmonary resuscitation immediately.
g. Severe sinus bradycardia H.R. less than 40: give 0.8 mg Atropine IV push and call House Officer.
h. All other arrhythmias: call House Officer.
2. Comments:

N. COMMENTS

B 089 (1-78) SIC 600
Physician's Signature | Date & Time

---

**UNIVERSITY HOSPITAL**
University of California
Medical Center, San Diego

MYOCARDIAL INFARCTION
PHYSICIAN'S ORDERS
STANDARD ORDERS
Source | Date | Patient Identification

PHYSICIAN: Use ball point pen. Cross-off and initial nonapplicable orders. To reinstate or add additional orders after signing and dating this set, use a blank 151.031, Physician's Orders. EVERY page must be signed and dated.
NURSE: Remove Nursing and Pharmacy copies. Retain Nursing copy. Check drugs needed, then forward Pharmacy copy, whether or not medications are ordered or appear on that page.

ANOTHER GENERICALLY EQUIVALENT BRAND IDENTICAL IN DOSAGE AND CONTENTS OF ACTIVE
INGREDIENT(S) MAY BE DISPENSED AND ADMINISTERED UNLESS A DRUG IS SPECIFIED BY CIRCLING.

F. ACTIONS REQUIRED BY LAB RESULTS
Comments:

G. MEDICATIONS/DRESSINGS/THERAPY
1. Ted hose - remove for 30 min. bid.
2. Routine medications:
a. DOSS (Colace) 100 mg po prn hs
b. Flurazepam 30 mg hs prn.
c. MOM 30 cc hs prn.
3. Oxygen by nasal prongs at ___ L/min.
4. Heparin sodium 5000 units subcutaneously q 12 hr.
5. Other medications:

H. RADIOLOGICAL REQUESTS
1. Portable 6 foot PA chest x-ray on admission if patient able to sit, otherwise portable AP film upright.
2. Comments:

I. NOTIFY PHYSICIAN IF . . .
1. See individual items under Arrhythmia Treatment in Section M. OTHER STATEMENTS REQUIRED BY THE PROCEDURE.
2. Comments:

J. DIET
1. Day 1: 1 gm NA clear liquid diet. All fluids room temperature only. No caffeinated beverages. Bottled H2O only.
2. Day 2: Surgical soft, 1 gm NA, low cholesterol, high polyunsaturated fat diet. No temperature extremes. No caffeine.
3. Day 3: 2 gm Na, otherwise the same as Day 2.
4. Day 4 and on: 2 gm Na, low cholesterol and high polyunsaturated fat. No caffeine.
5. Comments:

K. ACTIVITY/AMBULATION/STIMULATION
1. Activity: [Physician should designate patient as class (1) or (2) below.] Check one:
a. Day 1:     Bed rest with commode for BM only.
b. Day 2: ___ (1) Up in chair once as tolerated.
               ___ (2) Same as Day 1.
c. Day 3: ___ (1) Up in chair bid.
               ___ (2) Up in chair once.
d. Day 4: ___ (1) Up in chair tid.
               ___ (2) Up in chair bid.

B 089 (1-78) SIC 600
Physician's Signature | Date & Time

**Fig. 7.1** Standard CCU orders used at University of California Medical Center, San Diego (UCSD).

The concept of early warning dysrhythmias versus primary ventricular fibrillation is discussed later in this chapter and in Chapter 16.

A large number of electronic monitoring systems of variable technologic sophistication are commercially available. Reliability of operation and convenience to the patient and nursing staff are prime considerations in selecting a system. Detailed discussion of technical details is beyond the scope of this section. The prospective buyer, however, is well advised to investigate in detail the operational characteristics of a monitoring system. Common and unexpected problems encountered with some types of monitoring systems include inability to properly sense a predominantly negative QRS complex, extremely sensitive alarms, and unstable baselines. The most common problem encountered in long-term ECG monitoring is the frequent occurrence of false alarms (usually a high-rate alarm) due to movement artifact. This problem is gradually being solved with the development of improved skin electrodes, recognition of the importance of meticulous skin preparation prior to the application of the electrodes, and improved sophistication of modern electronics which often have the capability to discriminate between artifact and true tachycardia.

At the University of California Medical Center, San Diego, rhythm monitoring is carried out by means of an integrated, hardwire bedside and central station system.[7] The patient's rhythm is displayed at a bedside monitoring oscilloscope which includes a digital rate meter and the appropriate high and low rate alarms (Fig. 7.2). The central station includes a multichannel persistence oscilloscope with a 16-second electronic memory mode to facilitate documentation of the onset of each dysrhythmic episode (Fig. 7.3). A heated stylus electrocardiograph provides hardcopy capability at the

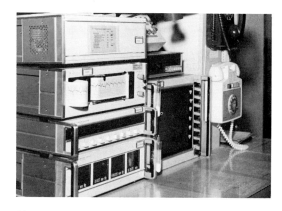

Fig. 7.3 Central Station monitoring equipment includes a 6-channel persistence oscilloscope with 16-second electronic memory, a heated stylus electrocardiograph, and digital readout of selected pressures monitored at bedside.

central station. Rhythm monitoring is carried out by visual inspection of the central station's oscilloscope performed continuously by a nursing staff member.[8,9] The question of computerized vs. visual monitoring techniques is discussed in Chapter 5.

Documentation of the patient's rhythm is performed by the monitoring staff member upon admission of the patient to the unit, every two hours thereafter, and at any time that changes in rhythm occur, ectopy develops, or lead placement is changed. The rhythm strips are analyzed for heart rate, PR, QRS, and QT intervals. The basic rhythm and the type and number of ectopic beats are also documented. All the above data are entered on a form maintained in the patient's rhythm folder at the central station separately from the medical record (Fig. 7.4). Rhythm strips are recorded on each patient at least once every 8 hours or whenever a change in rhythm occurs or ectopy develops. Rhythm strips are mounted and maintained at the central station arrhythmia folder. Visual monitoring by a single member of the nursing staff is advantageous in that it allows other nursing personnel to move about the unit rendering patient care without being obligated to monitor their patient's rhythm. By the same token, rhythm monitoring is a tiring task, and the monitoring person must be relieved regularly. It is now generally accepted that continuous moni-

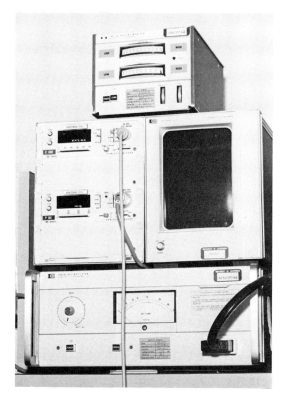

Fig. 7.2 Modular bedside monitoring equipment. This example includes: a two-channel persistence oscilloscope, ECG and pressure amplifiers with digital readouts, an additional pressure amplifier with analog readout and a defibrillator.

| Date Time | Atrial Rate | Ventricular Rate | P-R (.12-.20) | Q-T (.32-.40) | QRS (.06-.10) | PVC (min.) | Arrhythmia | Meds | Lidocaine Quinidine Digoxin Atropine |
|---|---|---|---|---|---|---|---|---|---|
|  |  |  |  |  |  |  |  |  |  |
|  |  |  |  |  |  |  |  |  |  |
|  |  |  |  |  |  |  |  |  |  |
|  |  |  |  |  |  |  |  |  |  |
|  |  |  |  |  |  |  |  |  |  |
|  |  |  |  |  |  |  |  |  |  |
|  |  |  |  |  |  |  |  |  |  |
|  |  |  |  |  |  |  |  |  |  |
|  |  |  |  |  |  |  |  |  |  |
|  |  |  |  |  |  |  |  |  |  |
|  |  |  |  |  |  |  |  |  |  |
|  |  |  |  |  |  |  |  |  |  |
|  |  |  |  |  |  |  |  |  |  |
|  |  |  |  |  |  |  |  |  |  |
|  |  |  |  |  |  |  |  |  |  |
|  |  |  |  |  |  |  |  |  |  |
|  |  |  |  |  |  |  |  |  |  |
|  |  |  |  |  |  |  |  |  |  |
|  |  |  |  |  |  |  |  |  |  |
|  |  |  |  |  |  |  |  |  |  |

D 081 (11-77) SIC 600

Fig. 7.4  Rhythm monitoring documentation form used at UCSD.

tor surveillance is nearly impossible, even in the best organized and staffed CCUs.[10] Estimates of effective visual monitor surveillance range from 20 to 50 percent of monitoring time. As the number of patients being monitored increases, the demands on the monitoring person also increase, and distractions must be minimized. The monitoring person should not be required to answer telephones or be responsible for additional paperwork. A unit secretary or ward clerk is invaluable in handling telephone calls and paperwork, and in directing traffic. Accuracy and detailed notation of rhythm changes are mandatory to insure proper intervention when a dysrhythmia develops and to document dysrhythmias which required treatment.

Electrocardiographic monitoring commonly requires three chest electrodes. These are usually placed on the two infraclavicular areas and over the right sternal edge away from large muscle masses in an effort to minimize muscle artifact. In this configuration, a modified limb lead

I or limb lead II is obtainable. We prefer to use a modified lead V1 (MCL-1), as advocated by Marriott, since this lead usually provides good P waves for dysrhythmia analysis, as well as a QRS complex which can be easily analyzed for the presence of intraventricular conduction defects.[11] An additional advantage of this lead configuration is its flexibility. If additional electrodes are placed in position V6 or on the left subcostal area, the change of the positive lead to these positions instantaneously provides a modified lead V6 (MCL-6) and a modified lead III (M-III), respectively (Fig. 7.5). Frequently, monitor strips will not provide adequate basis for the diagnosis of a complex dysrhythmia, and a 12-lead electrocardiogram (preferably with a multichannel machine) will be necessary.[12] Occasionally, special leads, such as a modified Lewis lead or an esophageal lead, are necessary to identify atrial activity. The modified Lewis lead is a bipolar lead I with the right arm electrode on the manubrium and the left arm electrode at the right sternal border in the fourth or fifth interspace.

It is the practice in the CCU of the University of California Medical Center, San Diego, to obtain a standard 12-lead electrocardiogram im-

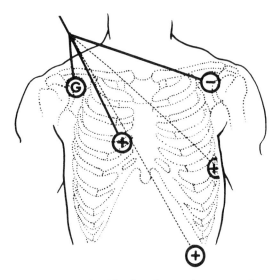

Fig. 7.5  ECG lead hookup for continuous monitoring with MCL-1 (solid lines) and alternative placement of electrodes to monitor MCL-6 or M-III (dashed lines) according to Marriott.[11] (By permission of the American Heart Association, Inc. and the author.)

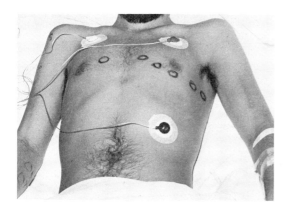

Fig. 7.6 Torso of patient being monitored via lead MIII and showing chest wall markings for accurate positioning of six standard precordial lead electrodes.

mediately upon admission to the unit and routinely every morning during the patient's stay in the unit. Additional 12-lead ECGs are obtained any time the patient complains of new onset chest pain or when changes are noted on the monitor suggesting alterations in intraventricular conduction. The ECGs are cut and mounted on a standard ECG board and kept in the arrhythmia folder at the central nursing station. When the patient is transferred out of the CCU, copies of these ECGs are placed in the patient's record. To avoid apparent changes due to precordial lead misplacement, the patient's anterior chest wall is marked with a felt-tip pen localizing the position of V1 to V6, thus insuring constant lead placement while the patient is in the unit (Fig. 7.6).

The need for constant rhythm monitoring, chest markings, etc., as well as the general concept of coronary care are explained to the patient and his family in simple terms as soon after admission as practicable. A reference booklet covering the salient features of coronary care and unit policy is provided to the patient and has been found to be a valuable aid in promoting understanding and allaying anxiety.[13]

## DIET

During the first 24 hours after admission, diet is limited to clear liquids containing no more than 1 g of sodium. Fluid intake is limited to between 1500 ml and 2000 ml for the first 24 hours to maintain urinary output of 800 to 1000 ml. The main purpose of the clear liquid diet is to minimize the risk of aspiration, should a cardiac arrest develop and resuscitation be required. Since this explanation may well be too unsettling for the patient, the alternative explanation that liquids require less work in consuming and digestion is a reasonable one and is usually well accepted by patients. It has been customary to offer the patient only tepid liquids avoiding extremes of temperature. However, recent studies have shown that hot and cold liquids in the immediate postinfarction period do not produce deleterious effects.[14] If the patient is nauseated—as is often the case following acute inferior myocardial infarction or as a result of narcotic analgesic administration—oral intake of fluids is limited and an intravenous infusion of 1500 ml of 5 percent glucose in normal saline is substituted.

In the patient with uncomplicated myocardial infarction, diet is advanced to a soft, low-sodium, low-cholesterol, balanced polyunsaturated/saturated fat diet on the second day. Patients with coronary atherosclerotic disease are often in need of dietary reeducation. Their initial stay in a CCU often provides the necessary motivation to learn and adhere to such a diet. The services of a good dietitian are utilized to help with patient instruction and eventually develop a regular diet which the patient will be able to follow after discharge. Obviously, the elderly patient sustaining a second or third infarct or the patient who is not overweight and whose lipid profile is in the normal range need not be made to adhere to a rigid diet. If, by day four postinfarction, the patient continues to pursue an uncomplicated course, his diet should be advanced to a regular one with sodium and fat restrictions as outlined above.

It has been customary to delay measurement of serum cholesterol and triglycerides, as these lipid values are often altered during the acute phase of a myocardial infarction and reliable measurements cannot be obtained until the convalescent phase. One recent study, however, indicated that the reduction in serum lipid levels which is often seen in the acute phase of myocardial infarction occurred approximately 36 hours after the onset of symptoms.[15] According to this study, serum lipid levels obtained the morning after the development of the acute infarction correlated well with those measured three months later. It appears reasonable, therefore, to obtain the patient's lipid phenotype soon after admission to the CCU and to tailor his subsequent diet accordingly.

Coffee and tea are not included in the diet of patients while in the CCU because of the positive chronotropic and inotropic effects of methylated xanthines and their potential for the production of dysrhythmias.[16] Decaffeinated coffee is allowed with meals. The use of tobacco in the CCU is strictly prohibited. Patients with acute myocardial infarction must discontinue the use of tobacco because of the acute circulatory response to cigarette smoking which commonly results in mobilization of catecholamines. Additionally, the long-term use of cigarettes has been clearly implicated as an important risk factor in the development of atherosclerotic vascular disease.[17] Since most patients in the CCU are receiving narcotic analgesics and/or tranquilizers, there is little tendency to complain about the lack of cigarettes. In fact, the immediate postinfarction period while the patient is confined in the CCU may, be the optimal time to eliminate the tobacco habit. Alcoholic beverages are usually denied to patients in the CCU and during subsequent hospitalization. However, there is no clear medical reason why small amounts of alcohol should not be permitted to carefully selected patients. A common-sense approach must be utilized.

## HEPARIN LOCK

All patients in the CCU must have a patent intravenous line for the administration of emergency and nonemergency medications. In fact, all parenteral medications are routinely administered intravenously while the patient is in the CCU. The use of a "heparin lock" has been found to have distinct advantages in the CCU patient. A #18G short plastic cannula (Angiocath and others) is usually inserted under strict aseptic precautions in a peripheral vein of the lower arm, avoiding the antecubital fossa and the area of the wrist in order to allow the patient full range of motion of his extremities. A 3-way stopcock is placed at the end of the cannula, and the openings are covered with Luer lock caps to maintain sterility. At the time the line is established, it is flushed with 2 ml of heparin flush solution, which is prepared in the pharmacy according to the standing orders (Fig. 7.1, item D3). The flush process is repeated every four hours, each time after a medication has been given, and after each collection of blood samples.

The heparin lock is a painless means of obtaining the multiple blood samples required in the CCU patient.[18] To obtain a blood sample, a tourniquet is applied to the arm above the cannula site and 2 ml of blood are withdrawn and discarded. The discarding of blood is necessary to prevent dilution of collected samples by the heparin flush solution remaining in the cannula. Clotting studies (prothrombin time, platelets, and partial thromboplastin time) are never drawn from the heparin lock because of the risk of contamination of the sample by the heparin in the flush solution.

Heparin locks are changed every three days to minimize the risk of phlebitis,[19] or more often if there is local tenderness, if the patient complains of any discomfort, or if phlebitis is suspected. The cannula site is redressed aseptically every day and an antimicrobial ointment such as Betadine ointment is applied to the skin puncture site. With this technique, the patient has freedom from connecting tubings and the risk of an inadvertent fluid overload is avoided, while at the same time an intravenous portal of entry is always available.

## BEDREST/ACTIVITY

Few topics have generated more controversy over the years than the topic of activity allowed the patient hospitalized with acute myocardial infarction. The abuse of absolute bedrest was emphasized by Samuel Levine and Bernard Lown in their classic paper on the chair treatment of coronary thrombosis.[20] Since then, there has occurred a gradual shortening of both length of bedrest and length of hospital stay for myocardial infarction patients. Recent studies have shown that uncomplicated cases may be discharged as early as one week after acute myocardial infarction,[21] with a low incidence of late serious complications at six months followup. At the University of California Medical Center, San Diego, patients with acute myocardial infarction are admitted and kept in the CCU for three to five days or for at least 48 hours after their last major complication. Following discharge from the CCU, patients are transferred to an intermediate care unit with rhythm monitoring continuing by means of radiotelemetry transmitters. Patients with transmural uncomplicated myocardial infarctions are discharged from the hospital 12 to 14 days after admission, whereas patients with uncomplicated nontransmural myocardial infarctions are kept only 8 to 10 days.

Upon admission to the coronary care unit, all patients are maintained on modified bedrest in accordance with the physician's classification designated in the standing orders (Fig. 7.1, item K). While on this regimen, the patient is instructed by the nursing staff to use the footboard and to perform deep-breathing and coughing exercises. The nursing staff performs passive range-of-motion extremity exercises when the patient is unable or too ill to do so himself. Antiemboli stockings (Tedhose) are applied and removed for 30 minutes twice daily. Daily weights are obtained initially by lifting the patient onto a bedside scale. This places minimal demands on the patient; more importantly, it allows the nursing staff to control and safely maintain indwelling lines or catheters. Usually by the third postinfarction day, the uncomplicated patient can be assisted to a standing scale at the bedside after a period of sitting sit up with his legs dangling over the edge of the bed. Except for patients in cardiogenic shock, all patients are permitted and encouraged to utilize the bedside commode for bowel movements from day one. The patient is assisted but not lifted onto the commode. It has been clearly shown that use of a bedside commode offers distinct advantages, as it is less strenuous and less likely to induce vagal stimulation that frequently occurs with the use of the bedpan.[22]

In the absence of cardiogenic shock, severe heart failure, postural hypotension, serious ventricular dysrhythmias, or advanced heart block, the patient is assisted and allowed to sit in a comfortable bedside chair on day two of the CCU hopitalization. It has been found that comfort is enhanced if patients sit on a highback chair with armrests and their feet are propped up on a foot stool. Patients are instructed never to cross their legs at the knees or ankles. The length of time out of bed increases progressively and is dependent upon the patient's response and development of fatigue. General guidelines for out-of-bed activity are listed in the standing orders (Fig. 7.1, item K).

From day two, the patient with uncomplicated myocardial infarction is allowed such personal activities as feeding himself, washing his hands and face, shaving with an electric shaver, and brushing his teeth. Bathing and brushing of hair are carried out by the nursing staff through day three, and then the patient is assisted with these activities. The subject of postmyocardial infarction ambulation and exercise is treated more extensively in Chapter 38.

## ANTIARRHYTHMIC THERAPY— PROPHYLACTIC OR FOR INDICATIONS?

It is generally accepted that the most common cause of death in human myocardial infarction is the development of cardiac arrhythmias. As a result, the focus of coronary care during the past 15 years has been directed to the area of arrhythmia prevention and treatment. The initial studies of Lown [23] clearly demonstrated a marked reduction of ventricular arrhythmias by the use of antiarrhythmic agents, primarily lidocaine. Aggressive approaches to rhythm management in the CCU have been associated with a reduction of the in-hospital mortality below 20 percent [24] and a stated goal of further reduction of in-hospital CCU mortality to less than 10 percent.[5,25]

It was initially suggested that all patients who experienced ventricular fibrillation or other life-threatening ventricular arrhythmias in a setting of acute myocardial infarction had premonitory or "warning arrhythmias"—for example, frequent premature ventricular contractions (PVCs), multiform or multifocal ventricular beats, PVCs demonstrating the R-on-T phenomenon, or couplets or short runs of ventricular tachycardia.[23] Furthermore, the thrust of Lown's investigation was that these premonitory arrhythmias could be suppressed with subsequent complete prevention of ventricular fibrillation. Treatment protocols utilizing lidocaine were subsequently developed and widely used in CCUs.[26,27] The protocol outlined in Fig. 7.1, item M, is based on these observations.

More recently, the concept of "warning ventricular arrhythmias" has been investigated and, as a result, seriously questioned. Recent studies indicate that, although many episodes of ventricular fibrillation are preceded by "warning arrhythmias," approximately 25 to 50 percent of patients in the CCU demonstrate no warning arrhythmias before their first episode of ventricular fibrillation.[28,29] Furthermore, Dhurandar et al. pointed out that, during the initial 12 hours after myocardial infarction, fewer instances of warning arrhythmias were recorded and the time interval from the first such arrhythmia to ventricular fibrillation was much shorter—frequently only a matter of minutes.[28] In addition, the significance of the R-on-T phenomenon has recently been questioned. Roberts et al. reported that repetitive ventricular activity was initiated more often by late rather than by early PVCs.[30]

A number of recent studies have investigated the efficacy and reliability of visual monitoring in detecting arrhythmias in the coronary care unit. Romhilt et al. compared the detection of arrhythmias by the nursing staff of their coronary care unit with those recorded on magnetic tape and analyzed by a computer system, with the computer analysis subsequently validated by physician review.[31] It is of interest that the computer system detected 97 percent of premature ventricular contractions, as opposed to only 45 percent detected by the coronary care unit staff. The corresponding figures for serious ventricular arrhythmias were 93 and 16 percent, respectively. Similar discrepancies between automated and visual arrhythmia detection have been recorded by other investigators.[32,33]

These observations have led to the conclusions that (1) during the first 48 hours after acute myocardial infarction, 95 to 100 percent of patients demonstrate some evidence of ventricular ectopy, and (2) only 50 to 75 percent of such patients have "warning arrhythmias," and less than half of these are detected by the staff of a conventional CCU.[34] These findings have led a number of investigators and physicians to recommend the routine administration of lidocaine prophylaxis in patients hospitalized after acute myocardial infarction.[4,34,35] In a double-blind randomized study of 212 consecutive patients, Lie and coworkers supported this view by demonstrating a definite reduction in the incidence of primary ventricular fibrillation in patients treated prophylactically with adequate doses of lidocaine, compared with those not so treated.[36] In previous studies which failed to demonstrate a salutary effect from prophylactic lidocaine, inadequate doses of the drug were probably employed.[37,38] In the study of Lie et al., side effects occurred in 16 out of 107 patients receiving lidocaine. These adverse reactions were limited to central nervous system symptoms and included drowsiness, numbness of the tongue and lips, speech disturbances, and dizziness. It was necessary to halve the rate of lidocaine infusion in seven of the 16 patients. Other investigators have reported focal and grand-mal seizures and even respiratory arrest occurring as complications of lidocaine therapy, especially when the plasma levels exceeded 9 $\mu$g/ml, with the usual therapeutic level being 1.4 to 6.0 $\mu$g/ml.[39] The pharmacokinetics and current recommendations regarding lidocaine dosage and administration are discussed in detail in Chapter 14.

Despite the favorable reports cited above, a note of caution must be sounded. In general, the routine use of any prophylactic agent must be based on incontrovertible evidence of its efficacy. Additional, carefully designed clinical trials of routine lidocaine administration must be carried out to determine whether the data obtained by Lie et al. are reproducible. Although side effects from lidocaine administration may be minimized by determining plasma levels and following recommendations to reduce dosage by half in the presence of shock, heart failure, and hepatocellular disease, it can be expected that, with routine lidocaine use, the incidence of its side effects will increase. Therefore, it appears prudent to reserve decision as to the use of prophylactic lidocaine based on local policy and personnel considerations. It has been stated that the need for prophylactic antiarrhythmic drug administration is inversely proportional to the sophistication of the therapeutic environment.[40] In many large CCUs where adequate staffing and large numbers of highly trained personnel, including house officers, are available, it may not be necessary or even prudent to use prophylactic lidocaine routinely in the treatment of uncomplicated acute myocardial infarction.[41]

In addition to the above-cited considerations of lidocaine's efficacy in preventing primary ventricular fibrillation as well the side effects of this agent, other factors enter into a decision of whether to treat all patients admitted to the CCU with lidocaine routinely or not. It has been shown that the risk of primary ventricular fibrillation is highest during the first four hours following the onset of myocardial infarction, being many times greater at this time than between four and 12 hours.[42] For this reason, patients admitted to a CCU several hours after the onset of chest pain may well be beyond the most critical period for the occurrence of primary ventricular fibrillation and, therefore, may not require routine antiarrhythmic prophylaxis. Similarly, it has been suggested by some investigators [36] that primary ventricular fibrillation occurs less commonly in patients over 70 years of age who develop acute myocardial infarction. Patients in this age group, therefore, could be reasonably excluded from a routine antiarrhythmic prophylaxis protocol. Finally, decision as to the use of a routine antiarrhythmic prophylactic regimen will depend upon the relative proportion of proven acute myocardial infarctions among all CCU admissions. Using antiarrhythmic prophylaxis in all patients admitted to the CCU for possible myocardial infarction will result in its administra-

tion to many patients who are later found not to have had an infarct. It has been argued that, since many of these patients do have unstable ischemic heart disease and are at high risk for the development of ventricular arrhythmias, the administration of lidocaine is not detrimental.[34] Nevertheless, in our opinion, the unnecessary administration of a drug may introduce serious therapeutic and ethical problems.

In summary, there is definite accumulating evidence that the concept of "warning arrhythmias" in patients with acute myocardial infarction leaves much to be desired and that the prophylactic administration of lidocaine may be the preferred mode of treatment. The evidence, however, is not totally convincing and additional studies are eagerly awaited. Furthermore, it is important to keep in mind that when lidocaine is administered—whether prophylactically or for specific indications—it should be administered in accordance with current recommendations based on the recently understood pharmacokinetic principles of distribution.[34,39] For additional discussion of this issue, see Chapters 14 and 16.

## ANALGESICS AND SEDATIVES

Immediate relief of the pain and anxiety associated with acute myocardial infarction remains a prime mode of therapy. Although most patients will have received some analgesic medication by the time they are admitted to the CCU, many of them will have recurrent or residual chest discomfort, as discussed in Chapter 8. Furthermore, most patients experience intense anxiety—resulting both from their symptoms and from their recognition of the implications of the suspected diagnosis. The term "impending doom" aptly describes the feelings of discomfort and anxiety experienced by many patients with acute myocardial infarction. Morphine sulfate, therefore, continues to be the drug of choice for the initial treatment of pain and anxiety of acute myocardial infarction.[4,35,43]

It is important to recognize that, in many patients early during the course of acute myocardial infarction, there exists a state of autonomic nervous system imbalance.[44] This may result in either parasympathetic overactivity associated with bradycardia and hypotension or with sympathetic overactivity characterized by tachycardia and mild hypertension. The choice of analgesic will depend to some extent on the presence or absence of these autonomic nervous system syndromes. It is well recognized that pain and anxiety can produce coronary arterial spasm, as well as stimulate secretion of catecholamines which further increase heart rate, cardiac output, cardiac work, and, in fact, may precipitate lethal dysrhythmias.[45] It is for these reasons that prompt treatment of pain and anxiety is indicated. In the presence of parasympathetic nervous system overactivity with bradycardia and hypotension, morphine sulfate—a parasympathomimetic agent—should be given with caution if at all. In this clinical situation, it has been recommended that atropine be administered in conjunction with morphine sulfate or that meperidine—a vagolytic agent—be substituted. Conversely, in the presence of sympathetic overactivity associated with anxiety, tachycardia, and hypertension, morphine sulfate will effectively combat this syndrome.

Morphine sulfate has been found to be remarkably well tolerated by patients with coronary artery disease. In fact, large doses of intravenous morphine sulfate have been widely utilized to provide profound analgesia during cardiac surgery, precisely because of the lack of circulatory depression.[46] In a clinical study of patients with chronic stable angina undergoing surgery, measurements were taken of right and left heart pressures, cardiac output, and vascular resistances during incremental intravenous morphine administration.[47] The results indicated that morphine, administered intravenously in doses of up to 2 mg/kg, was well tolerated with no significant increase in left and right ventricular filling pressures while reductions in heart rate and rate-pressure product were documented. On the negative side, morphine often decreases alveolar ventilation, increases right-to-left shunting, and decreases arterial oxygen tension.[4] Focal atelectasis and ventilation-perfusion abnormalities may occur because of the reduction in the rate and depth of respiration resulting from the direct depres-

sant effect of morphine on the brain stem respiratory centers.[48] Furthermore, morphine has been reported to produce hypotension through venous and arteriolar dilatation and pooling of blood in the venous capacitance system.[49] For these reasons, morphine is best administered in small doses, which can be repeated as necessary, in preference to a single large dose. It is good to remember that, in acute myocardial infarction, the minimal dose of morphine that will produce the desired analgesic effect should be used. Current recommendations are to administer several small increments of morphine in doses of 2 to 4 mg. Since the peak effect of intravenously administered morphine occurs within 20 minutes,[50] the patient may be titrated to the appropriate level of analgesia with less risk of respiratory depression.

The most bothersome side effects of morphine relate to the nauseant and emetic actions it produces by stimulating the chemoreceptor trigger zone. Morphine-induced nausea and vomiting may be minimized by the concomitant administration of 0.5 to 0.8 mg of atropine intravenously, or the administration of a phenothiazine compound. Great care, however, should be exercised because of the synergistic effect of phenothiazines and narcotic analgesics. Similarly, the effect of morphine on smooth muscle often enhances the urinary bladder sphincter tone and may result in urinary retention, which in turn may require catheterization for relief. Certain groups of patients are particularly sensitive to morphine administration, and special care must be exercised in administering this drug. This is particularly true of patients with severe chronic obstructive pulmonary disease, who may prove to be more sensitive to the respiratory depressant action of the drug. Similarly, older patients, and especially those on chronic diuretic therapy who may be volume depleted, may evidence a significant hypotensive reaction to the intravenous administration of morphine and must be carefully observed. The duration of action of morphine may be prolonged in patients with hepatocellular dysfunction, since inactivation of the drug occurs by conjugation in the liver.

Other drugs have been used for the relief of the pain and anxiety of acute myocardial infarction. Heroin has been reported to be an excellent such drug, but it is currently not available for prescription in the United States.[51] Meperidine (Demerol) has also been used; but, according to general experience, it is much less effective in relieving the severe discomfort and anxiety of acute myocardial infarction. Because of its vagolytic properties, meperidine may be advantageous in the patient with diaphragmatic myocardial infarction and associated sinus bradycardia. However, it is our preference in this situation to administer morphine in combination with atropine. When meperidine hydrochloride is administered parenterally, a dose of 75 mg provides analgesia approximately equivalent to 8 to 10 mg of morphine sulfate.

Since its introduction in 1967, pentazocine lactate (Talwin) was promoted as a safe and effective drug for control of pain in acute myocardial infarction, devoid of the potential hypotensive effects associated with the use of other narcotic agents. However, several studies indicate that pentazocine may elevate left ventricular filling pressures and raise systemic vascular resistance, resulting in increased myocardial oxygen requirements, a distinctly detrimental action in the face of ongoing myocardial ischemia.[52]

Nalbuphine-HCl is a new analgesic drug recently released and promoted for use in acute myocardial infarction. The advantages of this agent, when compared to morphine, are absence of cardiac depressant effects and lower incidence of respiratory depression and vomiting. At this time, available data do not allow a firm judgment on the merits of nalbuphine-HCl as an analgesic agent.

If a patient remains restless and anxious following relief of chest pain, mild sedation during the first 24 to 48 hours after admission is indicated and often necessary. The currently preferred sedative is diazepam (Valium). This drug is preferable to barbiturates because of its lesser CNS depressant action and the fact that it does not interfere with warfarin action. In addition, hemodynamic studies have indicated that diazepam reduces left ventricular filling pressure and systemic arterial pressure, thereby exerting a beneficial effect on depressed left ventricular function.[53] Other studies have concluded that

diazepam given intravenously reduces excretion of catecholamines and may in fact diminish the incidence of ventricular arrhythmias in the setting of acute myocardial infarction.[54] In the absence of hypotension and mental confusion, 5 to 10 mg of diazepam given orally three times a day has proven to be an effective tranquilizer. Flurazepam (Dalmane), a related compound, may be used as a bedtime hypnotic in doses of 15 to 30 mg orally.

In summary, morphine sulfate in small, incremental intravenous doses remains the analgesic drug of choice in a setting of acute myocardial infarction. In general, its hemodynamic effects are beneficial. Respiratory depression and hypotension can be minimized by using the smallest dose possible to achieve adequate analgesia. Certain groups of patients who may be more prone to exhibit exaggerated respiratory or hemodynamic responses must be treated with caution. The intravenous route of administration provides the most rapid and reliable onset of action and avoids the uncertainty of absorption from intramuscular or subcutaneous injections. Diazepam is an effective tranquilizing agent with apparently beneficial hemodynamic and metabolic effects in a setting of acute myocardial infarction. Finally, one should keep in mind that opiates and sedatives should be administered with great care to confused and restless patients who are suffering from CNS dysfunction due to hypotension or heart failure. The use of nitrous oxide analgesia in acute myocardial infarction is covered in the appendix to this chapter.

## ANTICOAGULANT THERAPY

The use of anticoagulant agents in acute myocardial infarction remains controversial 31 years after Irving Wright and coworkers reported the results of the first major clinical trial conducted for the American Heart Association.[55] In that landmark study, it was reported that anticoagulants apparently reduced the case fatality rate from 24 percent in the control to 50 percent in the treatment group, and that the thromboembolic complication rate was similarly reduced from 36 to 14 percent.

Although major problems existed with the statistical design of this study, its conclusions resulted in the widespread acceptance of anticoagulant therapy in acute myocardial infarction.

During the subsequent two decades, numerous studies were reported concerning the effectiveness of anticoagulant drugs in acute myocardial infarction. The reported results have been conflicting. Gifford and Feinstein [56] in 1969 reviewed 32 previous reports relating to the use of anticoagulation in myocardial infarction published between 1948 and 1966. The adequacy of the experimental protocol, methodology, and statistics was evaluated in detail. They concluded that none of the 32 studies reviewed fulfilled the criteria established by the reviewers for statistical and scientific accuracy. Furthermore, those studies demonstrating beneficial effects of anticoagulant therapy were reported to have fulfilled fewer of the reviewers' criteria than those demonstrating that anticoagulants had no effect.

More recently, two large-scale trials with improved experimental design have been reported. In the multicenter study by the Working Party of the British Medical Research Council [57] results were compared in 1,427 patients with acute myocardial infarction who were randomly assigned to one of two treatment groups: One group was treated with heparin plus phenindione, while the other was given phenindione alone. The conclusions of the study were that, although the death rates were similar in the two groups, clinically recognized thromboembolic phenomena were clearly reduced in the group of patients who had been treated with heparin. Similarly, in the Veterans Administration Cooperative Study [58] of 999 men with acute myocardial infarction, no significant reduction in mortality rate was observed among anticoagulated patients. However, clinical thromboembolic events (both pulmonary and systemic) and necropsy evidence of fatal embolization were significantly reduced in the anticoagulated patients when compared with the controls. Furthermore, two recent large studies which employed historical controls with attempted matching [59,60] reported significant decreases in case fatality rates in the patients treated with anticoagulants. Chalmers et al.,[61]

in 1977, again reviewed the published reports of clinical trials investigating the use of anticoagulant agents in acute myocardial infarction. Pooling of the results of all randomized controlled trials reviewed resulted in a case fatality rate of 19.6 percent for the controls and 15.4 percent for the anticoagulant-treated group, giving a relative reduction of mortality rate of 21 percent. These investigators commented on the marked preponderance of positive (beneficial) results of anticoagulant therapy, and suggested that significant differences in favor of anticoagulant therapy were apparently too small to be revealed by any but the largest of the individual trials. It was, therefore, concluded that patients who presented no specific contraindication should receive anticoagulant therapy during hospitalization for acute myocardial infarction.

Many reasons have been cited for the conflicting results reported in the numerous clinical trials of anticoagulant therapy in myocardial infarction: (1) In some studies, experimental design was inadequate and sample size was small.[56,61] (2) In other studies, anticoagulation was inadequate and the laboratory control of anticoagulant therapy was performed with inadequate thromboplastins.[62] (3) Although thromboembolism has a high prevalence rate in the postmyocardial infarction period, the associated morbidity and mortality are low;[63] therefore, factors affecting the development of thromboembolic complications are not appropriately reflected in the case fatality rates of the clinical studies. (4) Finally, it must be kept in mind that the early studies on the efficacy of anticoagulant therapy in acute myocardial infarction were conducted at a time when other aspects of therapy were changing profoundly. This is particularly true with respect to length of bedrest and immobilization after acute myocardial infarction.[64]

## Rationale for the Use of Anticoagulant Therapy

The classical reasons advanced in support of the use of anticoagulant therapy in acute myocardial infarction are: (1) prevention of peripheral venous thrombosis with subsequent pulmonary embolization; (2) prevention of mural thrombus formation with subsequent systemic embolization; (3) prevention of extension of myocardial necrosis and reduction of long-term recurrences of myocardial infarction, and (4) reduction of myocardial infarction-related mortality.

The recent development of [125]I-labeled fibrinogen scanning of the lower-extremity veins for evidence of peripheral thrombosis has greatly extended the ability to diagnose subclinical or early thrombus formation. The incidence of deep leg vein thrombosis after acute myocardial infarction has been reported to range from 32 to 37 percent [64] when the [125]I-fibrinogen scanning technique is used. The incidence of postoperative deep vein thrombosis has been reported to be in the same range.[65] By contrast, patients with suspected myocardial infarction who are admitted to a coronary care unit but proven not to have sustained myocardial damage appear to develop this complication at a much lower rate. Murray and coworkers [66] investigated 50 patients admitted with chest pain, with the diagnosis of myocardial infarction being confirmed in 35. The incidence of deep vein thrombosis was 34 percent in the infarction group and only 7 percent in the group who turned out not to have an infarct. It has been suggested that the higher incidence of deep vein thrombosis in the infarct group may be the result of a hypercoagulable state which may develop in the postmyocardial infarction period. An alternative explanation is that, in certain patients with an acute myocardial infarction, cardiac output is depressed and venous stasis contributes to the formation of deep leg vein thrombosis. In support of this latter theory are the findings that the incidence of deep leg vein thrombosis increases to 40 to 50 percent in the presence of left ventricular failure and rises to 50 or 60 percent in the presence of cardiogenic shock.[67] Other factors associated with a higher incidence of leg vein thrombosis in the postmyocardial infarction period are preexisting angina pectoris, age over 70, obesity, varicose veins, and a prior history of myocardial infarction or thromboembolism.[67] These observations, therefore, suggest that it may be possible to identify a high-risk subgroup of patients in whom anti-

coagulation would be particularly beneficial and effective in preventing deep leg vein thrombosis. A number of studies have convincingly substantiated that anticoagulant therapy in the postmyocardial infarction period is highly effective in preventing deep leg vein thrombosis and in reducing clinical pulmonary thromboembolic complications.[55,57,58,68,69]

Embolization from a ventricular mural thrombus to arteries of the extremities, brain, or kidneys usually constitutes a dramatic clinical event which is much easier to recognize than pulmonary embolism. Although the mechanism of thrombogenesis in the arterial side of the circulation is thought to be different from that in the venous system,[70] a number of clinical studies have demonstrated a significant reduction in the incidence of systemic thromboembolic complications with the use of anticoagulant therapy. Thus, the British Working Party study [57] documented a 3.4 percent incidence of systemic embolization in the phenindione-treated group, while the incidence was only 1.3 percent among those who were treated with a combination of heparin and phenindione. In the cooperative Veterans Administration trial,[58] anticoagulant therapy reduced the total number of clinical cerebrovascular accidents from 3.8 percent in the control group to 0.8 percent in the treated group. There were no emboli to the kidneys or lower extremities among the treated patients, although the incidence of systemic embolization was 0.6 percent in the untreated patients. Anticoagulation also reduced by half the frequency of mural thrombi and peripheral emboli found at necropsy.

In contrast to the fairly convincing evidence cited above regarding the effects of anticoagulant therapy on the incidence of pulmonary and systemic thromboembolic complications, no good evidence exists to support the thesis that anticoagulant therapy prevents the extension of myocardial necrosis or reduces the reinfarction rate. In both the British Working Party study and the Veterans Administration cooperative trial,[57,58] the incidence of both in-hospital and late reinfarction was the same for both anticoagulated and control groups. In a recent experimental study, however, Saliba et al.[71] found that heparin in large doses (60,000 units) reduced the extent of ischemic injury after acute coronary occlusion in the dog. This conclusion was reached by demonstrating significant reductions in ST segment elevation levels and myocardial creatine kinase depletion after heparin administration. In a subsequent *clinical* study, however, heparin in the usual anticoagulant doses failed to modify cardiac enzyme levels.[72] The entire question, therefore, of heparin efficacy in modifying acute ischemic injury still remains under study.

As outlined earlier in this section, the efficacy of anticoagulants in reducing in-hospital mortality following acute myocardial infarction has remained controversial. The best designed prospective studies failed to demonstrate reduction in short-term mortality rates. The two recent retrospective studies [59,60] and the most recent reevaluation of previously reported studies [61] have again fanned the controversy. Firm conclusions appear destined to remain elusive; it has been calculated by Wessler [73] that, because of the low mortality rate from thromboembolism after myocardial infarction, a sample population of 38,000 would be required to demonstrate a statistically significant effect of anticoagulant therapy on total mortality. It appears highly unlikely that a study of this magnitude can now be undertaken.

## Complications of Anticoagulant Therapy

The major complication of conventional anticoagulation with heparin and/or warfarin is hemorrhage. The risk of hemorrhage must, therefore, be weighed against any advantageous effects that anticoagulants may bring to play in reducing the incidence of deep vein thrombosis, pulmonary embolism, and systemic arterial embolism following acute myocardial infarction. The magnitude of this risk cannot be easily determined from published reports. Investigators have used widely varying anticoagulant regimens, have monitored anticoagulant effects with different laboratory procedures (some nonstandardized), and have maintained variable levels of anticoagulation. The issue is further complicated by evidence suggesting that USP heparin is 10 to 15 percent more potent than

heparin whose activity is measured in international units.[63] Studies conducted in the United States, therefore, are not strictly comparable to European and Canadian studies.

In most studies, patients with preexisting hemorrhagic diathesis, gastrointestinal ulcer disease, severe systemic hypertension, malignancy, or hepatic disease, and those over age 70 were excluded from anticoagulation. This selection process appears to reduce the danger of serious hemorrhage. In the Veterans Administration cooperative trial,[58] major gastrointestinal hemorrhage occurred in 0.6 percent of both groups with no resultant mortality. The British Working Party study [57] found clinical evidence of major hemorrhagic complications in 4.3 percent of patients receiving both heparin and phenindione, and in only 1.1 percent in patients receiving phenindione alone. At necropsy, the incidence of hemopericardium, subintimal hemorrhage, and hemorrhagic infarction was the same in both study groups. Nevertheless, it is common practice to withhold anticoagulant therapy for a day or two when a pericardial friction rub develops in an anticoagulated postinfarction patient. Microscopic hematuria is the commonest form of hemorrhage caused by anticoagulant therapy and is usually of little clinical importance. Other hemorrhagic complications which have been reported include bleeding in the skin and muscles, bleeding in the intestinal wall with resulting intestinal obstruction, adrenal hemorrhage, spontaneous subdural hematoma, and spontaneous retroperitoneal bleeding.[62] Although the incidence of hemorrhagic complications is relatively low, it is a matter of some concern that laboratory control of anticoagulant therapy is not totally reliable. Bleeding complications of conventional (full)-dose heparin therapy were reported to correlate poorly with the results of conventional laboratory tests.[74] As a result, controversy continues as to which is the most appropriate test for laboratory control of heparin therapy.[64]

An additional major difficulty with anticoagulant therapy is the large number of drug interactions one is bound to encounter during anticoagulation with oral warfarin. Although the subject of drug interactions is treated extensively in Chapter 40, Table 7.1 lists drugs and

**Table 7.1   Pathophysiologic and Pharmacologic Interactions of Warfarin**

| A. Potentiation of Warfarin Effects | B. Antagonism of Warfarin Effects |
|---|---|
| Alcohol | Antacids |
| Allopurinol | Barbiturates |
| Anabolic steroids | Cholestyramine |
| Antibiotics (especially oral broad-spectrum) | Chlordiazepoxide |
| | Corticosteroids |
| Chlorpropamide | Diabetes mellitus |
| Clofibrate | Griseofulvin |
| Congestive heart failure | Haloperidol |
| Diarrhea | Hereditary resistance to warfarin |
| Fever | High vitamin K diet |
| Hepatobiliary disease (hepatitis, obstructive jaundice) | Hyperlipidemia |
| High temperature environment | Hypothyroidism |
| Indomethacin | Massive edema |
| Phenylbutazone | Meprobamate |
| Propylthiouracil | Mineral oil |
| Salicylates | Multivitamin preparations |
| Tolbutamide | Oral contraceptive agents |
| Visceral malignancies | Pregnancy |
| Vitamin K deficiency states | Vitamin C |

certain pathophysiologic states which can commonly interact with warfarin.

Proper patient selection may, in fact, be the answer to minimizing hemorrhagic complications from anticoagulant therapy.[64] Elderly patients with complicated infarctions who fall in the "poor risk" category and who are expected to be at bedrest for prolonged periods of time are at greatest risk for thromboembolic complications; therefore, they are most likely to benefit from anticoagulant therapy. Conversely, in patients with high likelihood of hemorrhage, anticoagulation is best avoided.

## "Low-Dose" Heparin Therapy

The concept of low-dose heparin therapy represents a relatively recent departure in anticoagulant therapy and holds at the same time promise of eliminating the risk of significant hemorrhagic complications, as well as the need for continuous drug therapy monitoring. The studies of Sharnoff[75] introduced in 1962 the use of small, subcutaneous doses of heparin for the prevention of venous thrombosis in postoperative patients. Discussion of the precise molecular basis for the antithrombotic action of heparin is beyond the scope of this chapter. It should be recognized, however, that the clinical efficacy of low-dose heparin regimens rests on the observation that small quantities of the drug greatly increase the rate at which antithrombin-3 combines with and inactivates activated factor X (Xa).[76] In vitro studies have shown that 1 microgram of antithrombin-3, by neutralizing 32 units of activated factor X (Xa), indirectly blocks the potential generation of at least 1600 NIH units of thrombin.[63] If coagulation were not blocked, to neutralize this amount of thrombin, 1000 micrograms of antithrombin-3 would be required. These observations lead to the reasonable conclusion that, if a tendency to thrombosis were treated before intravascular coagulation had been initiated, less antithrombin-3 would be required than if therapy were begun after thrombin formation had occurred. By the same token, it is now clear that small doses of heparin are effective only if thrombin formation has not already occurred, and that they will not halt an ongoing thrombotic process.[63]

Once the efficacy of low-dose heparin in preventing deep vein thrombosis after major surgery was clinically demonstrated,[77] several controlled trials were undertaken to evaluate its efficacy in patients with suspected myocardial infarction.[78] Although one trial showed no benefit, it was limited by its methodology, which allowed heparin treatment only for seven days while leg scanning for thrombus formation was continued to 14 days. Two other trials involving large numbers of patients concluded that low-dose heparin provided a significant benefit in the prophylaxis of venous thrombosis. Gallus and associates [79] studied low-dose heparin administered to 78 patients with suspected myocardial infarction; they reported an incidence of venous thrombi of only 12.6 percent in treated patients as opposed to 22.5 percent in the controls. Therapy appeared to be particularly advantageous in patients with congestive heart failure. Subsequent venography revealed not only a reduction in the incidence of calf vein thrombosis, but also in the rate of propagation of the thrombus to the iliofemoral vessels.

It must, therefore, be concluded that heparin in small doses is effective in practically eliminating deep vein thrombosis in postmyocardial infarction patients without increasing the danger of hemorrhage, even in high-risk individuals. No evidence is currently available as to whether low-dose heparin will reduce the incidence of pulmonary emboli in myocardial infarction, although the above-cited studies suggest that it may. Similarly, there is no available information regarding the efficacy of low-dose heparin in reducing the incidence of mural thrombus and systemic embolization.

## Current Practice

In view of the controversy, the conflicting evidence, and the risk of hemorrhagic complications associated with the use of anticoagulants in acute myocardial infarction, proper selection of patients [64,80] appears to offer the most reasonable current approach.

In general, all patients admitted to the CCU of the University of California Medical Center in San Diego with documented or suspected acute myocardial infarction are given low-dose heparin therapy consisting of 5000 units subcutaneously every 12 hours (Fig. 7.1, Section G). The only contraindications to low-dose heparin are: (1) Active bleeding diathesis; (2) active GI or GU bleeding, and (3) recent central nervous system or ocular surgery. Low-dose heparin is continued until the patient is ambulating actively, usually to day seven after admission.

Full-dose anticoagulation in our institution initially consists of continuous heparin infusion in doses sufficient to maintain the activated partial thromboplastin time at between 2 and 3 times the control value, followed by warfarin therapy in doses sufficient to maintain the prothrombin time at twice the control value. Full-dose anticoagulation is employed in those patients with documented or suspected acute myocardial infarction who are under the age of 70 and who are thought to be at an increased risk for thromboembolic complications [64,81] (Table 7.2). Anticoagulation is again continued until the patient is fully ambulatory and discontinued at the time of discharge from the hospital. In the presence of compelling contraindications to

**Table 7.2   Indications for Full-dose Anticoagulation in Acute Myocardial Infarction**

1.  Chronic anticoagulant therapy
2.  History of previous pulmonary or systemic embolization
3.  Active venous thrombosis
4.  History of previous transient ischemic attacks
5.  Massive cardiac enlargement
6.  Left ventricular aneurysm
7.  Cardiogenic shock
8.  Congestive heart failure
9.  Atrial fibrillation
10. Massive obesity
11. Inability to ambulate
12. Extensive varicosities of lower extremities

**Table 7.3    Contraindications to Full-dose Anticoagulation in Acute Myocardial Infarction**

1. Active bleeding problem (GI, GU, etc.)

2. Hemorrhagic diathesis (congenital, hepatic, or drug-induced)

3. Active peptic ulcer disease

4. Recent neurosurgery or ocular surgery

5. Presence of purpura

6. Hepatic or renal insufficiency (severe)

7. Severe hypertension (sustained BP > 190/110)

8. Open wounds

9. Sepsis, especially infective endocarditis

10. Lack of adequate laboratory support

11. Anticipated invasive bedside procedures [73] (thoracentesis, subclavian vein puncture, Swan-Ganz insertion, etc.)

full-dose anticoagulation (Table 7.3), our patients receive low-dose heparin therapy. The risks of invasive procedures in the face of full-dose anticoagulation are discussed in Chapter 27.

## β-ADRENERGIC BLOCKADE

### Theoretical Considerations

The use of β-adrenoreceptor blocking agents in acute myocardial infarction has been advocated because of their myocardial oxygen-sparing effects and their antidysrhythmic properties. Both subjects are dealt with extensively in other chapters and will be covered only briefly here.

Considerable evidence has accumulated in recent years that, following acute myocardial infarction, ultimate prognosis is directly related to the size of the infarct—i.e., the amount of damaged myocardium.[83] The early experimental studies of Maroko et al.[84] suggested that the development of myocardial damage is a dynamic event, and therapeutic interventions that favorably alter the relationship between oxygen supply and demand in the ischemic area surrounding the central infarct zone may result in salvage of viable myocardium and minimize ultimate infarct size. Furthermore, it has been

known for many years that myocardial infarction is an acute physiologic and psychologic stress during which sympathetic nervous system activity increases, with a resultant increase in plasma and urinary catecholamine levels.[85] In addition, it has been shown by Mueller that, in experimental myocardial infarction, the norepinephrine content of coronary venous blood is increased, indicating catecholamine release by the ischemic myocardium.[86] This high local catecholamine environment may be expected to exert positive chronotropic and inotropic effects that wastefully increase myocardial oxygen requirements and may lead to extension of the infarct. Additionally, it has been recently pointed out that the potential for the induction of reentrant ventricular dysrhythmias is enhanced by increased local catecholamine concentrations.[87] Based on the above observations, it appears reasonable to expect that blockade of β-adrenoreceptors in the acutely infarcted myocardium will be beneficial both in decreasing myocardial oxygen requirements and in providing a degree of dysrhythmia protection.[88]

On the other hand, recent studies [89,90] have suggested that coronary arterial spasm may be an important pathogenetic mechanism in acute myocardial infarction. Although regulation of coronary blood flow appears to be primarily via sympathetic β-receptor activated vasodilatation, it has been shown that, when the β-receptors are experimentally blocked, α-receptor stimulation will produce vasoconstriction.[91] In fact, reductions in total coronary blood flow have been reported to result from β-adrenergic blockade, perhaps due to such an unmasking of unopposed α-adrenergic agonist (constricting) influences on the coronary arteries.[92,93] It is, therefore, reasonable to conclude that, in a setting of spontaneous coronary arterial spasm, β-adrenergic blockade may, in fact, be deleterious. However, the issue is further complicated by observations suggesting the operation of paradoxical β-adrenergic vasoconstrictor mechanisms in the coronary arteries of acutely ischemic myocardium.[94] If this is, in fact, so, the administration of β-adrenergic blocking agents would be beneficial by blocking the paradoxic constrictor influences and by allowing α-adrenergic constriction to take place in primarily nonischemic beds, thereby diverting critical blood flow to the ischemic areas which are undergoing maximal dilatation in response to the metabolic changes of hypoxia.[95]

## Clinical Considerations

Clinical studies reported to date are not in full agreement regarding the efficacy of propranolol in acute myocardial infarction. Snow was the first to report, from a nonrandomized study, reduction in mortality from acute myocardial infarction in patients treated with propranolol.[96] Subsequent randomized studies have failed to confirm improved survival in patients with acute myocardial infarction treated with propranolol but did suggest that dysrhythmias were better controlled in the early phases of infarction with this therapy.[97] More recently, clinical studies have been undertaken to determine whether the administration of propranolol early in the course of an uncomplicated myocardial infarction can in fact reduce infarct size. In general, studies reported indicate that propranolol administered intravenously early in the course of acute myocardial infarction does reduce myocardial injury, whether such injury was assessed electrocardiographically (sum of ST segment elevations)[98] or by measurement of peak CK levels.[99] Unfortunately, these and other similar clinical studies are all limited by the relative lack of precision of available clinical methods to measure infarct size.[100] It should further be noted that not all experimental studies are in agreement regarding the efficacy of β-adrenergic blockade in reducing myocardial injury after experimental infarction. In a recent study, Peter et al. were unable to demonstrate differences in loss of CK activity from the border and center zones of an experimentally induced infarct in control dogs compared with animals pretreated with propranolol.[101]

Potential disadvantages of β-adrenergic blockade in acute myocardial infarction include the above-cited unmasking of α-adrenergically mediated coronary vasoconstriction, development of atrioventricular conduction delay, development of bronchoconstriction, preservation of dysrhythmogenic islands of viable myocar-

dium in the infarcted area, and precipitation of congestive heart failure. Of these, the potential to further impair ventricular performance and precipitate congestive heart failure has been the factor that has deterred most clinicians from using propranolol widely in acute myocardial infarction. It appears, however, that this fear has been exaggerated. Balcon reported a greater tendency toward heart failure in the treated group than the control group.[97] However, critically ill patients were not excluded from this study. Early clinical studies utilizing hemodynamic measurements revealed that the administration of propranolol in a setting of acute myocardial infarction resulted in consistent reductions of stroke volume and heart rate, but in only slight increases in left ventricular filling pressures.[102] In subsequent studies, Mueller demonstrated that patients with acute myocardial infarction tolerated well the administration of propranolol at doses of 0.1 mg/kg intravenously; she also noted a paradoxical fall in pulmonary artery wedge pressure in six of the patients who had pulmonary artery wedge pressures above 16 mmHg.[103] These findings suggest that elevated left ventricular filling pressures may often result from increased stiffness of the ischemic ventricle. It appears that in this setting propranolol may operate more by reducing ischemia and improving ventricular compliance and less by impairing ventricular performance. In higher doses, however, propranolol has been shown to consistently elevate left ventricular filling pressures. Cairns and Klassen initially administered propranolol in doses of 0.15 mg/kg intravenously and followed this with a continuous infusion of 0.03 mg/kg/h in the early phases of myocardial infarction.[104] At these dosages, pulmonary artery wedge pressure rose while heart rate and blood pressure declined, but this was usually a transient phenomenon. In another clinical study, Malleck et al. administered the "cardioselective" β-blocking agent metoprolol to patients within the first 24 hours after the onset of acute myocardial infarction.[105] These investigators demonstrated reductions in heart rate, systolic blood pressure, and cardiac output, with no significant changes in stroke volume and diastolic blood pressure. The pulmonary artery end-diastolic pressure, used as an index of left ventricular filling pressure, did not change significantly, except for reductions in three of four patients with initially elevated values.

Although several promising studies have been reported, a number of questions remain yet to be answered before β-adrenergic blockade can be recommended as standard treatment in patients with *uncomplicated* myocardial infarction. For example, it has been postulated that, from a clinical standpoint, a propranolol-treated infarct may not be "reduced," but only "postponed." [43] Questions have also been raised as to whether such interrupted infarction is a stable condition, or whether these patients will require subsequent angiography and myocardial revascularization procedures to forestall later completion of the process. For these reasons, and until additional clinical studies—such as the ongoing multicenter clinical trial—better define the role of β-blockade in acute myocardial infarction, we do not administer propranolol routinely to patients with uncomplicated infarcts. Our current indications (except for dysrhythmias) for the use of β-adrenergic blockade in acute myocardial infarction are: (1) persistent ischemic pain, not relieved by usual analgesic therapy; (2) hypertension which persists following adequate analgesia and sedation, and (3) persistent sinus tachycardia in the face of normal left ventricular filling pressures and increased stroke work.[106] In the absence of contraindications (see below), patients who have been on chronic propranolol therapy prior to development of acute myocardial infarction are continued on the drug. Although the problem of propranolol withdrawal "rebound" is relatively uncommon,[107] Cairns and Klassen noted evidence of extension of the infarct after propranolol withdrawal in two of their patients.[104]

## β-Adrenergic Blockade in the Treatment of Arrhythmias

As described in greater detail in Chapter 14, recent studies have identified two major mechanisms for the antiarrhythmic actions of β-adrenergic antagonists: [108]

(1) The depressant effect of β-blockade on cardiac pacemaker potentials forms the basis for the control of arrhythmias arising from enhanced automaticity; at relatively low β-blocking concentrations, these agents effect a reduction in the dV/dt of pacemaker potentials, whether sinus or ectopic, especially when increased by catecholamines or digitalis.

(2) The membrane effect (previously called the quinidine-like effect). This effect results in reduction in the dV/dt of the transmembrane action potential and, consequently, in elevation of threshold excitability, delay in conduction velocity, and an increase in effective refractory period.

The relative importance of these two antiarrhythmic mechanisms of β-blocking agents has not been precisely defined; however, it seems likely that, in doses generally used clinically, β-blockade is the primary factor. This statement is supported by observations that dysrhythmias can be suppressed by plasma propranolol concentrations much below those necessary to exert the membrane-depressant effect on isolated cardiac muscle.[109] They are also supported by observations that practolol, which is a pure β-adrenergic blocking drug not possessing membrane-depressant activity, is an effective antiarrhythmic agent.[108]

Lemberg et al. were the first to report on the clinical use of propranolol in treating tachyarhythmias developing in patients with acute myocardial infarction complicated by mild-to-moderate congestive heart failure.[110] Forty-three episodes of tachyarrhythmias developing in 34 patients were treated with propranolol in incremental doses of 0.5 to 0.75 mg intravenously, given at two-minute intervals, until sinus rhythm returned or the ventricular rate slowed to 80 beats per minute. The tachyarrhythmias treated included atrial fibrillation, atrial flutter, supraventricular tachycardia and ventricular tachycardia, all with heart rates in excess of 140 beats per minute. The majority of patients responded to a total intravenous dose of propranolol of less than 5 mg, although in five patients the total dose was between 5 and 15 mg. None of the patients so treated showed an increase in the clinical severity of heart failure. It was postulated that slowing of the heart rate was the most important factor in reducing myocardial oxygen requirements and improving the clinical state. Similar favorable results have also been reported with the use of other $\beta$-adrenergic blocking agents such as oxprenolol, alprenolol, and practolol (the last no longer being available for human use).[103] Several additional important points emerge from the report of Lemberg et al.: (1) the fact that relatively small amounts of propranolol were necessary to slow ventricular response in supraventricular tachyarrhythmias if digitalis had been given previously; (2) the occasional occurrence of marked ventricular slowing and/or AV dissociation requiring treatment with atropine, isoproterenol, or temporary transvenous pacing; (3) the effectiveness of propranolol in slowing ventricular response in a number of patients when more conventional therapy had failed; and (4) the absence of significant hypotension as a result of propranolol therapy.

Our current indications for the use of $\beta$-adrenergic blocking agents in arrhythmias after myocardial infarction include atrial fibrillation, atrial flutter, atrial tachycardia, frequent atrial or ventricular premature contractions, and recurrent ventricular tachycardia or ventricular fibrillation.

(1) When a patient with recent myocardial infarction develops atrial fibrillation, atrial flutter, or atrial tachycardia with rapid ventricular response, $\beta$-adrenergic blocking drugs provide an important adjunct to digitalis preparations in controlling the heart rate. This is particularly true if the ventricular response is over 140 beats per minute and there is evidence of hemodynamic impairment such as congestive heart failure, hypotension, or recurring angina. Although direct current cardioversion of supraventricular tachyarrhythmias is also an effective mode of therapy, the requirement for patient sedation, as well as the probability of recurrence of the tachyarrhythmia, suggest the combination of digitalis and propranolol may be preferable. The use of $\beta$-adrenergic blockade is particularly useful in treating atrial tachycardia due to digitalis excess—a situation in which DC cardioversion is contraindicated. Similarly, $\beta$-adrenergic blockade and digitalis constitute the treatment of choice for recurring paroxysmal atrial fibrillation.

(2) The occurrence of frequent premature atrial contractions, particularly when they have a short coupling interval to the previous normal atrial complex, suggests a high probability for the development of atrial fibrillation and the use of $\beta$-blocking agents may be useful in preventing this occurrence.

(3) Ventricular premature contractions in a setting of acute myocardial infarction must be treated if they are frequent, multiform, or of the R-on-T variety. Lidocaine continues to be the treatment of choice for the management of these dysrhythmias; procainamide is the second drug of choice. If both drugs are ineffective, $\beta$-adrenergic blockade has been found to be helpful and is recommended.

(4) In repetitive ventricular tachycardia and ventricular fibrillation not suppressed by lidocaine or procainamide therapy, $\beta$-adrenergic blockade provides a rational alternative to bretylium tosylate therapy. Similarly, in ventricular fibrillation resistant to direct current shock, propranolol is a useful adjunct to the standard drugs lidocaine, procainamide, and bretylium.

When propranolol is used acutely for the control of tachyarrhythmias in a setting of acute myocardial infarction, it must be given intravenously. It is usually administered in 0.5 to 0.75 mg doses at intervals of 2 to 3 minutes until conversion of the tachyarrhythmia to sinus rhythm has taken place, or the ventricular response has slowed to 80 beats per minute or less. It is rarely necessary to exceed cumulative doses of 5 mg intravenously. Whenever propranolol is administered intravenously in a setting of acute myocardial infarction, atropine and isoproterenol infusions should be available for immediate use, should excessive ventricular slowing occur. Similarly, the capability for urgent insertion of a temporary transvenous pacemaker should exist whenever this form of therapy is undertaken. Maintenance oral propranolol therapy for suppression of chronic dysrhythmias in the CCU usually consists of a dose of from 10 to 30 mg orally every six hours.

Several contraindications exist to the use of $\beta$-blocking agents as antidysrhythmic drugs in a setting of acute myocardial infarction:

(1) The presence of any degree of atrioventricular block prior to the onset of the dysrhyth-

mia constitutes a definite contraindication to the use of propranolol, except in the presence of a ventricular pacemaker.

(2) Chronic obstructive airways disease is a definite contraindication to the use of all β-blocking agents, with the possible exception of the cardioselective drug, metoprolol. It should be kept in mind, however, that metoprolol is only relatively cardioselective and, in the face of broncho-obstructive symptoms and signs, should also be administered with extreme caution.

(3) When the basic sinus rhythm rate is less than 60 per minute, β-blockade is of little value in the treatment of ventricular premature contractions. As a matter of fact, increasing the degree of bradycardia by β-blockade may further facilitate the development of reentrant dysrhythmias and increase the frequency of premature contractions.

(4) The presence of overt left ventricular failure has been considered to be the major contraindication to the administration of β-adrenergic blocking agents because of their negative inotropic action and their potential for further reducing ventricular performance. Nevertheless, as the study of Lemberg et al. demonstrates,[110] in a setting of rapid ventricular rate with hemodynamic impairment, the net effect of propranolol administration is salutary because the benefits of slowing of the heart rate far outweigh the danger of additional depression of left ventricular function. Furthermore, conversion—for example, from atrial fibrillation to regular sinus rhythm—with reestablishment of mechanical atrial contribution will further improve ventricular performance. However, in the presence of myocardial infarction, propranolol should be administered cautiously, and low dosage schedules should be used as discussed above.

## OXYGEN THERAPY

Oxygen inhalation therapy has been customary and in widespread clinical use for many years in patients with acute myocardial infarction. Its beneficial effects must be considered from both cardiac and systemic points of view. In ischemic myocardial regions, profound re-

ductions in tissue $PO_2$ are found along with lactate production, which in turn further reduces energy delivery from anaerobic sources. In addition, patients with acute myocardial infarction have been commonly found to have hypoxemia, which tends to be more severe when left ventricular failure or cardiogenic shock complicate the infarct.[111] A variety of pathophysiologic mechanisms have been proposed to explain the occurrence of hypoxemia: (1) ventilation-perfusion abnormalities in the lung; [112] (2) collapse of small airways with right to left shunting; and (3) interstitial and/or alveolar pulmonary edema. It has been stated that oxygen therapy will reverse the hypoxemia toward normal more readily in uncomplicated infarction cases than in cases of left ventricular failure or cardiogenic shock; at the same time, systemic vascular resistance and systemic arterial pressure will rise and cardiac output will fall.[113] As a result of the above theoretical reasons, routine use of oxygen in patients with myocardial infarction who are not in left ventricular failure has come under recent attack.[114] In a controlled study of oxygen therapy in uncomplicated myocardial infarction, Rawles and Kenmore were unable to document any differences in mortality rate, incidence of dysrhythmias, or systolic time intervals in patients receiving oxygen vs. those breathing room air.[115] Furthermore, Rawles and Kenmore documented a slight increase in heart rate in patients receiving oxygen inhalation therapy. Early studies by Thomas et al. and Sukumalchantra et al. documented that oxygen administered to patients with acute myocardial infarction resulted in modest reductions of cardiac output and increases in arterial pressure, thought to be the result of oxygen mediated systemic vasoconstriction.[114,116] However, more recent studies by Loeb et al. failed to document physiologically meaningful interference with ventricular performance as measured by left ventricular pressures, stroke work, or systolic time intervals when patients with acute myocardial infarction were given oxygen at 6 liters per minute through a nasal cannula or a face mask.[117] They were able, however, to confirm slight increases in arterial pressure and decreases in cardiac output during oxygen administration. Arterial blood gas determinations did reveal that significant hypoxemia was commonly present and was corrected with low-flow oxygen administration. These clinical findings were consistent with the experimental work of Maroko et al.,[118] who found a significant reduction in the extent of acute ischemic injury and in the size of experimental myocardial infarction when the animal was breathing 40 percent oxygen. These same investigators also demonstrated in another study that the presence of hypoxemia ($PO_2$ below 45 mmHg) substantially increases myocardial damage.[119] In a clinical trial, Madias et al. demonstrated that the administration of 100 percent oxygen via a snug fitting mask early in the course of acute myocardial infarction resulted in a small but significant decrease in both ST segment elevations in precordial maps and in the number of sites showing significant ST segment elevation.[120] They concluded that their study demonstrated reduction of ischemic injury during oxygen inhalation, especially since they were able to document significant reelevation of the ST segments following discontinuation of the oxygen therapy.

In our current practice, we continue to administer low-flow oxygen to all patients with acute myocardial infarction. Our expectation is that even a minimal increase of oxygen delivery to the marginal myocardium will outweigh any increases in myocardial oxygen requirements produced by the slight elevation in arterial pressure secondary to the peripheral vasoconstrictor effects of increased arterial oxygen tension. Oxygen can be conveniently delivered through a nasal cannula at a rate of 4 to 5 liters per minute. Drying of nasal and pharyngeal secretions can be minimized with adequate humidification of inspired oxygen. Patients with more severe left ventricular failure may benefit from intermittent positive pressure breathing with 40 to 100 percent oxygen enriched mixtures. Obtunded or comatose patients may require endotracheal intubation with mechanical ventilatory assistance. Positive end-expiratory pressure (PEEP) breathing has been used recently to treat severe cardiopulmonary failure.[121] This technique can recruit atelectatic alveoli for gas exchange, increase functional residual capacity and lung compliance, raise ar-

terial oxygen tension, and increase oxygen transport to ischemic tissues. However, close monitoring of cardiac output and other hemodynamic parameters is essential because PEEP may, in fact, decrease cardiac output by obstructing venous return to the heart. The subject is dealt with in more detail in Chapter 32.

Oxygen therapy should be administered with extreme caution to patients with chronic obstructive lung disease and potential carbon dioxide retention. In such individuals, oxygen administration may eliminate the hypoxic respiratory drive and thereby further contribute to the retention of carbon dioxide by depressing respiratory rate and depth. In these patients, we administer oxygen only at rates of 1 to 2 liters per minute by nasal cannula and monitor arterial blood gases frequently. Adjustment of inspired oxygen flow rate and concentration must be carefully regulated by repeated arterial $PO_2$ and $PCO_2$ measurements.

## NITRATES AND OTHER VASODILATORS

The use of nitroglycerin in acute myocardial infarction has traditionally been thought to be contraindicated because of the risk that it may provoke hypotension and thereby increase the area of infarction.[122] In recent years, however, vasodilators have been utilized with increasing frequency in this clinical setting. Two theoretical concepts have provided the impetus for this approach: (1) Vasodilators act as afterload reducing agents and thereby improve the efficiency of the heart as a pump; and (2) vasodilators may in fact decrease myocardial ischemic injury and limit infarct size.[123] Several groups of investigators working independently have reported that vasodilator therapy is hemodynamically beneficial to patients with acute myocardial infarction and left ventricular failure. In this setting, vasodilator therapy will diminish left ventricular filling pressures and increase cardiac output.[124,125,126] These hemodynamic alterations may be expected to occur consistently with any one of several vasodilators available such as nitroglycerin, sodium nitroprusside, and phentolamine.[123] These changes are accompanied by modest declines in mean systemic arterial pressure. On the other hand, when vasodilators are administered to patients with normal left ventricular filling pressures, cardiac output consistently declines.[124,126]

Both animal and human studies have suggested that nitroglycerin alone is of minimal value in decreasing myocardial ischemic injury, but that this effect can be greatly enhanced if the reflex tachycardia and hypotension which accompany the use of nitroglycerin are eliminated with the simultaneous administration of a pressor agent such as methoxamine or phenylephrine.[127,128] This type of pharmacologic and hemodynamic intervention, however, appears to be (by today's standards at least) too complex and too aggressive for the patient with *uncomplicated* myocardial infarction. Not only does it require continuous monitoring of systemic arterial and left ventricular filling pressures as well as serial determinations of cardiac output, but also—if perfect balance is not achieved—enhances the potential for increasing ischemic injury. Furthermore, it appears that the nitroglycerin dose is of critical importance. Thus, in the study of Bussman et al.,[126] nitroglycerin at a dose of 6 mg/h given intravenously was less effective in reducing the extent of myocardial ischemia than the lower dose of 3 mg/h, despite the beneficial hemodynamic effects of the drug in both dosage groups. These observations support the view expressed several years ago that an improvement in hemodynamics does not necessarily result in reduction of the ischemic injury.[129] In a recent study, however, Kim and Williams documented the beneficial effects of large doses of sublingual nitroglycerin in acute myocardial infarction.[129a] Administered to patients with *persistent* ischemic pain in divided doses of up to 23.7 ± 10.6 mg over a 1- to 3-hour period, sublingual nitroglycerin was as effective as morphine in relieving pain. Furthermore, significantly fewer Q waves developed in patients treated with nitroglycerin than in those treated with morphine, suggesting that nitroglycerin reduced myocardial ischemic injury.

Sodium nitroprusside is a vasodilator agent that has been widely used in the treatment of left ventricular failure and mitral regurgitation.[130] However, its usefulness in uncomplicated myocardial infarction remains highly controversial.[43] A number of studies have suggested that sodium nitroprusside and nitroglycerin have different sites of action on the coronary vasculature: it appears that sodium nitroprusside primarily affects nondilated resistance vessels, whereas nitroglycerin affects primarily conductance vessels, especially the larger coronary epicardial arteries.[131,132] Recent clinical studies suggest that sodium nitroprusside may in fact increase the area of myocardial injury by producing a "steal" phenomenon away from the ischemic area, thereby enlarging the infarct rather than limiting its size.[133,134] For these reasons, sodium nitroprusside should not be administered during the early hours of an uncomplicated myocardial infarction and should be administered with caution for appropriate indications (left ventricular failure, acute mitral regurgitation, etc.) in a setting of recent myocardial infarction.

The effects of nitrate administration in acute myocardial infarction have been evaluated primarily by observing the effects of the drugs on ST segment abnormalities in precordial "surface map" ECGs. There are no well-documented data on the effect of nitrates on mortality and morbidity of patients with an acute myocardial infarction. Preliminary studies, however, suggest that, in a limited, properly selected group of patients, prolonged nitroglycerin infusion starting within 24 hours of the onset of the chest pain reduced hospital mortality to a statistically significant degree.[133] In the same study, the incidence of ventricular tachycardia and ventricular fibrillation was similarly reduced in the treatment group in comparison to the control group. Nitroglycerin is not currently available commercially in the United States in a parenteral form. However, it appears that nitrates administered by other routes (oral, sublingual, or transcutaneous) all have similar hemodynamic effects.[136,137,138]

The usual adverse reactions of nitrates are headache, syncope, flushing, and palpitations.[139] Other, more important side effects are: (1) the potential of nitrates to induce hypotension with reflex tachycardia, and (2) the potential of nitrates to (theoretically, at least) cause augmentation of myocardial oxygen demands while at the same time causing reduced coronary perfusion pressure and diastolic perfusion period.[141] Come et al. have reported the occurrence of severe hypotension and bradycardia induced by sublingual or parenteral nitroglycerin in a setting of acute myocardial infarction.[140] Elevation of the legs and administration of parenteral atropine as well as cessation of nitroglycerin administration were associated with the return of heart rate and hemodynamics to baseline. The exact mechanisms responsible for the bradycardia and hypotension during nitroglycerin administration are not known. However, the occurrence of these adverse reactions emphasizes the need for careful and continuous rhythm and hemodynamic monitoring during the administration of any vasodilator agent to patients with acute myocardial infarction.

In view of the conflicting reports quoted above, our current practice does not include the routine administration of vasodilators in patients with *uncomplicated* acute myocardial infarction. Patients with persistent chest pain unrelieved by seemingly adequate analgesics are treated preferentially with $\beta$-adrenergic blocking agents as discussed above. However, nitrate administration is warranted if a patient demonstrates recurrent chest pain, and especially if one suspects that coronary arterial spasm is intermittently present (as evidenced by fluctuating ST segment shifts).[90] In this setting, we administer nitroglycerin 0.3 to 0.4 mg sublingually. If there is a clear therapeutic effect, the patient is started on long-term nitrate therapy in the form of isosorbide dinitrate orally 10 to 20 mg every 6 hours—or, preferably, in the form of 2 percent nitroglycerin paste transcutaneously every 6 to 8 hours. In either case, careful monitoring of rhythm and arterial blood pressure are maintained. A flow-directed Swan-Ganz catheter is inserted into the pulmonary artery for monitoring of left ventricular filling pressure if there is any question regarding the hemodynamic stability of the patient. The use of vasodilator agents for their "afterload reducing" properties in *complicated* myocardial infarction is discussed in Chapter 22.

## BLADDER AND BOWEL CARE

Elderly patients receiving opiate analgesics and/or atropine often develop urinary retention.[4] If, in addition, a patient is moderately obtunded, he may suffer severe distress from a distended urinary bladder before communicating this problem to the coronary care unit staff. Careful monitoring, therefore, of urinary output and for urinary bladder distention is essential in all patients during the early hours of their hospitalization. If urinary retention develops early on, our current practice is to proceed with straight urinary bladder catheterization to relieve the distention, in the hope that it is a one-time occurrence. If retention recurs, whether due to repeated analgesic administration or to intrinsic genitourinary tract problems, an indwelling catheter is recommended for a few days. Similarly, if left ventricular failure or cardiogenic shock complicate the acute infarct, close monitoring of urinary output is critical and an indwelling catheter which allows hourly urinary output determination is essential.

Constipation is another common problem facing patients with acute myocardial infarction and is due to inactivity, change of diet, and the administration of opiate analgesics. To prevent the discomfort of constipation and later straining at stool, our current practice includes the routine administration of 100 mg of the stool softener dioctyl sodium sulfosuccinate (Colace, Doss, and others) along with 30 ml of milk of magnesia daily. More potent cathartics and enemas are avoided. Bowel function is helped by allowing the patients to use a bedside commode from day one of admission. The use of a bed pan is vigorously discouraged, since it is uncomfortable and in all likelihood subjects the patient to increased strain.

The question of whether a rectal digital examination in patients with acute myocardial infarction is dangerous or not has been recently studied.[142] In a series of 86 patients with acute myocardial infarction, Earnest and Fletcher performed a gentle rectal digital examination within 24 hours of admission. With the patient being monitored continuously, no adverse clini-

cal or electrocardiographic effects were observed and no angina was induced. Conversely,
the detection of unsuspected fecal or occult
blood, prostatic enlargement, and voluminous
hard stool in the rectum was common enough
to make the rectal examination an important
part of the initial patient evaluation. In view
of the above findings as well as the absence
of documented support for the previously held
belief that a rectal examination in this setting
is dangerous, we routinely include a rectal digital examination in the admission physical evaluation of the patient.

## HYPERTENSION IN ACUTE MYOCARDIAL INFARCTION

Many patients with acute myocardial infarction will be hypertensive on admission to the
CCU. Moderate hypertension with systolic
blood pressures in the range of 180 to 190
mmHg will frequently respond well to pain relief and sedation. More resistant cases of hypertension will often subside with the addition of
a mild vasodilator such as nitroglycerin administered either sublingually or transcutaneously.[4]
When hypertension is part of the syndrome of
sypathetic overactivity associated with the early
phases of acute myocardial infarction,[44,106] $\beta$-
adrenergic blocking agents constitute the treatment of choice. However, caution must be exercised in such cases, since the tachycardia and
mild hypertension may in fact be the cardiovascular system's response to left ventricular dysfunction rather than merely a manifestation of
sympathetic overactivity. Clinical clues that
tachycardia and hypertension are not due to
left ventricular dysfunction are the presence of
a loud first heart sound, wide pulse pressure,
and absence of tachypnea.[43] If any question remains regarding the cause of persistent tachycardia and hypertension, measurement of left
ventricular filling pressure should be undertaken before $\beta$-adrenergic blocking agents are
administered. As mentioned previously, the
sympathetic overactivity syndrome can often
be treated successfully with morphine sulphate
alone; $\beta$-adrenergic blockade need not be insti-

tuted unless tachycardia and hypertension persist for several hours after the onset of infarction.

Patients who are markedly hypertensive
(BP > 180/110 mmHg, for example) despite
sedation and analgesia and who do not respond
to sublingual nitroglycerin administration require aggressive pharmacologic intervention for
the treatment of their hypertension. In the absence of commercially available parenteral
nitroglycerin preparations, our current practice
is to cautiously administer an infusion of sodium nitroprusside, despite reports that this
agent may have caused extension of infarction
when given to moderately hypertensive
patients.[133] This practice is based on the assumption that treatment of severe hypertension
will result in greater reduction of myocardial
oxygen requirement than reduction of myocardial oxygen supply stemming from the potential
"coronary steal" possibly associated with nitroprusside use.[134] An alternative method of treatment of severe persistent hypertension is the
intravenous infusion of trimethaphan (Arfonad)
100 to 1000 $\mu$g/minute.[143] Trimethaphan has
been used successfully in patients with acute
or chronic hypertension and acute myocardial
infarction and has been shown to reduce one-
month mortality. Because of its mechanism of
action (ganglionic blockade), it is less likely to
produce reflex tachycardia than the directly acting vasodilators. In general we do not employ
other hypotensive agents such as hydralazine,
alphamethyldopa, or clonidine because of their
side effects and especially because of their
slower onset of action and potentially persistent
hypotensive effects.

The classic prognostic studies of Peel [144] and
Norris et al.[145] did not conclude that hypertension is a definite, adverse prognostic factor in
the outcome of acute myocardial infarction. On
the other hand, recent reports indicate that hypertension plays an important role not only in
the etiology of acute myocardial infarction but
also in the outcome. Beck et al. recently reported that mortality after myocardial infarction was significantly higher in their hypertensive patients (37 percent) than in their
normotensive patients (24 percent).[146] For these

reasons, it is our practice to aggressively attempt to return patients to the normotensive range in the early hours after the onset of acute myocardial infarction. A possible exception to this practice involves patients with bradycardia and hypertension. It has been shown that, in the face of bradyarrhythmias, patients with normal or elevated blood pressure have improved survival rates whether treated with atropine or not, in comparison to patients with bradycardia and hypotension.[147]

## THE ROLE OF THE NURSE IN CORONARY CARE

### Nursing Responsibilities

CCU nurses must be skilled in all aspects of critical care and should have previous training or classes in arrhythmia recognition. Skills should include knowledge of arrhythmias, disease entities, methods of treatment, drug actions and interactions, institution of intravenous lines, arterial blood gas drawing, cardiopulmonary resuscitation, defibrillation, principles of cardioversion, use of pacemakers, interpretation of blood tests, and determination of arterial blood gas tensions.[18] The nurses must be trained in policies and procedures specific to the institution and unit. Return demonstration of skills should be documented and reviewed periodically. The nursing staff must also be knowledgeable in the various methods of invasive pressure monitoring [148,149] and demonstrate mastery of both theory and safe practice. The nurse assumes the responsibility of handling life-threatening situations in the absence of a physician.[150] It is essential that dysrhythmias be properly identified and recorded and that subsequent interventions follow standing orders. Nurses function under procedures outlined in the standing orders section of "Arrhythmia Treatment" and are held responsible for their actions.

Aside from the technical skills, the nursing staff must be trained to handle the emotional, social, and family aspects of patient care.[151] The staff must have a broad base of knowledge in disease entities and modalities of treatment which can be discussed with the patient and family [150] according to the patient's status. The nurse consults with the physician [152] and establishes what has been discussed with the patient and family and when teaching will begin. A checklist of items to be covered in patient education sessions is a valuable procedural adjunct (Fig. 7.7). Visiting hours are defined in the standing orders. However, nursing discretion is imperative in restricting or liberalizing these rules. Depending upon patient and family acceptance, it is often beneficial to allow family members to be present more often than the rules state. Families are allowed and encouraged to call the CCU directly, at any time, for patient information. Messages are promptly relayed, since patients do not have telephones at their bedside.

### Emergency Care Aspects

Knowledge of drug side effects, interactions, and contraindications is essential for the R.N. functioning in the CCU. Documentation and justification of why a particular treatment was instituted are mandatory. An R.N. in the CCU is expected to have appropriate norms of treatment memorized and be able to institute treatment rapidly.[18] When ventricular ectopy requires suppression, lidocaine is the drug of choice. The nurse will proceed with administration of the drug while a physician is being contacted. If ventricular tachycardia arises and the patient shows hemodynamic compromise (in the absence of a physician), the nurse will defibrillate the patient up to three times and institute CPR if the arrhythmia persists.[153] Ventricular fibrillation is always and immediately treated with electrical defibrillation. A written examination has been devised in our Unit which must be completed by each R.N. before she is authorized to defibrillate patients. An oral quiz is also used, and demonstration of technique is required. The test and certification of clearance to defibrillate are kept on file and reviewed periodically.

Nurses accompany all patients out of the CCU for tests which cannot be performed in the Unit. The patient is continuously monitored with portable equipment which includes a defibrillator. A specially designed kit of emergency

**University of California Medical Center**
**San Diego**
**University Hospital**

**Patient Education Program**

Topic: **Myocardial Infarction—Heart Attack**

| Content | Date Time | Init | Need for Teaching | | Comments |
|---|---|---|---|---|---|
| | | | Yes | No | |
| How the Heart Functions: Anatomy and Physiology | | | | | |
| Development of A.S.H.D. | | | | | |
| Identification and Role of Risk Factors | | | | | |
| Myocardial Infarction Warning Symptoms | | | | | |
| Effect of Disease | | | | | |
| Treatment of Disease | | | | | |
| Physical Activity and Exercise | | | | | |
| Psychological Effect | | | | | |
| When to Call the Doctor | | | | | |
| Medications | | | | | |
| Diet | | | | | |
| Home Instruction and Activity Sheet | | | | | |

Fig. 7.7  Checklist for patient education program used at UCSD.

supplies accompanies the patient in transit. This kit is designed to assist in handling unexpected situations and is not to be considered complete for a total rescue situation. Included in the kit are lidocaine and atropine, an airway, a padded tongue blade, a blood pressure cuff, a stethoscope, extra Angiocaths, various tapes, alcohol and Betadine swabs, a bag of intravenous fluid, a tourniquet, and a tube of conducting gel for defibrillation. All CCU nurses are also trained as members of the cardiopulmonary resuscitation team and are thoroughly versed in the priorities of an arrest situation.

## Nursing Care Plans

A patient history [152] is taken upon admission [151] as quickly and briefly as possible. Family members are utilized if the patient is unconscious or too ill to be questioned. If the patient is in pain or distress, the nurse will es-

**Table 7.4   Progressive Ambulation Protocol for 14-Day Acute Myocardial Infarction Hospitalization**

| Postinfarct Day | Stage | Date | Activity |
|---|---|---|---|
| | 1. | | Bed rest all of the day. Use of bedside commode once with assistance. May help wash face and arms. May dangle at side of bed 1 to 2× a day. May flex and extend ankles. |
| | 2. | | With chair near bed, begin sitting in chair for short period 2× a day. |
| | 3. | | Sit in chair 30 min 3× a day. May help with bed bath. May shave while sitting in chair. May walk with assistance to bathroom 1× a day. Avoid any straining at any activity. Have staff open windows or move chairs. |
| | 4. | | Sit in chair 1 hour 4× a day. Walk to bathroom 2× a day. While in chair, exercise legs and arms with swinging motion. Avoid raising arms above shoulder level. Avoid any exercise that is resistant or isometric. While exercising breathe slowly in and out and never hold your breath while exercising. |
| | 5. | | May walk to bathroom as needed. Begin to walk in room-hall one minute with supervision 1× a day. |
| | | | Rest for at least 30 minutes after eating or between any exercise or activity. If you develop any chest discomfort or difficulty breathing, rest immediately and notify the nurse. |
| | | | Slowly walk for 1 minute 2 to 4× a day. While sitting in chair may bathe self. |
| | 6. | | Once a day with supervision do standing warm-up exercise. Arms at side, swing in circular motion 10 times. Holding on to a chair do right leg exercises. Bend R. knee and circle right leg and foot 2 times outward and 2 times inward. Repeat with left leg. Standing, raise on the toes 4×. Walk 1 minute 2 to 4× a day. |
| | 7. | | Walk 1 to 2 minutes 2 to 3× a day. May shower. Avoid using very hot or cold water as it could be harmful to your circulation. Continue previous exercise 2× a day. |
| | 8. | | Walk 2 to 3 minutes 2 to 3× a day. Once a day, do standing exercise under supervision (lateral side bends and trunk twists 2× each). |
| | | | Walk 3 to 4 minutes 3 to 4× a day. |
| | 9. | | Continue as above. With supervision, climb down one flight of stairs. |
| | 10. | | Walk 4 to 5 minutes at least 4× a day. With supervision climb up one flight of stairs. |
| | | | Walk at moderate pace for 4 to 5 minutes 4 to 6× a day. |

Table 7.5 Progressive Ambulation Protocol for 10-Day Acute Myocardial Infarction Hospitalization

| Postinfarct Day | Stage | Date | Activity |
|---|---|---|---|
| | 1. | | Bedrest all of day. Use of bedside commode once with assistance. May bathe face and arms. Passive exercise to feet and legs 2× a day. Avoid crossing ankles or legs, as it limits the blood circulation. |
| | 2. | | With chair near bed, begin sitting in chair for short periods 2× a day. |
| | 3. | | Sit in chair 1 hour 3× a day. Shave self while sitting in chair. Walk to bathroom with help 2× a day. While in chair, may exercise arms and legs with swinging motion. |
| | 4. | | Walk slowly 1 minute 1× a day with help. Sit in chair 1 hour 5× a day. |
| | 5. | | Walk slowly 1 minute 1 to 4× a day. Bathe self using sink in room. |
| | 6. | | Walk in hall as before but going at a quicker pace. |
| | 7. | | Walk in hall 2 minutes 3 to 4× a day. May shower. |
| | 8. | | Walk in hall 3 minutes 3 to 4× a day. |
| | 9. | | Walk in hall 4 minutes 4 to 6× a day. Climb down 1 flight of stairs with supervision. |
| | 10. | | Climb up 1 flight of stairs with supervision only. |

tablish essential information such as medications taken prior to admission and any allergies, significant health problems, and special needs the patient may have. It is very important for patients to know the staff will make phone calls for them and follow up on situations that may be stressful,[154] including unattended children or pets at home. Any aspect of nursing care which can produce comfort is considered and included.[155]

The nursing staff must move quickly yet calmly upon admission of a patient to the CCU. The nurses introduce themselves on a first-name basis and establish what title the patient is most comfortable being addressed with. The nurses explain what will happen in the initial phases of the admission and keep the patient continually informed. As soon as the nurse can be spared from the bedside, she addresses the family [150] and establishes rapport on a one-to-one basis. The unit phone number is given to the family along with the names of contact persons they may request to speak with.[156]

All admission data are recorded and updated according to the patient's condition. Target dates are defined for the physical, emotional, social, and educational care of the patient. Educational programs are clearly defined and instituted as soon as the patient is able to accept his myocardial infarction and is amenable to teaching.[157] The patient education program [158] (Fig. 7.7) begins at the basic level with presentations of cardiac anatomy and physiology. A heart model, displaying arteries and opened to reveal valves and chambers, is used in the program. The patient is encouraged to ask questions liberally, and the needs for further teaching are noted. Once the patient understands elementary anatomy and physiology, the program advances and includes not only knowledge concerning myocardial infarction but education about aspects of life after infarction.[159] The development of atherosclerosis is described, and the identification and role of risk factors is covered. The patient is taught the warning symptoms of myocardial infarction, the effects of the disease, and its treatment. Psychological effects are discussed, and potential problems are explored on an individual basis.[151]

The institution of physical activity and exercise are programmed for the patient according to the size of the infarction and the severity of complications.[159] Protocols have been designed to progressively ambulate and exercise patients on an individual basis (Tables 7.4, 7.5). In preparation for home life, patients are told when to call the doctor, given explanations regarding their medication and diet, and instructed to utilize the home-activity protocol geared specifically to their needs (Fig. 7.8). A list of general instructions and guidelines to be observed during the convalescence phase of acute myocardial infarction is also given to patients prior to discharge from the hospital (Fig. 7.9). When a person becomes a patient due to

UNIVERSITY HOSPITAL
University of California
Medical Center, San Diego

ACTIVITY PROGRAM AFTER A HEART ATTACK

From: ______

1. Rest frequently, either in bed or sitting in a chair.
May walk in house every two hours, for ______ minutes at a time.
May shower, preferably with a shower chair.
No tub bath.
No physical strain - No lifting of heavy objects (over 12 pounds).
No climbing of stairs if at all possible.
No bending or stooping.

From: ______

2. May walk out in yard. Increase length of walk every two days. Increase number of times you walk in yard daily. (Example: the first day only go outside once and the second day walk in yard twice for short distances.)
May go for auto rides.
May do knitting, sewing, drying dishes, or similar activity that you can sit to do.
May visit with friends or other social entertainment (meetings, movies, church, etc.).
You should be walking ______ minutes ______ times per day.
Avoid walking in very hot or very cold weather.

From: ______

3. May walk in blocks, increasing length and number of walks every two days. Walk slowly. Do not climb hills. Remember to walk daily. You should be walking ______ minutes ______ times per day.
May go fishing or attend sports games; if you take it easy.
May do light housework. Avoid changing the linen on the beds.
May do light gardening. Avoid hoeing or shoveling. May do pruning, weeding, planting.
May cook easy meals. Organize your equipment to save steps. Avoid reaching above the shoulder level for dishes or cooking equipment.

From: ______

4. May drive car for short distances. Avoid the stress of traffic.
May go shopping in stores. Do not lift heavy objects.
May resume sexual intercourse, with your partner taking the more active role.
You should be walking ______ minutes ______ times per day or ______ blocks per day.

From: ______

5. May do repair work around the house.
Do not raise arms above head during your activities.
May cook meals.
May wash and dry clothes in a machine. Avoid hanging the clothes out on a clothesline unless you are working at waist level.
May cut grass if you have a power lawn mower. May rake yard for brief intervals.

From: ______

6. May do vacuuming, sweeping the house or yard.
May drive car for long distances. Avoid high altitudes above 4,000 feet for long periods of time.
May travel by plane.
Avoid heavy duty cleaning or mowing lawn by hand until at least four to six months after your heart attack and with your physician's approval.
You should be walking ______ miles daily.

D 657 (10-75) SIC 300

Fig. 7.8 Activity guidelines given AMI patients at the time of discharge from UCSD.

UNIVERSITY HOSPITAL
University of California
Medical Center, San Diego

GUIDELINES TO HELP YOU RECUPERATE FROM YOUR HEART ATTACK

SECTION I — Space your activities to allow time for you and your heart to rest.

A. Plan your day's work. Spread out difficult tasks between rest periods. Alternate an easy task with a hard one.

B. If you get tired, no matter what you are doing, stop and rest for 15 to 30 minutes. Don't push yourself to wash the last few dishes or watch the last 45 minutes of that T.V. program.

C. Space your activities throughout the day. Rest in between activities and/or excercises.

D. Avoid being in a rush. Plan your day so that you can get everything done in an efficient manner.

E. Try to get at least six to eight (6 - 8) hours of sleep daily.

SECTION II — If you do house work, the following are helpful suggestions:

A. Eliminate unecessary tasks, for example dry dishes on a drainboard, avoid actively drying dishes.

B. Finish cleaning one room before you go to the next.

C. Have someone move your furniture when you plan to do your heavy cleaning.

D. Make-up one side of the bed completely and then go to the other side. This will cut down on the number of times you have to walk around the bed.

E. Do as many tasks as possible while sitting down.

F. Arrange your work activities so that you don't have to raise your arms over your head. Working with your arms above shoulder lever is hard on your heart. It will also cause you to tire very quickly. Have someone rearrange the cabinet contents so that things you use often are at shoulder or waist level. If you must have things in high cabinets, place items you use most often in the front of the cabinet.

G. Avoid trying to open a stuck window or unscrewing a jar lid. (Both activities are similar to isometric exercises.)

SECTION III — Exercise and activity programs will help promote good circulation.

A. Avoid lifting heavy objects. Remember to pick up objects from the floor by squatting and retreiving the objects or by sitting in a chair and reaching to the floor.

B. Bending at waist level to pick up objects increases the strain on the heart.

C. Avoid isometric exercises. For example, sit-ups, push-ups, or opposing muscle exercises, i.e., leaning against the wall and pushing your body away from the wall.

D. Walking daily is the best exercise for your heart and your circulation. For the first two to three (2 - 3) months after a heart attack, it is best to walk slowly in gradually increasing length of walks per day. Your physician will help guide you in an exercise regime as you continue your convalescence. Generally speaking though, most patients can perform the following activities in the later stages of their convalescence:

1. Billiards - Pool: 1 - 2 months after heart attack
2. Swimming: 2 - 4 months after heart attack
3. Golfing: 2 - 4 months after heart attack
4. Bowling: 3 - 5 months after heart attack
5. Running: 5 - 7 months after heart attack
6. Jogging: avoid this activity unless your doctor specifically authorizes it.
7. Tennis: 8 - 10 months after heart attack.

E. When starting any exercise or strenuous activity regime, one should begin slowly and build up their physical tolerance over a long period of time.

SECTION IV — Returning to work after recuperation from a heart attack:

A. Start back to work part-time (2 - 3 hours per day) and gradually increase your working hours over a three week period.

B. Organize your office work to reduce physical and emotional stress.

C. Continue to do your physical exercises at least four (4) times a week.

D. Continue to avoid further RISK factors for heart disease. For example: smoking, high blood pressure, obesity, dietary indiscretion, i.e. food that is too salty or too rich in fatty foods.

SECTION V — What to do in case you develop chest pain:

A. If you develop chest pain or pain that goes into your arm, hand, neck or jaw, do stop what you are doing. Take your Nitroglycerin tablets and rest for fifteen to twenty (15 20) minutes. When the discomfort disappears, continue what you were doing, but at a slower rate. Increased activity will cause some shortness of breath but resting will eliminate this symptom.

B. Notify your physician or go to the nearest Emergency Room if you have:
1. Chest pain or pressure or squeezing feeling in your chest. This discomfort may go into your arms or into your neck. This pain IS NOT relieved with the use of Nitroglycerin tablets (total of 4 tablets in 20 minutes or one tablet every five minutes).
2. Severe chest pain along with nausea, vomiting, sweating
3. Severe shortness of breath
4. Fainting

D 655 (10-75) SIC 300

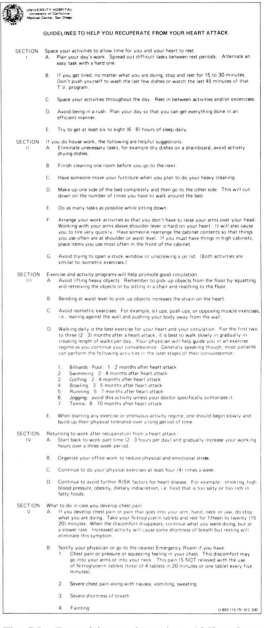

Fig. 7.9 General instructions given AMI patients at the time of discharge from UCSD.

acute myocardial infarction, the nursing care must be comprehensive.[154] The nurses must be capable of providing safe care in a confident manner and must realize the specific needs of each patient. Assisting the patient through the initial event is extremely important; however, preparing the patient for the future can begin early and must be considered in each case.

## REFERENCES

1. Pantridge JF, Adgey AAJ: Pre-hospital coronary care. Am J Cardiol 24:666, 1969.
2. Hackett TP, Cassem NH: Coronary care: patient psychology. Am Heart Assoc, NY, 1975.
3. Bloom BS, Peterson OL: End results, cost and productivity of coronary care units. N Engl J Med 228:72, 1973.
4. Gazes PC, Gaddy JE: Bedside management of acute myocardial infarction. Am Heart J 97:782, 1979.
5. Hugenholtz PG, Laird-Meeter K, Balakumaran K, Ritsema Van Eck HJ, Hagemeijer F: Reflections on current coronary care. Intensive Care Med 4:1, 1978.
6. Hultgren HN, Shettiger UR, Specht DJ: Clinical evaluation of a new computerized arrhythmia monitoring system. Heart & Lung 4:241, 1975.
7. Degner AR, Craddock LD, Wolf PS: Management modalities: cardiovascular system, in Critical Care Nursing, Ed by Hudak CM, Lohr TS, Gallo BM. Lippincott, Philadelphia, 1977.
8. Lindsay J Jr, Bruckner NV: Conventional coronary care unit monitoring. JAMA 232:51, 1975.
9. Lustig K, Cohen SI, Kansil BJ, Abelmann WH: Detection of ventricular premature contractions by a computerized arrhythmia monitoring system. Heart and Lung 7:72, 1978.
10. Turner GO: The cardiovascular care unit. Wiley Medical Publications, New York, 1978.
11. Marriott HJL, Fogg E: Constant monitoring for cardiac dysrhythmias and blocks. Mod Concepts Cardiovasc Dis 39:103, 1970.
12. Friedman HH: Diagnostic electrocardiography and vectorcardiography. McGraw-Hill Book Co, New York, 1977.
13. Inside the coronary care unit. A guide for the patient and his family. Pamphlet published by Amer Heart Assoc, Dallas.
14. Cohen IM, Alpert JS, Francis GS, Vieweg WVP, Hagan AD: Safety of hot and cold liquids in patients with acute myocardial infarction. Chest 71:450, 1977.
15. Fyfe T, Baxter RH, Cochran KM, Booth EM: Plasma-lipid changes after myocardial infarction. Lancet 2:997, 1971.
16. Ritchie JM: Central nervous system stimulants. II. The xanthines, in The Pharmacological Basis of Therapeutics, edited by Goodman LS, Gilman A, 3rd edition, The MacMillan Co, New York, 1965.
17. Doyle JT: Tobacco and the cardiovascular system, in The Heart, Ed Hurst JW, 4th edition, McGraw-Hill, New York, 1978.
18. Piergeorge AR: Basic philosophy utilized in development of the intensive care unit-coronary care unit concept. J Clin Engin 3:55, 1978.
19. Ferguson RL, Rosett W, Hodges GR, Barnes WG: Complications with heparin-lock needles. A prospective evaluation. Annals Int Med 85:583, 1976.
20. Levine SA, Lown B: The "chair" treatment of coronary thrombosis. Trans Assoc Am Physicians 64:316, 1951.
21. Mc Neer JF, Wagner GS, Ginsburg PB, Wallace AG, McGrants CB, Conley MJ, Rosati RA: Hospital discharge one week after acute myocardial infarction. N Engl J Med 298:229, 1978.
22. Goldberger E: Treatment of cardiac emergencies. C V Mosby Co, St Louis, 1974.
23. Lown B, Fakhro AM, Hood WB, Thorn GW: The coronary care unit; new perspectives and directions. J Am Med Assoc 199:188, 1967.
24. Burch GE, Oei H, Dillenkoffer RL: Survival in a coronary care unit. South Med J 68:947, 1975.
25. O'Rourke MF, Walsh B, Fletcher M, Crowley A: Impact of the new generation coronary care unit. Br Med J 2:837, 1976.
26. Grace WJ: Protocol for the management of arrhythmias in acute myocardial infarction. Critical Care Med 2:235, 1974.
27. Collinsworth KA, Kalman SM, Harrison DC: The clinical pharmacology of lidocaine as an antiarrhythmic drug. Circulation 50:1217, 1974.
28. Dhurandar RW, MacMillan RL, Brown KWG: Primary ventricular fibrillation complicating acute myocardial infarction. Am J Cardiol 27:347, 1971.
29. Lie KI, Wellens HJ, Durrer D: Characteristics and predictability of primary ventricular fibrillation. Europ J Cardiol 1:379, 1974.
30. Roberts R, Ambos HD, Loh CW, Sobel BE: Initiation of repetitive ventricular depolarizations by relatively late premature complexes in patients with acute myocardial infarction. Am J Cardiol 41:678, 1978.
31. Romhilt DW, Bloomfield SS, Chou TC, Fowler NO: Unreliability of conventional electrocardiographic monitoring for arrhythmia detection in coronary care units. Am J Cardiol 31:457, 1973.
32. Holmberg S, Ryden L, Waldenstrom A: Efficiency of arrhythmia detection by nurses in a

coronary care unit using a decentralized monitoring system. Br Heart J 39:1019, 1977.

33. Vetter NJ, Julian DG: Comparison of arrhythmia computer and conventional monitoring in coronary care units. Lancet 1:1151, 1975.

34. Harrison DC: Should lidocaine be administered routinely to all patients after acute myocardial infarction? Circulation 58:581, 1978.

35. Whiting RB, Martin RH: Coronary care—1978. Missouri Med 75:503, 1978.

36. Lie KI, Wellens HJ, Van Capelle FJ, Durrer D: Lidocaine in the prevention of primary ventricular fibrillation. N Engl J Med 291:1324, 1974.

37. Darby S, Bennett MA, Cruickshank JC, Pentecost BL: Trial of combined intramuscular and intravenous lignocaine in prophylaxis of ventricular tachyarrhythmias. Lancet 1:817, 1972.

38. Church G, Biern R: Prophylactic lidocaine in acute myocardial infarction. Circulation 46: Suppl 2:139, 1972.

39. Harrison DC, Meffin PJ, Winkle RA: Clinical pharmacokinetics of antiarrhythmic drugs. Progr in Cardiovasc Dis 20:217, 1977.

40. Koch-Weser J: Antiarrhythmic drugs for ischemic heart disease. Postgrad Med 59:168, 1976.

41. Karliner JS: Should antiarrhythmic agents be used prophylactically in patients with uncomplicated myocardial infarction? Pract Cardiol 9:159, 1978.

42. Pantridge JF, Webb SW, Adgey AAJ, Geddes JS: The first hour after the onset of acute myocardial infarction. In Progress in Cardiology, Lea & Febiger, Philadelphia, vol 3, 1974.

43. Gunnar RM, Loeb HS, Scanlon PJ, Moran JF, Johnson SA, Pifarre R: Management of acute myocardial infarction and accelerating angina. Progr in Cardiovasc Dis 22:1, 1979.

44. Webb SW, Adgey AAJ, Pantridge JF: Autonomic disturbances at onset of acute myocardial infarction. Br Med J 3:89, 1972.

45. Lown B, Verrier RL, Rabinowitz SH: Neural and psychologic mechanisms and the problem of sudden cardiac death. Am J Cardiol 39:890, 1977.

46. Lowenstein E: Morphine "anesthesia"—a perspective. Anesthesiology 35:563, 1971.

47. Lappas DG, Geha D, Fischer JE, Laver MB, Lowenstein E: Filling pressures of the heart and pulmonary circulation of the patient with coronary artery disease after large intravenous doses of morphine. Anesthesiology 42:153, 1975.

48. Jaffe JH: Narcotic analgesics, in The Pharmacological Basis of Therapeutics, ed by Goodman LS, Gilman A, 3rd edition, The MacMillan Co, New York, 1965.

49. Vasco JS, Henney RP, Oldham HM, Brawley RK, Morrow AG: Mechanisms of action of morphine in the treatment of experimental pulmonary edema. Am J Cardiol 18:876, 1966.

50. Alderman EL: Analgesics in the acute phase of myocardial infarction. J Am Med Assn 229:1646, 1974.

51. MacDonald HR, Rees HA, Muir AL, Lawrie DM, Burton JL, Donal KW: Circulatory effects of heroin in patients with myocardial infarction. Lancet 1:1070, 1967.

52. Lee G, De Maria AN, Amsterdam EN: Comparative effects of morphine, meperidine, and pentazocine on circulatory dynamics in patients with acute myocardial infarction. Am J Med 60:949, 1976.

53. Côte P, Campeau L, Bourassa MG: Therapeutic implications of diazepam in patients with elevated left ventricular filling pressure. Am Heart J 91:747, 1976.

54. Melsom M, Andreassen P, Melsom H, Hansen T, Grendahl H, Hillestad LK: Diazepam in acute myocardial infarction. Br Heart J 38:804, 1976.

55. Wright IS, Marple CD, Beck DF: Report of the committee for the evaluation of anticoagulants in the treatment of coronary thrombosis. Am Heart J 36:801, 1948.

56. Gifford RH, Feinstein AR: A critique of methodology in studies of anticoagulant therapy for myocardial infarction. N Engl J Med 280:351, 1969.

57. Report of the working party on anticoagulant therapy in coronary thrombosis to the medical research council: Assessment of short-term anticoagulant administration after cardiac infarction. Br Med J 1:335, 1969.

58. Veterans administration cooperative clinical trial: Anticoagulants in acute myocardial infarction. JAMA 225:724, 1973.

59. Modan B, Shani M, Schor S, Modan M: Reduction of hospital mortality from acute myocardial infarction by anticoagulant therapy. N Engl J Med 292:1359, 1975.

60. Tonascia J, Gordis L, Schmerler H: Retrospective evidence favoring use of anticoagulants for myocardial infarction. N Engl J Med 292:1362, 1975.

61. Chalmers TC, Matta RJ, Smith H, Kunzler A-M: Evidence favoring the use of anticoagu-

lants in the hospital phase of acute myocardial infarction. N Engl J Med 297:1091, 1977.

62. Vreeken J: Anticoagulant therapy in myocardial infarction, in Textbook of Coronary Care, ed by Meltzer LE and Dunning AJ. Charles Press, Philadelphia, 1972.

63. Wessler S: Prevention of venous thromboembolism by low-dose heparin. Mod Concepts of Cardiovasc Dis 45:105, 1976.

64. Ribner HS, Frishman WH: Anticoagulation in myocardial infarction: New approaches to an old problem. Cardiovasc Med 2:787, 1977.

65. Prevention of fatal postoperative pulmonary embolism by low doses of heparin: An international multicenter trial. Lancet 2:45, 1975.

66. Murray TS, Cox FC, Lorimer AR, Lawrie TDV: Leg vein thrombosis following myocardial infarction. Lancet 2:792, 1970.

67. Simmons AV, Sheppard MA, Cox AF: Deep-vein thrombosis after myocardial infarction: Predisposing factors. Br Heart J 35:623, 1973.

68. Handley AJ, Emerson PA, Fleming PR: Heparin in the prevention of deep-vein thrombosis after myocardial infarction. Br Med J 2:436, 1972.

69. Wray R, Maurer B, Shillingford J: Prophylactic anticoagulant therapy in the prevention of calf-vein thrombosis after myocardial infarction. N Engl J Med 288:815, 1973.

70. Deykin D: Thrombogenesis. N Engl J Med 276:622, 1967.

71. Saliba MJ, Covell JW, Bloor CM: Effects of heparin in large doses on the extent of myocardial ischemia after acute coronary occlusion in the dog. Am J Cardiol 37:599, 1976.

72. Saliba MJ, Kuzman WJ, Marsh DG, Lasry JE: Effect of heparin in anticoagulant doses on the electrocardiogram and cardiac enzymes in patients with acute myocardial infarction. Am J Cardiol 37:605, 1976.

73. Wessler S, Kleiger RE, Cornfield J, Teitelbaum SL: Coumadin therapy in acute myocardial infarction. Arch Int Med 134:774, 1974.

74. Sherry S: Low dose heparin for the prophylaxis of pulmonary embolism. Am Rev Resp Dis 114:661, 1976.

75. Sharnoff JG, Kass HH, Mistica BA: A plan of heparinization of the surgical patient to prevent postoperative thromboembolism. Surg Gyn Obst 115:75, 1962.

76. Biggs R, Denson KWE, Akman N, Borrett R, Hadden M: Antithrombin III, antifactor Xa, and heparin. Br J Haematol 19:283, 1970.

77. Kakkar VV, Spindler J, Flute PT, Corrigan T, Fossard DP, Crellin RQ: Efficacy of low doses of heparin in prevention of deep-vein thrombosis after major surgery. Lancet 2:101, 1972.

78. Fratantoni J, Wessler S (Eds): Prophylactic therapy of deep vein thrombosis and pulmonary embolism. DHEW Public No (NIH) 76–866, 1975.

79. Gallus AS, Hirsh J, Tuttle RJ, Trebilcock R, O'Brien SE, Caroll JJ, Minden JH, Hudeckin SM: Small subcutaneous doses of heparin in prevention of venous thrombosis. N Engl J Med 288:545, 1973.

80. Russek HI: Anticoagulants should not be used routinely for acute myocardial infarction. Cardiovasc Clinics 8:123, 1977.

81. Hurst JW, Logue RB, Walter PF: The clinical recognition and management of coronary atherosclerotic heart disease, in The Heart, Ed Hurst JW et al, 4th Ed, McGraw-Hill, New York, 1978.

82. Page DL, Caulfield JB, Kastor JA, De Sanctis RW, Sanders CA: Myocardial changes associated with cardiogenic shock. N Engl J Med 285:133, 1971.

83. Alonso DR, Scheidt S, Post M, Killip T: Pathophysiology of cardiogenic shock. Circulation 48:588, 1973.

84. Maroko PR, Kjekshus JK, Sobel BE, Watanabe T, Covell JW, Ross J Jr, Braunwald E: Factors influencing infarct size following experimental coronary artery occlusions. Circulation 43:67, 1971.

85. Klein RF, Troyer WG, Thompson HK, Bogdonoff MD, Wallace AG: Catecholamine excretion in myocardial infarction. Arch Int Med 86:470, 1968.

86. Mueller H: Propranolol in acute myocardial infarction in man. Effects on hemodynamics and myocardial oxygenation. Acta Med Scand Suppl 587:177, 1976.

87. Wit AL, Hoffman BF, Rosen MR: Electrophysiology and pharmacology of cardiac arrhythmias IX. Cardiac electrophysiologic effects of beta adrenergic stimulation and blockade. Am Heart J 90:521, 1975.

88. Lee RJ: Beta adrenergic blockade in acute myocardial infarction. Life Sciences 23:2539, 1978.

89. Oliva PB, Breckenridge JC: Arteriographic evidence of coronary arterial spasm in acute myocardial infarction. Circulation 56:366, 1977.

90. Maseri A, L'Abbate A, Baroldi G, Chierchia S, Marzilli M, Ballestra AM, Severi S, Parodi O, Biagini A, Distante A, Pesola A: Coronary

vasospasm as a possible cause of myocardial infarction. N Engl J Med 299:1271, 1978.

91. Feigl EO: Sympathetic control of coronary circulation. Circ Res 20:262, 1967.

92. Marchetti G, Merlo L, Noseda V: Mechanism of the decrease in coronary blood flow after beta-blockade in conscious dogs. Cardiovasc Res 16:532, 1972.

93. Pitt B, Elliot EC, Gregg DE: Adrenergic receptor activity in the coronary arteries of the unanesthetized dog. Circ Res 21:75, 1967.

94. Borda L, Suchleib R, Henry P: Beta-adrenergic coronary arterial constriction during hypoxia. Clin Res 25:210A, 1977.

95. Pitt B, Craven P: Effect of propranolol on regional myocardial blood flow in acute ischemia. Cardiovasc Res 4:176, 1970.

96. Snow PJD: Effect of propranolol in myocardial infarction. Lancet 2:551, 1965.

97. Balcon R, Jewitt DE, Davies JPH, Oram S: A controlled trial of propranolol in acute myocardial infarction. Lancet 2:917, 1966.

98. Gold HK, Leinbach RC, Maroko PR: Propranolol-induced reduction of signs of ischemic injury during acute myocardial infarction. Am J Cardiol 38:689, 1976.

99. Peter T, Norris RM, Clarke ED, Heng MK, Singh BN, Williams B, Howell DR, Ambler PK: Reduction of enzyme levels by propranolol after acute myocardial infarction. Circulation 57:1091, 1978.

100. Roberts R: Can we clinically measure infarction size? JAMA 242:183, 1979.

101. Peter T, Heng MK, Singh BM, Ambler P, Nisbet H, Elliot R, Norris RM: Failure of high doses of propranolol to reduce experimental myocardial ischemic damage. Circulation 57: 534, 1978.

102. Amsterdam EA, Hilliard G, Williams DO, Caudill C, Vismara L, Massumi RA, Mason DT: Hemodynamic effects of propranolol in acute myocardial infarction. Circulation 47–48 Suppl IV:138, 1973.

103. Mueller HS, Ayres SM: The role of propranolol in the treatment of acute myocardial infarction. Progr CV Dis 19:405, 1977.

104. Cairns JA, Klassen G: Modification of acute myocardial infarction by IV propranolol. Circulation 51–52 Suppl II:107, 1975.

105. Malek I, Waagstein F, Hjalmarson A, Helmberg S, Swedberg K: Hemodynamic effects of the cardioselective beta-blocking agent metoprolol in acute myocardial infarction. Acta Med Scand 204:195, 1978.

106. Chatterjee K, Swan HJC: Hemodynamic profile of acute myocardial infarction. In Myocardial Infarction, Corday E and Swan HJC (Eds), Baltimore, Williams & Wilkins Co, 1973.

107. Shiroff RA, Mathis J, Zelis R, Schneck DW, Babb JD, Leaman DM, Hayes AH: Propranolol rebound—a retrospective study. Am J Cardiol 41:778, 1978.

108. Jewitt DE, Singh BN: The role of $\beta$-adrenergic blockade in myocardial infarction. Prog CV Dis 16:421, 1974.

109. Coltart DJ, Gibson DG, Shand DG: Plasma propranolol levels associated with suppression of ventricular ectopic beats. Br Med J 1:490, 1971.

110. Lemberg L, Castellanos A, Arcebal AG: The use of propranolol in arrhythmias complicating acute myocardial infarction. Am Heart J 80:479, 1970.

111. Oxygen in myocardial infarction. Editorial. Br Med J 1:731, 1976.

112. Pace JB, Gunnar RM: Influence of coronary occlusion on pulmonary vascular resistance in anesthetized dogs. Am J Cardiol 39:60, 1977.

113. McNicol MW, Kirby BJ: Oxygen therapy in myocardial infarction, in Textbook of Coronary Care, Ed Meltzer LE and Dunning AJ, Amsterdam, Exerpta Medica, 1972.

114. Sukumalchantra Y, Danzig R, Levy SE, Swan HJC: The mechanism of arterial hypoxemia in acute myocardial infarction. Circulation 41: 641, 1970.

115. Rawles J, Kenmore ACF: Controlled trial of oxygen therapy in uncomplicated myocardial infarction. Br Med J 1:1121, 1976.

116. Thomas M, Malmcrona R, Shillingford J: Hemodynamic effects of oxygen in patients with acute myocardial infarction. Br Heart J 27:401, 1965.

117. Loeb HS, Chuquimia R, Sinno MZ, Rahimtoola SH, Rosen KM, Gunnar RM: Effects of low-flow oxygen on the hemodynamics and left ventricular function in patients with uncomplicated acute myocardial infarction. Chest 60:352, 1971.

118. Maroko PR, Radvany P, Braunwald E, Hale SL: Reduction of infarct size by oxygen inhalation following acute coronary occlusion. Circulation 52:360, 1975.

119. Radvany P, Maroko PR, Braunwald E: Effects of hypoxemia on the extent of myocardial necrosis after experimental coronary occlusion. Am J Cardiol 35:795, 1975.

120. Madias JE, Hood WB Jr: Reduction of precor-

dial ST segment elevation in patients with acute myocardial infarction by oxygen breathing. Circulation 53 (Suppl I):198, 1976.

121. Suter PM, Fairley B, Isenberg MD: Cardiopulmonary effects of PEEP in respiratory failure. N Engl J Med 292:284, 1975.

122. Nitroglycerin in acute myocardial infarction. Med Let 18:37, 1976.

123. Epstein SE, Kent KM, Borer JS, Goldstein RE, Smith HJ, Capuro NL: Vasodilators in the management of acute myocardial infarction. Adv Cardiol 22:138, 1978.

124. Chatterjee K, Parmley WW, Ganz W, Forrester J, Walinsky P, Crexells C, Swan HJC: Hemodynamic and metabolic responses to vasodilator therapy in acute myocardial infarction. Circulation 48:1183, 1973.

125. Flaherty JT, Reid PR, Kelly DT, Taylor DR, Weisfeldt ML, Pitt B: Intravenous nitroglycerin in acute myocardial infarction. Circulation 51:132, 1975.

126. Bussman W-D, Schofer H, Kaltenbach M: Effects of intravenous nitroglycerin on hemodynamics and ischemic injury in patients with acute myocardial infarction. Europ J Cardiol 8:61, 1978.

127. Hirshfeld JW Jr, Borer JS, Goldstein RE, Barrett MJ, Epstein SE: Reduction in severity and extent of myocardial infarction when nitroglycerin and methoxamine are administered during coronary occlusion. Circulation 49:291, 1974.

128. Borer JS, Redwood DR, Levitt B, Cagin N, Bianchi C, Vallin H, Epstein SE: Reduction in myocardial ischemia with nitroglycerin or nitroglycerin plus phenylephrine administered during acute myocardial infarction in man. N Engl J Med 293:1008, 1975.

129. Epstein SE: Hypotension, nitroglycerin, and acute myocardial infarction. Circulation 47:729, 1973.

129a. Kim YI, Williams JF Jr: Relief of chest pain and reduction of Q-wave evolution in acute myocardial infarction by large-dose sublingual nitroglycerin. Am J Cardiol 45:483, 1980.

130. Chatterjee K, Parmley WW, Swan HJC, Berman G, Forrester J, Marcus HS: Beneficial effects of vasodilator agents in severe mitral regurgitation due to dysfunction of subvalvular apparatus. Circulation 48:684, 1973.

131. Cohen MV, Kirk ES: Differential response of large and small coronary arteries to nitroglycerin and angiotensin. Autoregulation and tachyphylaxis. Circ Res 33:445, 1973.

132. Miller RR, Vismara LA, Williams DO, Amsterdam EA, Mason DT: Pharmacologic mechanisms for left ventricular unloading in clinical congestive heart failure. Differential effects of nitroprusside, phentolamine, and nitroglycerin on cardiac function and peripheral circulation. Circ Res 39:127, 1976.

133. Chiarello M, Gold HK, Leinbach RC, Davis MA, Maroko PR: Comparison between the effects of nitroprusside and nitroglycerin on ischemic injury after acute myocardial infarction. Circulation 54:766, 1976.

134. Mann T, Holman BL, Green LH, Phillips DA, Markis JE, Cohn PF: Effect of nitroprusside on regional myocardial blood flow and comparison with nitroglycerin in patients with coronary artery disease. Circulation 55–56 (Suppl III):33, 1977.

135. Derrida JP, Sol R, Chiche P: Favorable effects of prolonged nitroglycerin infusion in patients with acute myocardial infarction. Am Heart J 96:833, 1978.

136. Bussman, W-D, Lohner J, Kaltenbach M: Orally administered isosorbide dinitrate in patients with and without left ventricular failure due to acute myocardial infarction. Am J Cardiol 39:91, 1977.

137. Armstrong PW, Mathew MT, Boroomand K, Parker JO: Nitroglycerin ointment in acute myocardial infarction. Am J Cardiol 38:474, 1976.

138. Baxter RH, Tait CM, McGuiness JB: Vasodilator therapy in acute myocardial infarction. Use of sublingual isosorbide dinitrate. Br Heart J 39:1067, 1977.

139. Dobbs W, Povalsky HJ: Coronary circulation, angina pectoris, and antianginal agents, in Cardiovascular Pharmacology, Ed by Antonaccio MJ, Raven Press, New York NY, p 493, 1977.

140. Delgado OE, Pitt B, Taylor DR, Weisfeldt ML, Kelly DT: Role of sublingual nitroglycerin in patients with acute myocardial infarction. Br Heart J 37:392, 1975.

141. Come PA, Pitt B: Nitroglycerin induced severe hypotension and bradycardia in patients with acute myocardial infarction. Circulation 54:624, 1976.

142. Earnest DL, Fletcher GF: Danger of rectal examination in patients with acute myocardial infarction—fact or fiction? N Engl J Med 281:238, 1969.

143. Shell WE, Sobel BE: Protection of jeopardized ischemic myocardium by reduction of ventricular afterload. N Engl J Med 291:481, 1974.

144. Peel AAF, Semple T, Wang I, Lancaster WM, Doll JLG: A coronary prognostic index for grading the severity of infarction. Br Heart J 24:745, 1962.
145. Norris RM, Brandt PWT, Caughey DE, Lee AJ, Scott PJ: A new coronary prognostic index. Lancet 1:274, 1969.
146. Beck AO, Hochrein H: Clinical course and prognosis of myocardial infarction in hypertensives. Dtsch Med Wochenschr 99:815, 1974.
147. Warren JV, Lewis RP: Beneficial effects of atropine in the pre-hospital phase of coronary care. Am J Cardiol 37:68, 1973.
148. Rosner MI, Comiskey WM, Lannuti PQ, Fuller RS: Critical cardiac care. JAOA 77:222, 1977.
149. Carabello B, Cohn P, Alpert JS: Hemodynamic monitoring in patients with hypotension after myocardial infarction. Chest 74:5, 1978.
150. Bilodeau C: The nurse and her reactions to critical care nursing. Heart and Lung 2:358, 1973.
151. Hackett TP, Cassem NH, Wishnie HA: The coronary care unit: An appraisal of its psycho-logic hazzards. N Engl J Med 279:1365, 1968.
152. Zuzich AM: Physicians and nurses planning together will best promote welfare of the patient. Mich Med 77:404, 1978.
153. Thierer J: Standards of care for the critically ill patient. Heart and Lung 7:731, 1978.
154. Cassem NH, Hackett TP, Bascom C, Wishnie HA: Reactions of coronary patients to the CCU nurse. Am J N 70:319, 1970.
155. Hoffman M, Donchers S, Hauser M: The effect of nursing intervention on stress factors perceived by patients in a coronary care unit. Heart and Lung 7:804, 1978.
156. Cowper-Smith T: Intensive care needed for all in the ICUs. Nurs Times 74:1158, 1978.
157. Cohen NH, Lemberg L: Cardiac rehabilitation in the coronary care unit. Part II. Heart and Lung 7:861, 1978.
158. Cohen NH, Lemberg L: Cardiac rehabilitation in the coronary care unit. Part I. Heart and Lung 7:667, 1978.
159. McCoy P: Rehabilitation after uncomplicated myocardial infarction. Phys Ther 64:183, 1978.

# Appendix: Nitrous Oxide Analgesia in Patients with Acute Myocardial Infarction

## Joseph S. Alpert, M.D.

Nitrous oxide has been employed as an inhalational analgesic agent for decades.[160-162] Recently, nitrous oxide has been used in coronary care units to provide relief from the pain and anxiety of acute myocardial ischemia.[163-166] Opiate analgesics can produce potentially harmful hemodynamic and respiratory actions. For example, the most commonly employed analgesic agent in the coronary care unit, morphine sulfate (see above), causes increased vagal tone, which can predispose the patient to ventricular dysrhythmias, nausea, and vomiting. Central respiratory center depression with resultant hypoventilation can also occur. Inhalation of nitrous oxide, on the other hand, has none of these potentially deleterious effects. Indeed, nitrous oxide inhalation provides effective relief from mild to moderate ischemic discomfort without observable alteration in hemodynamic, respiratory, or gastrointestinal function.[166]

## CARDIOVASCULAR ACTIONS OF NITROUS OXIDE

Studies on the cardiovascular effects of nitrous oxide have produced conflicting results regarding the agent's hemodynamic actions. Some animal studies, including observations made on isolated papillary muscle preparations, have demonstrated myocardial depression secondary to nitrous oxide.[167-171] Other, equally well-designed investigations have failed to document negative inotropic effects secondary to nitrous oxide.[172-174] The disagreement between these studies is probably the result of two factors: the use of different animal species in the various experiments and the frequent use of other anesthetic agents together with nitrous oxide.

Mild depression of myocardial function has been seen in patients inhaling nitrous oxide.[175-179] Eisele and Smith studied ten volunteer subjects by means of ballistocardiography and dye-dilution curves.[178] These investigators noted depression of myocardial function during nitrous oxide inhalation. Others have noted depressed left ventricular function in anesthetized patients undergoing coronary arterial surgery and in conscious patients with coronary artery disease undergoing cardiac catheterization.[177-179] In the latter investigation, however, patients were studied following injection of contrast media, thereby rendering interpretation of the results difficult.[179]

Other studies in conscious patients with coronary artery disease with and without acute myocardial infarction have demonstrated either insignificant or absent depression of left ventricular function secondary to inhalation of nitrous oxide.[163,180] Thus, heart rate, arterial blood pressure, and cardiac index decrease slightly during administration of 50 percent nitrous oxide and 50 percent oxygen.[163,180] This decrease in heart rate and systemic blood pressure produces a modest decline in the pressure-rate product, an indirect measure of myocardial oxygen consumption (Table 7.6). Left ventricular stroke work index and peak dP/dt also decline modestly, but ejection fraction remains unchanged during nitrous oxide inhalation (Table 7.7). Noninvasive parameters of left ventricular function also remain unchanged in individuals who inhale 30 to 50 percent nitrous oxide in oxygen.[181] In one study, end-systolic volume index, cardiac index, ejection fraction, and normalized wall velocity (all determined echocardiographically) and the ratio of preejection period to ejection time were unaltered after 30 minutes of nitrous oxide inhalation.[181] In this study,

**Table 7.6   Hemodynamic Effects of Nitrous Oxide**

|  | n | Control (mean ± SEM) | N₂O (mean ± SEM) | p |
|---|---|---|---|---|
| Heart Rate (beats/min) | 30 | 64 ± 2 | 59 ± 2 | <0.001 |
| Aortic Systolic Pressure (mmHg) | 30 | 144 ± 4 | 141 ± 4 | NS |
| Mean Aortic Pressure (mmHg) | 30 | 100 ± 2 | 97 ± 2 | <0.05 |
| LV End Diastolic Pressure (mmHg) | 28 | 17 ± 1 | 17 ± 1 | NS |
| Pressure-Rate Product (mmHg-beats/min) | 30 | 9237 ± 432 | 8444 ± 378 | <0.001 |

LV = Left ventricular; $N_2O$ = nitrous oxide; n = number of subjects studied
(Wynne J, Mann T, Alpert JS, Grossman W: Effects of nitrous oxide on left ventricular performance in man. In press.)

**Table 7.7   Effects of Nitrous Oxide on Left Ventricular Performance**

|  | n | Control (mean ± SEM) | N₂O (mean ± SEM) | p |
|---|---|---|---|---|
| Cardiac index (L/min/M²) | 16 | 2.8 ± 0.1 | 2.5 ± 0.1 | <0.001 |
| End diastolic volume index (ml/M²) | 3 | 77 ± 6 | 79 ± 6 | NS |
| End systolic volume index (ml/M²) | 5 | 30 ± 5 | 32 ± 5 | <0.05 |
| Stroke volume index (ml/M²) | 16 | 46 ± 2 | 44 ± 2 | <0.05 |
| Ejection fraction | 5 | 0.62 ± 0.05 | 0.61 ± 0.04 | NS |
| LV stroke work index (gram-meters/M²) | 16 | 51 ± 3 | 47 ± 3 | <0.001 |
| LV minute work index (kg-meters/M²/min) | 16 | 3.1 ± 0.2 | 2.6 ± 0.2 | <0.001 |
| LV peak dP/dt (mmHg/sec) | 8 | 2056 ± 83 | 1876 ± 69 | <0.05 |

LV = Left Ventricular; $N_2O$ = nitrous oxide; n = number of subjects studied
(Wynne J, Mann T, Alpert JS, Grossman W: Effects of nitrous oxide on left ventricular performance in man. In press.)

heart rate and blood pressure declined modestly during nitrous oxide administration.[181] Thus, inhalation of a mixture of 50 percent nitrous oxide and 50 percent oxygen would seem to produce barely measurable depression of left ventricular function, with a resultant small decline in myocardial oxygen consumption.

No arrhythmias or conduction disturbances have been noted during administration of nitrous oxide to patients with myocardial infarction.[166,180]

## EFFECTS OF NITROUS OXIDE ON OTHER ORGAN SYSTEMS

Unlike other analgesic agents, nitrous oxide does not depress respiration—a fact which makes it a particularly useful drug in patients with marginal cardiac and respiratory status. Indeed, Kerr et al. demonstrated significant increases in arterial $PO_2$ and unchanged arterial $PCO_2$ and pH during inhalation of 50 percent nitrous oxide and 50 percent oxygen in patients with acute myocardial infarction.[163] Occasional patients experience slight nausea and/or dizziness during inhalation of the anesthetic. These unpleasant side effects rapidly abate when patients discontinue inhalation of nitrous oxide. Bone marrow depression has been reported in patients with tetanus who inhaled nitrous oxide continuously for prolonged periods of time (48 hours or more).[182] Patients with myocardial ischemic pain rarely if ever require such prolonged administration of analgesic agents; consequently, no evidence of bone marrow depression has ever been noted in infarction patients.[163,166]

## ANALGESIC PROPERTIES OF NITROUS OXIDE IN PATIENTS WITH ACUTE MYOCARDIAL INFARCTION

In patients with mild to moderate ischemic discomfort, nitrous oxide may be the only analgesic required for complete relief of pain.[164,166] Patients with moderate to severe discomfort may obtain complete relief of pain from nitrous oxide alone; however, such individuals frequently require concomitant administration of opiate analgesics in moderate dosage. In a double-blind study, Thompson and Lown compared inhalation of 35 percent nitrous oxide in oxygen to 100 percent oxygen alone for relief of the pain of myocardial infarction. A significant reduction in pain occurred in 74 percent of patients who received nitrous oxide, as compared with 29 percent of individuals who received only oxygen.[166] Complete relief of pain occurred in approximately 40 percent of patients treated with nitrous oxide. There were no individuals who obtained complete relief of pain with 100 percent oxygen.[166] In this study, nitrous oxide proved particularly effective in patients with recurrent, prolonged episodes of chest pain. Moreover, the agent was also very effective in patients with unstable angina in whom ischemic discomfort and anxiety were both relieved.

## METHODS FOR THE ADMINISTRATION OF NITROUS OXIDE

A number of different systems have been employed in coronary care units for the administration of nitrous oxide, including nasal prongs, various types of hospital rebreathing masks, and, recently, commercially available airline rebreathing masks. Only the airline rebreathing mask (Sierra * Model PN–289–701, BAC 10–60137–26) delivers appropriate inspiratory concentrations of nitrous oxide.[181] Such masks can be gas sterilized and reused numerous

---

\* Sierra Engineering Company, Sierra Madre, California

**Table 7.8   Nitrous Oxide Protocol**

1. The $N_2O$ tank and blender * are portable and are brought into the patient's room when needed after explaining both purpose and procedure to the patient.

2. To avoid suggestion, side effects are not discussed.

3. The oxygen hose from the blender is then connected directly to a wall $O_2$ outlet, and the $N_2O$ hose is connected to the tank. The $O_2$ and $N_2O$ valves must be opened simultaneously to avoid sounding the alarm whistle which warns of unequal pressures.

4. A dial on the blender allows easy adjustment of the percentage $N_2O$ delivered to the patient.

5. Dosage is regulated according to the patient's needs. 70 percent $N_2O$ mixed with 30 percent oxygen is the maximum amount that may be administered without danger of hypoxia. Patients experiencing severe chest pain are initially given 50 to 60 percent $N_2O$.

6. Following relief of pain, the inspiratory $N_2O$ concentration is tapered to a lower level. An adequate maintenance range is 30 to 40 percent $N_2O$.

7. If pain recurs, the dosage may be increased again according to need.

8. When the patient has remained pain-free for six hours or more on a maintenance level of $N_2O$, the anesthetic may be discontinued and replaced by $O_2$ via nasal prongs.

9. When $N_2O$ is used for sedation alone, 30 to 40 percent is usually adequate.

10. The $N_2O$ dosage may need to be decreased or discontinued if side effects such as nausea, vomiting, hyperexcitability, or obtundation develop.

11. The physician is responsible for the written order to initiate treatment with $N_2O$. The CCU nurse titrates the dose according to the patient's response, and records times and changes in dose on a frequent observation sheet. Respiratory Therapy changes the $N_2O$ tanks as necessary.

---

\* Manufactured by Bird Respiratory Company.

times. Various inspiratory concentrations of nitrous oxide and oxygen are delivered by means of a constant ratio-mixing blender with attached flowmeter and humidifier ** connected to a standard tank of nitrous oxide and the routine hospital oxygen delivery system. Inspiratory nitrous oxide concentration is usually set between 30 and 50 percent. A typical protocol for employing nitrous oxide in the coronary care unit is given in Table 7.8. Nitrous oxide analgesia is both safe and effective when the described equipment and protocol are employed. Nitrous oxide is a particularly attractive analgesic agent for use in the CCU because of its relative ease of administration, rapid onset of action, rather prompt elimination, lack of respiratory depression, and minor but possibly beneficial effects on the cardiovascular system.

## REFERENCES

160. Clement FW: Nitrous Oxide—Oxygen Anesthesia. Philadelphia, Lea and Febiger, 1951, p. 30.
161. Ruben H: Nitrous oxide analgesia for dental patients. Acta Anesthesiol Scand (Suppl 25): 419–420, 1966.
162. Parbrook GD: Therapeutic uses of nitrous oxide. Br J Anaesth 40:365–471, 1968.
163. Kerr F, Ewing DJ, Irving JB, Kirby BJ: Nitrous oxide analgesia in myocardial infarction. Lancet 1:63–66, 1972.
164. Kerr F, Hoskins M, Brown MB, Ewing DJ, Irving JB, Kirby BJ: A double-blind trial of patient-controlled nitrous oxide/oxygen analgesia in myocardial infarction. Lancet 1:1397–1400, 1975.
165. Kerr F, Donald KW: Analgesia in myocardial infarction. Br Heart J 36:117–121, 1974.
166. Thompson PL, Lown B: Nitrous oxide as an analgesic in acute myocardial infarction. JAMA 235:924–927, 1976.
167. Fisher CW, Bennett LL, Allahwala A: The effect of inhalational anesthetic agents on the myocardium of the dog. Anesthesiology 12:19–26, 1951.
168. Price HL, Helrich M: The effect of cyclopropane, diethyl ether, nitrous oxide, thiopental and hydrogen ion concentration on the myocar-

dial function of the heart-lung preparation. J Pharmacol Exp Ther 115:206–216, 1955.
169. Craythorne, NWB, Darby TD: The cardiovascular effects of nitrous oxide in the dog. Br J Anaesth 37:560–565, 1965.
170. Eisele JH, Trenchard D, Stubbs J, Guz A: The immediate cardiac depression by anesthetics in conscious dogs. Br J Anaesth 41:86–93, 1969.
171. Price HL: Myocardial depression by nitrous oxide and its reversal by $Ca^{++}$. Anesthesiology 44:211–215, 1976.
172. Lundborg RO, Milde JH, Theye RA: Effect of nitrous oxide on myocardial contractility of dogs. Can Anaesth Soc J 13:361–367, 1966.
173. Smith NT, Corbascio AN: The cardiovascular effects of nitrous oxide during halothane anesthesia in the dog. Anesthesiology 27:560–566, 1966.
174. Goldberg AN, Sohn YZ, Phear WPC: Direct myocardial effects of nitrous oxide. Anesthesiology 37:373–380, 1972.
175. Thornton JA, Fleming JS, Goldberg AD, Baird D: Cardiovascular effects of 50% nitrous oxide and 50% oxygen mixture. Anaesthesia 28:484–489, 1973.
176. McDermott RW, Stanley TH: The cardiovascular effects of low concentrations of nitrous oxide during morphine anesthesia. Anesthesiology 41:89–91, 1974.
177. Lappas DG, Buckley MJ, Laver MB, Daggett WM, Lowenstein E: Left ventricular performance and pulmonary circulation following addition of nitrous oxide to morphine during coronary artery surgery. Anesthesiology 43:61–69, 1975.
178. Eisele JH, Smith NT: Cardiovascular effects of 40 percent nitrous oxide in man. Anesth Analg 51:956–963, 1972.
179. Eisele JH, Reitan JA, Massumi RA, Zellis RF, Miller RR: Myocardial performance and $N_2O$ analgesia in coronary artery disease. Anesthesiology 44:16–20, 1976.
180. Wynne J, Mann T, Alpert JS, Grossman W: Effects of nitrous oxide on left ventricular performance in man. In press.
181. Lichtenthal P, Philip J, Sloss LJ, Gabel R, Resch M: Administration of Nitrous Oxide in Normal Subjects. Evaluation of systems of gas delivery for their clinical use and hemodynamic effects. Chest 72:316–322, 1977.
182. Lassen HCA, Henriksen E, Neukirch F, Kristensen HS: Treatment of tetanus: Severe bone marrow depression after prolonged nitrous oxide anesthesia. Lancet 1:527–530, 1956.

** Bird Corporation, Palm Springs, California

# Section 4
# DIAGNOSIS OF
# ACUTE MYOCARDIAL
# INFARCTION

# 8 | *History and Differential Diagnosis of Acute Myocardial Infarction*

*Richard A. Walsh, M.D.*
*Robert A. O'Rourke, M.D.*

Despite the availability of sophisticated biochemical, electrophysiologic, and radioisotopic techniques for the determination of myocardial necrosis, the clinician must rely initially on the patient's history to make important diagnostic and therapeutic decisions regarding potential victims of acute myocardial infarction. Accordingly, this discussion will focus on the value and limitations of the history in the diagnosis of both typical and atypical presentations of prolonged myocardial ischemia or infarction.

Adam Hammer described the first patient with a correct antemortem diagnosis of acute myocardial infarction in 1878; the initial complete description of the disease was published in 1910 by Obrastzow and Straschesko.[1] However, James Herrick is credited appropriately as the first physician in the western hemisphere to emphasize the importance of myocardial infarction as a distinct clinical entity in his classic paper entitled "Clinical Features of Sudden Obstruction of the Coronary Arteries."[2] The nosologic difficulties to be encountered in clinical subsets of patients with acute or chronic ischemic heart disease were clearly anticipated in this landmark work: "The clinical manifestations of coronary obstruction will evidently vary greatly depending on the size, location, and number of vessels occluded. No simple picture of the condition can therefore be drawn. All attempts at dividing these clinical manifestations into groups must be artificial and more or less imperfect."

## CARDIAC CHEST PAIN

### Ischemic Causes

The most common symptom present in patients with ischemic heart disease is chest pain which occurs either at rest or with exercise. Therefore, the initial dilemma faced by the physician when confronted with a patient complaining of chest pain is whether the pain is cardiac or noncardiac in origin (Fig. 8.1). If the pain is cardiac, then it is obviously important to know whether it is ischemic or nonischemic in etiology. Ischemic pain is invariably produced by a transient or prolonged disparity between myocardial oxygen supply and oxygen demand. This may result from a sudden decrease in coronary blood flow (e.g., coronary thrombosis or spasm) and/or from the inability to increase coronary blood flow sufficiently to meet an increment in myocardial oxygen demand as occurs during exercise (e.g., severe coronary narrowing due to atherosclerosis). Such pain may occur in the absence of coronary occlusive disease when coronary perfusion pressure is low (e.g., hypotension) or when oxygen demands are greatly elevated (e.g., aortic stenosis).

The pain of myocardial ischemia is characterized by the abrupt or gradual onset of substernal discomfort—frequently described as deep, visceral and squeezing in nature. The words "pressure," "tightness," "heavy," "burning," "ach-

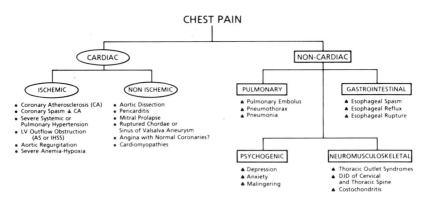

Fig. 8.1 Schematic representation of an approach to differential diagnosis of chest pain. AS = aortic stenosis; IHSS = idiopathic hypertrophic subaortic stenosis; and DJD = degenerative joint disease.

ing," "strangling," or "constricting" are frequently used modifiers for the type of pain experienced by the patient. Many patients with myocardial ischemia will deny the presence of chest "pain" but readily admit the existence of severe chest "discomfort." The clinician must realize the important influence of intelligence, education, and sociocultural background of the patient upon the descriptive quality of precordial discomfort. Facial expression and gestures may provide important clues to the ischemic etiology of the pain.[3] One or two clenched fists held by the patient over the sternal area (Levine's sign) is much more suggestive of ischemic pain than is a pointed finger circumscribing a small area in the left inframammary region.[4] Although the pain is usually localized to the mid chest, primary discomfort in the epigastric region is a well-recognized presentation, particularly of inferior myocardial infarction. Individual cases have been witnessed where the pain was completely extrathoracic (occiput, jaw, arms) or localized to the back, but these are unusual.[5] The pain may remain localized to the chest or epigastrium or radiate to one or both inner arms and/or the neck and jaw. Chest discomfort resulting from ischemia at rest (i.e., unstable angina) is qualitatively similar to that arising from acute myocardial infarction.[6] The dividing line between pain resulting from severe myocardial ischemia and that which occurs due to myocardial necrosis is usually impossible to determine from the history alone. Pain associated with transmural myocardial infarction is usually more severe, of longer duration (i.e.,

greater than 30 minutes), unrelieved by nitroglycerin, and often associated with nausea, vomiting, and diaphoresis. If the physician is present during an episode of rest pain, the response to various simple maneuvers may help discern the difference between ischemic and nonischemic causes of chest discomfort (Fig. 8.2). The performance of the Valsalva maneuver has frequently been observed to relieve cardiac ischemic rest pain, presumably by a reduction of left ventricular wall tension secondary to decreased systemic venous return during the strain phase.[10] Carotid sinus massage may also ameliorate ischemic rest pain through the decrease in myocardial oxygen demand accompanying the reflex bradycardia. Sublingual nitroglycerin in the hypertensive or normotensive patient may provide complete or partial relief of ischemic chest pain. Failure to relieve chest pain by any of these three bedside maneuvers, which may be performed while the patient is being attached to ECG leads, provides evidence for either a noncardiac etiology or pain secondary to acute myocardial infarction. These maneuvers should not be performed in patients with obvious acute myocardial infarction by history and observation, in patients with unstable hemodynamics, or in patients with bradycardia.

Depending on the size and location of the infarct, other noncardiac symptoms may be present. With large infarcts, symptoms of pulmonary venous congestion (dyspnea and orthopnea) may be associated with, or shortly follow the onset of, chest pain. With even greater

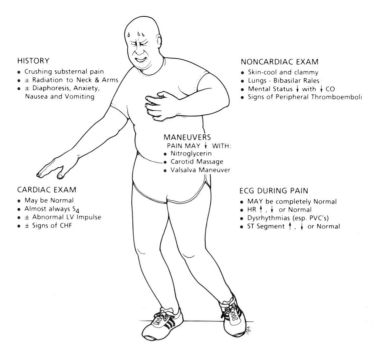

**HISTORY**
- Crushing substernal pain
- ± Radiation to Neck & Arms
- ± Diaphoresis, Anxiety, Nausea and Vomiting

**NONCARDIAC EXAM**
- Skin-cool and clammy
- Lungs - Bibasilar Rales
- Mental Status ↓ with ↓ CO
- Signs of Peripheral Thromboemboli

**MANEUVERS**
PAIN MAY ↓ WITH:
- Nitroglycerin
- Carotid Massage
- Valsalva Maneuver

**CARDIAC EXAM**
- May be Normal
- Almost always S₄
- ± Abnormal LV Impulse
- ± Signs of CHF

**ECG DURING PAIN**
- MAY be completely Normal
- HR ↑, ↓ or Normal
- Dysrhythmias (esp. PVC's)
- ST Segment ↑, ↓ or Normal

Fig. 8.2 Summary of baseline data which may be present in the typical patient with acute myocardial infarction. $S_4$ = fourth heart sound; CHF = congestive heart failure; and CO = cardiac output.

degrees of myocardial necrosis, low-output symptoms (fatigue, weakness) may be observed. The patient who presents with a history of chest pain and syncope or presyncope represents a particularly perplexing problem for the physician. If this symptom complex is of long standing, the etiology is often functional. However, it should be noted that recurrent syncope associated with chest pain has been reported in the setting of symptomatic coronary artery disease and with pure vasopastic Prinzmetal's angina, as a result of AV block due to myocardial ischemia affecting the conduction system.[7,8] Transient, self-limited ventricular dysrhythmias may also contribute to syncope in the setting of acute myocardial infarction.

Questions relating to a prior history of ischemic heart disease are helpful in that approximately 60 percent of patients presenting with acute myocardial infarction will have a history of prior infarction or exertional angina.[9]

In addition, a history of classic exertional angina accurately predicts the presence of coronary artery disease at selective coronary angiography in 90 percent of patients. By contrast, a history of rest pain alone that qualitatively

seems ischemic in origin is a much less perfect diagnostic tool with an accuracy of only 50 to 60 percent when correlated with angiography.[11] All interviews of patients with chest pain of potential ischemic etiology and/or with their relatives should include a careful search for the presence of known risk factors for coronary artery disease. Established independent coronary risk factors include: increasing age, male sex, hypercholesterolemia, cigarette smoking, diabetes, and hypertension; potential risk factors include: obesity, sedentary life-style, family history of premature coronary artery disease, Type A personality, hypertriglyceridemia, and hyperuricemia. The Framingham study concluded that patients with a combination of increased serum cholesterol, hypertension, and a history of cigarette smoking had an incidence of coronary disease eight times that of the general population. However, some clinical investigations have indicated that as many as 40 percent of patients presenting with acute myocardial infarction have no known risk factors. Thus, negative information related to the presence of risk factors may be of little value in the individual patient if the history is otherwise suggestive of ischemic rest pain. It should be emphasized that cardiac conditions other than fixed and/or vasopastic coronary artery disease may also produce pain of ischemic origin, qualitatively similar to that which we have discussed. Severe systemic or pulmonary hypertension, left ventricular outflow obstruction (e.g., aortic stenosis or hypertrophic cardiomyopathy), aortic regurgitation, and severe anemia or hypoxia may all produce exertional chest pain. Little difficulty arises in excluding these entities from the differential diagnosis of acute myocardial infarction, since prolonged rest pain is uncommonly observed in these disorders.

### Nonischemic Causes

Nonischemic cardiac causes of chest pain at rest (Fig. 8.1) may at times be confused with acute myocardial infarction. Foremost among these is dissection of the aorta. Typically, the pain is of sudden onset, with the severity greatest at the onset of symptoms—in contrast with pain due to myocardial ischemia, which builds in intensity with time. Patients frequently describe the pain as excruciating—the most intense pain they have experienced—and as having a tearing quality. The pain may have wide radiation into the neck, back, flanks, and legs, depending on the location of the dissection and the degree of luminal compression. Syncope and neurologic symptoms may occur when dissection involves the cerebral vessels. With the exception of those patients with Marfan's syndrome or idiopathic cystic medial necrosis, the majority of patients with aortic dissection will have a history or clinical evidence of severe, longstanding hypertension. Coronary luminal occlusion with resultant myocardial infarction is a recognized complication of Type I aortic dissection, particularly when the latter is associated with hemopericardium and acute aortic regurgitation.[12]

Acute pericarditis is another nonischemic cardiac cause of chest pain at rest. However, the diagnostic hallmark of pain due to pericardial disease is its frequent aggravation by changes in body position, breathing and occasionally swallowing. Although the pain is most often sharp and cutting in quality, it may at times resemble ischemic rest pain. Radiation of the central precordial pain to the shoulders, upper back, and neck because of diaphragmatic pleural irritation may cause further diagnostic confusion. Because of the frequent association of acute pericarditis with myocardial infarction and aortic dissection, proper diagnosis depends on a careful synthesis of the history, physical, ECG, and echocardiographic findings.[13]

Either acute mitral regurgitation secondary to ruptured chordae tendineae, or acute aortic regurgitation secondary to ruptured sinus of Valsalva aneurysm, may initially present with features suggestive of acute myocardial infarction in that the patient may have a history of chest pain and clinical findings of pulmonary and/or systemic venous congestion. However, the physical examination coupled with serial ECGs and serum enzyme determinations should readily separate these entities. Chest pain occurring as a feature of the mitral valve prolapse syndrome is rarely confused with rest pain of ischemic origin because there is no exertional component to the pain, and the quality is usually atypical. The syndrome of massive pulmonary embolism with associated acute pulmonary hypertension and low cardiac output may occasionally simulate acute myocardial infarction, since myocardial ischemia is present in both conditions. The quality of chest pain may be identical to that of patients with nonradiating ischemic rest pain. However, the associated signs of severe dyspnea, tachypnea, and intense cyanosis associated with profound anxiety and agitation favor the diagnosis of pulmonary embolism. The clinical setting may be helpful because of the known frequency of pulmonary embolism associated with the postpartum or postoperative state, long trips, congestive heart failure, and peripheral edema or acute deep vein thrombophlebitis.

## NONCARDIAC CHEST PAIN

Diffuse esophageal spasm (DES) is the noncardiac condition that may most closely simulate rest pain due to myocardial ischemia. Most patients who present with DES are between the ages of 50 and 60 years. The pain is almost always substernal and may be described as squeezing or aching with radiation to one or both arms. Some patients describe pain that is precipitated by exercise. Many patients obtain relief of their chest discomfort with nitroglycerin because of its generalized smooth muscle relaxing properties.[14] Helpful features which may differentiate DES from ischemic rest pain include its frequent association with dysphagia, pain on swallowing, and regurgitation of gastric contents. The pain is frequently precipitated by either extremely hot or cold drinks, or emotional upset. The definitive diagnosis of DES depends upon the demonstration of abnormal esophageal motility by cine-esophagograms or by esophageal manometry.

Acute esophageal perforation (Boerhaave's syndrome) may produce severe retrosternal pain secondary to chemical mediastinitis due to leakage of gastric contents. Differentiating this cause of chest pain from acute myocardial infarction is rarely difficult, since esophageal rupture usually occurs during or after a prolonged bout of wretching or emesis and is a recognized iatrogenic complication of esophageal instrumentation. Peptic ulcer disease and biliary colic are rarely confused with chest pain of cardiac origin, although the latter may also be relieved at times by nitroglycerin.

Reflux esophagitis results from mucosal irritation produced by failure of the lower esophageal sphincter to prevent regurgitation of highly acidic gastric contents into the distal esophagus. The pain is most often epigastric or substernal and is burning in character. The patient will frequently describe indigestion or "heartburn" precipitated after meals or at bedtime upon assumption of the recumbent posture. Nocturnal or postprandial eructation and regurgitation of gastric juices are commonly noted by the patient. Many patients are obese and will report relief of discomfort by food, antacids, and/or elevation of the head of the bed. Dysphagia may occur as a result of esophageal stricture formation secondary to longstanding esophageal reflux. With massive lower esophageal sphincter incompetence, the patient may have a history of recurrent aspiration pneumonia similar to that observed with achalasia or Zenker's diverticulum.

The various thoracic outlet syndromes may at times produce symptoms which are confused with cardiac chest pain. Axillary neurovascular bundle compression by a cervical rib or the scalenus anterior muscle may cause discomfort involving the chest, neck, and/or ulnar surface of either arm. Helpful differential features from ischemic chest pain include the prominence of associated paresthesias, the lack of clear relation of the discomfort to physical exercise and its aggravation in certain body positions. Idiopathic costochondritis is an occasional cause of anterior chest wall pain which is aggravated by movement and deep breathing. This condition is frequently overdiagnosed on the basis of localized tenderness to palpation at the costochondral junction; perhaps a more definitive diagnosis requires immediate relief of pain by local injection of lidocaine and salutary response to salicylates. The demonstration of costochondral tenderness to palpation does not rule out the presence of coincident chest discomfort resulting from myocardial ischemia or infarction. Degenerative arthritis of the cervical and thoracic spine may cause band-like pain confined to the chest, neck, or back which often radiates to the arms. Radiographic evidence of degenerative changes involving the cervical and thoracic vertebrae is frequently observed in asymptomatic elderly patients. More valuable information to support the diagnosis of chest pain secondary to vertebral disease is the production or intensification of the pain by movement, sneezing, coughing, and various body positions coupled with a careful neuromusculoskeletal examination. Another cause of band-like chest pain, which may at times be misdiagnosed as ischemic rest pain, is the prevesicular phase of herpes zoster. The elderly age of the patient, the frequent presence of hyperesthesia in a dermatomal distribution on physical examination, and the eventual eruption of typical lesions three or four days after the onset of symptoms will eliminate any diagnostic difficulties.

Undoubtedly, the most frequent cause of chest pain is anxiety. Although it is essential to realize that anxiety can coexist with and aggravate discomfort due to myocardial ischemia, there are certain characteristics that aid in differentiating the two conditions. Psychogenic chest pain is frequently stabbing in character, left inframammary in location and sharply circumscribed. Words such as "needle-like," "knife-like," or "lightning-like" are frequently used by the patient as descriptions. Duration of the pain is helpful, since it is frequently either extremely evanescent (seconds to one minute) or protracted, and may last for days. Patients often note pain after rather than during activity, or in the evening after work. In addition, other indicators such as a flat or saddened facial expression, retarded motor activity, and hand wringing coupled with a history of insomnia, loss of appetite, and crying spells may point to depression as the source of the chest discomfort. Associated symptoms such as air hunger, circumoral paresthesia, globus hystericus, and chronic fatigue coupled with multiple other somatic complaints also point toward a potential psychogenic basis for the chest pain. Of note is the fact that many patients with mitral valve prolapse also have such "neurasthenic" symptoms. A careful physical examination may reveal the presence of a midsystolic click and/or late systolic murmur indicating that the atypical chest pain is part of the prolapsing mitral valve leaflet(s) syndrome.

## ATYPICAL PRESENTATIONS OF MYOCARDIAL INFARCTION

Although the classic clinical presentation of acute myocardial infarction is well recognized, certain atypical presentations (Table 8.1) may be less widely appreciated. The common denominators of these atypical clinical patterns of myocardial infarction are either the absence or the unusual location of the pain produced by myocardial necrosis. The incidence of acute myocardial infarction in the absence of chest pain ranges from 4 to 30 percent in various clinical series.[9] In one study [9] involving 250 consecutive patients with acute transmural myocardial infarction, only 4.8 percent of patients had no chest pain in the first 24 hours of observation. However, 18 percent of patients in this group over age 60 had painless transmural infarction. In another study of 258 diabetic patients with acute transmural myocardial

**Table 8.1   Atypical Presentations of Myocardial Infarction**

Nausea and vomiting alone

Atypical location of pain (e.g. arms, back, jaw, occiput only)

Profound fatigue of rapid onset ± syncope

Sudden onset pulmonary edema

Cerebral or peripheral embolus

Pericarditis

Abnormal ECG in the mentally obtunded patient (e.g. perioperative infarct, diabetic ketoacidosis, etc.)

Severe ventricular dysrhythmias

infarction, 25 percent experienced no chest discomfort.[15] Thus, it seems that both advanced age and the presence of diabetes mellitus predispose one to a higher incidence of painless myocardial infarction. Of interest, however, is a recent study demonstrating a higher percentage of diseased vessels present at selective coronary angiography in diabetic patients with anginal chest pain, when compared with anginal controls (68 percent and 46 percent, respectively).[16] Although the mechanism of "silent" infarction in most diabetic and nondiabetic patients is unknown, mental obtundation of any cause may obscure this diagnosis. This is particularly true of the surgical patient at high risk, in whom anesthesia and/or narcotic analgesics given in the perioperative period may prevent recognition of chest pain due to myocardial necrosis. The only clue to the diagnosis in this setting may be the onset of pulmonary edema, ventricular dysrhythmias, or hypotension unexplained by intravascular volume depletion. Another clinical situation in which altered mental status may obscure the diagnosis occurs when the stress of acute myocardial infarction precipitates severe diabetic ketoacidosis and coma. Nausea and vomiting with "indigestion" is a relatively frequent atypical presentation of acute inferior myocardial infarction. Transmural or subendocardial infarction must be considered in any patient presenting with pulmonary edema of unknown etiology, since the severe respiratory distress may overshadow perception of chest pain. An occasional patient may present with profound fatigue with or without syncope, due to severe ventricular dysrhythmias or A-V block.

## DIFFERENTIAL DIAGNOSIS OF MYOCARDIAL INFARCTION

During the past decade, basic investigations utilizing animal models of ischemia and the use of enzymatic and electrophysiologic methods with increased sensitivity for detecting myocardial necrosis have established myocardial infarction as a dynamic process which evolves at varying rates dependent upon multiple factors. Therefore, patients with recent rather than acute infarction may present with chest pain due to extension of the necrotic area. Likewise, patients with myocardial infarction may present with chest pain because of symptoms and physical findings due to a cerebral or peripheral embolus secondary to dislodgement of an endocardial mural thrombus. They are often admitted to a neurology or vascular surgical service with the myocardial infarction undiagnosed and even unsuspected until an ECG reveals a recent transmural or, less commonly, subendocardial infarction. In patients with severe cerebrovascular atherosclerosis, a decrease in arterial blood pressure and cardiac output due to acute myocardial infarction may precipitate neurological symptoms in the absence of cerebral embolism. Recent myocardial infarction must also be considered in the differential diagnosis of any patient at risk presenting with clinical features of acute pericarditis. The latter may represent direct pericardial irritation from an otherwise silent acute transmural infarction or Dressler's syndrome secondary to a recent (though usually greater than one week old) coronary event. The most common cause of transient pericarditis is acute myocardial infarction; in our experience, pericarditis is a more common cause than infarct extension for recurrent chest discomfort during the first three days postinfarction. This pain is often associated with further ST segment elevation and commonly increases with inspiration and diminishes when the patient sits upright.[17]

Although a compulsively taken history is usually extremely valuable in identifying the underlying etiology of chest pain or restricting the diagnostic possibilities, at times it is not helpful or frankly misleading. There are two principal variables which, operating alone or in concert, may result in an ambiguous history. First, physicians may vary in their ability to elicit an accurate history. Second, patients differ in their competence, particularly regarding the qualitative description of symptoms, as a function of their intelligence, sociocultural background, and psychological makeup. For example, patients often minimize their symptoms for economic reasons, job security, or because of a stoical personality; other patients may exaggerate or manufacture symptoms in order to achieve disability or other secondary gains.

Even the time-honored response of chest pain to sublingual nitroglycerin may be misleading because of the placebo effect. The latter has three recognized components: the beliefs and expectations of the physician, the beliefs and expectations of the patient, and the physician-patient relationship.[18] These three components are, of course, maximized when the physician is present during the therapeutic intervention. Despite these recognized vagaries of physician-patient communication, a carefully obtained history remains the keystone in the initial evaluation of chest discomfort which may be due to myocardial ischemia. Therefore, the initial disposition of the patient should never be based on a normal resting electrocardiogram taken during or after an episode of chest discomfort when the history is suggestive of angina at rest or acute myocardial infarction. Rather, the disposition should be a result of sound clinical judgment, derived from a synthesis of information gained from the patient's history, physical examination, and resting electrocardiogram (Fig. 8.2).

## REFERENCES

1. Leibowitz JD: The history of coronary heart disease. Berkeley, University of California Press 1970, p. 135–145.
2. Herrick JB: Clinical features of sudden death. JAMA 59:2015, 1912.

3. Martin WB: Patient's use of gestures in the diagnosis of coronary insufficiency disease. Minn Med 40:691, 1957.

4. Levine SA: Coronary thrombosis—the variable clinical features. Medicine 8:245, 1929.

5. Sampson JJ, Cheitlin M: Pathophysiology and differential diagnosis of cardiac pain. Prog in Cardiovasc Dis 13:507, 1971.

6. Fischl SJ, Herman MV, Gorlin R: The intermediate coronary syndrome: Clinical angiographic and therapeutic aspects. N Engl J Med 288:1193, 1973.

7. Cheike P, Haist Steff P: Angina pectoris with syncope due to transient atrioventricular block. Br Heart J 36:577, 1974.

8. Harper R, Peter R and Hunt P: Syncope in association with Prinzmetal's variant angina. Br Heart J 37:771, 1975.

9. Chazov EI: Main clinical syndromes of acute myocardial infarction. In Myocardial Infarction, ed, Chazov EI, Moscow, MR Publishers 1976, p. 140.

10. Pepine CJ, Weiner L: Effects of the Valsalva maneuver on myocardial ischemia in patients with coronary artery disease. Circulation 59:1304, 1979.

11. Proudfit WL, Shirey EK, Sones FM Jr.: Selective cine coronary arteriography: Correlation with clinical findings in 1000 patients. Circulation 33:90, 1966.

12. Slater E, De Sanctis R: The clinical recognition of dissecting aortic aneurysm. Am J Med 60:625, 1976.

13. Walsh RA, O'Rourke RA: Clues to the evaluation of chest pain in the patient's history. Practical Cardiol 4:41, 1978.

14. Orlando RC, Bozymski EM: Clinical and manometric effects of nitroglycerin in diffuse esophageal spasm. N Engl J Med 289:23, 1973.

15. Partamian J, Bradley RF: Acute myocardial infarction in 258 cases of diabetes: immediate mortality and five year survival. N Engl J Med 273:455, 1965.

16. Dortimer AC, Shenoy PN, Shiroff RA, Leaman DM, Bebb JD, Liedke AJ, Zielis R: Diffuse coronary artery disease in diabetic patients. Fact or fiction? Circulation 57:322, 1978.

17. Hardarson T, Henning H, O'Rourke RA, Karliner JS, Ryan W and Ross J Jr.: Variability, reproducibility and application of precordial ST segment mapping following acute myocardial infarction. Circulation 57:1096, 1978.

18. Benson H, McCallie DP: Angina pectoris and the placebo effect. N Engl J Med 300:1424, 1979.

# 9 | The Physical Examination in Acute Uncomplicated and Complicated Myocardial Infarction

*Richard A. Walsh, M.D.*
*Robert A. O'Rourke, M.D.*

The physical signs present in patients with acute myocardial infarction are critically dependent upon the time course of ischemic necrosis and the presence or absence of electrical or mechanical complications. Accordingly, the physical findings associated with acute myocardial infarction will be discussed in the following four categories: (1) the early uncomplicated acute infarction; (2) the early (less than 48 hours) complicated infarction; (3) the late (greater than 48 hours) complicated infarction; and (4) important noncardiac physical findings which may be observed in the course of acute myocardial infarction.

## EARLY UNCOMPLICATED MYOCARDIAL INFARCTION

The general appearance of the patient presenting with acute myocardial infarction is causally related to an interplay of several variables. The presence and intensity of chest discomfort, coupled with the patient's reaction to pain, result in a spectrum of overall findings on inspection. In general, the patient appears quiet, introspective, and slightly anxious, usually without agitation and excessive movement. Autonomic dysfunction and/or transiently reduced left ventricular performance may result in diaphoresis, nausea, vomiting, peripheral cyanosis, and varying degrees of dyspnea.[1] Conversely, other patients may appear completely normal. Occasionally, because of the intensity of pain or the reaction to it, the patient may appear restless and even insist on walking about.

The heart rate and blood pressure during acute myocardial infarction are dependent upon the time at which the patient is observed after the onset of symptoms and the extent of myocardial necrosis. With the advent of mobile coronary care units, many physicians are seeing patients earlier than previously in the course of their illness. Webb et al.[2] reported on the frequency of autonomic overactivity in a group of 78 patients observed within 30 minutes of the onset of chest pain. Over 90 percent of these individuals had signs of autonomic imbalance. The majority of the 42 patients with anterior infarcts (54 percent) had evidence of excess sympathetic tone (heart rate greater than 100 beats per minute and blood pressure greater than 160/100 mmHg), while most (77 percent) of the 44 patients with inferior and/or true posterior myocardial infarctions demonstrated excess parasympathetic tone (heart rate less than 60 beats per minute, systolic blood pressure less than 100 mmHg, or atrioventricular block). In areas where mobile coronary care units are unavailable, the interval between the onset of symptoms and admission to the coronary care unit is considerably greater (frequently 6 to 8 hours), and the influence of autonomic imbalance on the initial physical findings is correspondingly less. In these patients, the blood pressure and heart rate are more dependent upon the size of the infarct, the presence of dysrhythmias, and the existence of previous cardiovascular disease.

Inspection of the precordium in the asthenic patient or palpation in many patients may reveal the presence of abnormal precordial pulsations. The systolic apical impulse may be diffuse and delayed or frankly dyskinetic. It is difficult to distinguish a prominent apical impulse due to abnormal wall motion in patients with acute or recent infarction from the sustained systolic impulse of left ventricular pressure overload when coincident hypertension is present. In addition, a palpable left ventricular presystolic filling wave ("a" wave of apexcardiogram) often is present, which corresponds in timing to an audible fourth heart sound. Less frequently, one can palpate an early left ventricular diastolic rapid filling wave, which is associated with an audible third heart sound. Patients with large transmural anterior infarcts often have transient early, mid, or late systolic impulses, which are palpable medial and superior to the point of maximal impulse. Persistence of such dyskinetic areas for more than eight weeks postinfarction may provide a clue to the presence of an anteroapical aneurysm.

## Jugular Venous Pulse

In the absence of previous cardiopulmonary disease or associated right ventricular infarction (see below), the jugular venous pulse contour and pressure are almost invariably normal in the early uncomplicated infarction patient (Fig. 9.1). However, since the jugular venous pulse normally reflects the pressure changes in the right atrium, inspection of its contour may reveal the presence and nature of atrial or ventricular dysrhythmias, when ECG monitoring has not yet been initiated or is unavailable. For example, in some rhythm disorders, atrial systole (ECG "p" wave) may occur during ventricular systole (ECG Q-T interval) and produce "cannon" A waves because of right atrial contraction against a closed tricuspid valve. Irregular cannon A waves may be observed during ventricular tachycardia when there is A-V dissociation, or simply with premature ventricular

contractions which are unassociated with retrograde atrial capture.[3]

The first heart sound is diminished in intensity (Fig. 9.1) in approximately 24 percent of patients with acute myocardial infarction.[1] This may be a result of decreased left ventricular performance and diminished LV dP/dt in patients with large infarcts, or may be due to the presence of first degree A-V block associated with ischemia or increased vagal tone in the proximal conduction system, particularly in patients with inferior infarction. Paradoxic or reversed splitting of the second heart sound has been observed during acute myocardial infarction or reversible ischemia.[4] Two mechanisms that have been evoked as an explanation for reversed splitting of S2 are transient left ventricular conduction abnormalities or prolongation of electromechanical systole produced by ischemia or infarction. In our experience, reversed splitting of the second heart sound is rarely observed in acute or chronic ischemic heart disease in the absence of left bundle branch block. There are no large studies using simultaneous phonocardiograms and indirect carotid pulse tracings or aortic valve echograms to document the true incidence of this auscultatory finding. Leatham's admonition is relevant to the evaluation of patients with acute myocardial infarction: namely that a frequent reason for misdiagnosis of reversed splitting is the disappearance of the pulmonic component of the second heart sound during inspiration in patients with chronic obstructive pulmonary disease who have increased anteroposterior chest diameters.

## Left Ventricular Diastolic Gallop Sounds

Left ventricular diastolic gallop sounds are frequently present during transient ischemia or acute myocardial infarction (Fig. 9.1). These are low-pitched sounds which are best heard with the bell of the stethoscope lightly applied to the left ventricular apex with the patient turned to the left lateral decubitus position. Right ventricular diastolic gallops may be auscultated in the same manner, are loudest at the lower left sternal border or subxiphoid area, and frequently increase in intensity with inspi-

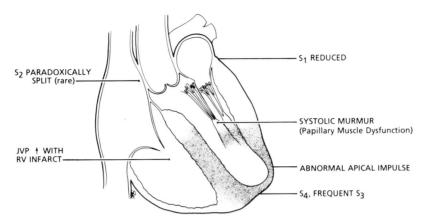

Fig. 9.1 Schematic representation of cardiac physical findings which may be present in acute uncomplicated myocardial infarction. $S_1$, $S_2$, $S_3$, $S_4$ = first through fourth heart sound, respectively; JVP↑ = increase in jugular venous pressure; RV = right ventricle. Right ventricular infarction is included in this diagram to indicate it is a specific entity, even though it more commonly occurs in patients with a complicated left ventricular infarction.

ration. The fourth heart sound is most likely due to the reduced compliance of the left ventricular cavity resulting from ischemia or infarction. One study documented the presence of a fourth heart sound in 98 percent of 107 patients evaluated during the first 24 hours after acute myocardial infarction by serial auscultation, phonocardiograms, and simultaneous apexcardiograms.[5] Thus, the absence of this sound on careful auscultation in a patient with chest pain and in sinus rhythm makes the diagnosis of acute myocardial infarction less likely. However, auscultation may be difficult in obese patients and those with chronic obstructive lung disease, and a fourth heart sound may not be detected in such patients despite acute infarction and sinus rhythm.

Ventricular diastolic gallops (S3) are somewhat less common in acute myocardial infarction. The third heart sound is considered by many to be the auscultatory hallmark of left-sided heart failure and is thought to result from an imbalance between the volume of left ventricular inflow during the rapid filling phase of diastole and the ability of the ventricle to accommodate this inflow. Riley et al.[6] noted the presence of a third heart sound in 40 percent of 156 patients at the time of admission with acute myocardial infarction. The presence of a third heart sound was predictive of an elevated pulmonary artery diastolic or left ventricular

end-diastolic pressure in 25 of 27 patients. However, a substantial number of patients with elevated left-sided filling pressures had no audible S3. The prognostic importance of this physical finding was indicated by the fact that patients with acute anterior infarctions and audible third heart sounds on admission to the CCU had twice the mortality of patients with anterior infarction and no third heart sounds on admission. Another study[5] performed with auscultation and serial phonocardiograms documented a somewhat higher incidence of third heart sounds at the time of the initial physical examination in patients with acute myocardial infarction (65 percent). However, the majority (60 percent) of these third heart sounds disappeared during the first three days of hospitalization. Having the patient cough several times causes a transient rise in pulmonary venous pressure and a slight increase in heart rate, and often brings out or accentuates a third or fourth heart sound when no definite S3 or S4 are present at rest. Auscultation over the subclavian and carotid arteries may detect transmitted left ventricular fourth and third heart sounds in certain patients in whom precordial auscultation is limited by obesity, increased anteroposterior chest diameter, or respiratory sounds such as wheezing.[7] Up to 50 percent of left-sided fourth heart sounds and 25 percent of third sounds can be detected in this manner.

The most common cause of a systolic murmur during acute myocardial infarction is papillary muscle dysfunction (Fig. 9.1). In a prospective study of 210 patients with acute myocardial infarction,[8] Heikkila found that 56 percent developed a new systolic murmur within five days after admission. Although there is no characteristic configuration of the murmur, it is frequently holosystolic, is best heard at the apex, and may have a crescendo quality due to progressive retroversion of one or both mitral leaflets during systole. This crescendo configuration may be produced by the failure of effective papillary muscle contraction to tighten the chordae tendineae as the ventricle shortens along its long axis during systole. Another common mechanism for the production of a systolic murmur during complicated acute myocardial infarction is left ventricular cavity dilatation which leads to papillary muscle-chordae malalignment, thus preventing optimal coaptation of the mitral leaflets. The murmur of papillary muscle dysfunction resulting from myocardial ischemia and/or infarction may be early, mid, late, or holosystolic, depending on whether one or both papillary muscles are ischemic, necrotic or fibrosed, and on the geometry of the left ventricle and the left atrium. The systolic murmur of papillary muscle dysfunction, papillary muscle rupture (see below) or an acquired ventricular septal defect (see below) can often be distinguished from the systolic murmur due to flow across a normal or obstructed aortic outflow tract in patients with spontaneous PVCs or with changing cardiac cycle length due to atrial fibrillation. Mid-systolic murmurs of semilunar valve origin increase in intensity in the beat following a PVC or a long cycle length when atrial fibrillation is present. Murmurs due to mitral regurgitation or a ventricular septal defect often change in duration but not in intensity.[9]

## EARLY COMPLICATIONS OF MYOCARDIAL INFARCTION

Current hospital therapy of acute myocardial infarction is directed toward either the prevention or the prompt and effective treatment of the electrical and mechanical sequelae of regional myocardial ischemia or infarction, while preserving jeopardized ischemic myocardium. With the advent of coronary care units and continuous ECG monitoring, the mortality due to dysrhythmic consequences of myocardial ischemia and infarction has declined considerably. Mechanical complications are now the most common cause of death in the hospitalized patient with acute or recent infarction. The availability of new inotropic agents, external and internal circulatory assist devices, and improved surgical techniques should encourage the early identification of these problems, and careful attention to physical findings may provide the first clue to their presence. Although these complications will be divided into early (less than 48 hours after onset of symptoms) and late (greater than 48 hours) categories, it should be noted that this classification is somewhat arbitrary and that some overlap in presentation will occur between subsets of patients.

### Right and Left Ventricular Infarction

Right ventricular (RV) infarction in addition to left ventricular (LV) infarction has recently emerged as a distinct clinical entity. In some patients, right ventricular infarction may be the dominant lesion. RV infarction has been identified in 8 percent of 78 patients presenting with acute infarction.[10] Two necropsy series have reported an even higher incidence of 14 percent.[11-12] Both clinical and necropsy series have confirmed the invariable association of inferior or posterior infarction of the left ventricle in the majority of these patients. The clinical hallmark of RV infarction is the presence of right ventricular failure disproportionate to left ventricular failure. These patients usually have distended neck veins, right-sided third and fourth heart sounds and hypotension. Frequently, they also present with the physical findings of tricuspid regurgitation as indicated by a large "V" wave and rapid "Y" descent in the jugular venous pulse and a holosystolic murmur at the lower left sternal border that increases with inspiration. Kussmaul's sign (an increase or failure to decline of the jugular venous pressure on inspiration) has also been observed in this setting. This combination of hypotension and distended neck veins may resemble cardiac tamponade. Although the absence of pulsus paradoxus (systolic blood pressure fall of greater than 10 mmHg on inspiration) may be a helpful differential feature between these conditions, the definitive diagnosis of RV infarction may be dependent upon the noninvasive demonstration of RV dilatation without cardiac compression due to pericardial effusion by M-mode echocardiography[13] or the typical hemodynamic profile of disproportionate elevation of right atrial pressure relative to pulmonary capillary wedge pressure present by right heart catheterization. The recognition of this entity is important, since intravascular volume expansion is necessary to maintain cardiac output and restore normal systemic blood pressure despite the elevated jugular venous pressure.

## Left Ventricular Decompensation

Left ventricular decompensation is the most common mechanical complication and the most frequent cause of death in the hospitalized patient with acute myocardial infarction. The degree of failure is a function of the amount of ischemic or necrotic myocardium and the presence or absence of preexisting heart disease. The clinical spectrum of failure in myocardial infarction has been classified[14] and has been shown to correlate with survival and invasively determined hemodynamic profiles.[15] Killip categorized myocardial infarction patients into four subgroups: Class I–no pulmonary rales or S3; Class II–bibasilar rales persistent after coughing, and/or a third heart sound; Class III–rales over one-half of the lung fields bilaterally with radiographic evidence for pulmonary edema; and Class IV–pulmonary congestion as in Class III associated with hypotension and signs of reduced peripheral perfusion (depressed mental status, peripheral cyanosis with cool, clammy extremities, and oliguria). There is often clinical confusion concerning the pulmonary or cardiac origin of rales in the dyspneic patient with both acute myocardial infarction and chronic obstructive pulmonary disease. Rales of purely pulmonary origin frequently clear on coughing and are independent of posture. Cardiac rales occur as a result of the tran-

sudation of fluid into the pulmonary interstitial or interalveolar space secondary to the elevation of pulmonary venous pressure produced by ischemic left ventricular dysfunction. The postural nature of these cardiac rales may be diagnosed by placing the patient on one side for one half hour and noting the increase in rales in the dependent lung field. At times, the physical examination may be misleading after the initiation of therapy for congestive failure in acute infarction. This occurs because of a recognized phase lag of as much as 48 hours between invasively determined hemodynamic stabilization (pulmonary wedge pressure decreasing to normal) and the resolution of abnormal physical and radiologic signs.[16]

Another valuable bedside clue to the presence of left ventricular dysfunction, commonly severe, is the presence of pulsus alternans—an alternation in the amplitude of the arterial pulse on every other beat in the presence of regular sinus rhythm. In patients with left ventricular failure, pulsus alternans is often present transiently after premature beats, but may be sustained. It is best appreciated in the more peripheral arterial pulses (e.g., radial or femoral) where the pulse pressure is usually greater than central pulses (e.g., carotids). The mechanism of pulsus alternans remains controversial. Some feel this phenomenon may relate to alternating end-diastolic volumes and resultant alternation of the force of ventricular contraction (i.e., a Starling effect). Other data point to the possibility of alternating failure of electromechanical coupling. Cardiogenic shock (Killip Class IV) is the most severe form of left ventricular dysfunction secondary to acute infarction (Fig. 9.2). It may be present in 10 to 20 percent of patients with acute myocardial infarction and carries an in-hospital mortality rate of approximately 85 percent with conventional medical therapy. One-half of these patients develop the syndrome within 24 hours of admission; however, the onset of cardiogenic shock was delayed for one week in 13 percent of patients in one large series.[17] Physical findings are usually consistent with severe left ventricular dysfunction—i.e., hypotension (systolic BP less than 90 mmHg), diastolic gallops (S3 and S4), a laterally displaced and frequently dyskinetic apical

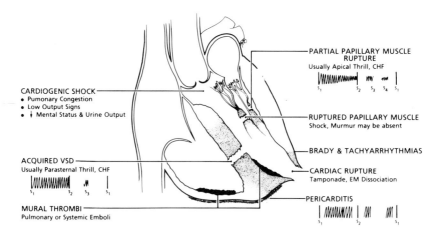

Fig. 9.2   Summary of cardiac examination in complicated myocardial infarction. CHF = congestive heart failure; EM = electromechanical. Other abbreviations as in Fig. 9.1.

impulse, and signs of pulmonary congestion (bilateral rales and/or pleural effusion). Direct and reflex mediated signs of systemic arterial hypoperfusion include: acrocyanosis; cool, clammy extremities; altered mental status; and oliguria. Sinus tachycardia is usual, but atrial tachyrhythmia and premature beats are also common. Necropsy studies have demonstrated ischemic necrosis of more than 40 percent of the left ventricular wall in such patients. However, a lesser amount of myocardial necrosis may produce the same hemodynamic result in patients with prior infarctions (old + new infarct = 40 percent). A major task of the clinician is to separate cardiogenic shock from more readily correctable causes of hypotension in the postinfarction patient, such as intravascular volume depletion. This usually requires bedside right heart catheterization with determination of filling pressures and cardiac output (see Ch. 27).

Two types of pericarditis may be observed during the course of acute myocardial infarction and must be differentiated from other causes of chest pain in the postinfarction patient (i.e., infarct extension, pulmonary embolus, and esophageal reflux produced by recumbency). The more common of these causes of pericarditis is a direct result of pericardial inflammation produced by adjacent necrotic myocardium; it is present in 7 to 42 percent of patients with acute myocardial infarction in various series.[18] A pericardial rub may be present on admission

in patients with a large transmural infarct; more commonly, it develops during the first four days of hospitalization. The diagnosis of acute myocardial infarction is suggested by the presence of a pericardial rub on cardiac auscultation, as well as by the characteristic history (see Ch. 8) which is obtained in approximately one-half of these patients. The pericardial rub is usually best elicited with the diaphragm of the stethoscope firmly applied to the precordium while the patient is sitting up and leaning forward. The typical pericardial rub is superficial and scratching or crunching in quality, and may have three components which correspond to the times of maximal heart motion within the cardiac cycle. One component occurs during early diastole at the time of rapid passive ventricular filling; another occurs during late diastole at the time of atrial contraction; and the final component occurs during ventricular systole. Respiratory variation of the intensity of the sounds is frequent. Any or all of these components of a pericardial rub may be absent at various times; the hallmark of the pericardial rub associated with acute myocardial infarction is its evanescence. Another type of postinfarction pericarditis, Dressler's syndrome, usually occurs later and is believed to have an autoimmune basis (see below).

Fever may accompany large transmural infarcts within the first 24 to 48 hours, but it is usually less than 38°C. The fever due to myocardial necrosis must be differentiated from other common causes of hyperthermia noted in the CCU setting, such as postcardiac arrest aspiration pneumonia, cystitis or pyelonephritis from indwelling Foley catheters, thrombophlebitis, bacteremia from indwelling arterial or venous lines, pulmonary emboli, or pericarditis.

## LATE COMPLICATIONS OF ACUTE MYOCARDIAL INFARCTION

### Cardiac Rupture

After dysrhythmias and cardiogenic shock, rupture of the left ventricular free wall is the third most common fatal complication of myocardial infarction, accounting for 9 percent of fatal myocardial infarcts.[19] Most patients are elderly females, with a peak incidence among patients in their seventies. Cardiac rupture is more common with first infarctions, and there is frequently a history of systemic hypertension. Anecdotal reports implicate, as a possible potentiating factor, vigorous physical activity such as straining with bowel movements early after myocardial infarction. This complication usually occurs within the first ten days after infarction, and one of three clinical patterns is likely to emerge. In the more typical group of patients, prolonged chest pain recurs during the first few days postinfarction, followed by the abrupt onset of dyspnea associated with hypotension, and neck vein distension that rapidly deteriorates to electromechanical dissociation and death.

A second, less common group of patients presents with a more gradual onset of features suggesting cardiac tamponade. Over a period of hours, usually within a single day, these patients develop distended neck veins, tachycardia, systemic hypotension, and pulsus paradoxus. Pulsus paradoxus is an accentuation of the usual inspiratory decline in systolic arterial pressure which is normally less than 10 mmHg. It is best determined by using the cuff sphygmomanometer during normal respiration and noting: (1) the arterial pressure at which Korotkoff sounds are heard only with expiration, and (2) the lower arterial pressure at which the sounds are heard during both inspiration and expira-

tion. When the paradox is greater than 20 mmHg, there is usually a palpable diminution in the peripheral arterial pulses during inspiration. Pulsus paradoxus may not be evident despite cardiac tamponade in the presence of profound systemic hypotension (systolic blood pressure less than 80 to 90 mmHg). It is important to recall that pulsus paradoxus may occur in patients with acute or chronic respiratory distress, hypovolemic shock, and massive pulmonary embolism as well as in intubated patients undergoing positive pressure ventilation.

A final presentation of cardiac rupture occurs with the formation of a left ventricular pseudoaneurysm. The LV pseudoaneurysm represents a partially contained cardiac rupture which is usually connected to the left ventricle through a narrow neck. Therefore, the walls of a pseudoaneurysm are made entirely of organized clot and fibrous connective tissue, while the walls of a true ventricular aneurysm may contain variable amounts of endocardium, myocardium, and epicardium. The to-and-fro movement of blood through the neck of the aneurysm may produce systolic and/or diastolic murmurs. Cross-sectional (2D) echocardiography and radionuclide blood pool scans may prove to be valuable noninvasive techniques for the diagnosis of ventricular pseudoaneurysm, which usually requires angiographic definition. Recognition of this complication of infarction is important because, unlike true left ventricular aneurysms due to ischemic heart disease, pseudoaneurysms may rupture.[20]

Electromechanical dissociation refers to a sudden loss of consciousness, not preceded by symptoms of respiratory failure or cardiac dysrhythmia, associated with regular sinus rhythm on ECG, but without palpable pulse or audible heart sounds. This complication occurred in 2.3 percent of 663 hospitalized patients with acute myocardial infarction in one series.[21] The gravity of this condition is emphasized by the fact that all 15 patients in this series who developed electromechanical dissociation died. Also, none of 514 consecutive survivors of acute myocardial infarction had required resuscitation because of a nonarrhythmic cardiac arrest.[21]

In addition to cardiac rupture, other causes of electromechanical dissociation include extension of infarction, reflex inhibition of sympathetic tone, or enhancement of vagal tone.

## Mitral Regurgitation

Mitral regurgitation resulting from myocardial infarction is produced by a loss of the structural or functional integrity of the papillary muscle apparatus. The primary chordae tendineae originate from the heads of the anterolateral and posteromedial papillary muscles of the left ventricle and give rise to secondary and tertiary chordae which attach to each of the mitral valve leaflets. Each leaflet receives chordae from both papillary muscles. Thus, interference with the structure or function of either papillary muscle may result in dysfunction of both leaflets of the mitral valve. As previously mentioned, the occurrence of mitral regurgitation is frequently due to either papillary muscle dysfunction or left ventricular cavity dilatation. The diagnosis of mitral regurgitation is usually determined by auscultation because of a new, usually hemodynamically unimportant, systolic murmur occurring in the postinfarction period.

An additional and more severe form of mitral regurgitation, arising as a complication of myocardial infarction, is rupture of the head or body of a papillary muscle (Fig. 9.2). The incidence of papillary muscle rupture observed at autopsy varies between less than 1 percent to 5 percent of cases.[22,23] A recent study [23] has indicated that less than 25 percent of the left ventricle was infarcted at necropsy in the majority (10 of 13) of these patients; and in all instances, the myocardium around the mitral annulus was not infarcted. These findings indicate the feasibility of early mitral valve replacement in this condition, which carries a medical mortality of 50 percent in the first 24 hours and 93 percent by two months after the onset of symptoms.[22] Papillary muscle rupture usually occurs in the first two to four days after myocardial infarction and is two and one-half times as frequent in patients with inferior wall necrosis as it is in those with anterior infarction. This disparity in frequency, based on the localization of the myocardial infarct, may relate to the dual blood supply of the anterolateral papillary muscle (circumflex and left anterior descending coronary arteries) contrasted with the single blood supply to the posteromedial papillary muscle from the right coronary artery. Two clinical presentations occur as a consequence of papillary muscle rupture, depending on whether a head or the entire body of the papillary muscle is involved. Rupture of the papillary muscle body is generally heralded by the precipitous development of intractable pulmonary edema and shock. The murmur of mitral regurgitation may be unimpressive because of equalization of a reduced left ventricular and an elevated left atrial pressure early in systole resulting from severe mitral regurgitation coupled with marked left ventricular dysfunction.

Rupture of one head of a papillary muscle generally produces hemodynamically severe mitral regurgitation that may be responsive to initial medical treatment with inotropic agents, diuretics, and vasodilators. The systolic murmur may have the characteristics which are observed in acute mitral regurgitation of any cause, being holosystolic with a decreasing intensity in late systole due to equilibration of left ventricular and left atrial pressures at the time of the left atrial "V" wave. A prominent left-sided fourth heart sound may be observed in patients with sinus rhythm due to a vigorous left atrial contraction. A systolic parasternal lift may be appreciated at the lower left sternal border. If early and sustained, this may result from a right ventricular impulse due to severe secondary pulmonary hypertension. If late and more dynamic, the parasternal lift may be secondary to distension of a noncompliant left atrium by the torrential regurgitant jet and corresponds in timing with a large left atrial "V" wave on cardiac catheterization.

There is often a systolic thrill present at the left ventricular apex. This finding may be helpful in differentiating papillary muscle rupture from a post-infarction ventricular septal defect (VSD), which is another cause for the development of a postmyocardial infarction holosystolic murmur associated with signs of pulmonary venous congestion with or without associated systemic arterial hypotension. Post-infarction ventricular septal defects usually produce a systolic thrill which is maximum at the lower left sternal border. It must be emphasized that the presence and location of a thrill is merely a diagnostic aid in differentiating ruptured papillary muscle from acquired postinfarction ventricular septal defect. A thrill may be absent due to severely impaired left ventricular function or the large size of the regurgitant orifice or septal defect. Also, papillary muscle rupture more commonly involves the posteromedial papillary muscle, and the regurgitant jet may be directed anteriorly and superiorly to the posterior aortic–left atrial junction. This may produce a thrill at the lower left sternal border or base of the heart. Furthermore, acquired ventricular septal defects due to acute myocardial infarction involve the muscular septum, not the membranous septum, as is true in most congenital defects. Accordingly, the systolic murmur of an acquired ventricular septal defect is well heard at the left ventricular apex and may even be loudest at this site.

Right heart catheterization with oximetry usually provides the proper diagnosis with a significant oxygen step-up in the right ventricle or pulmonary artery noted in association with an acquired ventricular septal defect or with giant "V" waves observed with acute severe mitral regurgitation secondary to papillary muscle rupture.[24] Angiography should be performed preoperatively in all patients, since oxygen step-ups at the pulmonary artery level have been reported to occur in the presence of acute severe mitral regurgitation due to the massive reflux of oxygenated blood produced by the regurgitant wave.[25] Additional features which may help to distinguish postinfarction VSD from complete or partial papillary muscle rupture include:

1. With anterior infarction, VSD is a more common complication than papillary muscle rupture; however, with interior infarction, papillary muscle rupture is more common.

2. Axillary transmission of the murmur is distinctly uncommon in acquired VSD.

3. Conduction abnormalities are more common with septal as opposed to papillary muscle rupture.

Another later complication of myocardial infarction is postmyocardial infarction or Dressler's syndrome. This form of pericarditis, believed to have an autoimmune origin, was initially not thought to occur until a few weeks postinfarction. More recent evidence and clinical experience have indicated that it may occur as early as the first week after myocardial infarction and persist for as long as two years.[27] This entity may be differentiated from the more common peri-infarction pericarditis by its later onset and frequent association with fever, leukocytosis, and left pleural effusion.

## Mural Thrombi

Finally, mural thrombi are recognized sequelae of ventricular aneurysms, transmural infarcts, and, less commonly, subendocardial infarcts (Fig. 9.2). Peripheral embolization to the cerebral or systemic circulation may occur secondary to dislodgement of these mural thrombi within the first weeks to months postinfarction. As mentioned in the previous chapter, some of these patients may be admitted initially to the neurology service with a cerebrovascular accident. The presence of a recent, otherwise silent myocardial infarct may be evident only from the admission electrocardiogram. Other patients may develop evidence for sudden arterial insufficiency in one or both lower extremities. The hallmark of arterial as opposed to venous insufficiency is the sudden onset of a cold extremity or digit associated with the "five P's": pulselessness, pallor, paresthesias, paralysis, and pain.[28]

## IMPORTANT NONCARDIAC PHYSICAL FINDINGS IN THE POSTINFARCTION PATIENT

Careful serial pulmonary auscultation is mandatory in the postmyocardial infarction patient, because of various noncardiac physical problems that may develop during the peri-infarction period (Fig. 9.3). Currently, pulmonary embolism occurs much less commonly after acute infarction because of earlier mobilization of the patient, but must be considered in the differential diagnosis of chest pain in the coronary care unit. Dullness to percussion at one or both lung bases due to pleural effusion may be present in patients with pulmonary infarc-

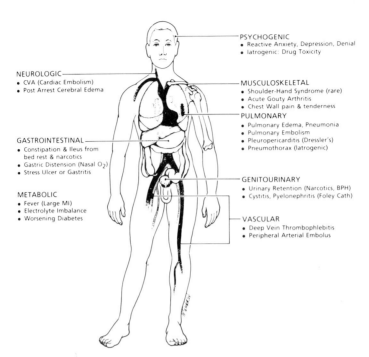

Fig. 9.3 Visual summary of important noncardiac physical findings which may develop during the peri-infarction period. CVA = cerebral vascular accident; MI = myocardial infarction; and BPH = benign prostatic hypertrophy.

tion. A pleural rub may be heard in this setting or with Dressler's syndrome. However, the most common auscultatory finding in patients with documented pulmonary embolism is non-specific atelectatic rales. Thus, the physical examination is much less helpful in the diagnosis of pulmonary embolism or infarction than are more specific laboratory tests such as arterial blood gas determinations and ventilation-perfusion lung scans.[29] This diagnosis must be considered in any patient who has chest pain with associated tachypnea, tachycardia, or fever in the intensive care unit setting. Pulmonary infarction is a recognized complication of indwelling right heart balloon flotation catheters, particularly if the balloon has been left inflated or the catheter has been in place for more than 72 hours.[30] Unilateral diminished or absent breath sounds may be the first clue to the presence of a pneumothorax produced by the insertion of a subclavian venous line. Signs of pulmonary consolidation may be present in patients with hypostatic pneumonia or pneumonia secondary to postcardiac arrest aspiration. The phase lag between hemodynamic and clinical

or radiographic improvement during treatment of pulmonary congestion due to postinfarction congestive failure has previously been discussed.

Gastrointestinal discomfort is common in patients hospitalized in the CCU and may arise from multiple causes, including gastric distension from nasal $O_2$ administration or improper endotracheal intubation (left upper quadrant tympany to percussion), constipation and ileus due to bed rest and narcotic analgesics (decreased bowel sounds and fecal masses on abdominal palpation), activation of peptic ulcer disease from stress, or aggravation of esophageal reflux by recumbency (epigastric tenderness to palpation, response to antacids).

Focal neurologic findings may arise at any time during the peri-infarction period as a result of decreased cerebral perfusion from low cardiac output in patients with intrinsic cerebrovascular disease, or from systemic embolization of a mural thrombus. Patients who have been resuscitated successfully often have transient neurologic findings due to post-arrest cerebral edema, including obtundation and transient focal neurologic signs. Alterations in mental status are common in patients hospitalized in the coronary care unit setting. Reactive anxiety, depression, denial, and/or hostility are frequent by-products of the psychogenic stress associated with myocardial infarction. These by-products must be distinguished from iatrogenically induced mental status changes produced by drugs (e.g., lidocaine-induced hallucinations or seizures; digitalis toxicity; paradoxic agitation from sedatives or hypnotics in the elderly). At times, a reduction in mental alertness may be the first sign of deteriorating left ventricular function.

Genitourinary problems may be encountered because of drug administration or bladder instrumentation. Urinary retention in the elderly male patient with benign prostatic hypertrophy is frequently precipitated by narcotic analgesics. Careful suprapubic palpation and percussion may disclose a distended bladder in the patient with a "low" urine output. Cystitis and pyelonephritis are recognized complications of chronic indwelling Foley catheters. Suprapubic tenderness and/or costovertebral angle tenderness are helpful physical signs which should be elicited if a urinary tract infection is suspected.

The most specific of the musculoskeletal complications of myocardial infarction, the shoulder-hand syndrome, is largely of historical interest and has rarely occurred since early mobilization of the infarction patient became commonplace therapy. However, a nonspecific "chest wall syndrome" has been noted in many patients with large infarcts. This poorly understood phenomenon is characterized by generalized tenderness over the left precordium and poorly characterized chest pain lasting from seconds to days. Acute gouty arthritis with its usual clinical manifestations may be precipitated by the dehydration and stress experienced following myocardial infarction.

Deep-vein thrombophlebitis should be carefully and recurrently excluded by daily examination of the extremities. Calf tenderness or asymmetry with or without palpable chords are much more valuable diagnostically than a negative Homan's sign (pain in the calf on rapid passive dorsiflexion of the foot), which is neither sensitive nor specific for this diagnosis. Portable Doppler probes are useful but insensitive, widely available, noninvasive, ancillary diagnostic aids. Evidence of chronic arterial insufficiency should be noted on admission (e.g., diminished or asymmetric pulses, vascular bruits, trophic skin changes in the lower extremities) so that appropriate nursing care may be implemented.

Metabolic problems are frequent and may be either a spontaneous result of the physiologic stress of myocardial infarction or iatrogenically induced. Polydipsia and polyuria may be the first clue to an aggravation of latent or previously controlled diabetes. Leg cramps may be the first clue to the presence of diuretic-induced hypokalemia; changes in mental status may be the first clue to the presence of diuretic-induced hyponatremia.

## REFERENCES

1. Fowler NO: Physical signs in acute myocardial infarction and its complications. Prog Cardiovasc Dis 10:287, 1968.
2. Webb SW, Adgey AA, Pantridge FJ: Autonomic disturbances at onset of acute myocardial infarction. Br Med J 3:89, 1972.
3. Harvey WP, Ronan JA: Bedside diagnosis of arrhythmias. Prog Cardiovasc Dis 8:419, 1966.
4. Yurchak PM, Gorlin R: Paradoxic spitting of the second heart sound in coronary artery disease. N Engl J Med 269:741, 1963.
5. Hill JC, O'Rourke RA, Lewis RP, McGranahan GM: The diagnostic value of the atrial gallop in acute myocardial infarction. Am Heart J 78:194, 1969.
6. Riley CP, Russel RO, Rackly CE: Left ventricular gallop sound and acute myocardial infarction. Am Heart J 86:598, 1973.
7. DiDonna GJ, Karliner JS, Peterson KL, O'Rourke RA: Transmission of audible precordial gallop sounds to the right supraclavicular fossa. Br Heart J 37:1277, 1975.
8. Heikkila J: Mitral incompetence complicating acute myocardial infarction. Br Heart J 29:162, 1967.
9. Karliner JS, O'Rourke RA, Kearney DJ, Shabetai R: Haemodynamic explanation of why the murmur of mitral regurgitation is independent of cycle length. Br Heart J 35:397, 1973.
10. Cohn JN, Guiha NH, Broden MI, Limas CJ:

Right ventricular infarction-clinical and hemodynamic features. Am J Cardiol 33:209, 1974.

11. Wartman WB, Hellerstein HK: The incidence
of heart disease in 2000 consecutive autopsies.
Ann Int Med 28:41, 1948.

12. Isner JM, Roberts WC: Right ventricular infarction complicating left ventricular infarction secondary to coronary artery disease. Am J Cardiol
42:885, 1978.

13. Sharpe DN, Botvinick EH, Shames DM, Schiller
NB, Massie BM, Chatterjee K, Parmley WW:
The non-invasive diagnosis of right ventricular
infarction. Circulation 57:483, 1978.

14. Killip T, Kimball JT: Treatment of myocardial
infarciton in a coronary care unit. Am J Cardiol
20:457, 1967.

15. Forrester, JS, Diamond G, Chatterjee K, Swan
HJC: Medical therapy of myocardial infarction
by application of hemodynamic subsets. N Engl
J Med 295:1356, 1976.

16. McHugh TJ, Forrester JS, Adler L et al: Pulmonary vascular congestion in acute myocardial infarction; hemodynamic and radiologic correlations. Ann Int Med 76:29–33, 1972.

17. Scheidt S, Ascheim R, Killip T III: Shock after
acute myocardial infarction: a clinical and hemodynamic profile. Am J Cardiol 26:556, 1970.

18. Thadani U, Chopra MP, Aber CP, Portal RW:
Pericarditis after acute myocardial infarction. Br
Med J 2:135, 1971.

19. Mundth E: Rupture of the heart complicating
myocardial infarction. Circulation 46:427, 1972.

20. Vlodaver A, Coe JI, Edwards JE: True and false
left ventricular aneurysms. Propensity for the
latter to rupture. Circulation 51:567, 1975.

21. Raizes G, Wagner GS, Hackel DB: Instantaneous non-arrhythmic cardiac death in acute
myocardial infarction. Role of electromechanical
dissociation. Am J Cardiol 39:1, 1977.

22. Fox AC, Glassman E, Isom OW: Surgically re-
mediable complications of myocardial infarction.
Prog in Cardiovasc Dis 21:961, 1979.

23. Wei JU, Hutchins GM, Bulkley BH: Papillary
muscle rupture in fatal acute myocardial infarction. Ann Int Med 90:149, 1979.

24. Meister SG, Helfant RH: Rapid bedside differentiation of ruptured intraventricular septum from
acute mitral insufficiency. N Engl J Med
287:1029, 1972.

25. Tatooles CJ, Gault JH, Mason T, Ross J Jr:
Reflux of oxygenated blood into the pulmonary
artery in severe mitral regurgitation. Am Heart
J 75:102, 1968.

26. Vlodaver Z, Edwards JE: Rupture of ventricular
septum or papillary muscle complicating myocardial infarction. Circulation 55:815, 1977.

27. Kassowsky WA, Epstein PJ, Levine RS: Post
myocardial infarction syndrome: an early complication of acute myocardial infarction. Chest
63:35, 1973.

28. Thompson, JE: Acute peripheral arterial occlusions. N Engl J Med 290:950, 1974.

29. Scucs MM Jr, Brooks HL, Grossman W, Banas
JS Jr, Merster SG, Dexter L, Dalen JE: Diagnostic sensitivity of laboratory findings in acute pulmonary embolism. Ann Intern Med 74:161–166,
1971.

30. Joote GA, Schabel SJ, Hodges M: Pulmonary
complications of the flow-directed balloon tipped
catheter. N Engl J Med 290:927, 1974.

# 10 | *Electrocardiogram in Acute Myocardial Infarction*

## *Ary L. Goldberger, M.D.*

The diagnosis of myocardial ischemia and infarction is one of the most important aspects of clinical electrocardiography. Familiarity with these ECG patterns is essential for those involved in coronary care. The purpose of this chapter is to review this topic with particular emphasis on the uses and limitations of the ECG in diagnosing myocardial infarction (MI). The vectorcardiographic (VCG) diagnosis of infarction is also briefly described. Dysrhythmias and conduction disturbances complicating MI are discussed separately in Chapters 15 through 18.

## THE NORMAL ECG AND VCG

The standard 12-lead ECG records electrical potentials generated by cardiac cells. These electrical potentials are produced by two sequential processes: myocardial depolarization (activation) and myocardial repolarization (recovery). Atrial depolarization produces the P wave. Atrial repolarization begins during the PR segment and is generally obscured by the QRS complex which represents ventricular depolarization. Ventricular repolarization is recorded by the ST-T complex.

Infarction of the left ventricle may produce distinctive changes in both depolarization (QRS) and repolarization (ST-T) waveforms. Ventricular ischemia without actual infarction generally produces ST-T changes alone. (Infarc-

tion of the atria and right ventricle are discussed separately below). Before examining in detail the ECG changes in acute MI, normal ECG and VCG patterns will be briefly reviewed.

An example of a normal ECG is shown in Fig. 10.1. One of the key landmarks in ECG analysis is the QRS pattern in the chest (transverse plane) leads. Normally, the interventricular septum is the first part of the ventricles to depolarize, and septal depolarization is directed from left to right. These initial depolarization forces, therefore, produce a small positive deflection (r wave) in the right chest leads, and a small negative deflection (septal q wave) in the left chest leads. The second and major phase of ventricular activation is dominated by the left ventricle. The vector representing this main phase of ventricular depolarization, therefore, points posteriorly and leftward, resulting in a deep, negative deflection (S wave) in the right chest leads and a tall, positive R wave in the left chest leads. The T wave is normally positive (upright) from leads $V_3$-$V_6$ in most adults.

The normal QRS pattern in the extremity (frontal plane) leads is variable, depending on the mean *electrical axis*. The electrical axis refers to the mean orientation of the QRS vector in the frontal plane. With a relatively "vertical" QRS axis, leads II, II, and aVF will show qR-type complexes. With a relatively "horizontal" QRS axis, leads I and aVL will show qR-type complexes. The QRS and T wave vectors are

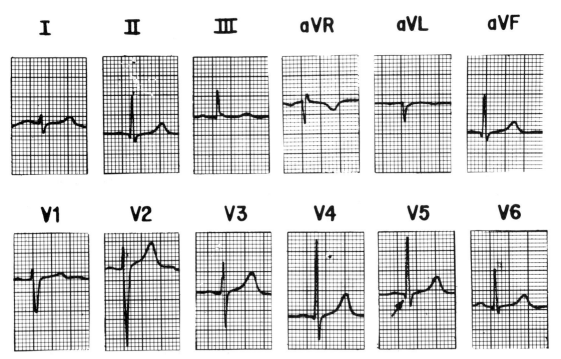

Fig. 10.1 Normal ECG. Note normal "septal" q wave in leads II, III, aVF, $V_5$ (arrow), $V_6$ and normal R wave progression in chest leads ($V_1$–$V_6$), with small r waves in right chest leads and prominent R-waves in left chest leads.

normally concordant in the frontal plane leads. Therefore, leads showing positive QRS complexes, with relatively tall R waves, will show upright T waves.

The cardiac potentials can also be recorded on a three-dimensional display by means of the VCG. A vector is a quantity with both magnitude and direction. Cardiac depolarization and repolarization forces are vectors with a specific magnitude, measured in millivolts, and a direction which can be plotted spatially on a three-dimensional grid. Basically, the VCG records the instantaneous cardiac potentials using three leads: X, Y, and Z. These three leads are *orthogonal*—oriented at right angles to each other. Therefore, vector leads can be used to determine the orientation of cardiac potentials in the three planes of the body: *frontal, transverse,* and *sagittal*. Lead X is similar in orientation to lead I; lead Y is similar to aVF, and lead Z is similar to $V_2$ (Fig. 10.2).

The frontal plane of the body, which cuts it into front and back halves, is represented by the X and Y leads. The transverse plane, which cuts the body into top and bottom halves,

is represented by the X and Z leads. Finally, the sagittal plane, which cuts the body into right and left sides, is represented by the Y and Z leads (Fig. 10.2).

The standard VCG consists of three loops representing atrial depolarization, ventricular depolarization, and ventricular repolarization. These loops are inscribed by a moving oscilloscopic line which records the instantaneous cardiac vector in relation to the three lead axes. A schematic example of a normal VCG is drawn in Fig. 10.3. For clarity, the P wave vector has been omitted. In the transverse plane, the normal QRS vector is inscribed in a counterclockwise direction. The initial forces are oriented anteriorly and rightward, reflecting the direction of early septal depolarization. The remainder of the horizontal plane loop moves posteriorly and leftward, due to the electrical predominance of the left ventricular free wall.

The normal frontal plane QRS loop (Fig. 10.3) may have a variable pattern depending on the electrical axis. In most normal subjects with a relatively vertical electrical axis, the frontal plane QRS loop is inscribed in a clockwise

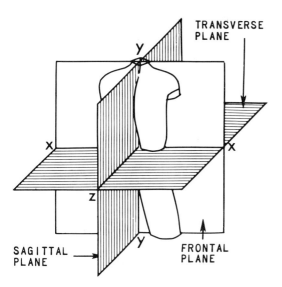

Fig. 10.2 Leads X, Y, and Z are orthogonal (oriented at right angles to each other) and can be used to determine the orientation of the cardiac vector in frontal, sagittal, and transverse (horizontal) planes. (Winsor T: Primer of Vectorcardiography. Lea and Febiger, Philadelphia, 1972.)

direction, as shown in Fig. 10.3. Some normal subjects, with a relatively horizontal QRS axis, will have counterclockwise inscription of the frontal plane loop.

In the right sagittal plane (Fig. 10.3), the early ventricular depolarization forces are oriented anteriorly and superiorly. The remainder of the loop moves clockwise in an inferior and posterior direction. The effect of transmural MI in various locations on these VCG patterns is described below.

## ECG PATTERNS OF ISCHEMIA AND INFARCTION: AN OVERVIEW

There is no single ECG pattern associated with myocardial ischemia or infarction. Rather, depending on the duration of the ischemic injury (acute vs. chronic) and the location of the affected myocardium (transmural vs. subendocardial), the ECG may show a wide variety of QRS and ST-T changes (Fig. 10.4). For example, with classic transmural infarction (Fig. 10.5) involving a full thickness of ventricular wall, the ECG generally shows a distinctive pat-

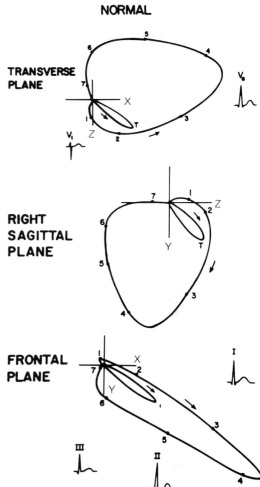

Fig. 10.3 Normal VCG. See text for details. Note that in the transverse (horizontal) plane initial QRS forces are oriented anteriorly and the vector loop moves posteriorly and to the left in a counterclockwise direction. The numbers on the loops indicate the orientation of the cardiac vector at 10 msec intervals. (Modified from Chou TC, Helm RA, Kaplan S: Clinical Vectorcardiography, 2nd ed. Grune and Stratton, New York, 1974. By permission.)

tern of new Q waves with an evolving sequence of ST-T changes (Figs. 10.6, 10.7). When transient transmural ischemia without infarction occurs, ST segment elevation without Q waves may appear—Prinzmetal's variant angina pattern. Infarction or ischemia limited to the inner half of the ventricular wall (subendocardium) (Fig. 10.5) generally does not affect depolarization but may be associated with marked repolar-

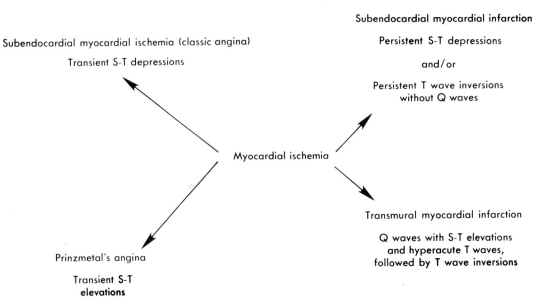

Fig. 10.4 Diversity of ECG changes with myocardial ischemia. (Goldberger A, Goldberger E: Clinical Electrocardiography. The C V Mosby Company, St. Louis, 1977.)

ization changes, including ST segment depressions and/or deep T wave inversions. These ECG changes are described in greater detail below.

## ECG TRANSMURAL INFARCTION PATTERNS

Transmural MI produces a characteristic sequence of QRS and ST-T changes, as illustrated in Figs. 10.6 and 10.7. The ECG hallmark of infarction involving a full or nearly transmural thickness of myocardium is the appearance of pathologic Q waves. A Q wave by definition is an initial negative deflection of the QRS complex. An entirely negative QRS deflection is referred to as a QS wave. Q waves may occur normally in any of the 12 standard ECG leads. In addition, abnormal, noninfarctional Q waves may occur in a variety of other settings (e.g., ventricular hypertrophy, nonischemic myocardial injury, ventricular conduction disturbances). The differential diagnosis of such "pseudoinfarctional" Q waves will be discussed later.

The appearance of Q waves in such non-infarctional settings reflects the limited *specificity*

of the ECG in diagnosing "transmural" MI. Furthermore, as indicated below, nontransmural MI occasionally produces pathologic Q waves. In addition, it should be emphasized that the *sensitivity* of the ECG is limited because acute MI may not always be associated with diagnostic QRS or ST-T changes.

With acute transmural infarction, new Q

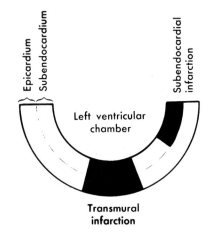

Fig. 10.5 Transmural infarction involves a full thickness of the ventricular wall. Subendocardial (nontransmural) MI is limited to inner layer of wall. (Goldberger A, Goldberger E: Clinical Electrocardiography. The C V Mosby Company, St. Louis, 1977.)

**ECG SEQUENCE WITH ANTERIOR WALL INFARCTION**

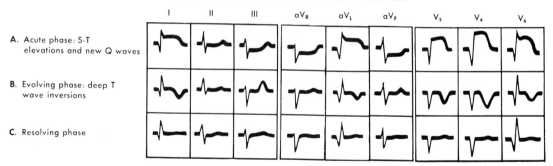

Fig. 10.6 Sequential changes with acute anterior wall MI. See text for details. (Goldberger A, Goldberger E: Clinical Electrocardiography. The C V Mosby Company, St. Louis, 1977.)

waves, as part of QS or Qr complexes, generally appear within the first day or two. These pathologic Q waves are usually wide, 0.04 sec or more in duration, in contrast to the "narrow" septal Q waves which are seen normally in the left chest and extremity leads (Fig. 10.1). The amplitude of these pathologic Q waves is sometimes, but not always, increased. In general, Q waves which are 25 percent or more of the R wave height in the left chest leads ($V_4$-$V_6$) are abnormal.[1] Similarly, Q waves exceeding 25 percent of the R wave height in leads II, III, and aVF are pathologic. However, as noted below, relatively deep, wide Q waves may sometimes occur in leads III and aVF as normal variants. In some leads, infarctional Q waves may show a QS or W-shaped morphology.

The pathogenesis of infarctional Q waves is best conceptualized in terms of vectorial theory. When necrosis of a portion of heart muscle occurs, the electrical potentials (forces) generated by this segment are lost. Consequently, the balance of depolarization forces will be shifted away from the infarcted region. Orientation of the initial depolarization vector away from the infarcted zone results in the appearance of negative initial forces (Q waves) in selected ECG leads.

A more concrete model of Q wave pathogenesis was initially proposed by Wilson and his colleagues.[2] According to their classic theory, infarctional Q waves were viewed as equivalent to the left ventricular (LV) cavity potential. An electrode placed in the LV cavity will normally record an entirely negative QS potential. Wilson proposed that a transmural MI creates a figurative "window" or "hole" in the heart, allowing the negativity of the LV cavity to be recorded by surface leads. In cases of incomplete infarction, with an admixture of living and necrotic tissue, QR complexes rather than QS complexes might be recorded.

**ECG SEQUENCE WITH INFERIOR WALL INFARCTION**

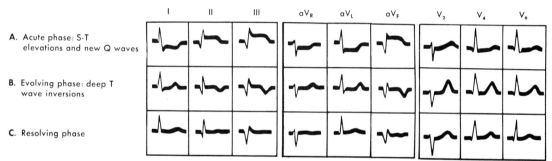

Fig. 10.7 Sequential changes with acute inferior wall MI. See text for details. (Goldberger A, Goldberger E: Clinical Electrocardiography. The C V Mosby Company, St. Louis, 1977.)

Infarctional Q waves will appear in different leads depending on the location of the infarct. In simplest terms, infarctions can be topographically divided by *anterior* wall or *inferior* (diaphragmatic) wall involvement (Fig. 10.8). This localization of injury is a result of the regional distribution of the coronary arteries (see Ch. 3). When MI involves the anterior wall of the left ventricle, pathologic Q waves and associated ST-T changes will appear in one or more of leads I, aVL, $V_1$-$V_6$ (Fig. 10.6). The inferior wall is reflected by leads II, III, and aVF (Figs. 10.7, 10.9). Anterior wall infarcts can be further subdivided into *anteroseptal* with Q waves in leads $V_1$-$V_3$ (Fig. 10.10), and *anterolateral,* with Q waves in leads $V_4$-$V_6$ (Fig. 10.11). High lateral infarcts may only produce changes in leads

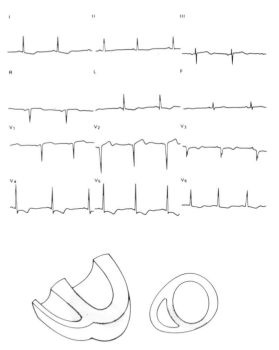

Fig. 10.10 Anteroseptal MI. Note loss of normal septal r waves in right chest leads, resulting in pathologic QS waves in $V_1$–$V_3$. In addition, there are diffuse anterior ischemic T wave inversions. Stippled areas in diagram below indicate region of infarcted myocardium. (Reproduced with permission from Karliner, JS: Noninvasive Evaluation of the Patient with Suspected Coronary Artery Disease, in Harvey, W. P., et al. (eds.): CURRENT PROBLEMS IN CARDIOLOGY. Copyright © 1978 by Year Book Medical Publishers, Inc., Chicago.)

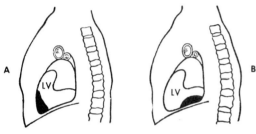

Fig. 10.8 Myocardial infarcts are generally localized to either the anterior, *A,* or inferior (diaphragmatic), *B,* portions of the left ventricle. (Goldberger A, Goldberger E: Clinical Electrocardiography. The C V Mosby Company, St. Louis, 1977.)

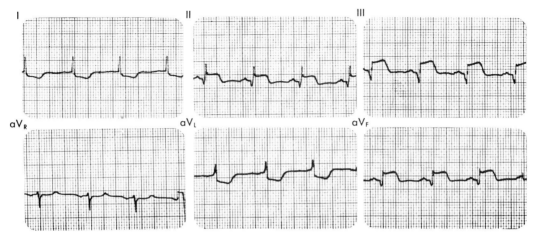

Fig. 10.9 Acute inferior MI. Note ST elevations with Q waves in leads II, III, and aVF with reciprocal ST depressions in leads I and aVL. (Goldberger A, Goldberger E: Clinical Electrocardiography. The C V Mosby Company, St. Louis, 1977.)

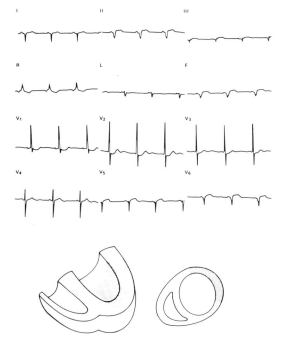

Fig. 10.11 Extensive inferior, posterior, lateral MI. Note pathologic Q waves in I, II, III, aVF, V₅, V₆. In addition, Leads V₁–V₂ show permanent tall R waves due to loss of posterior and lateral potentials. Stippled areas in diagram below indicate extent of infarcted myocardium. (Reproduced with permission from Karliner JS: Noninvasive Evaluation of the Patient with Suspected Coronary Artery Disease, in Harvey, W.P., et al. (eds.): CURRENT PROBLEMS IN CARDIOLOGY. Copyright © 1978 by Year Book Medical Publishers, Inc., Chicago.)

I and aVL. Infarction of the left ventricular apex is generally reflected in the lateral chest leads $V_4$-$V_6$.

Infarction localized to the true posterior portion of the left ventricle may not produce Q waves in any of the 12 standard leads. Instead, the diagnosis of true posterior MI must be made on the basis of a reciprocal increase in R wave height in leads $V_1$-$V_2$, opposite to the infarcted region (Fig. 10.11).[3]

Myocardial infarction may involve more than one surface of the heart, in a contiguous or noncontiguous fashion. For example, it is not uncommon to see evidence of inferolateral MI with Q waves and ST-T changes in leads II, III, and aVF, as well as in leads $V_5$-$V_6$. Multiple serial infarcts may also result in Q waves in anterior and inferior leads.

In the weeks or months following acute MI, these pathologic Q waves may show a variety of changes. In some cases, Q waves may persist indefinitely. In others, Q waves may regress in size or even disappear entirely. Disappearance of Q waves is most common following relatively small inferior infarcts. Therefore, the absence of Q waves or even a normal ECG [4] does not exclude prior transmural infarction. Even patients with ischemic cardiomyopathy may not show pathologic Q waves.[5]

There are several possible causes of Q wave regression following MI.[6] In some cases, the final scar that forms in the infarcted zone may have a smaller area than the original precinct of injury. In other cases, new intraventricular conduction disturbances may alter activation pathways and mask prior Q waves. For example, the pattern of anterior or inferior infarction may be masked by a new left bundle branch block (LBBB). Left anterior hemiblock, which produces inferior orientation of initial depolarization forces, may also mask the Q waves of inferior infarction.[7] Finally, a second MI involving the contralateral portion of the ventricle may cause an apparent regrowth of R waves over the area of the first infarct—"contrecoup effect."[8]

Transmural MI also produces a characteristic

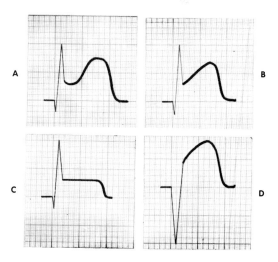

Fig. 10.12 S-T segment elevation seen with acute infarction may have variable shapes, as shown in A to D. (Goldberger A: Myocardial Infarction: Electrocardiographic Differential Diagnosis, 2nd ed. The C V Mosby Company, St. Louis, 1979.)

sequence of repolarization changes associated with these Q waves. The earliest ECG sign of acute transmural ischemia, which usually precedes the appearance of Q waves, is elevation of the ST segment—*current of injury* pattern. This ST elevation is sometimes accompanied by tall, positive "hyperacute" T waves. These acute ST-T changes are followed within hours or days by resolution of the ST elevations and the appearance of deep T wave inversions (evolving or chronic phase).

Figure 10.12 illustrates the variable appearance of ST segment elevation with acute MI. In some cases, the ST segment is concave; in others it has a convex shape. In some cases, the ST segment may have a flattened plateau appearance.

With acute anterior MI, ST segment elevation will be seen in one or more of leads I, aVL, $V_1$-$V_6$. At the same time, reciprocal ST segment depressions will be recorded in the inferior leads: II, III, and aVF (Fig. 10.6). With acute inferior MI, the primary ST elevations are seen in leads II, III, and aVF, with reciprocal ST depression in one or more of the anterior leads (Fig. 10.9). The presence of reciprocal ST depressions with acute MI is a key feature and is particularly helpful in distinguishing these changes from the diffuse ST elevations seen with acute pericarditis or early repolarization (Fig. 10.28).

The ST segment elevations are sometimes accompanied or preceded by tall, positive T waves,[9] so-called "hyperacute T waves of in-

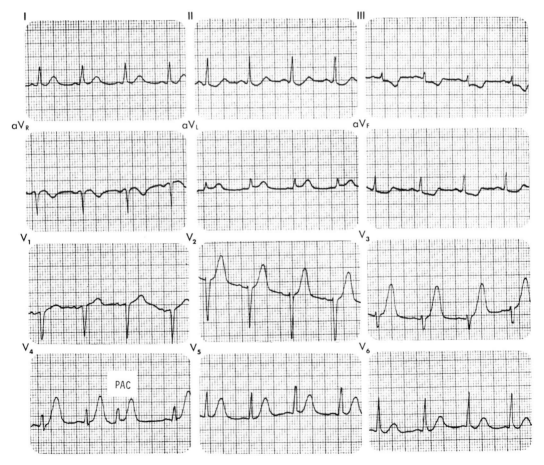

Fig. 10.13 Hyperacute T waves with anterior MI. Note very tall T waves in $V_2$–$V_5$, with slight ST segment elevation in aVL and reciprocal ST depression in leads II, III, aVF. Patient was complaining of severe chest pain and evolved an extensive anterior MI. PAC = premature atrial contraction. (Goldberger A, Goldberger E: Clinical Electrocardiography. The C V Mosby Company, St. Louis, 1977.)

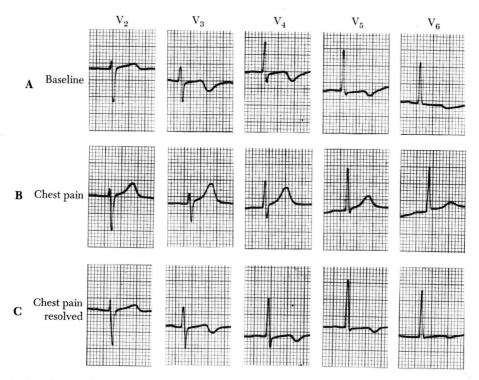

Fig. 10.14.   Paradoxic normalization of T waves. Baseline ECG *(A)* shows ischemic T wave inversions. With chest pain *(B),* T waves normalized transiently, returning to baseline, *(C),* following resolution of angina. Courtesy of Dr. Christine Simonelli.

farction" (Fig. 10.13). These hyperacute T waves may be symmetric or asymmetric and preceded by elevated, isoelectric, or even depressed ST segments. In some cases, the earliest phase of MI may be heralded by T waves which are only relatively increased in amplitude or even by the *paradoxical normalization* [10] of previously inverted T waves (Fig. 10.14).

Following the hyperacute-acute phase of MI, the T waves in leads reflecting the injured area

become deeply inverted (Fig. 10.6*B*). The terms "cove-plane" [11] and "coronary" T wave [12] have been used to describe these ischemic T waves (Fig. 10.15). Cove-plane T waves are T wave inversions preceded by an elevated ST segment. Coronary T waves are inverted T waves preceded by an isoelectric ST segment. At the same time that these ischemic T wave inversions appear, leads reflecting the uninjured surface of the heart will show reciprocally symmetrical,

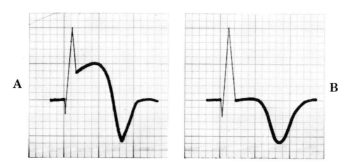

Fig. 10.15   *(A)* Cove-plane T waves are preceded by ST segment elevation. *(B)* Coronary T waves have an isoelectric ST segment followed by deep symmetrical inversion of the T-wave.

positive T waves (Fig. 10.6*B*). For example, during the evolving phase of an inferior wall MI, leads II, III, and aVF will show deeply inverted T waves, while one or more of the anterior leads I, aVL, and $V_1$-$V_6$ will show tall, positive T waves as a reciprocal change.

In the weeks or months following MI, these ST-T changes may have a variable course. In some cases, the repolarization abnormalities may regress entirely. Other cases are marked by persistence of relatively nonspecific ST-T alterations, with slight T wave inversion or flat-

tening. In still other cases, the T waves may remain deeply inverted for an indefinite time. Finally, persistence of ST segment elevation following acute MI sometimes occurs and is generally indicative of underlying ventricular aneurysm.[13]

Mills et al.[14] studied the natural history of ST segment elevation after acute MI and found that ST segment elevation persisting for two weeks or longer was likely to last indefinitely. Their analysis of data from other cases indicated that such persistent ST elevation was a

THEORETICAL BASIS OF ST ELEVATION

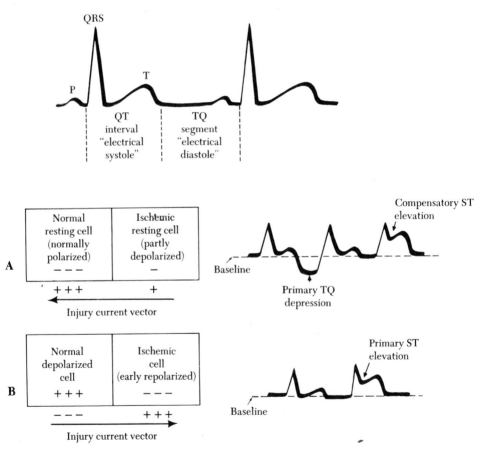

Fig. 10.16  Theoretical basis of ST elevation with acute infarction. *(A)* Diastolic injury current results from depolarization of ischemic cell membranes during electrical diastole (T-Q segment). As a result, the injury current (ST) vector points away from ischemic zone, causing primary depression of the T-Q baseline. However, AC coupled ECG recorders automatically compensate for the negative baseline shift, producing apparent ST elevation. *(B)* Systolic injury current may result in part from early repolarization of infarcting cells, making them electropositive. Consequently, the injury current (ST) vector will be directed toward the infarcted zone causing true ST elevation. (Goldberger A: Myocardial Infarction: Electrocardiographic Differential Diagnosis, 2nd ed. The C V Mosby Company, St. Louis, 1979.)

relatively specific but *not* a highly sensitive indicator of ventricular aneurysm. Thus, finding ST elevation several weeks following acute infarction suggests an underlying ventricular wall motion disorder. However, this sign will be present in only about two-thirds of patients with ventricular aneurysm.[14] Another sign that has been reported with ventricular aneurysm is an rsR-type complex in the left chest leads.[15]

The pathophysiology of the evolutionary ST-T changes with acute transmural MI continues to be a topic of ongoing investigation.[16] In most basic terms, the ST segment deviations seen with acute myocardial ischemia are produced by a *current of injury* which flows between healthy and infarcting zones (Fig. 10.16). Normally, the ST segment is isoelectric, neither positive nor negative, due to the fact that myocardial cells attain the same membrane potential during the early phase of repolarization—the plateau phase of the action potential. Acute MI alters both the resting membrane potential and the action potential duration of cardiac cells in a localized area. As a result, there will be a voltage gradient between normal and infarcting tissue and a current of injury will flow between these regions.

Recent data suggest that this injury current flows both during electrical systole (Q-T interval) and during electrical diastole (T-Q segment).[17,18] The systolic current of injury is probably the result of paradoxical shortening of repolarization time in the acutely infarcting zone.[17] The ischemic cells, which repolarize earlier, become electrically positive relative to the normal cells. As a result, the injury current vector will be directed toward the electropositive ischemic region, causing primary ST elevation and tall, positive, hyperacute T waves.

The diastolic current of injury results from a lowering of the membrane resting potential of acutely infarcting cells, probably caused by a leakage of intracellular potassium.[19] This diastolic depolarization tends to make the ischemic cells relatively negative. Therefore, the injury current vector will be oriented away from the electronegative infarcting zone, resulting in depression of the diastolic T-Q baseline. However, conventional alternating current ECG recorders automatically compensate for this shift of the diastolic baseline, resulting in apparent ST segment elevation (Fig. 10.16).

The degree of ischemic ST elevation recorded in any particular lead is a function of two key variables.[20] The magnitude of ST elevation is related in part to the spatial relation of the recording electrode to the ischemic zone. According to *solid angle* theory,[19] the magnitude of ST elevation will be proportional to the angle subtended by the border of the infarct and the recording electrode. The second determinant of ST segment magnitude is the voltage gradient between normal and ischemic zones. The greater the difference in membrane potential during electrical systole and/or diastole, the greater the resulting injury current.

The deep ischemic T wave inversions observed during the evolving chronic phase of infarction are due to regional delay in repolarization, with local prolongation of the action potential.[20] As a result, chronically ischemic cells, in contrast to the cells that repolarize early in the acutely infarcting zone, become electrically negative. The ST-T vector will point away from this negative zone, resulting in T wave inversion.

## VCG PATTERNS OF TRANSMURAL MI

### Anteroseptal MI

The VCG diagnosis of anteroseptal MI is made from the horizontal plane QRS loop. Normally, the initial QRS forces in this plane are directed anteriorly and rightward (Fig. 10.2), reflecting normal septal activation. Infarction of the interventricular septum results in loss of these normal anterior forces. The VCG diagnosis of septal MI is made on the basis of posterior orientation of the 20 msec QRS vector in the horizontal plane (Fig. 10.17).[21]

### Anterolateral MI

With infarction of the anterolateral aspect of the left ventricle, the initial rightward and anterior "septal" forces in the horizontal plane are preserved (Fig. 10.18). However, loss of free wall depolarization forces results in abnormal

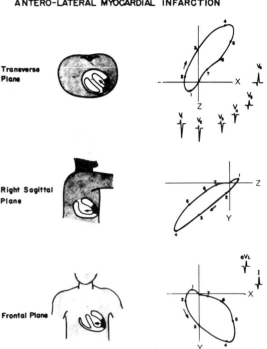

ANTERO-LATERAL MYOCARDIAL INFARCTION

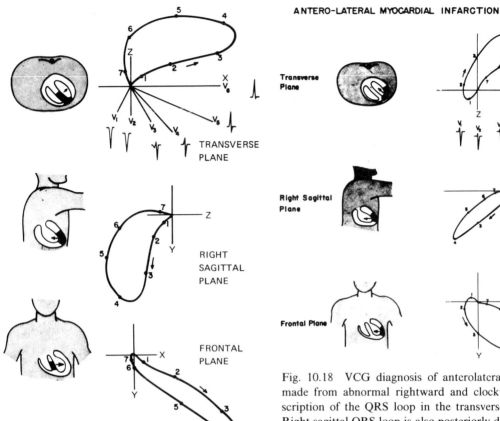

TRANSVERSE
PLANE

RIGHT
SAGITTAL
PLANE

FRONTAL
PLANE

Transverse
Plane

Right Sagittal
Plane

Frontal Plane

**ANTERO-SEPTAL INFARCTION**

Fig. 10.17 Anteroseptal MI causes posterior orientation of the 20 msec QRS vector in the transverse (horizontal) plane, resulting in abnormal Q waves in leads $V_1$–$V_3$ (Fig. 10.10). Numbers on loops indicate position of the cardiac vector at 10 msec intervals. (Modified from Chou TC, Helm RA, Kaplan S: Clinical Vectorcardiography, 2nd ed. Grune and Stratton, New York, 1977. By permission.)

rightward and clockwise inscription of the QRS loop in the horizontal plane. The sagittal plane may also show posterior displacement of the QRS loop. In the frontal plane, the initial forces may be directed abnormally rightward (> 22 msec), reflected on the scalar ECG by prominent Q waves in leads I and aVL.[21]

## Inferior Wall MI

Inferior MI causes superior displacement of the initial QRS forces in the frontal and sagittal

Fig. 10.18 VCG diagnosis of anterolateral MI is made from abnormal rightward and clockwise inscription of the QRS loop in the transverse plane. Right sagittal QRS loop is also posteriorly displaced and initial forces in the frontal plane are deviated to the right, resulting in abnormal Q waves in leads I and aVL. Numbers on loops indicate position of the cardiac vector at 10 msec intervals. (Modified from Chou TC, Helm RA, Kaplan S: Clinical Vectorcardiography, 2nd ed. Grune & Stratton, Inc., New York, 1977. By permission.)

planes (Fig. 10.19). In the frontal plane, diagnosis of inferior MI can be made on the basis of superior orientation of the 25 msec QRS vector.[21] The horizontal plane loop is not affected by pure inferior MI. More detailed criteria for VCG recognition of inferior MI have recently been proposed.[22]

## Posterior Wall MI

With infarction of the true posterior wall (Fig. 10.20), the QRS loop will be displaced anteriorly in the horizontal and sagittal planes. Diagnostic criteria for true posterior MI include anterior orientation of the 40 msec QRS vector in the horizontal plane and anterior orientation

INFERIOR MYOCARDIAL INFARCTION

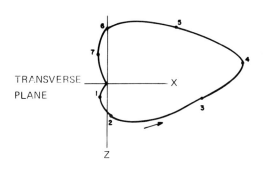

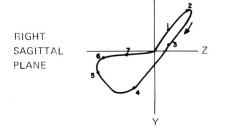

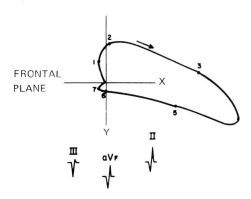

Fig. 10.19 Inferior MI results in abnormal superior displacement of the initial QRS vector in the frontal and sagittal planes. Numbers on loops indicate position of the cardiac vector at 10 msec intervals. (Modified from Chou TC, Helm RA, Kaplan S: Clinical Vectorcardiography, 2nd ed. Grune & Stratton, Inc., New York, 1977. By permission.)

of 50 percent of the horizontal plane QRS area.[23] The specificity of these findings, however, is limited because anterior displacement of QRS forces is also seen with right ventricular hypertrophy, as well as in some normal subjects.[24]

The relative sensitivity and specificity of the

ECG vs. VCG in diagnosing MI remains unsettled. Early studies suggested that both tests were of relatively equal diagnostic accuracy. More recent studies [22,25] using quantitative vector analysis suggest that the VCG may be both more sensitive and more specific, particularly in the diagnosis of inferior wall MI. For example, in one recent study [25] of patients with inferior wall motion abnormalities, the diagnostic sensitivity for the ECG was 63 percent, compared with 81 percent for the VCG. The VCG is particularly helpful in differentiating pathologic and "positional" Q waves and also in evaluating borderline or equivocal Q waves seen in one or more of the inferior limb leads.

The VCG does have significant limitations which make the scalar ECG more useful in the day-to-day management of patients with MI. Repolarization changes are more easily evaluated and followed with the standard ECG, as are dysrhythmias. Furthermore, conditions which cause pseudoinfarct patterns (e.g., left or right ventricular hypertrophy, chronic cor

STRICTLY POSTERIOR INFARCTION

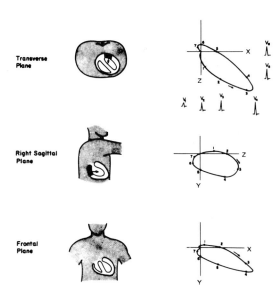

Fig. 10.20 Posterior MI causes abnormal anterior displacement of QRS forces in the sagittal and transverse planes. Numbers on loops indicate position of the cardiac vector at 10 msec intervals. (Modified from Chou TC, Helm RA, Kaplan S: Clinical Vectorcardiography, 2nd ed. Grune & Stratton, Inc., New York, 1977. By permission.)

pulmonale, hypertrophic and congestive cardiomyopathy, etc.), will also simulate the VCG pattern of infarction.

## DIAGNOSIS OF MI WITH BUNDLE BRANCH BLOCK AND PREEXCITATION

Alterations in ventricular activation may obscure the diagnosis of MI. With left bundle branch block (LBBB), changes in the orientation of initial depolarization forces may both mask and mimic infarction. In some cases, the Q waves of anterior or inferior MI may be masked by LBBB. Similarly, the secondary ST-T changes associated with LBBB often hide primary ischemic repolarization abnormalities. In certain cases, the diagnosis of underlying *septal* infarction with LBBB can be made by the presence of Q waves as part of QR complexes appearing paradoxically in the *lateral* chest leads.[26] These prominent lateral Q waves may represent early right ventricular forces, unmasked by the septal infarct (Fig. 10.21).

In contrast to LBBB, right bundle branch block (RBBB) primarily affects the terminal portion of the QRS and generally does not interfere with the diagnosis of MI (Fig. 10.22). However, the Wolff-Parkinson-White (WPW) preexcitation pattern may obscure both the Q waves and ST-T changes of acute or chronic MI. In addition, as mentioned below, the WPW pattern frequently simulates inferior wall MI. Finally, as noted earlier, left anterior hemiblock (LAHB) may produce small r waves in the inferior limb leads, masking the diagnosis of inferior MI.

Occasionally, MI can be diagnosed from premature extrasystoles, which may show pathologic Q waves not apparent in normally conducted beats.[26] The diagnosis of MI should be suspected when the premature beat shows a QR or QRS morphology in one or more leads excluding aVR and V$_1$.

## SUBENDOCARDIAL INFARCTION

Because its blood supply is directly impeded by the high pressure of the ventricular cavity, the subendocardium is particularly susceptible to ischemia. Furthermore, the vasodilatory reserve of the subendocardium appears to be limited.[27] Therefore, subendocardial ischemia and even infarction may occur while epicardial perfusion is relatively well preserved.

The ECG diagnosis of subendocardial isch-

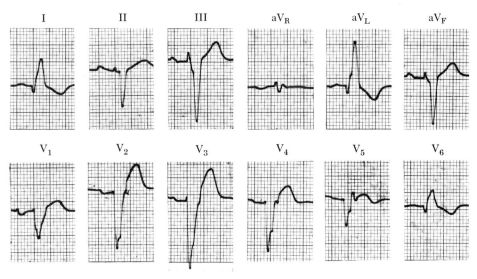

Fig. 10.21 Anterior wall MI with LBBB. QS type complexes are commonly seen with LBBB in the absence of infarction. However, QR complexes in the lateral chest leads are often indicative of underlying infarction. See text for details. (Goldberger A: Myocardial Infarction: Electrocardiographic Differential Diagnosis, 2nd ed. The C V Mosby Company, St. Louis, 1979.)

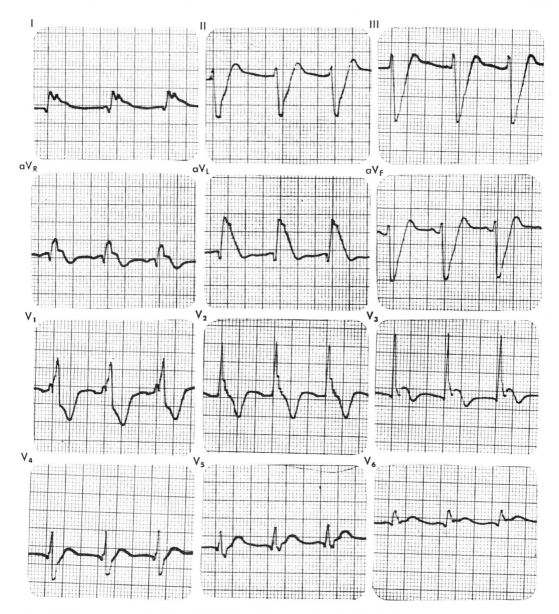

Fig. 10.22  Acute anterior MI with RBBB and left anterior hemiblock (LAHB). Note broad rsR′ in V₁ with ST elevations and Q waves in leads I and aVL, as well as Q waves in the lateral chest leads. Marked left axis deviation is present consistent with left anterior hemiblock. The combination of RBBB and left anterior hemiblock with acute anterior MI often presages complete heart block. (Goldberger A, Goldberger E: Clinical Electrocardiography. The C V Mosby Company, St. Louis, 1977.)

emia and infarction is inferred from repolarization changes, including ST segment depression (Fig. 10.23) and/or T wave inversion (Fig. 10.24). Experimental [28] and clinical [29] data suggest that pure localized subendocardial infarction, unlike transmural injury described above, generally does not produce pathologic Q waves.

However, nontransmural infarction involving more than half the ventricular wall may produce new Q waves.[30]

The ST segment depression associated with subendocardial ischemia has a characteristic "squared-off" appearance, with a horizontally depressed or downsloping ST segment (Fig.

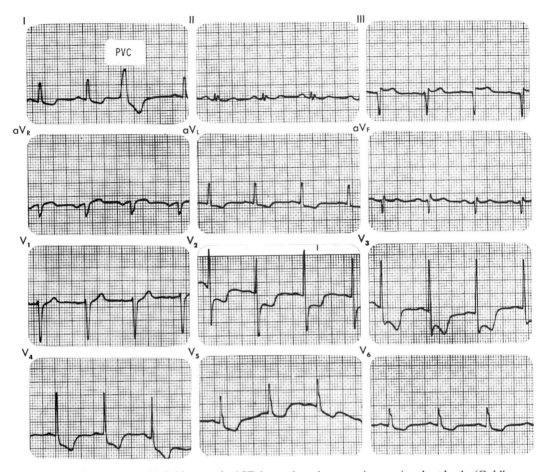

Fig. 10.23  Subendocardial MI. Note marked ST depressions, best seen in anterior chest leads. (Goldberger A, Goldberger E: Clinical Electrocardiography. The C V Mosby Company, St. Louis, 1977.)

10.23). This pattern of ST segment depression may occur with transient subendocardial ischemia, for example, in the context of typical angina pectoris or during exercise treadmill testing. When actual subendocardial infarction occurs, the ST segment depression tends to be more persistent. These ST depressions may be seen in anterior and/or inferior leads. ST segment elevation is usually seen concomitantly in lead aVR. In other cases, subendocardial infarction is associated with deep T wave inversions, with or without ST segment depression (Fig. 10.24).

The pathogenesis of the repolarization changes with subendocardial ischemia is not fully explained. The most widely held theory is that the ST segment depressions recorded by surface leads are reciprocal to a primary

subendocardial injury current which will produce ST elevation in leads reflecting the ventricular cavity (e.g., lead aVR).[31] The T wave inversions seen in some cases of subendocardial infarction probably reflect transmural ischemia.[32] However, in such cases only the subendocardium, because of its greater hemodynamic vulnerability, actually becomes infarcted.[32]

An alternate explanation for the ST segment depressions associated with subendocardial infarction was proposed by Prinzmetal and his colleagues.[33] They suggested that these ST depressions actually reflect a primary epicardial injury current and are not reciprocal to subendocardial ST elevation. According to their theory, relatively mild degrees of epicardial ischemia result in epicardial hyperpolarization (in-

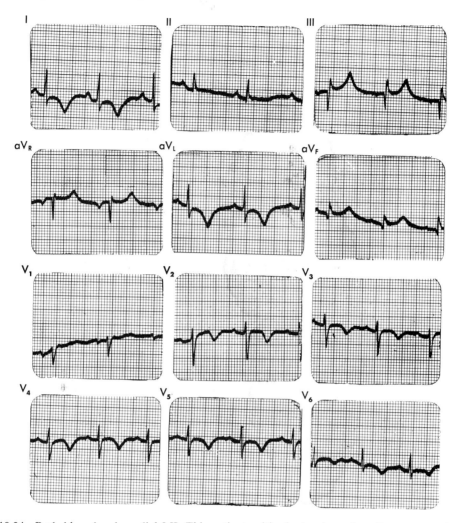

Fig. 10.24 Probable subendocardial MI. This patient, with chest pain and cardiac enzyme elevation, showed new deep T wave inversions in leads I, aVL and $V_2$–$V_6$. Prominent Q waves in leads aVF reflected prior inferior MI. Subendocardial (nontransmural) infarction may cause ST segment depression and/or deep T-wave inversions. (Goldberger A, Goldberger E: Clinical Electrocardiography. The C V Mosby Company, St. Louis, 1977.)

creased cell membrane potential), causing ST segment depression, while severe epicardial ischemia causes epicardial depolarization (decreased cell membrane potential) and ST elevation.

In summary, the diagnosis of subendocardial *ischemia* is inferred from the ECG pattern of ST segment depression and/or T wave inversions without new Q waves. The diagnosis of actual subendocardial *infarction* requires other confirmatory evidence of myocardial necrosis (e.g., cardiac enzyme elevations).

## ATRIAL AND RIGHT VENTRICULAR INFARCTION

Infarction of the left or right atrium sometimes occurs in association with ventricular infarcts. In such cases, the ECG may show alterations in P wave morphology, deviation of the PR segment due to an atrial injury current and atrial arrhythmias.[34] Patients with right ventricular infarction generally show the ECG pattern of inferior MI with Q waves and ST-T changes in the leads II, III, and aVF.[35]

## DIFFERENTIAL DIAGNOSIS OF MI (PSEUDOINFARCT PATTERNS)

The ECG diagnosis of myocardial ischemia and infarction, as noted above, is based on ventricular depolarization and repolarization changes including Q waves, ST segment elevations, ST segment depressions, T wave inversions, and tall, positive (hyperacute) T waves. Unfortunately, none of these patterns is entirely specific for ischemia. In fact, all of these signs may be caused by a variety of other factors, including both normal variants and a number of abnormal, nonischemic conditions.[6]

Q waves may be produced by four basic mechanisms:

1. Positional or physiologic Q waves result from variations in cardiac orientation or depolarization. For example, normal variant QS complexes may be seen in lead $V_1$, and occasionally in $V_1$ and $V_2$, simulating anteroseptal MI. Normal variant QS or QR complexes may also appear in leads III and aVF. Both pathologic and normal variant positional Q waves in the inferior leads may decrease in size during inspi-

ration. Therefore, respiratory maneuvers cannot be used reliably to differentiate these patterns.[36] The VCG (Fig. 10.19) may be particularly helpful in differentiating such positional inferior lead Q waves, which are due to leftward orientation of initial QRS forces in the frontal plane, from inferior MI, which causes abnormal superior displacement of initial QRS forces. Normal variant QS and QR complexes may appear in lead aVL. Relatively narrow (< 0.04 sec) Q waves, representing septal depolarization, are regularly seen in the left chest leads ($V_5$-$V_6$) and one or more of the extremity leads (Fig. 10.1). Positional Q waves due partly to rightward mediastinal shift may occur in the chest leads with left pneumothorax.[37] Poor R wave progression is not uncommon with pectus excavatum.[38] In patients with complete corrected transposition of the great vessels, reversed direction of septal activation and altered septal orientation may result in both inferior and anterior pseudoinfarct patterns.[39] Dextrocardia may also simulate extensive anterior wall MI with apparent loss of QRS forces in the left chest leads.

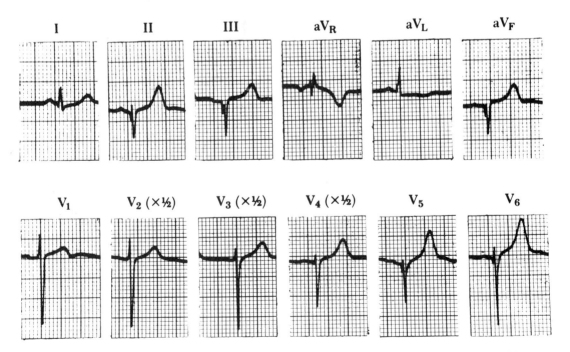

Fig. 10.25   Pseudoinfarction pattern with IHSS. Note bizarre W-shaped Q waves in inferolateral leads. (Goldberger A: Myocardial Infarction: Electrocardiographic Differential Diagnosis, 2nd ed. The C V Mosby Company, St. Louis, 1979.)

2. Q waves may also be associated with ventricular enlargement. Left ventricular hypertrophy frequently produces poor R wave progression in the right to mid-chest leads. With right ventricular hypertrophy, QR waves may appear in the right chest leads. Deep pseudoinfarctional Q waves are often a striking feature of the ECG in patients with idiopathic hypertrophic subaortic stenosis (IHSS) (Fig. 10.25).[40] Acute cor pulmonale, usually due to massive pulmonary embolism, may simulate the ECG patterns of anterior and/or inferior MI. Acute right ventricular dilatation may cause loss of normal R wave progression in the chest leads, along with T wave inversions due to right ventricular "strain." The S1Q3T3 pattern, which has been noted in occasional cases of massive pulmonary embolism, consists of noninfarctional Q waves in leads III and aVF with inferior T waves inversions.[41] Chronic cor pulmonale (pulmonary emphysema) is also a common cause of poor precordial R wave progression simulating anterior MI. This pattern may be related to inferior displacement of the heart and in some cases to right ventricular dilatation.

3. Q waves may result from any process,

ischemic or nonischemic, which causes significant replacement of or injury to myocardial fibers,[6] including myocarditis, amyloidosis, chronic constrictive pericarditis, cardiac tumors, and various cardiomyopathies such as Duchenne muscular dystrophy,[42] myotonia atrophica,[42] idiopathic congestive cardiomyopathy (Fig. 10.26) and Friedreich's ataxia. (In some cases the Q waves in Friedreich's ataxia may reflect underlying hypertrophic cardiomyopathy).[43] Transient Q waves may also occur in the context of severe, but temporary, metabolic insults. Such transient noninfarctional Q waves have been reported with marked hyperkalemia,[45] hypoglycemia,[46] hypotension,[47] and phosphorus ingestion,[48] as well as with noninfarctional ischemia.[49]

4. Finally, Q waves may be the result of altered ventricular activation. Left bundle branch block commonly causes loss of precordial R wave progression and sometimes inferior lead Q waves due to abnormal right-to-left septal activation. The WPW pattern, Type A or B, frequently produces pseudoinfarctional Q waves in the inferior limb leads (Fig. 10.27). In some cases of RBBB, the initial r wave in

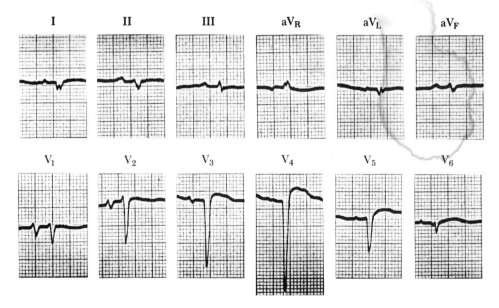

Fig. 10.26    Pseudoinfarction pattern with idiopathic congestive cardiomyopathy. Note extensive Q waves as well as left atrial enlargement, first degree AV block, low voltage and right axis deviation. Patient had dilated cardiomyopathy with normal coronary arteries at catheterization. (Goldberger A: Myocardial Infarction: Electrocardiographic Differential Diagnosis, 2nd ed. The C V Mosby Company, St. Louis, 1979.)

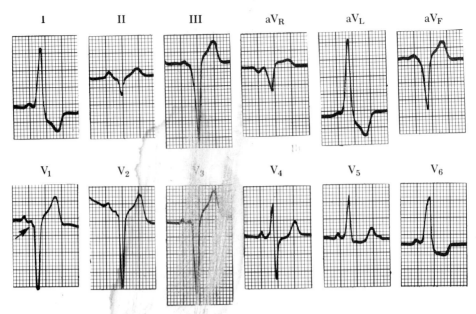

Fig. 10.27   Type B WPW pattern simulating inferior and anteroseptal MI. Note wide QRS, short PR interval and delta wave (arrow in $V_1$) characteristic of the preexcitation pattern. Noninfarction Q waves (II, III, aVF, $V_1$–$V_3$) are due to altered ventricular activation. (Goldberger A: Myocardial Infarction: Electrocardiographic Differential Diagnosis, 2nd ed. The C V Mosby Company, St. Louis, 1979.)

leads $V_1$-$V_2$ may not be apparent, resulting in noninfarctional QR waves in these leads. Finally, LAHB may cause small q waves as part of qrS complexes in the right precordial leads. These small q waves have been ascribed to selective inferoposterior activation of the left ventricle and typically disappear in leads recorded one interspace below the usual positions.[7]

The diagnosis of true posterior wall MI, as described above, is supported by tall R waves in the right chest leads. However, a similar pattern may occur in a number of other settings, including normal variants, congenital dextroversion, right ventricular hypertrophy, RBBB, IHSS, WPW pattern Type A, Duchenne muscular dystrophy, and, rarely, chronic constrictive pericarditis.[59]

Pseudoinfarct patterns with Q waves and ST-T changes identical to those of transmural infarction have also been reported with acute pancreatitis.[51] However, most of the patients reported with this pattern have been hypotensive, which may account for the transient infarct patterns.[6] Furthermore, acute pancreatitis is a relatively common disease and pseudoinfarct patterns have been reported only rarely.

Therefore, until further evidence is available, the validity of this association remains questionable. Similarly, acute biliary disease probably does not cause actual pseudoinfarct patterns.[52]

ST segment elevation may also result from a variety of nonischemic factors. Normal variant ST segment elevation is commonly encountered in the right or left chest leads as part of the functional *early repolarization pattern* (Fig. 10.28). This pattern is particularly common in athletic young adult males. Acute pericarditis causes diffuse ST elevations (e.g., in leads I, II, aVL, aVF, $V_2$-$V_6$) in contrast to the more localized injury current with reciprocal changes seen in acute MI. Systemic hypothermia may cause unusual convex elevation of the J point (Osborn wave).[6] Hyperkalemia may induce ST elevation, most marked in the right chest leads.[6] Nonischemic ST elevation is also commonly seen in the right chest leads with LBBB or left ventricular hypertrophy with strain, reciprocal to ST depressions seen in the lateral chest leads.

The differential diagnosis of ST segment depression includes functional causes (e.g., hyperventilation, orthostatic change) as well as digitalis effect, hypokalemia, and left ventricular strain. Secondary ST depressions are frequently seen in the left precordial leads with LBBB. Slight ST segment depression and sometimes T wave inversions simulating ischemia are often observed in the inferolateral leads with mitral valve prolapse.[53]

Deep T wave inversions may be seen as a normal variant in the right chest leads as part of the persistent "juvenile" T wave pattern in some adults. Left precordial T wave inversions may be seen in association with the early repolarization variant, particularly in athletic young adult males (Fig. 10.29).[54] Friedreich's ataxia may also be associated with prominent lateral T wave inversions. Diffuse T wave inversions are seen during the evolving phase of pericarditis. Very deep T wave inversions, with pronounced Q-T prolongation, are seen in some cases of cerebrovascular accident,[55] particularly with subarachnoid hemorrhage (Fig. 10.30). These "CVA T waves" are probably caused by alterations in autonomic tone. Deep T wave inversions simulating infarction have also been reported in some normal subjects following bouts of tachyarrhythmia *(posttachycardia T wave pattern)*.[56] Noninfarctional T wave inversions may also occur after electronic ventricular pacing *(postpacemaker T wave pattern)* [57] or following Stokes-Adams attacks.[58] Deep T wave inversions are also common with left and right ventricular strain patterns.

Secondary T wave inversions are seen in the right chest leads with RBBB, associated with an rSR' complex, and in the left chest and selected limb leads with LBBB associated with R waves. Recently, deep T wave inversions in the right and midprecordial leads have been reported with intermittent LBBB in normally conducted beats.[59] The mechanism of these repolarization changes is uncertain.

Tall, positive T waves simulating the hyperacute phase of infarction may also occur in a variety of nonischemic settings including normal variants, hyperkalemia (tall, narrow T waves), and some cases of cerebrovascular accident (tall, wide T waves). Tall T waves with a high ST segment take-off are frequently seen in the right precordial leads with LBBB and also left ventricular hypertrophy.

In summary, a wide variety of conditions may

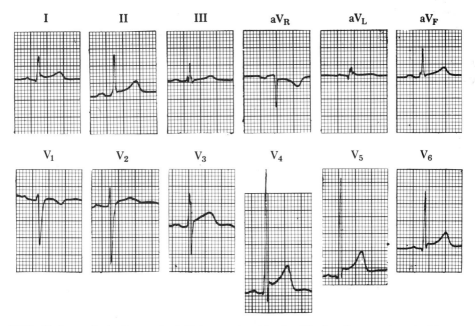

Fig. 10.28 Early repolarization variant. Note prominent benign ST elevations most marked in precordial leads. In addition, QRS complex shows characteristic notching at J junction, giving the appearance of an RSr' configuration ($V_4$–$V_6$). Reciprocal ST depression is seen in lead aVR. (Goldberger A: Myocardial Infarction: Electrocardiographic Differential Diagnosis, 2nd ed. The C V Mosby Company, St. Louis, 1979.)

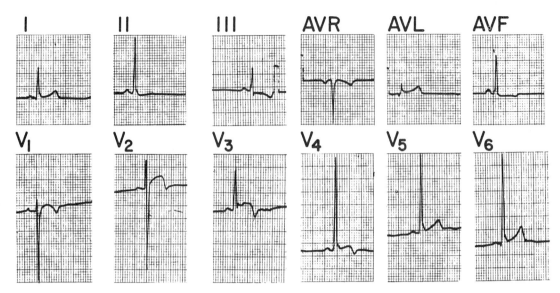

Fig. 10.29  Benign T wave inversion associated with early repolarization variant. ECG from trained athlete showing functional ST-T change simulating acute MI. In addition, prominent chest lead QRS voltage may reflect "physiologic" left ventricular hypertrophy in response to athletic training. (Lichtman, J et al: The electrocardiogram of the athlete: alterations simulating those of organic heart disease. Arch Intern Med 132:763, 1973.)

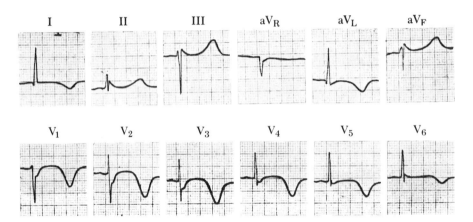

Fig. 10.30  Deep T wave inversion associated with subarachnoid hemorrhage. Note marked prolongation of Q-T interval. (Goldberger A: Myocardial Infarction: Electrocardiographic Differential Diagnosis, 2nd ed. The C V Mosby Company, St. Louis, 1979.)

simulate ECG patterns of MI and ischemia. Particular care must be taken not to overinterpret ubiquitous "nonspecific ST and T wave changes," which include slight ST segment deviations and flattening or minimal inversion of the T wave. While relatively minor ST-T changes may be the only evidence of myocardial ischemia in certain cases, similar patterns may result from a myriad of factors including normal variants, drug effects, and metabolic factors, as well as other forms of organic heart disease.

## ACKNOWLEDGMENT

Supported in part by the NIH Graduate Training Grant HL-05846, awarded by the National Heart, Lung and Blood Institute.

## REFERENCES

1. Goldberger E: Unipolar Lead Electrocardiography and Vectocardiography, Lea and Febiger, 3rd edition, Philadelphia, 1953, p. 280.

2. Wilson FN, Johnston FD, Hill IGW: The form of the electrocardiogram in experimental myocardial infarction. IV. Additional observations on the later effects produced by ligation of the anterior descending branch of the left coronary artery. Am Heart J 10:1025, 1933.

3. Perloff JK: The recognition of strictly posterior myocardial infarction by conventional scalar electrocardiography. Circulation 30:706, 1964.

4. Kaplan BM, Berkson DM: Serial electrocardiograms after myocardial infarction. Ann Intern Med 60:430, 1964.

5. Johnson AD, Laiken SL, Shabetai R: Non-invasive diagnosis of ischemic cardiomyopathy by fluoroscopic detection of coronary artery calcification. Am Heart J 96:521, 1978.

6. Goldberger AL: Myocardial Infarction: Electrocardiographic Differential Diagnosis. The C V Mosby Company, 2nd edition, St. Louis, Mo, 1979.

7. Rosenbaum M, Elizari MD, Lazzari JO: The Hemiblocks. Tampa Tracings, Oldsmar, Fla., 1970, p. 222.

8. Evans W: Cardiac contrecoup in the course of cardiac infarction. Br Heart J 24:713, 1963.

9. Dressler W, Roesler H: High T waves in the earliest stage of infarction. Am Heart J 34:627, 1947.

10. Noble RJ, Rothbaum DA, Knoebel SB, McHenry PL, Anderson GJ: Normalization of abnormal T waves in ischemia. Arch Intern Med 136:391, 1976.

11. Rothschild MA, Mann H, Oppenheimer BS: Successive changes in the electrocardiogram following acute coronary artery occlusion. Proc Soc Exp Biol Med 23:253, 1926.

12. Pardee HEB: Heart disease and abnormal electrocardiograms, with special reference to coronary T wave. Am J Med Sci 169:770, 1925.

13. Gorlin R, Klein MD, Sullivan JM: Prospective correlative study of ventricular aneurysm: mechanistic concept and clinical recognition. Am J Med 42:512, 1967.

14. Mills RM Jr, Young E, Gorlin R, Lesch M: Natural history of S-T segment elevation after acute myocardial infarction. Am J Cardiol 35:609, 1975.

15. El-Sherif N: The rsR pattern in left surface leads in ventricular aneurysm. Br Heart J 32:440, 1970.

16. Ross J Jr: Electrocardiographic ST-segment analysis in the characterization of myocardial ischemia and infarction. Circulation 53 (Suppl IV):I-73, 1976.

17. Samson WE, Scher AM: Mechanism of S-T segment alteration during acute myocardial injury. Circ Res 8:780, 1960.

18. Vincent GM, Abildskov JA, Burgess MJ: Mechanisms of ischemic ST-segment displacement: evaluation by direct current recordings. Circulation 56:559, 1977.

19. Prinzmetal M, Toyoshima H, Eckmekci A, Mizuno Y, Nagaya T: Myocardial ischemia: nature of ischemic electrocardiographic patterns in the mammalian ventricles as determined by intracellular electrographic and metabolic changes. Am J Cardiol 8:493, 1961.

20. Holland RP, Brooks H: TQ-ST segment mapping: critical review and analysis of current concepts. Am J Cardiol 40:110, 1977.

21. Chou TC, Helm RA, Kaplan S: Clinical Vectorcardiography, Grune and Stratton, 2nd edition, New York, NY, 1974, pp. 187–254.

22. Starr JW, Wagner GS, Behar VS, Walston A, Greenfield JC Jr: Vectorcardiographic criteria for the diagnosis of inferior myocardial infarction. Circulation 49:829, 1974.

23. Benchimol A: Vectorcardiography. Williams and Wilkins Company, Baltimore, MD, 1973, p. 115.

24. Ha D, Kraft, DI, Stein PD: The anteriorly oriented horizontal vector loop: the problem of distinction between direct posterior myocardial infarction and normal variation. Am Heart J 88:408, 1974.

25. Howard PF, Benchimol A, Desser KB, Reich FD, Graves C: Correlation of electrocardiogram and vectorcardiogram with coronary occlusion and myocardial contraction abnormality. Am J Cardiol 38:582, 1976.

26. Sodi-Pallares D, Cisneros F, Medrano GA, Bisteni A, Testelli MR, deMicheli A: Electrocardiographic diagnosis of myocardial infarction in the presence of bundle branch block (right and left), ventricular premature beats and Wolff-Parkinson-White syndrome. Prog Cardiovasc Dis 6:107, 1963.

27. Guyton RA, McClenathan JH, Newman GE, Michaelis LL: Significance of subendocardial S-T segment elevation caused by coronary stenosis in the dog. Am J Cardiol 40:374, 1977.

28. Massumi RA, Goldmar A, Rakita L, Kuramoto K, Prinzmetal M: Studies on the mechanism of ventricular activity. XVI. Activation of the human ventricle. Am Heart J 19:832, 1955.

29. Yu PNG, Stewart JM: Subendocardial myocardial infarction with special reference to the electrocardiographic changes. Am Heart J 39:862, 1950.

30. Cook, RW, Edwards JE, Pruitt RD: Electrocardiographic changes in acute subendocardial infarction. I. Large subendocardial and nontransmural infarcts. Circulation 18:603, 1958.

31. Wolferth CC, Bellet S, Livezy MM, Murphy FD: Negative displacement of the electrocardiogram and its relationships to positive displacement: an experimental study. Am Heart J 29:220, 1945.

32. Pruitt RD: Certain clinical states associated with deeply inverted T waves in the precordial electrocardiogram. Circulation 11:517, 1955.

33. Ekmeckci A, Toyoshima H, Kwoczynski JK, Nagaya T, Prinzmetal M: Angina pectoris. IV. Clinical and experimental difference between ischemia with S-T evaluation and ischemia with S-T depression. Am J Cardiol 7:412, 1961.

34. Liu CK, Greenspan G, Piccirillo RT: Atrial infarction of the heart. Circulation 23:331, 1961.

35. Cohn JN, Guiha NH, Broder MI, Limas CJ: Right ventricular infarction. Clinical and hemodynamic features. Am J Cardiol 33:209, 1974.

36. Shettigar UR, Hultgren HN, Pfeiter JF, Lipton MJ: Diagnostic value of Q-waves in inferior myocardial infarction. Am Heart J 88:170, 1974.

37. Copeland RB, Omenn GS: Electrocardiogram changes suggestive of coronary disease in pneumothorax. Arch Intern Med 125:151, 1970.

38. Dressler W, Roesler H: Electrocardiographic changes in funnel chest. Am Heart J 40:877, 1950.

39. Perloff JK: Clinical Recognition of Congenital Heart Disease, W B Saunders Company, Philadelphia, 1970, p. 52.

40. Frank S, Braunwald E: Idiopathic hypertrophic subaortic stenosis: clinical analysis of 126 patients with emphasis on the natural history. Circulation 37:759, 1968.

41. McGinn S, White PD: Acute cor pulmonale resulting from pulmonary embolism: its clinical recognition. JAMA 104:1473, 1935.

42. Perloff JK: Cardiomyopathy associated with heredofamilial neuromyopathic diseases. Mod Concepts Cardiovasc Dis 40:23, 1971.

43. Gach JV, Andriange M, Franck G: Hypertrophic obstructive cardiomyopathy and Friedreich's ataxia. Report of a case and review of literature. Am J Cardiol 27:436, 1971.

44. Levine HD: Myocardial fibrosis in constrictive pericarditis. Electrocardiographic and pathologic observations. Circulation 48:1268, 1973.

45. Nora TR, Pilz CG: Pseudo-infarction pattern associated with electrolyte disturbance. Ann Intern Med 104:300, 1959.

46. Shugoll GI: Transient QRS changes simulating myocardial infarction associated with shock and severe metabolic stress. Am Heart J 74:402, 1967.

47. DePasquale NP, Burch GE, Phillips JH: Electrocardiographic alterations associated with electrically "silent" areas of myocardium. Am Heart J 68:697, 1964.

48. Pietras RJ, Staverato C, Gunnar RM, Tobin JR Jr: Phosphorus poisoning simulating acute myocardial infarction. Arch Intern Med 122:430, 1968.

49. Haiat R, Chiche P: Transient abnormal Q waves in the course of ischemic heart disease. Chest 65:140, 1974.

50. Chester E, Mitha AS, Matisonn RE: The ECG of constrictive pericarditis: pattern resembling right ventricular hypertrophy. Am Heart J 91:420, 1976.

51. Fulton MC, Marriott HJ: Acute pancreatitis simulating myocardial infarction in the electrocardiogram. Ann Intern Med 59:730, 1963.

52. Friedman GD: The relationship between heart disease and gallbladder disease: a critical review. Ann Intern Med 68:222, 1968.

53. Jeresaty RM: Mitral valve prolapse-click syndrome. Prog Cardiovasc Dis 15:623, 1973.

54. Goldman MJ: Normal variants in the electrocardiogram leading to cardiac invalidism. Am Heart J 59:71, 1960.

55. Burch GE, Meyers R, Abildskov JA: A new electrocardiographic pattern observed in cerebrovascular accidents. Circulation 9:719, 1954.

56. Smith LB: Paroxysmal ventricular tachycardia followed by electrocardiographic syndrome with a report of a case. Am Heart J 32:257, 1946.

57. Chatterjee K, Harris AN, Davies JG, Leatham A: Electrocardiographic changes subsequent to artificial ventricular depolarization. Br Heart J 31:770, 1969.

58. Jacobson D, Schrire V: Giant T wave inversion. Br Heart J 28:768, 1966.

59. Denes P, Pick A, Miller RH, Pietras RJ, Rosen KH: A characteristic precordial repolarization abnormality with intermittent left bundle branch block. Ann Intern Med 89:55, 1978.

# 11 | Serum Enzyme Determinations in the Diagnosis of Acute Myocardial Infarction

*Robert Roberts, M.D.*

The diagnosis of myocardial infarction has undergone considerable evolution in the past ten years. The development of new diagnostic techniques and improvement of existing methods have not only provided new means of assessing infarction but also provided a more critical evaluation of existing diagnostic methods. Included in these developments are the widespread use of creatine kinase (CK) isoenzymes, the development of the first quantitative assay for plasma CK isoenzymes,[1] development of a prognostic index for patients with myocardial infarction based on enzymatic estimate of the extent of myocardial damage,[2,3] and the introduction of several radioisotopes for the diagnosis and quantitative assessment of myocardial infarction and its effect on left ventricular function.[4]

Diagnosis of myocardial infarction conventionally has been confirmed by either the development of new Q waves on the electrocardiogram (ECG), or the elevation of certain plasma enzymes, namely SGOT or LDH, as outlined by the World Health Organization.[5] Several studies, however, have shown that myocardial infarction documented at necropsy frequently had occurred without development of Q waves;[6,7] this has led to the use of the term subendocardial infarction, which refers to ST-T changes on ECG and the presence of elevated enzymes. There is, however, no standard agreement on the precise criteria for the diagnosis of subendocardial infarction. The transient ST-T changes on ECG associated with this entity are nonspecific and are frequently observed in situations unassociated with myocardial infarction. The latter problem, coupled with coexisting ECG abnormalities that mask the development of Q waves on ECG, has led the clinician to rely very heavily on elevation of plasma enzymes as confirmatory evidence of myocardial infarction. The diagnostic criteria described by the World Health Organization were formulated before the concept of isoenzymes. The plasma enzymes conventionally used for the diagnosis of myocardial infarction consist of aspartic transaminase (AST), previously referred to as SGOT; lactate dehydrogenase (LDH); and CK. However, these enzymes can be elevated in many conditions other than myocardial infarction. The development of assays for isoenzymes has substantially improved diagnostic specificity and the future trend will probably be to replace enzyme estimation with isoenzyme determinations as a more reliable criterion for diagnostic confirmation of myocardial infarction.

## HISTORICAL PERSPECTIVE OF CLINICAL ENZYMOLOGY

In 1908, Wohlgemuth[8] demonstrated that human serum exhibited considerable amylase activity and concluded that it was released from the pancreas or the parotid gland. In 1922,

Robison demonstrated that bone extracts were rich in phosphatase activity and showed that this activity may be released into the serum.[9,10] Gutman et al.[11] showed that patients with carcinoma of the prostate gland having metastasis to other organs exhibited elevated alkaline phosphatase activity in the serum, and that this could be used as a diagnostic test. Despite these early observations, the incorporation of enzymatic diagnostic tests in clinical chemistry was slow, but was accelerated when Bodansky[12] and King and Armstrong[13] developed convenient assays for the determination of serum alkaline phosphatase. Other enzymes were added to the diagnostic array when Warburg and Christian[14] demonstrated elevated serum levels of aldolase and phosphohexose isomerase in rats with tumors. The year 1954 turned out to be a watershed for clinical enzymology—particularly for cardiology—when LaDue et al.[15] demonstrated elevated serum glutamic oxaloacetic transaminase (SGOT) in patients with myocardial infarction. This was followed shortly thereafter by the observation that LDH is also elevated in patients with myocardial infarction. It had by then been widely demonstrated that organs undergoing necrosis would release their intracellular enzymes into the interstitial fluids and into the vascular compartment. In 1959, Ebashi et al.[16] demonstrated that elevated plasma CK activity is an extremely sensitive index of skeletal muscle disease. One year later, Dreyfus et al.[17] demonstrated markedly elevated plasma CK activity in patients with myocardial infarction. It might be appropriate to indicate why creatine phosphokinase (CPK) is now referred to as creatine kinase (CK): All energy-transferring enzymes must transfer phosphorus, since it is the only utilizable form of energy; thus, the P is redundant and by international agreement has been dropped.

The concept of isoenzymes had been referred to by many investigators dating back to Fischer in 1895.[18] However, the wider recognition of isoenzymes and their application to clinical medicine did not come until 1957, when it was shown by Vesell and Bearn[19] that LDH, from various human and animal tissues, consisted of several different forms which could be separated by electrophoresis. This led to wide-spread recognition of the occurrence of enzymes in multiple molecular forms and their application to clinical medicine, which markedly improved diagnostic specificity. CK was shown to exist in three molecular forms; their use in the diagnosis of myocardial infarction was first reported by Van der Veen and Willebrands in 1966.[20] The full potential of CK isoenzymes as a diagnostic marker of myocardial infarction, however, was not realized until the early 1970s, in part because of the lack of a quantitative assay. The first quantitative assay for plasma CK isoenzymes was developed in 1974.[1] Since that time, several more convenient and rapid quantitative assays have been developed; and their application will soon be routine in the diagnosis of myocardial infarction. At the present time, there is still no available, convenient quantitative assay for plasma LDH isoenzymes; however, considerable progress is being made, and it is anticipated that a convenient assay will be available in the future.

## ENZYMES, THEIR FUNCTION AND ANALYSIS

An enzyme is an organic catalyst whose function is to speed up the rate of a biochemical reaction. It does not initiate or terminate the reaction; furthermore, the enzyme itself is neither created nor destroyed during the process. All enzymes are proteins composed of amino acids woven together in a complex fashion in which the precise spatial configuration is as important in performing its function as is the amino acid sequence and composition. The reaction catalyzed by an enzyme is almost always reversible under appropriate conditions. Some of the properties of enzymes are perhaps best discussed by using a specific example:

$$CP + ADP \overset{CK}{\rightleftharpoons} C + ATP$$

In this reaction, the enzyme CK acts on its specific substrate creatine phosphate (CP), and its function is to speed up the transfer of a high-energy phosphate from CP to that of adenosine diphosphate (ADP) to produce adenosine triphosphate (ATP). CP and ADP are referred to as the reactants; C and ATP are referred to as the products generated. However, as indicated by the arrows, CK will also speed up the reaction from right to left, transferring the P from ATP to C under specified conditions. In the body, depending on the conditions, CK can and does accelerate the reaction in both directions. One of the factors which determines in which direction the reaction will go is the relative concentration of the reactants on either side of the equation. If the reaction proceeds from left to right, it will do so until an equilibrium state is reached and the rate of formation of ATP equals the rate of formation of ADP. The enzyme speeds up the reaction by promoting a higher energy state of the reactants which is less stable; thus, it promotes the transfer of the high-energy phosphate to its receptor, namely ADP, leading to the formation of ATP.

Certain features that make enzymes appropriate diagnostic markers relate to their biochemical nature. First, in the above equations CK only reacts with a specific substrate—namely, CP for the rightward reaction or ATP for the leftward reaction. This is a highly specific feature in that CK will not react with other molecules. This characteristic is true of all enzymes in that each has its own specific substrate. Thus, by selecting the enzyme's specific substrate, one can assay the particular enzyme of interest even though hundreds of other enzymes may be present in the sample, as is always the case with blood samples. The second feature important in the diagnostic interpretation of elevated plasma enzymes is that one does not use enzymatic assays to measure the concentration of enzyme protein as one does, for example, with plasma albumin or gamma globulins; rather, one measures the rate of the reaction which is referred to in units of activity. To measure the rate of activity, one determines how much product is generated per substrate utilized per unit of time. To standardize the procedure and make it possible to compare results from one laboratory to another, the International Convention on Biochemistry has defined an international unit to be the generation of one micromole of product from one micromole of substrate per minute, with the reaction being performed under a given set of conditions at 30°C. This can be confusing and must be taken into account, since some laboratories perform their reactions at 37°C and others at 26°C rather than at the prescribed international standard of 30°C. The importance of temperature emphasizes a third feature of enzymatic assays—namely, the temperature-dependent nature of enzymes. Enzymes are particularly sensitive to temperature; in general, an increase in temperature of 1°C will increase the activity of most enzymes by about 10 percent. Thus, if the CK activity is reported to be 60 IU/l at 30°C, its value if performed at 37°C would be approximately 102 IU/l.

For the reaction to accurately reflect the amount of enzyme present in the blood sample, certain conditions must be met and standardized—namely, the substrate and other reactants must be in excess and product inhibition must be avoided so that the only rate-limiting step is the amount of enzyme present. Often, enzymes require cofactors for optimal activity. Examples of this are magnesium for CK and zinc for LDH. If the blood sample is collected in EDTA, the latter may chelate the magnesium; thus, the activity measured may be less than the activity actually present. Similarly, collection and storage of enzymes may lead to denaturation or proteolysis of the enzyme and give falsely low values. Similarly, inhibitors in the blood or inhibitors introduced during its analysis may also give erroneous values. Another consideration in enzyme analysis is the actual product being monitored or assayed. Although ATP is generated by CK and is preferably the product to be measured as a reflection of CK activity, it is particularly cumbersome and difficult to measure. Thus, enzymatic assays have been developed that measure the formation of NADH or NADPH, which requires linking another reaction to that of ATP so that the formation of NADH is proportional to the amount of ATP generated—which, in turn, is proportional to the amount of CK activity. Similarly, in assays for lactate dehydrogenase (LDH), the end product monitored is also NADH. The reaction coupled to the initial reaction must also satisfy the requirements of substrate excess, linearity with respect to temperature, pH, and other cofactors. NADH, the reduced form of NAD, is a convenient molecule to monitor, since it specifically absorbs light at a wavelength of 340 nanometers. However, other chromogens may also be present in the sample and absorb light at that particular wavelength; this could lead to erroneous values and so is another variable that must be properly controlled.

## ISOENZYMES

The term isozyme—first used by Markert and Moller in 1959 [21] and more recently referred to as isoenzyme (although the terms may be used interchangeably)—refers to different molecular forms of the same parent enzyme. The discovery of enzymes having different molecular forms provided one of the greatest advances in clinical enzymology—namely, organ specificity. The ability to pinpoint the source of a particular plasma enzyme elevation is related to the plasma isoenzyme profile. This particular property of an enzyme will be discussed in greater detail under each separate enzyme. For the present, it will suffice to define an isoenzyme: Isoenzymes are different molecular forms of the same parent enzyme having the same molecular weight, the same specific substrate, and, in general, similar catalytic properties. However, there is enough difference in the physical or chemical properties that one can, by conventional chemical means, detect and assess the individual isoenzymes. The diagnostic advantage is that each organ has a preference for a particular isoenzyme or combination of isoenzymes, which affords us the ability to detect which organ is responsible for a particular isoenzyme elevation. Unfortunately, the ideal specific marker has not yet been found; but the increased specificity afforded by isoenzymes is substantial and, in general, allows one to diagnose myocardial injury with reasonable precision and accuracy.

## RELEASE OF ENZYMES FROM TISSUES

Many enzymes and other compounds are present normally in the blood in relatively low concentrations and in general reflect breakdown of cells as a result of normal wear and tear. In the presence of acute cellular injury such as myocardial infarction, there is an explosive release of cellular contents with a corresponding increase above the normal plasma level. In the case of ischemic myocardial injury, the damage may be reversible if the duration of ischemia is short, as in angina, or irreversible, as in myocardial infarction. Even during transient ischemia, small ions such as potassium and inorganic phosphate are released within minutes of onset; as damage proceeds, large macromolecules such as enzymes are released. Elevated levels of plasma enzymes such as CK or LDH are regarded as markers of irreversible damage and reflect myocardial necrosis. It has not yet been definitively determined whether transient ischemia of the heart is associated with release of CK or LDH.

After the myocardial cell is irreversibly injured—a process which requires probably 30 to 60 minutes of sustained ischemia—the cell membrane integrity is markedly impaired and enzymes migrate from their intracellular position through the cell membrane into the interstitial fluid. Access to the blood requires further passage through the vascular walls, which may occur as a result of impaired vascular integrity or by diffusion through normal vascular walls. As the enzymes accumulate in the interstitial fluid, entry into the lymph may initially precede entry into the blood vessels; thus, transport may occur, via the right atrium, to the systemic circulation. The result is a delay between the onset of cellular injury and the appearance of enzymes in the blood. The duration of this lag phase will in part depend on the size of the enzyme molecule, regional myocardial blood flow, lymph flow, the concentration gradient between the intracellular constituents, and the concentration gradient of the interstitial fluid, lymph, and blood. Clinically and experimentally, it has been shown that myoglobin with a molecular weight of 17,000 appears slightly earlier in the blood than CK with a molecular weight of 84,000, and that both appear before LDH with a molecular weight of 135,000. It is likely that an enzyme present in the cytosol will gain access to the bloodstream before its counterpart present in the mitochondria.

## ENZYMES AS DIAGNOSTIC MARKERS

The preceding discussion has provided a brief background to the understanding of the basis of utilizing plasma enzyme elevations as diagnostic markers. It is appropriate now to summarize the factors that should be considered before making a clinical decision based on elevated plasma enzyme activity:

(1) Enzyme determinations are assays of activity, not of the amount or concentration of the specific enzyme protein; enzyme activity may be influenced not only by substrate concentration but also by the presence of inhibitors, cofactors, activators, by end product inhibition, and by nonspecific chromogens which may simulate the end product being measured.

(2) The nature of the assay procedure used, which may influence results profoundly; and, whether the data obtained are quantitative or qualitative; for instance, assays based on continuous monitoring are generally superior to those based on two-point determinations of end products.

(3) The abundance of the enzyme activity in the tissue under question and the concentration gradient between the tissue and the blood.

(4) The tissue distribution of enzyme activity and the tissue isoenzyme profiles, which are most important in the interpretation of diagnostic sensitivity and specificity.

(5) The appropriate frequency of sampling with respect to the temporal profile of plasma enzyme activity—namely, the time of initial elevation, peak elevation, and return to normal in relation to the onset of symptoms.

(6) The appropriate conditions for storage and preservation of enzyme and isoenzyme activity.

(7) The time course of depletion of enzyme activity in the damaged organ generally, but not always, correlates with the time course of increase in plasma activity.

(8) The change in plasma enzyme activity as reflected by plasma enzyme activity curves occurs as a result of two competing processes—namely, the rate of release of enzymes from the damaged organ and the rate of disappearance of enzyme activity from the circulation. Recent studies [23] have documented the enzyme disappearance rate to be specific for each enzyme and also for each species but within each species there is also marked variation in the disappearance rate from patient to patient or animal to animal.

(9) The relative diagnostic value of enzyme determination in a specific disease depends on sensitivity and specificity. A method is highly sensitive if the ratio of true positives to false negatives is high and the incidence of false negatives is low; it is highly specific when the ratio of true positives to false positives is high. Obviously, sampling time and frequency will influence the apparent sensitivity and specificity.

(10) The normal range of activity for each plasma enzyme must be established under the assay conditions applied and is usually defined as the mean $\pm 2$ standard deviations of values in the control population, with confidence levels of 95 percent. Stated another way, abnormal values for plasma enzyme activity will be obtained in 5 percent of normal individuals. Thus, an "abnormal" value does not necessarily imply that the patient harbors the disease. Enzymes vary with age, sex, and physical activity. It is preferable, therefore, that the normal range established for each laboratory be based on a population which is comparable in age and sex to the one in which the test is being applied diagnostically.

## CHOICE OF ENZYME MARKERS

Historically, aspartic transaminase (SGOT) was the first enzyme used in the diagnosis of myocardial infarction, followed by LDH. Several other enzymes have since been explored as possible diagnostic markers, at least in a preliminary fashion. There is a long list of potential candidates, but only a few have been assessed even in a preliminary fashion. These include: aspartic transaminase, lactate dehydrogenase, glutamic dehydrogenase, glutamic pyruvate transaminase, creatine kinase, aldolase, malate dehydrogenase, glyceraldehyde phosphate dehydrogenase, glycogen phosphorylase, adenylate kinase, triosephosphate isomerase, isocitrate dehydrogenase, gamma glutamyl transpeptidase, pyruvate kinase, n-acetyl-beta-glucosaminidase, n-acetyl-beta-galactosaminidase, acid phosphatase, beta-galactosidase, beta-gluc-uronidase, and cathepsin-c. Aldolase and phosphohexoisomerase activities are only tran-siently elevated following infarction, and analy-sis has been plagued with some technical diffi-culties. Serum adenylate kinase activity is extremely ubiquitous and lacks specificity. Simi-larly, lack of specificity applies to glyceralde-hyde phosphate dehydrogenase, which Karliner et al.[24] found to be elevated in patients with myocardial infarction.

Only three enzymes have been used on a rou-tine basis—namely, AST (SGOT), LDH, and CK. Despite the historical significance of SGOT, it has been shown to be relatively insen-sitive and also nonspecific, and should not be included in the diagnostic assessment of heart disease. LDH, CK, and their isoenzymes are at present the routine armamentarium for the diagnostic assessment of myocardial infarction. In view of these considerations and the present state of the art, CK, LDH, HBD and myoblogin will be discussed.

## CHARACTERISTICS OF CREATINE KINASE

Creatine kinase is a dimeric molecule with a molecular weight of approximately 84,000, consisting of two polypeptides referred to as subunits of either the B or the M type. The subunits are so named because M is the predom-inant subunit in muscle and B is the predomi-nant subunit in brain. The enzyme participates in a reversible reaction transferring high energy phosphate from CP to ADP to produce ATP, as illustrated below.

$$CP + ADP \xrightarrow{\text{CK}} ATP + C$$

An arginine residue appears to be the site for binding the magnesium-ATP or -ADP complex which is necessary for the reaction. Each sub-unit contains one sulphydryl group which is thought to be necessary for activity. Three CK isoenzymes have been recognized in plasma; based on their subunit composition, they are referred to as BB, MM, and MB, as illustrated in Fig. 11.1. All three isoenzymes are present

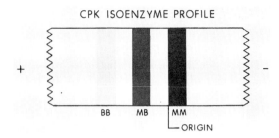

CPK ISOENZYME PROFILE

Fig. 11.1 The migratory pattern of MM, MB, and BB CK isoenzymes following electrophoresis at a pH of 8.0. MM CK, which is essentially neutral, remains at the origin. MB CK and BB, which are negatively charged, migrate toward the positive elec-trode. BB migrates further than MB, indicating that the negative charges are carried primarily by the B subunits.

in the cytosol of the cytoplasm; however, MM has been shown to be the predominant protein of the so-called M band in muscle tissue ob-served by electron microscopy.

### Collection, Storage and Analysis of CK Activity

Samples for CK activity may be collected as serum or plasma, since activity is similar and is not affected by therapeutic concentra-tions of heparin or coumarin compounds. How-ever, if plasma is collected, it should be in EGTA rather than EDTA, since magnesium required for enzymatic activity may be seques-tered by EDTA. EGTA, which has a much higher affinity for calcium ions, tends to be satu-rated with calcium with little remaining binding capacity for magnesium. Stability of CK during storage varies with the isoenzyme profile in the sample. MM CK collected in EGTA (10 mM) and mercaptoethanol (10 mM) is stable at room temperature for 48 hours, but MB and BB are less stable. With refrigeration, MM is stable for at least six days and MB for 24 hours when collected in EGTA and mercaptoethanol.[25,26] EGTA has been shown to afford a protective effect on CK activity independent of mercapto-ethanol and should be included in the storage of samples even if not collected as plasma. With fast freezing and storage at −20°C or −70°C in the presence of mercaptoethanol and EGTA, MM and MB are stable for years. However, if samples are repeatedly frozen and thawed,

CK activity will decline despite EGTA and mercaptoethanol, due to denaturation.

The conventional assay for CK activity consists of a coupled enzyme approach, with the generation of NADPH based on the Rosalki modification of the original Oliver assay.[27] The reaction is that of the backward approach in which creatine phosphate is converted to ATP. The assay is outlined below. The reagents are now available in a single vial supplied by several manufacturers in kit form and consistently give reproducible results as long as reasonable precautions are taken for quality control.

$$CP + ADP \xrightleftharpoons{CK} P + ATP$$

$$Glucose + ATP \xrightleftharpoons{Hexokinase} G - 6 - P + ADP$$

$$G - 6 - P + NADP \xrightleftharpoons{G-6-P} NADPH + 6 - Phosphogluconate + H^+$$

AMP is also included in the reagents to inhibit the formation of ATP from adenylate kinase (AK), which might be present, particularly in serum samples obtained after myocardial infarction. The reaction catalyzed by adenylate kinase (AK) is shown below which is:

$$ADP + ADP \xrightleftharpoons{AK} ATP + AMP$$

The inclusion of AMP inhibits this reaction. Unless large amounts of AK are present, this reaction does not occur and, thus, is not a source of error. However, occasionally in a hemolyzed specimen, the red cells, which are rich in adenylate kinase, will generate considerable activity. When the assay is performed without CP (the specific substrate for CK), the activity will be shown to be due to adenylate kinase. Creatine kinase activity is expressed in international units (IU) per liter. In our laboratory, the upper limit of normal for total CK is 75 IU/l and 65 IU/l for male and female subjects, respectively.

## Tissue Distribution of CK Activity

Since CK is an energy-transferring enzyme, it is not surprising that it is most abundant in highly contractile muscular tissues.[28] As illustrated in Fig. 11.2, CK occurs with abundance in only two tissues: skeletal muscle and heart. CK occurs in significant amounts, but several-fold less, in brain and the gastrointestinal tract. Other tissues have only minimal CK activity, and red blood cells are essentially devoid of CK activity. However, trace amounts can be detected at least in platelets with sensitive assays. The high abundance of CK activity in skeletal and cardiac muscle provides a tremendous concentration gradient between the tissue and the blood and accounts for the high diagnostic sensitivity of CK in disease involving these tissues.

The total CK activity and the isoenzyme profiles shown for tissues in Fig. 11.2 were obtained utilizing the quantitative fluorometric elution assay for CK isoenzymes.[28] Human tissues were removed at the time of surgery and assayed immediately prior to freezing with and without creatine phosphate to exclude apparent activity due to moieties other than CK. As shown in Fig. 11.2, myocardium was found to contain predominately MM, with MB representing approximately 15 percent of total CK activity. Skeletal muscles analyzed included deltoid, pectoralis major and minor, and gastrocnemius and rectus abdomini, all of which contained essentially MM CK. Any MB CK that would have been present in these tissues must have been

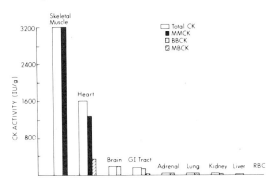

Fig. 11.2 Bar graph illustrating the abundance of total CK activity in the various organs (indicated by the open bar) and the isoenzyme profile of each tissue (indicated by the code in the upper right hand corner). As shown here, the only organs rich in CK activity are skeletal muscle and heart. Of particular significance is the specificity of MB CK for the heart, which is the only organ which has other than trace amounts of MB CK.

in trace amounts of less than one percent, since the sensitivity of the assay was about 2 to 5 IU/l. Lung, kidney and spleen contain predominately BB CK with no MB, and red blood cells were essentially devoid of CK activity. The small intestine contained trace amounts of MB (less than 3 percent of total CK activity), and trace amounts of MB were observed in the prostate and the urethra; but the myocardium is the only tissue containing more than trace amounts of MB CK. Subsequent development of more rapid and convenient quantitative assays for CK isoenzymes confirms that, of the total CK activity in human myocardium, 15 to 20 percent is MB CK, and that skeletal muscle contains essentially only MM.[29-34]

Recent studies by other investigators have analyzed tissue CK isoenzyme profiles with quantitative assays in fresh human tissues obtained at the time of surgery. The results obtained are virtually identical to those shown in Fig. 11.2.[35,36]

The lack of significant MB CK activity in skeletal muscle deserves further comment. Earlier studies have shown varying amounts of MB CK in skeletal muscle ranging from 0 to 30 percent of the total CK activity.[25] Since there are numerous skeletal muscles in the body, analysis of the CK isoenzyme profile of each skeletal muscle group is not practical; thus, possible heterogeneity of skeletal muscle isoenzyme profiles cannot be excluded. However, previous results showing varying amounts of MB CK activity present in skeletal muscle are probably explainable on the basis of several factors:[25] (1) Assays were performed with qualitative techniques that would overestimate trace amounts; (2) Tissues were obtained postmortem, and conformational changes or hybridization may have occurred; (3) In many of the studies, creatine phosphate was not excluded, and, thus, the possibility of fluorescence due to other moieties could not be excluded. While further investigation is needed in this area, it is unlikely that it represents a significant problem; several studies have documented that serial analysis of plasma MB CK activity in patients after intramuscular injections, noncardiac surgery, or trauma shows no significant elevation in plasma MB CK activity despite several-fold elevations in to-

tal plasma CK activity due to release of MM CK from skeletal muscle.[25,29,34] Caution, however, must be exercised until further data are available, particularly with respect to the human diaphragm. Since diaphragmatic muscle has characteristics of both skeletal and cardiac muscle it may be rich in MB CK activity. The only studies available on the human diaphragm have been postmortem, and in some studies MB has been documented as well as MM. At the present time, the author is unaware of any studies performed on fresh human diaphragm with a quantitative assay for CK isoenzymes.

## Plasma CK Time-Activity Curves After Myocardial Infarction

Elevated plasma CK activity as a marker of myocardial infarction was first described by Dreyfus and coworkers, who showed it to be a sensitive index for acute myocardial injury with significant elevation in 95 to 100 percent of patients with myocardial infarction.[17] Results of comparative studies in patients led Smith to conclude that plasma CK was the most sensitive index for diagnosing myocardial injury.[33] Total plasma CK activity generally increases 4 to 8 hours after the onset of chest pain, peaks within 12 to 20 hours, and returns to normal within 72 to 96 hours.[28] It thus provides an extremely sensitive and rapid diagnosis of myocardial injury.

Despite its sensitivity, however, elevation of total plasma CK activity lacks specificity for the diagnosis of acute myocardial infarction, with a false positive incidence of 15 to 30 percent.[38] This is not surprising, since CK is so abundant in skeletal muscle—which, of course, is the tissue most commonly undergoing injury and the most likely to be confused with myocardial infarction, particularly in patients receiving intramuscular injections or minor trauma. Total plasma CK activity increases in association with many noncardiac disorders. As comprehensively reviewed by King and Zapf,[39] these disorders include: muscular dystrophy; inflammatory disease of muscle; trauma or intramuscular injections (particularly of morphine, phenothiazines, and barbiturates, even without overt signs of injury); cerebral disease; alcohol intoxication; convulsions; and diabetes mellitus with and without ketosis. In addition, increases in plasma CK occur with shock, myxedema, pulmonary emboli, pneumonia, radiotherapy, chronic lung disease, surgery, and exercise.

Several cardiac conditions besides myocardial infarction may give rise to elevated total plasma CK activity. Although plasma CK does not generally increase in patients with mild congestive heart failure, it may do so in patients with pulmonary edema and severe hepatic congestion. Pericarditis, myocarditis, electrical cardioversion, and cardiac catheterization may lead to increased CK due to release from skeletal muscle or other organs besides the heart.[25]

## Plasma CK Isoenzymes and Myocardial Infarction

At the present time, plasma MB CK is the most specific and rapid enzymatic indicator of myocardial injury. The plasma MB CK isoenzyme time-activity curve is very similar to that of MM CK: It becomes elevated within 4 to 6 hours after chest pain, and reaches a peak at 12 to 20 hours; but, because of a faster disappearance rate, it returns to normal earlier than that of MM CK, and it generally falls back within normal limits within 48 to 72 hours. However, on occasion patients presenting between 36 and 72 hours after the onset of infarction may have an elevated MB CK in the presence of a normal total CK which has fallen from previously raised values. Interpretation is often clarified by a further decline in total CK and disappearance of MB CK activity.

CK isoenzymes were first utilized in the diagnosis of myocardial infarction in 1966.[20] The results show that MB CK provided a more sensitive index of myocardial infarction than total plasma CK activity. Increased plasma MB CK activity has been consistently observed in patients with acute myocardial infarction.[25,29-34] In contrast, MB CK is not increased in patients with chest pain and only transient nonspecific electrocardiographic changes. Normal plasma MB CK has been reported in numerous studies of patients with angina without infarction; so has the absence of MB CK elevation after transitory coronary occlusion in experimental animals subjected to ischemia insufficient to produce infarction. These findings support the view that MB CK is released from the myocardium only when necrosis occurs.[40] In addition, ischemia induced by treadmill exercise and documented electrocardiographically in patients with coronary artery disease [41] does not lead to increased plasma MB CK activity, despite elevated total CK from noncardiac sources. Studies performed in patients with unstable angina who have prolonged episodes of chest pain without the development of Q waves or other evidence for myocardial infarction have consistently exhibited normal plasma MB CK activity.[42] In one such study, patients with unstable angina were operated on within 24 hours if the plasma MB CK activity was normal; in 47 such patients, operative mortality associated with coronary bypass grafting was less than 4 percent, markedly less than the mortality of 40 percent observed in patients undergoing surgery during evolving myocardial infarction.[42] Thus, selection of candidates for surgery by exclusion of apparent infarction based on the lack of elevated MB CK avoids the excessive mortality associated with surgery in patients with evolving infarction, suggesting that absence of elevated MB CK does indeed reflect absence of infarction.

Studies performed in patients after noncardiac surgery have shown that, despite marked increases in total plasma CK activity, MB CK remains normal. These studies are summarized in a recent review.[25] The advantage of plasma MB CK activity over that of total CK is illustrated in Fig. 11.3, which shows the marked increase in total plasma CK activity due to intramuscular injections of morphine but with the plasma MB CK activity curve returning to normal. Patients undergoing cardiac catheterization without complicating myocardial injury may exhibit marked elevation in total plasma CK due to release from skeletal muscle, but MB CK remains normal as illustrated in Fig. 11.4. The diagnostic implication of plasma MB CK in patients with myocardial infarction and cardiogenic shock is illustrated in Fig. 11.5. As shown in the top curve, total plasma CK activity continues to increase while MB CK begins to decrease. The total CK reflects in-

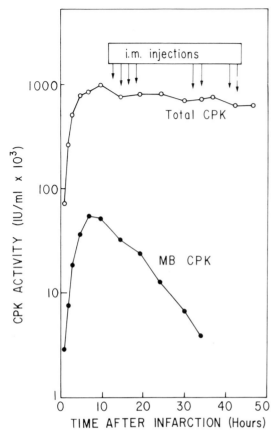

Fig. 11.3  Serial changes in MB CK and total CK activity in samples from a patient with acute myocardial infarction complicated by frequent intramuscular injections (indicated by the arrows). Despite continuing release of MM CK from skeletal muscle, MB CK returned to normal levels as seen in patients with uncomplicated myocardial infarction.

creasing release of MM CK from skeletal muscle due to hypoperfusion while MB CK indicative of myocardial necrosis is beginning to decrease despite the increasing total CK activity due to MM CK. Thus, elevated plasma MB CK activity is virtually specific for myocardial injury in man and appears to differentiate myocardial infarction from ischemia.

MB CK is particularly useful as a diagnostic index of myocardial infarction occurring in patients after noncardiac surgery.[31] Conventionally measured enzymes are elevated, and LDH isoenzyme analysis may not be helpful since hemolysis leads to increases in $LDH_1$ and

$LDH_2$, simulating the isoenzyme pattern resulting from myocardial infarction. Mortality associated with infarction after noncardiac surgery is high, sometimes as high as 40 percent,[42] possibly reflecting delay in initiating appropriate therapy because of delayed recognition of infarction. Postoperative infarction is most common in elderly patients and those with cardiac diseases, and definitive electrocardiographic diagnosis is often most difficult. For these reasons, differentiation between ischemia and infarction within the first few hours after the operation is difficult in these patients and may best be achieved by analysis of plasma MB CK activity.[43]

On the other hand, analysis of plasma MB CK activity after cardiac surgery does not help to establish the presence or absence or intra- or perioperative infarction, since MB activity is invariably elevated as a result of even minor surgical trauma to the heart.[44] Furthermore, since the proportion of myocardial MB CK appearing in the circulation after surgical trauma is too variable to be helpful, even quantitative evaluation of MB activity in plasma may not be useful. The appearance of Q waves on the electrocardiogram and/or new abnormalities on myocardial scintigrams obtained with [99m]Tc-

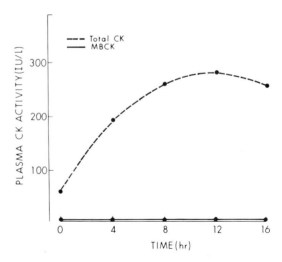

Fig. 11.4  The CK time-activity curves for total and MB CK in plasma samples obtained from a patient after cardiac catheterization. Total CK activity is markedly increased to 290 IU/l, but plasma MB CK activity remains normal.

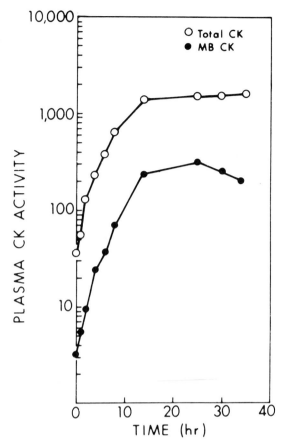

Fig. 11.5  Serial changes in total plasma CK (upper curve, open circles) and MB CK (lower curve, solid circles) in a patient with myocardial infarction and cardiogenic shock. Despite plasma MB CK activity having reached a peak and already significantly decreasing, total CK activity continues to increase illustrating the specificity of MB CK for myocardium. The MM CK presumably reflects continuing release from skeletal muscle due to hypoperfusion.

pyrophosphate appear to be the most useful diagnostic criteria of infarction in this setting.[44,45]

Plasma MB CK activity appears to remain normal in patients with pneumonia, chronic lung disease, and pulmonary emboli even when total plasma CK is increased, although elevated plasma MB CK might be anticipated if ischemia leads to right ventricular infarction. Pericarditis has not been associated with elevated plasma MB CK,[46] but extensive associated epicarditis might be expected to release MB CK into the circulation.

## Plasma MB CK in Noncardiac Conditions

Minor increases in plasma total CK activity may be observed in patients with hypothyroidism. Recent evidence suggests that this is because of increased MM CK that presumably accumulates due to decreased clearance.[47] However, on occasion MB CK may be elevated for the same reason, but such an increase would be very minor, and its cause would be easy to differentiate from myocardial ischemia. Both MM and MB CK are consistently elevated in patients with congenital muscular dystrophy. This appears to result from failure of the muscles to undergo normal differentiation and, hence, failure of the normal progression of isoenzyme profiles within the tissue, from BB initially to MM and MB at or before term to MM alone by birth or during the neonatal period. In addition, elevated plasma MB CK in patients with muscular dystrophy may reflect release from the dystrophic heart. Among patients with polymyositis, elevated plasma MB CK, though recognized, appears to be much less consistent. Patients with malignant hyperthermia may exhibit elevations of MM, MB, and BB CK, presumably from cardiac involvement, as is the case in Reye's syndrome,[25] a viral systemic illness involving the heart which affects children primarily. It has been postulated that elevated MB CK in patients with acquired muscle disease may be due to regenerative, undifferentiated muscle fibers which initially have BB, MB, and MM isoenzymes.

## Assays for MB CK Analysis

Analysis of plasma CK isoenzymes was plagued for some time with the same difficulty that still besets LDH isoenzymes and other conventional isoenzymes—namely, the lack of a precise quantitative assay. The development of the first quantitative assay in 1974,[1] the kinetic fluorometric elution technique, was extremely tedious, cumbersome, and not applicable to routine clinical use. However, it has provided an important technique for the assessment of tissue isoenzyme profiles and a standard for the development of more convenient and rapid quantitative techniques. The development of several quantitative assays for CK isoenzymes has encouraged the widespread use of CK isoenzymes and has considerably enhanced their diagnostic sensitivity and specificity. Nevertheless, the quantitative assays available still require further improvement.

CK isoenzymes have been conventionally separated on the basis of electric charge. They have been visualized colorimetrically by incubation with a medium containing redox dyes, or fluorometrically by detection of fluorescence from NADPH generated during incubation. Their separation by electrophoresis is diagramatically illustrated in Fig. 11.1. The colorimetric method is relatively insensitive and is no longer used. Procedures based on detection of fluorescence with a scanning device have represented an important advance since they provide increased sensitivity.

Despite the claims that electrophoresis is quantitative, it is at best semiquantitative; perhaps it is more appropriately referred to as a qualitative test. The results obtained with scanning after electrophoresis must be interpreted with caution. This has recently been reviewed,[25] and it will be sufficient here to point out some of the reasons why this procedure is not quantitative: (1) Isoenzymes are usually distributed asymmetrically along the axis of scanning; (2) Diffusion of substrate in the supporting medium may be limited, thereby leading to underestimation of activity of specific isoenzymes; (3) NADPH or dye may be lost in the supporting medium—again leading to underestimation of isoenzyme activity; (4) The reaction associated with one or more isoenzymes may deviate from linearity to an unpredictable extent because of disparate activities of each isoenzyme in the sample; and (5) Individual isoenzymes may exhibit different affinities for specific reagents in the incubation medium. Although electrophoretic scanning techniques have significantly improved the diagnosis, a substantial number of false positives may occur, as was the case in early reports. Several moieties such as adenylate kinase may generate fluorescence in the MB area and thus be falsely interpreted as MB CK. This, of course, can be excluded by omitting creatine phosphate from the medium to determine whether the fluorescence is due to CK. Other problems relate to moieties that generate fluorescence, such as drugs, namely diazepam (Valium), high doses of aspirin, tricyclic compounds and chlordiezepoxide (Librium) which migrate with serum proteins and fluoresce in the region of MB CK giving rise to false positives. Nevertheless, electrophoresis will provide very sensitive and specific data when used appropriately in serial samples.

With the development of quantitative assays for plasma MB CK, it is hoped that electrophoresis will soon be superseded by the more rapid, convenient quantitative assays. Several methods based on the column chromatographic separation of isoenzymes are now available and provide quantitative data for CK isoenzymes. However, the sensitivity of these assays is between 5 and 10 IU/l, and there may be carryover of MM into the MB fraction, leading to false positives. It is anticipated in the near future that this difficulty will be minimized and that sensitivity will probably be increased. The method of Henry et al.[47a] utilizing glycophase-coated glass beads avoids the problem of MM carry-over; however, the lower limit of sensitivity is still around 5 IU/l. The MB CK inhibition technique of Rao et al.[47] is insensitive and nonspecific, and its use is not recommended. The immunoinhibition test[48] gives extremely errornerous values, and in its present form is not recommended. The test is based on selected B subunit inhibition by an antibody that inhibits BB and, to some extent, MB but not MM. The problem with the assay is that it attempts to measure the pebble on the mountain by measuring the mountain. Total activity is determined followed by the addition of the antibody with repeat assay of total activity, the difference being due to MB CK. Since the reliability of a spectrophotometric assay is ±5 percent and the amount of MB present will vary from 1 to 15 percent, the sensitivity is extremely low. Furthermore, there is no standard inhibition curve to account for variation in antisera and inhibition. Even if one overcomes the latter difficulties, the inherent problem of assaying activity spectrophotometrically with a background noise of 85 to 98 percent prohibits it from being a sensitive and reliable assay. The approach taken by Merck (Abbott Laboratories) of inhibiting the M subunit has similar problems.

Of the available quantitative assays, the column chromatographic method of Mercer or the glass bead method of Henry et al. are the most reliable and provide adequate sensitivity with good reproducibility. The advantages of the glass bead technique are that it is simple and rapid, and that it avoids the cumbersome problems of column chromatography which most clinical laboratories prefer to avoid. Furthermore, the glass beads do not require preparation and have essentially endless shelf life. However, techniques are not available whereby either the column or the glass bead technique could be automated and provide very rapid and reliable quantitative results.

### Radioimmunoassays for CK Isoenzymes

The first radioimmunoassay for plasma CK isoenzyme was recently developed.[49,50] Because it does in fact measure the concentration of enzyme protein and not enzyme activity, it would avoid some of the problems associated with enzymatic assays, including substrate limitations, inhibition, activation, lack of linearity with respect to temperature, and pH or substrate problems. However, at the present time it is more a research tool than a routine diagnostic technique. Since the original radioimmunoassay, several other investigators have developed radioimmunoassays for CK isoenzymes and studies are underway for similar radioimmunoassays for LDH isoenzymes. It is too early yet to determine whether radioimmunoassay for CK isoenzymes will provide an improved technique for the diagnosis and assessment of myocardial infarction, but it does provide a very exciting alternative potential for the future.

### Routine Sampling and Assessment

In assessing myocardial infarction with plasma CK isoenzymes, it is important to realize that one must sample within the plasma temporal profile. In our experience, a blood sample obtained on admission and q12H × 3 for CK isoenzymes has been extremely beneficial and also cost effective. In the Barnes Coronary Care Unit five years ago, prior to the introduction of CK isoenzymes, the number of patients admitted per year was around 900. With the routine use of CK isoenzymes and no increase in the number of beds, 1250 patients are now admitted per year. Utilization of CK isoenzymes permits a more rapid turnover of patients and more prompt implementation of appropriate therapy. If the patient is admitted to the Coronary Care Unit more than 36 to 48 hours after the onset of symptoms, analysis of CK isoenzymes is inappropriate and one should rely on LDH isoenzymes or some other technique such as pyrophosphate scans.

## LACTATE DEHYDROGENASE

Lactate dehydrogenase (LDH) is widely distributed throughout nature and is one of the best studied enzymes. The enzyme catalyzes the reversible reaction of lactate to pyruvate as shown below:

$$\text{Lactate} + NAD^+ \overset{LDH}{\rightleftharpoons} \text{pyruvate} + NADH + H^+$$

LDH exists in most human and animal tissues in five electrically distinct forms.[51] In humans, the isoenzymes have essentially the same molecular weight of 135,000. The basic building block is that of two subunits designated H and M subunits, so designated because M is the predominate subunit in skeletal muscle and H is the predominate subunit in the heart.[52] Each LDH isoenzyme is a tetramer consisting of four subunits of the H or M type or various combinations giving rise to five isoenzymes. The isoenzymes have different charges and have conventionally been separated by electrophoresis. $LDH_1$, which is the most negatively charged and has the greatest electrophoretic mobility, consists of four subunits of the H type: $LDH_5$, which has the least electrophoretic mobility, consists of four subunits of the M type; $LDH_2$, three H subunits and one M subunit; $LDH_3$, two of each; and $LDH_4$, three M subunits and one H subunit. The striking difference in electric charge is believed to be due to the different amino acid content.[53] There is a gradual increase in the content of lysine and arginine and a decrease in aspartic and glutamic acid moieties proceeding from $LDH_1$ to $LDH_5$ which correlates with the changes in electrophoretic mobility. The subunits are believed to be inactive, and the catalytic property is found only in the intact tetrameric molecule.

## Collection, Storage, and Analysis of LDH

Quantitative assays for total LDH activity in tissue extracts from various body fluids have been available for some time. However, there has been considerable discussion as to whether the backward or forward reaction should be measured.[54] Lactate dehydrogenase catalyzes the reversible reaction:

$$Lactate + NAD^+ \overset{LDH}{\rightleftharpoons} pyruvate + NADH + H^+$$

The above reaction from left to right is considered the more physiological, since it is the predominant reaction in aerobic tissues like liver; thus, it has been referred to, as the forward reaction (L-P), whereas the backward reaction of pyruvate to lactate (P-L) takes place under anaerobic conditions in tissues like the heart. Lactate has no inhibitory effect on the reaction, but high concentrations of pyruvate inhibit the backward reaction, particularly for the isoenzymes rich in H subunits. Amador and colleagues[54] compared the two reactions and have found the rate of reaction linear for the L-P reaction but nonlinear for the P-L reaction.

The mechanisms of inhibition of pyruvate on LDH are now known.[55] LDH forms an abortive complex which inhibits enzymatic activity. The complex responsible for inhibition of enzyme activity in the presence of a high concentration of pyruvate consists of $NAD^+$, pyruvate and LDH which is illustrated in the following equation:

$$NADH + pyruvate + H^+ \overset{LDH}{\rightleftharpoons} NAD^+ + lactate$$

$$NAD^+ + pyruvate + LDH \rightleftharpoons ternary\ complex\ (enzymatically\ inactive)$$

NADH must first bind to LDH before pyruvate can bind to exhibit catalytic activity. In the P-L reaction, $NAD^+$ acts as an analog for NADH and binds the pyruvate which in turn binds to LDH. The complex is termed abortive because no catalyzed electron traffic can occur between the two oxidized subjects. Thus, as $NAD^+$ is formed, more complexes form. In the initial seconds there is very little inhibition, but the complex accumulates and the reaction proceeds. The complex formation occurs mainly for the H subunits being almost negligible for the M subunits. Thus, assays utilizing the pyruvate as substrate may encounter significant inhibition because of this complex formation.

Bowers et al.[56] have worked on a scheme by adjusting all the various parameters including pH, such that minimal variation occurs whether using the forward or backward reaction. Thus, it appears possible to use either reaction for determination of total LDH activity. However, it is generally agreed that one can detect more accurately smaller amounts of a substance formed than a slight decrease in the concentration of substances already present. In the forward reaction, one detects the appearance of NADH as opposed to its disappearance in the backward reaction. A further advantage of the forward reaction is the greater stability of NAD over NADH. Furthermore, NADH is also far more expensive. In general, the forward reaction is the preferred method in North America, but in Europe the backward reaction is more common.

The backward or forward reaction can be monitored spectrophotometrically at a wavelength of 340 nanometers by observing the appearance of NADH (forward reaction) or its disappearance (backward reaction). The other approach that has become popular, particularly with automated instruments, is coupling the reaction with various compounds that react with pyruvate to form a colored complex. Other colorimetric analyses use redox indicators that will form colored complexes on reduction. The oxidation of lactate to pyruvate causes a concomitant reduction of NAD to NADH. The hydrogen from NADH can be transferred to a suitable mediator, such as leuco-compounds, which become strongly colored on reduction.

One of the earlier agents used was phenazine methosulphate (PMS), but the most popular today is nitro blue tetrazolium (NBT). The NBT stain is also the most commonly used to visualize LDH isoenzymes following separation by electrophoresis.

Blood samples for LDH activity or LDH isoenzyme analysis are usually collected as serum and stored at room temperature. Refrigeration or freezing is associated with significant loss of activity of $LDH_5$ and the other isoenzymes rich in M subunits. Samples may be obtained as plasma following heparinization but if so, it is important to get rid of the platelets, a rich source of LDH activity. The major problem with collection of blood is hemolysis. Since red blood cells are abundantly rich in LDH activity, even minimal hemolysis precludes their use for LDH activity. Unlike CK, LDH is stable for days at room temperature; thus, it is the more appropriate means of storage.

### Tissue Distribution of LDH

Despite the tremendous interest in LDH isoenzymes and their diagnostic importance in clinical recognition of various disorders, a precise quantitative assay for individual LDH isoenzymes has not been developed. A quantitative assay for LDH isoenzymes is much more difficult than those of CK because of the existence of five isoenzymes rather than three and because tissues contain all five LDH isoenzymes rather than the usual distribution of CK isoenzymes in which most tissues usually have only two isoenzymes. As a result of these difficulties, many assays have been developed for LDH isoenzymes, all of which are semiquantitative and frequently give different results. Thus, despite the voluminous literature available on the distribution of tissue LDH isoenzymes, there are no available systematic studies on human tissues analyzed by a quantitative technique, performed on fresh tissue rather than material obtained at necropsy.[57] Necropsy material tends to favor $LDH_{1,2}$ because $LDH_{4,5}$ are much less stable. Comparison of total LDH activity from postmortem tissue can be very misleading. Not infrequently, the material was stored prior to analysis, which is also associated with loss of

LDH activity, particularly $LDH_{4,5}$. Appropriate controls without substrate are also frequently lacking. Thus, the results are best semiquantitative, and, because of the various techniques utilized, results vary considerably. It can, however, be stated that liver, skeletal muscle, kidney, erythrocytes, heart and lung, in decreasing order of activity, are abundantly rich in LDH activity.[7] The tissue isoenzyme profile is shown in Table 11.1. It must be kept in mind that the actual values for individual isoenzymes do vary with the assay, but that there is general agreement on the overall relative distribution and isoenzyme predominance. The predominant isoenzyme in the heart is $LDH_1$ and, to a lesser extent, $LDH_2$. In contrast, $LDH_5$ is the predominant LDH isoenzyme in skeletal muscle and liver. The organs with significant $LDH_{1,2}$ which may cause diagnostic confusion in the detection of myocardial injury are erythrocytes, kidney, brain, stomach, and, to a lesser extent, the pancreas. Based on very limited studies, Dawson et al.[58] postulated that fast-contracting (superficial) muscles contained predominately $LDH_5$, whereas slow-contracting muscles (generally found in the deeper muscle layers) contain $LDH_2$. Data on human skeletal muscle have not in fact borne out this hypothesis, and $LDH_5$ appears to be the predominant isoenzyme in skeletal muscle. However, it has been reported that the soleus muscle in man contains predominantly $LDH_1$. It must be kept in mind, however, that the development of quantitative assays in the future and analysis of fresh human tissues may exhibit different results.

### Plasma LDH Time-Activity Curves in Patients After Myocardial Infarction

The general temporal profile of LDH activity in serum after myocardial infarction is shown diagramatically in Fig. 11.6. LDH activity is elevated within 6 to 10 hours after myocardial infarction, reaches a peak within 24 to 48 hours, and may remain elevated for up to 10 to 14 days. The isoenzyme profile after myocardial infarction shows a predominance of $LDH_{1,2}$ activity over that of other isoenzymes and follows

Table 11.1  Distribution of LDH Isoenzymes in Human Tissues

| Tissue | LDH Isoenzyme Activity Percent of Total | | | | |
|---|---|---|---|---|---|
| | 1 | 2 | 3 | 4 | 5 |
| Colon | 2 | 20 | 40 | 27 | 9 |
| Heart | 51 | 36 | 9 | 1 | 1 |
| Lung | 10 | 20 | 32 | 22 | 14 |
| Gall Bladder | 7 | 22 | 40 | 23 | 7 |
| Esophagus | 5 | 18 | 40 | 24 | 13 |
| Duodenum | 3 | 19 | 32 | 29 | 15 |
| Mucosa | 18 | 21 | 16 | 83 | 35 |
| Kidney | 42 | 48 | 9 | 1 | 0 |
| Brain | 21 | 26 | 26 | 20 | 8 |
| Erythrocytes | 39 | 46 | 15 | 0 | 0 |
| Adrenal | 3 | 20 | 75 | 0 | 2 |
| Placenta | 12 | 18 | 15 | 30 | 25 |
| Lymph Node | 10 | 25 | 60 | 0 | 5 |
| Pancreas | 30 | 15 | 50 | 0 | 5 |
| Thymus | 10 | 11 | 30 | 28 | 21 |
| Thyroid | 12 | 25 | 55 | 0 | 8 |
| Prostate | 7 | 21 | 44 | 21 | 7 |
| Spleen | 10 | 25 | 40 | 20 | 5 |
| Leucocytes | 11 | 58 | 27 | 4 | 0 |
| Platelets | 13 | 43 | 39 | 4 | 0 |
| Muscle (skeletal) | 4 | 20 | 21 | 27 | 41 |
| Stomach (smooth) | 51 | 8 | 11 | 0 | 30 |
| Tongue | 24 | 19 | 19 | 0 | 38 |
| Diaphragm | 20 | 12 | 30 | 0 | 47 |
| Liver | 2 | 4 | 11 | 27 | 56 |
| Uterus | 5 | 25 | 44 | 22 | 4 |
| Uterus (gravid) | 2 | 5 | 28 | 45 | 20 |

a similar temporal sequence to that observed for total LDH activity. However, the plasma half-lives of $LDH_{1,2}$ are much longer being about four days as opposed to about 10 hours for $LDH_5$. $LDH_1$ isoenzyme predominates at about 24 hours and peaks at around 48 hours. The isoenzyme pattern in the latter days after infarction also demonstrates predominantly $LDH_1$. It is of interest that LDH activity may remain elevated for 10 to 14 days, as opposed to the short elevation of CK activity of 3 to 4 days. Part of the reason for the prolonged elevation of LDH activity is that of the longer half-life. Secondly, a part of the LDH activity released during infarction is from the infiltrate of inflammatory cells such as white blood cells, platelets, and, to a lesser extent, red blood cells, rather than myocardial cells. Thus, the more rapid test for diagnosis of myocardial infarction is that of plasma MB CK. However,

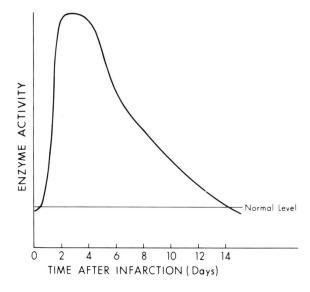

Fig. 11.6 The plasma LDH time-activity curve after myocardial infarction. Peak activity is reached at 48 to 96 hours and remains elevated for 10 to 14 days. Significant elevation is present about 12 hours after onset of symptoms.

LDH isoenzyme analysis is more appropriate in patients presenting more than 48 hours after onset of symptoms.

## LDH Isoenzymes In Noncardiac Conditions

As observed from the tissue LDH isoenzyme profile, myocardial infarction as expected would be associated with marked elevation in LDH activity; thus, the diagnostic test is a ratio of $LDH_1$ to $LDH_2$ of one or greater. However, it must be kept in mind that several other tissues may exhibit a plasma isoenzyme profile similar to that of myocardial infarction. It is often not possible to distinguish the plasma LDH isoenzyme profiles during injury to the kidney, red blood cells, pancreas, brain, or stomach from that of injury to myocardium. Since all of these tissues have a predominance of $LDH_{1,2}$ as well as the myocardium, the most common problem is hemolysis because red blood cells are abundant in LDH activity and contain predominately $LDH_{1,2}$. This is a common source of error due to artifactually induced hemolysis or hemolytic anemias. Even in patients after non-

cardiac surgery, the amount of trauma or induced hemolysis may in itself produce an LDH isoenzyme profile similar to that of myocardial injury. However, it must be emphasized that elevated LDH activity due to minor muscle injury is easily distinguished from that of myocardial injury.

Patients with congenital muscular dystrophy may also exhibit plasma LDH isoenzyme profiles similar to that of myocardial infarction. Elevations of serum $LDH_{1,2}$ have been consistently observed in patients with muscular dystrophy and tissue analysis of muscle biopsies from affected muscles in these patients showed a predominance of $LDH_{1,2}$ rather than $LDH_5$.[59] Several findings have also been observed in carriers of this disease as well as in their unaffected siblings.[60] This is felt to be due to a genetic deficiency in the synthesis of M subunits. During the embryonic period, skeletal muscle favors synthesis of the H subunits. As gestation proceeds, there is an increase in synthesis of H subunits with the formation of $LDH_5$. This process accelerates rapidly near term. In a few months after birth, the normal adult pattern of skeletal muscles is complete, with $LDH_5$ being the predominant isoenzyme. It is postulated that in muscular dystrophy there is a partial arrest of the process leading to $LDH_{1,2}$ being the predominant isoenzyme. A parallel to this is observed for CK isoenzymes in which the normal regression of the synthesis of B subunits by skeletal muscle is repressed with the emergence of the M subunit. In muscular dystrophy, an analogous repression of M subunit synthesis occurs resulting in the presence of BB and MB CK in muscles from patients with this disorder.

It is interesting that $LDH_5$ activity in skeletal muscles is markedly decreased in experimental animals following nerve resection.[61] Elevated $LDH_{1,2}$ levels in the serum have been observed in some acquired neuromuscular diseases which may reflect decreased synthesis of M subunits in the reparative process. Elevated serum levels of $LDH_{1,2}$ have been observed in several acquired neuromuscular diseases including polymyositis.[62] It is believed that dedifferentiation occurs in the pathological muscles leading to the defective synthesis of M subunits and, thus, to a preponderance of $LDH_{1,2}$ isoenzymes. Again, similar findings have been observed for CK isoenzymes.

## Assays for LDH Isoenzymes

As stated earlier, there is at present no quantitative assay available for individual LDH isoenzymes. Separation of the LDH isoenzymes by electrophoresis is by far the preferred approach both for quantitative and qualitative analysis utilizing as a support medium either agarose or, preferably,[63] cellulose acetate. During electrophoresis, however, there may be considerable loss of the more labile, slow-moving isoenzymes. Following separation, the strips are incubated with lactate and NAD to generate NADH, which in turn reduces phenazine methosulphate to a colored and soluable formazine at the site of the separated isoenzyme.[64] For qualitative assessment, one can visualize the bands from the intensity of the staining, or the intensity can be scanned and estimated by densitometry. The area of each peak obtained from densitometric scanning is integrated and expressed as a percentage of the total peak area. Factors which preclude precise quantitation are similar to those discussed for CK. Since there are five isoenzymes, activities of the individual isoenzymes are even more disparate and provide for less linearity than that of CK. However, for diagnostic purposes this method has substantially improved the specificity of LDH as a diagnostic marker of myocardial injury. Elution of the isoenzyme bands has not been practical for routine use.[64] Similar problems exist for quantitation of gels following spearation by isoelectric focusing.

Several approaches have been employed in an attempt to quantify LDH isoenzymes; these have been reviewed by Roman[57] and more recently by Rosalki.[64] However, it will be sufficient here to mention a few of these approaches and to indicate their inherent problems and why quantification has not been achieved.

Ion exchange chromatography has problems concerning loss of activity on the columns, overlap of isoenzymes, and insensitivity due to dilution. Mercer recently used minicolumns with DEAE-Sephadex and has improved the technique somewhat, but it remains to be determined whether this can become a routine quantitative method.[65] The various substrate inhibition assays all have in common differential inactivation of the H or M subunits and provide a quantitative assessment of the proportion of specific subunits present but not of individual isoenzymes.

The most popular of the inhibition assays is the use of 2-oxybutyrate substrate instead of pyruvate, which is the so-called HBD test. 2-oxybutyrate is preferentially reduced by the fast, electrophoretically moving LDH isoenzymes, which are rich in H subunits. Thus, myocardial injury will be manifested by high HBD levels since the myocardium is rich in $LDH_{1,2}$. However, again specificity will be lacking in separating injury to tissues such as kidney, brain, red blood cells, pancreas, and stomach from that of the heart because of the abundance of $LDH_{1,2}$ in the former tissues. But, HBD is much less specific than electrophoresis. This is because (1) there is some reduction by the M subunits, and (2) tissues such as skeletal muscle or liver rich in $LDH_5$ cannot be clearly separated from that of profiles associated with myocardial injury. HBD is elevated if there is a marked elevation even of $LDH_5$; thus, its lack of specificity has diminished its popularity. It was at first and still is in many centers considered the "poor man's" cardiac specific isoenzyme test, but its use is declining and should be replaced by isoenzyme analysis utilizing electrophoresis. Oxalate also preferentially inhibits the fast-moving isoenzymes. Heat inactivation at 56 to 65°C affects primarily slow-moving isoenzymes, which are the least stable isoenzymes, while antibodies developed to the H subunits selectively inhibit the slow moving isoenzymes.

The stop-flow technique is a recent development by Everse et al.[16] which measures the total LDH activity and the proportion of H and M subunits present in 10 seconds. LDH is assayed in a special stop-flow apparatus by the backward reaction at which the rate of reaction is determined between 0.2 and 0.4 seconds. This reflects the total LDH activity seen at this time because neither the H or M subunits are inhibited. A second interval is measured at 4 to 10 seconds, during which there is inhibition of the H subunits by the pyruvate-NAD complex but no inhibition of M subunits. The ratio of the two reflects the activity of the H subunits and is subtracted from the total activity reflecting the M subunit activity. The stop-flow technique offers great promise as a means of rapidly diagnosing myocardial infarction, but again it is not a quantitative test of a particular LDH isoenzyme.

In general, it can be said of the available methods that none provides precise quantitative data of the individual LDH isoenzymes, particularly $LDH_{2,3,4}$. All of the methods, particularly electrophoresis, are reliable in determining whether $LDH_1$ or $LDH_5$ is the dominant isoenzyme. However there is a tendency to overestimate the contribution of $LDH_{1,2}$ isoenzymes. Despite the lack of a quantitative assay for the individual LDH isoenzymes, the data provided by the semiquantitative methods, particularly by electrophoresis, offer improved specificity in the diagnosis of myocardial infarction.

### Routine Sampling of LDH Isoenzymes

Unlike CK, LDH isoenzymes reach a peak at 24 to 48 hours and may remain elevated for as long as 10 to 14 days. In some instances, however, the $LDH_{1,2}$ ratio may return to normal within the first few days after infarction. Thus, sampling for LDH isoenzymes is only required on a daily basis. It is the preferred enzymatic approach in patients presenting late after onset of symptoms, particularly after 48 to 72 hours. In general, patients presenting 24 to 48 hours after onset of symptoms should have serial CK isoenzymes performed as indicated earlier and a sample drawn for LDH isoenzymes. It is sufficient thereafter for LDH activity to be performed on a daily basis until adequate information is available to confirm or exclude the diagnosis of myocardial infarction.

## MITOCHONDRIAL CK ISOENZYME

The CK isoenzymes MM, MB, and BB are present in the cytosol. Jacobs et al.[67] showed that mitochondria are rich in CK activity and postulated that they contain a CK isozyme

different from the cytosolic isoenzymes MM, MB, and BB. Mitochondrial CK ($CK_m$) is positively charged at a pH of 8.0; in contrast with the other isoenzymes, it migrates toward the cathode in conventional electrophoretic systems.[68,69] Further characterization of $CK_m$ has been difficult because of its lability and the difficulty of isolating it in pure form. However, we have recently developed a method for purification[70] of mitochondrial CK from dog heart which results in a preparation that is devoid of other isoenzymes. Incubation of this preparation in 50 mM mercaptoethanol stabilizes the enzyme and permits storage at $-7°C$ for up to six weeks without loss of activity. We have shown that, by quick-freezing and thawing, mixtures of purified MM CK and BB give rise to the hybrid form.[71] In contrast mixtures of MM or BB with the $CK_m$ isoenzyme subjected to this treatment fail to form a hybrid. Furthermore, we have obtained a specific antibody to $CK_m$ which exhibits no cross-reactivity with MM, MB, or BB.[72] Based on this specific antibody, a radioimmunoassay is being developed to detect and quantify $CK_m$.[72] Mitochondrial CK has been shown to have a half-life of approximately 20 minutes in vitro, as opposed to approximately six hours for canine endogenous MM CK. In view of these and other properties of mitochondrial CK (lability, rapid disappearance rate, and intracellular location), the use of $CK_m$ in estimating infarct size may offer several potential advantages. Release of $CK_m$ into the plasma almost certainly would reflect irreversible myocardial damage. Thus, a comparative analysis should help to determine whether cystosolic isoenzymes are released under conditions other than those entailing cell death. Since $CK_m$ disappears rapidly, diffusion into the extravascular compartment is probably negligible due to the rapid rate of removal within the vascular compartment. Thus, reentry from the extravascular compartment is likely to be minimal compared to that observed with cytosolic isoenzymes. Accordingly, a plasma mitochondrial CK time-activity curve should more closely reflect the true enzyme disappearance rate and may provide an approach to clinical estimation of individual values of $k_d$. Since $CK_m$ is labile, local degradation is likely to be rapid, and washout or late release from zones of previous damage is unlikely to occur. Accordingly, the declining portion of the curve is unlikely to be influenced by late release. It is hoped that a radioimmunoassay can be developed for mitochondrial CK isoenzyme, which will provide not only a valuable diagnostic method for myocardial infarction but also a more precise assessment of the extent of myocardial damage than that obtainable with cytosolic CK isoenzymes.

## MYOGLOBIN AS A DIAGNOSTIC MARKER OF MYOCARDIAL INFARCTION

The use of myoglobin as a diagnostic marker of myocardial infarction has been proposed for over a decade. Myoglobin is a heme-containing protein with a molecular weight of only 17,000; it is found in abundance in skeletal and cardiac muscle but only sparsely in smooth muscle.[73,74] Serum myoglobin has a very low renal threshold and is rapidly cleared by the kidney. Earlier studies based on immunologic detection of myoglobin in the urine showed that the urinary concentration of myoglobin was markedly elevated in patients with myocardial infarction and disorders involving skeletal muscles such as trauma, myositis, surgically induced trauma, and a host of other conditions.[73] Its lack of specificity in part precluded its measurement from becoming a popular test. Immunologic detection of serum myoglobin has also been used previously by Jutzy et al.[75] in patients with acute myocardial infarction. Immunologic detection of myoglobin is based on an antibody that appears to have the same affinity for myoglobin released from either cardiac or skeletal muscle. Despite the nonspecificity of elevated myoglobinuria in differentiating skeletal muscle from cardiac disorders, the radioimmunoassay for serum myoglobin appears to have less interference from myoglobin released secondary to skeletal muscle trauma. This may in part be related to the rapid clearance of myoglobin by the kidney, which prevents high levels from developing unless extensive skeletal muscle necrosis has occurred. Thus, the apparent specificity

of serum myoglobin depends on the quantity of skeletal muscle in relation to the level of renal function.[74]

Recently, Stone et al.[76] reported on the potential value of elevated serum myoglobin in the diagnosis of myocardial infarction using a radioimmunoassay for serum myoglobin which is more sensitive than other radioimmunoassays for myoglobin and can detect levels as low as 0.5 ng/ml. Normal persons have a wide range varying from 6 to 85 ng/ml. Only 2 of 42 patients with chest pain without infarction had myoglobin levels outside the normal range.

In contrast, 62 of 64 patients with documented myocardial infarction had elevated serum myoglobin levels, half of which were elevated on admission, and developed a mean peak level of 528 ng/ml, which was attained within 4 hours of admission in most patients. Serum myoglobin was normal in 16 of 17 patients with congestive failure and in all 16 patients undergoing either cardiac catheterization (9 of 16) or stress testing (7 of 16). Patients with rhabdomyolysis and all of those undergoing cardiac surgery had elevated myoglobin levels. The possibility for a more prompt diagnosis than that afforded by CK was indicated by the occurrence of elevated myoglobin levels in 19 patients prior to an increase in plasma total CK.

The finding of an elevated serum myoglobin level is not likely to be as specific as elevations of MB CK and will probably not be an adjunct in the diagnosis of infarction after cardiac or noncardiac surgery.[74] Myoglobin is elevated within 2 to 4 hours after chest pain whereas plasma MB CK is elevated within 3 to 6 hours. This slight advantage of myoglobin is probably of moot value because this interval is often needed for many patients to reach the hospital. The failure of elevated serum levels of myoglobin to develop after moderate trauma to skeletal muscle may also be true for minor damage to the heart and preclude the detection of small infarcts. The most pressing but unanswered question is whether myoglobinemia is a specific index of myocardial infarction. Will it remain specific in conditions such as severe cardiac failure with vigorous respiratory muscle activity, cardiogenic shock, multiple intramuscular injections, or severe exercise (or even mild exercise) in the presence of impaired renal function? However, myoglobin may be an important adjunct along with MB CK in the detection of early extension of infarction, particularly if the extension has occurred before plasma MB CK activity has returned to normal. Since myoglobin disappears more rapidly, an extension would be manifested by a secondary peak as opposed to prolonged elevation in the case of MB CK.

Assessment of infarct size from serial changes in plasma myoglobin levels has not been attempted. One assumes that enzyme clearance is relatively constant when estimating infarct size enzymatically. MB CK is a large molecule with a molecular weight of 82,000; it is not removed by the kidney but is cleared exponentially, presumably by the reticuloendothelial system. Myoglobin, on the other hand, is cleared mainly by the kidney, and its rate of disappearance would be expected to vary with renal blood flow and renal function, both of which may vary throughout the course of myocardial infarction. Thus, theoretically, myoglobin would not appear to be as good a marker for estimating infarct size as CK. Further clinical testing is needed in disorders of cardiac and noncardiac origin to determine its diagnostic sensitivity and specificity. Until information from such studies is available, measurement of myoglobinemia as an adjunct in assessing myocardial infarction remains uncertain.

## ESTIMATION OF INFARCT SIZE

Recent concepts suggest that acute myocardial infarction is a dynamic process which is susceptible to favorable therapeutic modification and that the ultimate extent of infarction is an important determinant of prognosis.[77] These hypotheses stimulated the development of methods to quantify the extent of myocardial damage. This became necessary to determine the efficacy of pharmacological and physiological interventions in patients with myocardial infarction. The traditional use of mortality rates requires so many patients that it would be impractical except in large multicenter clinical trials performed over many years. Although infarction has been defined traditionally on the basis of morphological criteria, such criteria cannot be employed in intact animals or patients. Electrophysiological criteria, including ST segment elevation in epicardial or precordial recordings, are useful in reflecting the severity of regional ischemia in individual cases[77] but do not provide a quantitative estimate of the extent of infarction. Radionuclide imaging using technetium pyrophosphate or thallium-201 isotopes is useful in detecting injured myocardium,[4] but quantification is limited because of superimposition of overlapping regions of myocardium on two-dimensional displays, poor resolution, and limited contrast.[78] Although promising techniques such as positron emission transaxial tomography may overcome many of these difficulties,[79] calibration of results using independent criteria to estimate the overall extent of infarction will be necessary.

## Enzymatic Estimation of Infarct Size

CK is particularly advantageous for enzymatic assessment of myocardial ischemic injury. This is because, contrary to the case of a lower molecular weight species such as myoglobin, CK in plasma is not cleared by the kidney, and levels of plasma CK activity after myocardial infarction are independent of renal blood flow. In the heart, CK is virtually confined to myocardial components rather than other cellular elements such as connective tissue, white blood cells, and other participants in the inflammatory exudate or vascular endothelium. The importance of this consideration is underscored by the observation that after experimental myocardial infarction the total activity of enzymes such as lactate dehydrogenase (LDH) released into the plasma is frequently greater than that present in the heart prior to infarction—presumably because of substantial contributions from elements other than cardiac muscle, such as cells participating in the inflammatory response.[57] Elevated plasma MB CK is virtually specific for the heart and is also particularly useful for estimating infarct size because it is rapidly released; peak plasma values are reached in 12 to 24 hours; and it returns to normal within 36 to 58 hours.

Table 11.2  Sample Size Required for Mortality vs. Infarct Size as an Endpoint

| | Sample Size Per Group (To Detect 20% Difference) | |
|---|---|---|
| Power | Mortality | Infarct Size |
| .5 | 1105 | 113 |
| .667 | 1761 | 179 |
| .75 | 2197 | 223 |
| .8 | 2525 | 257 |
| .9 | 3497 | 355 |
| .95 | 4419 | 448 |

| | Sample Size Per Group (To Detect 30% Difference) | |
|---|---|---|
| Power | Mortality | Infarct Size |
| .5 | 465 | 41 |
| .667 | 740 | 65 |
| .75 | 923 | 81 |
| .8 | 1061 | 93 |
| .9 | 1470 | 128 |
| .95 | 1857 | 162 |

Enzymatic estimates of infarct size based on the amount of CK released into the plasma in patients with myocardial infarction have been shown to correlate closely with acute and long-term mortality,[80,81] impairment of left ventricular function,[82] hemodynamics,[83] regional wall motion abnormalities,[84] and ventricular dysrhythmia.[85] Enzymatic estimates of infarct size utilizing the CK method have been widely used by several investigators as a method for evaluating the effect of various interventions on ischemic myocardial damage.[81] The impact of enzymatic estimates of infarct size is summarized in Table 11.2, showing the marked reduction in the number of patients required to evaluate an intervention using infarct size as an endpoint versus that of mortality. To demonstrate a 30 percent reduction in mortality requires 1857 patients, as opposed to only 162 patients for a 30 percent reduction in infarct size. However, adequate interpretation of qualitative and quantitative changes in infarction induced by interventions requires delineation of the sensitivity, precision, and limitations of methods utilized. Despite the close correlation between enzymatic estimates of infarct size and other clinical parameters, there is still a need for further characterization of the various parameters used in this approach and to determine their sensitivity and limitations. Estimation of infarct size from plasma CK release depends on several factors, one of which is the fractional disappearance rate ($k_d$) for CK and another of which is the fractional release ratio from the tissues. There are considerable data available on these parameters,[86,87] and further investigations are ongoing which, it is hoped, will improve the sensitivity and precision of this technique.

## REFERENCES

1. Roberts R, Henry PD, Witteveen SAGJ and Sobel BE: Quantification of serum creatine phosphokinase (CPK) isoenzyme activity. Am J Cardiol 33:650, 1974.
2. Shell WE, Kjekshus JK and Sobel BE: Quantitative assessment of the extent of myocardial infarction in the conscious dog by means of analysis of serial changes in serum creatine phosphokinase activity. J Clin Invest 50:2614, 1971.
3. Roberts R, Henry PD and Sobel BE: An improved basis for enzymatic estimation of infarct size. Circulation 52:743, 1975.
4. Willerson JT, Parkey RW, Bonte FJ, Meyer SL, Atkins JM and Stokely EM: Technetium stannous pyrophosphate myocardial scintigrams in patients with chest pain of varying etiology. Circulation 51:1046, 1975.
5. World Health Organization Technical Report Series 168. Hypertension and coronary heart disease: Classification and criteria for epidemiological studies, p 3, 1959.
6. Cook RW, Edwards JE and Pruitt RD: Electrocardiographic changes in acute subendocardial infarction. I. Large subendocardial and large transmural infarcts. Circulation 18:603, 1958.
7. Abildskov JA, Wilkinson RS Jr, Vincent WA and Cohen W. An experimental study of the electrocardiographic effects of localized myocardial lesions. Am J Cardiol 8:485, 1961.

8. Wohlgemuth J: Unersuchungen über die Diastasen. Biochem Z 9:10, 1908.

9. Robinson R: A new phosphoric ester produced by the action of yeast juice on hexoses. Biochem J 16:809, 1922.

10. Martland M and Robison R: Possible significance of hexosephosphoric esters in ossification. VI. Phosphoric esters in blood plasma. Biochem J 20:847, 1926.

11. Gutman EB, Spraul EE and Gutman AB: Significance of increased phosphatase activity of bone at site of osteoblastic metastases secondary to carcinoma of the prostate gland. Am J Cancer 28:485, 1936.

12. Bodansky A: Phosphatase studies. II. Determination of serum phosphatase. Factors influencing the accuracy of the determination. J Biol Chem 101:93, 1933.

13. King EJ and Armstrong AR: A convenient method for determining serum and bile phosphatase activity. Canad Med Assoc J 31:376, 1934.

14. Warburg O and Christian W: Gärungsfermente im Blustserum von Tumor-Ratten. Biochem Z 314:399, 1943.

15. LaDue JS, Wroblewski F and Karmen A: Serum glutamic oxalacetic transaminase activity in human acute transmural myocardial infarction. Science 120:497, 1954.

16. Ebashi S, Toyakura Y, Momoi H and Sugita H: High creatine phosphokinase activity of sera of progressive muscular dystrophy. J Biochem 46:103, 1959.

17. Dreyfus JC, Schapira G, Resnais J and Scebat L: Serum creatinine kinase in the diagnosis of myocardial infarct. Rev Franc Etud Clin Biol 5:386, 1960.

18. Fischer E: Über den Einfluss der Coufiguration auf die Wirkung der Enzyme III. Ber Deutsch Chem Ges 28:1429, 1895.

19. Vesell ES and Bearn AG: Localization of lactic acid dehydrogenase activity in serum fractions. Proc Soc Exp Biol Med 94:96, 1957.

20. Van der Veen KJ and Willebrands AF: Isoenzymes of creatine phosphokinase in tissue extracts and in normal and pathological sera. Clin Chim Acta 13:312, 1966.

21. Market CL and Moller F: Multiple forms of enzymes: tissue, ontogenetic and species specific patterns. Proc Nat Acad Sci 45:753, 1959.

22. Jennings RB, Ganote CE and Reimer KA: Ischemic tissue injury. Am J Pathol 81:179, 1975.

23. Roberts R and Sobel BE: Effect of selected drugs and myocardial infarction on the disappearance of creatine kinase from the circulation in conscious dogs. Cardiovas Res 11:103, 1977.

24. Karliner JS, Gander MP and Sobel BE: Elevated serum glyceraldehyde phosphate dehydrogenase activity in patients with acute myocardial infarction. Chest 60:318, 1971.

25. Roberts R and Sobel BE: Creatine kinase isoenzymes in the assessment of heart disease. Am Heart J 95:521, 1978.

26. Morin LG: Improved separation of creatine kinase cardiac isoenzyme in serum by batch fractionation Clin Chem 22:92, 1976.

27. Rosalki SB: Improved procedure for serum creatine phosphokinase determination. J Lab Clin Med 69:696, 1967.

28. Roberts R, Gowda KS, Ludbrook PA and Sobel BE: The specificity of elevated serum MB CPK activity in the diagnosis of acute myocardial infarction. Am J Cardiol 36:433, 1975.

29. Mercer DW: Separation of tissue and serum creatine kinase isoenzymes by ion-exchange column chromatography. Clin Chem 20:36, 1974.

30. Yasmineh WG and Hanson NQ: Electrophoresis on cellulose acetate and chromatography on DEAE-Sephadex A-50 compared in the estimation of creatine kinase isoenzymes. Clin Chem 21:381, 1975.

31. Roberts R and Sobel BE: Elevated plasma MB creatine phosphokinase activity. A specific marker for myocardial infarction in perioperative patients. Arch Intern Med 136:421, 1976.

32. Dixon SH, Limbird LE and Roe CR: Recognition of post-operative acute myocardial infarction: Application of isoenzyme techniques. Circulation 48 (Suppl. III):III–137, 1973.

33. Smith AF, Radford D, Wong CP and Oliver MF: Creatine kinase MB isoenzyme studies in diagnosis of myocardial infarction. Br Heart J 38:225, 1976.

34. Roberts R, Sobel BE and Ludbrook PA: Determination of the origin of elevated plasma CPK after cardiac catheterization. Cath Cardiovasc Diag 2:329, 1976.

35. Tsung SH: Creatine kinase isoenzyme patterns in human tissues obtained at surgery. Clin Chem 22:173, 1976.

36. Ogunro EA, Hearse DJ and Shillingford JP: Creatine kinase isoenzymes: Their separation and quantitation. Cardiovasc Res 11:94, 1977.

37. Smith AF: Diagnostic value of serum creatine kinase in a coronary care unit. Lancet 2:178, 1967.

38. Goldberg DM and Windfield DA: Diagnostic accuracy of serum enzyme assays from myocardial infarction in a general hospital population. Br Heart J 34:597, 1972.

39. King JO and Zapf P: A review of the value of creatine phosphokinase estimations in clinical medicine. Med J Australia 1:699, 1972.

40. Ahmed SA, Williamson JR, Roberts R, Clark RE and Sobel BE: The association of increased plasma MB CPK activity and irreversible ischemic myocardial injury in the dog. Circulation 54:187, 1976.

41. Klein MS, Coleman RE, Roberts R and Weiss AN: $^{99m}$Tc(Sn) pyrophosphate scintigrams in exercise-induced angina and calcified valves. Am J Cardiol 37:149, 1976. (Abstract)

42. Klein MS, Ludbrook PA, Mimbs JW, Gafford FH, Gillespie TA, Weldon CS, Sobel BE and Roberts R: Perioperative mortality in patients with unstable angina selected by exclusion of myocardial infarction. J Thor Cardiovasc Surg 73:253, 1977.

43. Roberts R and Sobel BE: CPK enzymes in evaluation of myocardial ischemic injury. Hosp Prac 11:55, 1976.

44. Klein MS, Coleman RE, Weldon CS, Sobel BE and Roberts R: Concordance of electrocardiographic and scintigraphic criteria of myocardial injury after cardiac surgery. J Thor Cardiovasc Surg 71:934, 1976.

45. Righetti A, O'Rourke RA, Schelbert H, Henning H, Hardarson T, Daily PO, Ashburn W and Ross J Jr: Usefulness of preoperative and postoperative Tc-99m (Sn)-pyrophosphate scans in patients with ischemic and valvular heart disease. Am J Cardiol 39:43, 1977.

46. Fleg JL, Siegel BA, Williamson JR and Roberts R: Technetium-99m pyrophosphate imaging in acute pericarditis: A clinical and experimental study. Radiology 126:727, 1978.

47. Rao PS, Lukes JJ, Ayres SM and Mueller H: New manual and automated method for determining activity of CK isoenzyme MB by use of dithiothreitol: Clinical application. Clin Chem 21:1612, 1975.

47a. Henry PD, Roberts R, Sobel BE: Rapid separation of plasma creative kinase isoenzymes by batch adsorption with glass beads. Clin Chem 21:844, 1975.

48. Jockers-Wretou E, Grabert K and Pfleiderer G: Quantitative immunologische bestimmung der isoenzyme der creatinkinase im serum. Z Clin Chem 13:85, 1975.

49. Roberts R, Sobel BE and Parker CW: Radioimmunoassay for creatine kinase isoenzymes. Science 194:855, 1976.

50. Roberts R, Parker CW and Sobel BE: Detection of acute myocardial infarction with a radioimmunoassay for creatine kinase MB. Lancet 2:319, 1977.

51. Plagemann PGW, Gregory KF and Wroblewski F: The electrophoretically distinct forms of mammalian lactic dehydrogenase. I. Distribution of lactic dehydrogenases in rabbit and human tissues. J Biol Chem 235:2282, 1960.

52. Appella E and Markert CL: Dissociation of lactate dehydrogenase into subunits with guanidine hydrochloride. Biochem Biophys Acta 6:171, 1961.

53. Wieland T. and Pfleiderer G: Chemical differences between multiple forms of lactic acid dehydrogenase. Ann NY Acad Sci 94:691, 1961.

54. Amador E, Dorfman LE and Wacker WEC: Serum lactic dehydrogenase activity: analytical assessment of current assays. Clin Chem 9:391, 1963.

55. Kaplan NO, Everse J and Admiraal J: Significance of substrate inhibition of dehydrogenases. Ann NY Acad Science 151:400, 1968.

56. Gay RJ, McComb RB and Bowers GN Jr: Optimum reaction conditions of human lactate dehydrogenase isoenzymes as they affect total lactate dehydrogenase activity. Clin Chem 14:740, 1968.

57. Roman W: Quantitative estimation of lactate dehydrogenase isoenzymes in serum. I. Review of methods and distribution in human tissues. Enzymol 36:190, 1968.

58. Dawson DM and Kaplan NO: Factors influencing the concentration of enzymes in various tissues. J Biol Chem 240:3215, 1965.

59. Dreyfus JC, Demos J, Schapira F and Schapira G: La lacticodéshydrogénase musculaire chez le myopathe: persistance apparente du type foetal. CR Acad Sci (Paris) 254:4384, 1962.

60. Emery AEH: Electrophoretic pattern of lactic dehydrogenase in carriers and patients with Duchenne muscular dystrophy. Nature (London) 201:1044, 1964.

61. Brody IA: Effect of denervation on the lactate dehydrogenase isozymes of skeletal muscle. Nature (London) 205:196, 1965.

62. Schapira F, Dreyfus JC and Schapira G: Fetal-like patterns of lactic-dehydrogenase and aldolase isoenzymes in some pathological conditions. Enzym Biol Clin 7:98, 1966.

63. Wilkinson JH: The Principles and Practice of Diagnostic Enzymology. Year Book Medical Publishers Inc., Chicago, 1976.

64. Rosalki SB: Methods in the study of isoenzymes. Histochem J 6:361, 1974.

65. Mercer DW: Simultaneous separation of serum creatine kinase and lactate dehydrogenase isoenzymes by ion-exchange column chromatography. Clin Chem 21:1102. 1975.

66. Everse J, Reich RM, Kaplan NO and Finn WD: New instrument for rapid determination of activ-

ities of lactate dehydrogenase isoenzyme. Clin Chem 21:1277, 1975.

67. Jacobs H, Heldt HW and Klingenberg M: High activity of creatine kinase in mitochondria from muscle and brain and evidence for a separate mitochondrial isoenzyme of creatine kinase. Biochem Biophys Res Comm 16:516, 1966.

68. Jacobus WE and Lehninger AL: Creatine kinase of rat heart mitochondria. J Biol Chem 248:4803, 1973.

69. Sobel BE, Shell WE and Klein MS: An isoenzyme of creatine phosphokinase associated with rabbit heart mitochondria. J Mol Cell Cardiol 4:367, 1972.

70. Roberts R and Grace AM: Purification of mitochondrial creatine kinase: biochemical and immunological characterization. J Biol Chem 255:2870, 1980.

71. Grace A and Roberts R: Isolation of a unique mitochondrial creatine kinase isoenzyme. Clin Res 26:647A, 1978 (Abstract)

72. Roberts R and Sobel BE: Mitochondrial creatine kinase: An isoenzyme with unique properties demonstrable with a specific antibody. Clin Res 26:265A, 1978. (Abstract)

73. Kagen LJ: Myoglobin: biochemical, physiological and clinical aspects. New York, Columbia University Press, p 79, 1973.

74. Roberts R: Myoglobinemia as an index to myocardial infarction. Ann Intern Med 87:788, 1977.

75. Jutzy RV, Nevatt GW, Palmer RJ and Nelson JC: Radioimmunoassay of serum myoglobin in acute myocardial infarction. Am J Cardiol 35:147, 1975. (Abstract)

76. Stone MJ, Waterman MR, Harimoto D, Murray G, Willson N, Platt MR, Blomqvist G and Willerson JT: Serum myoglobin level as diagnostic test in patients with acute myocardial infarction. Br Heart J 39:375, 1977.

77. Maroko PR, Kjekshus JK, Sobel BE, Watanabe T, Covell JW, Ross J Jr and Braunwald E: Factors influencing infarct size following experimental coronary artery occlusion. Circulation 43:67, 1971.

78. Klein MS, Roberts R and Coleman RE: Radionuclides in the assessment of myocardial infarction. Am Heart J 95:659, 1978.

79. Ter-Pogossian MM: Limitations of present radionuclide methods in the evaluation of myocardial ischemia and infarction. Circulation 53 (Suppl. I):119, 1976.

80. Sobel BE, Bresnahan GF, Shell WE and Yoder RD: Estimation of infarct size in man and its relation to prognosis. Circulation 46:640, 1972.

81. Geltman EM, Ehsani AA, Campbell MK, Roberts R and Sobel BE: Determinants of prognosis after initial subendocardial compared to transmural myocardial infarction: the importance of infarct size. Am J Cardiol 43:370, 1979. (Abstract)

82. Kostuk WJ, Ehsani AA, Karliner JS, Ashburn WL, Peterson KL, Ross J Jr and Sobel BE: Left ventricular performance after myocardial infarction assessed by radioisotope angiocardiography. Circulation 47:242, 1973.

83. Bleifeld W, Mathey D, Hanrath P, Buss H and Effert S: Infarct size estimated from serial serum creatine phosphokinase in relation to left ventricular hemodynamics. Circulation 55:303, 1977.

84. Rogers WJ, McDaniel HG, Smith LR, Mantle JA, Russell RO Jr and Rackley CE: Correlation of CPK-MB and angiographic estimates of infarct size in man. Circulation 54 (Suppl. II):II–2. 1976. (Abstract)

85. Roberts R, Husain A, Ambos HD, Oliver GC, Cox JR Jr and Sobel BE: Relation between infarct size and ventricular arrhythmia. Br Heart J 37:1169, 1975.

86. Sobel BE, Markham J, Karlsberg RP and Roberts R: The nature of disappearance of creatine kinase from the circulation and its influence on enzymatic estimation of infarct size. Circ Res 41:836, 1977.

87. Sobel BE, Markham J and Roberts R: Factors influencing enzymatic estimates of infarct size. Am J Cardiol 39:130, 1977.

# 12 | Nuclear Cardiology Techniques

*Introductory Principles and Applications to Myocardial Imaging in the Diagnosis of Acute Myocardial Infarction*

*William L. Ashburn, M.D.*
*Kathryn F. Witztum, M.D.*

## DIAGNOSIS OF AMI BY NUCLEAR TECHNIQUES

Physicians are becoming increasingly aware of the utility of nuclear imaging techniques to assess myocardial perfusion and ventricular function in the setting of known or suspected acute myocardial infarction. The methods to be discussed in this and in Chapter 28 are similar in that they are nontraumatic and only minimally invasive in the sense that they involve nothing more arduous than the simple intravenous injection of a harmless amount of radiopharmaceutical tracer.

In this chapter we will consider nuclear cardiac diagnostic procedures designed to study several aspects of myocardial perfusion, including thallium-201 and technetium-99m pyrophosphate imaging. Before discussing these diagnostic procedures, however, we will review the fundamental principles of nuclear physics, radiopharmaceuticals, and the instrumentation necessary to record the distribution of radioactive drugs in the body.

In order to use wisely and appropriately any medical tool or technique, one must first have some comprehension of its potentials, limitations, applications, and reliability. As regards Nuclear Cardiology, this requires an understanding of the basic principles of atomic physics; radioactive decay; radiation interaction and detection; accumulation and analysis of nuclear data; and radionuclide imaging. While this chapter cannot hope to cover such complex topics in any great detail, nevertheless, we will attempt to present a simplified approach to this information, in order to introduce the vocabulary needed in subsequent discussion. For clarification and more in-depth material, the reader is referred to the several excellent texts and monographs listed in the reference portion of this chapter.[1-7]

## NUCLEAR MEDICINE PHYSICS

### The Atomic Model

The atomic theory states that all matter is composed of particles called atoms; or as the Greeks put it, "the only existing things are atoms and empty space."[1] In reality, however, an atom is composed of fundamental subunits, primarily protons, neutrons, and electrons. For nuclear medicine purposes, these three kinds of atomic particles may be considered to be arranged according to the modified Bohr Model of the atom,[1] represented schematically in Figure 12.1, in which a central atomic nucleus, composed of protons and neutrons, is surrounded by electrons moving at high velocity in fairly discrete orbits with different radii. The orbits of similar radius form bands or shells. These shells are labeled alphabetically, from inner to outer (in relation to the nucleus), as K,

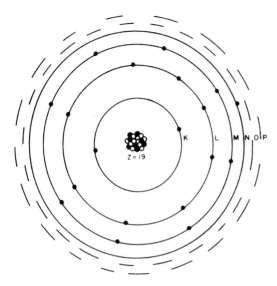

Fig. 12.1 Schematic diagram of the Bohr model of the atom for potassium (Z = 19). (Adapted from Hendee: Medical Radiation Physics, 2nd ed., 1979, by permission of Year Book Medical Publishers.)

L, M, and so on, and represent specific energy levels, containing restricted numbers of electrons, depending on the shell; e.g., the K shell contains no more than two electrons, the L shell no more than eight, and so on.

The nucleus of an atom contains the major mass of the atom. Each proton carries an electric charge of $1.6 \times 10^{-19}$ coulomb, defined as one unit of *positive* charge, and has a mass of $1.6724 \times 10^{-27}$ kg. Neutrons are uncharged particles with a mass of $1.6747 \times 10^{-27}$ kg. Each orbiting electron carries a charge equal but opposite to that of a proton and has a mass of $0.9108 \times 10^{-30}$ kg. For convenience, however, the mass of atomic particles is usually expressed in *atomic mass units* (amu), where one amu is defined as 1/12 the mass of the carbon atom (containing six protons, six neutrons, and six electrons); therefore, one amu is equal to $1.6605 \times 10^{-27}$ kg. The number of protons in a nucleus is called the *atomic number Z* and

determines the chemical identity of the atom and its relative position in the periodic table of elements. The number of neutrons in a nucleus is the *neutron number N.* The *mass number A* of a nucleus is the total number of *nucleons* (neutrons and protons). Thus $A = Z + N$. A summary of the above information is shown in Table 12.1.

## Nuclear Nomenclature

It is also important to define certain other standard nomenclature used to describe the status of an atomic nucleus, or *nuclide:*

1. *Isotopes* are atoms having the same number of protons, but a varying neutron content. For example, $^{12}_{6}C$, $^{14}_{6}C$, $^{11}_{6}C$ (and others) are isotopes of carbon. These are all the *same element* with the same chemical identity, because they all share the *same atomic (Z) number,* 6, noted above as a left subscript to the chemical symbol, C. The left superscript in each isotope above represents the *mass (A) number.* (The general form of these conventions is $^{A}_{Z}X$.) Therefore, one may determine the number of neutrons in each of the above examples by simply subtracting the subscript from the superscript (e.g., $12 - 6 = 6$), which is to say $N = A - Z$.

2. *Isotones* are atoms possessing the same *neutron* number but a different number of protons. Examples: $^{5}_{2}He$, $^{6}_{3}Li$, $^{9}_{6}C$. Here, $N = 5 - 2 = 3$, or $6 - 3 = 3$, and so on; in each case there are three neutrons.

3. *Isobars* have the same *mass (A) number,* but differing numbers of protons, e.g., $^{6}_{2}He$, $^{6}_{3}Li$, $^{6}_{4}Be$.

4. *Isomers* represent different *energy states* of nuclei of the *same A and Z number,* and may be distinguished by an asterisk after the chemical symbol of the "energetic" form (see further discussion below). For example, $^{12}_{6}C$ and $^{12}_{6}C^*$ are isomers.

Table 12.1.  **Summary of Atomic Particles**

| Atomic Particle | Location | Mass | Charge | Significant Number |
|---|---|---|---|---|
| Proton | Nucleus | 1.00727 amu | +1 | Z (atomic number) |
| Neutron | Nucleus | 1.00866 amu | 0 | N (neutron number) |
| Electron | Orbits | 0.00055 amu | −1 | |

### Nuclear Force and Binding Energy

Under certain unstable nuclear conditions (to be discussed further later), nucleons are capable of "transmutating" from one form to the other (i.e., from proton to neutron or visa versa), with the accompanying release of energy and of an appropriately charged particle. Also note that under "ordinary" circumstances, electrostatic repulsive forces exist between particles of similar charge. Hence, protons *repel* each other when separated by a distance greater than the diameter of the nucleus; but if the distance is *less* than the nuclear diameter, they remain together. This paradox has been explained by postulation of the existence of a *nuclear force,* which is stronger than electrostatic repulsive forces and binds the nucleons within the nucleus. Further, the mass of a nucleus is less than the sum of the masses of the separate nucleons, the mass difference being termed the *mass defect.* Einstein postulated a relationship between mass and energy, which he described by the classic formula $E = mc^2$, where E is the energy equivalent of a mass m, and c is a conversion factor equal to the speed of light *in vacuo* ($3 \times 10^8$ m/sec). The nuclear mass defect, therefore, is the mass-energy equivalent, which must be supplied to disintegrate the nucleus into its separate nucleons and is called the *binding energy of the nucleus.*

### Relationships Between the Nucleus and Orbiting Electrons

Another type of binding energy relates to the energy a nucleus exerts on its orbiting electrons. The concept is analogous to the differing forces exerted by the sun on each planet in our solar system (the farther away from the sun, the less the gravitational pull of the sun on the planet). Similarly, an electron in an inner shell of an atom is attracted or "bound" to the nucleus by a force greater than that which binds an electron in a more distant shell. Or conversely, the energy required to *remove* an electron from its shell and completely separate it from the atom, may be termed the binding energy ($E_B$) for the electron. The binding force exerted on an electron in a given shell (e.g., the K shell)

is greater from a larger nucleus with a larger positive charge, than from a smaller nucleus. Therefore, the binding energy for K-shell electrons (or those in any other shell) increases rapidly with increasing atomic (Z) number.

In the stable or "ground" state, electrons occupy the "highest" binding energy levels (or the lowest possible shells), since usually "nature likes to take the course of least resistance." On the surface, this may seem to be a contradictory statement, when one juxtaposes the phrases "highest binding energy level," and "lowest shell" or "least resistance." However, *binding energy* must be considered negative energy, in that energy must be "lost" into the system before an electron can be liberated. A K-shell electron requires *more input* (or *lost,* or *greater negative*) energy to be freed, than does an L-shell or an M-shell electron; while from the standpoint of the *nucleus,* the K-shell electrons are the most easily held, because they are closest to the influence of the nuclear positive charge. Consequently, if by some mechanism a "hole" is created in an electron shell of an atom having electrons in more distant shells as well, the vacancy will be promptly filled by an electron "cascade" from energy levels farther from the nucleus. As a result of this cascade phenomenon, energy is released, usually in the form of *electromagnetic radiation,* and most often as a *photon* or "packet of energy." If these packets of energy are not very "energetic," they fall on the scale of ultraviolet, visible, infrared, and so on. If they are more energetic ($>100$ eV), they are considered *X-rays.* (The symbol eV means *electron volt,* which is a unit of energy defined as the kinetic energy of an electron accelerated through a potential difference of one volt; 1 eV = $1.6 \times 10^{-19}$ joule; 1 keV = $10^3$ eV; 1 MeV = $10^6$ eV.) The electromagnetic spectrum is shown in Fig. 12.2. During the transition of a particular electron from one level to another—e.g., from L to K—the energy released equals the difference between the binding energies of the original and final energy levels of that electron. (That is, from L to K would yield an energy release = $E_{BK} - E_{BL}$.) This energy release is termed *characteristic radiation,* because specific photon energies are characteristic of differences in binding energies unique to

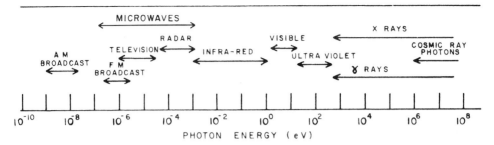

Fig. 12.2 The electromagnetic spectrum. (Ranges are approximate; no exact end points exist.) (Adapted from Hendee: Medical Radiation Physics, 2nd ed., 1979, by permission of Year Book Medical Publishers.)

the electrons of a specific atom. The radiation is also described as K-fluorescence, L-fluorescence, and so on, denoting the destination of the cascading electron. Occasionally the "cascade energy" may cause the ejection of an electron from the atom, usually from the same shell as the cascading electron. Such an ejected electron is called an *Auger electron,* and occurs more commonly from low Z-number atoms.

### Radionuclides: Excitation and Ionization

In order to change an atom from ground state to a state in which an electron cascade will occur, as described above, energy must first be imparted to an orbital electron (by mechanisms to be discussed later), so that it will move out of its "normal" shell. If sufficient energy is supplied only to cause the electron to move from a lower shell to an unoccupied site in a higher shell, the process is called *"excitation."* If the absorbed energy equals or exceeds the binding energy for that electron, so that it is completely removed from the atom, *"ionization"* is said to have occurred. This will be further mentioned in the discussion of radiation interactions to follow.

The majority of nuclei with atomic numbers above 82, and many with Z < 82, are unstable, either due to the arrangement of protons and neutrons, or to the neutron/proton (n/p) ratio. These unstable nuclides, or "radionuclides," eventually tend to seek a stable state by undergoing transitions such as nuclear fission (separation into two parts), or more frequently, by *radioactive decay,* in which the nucleus emits either electromagnetic radiation, charged particles, or both. Certain radionuclides occur natu-

rally; others may be produced artifically in nuclear reactors (by means of thermal neutron bombardment), or in high-energy accelerators such as cyclotrons (by means of positive-particle bombardment). Nuclides may also be raised to an "excited" state by energy absorption (analogous to that described above for electrons), or may "pass through" such an excited state during a series of decay transitions. These higher energy "excited" states are generally unstable, frequently very brief, and usually decay by emission of high-energy radiation. The proper term for such a radionuclide is *isomer,* as described above, because it has the same A and Z numbers as its stable-state form. These excited states are called "metastable states" if their half-lives exceed $10^{-6}$ seconds (see later discussion for definition of half-life), and may have individual durations of seconds, minutes, hours or in some cases, longer. A particular isomer of great importance to this discussion of nuclear cardiology is technetium–99m ($^{99m}$Tc, or Tc-99m). The letter "m" following the mass number indicates the metastable state, which is said to decay by "isomeric transition" (I.T.). Technetium–99m will be discussed more thoroughly in the section on radiopharmaceuticals.

### Modes of Radioactive Decay

The possible modes of radioactive decay include: alpha ($^4_2\alpha$); beta ($\beta^-$ or $_{-1}^0\beta$, also called negatron decay); gamma ($\gamma$); positron ($\beta^+$ or $_{+1}^0\beta$); electron capture (E.C.); and internal conversion (I.C.).

In order to determine which mode of decay has occurred in the case of a particular radionuclide, one must identify (a) the radiation emitted during decay and (b) the products remaining after decay. This is simplified by an awareness that in any "decay equation," the natural laws of conservation require the following:

1. The *sum of mass numbers* on one side of the equation must equal the sum of mass numbers on the other side.

2. *Total energy* at the beginning of the reaction must equal total energy at the end (including mass-energy equivalents, kinetic or motion energy, and electromagnetic energy).

3. *Total electric charge* must also remain constant during a radioactive process.

Each decay equation may be described diagramatically by a *decay scheme* (see subsequent examples) in which the *parent nuclide* is shown in relationship to all possible *daughter nuclides;* in cases where more than one decay path is possible, the percent of parent nuclei decaying by a particular path is shown as the *branching ratio* or *percent abundance for that path.* By convention, those decay paths that yield a *net loss* of *nuclear positive charge* (e.g., $\frac{4}{2}\alpha$-decay, $_{+1}^{0}\beta$-decay, E.C.), are shown as branching toward the *left.* Conversely, those paths that yield a *net gain* in *nuclear positive charge* (e.g., $_{-1}^{0}\beta$-decay) branch toward the *right.* When there is a net loss in *nuclear energy,* but *no change* in *nuclear charge* (e.g., as in $\gamma$-decay and I.C.), the energy transition is shown as a *vertical* branch, often represented as a "wavy" arrow in the case of $\gamma$-photons.

**Alpha Decay.** Alpha ($\alpha$) decay, or emission of a helium nucleus (two protons and two neutrons in a very stable configuration), was first described by Ernest Rutherford in 1899, and its particulate nature characterized in 1911 by Boltwood and Rutherford.[1] This type of transition occurs in radionuclides with a high Z number, and may be described by the general equation:

$$_Z^A X \longrightarrow {}_{(Z-2)}^{(A-4)}Y + {}_2^4He$$

Alpha decay releases nuclear energy as kinetic energy of the $\alpha$ particle, and each $\alpha$ particle from a specific nuclide is ejected with a *discrete energy.* The $\alpha$-decay scheme for $^{226}$Ra is shown in Figure 12.3.

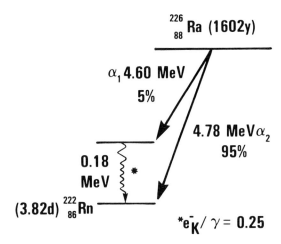

Fig. 12.3   Alpha decay scheme for $^{226}$Ra. (Radiologic Health Handbook, USPHS, revised edition, January, 1970.)

The information diagrammed in Figure 12.3 may be verbally interpreted as follows: $^{226}$Ra has a *half-life* of 1602 years, which means that it is radioactive and decays such that if we had n nuclei of $^{226}$Ra at time zero, it would take 1602 years for one-half of those nuclei to decay down to $^{222}$Rn, so that we would be left with ½n nuclei of $^{226}$Ra. $^{226}$Ra has two possible decay paths, with branching ratios of 5 percent and 95 percent as shown; 95 percent of the time the $^{226}$Ra nuclei decay by emitting only a single $\alpha$ particle with a kinetic energy of 4.78 MeV. The remaining 5 percent of the time, the nuclei decay emitting a 4.60 MeV $\alpha$ particle, with a "coincident" energy loss from the nucleus of 0.18 MeV, either as a $\gamma$-photon or as a conversion electron (e⁻), with a *coefficient of internal conversion* (see further description of I.C. later) of $e_K^-/\gamma = 0.25$. In this latter decay path, the "intermediary form" of $^{222}$Rn has a half-life too short to be considered metastable. $^{222}$Rn in turn, is radioactive, and decays with a half-life of 3.82 days (to $^{218}$Po, not shown). In all cases of decay of $^{226}$Ra, the *total transition or disintegration energy* is 4.78 MeV.

## Negatron Decay

Negatron decay (or negative beta, $_{-1}^{0}\beta$, decay), discovered by Henri Becquerel in 1896,[1] tends to occur in those radionuclides which have an n/p ratio that is too high for maximum nuclear stability. Thus, during this decay process, the n/p ratio is reduced by transmutation of a neutron to a proton, releasing an electron and energy. This transition may be expressed as:

$$_0^1n \longrightarrow _{+1}^1p + _{-1}^0\beta + \tilde{\nu}$$

Note that the negatron, $_{-1}^0\beta$, (which is really the same as an ordinary electron, but is denoted by $_{-1}^0\beta$ to indicate its *nuclear origin*) is considered to have essentially *no mass,* compared to the neutron and proton. However, as previously stated, the net mass-energy equivalents must be equal on both sides of the reaction. The fact that during these transitions, the *total disintegration energy* almost always exceeds the energy accounted for by the mass-energy equivalent of the negatron, the kinetic energy of the $_{-1}^0\beta$, and any photon energy released simultaneously, gave rise to the postulation in 1933 by Pauli, that a second "particle" must accompany the emission of a negatron. The energy unaccounted for in such transitions is possessed by this particle, called by Fermi an *antineutrino* (or $\tilde{\nu}$ above). This is an uncharged particle with vanishingly small mass, which interacts only rarely with matter, and the existence of which has been verified experimentally.[1] From the standpoint of the nucleus, negatron decay may be summarized as:

$$_Z^AX \longrightarrow _{Z+1}^AY + _{-1}^0\beta + \tilde{\nu}$$

Thus, there is an increase in Z number, but essentially no change in mass (A), so this may

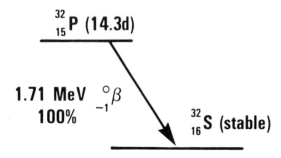

Fig. 12.4  Negatron decay scheme, $^{32}$P. (Radiologic Health Handbook, USPHS, revised edition, January, 1970.)

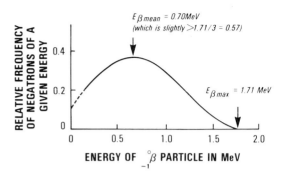

Fig. 12.5  Negatron energy spectrum from $^{32}$P. (Adapted from Hendee: Medical Radiation Physics, 2nd ed., 1979, by permission of Year Book Medical Publishers.)

properly be called an "isobaric transition." The negatron decay scheme for $^{32}$P is shown in Figure 12.4. It should be noted that the 100 percent in this decay scheme indicates the *branching ratio* (i.e., $^{32}$P only decays by $_{-1}^0\beta$ emission), and *not* the percent emitted $_{-1}^0\beta$'s having energy of 1.71 MeV. While negatrons emitted by a particular nuclide have *discrete maximum energies* ($E_\beta$max), most of the negatrons ejected during a particular transition have energies *less* than $E_\beta$max. As a result, each $_{-1}^0\beta$-decay path has a characteristic $E_\beta$max, a characteristic $_{-1}^0\beta$-*spectrum,* and a characteristic $E_\beta$*mean.* The $_{-1}^0\beta$-spectrum depicts the relative frequencies of negatrons emitted, with energies ranging from (a theoretical) zero to $E_\beta$max for that $_{-1}^0\beta$-decay path. The $E_\beta$mean for that path is usually the most commonly occurring negatron energy, and is approximately equal to $E_\beta$max/3. The negatron energy spectrum for the single $_{-1}^0\beta$-decay path of $^{32}$P is shown in Figure 12.5. It is apparent from the curve shown here that negatrons from $^{32}$P with energy $E_\beta$max, or 1.71 MeV, occur rarely, while those with $E_\beta$mean occur approaching 40 percent of the time.

## Positron Decay and Electron Capture

Emission of positively-charged "electrons," or positrons ($_{+1}^0\beta$), from radionuclides was first discovered by Anderson in 1932 in cosmic rays, and described in conjunction with artificial radioactivity in 1934 by Curie and Joliot.[1] Positron emitters have n/p ratios too low for maximum nuclear stability and, therefore, tend

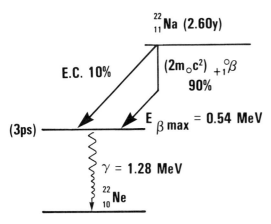

Fig. 12.6   Decay scheme for positron decay of $^{22}$Na. (Radiologic Health Handbook, revised edition, January, 1970.)

to increase the n/p ratio by means of the following nuclear change:

$$_{+1}^{1}\text{p} \longrightarrow {}_{0}^{1}\text{n} + {}_{+1}^{0}\beta + \nu$$

Again, the $_{+1}^{0}\beta$ indicates the positively charged nature and nuclear origin of the ejected positron; and the $\nu$ represents the accompanying *neutrino,* the postulated existence of which originates from the same line of reasoning as described above for the *antineutrino* in negatron decay. Also as with negatron decay, positrons are emitted with *characteristic energy spectra* and $E_\beta max$. The nuclear equation is summarized as,

$$_{Z}^{A}\text{X} \longrightarrow {}_{Z-1}^{A}\text{Y} + {}_{+1}^{0}\beta + \nu$$

where there is a decrease in Z and no change in A, again an isobaric transition. An example of positron decay is shown in Figure 12.6.

In Figure 12.6, the $2m_0c^2$, shown in parenthesis, with the positron decay pathway, represents the energy equivalent of the additional mass of the products of this type of decay, the neutron and positron, compared to the mass of the proton. This energy equivalent is 1.02 MeV, or $2m_0c^2$, where $m_0$ is the rest mass of an electron, 0.00055 amu, and c is the speed of light *in vacuo,* as noted earlier. From prior information and consideration of mechanical physics, the energy equivalent of 1 amu is calculated from:

$$1 \; amu = \frac{(1.66 \times 10^{-27}\text{kg/amu})(3 \times 10^8\text{m/sec})^2}{(1.6 \times 10^{-13}\text{ J/MeV})}$$
$$= 931 \; MeV$$

Thus:   $2\,(0.00055)\,(931) = 1.024 \; MeV$

Therefore, the transition energy of the nucleus must supply at least 1.02 MeV during positron decay. Radionuclides that do not produce this amount of transition energy, but still need to increase their n/p ratios for greater stability, decay by means of *electron capture* (E.C.), also shown in Figure 12.6. In this process, an electron is captured from orbit, usually from the K shell, which results in a nuclear transition summarized by:

$$_{+1}^{1}\text{p} + {}_{-1}^{0}\text{e} \longrightarrow {}_{0}^{1}\text{n} + \nu$$

Again, a neutrino is released, and the K shell vacancy is filled by electron cascade, releasing either X radiation or an Auger electron. If a particular radionuclide decays both by positron emission and by electron capture, in general, positron decay will occur more often than E.C., as illustrated by the branching ratios in Figure 12.6.

## Gamma Decay

When a radionuclide needs only undergo a loss of energy to become stable, without requiring a change in n/p ratio, an isomeric transition occurs, with release of *gamma* ($\gamma$) *radiation.* Gamma photons were described first in 1900 by Villard. It may be noted from Figure 12.2 that X and $\gamma$ radiation occupy the same general region in the electromagnetic spectrum. Indeed, they may be distinguished only by their different origins: $\gamma$ rays from nuclei, X-rays from electron orbits. Gamma decay may occur in conjunction with any of the above-described modes of radioactive decay and is illustrated in Figures 12.3 and 12.6. Gamma photons are discrete and characteristic of the particular nucleus of origin.

## Internal Conversion

On occasion, instead of releasing $\gamma$ photons, a nucleus undergoes *internal conversion* (I.C.), in which the excess nuclear energy interacts with an inner orbital electron, causing it to be ejected as a *conversion electron,* with a kinetic energy equal to the nuclear energy excess minus the binding energy of the electron. No $\gamma$ radiation is emitted, but subsequent electron cascade produces X-rays and/or Auger electrons. This type of decay is illustrated in Figure 12.3, and the *coefficient of internal conversion* (as noted above) is the ratio of the number of conversion electrons produced by a particular I.C. pathway to the number of $\gamma$ rays produced alternatively. Internal conversion tends to occur more often with increasing atomic number and with longer-lived excited nuclear states.

### Mathematics of Radioactive Decay

The rate of decay of a sample of radioactive material is referred to as the *activity* of the sample and is quantitated in curies, where one curie (Ci) is defined as follows:

$$1 \text{ Ci} = 3.7 \times 10^{10} \quad \text{disintegrations per second (dps)}$$
$$1 \text{ millicurie} = 1 \text{ mCi} = 3.7 \times 10^7 \text{ dps} = 10^{-3} \text{ Ci}$$
$$1 \text{ } \mu\text{Ci} = 10^{-6} \text{ Ci}$$
$$1 \text{ nCi} = 10^{-9} \text{ Ci}$$
$$\text{and } 1 \text{ pCi} = 10^{-12}\text{Ci}$$

(All of these subunits are defined according to standard metric terminology.) The original definition of the curie was the rate of decay of 1 g of radium, which was initially measured to be numerically as shown above. More recent determinations of this decay rate have established it as actually $3.61 \times 10^{10}$ dps; however, the classic numerical equivalent of the curie has been retained. A recently adopted new unit of radioactivity, which increasingly appears in the literature, is called the becquerel (Bq) and is defined as:

$$1 \text{ Bq} = 1 \text{ dps} = 2.7 \times 10^{-11} \text{ Ci}$$

Every radionuclide has a unique and characteristic fractional rate of decay over time, which has been established and defined as the *decay constant* for that radionuclide. The symbol for

a decay constant is a lambda ($\lambda$), which has units of inverse time ($sec^{-1}$, $min^{-1}$, and so on), and may be determined for a given radioactive sample from the following relationship:

$$A = \lambda N$$

where A is the activity (or radioactivity, as discussed above), which may be measured with various types of counting devices (see later); and N is the number of radioactive atoms in the sample. N may be calculated from the equation:

$$N = \frac{(\text{grams in sample}) (\text{atoms/g-atomic mass})}{(\text{grams/g-atomic mass})}$$
$$= \frac{(\text{grams in sample}) (6.02 \times 10^{25})}{(\text{atomic mass number})}$$

where $6.02 \times 10^{25}$ is Avogadro's number, and by definition one gram-atomic mass of a nuclide is equal to the mass number in grams. The relationship, $A = \lambda N$, indicates that the number of atoms (A) of a particular radionuclide, which will disintegrate in a given time interval, is dependent on the total number of atoms (N) in the sample and, therefore, $\lambda$ is a probability factor defining the likelihood that a single radioatom will decay per given unit of time. From this relationship, it may be shown that:

$$N_{t_1} = N_{t_0} e^{-\lambda t_1}$$

where $N_{t_0}$ is the number of atoms originally present in a sample at time zero ($t_0$), $t_1$ is a given elapsed time, $N_{t_1}$ is the number of atoms left in the sample after time $t_1$ has elapsed, and e is the exponential quantity 2.7183, which is the base of the natural (or Napierian) logarithm system.* It should be carefully noted that $t_1$ in this equation must be expressed in the same units of time as the inverse time units of $\lambda$ for the given radionuclide, so that appropriate unit "cancellations" may occur during these calculations. Therefore, for example, if $\lambda$ is given as

---

* Natural logs, denoted by "ln," are expressed in the form $\ln X = y$, such that $e^y = X$, and are related to common logs to base 10 by the equation $\ln X = 2.3026 \log X$.

Table 12.2.  Decay Characteristics of Some Radionuclides used in Nuclear Cardiology Studies *

| Radionuclide | Physical $T_{1/2}$ | Decay Mode † | Principal Useful Photons (Abundance) |
|---|---|---|---|
| $^{99m}$Tc | 6.0  hr | I.T. | 140 KeV (90%) |
| $^{201}$Tl | 73.0  hr | E.C. | 69–83 KeV (93%; $^{200}$Hg X-rays) |
| $^{133}$Xe | 5.3  d | $\beta^-$ | 81 KeV (35%) |
| $^{43}$K | 22.2  hr | $\beta^-$ | 373 KeV (85%) |
| $^{81}$Rb | 4.58 hr | $\beta^+$, E.C. | 511 KeV ‡ (2 photons, 33%) (daughter $^{81m}$Kr, 13 sec., 190 KeV$\gamma$,§ 65%) |
| $^{82}$Rb | 1.25 min | $\beta^+$, E.C. | 511 KeV (2 photons, 81%) |
| $^{13}$N | 10.0  min | $\beta^+$ | 511 KeV (2 photons, 100%) |
| $^{11}$C | 20.5  min | $\beta^+$ | 511 KeV (2 photons, 100%) |
| $^{15}$O | 2.0  min | $\beta^+$ | 511 KeV (2 photons, 100%) |

* Adapted from Budinger and Rollo: Principles of Cardiovascular Nuclear Medicine, 1978, by permission of Grune and Stratton, Inc.
† E.C. = electron capture; I.T. = isomeric transition; $\beta^+$ = positron decay; $\beta^-$ = negatron decay
‡ 511 KeV, 2 photons → emitted as result of $\beta^+$ annihilation after $\beta^+$ decay (see discussion of annihilation under interactions of radiation with matter).
§ $\gamma$ = gamma photon emitted during I.T.

hours $^{-1}$, then $t_1$ must also be expressed in hours of elapsed time. The more standard form of the above equation is:

$$N = N_0\, e^{-\lambda t}$$

and may also be stated as:

$$\boxed{A = A_0\, e^{-\lambda t}}$$

where $A_0$ and $A$ are initial and final activity. These relationships are referred to as the *exponential decay equations* and are fundamental to any work requiring the use of radionuclides. A further important term, introduced earlier, is the concept of half-life, or $T_{1/2}$. The *physical half-life* of a particular radionuclide is also unique, like its $\lambda$, and is defined simply as the time required for one-half of the atoms of a sample of that nuclide to decay away. The physical $T_{1/2}$ of a nuclide may be determined as follows:

$$N = \tfrac{1}{2}\, N_0 \text{ when } t = T_{1/2}$$

Therefore, by substitution:

$$\tfrac{1}{2}\, N_0 = N_0\, e^{-\lambda T_{1/2}}$$

$$\text{or} \quad (\tfrac{1}{2})\left(\frac{N_0}{N_0}\right) = e^{-\lambda T_{1/2}}$$

$$2 = e^{\lambda T_{1/2}}$$

$$\text{or} \quad \ln 2 = \lambda T_{1/2}$$

Since $\ln 2 = 0.693$, the very important resulting equation may be written:

$$\boxed{T_{1/2} = \frac{0.693}{\lambda}}$$

Both $\lambda$ and the physical $T_{1/2}$ of the above equation are well-established values for all known radioisotopes. Those radioisotopes employed in nuclear cardiology are shown, in part, in Table 12.2, along with their principal modes of decay, and their principal useful photons and relative abundances. The methodology of incorporating the more commonly used of these radionuclides into the substances utilized for the imaging procedures that constitute most of nuclear cardiology, will be discussed in the subsequent section on radiopharmaceuticals.

It seems appropriate to introduce the concept of *effective half-life* at this point. The actual

$T_{1/2}$-*elimination* of a radioactive substance from the body depends not only on the physical decay of the radionuclide, but also on the biologic elimination of the substance from the body by various potential excretory routes. Therefore, the effective half-life, or $T_{1/2\,eff}$, relates to $T_{1/2\,phys}$ and $T_{1/2\,biol}$ as follows:

$$\frac{1}{T_{1/2\,eff}} = \frac{1}{T_{1/2\,phys}} + \frac{1}{T_{1/2\,biol}}$$

The biologic $T_{1/2}$ is determined by the nature of the particular "pharmaceutical" to which the radionuclide is attached, which will be further discussed under radiopharmaceuticals. The significance of the $T_{1/2\,eff}$ will become apparent in the subsequent discussion of radiation safety and dosimetry.

## Radiation Interaction with Matter

### Particulate Radiation Interactions

In order to discuss the basic principles of nuclear medicine instrumentation, radiation safety, and dosimetry, we must introduce certain concepts concerning the kinds of interactions with matter which are possible for the emitted radiation produced during the above-described decay processes. The two major categories of radiation are *particulate* and *nonparticulate* or *photon* radiation. Of the types of radiation discussed earlier, $\alpha$-particles, positrons, and negatrons are all particulate; $\gamma$ and X radiation are photons, or nonparticulate radiation.

Heavy-charged particles, such as $\alpha$ particles (and also protons, deuterons, and so on), lose kinetic energy rapidly as they penetrate matter. The energy-transfer to the absorbing medium is accomplished primarily by interaction of electric fields, and "physical contact" of particles is not necessary. The energy imparted to the absorber may produce *excitation* of electrons, or ejection of *primary electrons* from orbits, which is *ionization*. The primary electrons may in turn cause the ejection of *secondary electrons*. The excited (nonejected) electrons will in turn release their energy as *characteristic* or *X-radia-*

*tion* (see earlier discussion also). An ejected electron and its residual positive ion are termed an *ion pair; in air,* an average energy of 33.7 eV must be expended by a charged particle for each ion pair produced, and on the average, *excitation* occurs 2.2 times per single *ionization*. The *specific ionization* (SI) is the total number of primary and secondary ion pairs produced per unit length of path of the particle in the absorbing medium. The *linear energy transfer* (LET) of a particle is the average loss of energy per unit path length, calculated by:

$$LET = (SI)(W)$$
(where $W$ = the energy expended per ion pair produced in the particular absorbing medium; e.g., W = 33.7 eV for $\alpha$ particles in air)

The *range* of an ionizing particle in an absorbing medium is the straight line distance it travels prior to stopping completely, and is defined in terms of initial energy, E, of the particle, and its LET:

$$Range = E/LET$$

LET is directly related to the density of the absorbing medium (i.e., the denser the medium, the more possible interactions can occur per unit path length and, therefore, the higher the SI, while W for a given medium remains essentially constant). However, *range* is *inversely* related to LET. Thus, it follows that the denser the medium, the shorter the range of a particle with a given energy. So that if we combine the above two equations:

$$Range = (E)/(LET)$$
$$and\ LET = (SI)(W)$$
$$therefore\ Range = (E)/(SI)(W)$$
$$or\ SI = (E)/(Range)(W)$$

it becomes apparent that a high energy particle, expending its energy over a short range in a relatively dense material (such as soft tissue) can produce a great deal of ionization and damage. The range of $\alpha$ particles of a few MeV or less is only a few microns in soft tissue. Therefore, this form of radiation is virtually useless in nuclear imaging but would be of potentially great harm, and so is of no further interest in this discussion.

Negatrons and positrons, impinging on an absorbing medium, may interact with either the orbiting electrons or the nuclei of the medium. If the kinetic energy of the incident particle ($E_k$) is relatively low (approximately 0 to 10 MeV), it is most likely to interact with orbiting electrons of the medium; and the probability of these "electron-electron" interactions increases proportionally with the Z number of the absorber. Such an interaction may produce one of two effects on the orbiting electron: (1) excitation or (2) ionization. In either case, the impinging electron consequently loses energy and is deflected or *scattered* at some angle with respect to its original path. Excitation is, as usual, followed by characteristic X-ray emission. When ionization occurs, the ejected orbital electron has imparted to it a certain total energy, which is divided between the binding energy necessary to cause ejection, and the remaining energy, which becomes the kinetic energy of the ejected electron. Subsequently, secondary electrons may also be ejected, as described under $\alpha$-particle interactions. The most significant differences between the interactions of these lower energy electrons compared to the lower energy $\alpha$ particles discussed above are apparent when we consider the relative specific ionizations (SI) and LETs of the two types of particles. For example, in air, with W-quantity of 33.7 eV required per ion pair produced, note the following:

For a negatron or positron of energy in the range of 0.1 MeV, the SI may be estimated by the equation:

$$\boxed{SI = \frac{45}{(v/c)^2}}$$

where $v$ = velocity of the incident electron and $c$ = speed of light *in vacuo*

In this case, SI = 150 ion pairs/cm, for the electron. For $\alpha$ particles, the SI in air averages 30,000 to 70,000 IP/cm. Therefore, from the formula for LET:

For the *electron* of about 0.1 MeV:

$$LET = (SI)(W)$$
$$= (150)(33.7)$$
$$= 5.06 \ KeV/cm$$

For an $\alpha$ *particle* of about 0.1 MeV (assuming SI = 30,000):

LET = (30,000)(33.7) = *1,011 KeV/cm* (or about three orders of magnitude greater than for the electron).

When a *positron* has expended its kinetic energy, it combines with an electron of the absorbing medium, and pair *annihilation* occurs, with their mass-energy equivalents being released as two 511 KeV photons emitted in opposite directions. It is this annihilation radiation from positron-emitting radionuclides that is utilized in the positron tomographic imaging devices currently being developed and refined.

When the kinetic energy of an impinging negatron or positron is higher (usually > 10 MeV), the particle is more likely to interact with the nuclei of the absorbing medium. The probability of such an "electron-nuclear" interaction is approximately proportional to $Z^2$ of the absorber. The impinging electron may be simply deflected with *reduced energy* away from the nucleus, called *elastic scattering,* which occurs with a probability approximately proportional to $1/E_k^2$, where $E_k$ is the original kinetic energy of the incident electron). Or the incident particle may interact via *inelastic scattering,* in which case the impinging electron is deflected with *reduced* velocity and the consequent release of electromagnetic radiation called *bremsstrahlung* (German for "braking" radiation). A *bremsstrahlung* photon may possess varying energies, up to the entire kinetic energy of the incident particle, and is predominantly emitted at right angles to the initial path of the electron. The angle of the bremsstrahlung photon narrows as the kinetic energy of the incident electron increases, and, similarly, the energy of the emitted photon approaches a higher maximum energy. Thus, bremsstrahlung emissions for a given fixed energy of incident electrons become a spectrum, as shown in Figure 12.7. The probability of bremsstrahlung

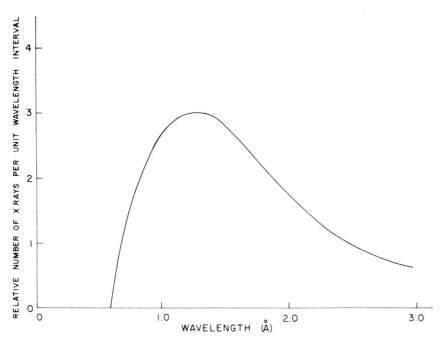

Fig. 12.7 Bremsstrahlung spectrum for a molybdenum target bombarded by electrons accelerated through 20 kV. (Hendee: Medical Radiation Physics, 2nd ed., 1979, by permission of Year Book Medical Publishers.)

production increases with $Z^2$ of the absorbing medium. The X-rays emitted by an X-ray tube, used for diagnostic radiology, are primarily the result of "boiling" electrons off a tungsten filament by means of an electric current in the filament, accelerating those electrons through a potential difference until they reach an optimum energy, and causing those accelerated electrons to "bombard" a tungsten target to produce the bremsstrahlung (or X-ray) photons, which are then allowed to exit the tube through a shielded narrow "window"; thus, the X-ray beam for production of X-ray images. High-energy electrons, moving through a medium at a velocity exceeding the speed of light in the medium, also lose a small fraction of their kinetic energy as visible light, called *Cherenkov radiation.*

## Nonparticulate Radiation Interactions

There are five major categories of interaction, which may occur between a gamma- or X-ray photon, and the medium through which it passes upon being emitted from a radionuclide:

coherent scattering, photoelectric absorption, Compton (incoherent) scattering, pair production, and photodisintegration. Of these potential interactions, photoelectric absorption, Compton scattering, and pair production are of greatest significance in nuclear medicine. *Coherent* or *classical scattering* occurs with photons of energies up to 150 to 200 KeV in high Z-number media, but in tissue occurs only with low-energy photons. This interaction is best described based on principles of classic physics, in which the incident photon interacts with an atom of the absorber by being deflected, with neligible energy loss, in a direction nearly back toward its origin. Coherent scattering is important only in that it may degrade the resolution of nuclear medicine images obtained from low-energy γ-emitters. *Photodisintegration,* at the other extreme, occurs when photons of very high energy interact with nuclei; this process becomes important primarily when considering shielding requirements for high-energy photon beams. Therefore, this subsequent discussion will be confined to the remaining three types of nonparticulate interactions with matter.

During *photoelectric absorption,* the total energy of the incident X- or γ-photon is transferred to an electron of an atom of the absorbing medium, which results in ejection of that electron from the atom with a kinetic energy equal to the original photon energy minus the binding energy of the ejected electron. Most photons interact preferentially with electrons having binding energies nearest to the energy of the incident photon. After such an interaction occurs, the resultant shell vacancy is filled by the usual electron cascade, with emission of characteristic radiation and/or Auger electrons, as previously discussed. Thus, if a monoenergetic beam of photons of known energy is aimed at a thin foil of a particular element, and the transmission of that beam of photons is measured while varying the beam energy by known amounts, the transmission of that beam through the foil (or conversely, the absorption of the beam) will change dramatically whenever the beam energy closely approximates the binding energy of a particular electron in a particular shell of that element; also, the characteristic radiation of that electron shell will be released. These dramatic changes are termed *absorption edges,* and may be used to characterize the energy configurations of the electron orbits of a particular element. We take advantage of the knowledge of specific absorption edges routinely in *radiology* by the use of iodine and barium as contrast media, having K-edges of 33 and 37 KeV, respectively, which allow a significant number of X-ray photons in the diagnostic range of 33 to 88 KeV to be absorbed, thus producing opacification on the radiograph of structures filled with such media. Also, since photoelectric interactions in soft tissue usually occur at photon energies *less* than 0.5 KeV, radionuclide emissions ordinarily used in nuclear medicine imaging (with photopeaks of 80 KeV or greater) stand a far better chance of having sufficient numbers of photons escape the soft tissue barrier to interact with the imaging detector (without being absorbed photoelectrically by the soft tissues). The electron ejected in a photoelectric interaction is called the *photoelectron,* and is ejected at a right angle to the incident photon for low-energy photons, and at increasingly narrower angles with increasing photon energy. The probability of photoelectric absorption *decreases* as photon energy increases, and *increases* as Z of the absorber increases. (Note that the effective Z-number of soft tissue is about 7.45.) Therefore:

$$\text{probability of photoelectric event} \propto \frac{Z^3}{(h\nu)^3}$$

where *hν* is the energy of the incident photon, and Z is the atomic number of the absorber. Photoelectrons may undergo secondary interactions of their own with the absorbing medium—the characteristic photons and Auger electrons usually have energies less than 0.5 KeV, and are absorbed rapidly by the immediate surrounding medium.

Emitted X- or γ-photons of energy between 30 KeV and 30 MeV interact in soft tissue primarily by *Compton scattering.* Compton interactions are *nearly independent of the Z number* of the absorbing medium, but are more directly related to its *electron density* (electrons per gram), because these interactions occur predominantly with loosely-bound electrons. Therefore, radiographs produced with high-energy photons show very poor contrast due to poor differential absorption in the different body tissues. Compton scatter also contributes very significantly to degradation of nuclear medicine images, as will become apparent in the following discussion. The incident photon in a Compton interaction impinges on a loosely bound electron (whose binding energy is assumed to be negligible); the electron is ejected at an angle θ, as a *Compton electron* with kinetic energy equal to the energy lost by the incident photon; the incident photon is also deflected, at an angle φ, with a residual energy equal to the initial energy minus the kinetic energy of the Compton electron. The deflected photon is termed the *Compton photon.* Both angles φ and θ tend to decrease with increasing energy of the incident photon; but while φ may assume *any* angular value from 0° to 180°, with respect to the incident photon path, the angle θ must be 90° or less, relative to the incident photon path. This latter fact is illustrated in Figure 12.8. Two

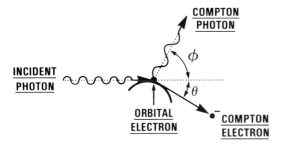

Fig. 12.8 Compton interaction of a "medium energy" X- or $\gamma$-photon with a loosely bound orbital electron. Note that $\phi$ may be any angle from 0°–180°, depending on the incident photon energy and *need not* be equal to $\theta$, which must be between 0°–90°.

additional relationships pertain in Compton scattering:

(1) $\quad\quad \Delta\lambda = 0.0243\,(1 - \cos\,\phi)$
and (2) $\quad\quad \lambda' = \lambda + \Delta\lambda$

where $\lambda$ is the wavelength in angstroms (Å) of the incident photon, $\lambda'$ is the wavelength (Å) of the Compton photon, and $\phi$ is the angle between the incident and Compton photons. Also it may be shown mathematically that:

(3) $\quad h\nu'\,(\text{KeV}) = \dfrac{12.4}{\lambda'\,(\text{Å})}$, or $h\nu = \dfrac{12.4}{\lambda}$

where $h\nu'$ is the energy of the scattered photon in KeV, $h\nu$ is the energy of the incident photon, while $\lambda$ and $\lambda'$ are the wavelengths in Å of the incident and scattered photons, respectively. In the case of a relatively high energy incident photon, $\lambda$ may be neglected compared to $\Delta\lambda$ and $\lambda'$ (since wavelength is inversely related to photon energy), so that,

$$\lambda' = \lambda + \Delta\lambda$$
becomes $\quad\quad \lambda' \approx \Delta\lambda$

Thus, for such a photon scattered at $\phi = 180°$,

$$\lambda' = \Delta\lambda = 0.0243\,[1 - \cos\,(180°)]$$
$$= 0.0243\,[1 - (-1)]$$
$$= 0.0486\ \text{Å}$$
and $\quad h\nu' = 12.4/\lambda' = 12.4/0.0486 = 255$ KeV

Therefore, for $\phi = 180°$, $h\nu' = 255$ KeV at maximum, no matter how much we may theoretically increase the energy of the incident photon. Similar calculations may be performed to show that maximum $h\nu'$ for a photon scattered at 90° is 511 KeV. Conversely, for incident photons of relatively low energy, such as the 80 KeV photon of $^{201}$Tl if we assume only a 10 percent energy loss in Compton scatter (or $80 - 8 = 72$ KeV):

$$h\nu' = \frac{12.4}{\lambda'}$$

therefore $\quad 72\ \text{KeV} = \dfrac{12.4}{\lambda'\,(\text{Å})}$

$$\lambda' = \frac{12.4}{72} = 0.172\ \mathring{A}$$

and $\quad\quad h\nu = \dfrac{12.4}{\lambda}$

$$80\ \text{KeV} = \frac{12.4}{\lambda\,(\mathring{A})}$$

$$\lambda = \frac{12.4}{80} = 0.155\ \mathring{A}$$
$$\Delta\lambda = \lambda' - \lambda = 0.172 - 0.155 = 0.017\ \mathring{A}$$
$$0.017 = 0.243\,[1 - \cos\,\phi]$$
$$1 - \cos\,\phi = (0.017/0.0243)$$
$$-\cos\,\phi = -1 + (0.017/0.0243)$$
$$\cos\,\phi = 1 - (0.017/0.0243)$$
$$= 1 - 0.6996$$
$$\cos\,\phi = 0.3004$$
$$\phi = 73°\ \text{(angle of Compton}$$
$$\text{photon)}$$

Whereas, for a slightly more energetic photon such as $^{99m}$Tc, a 10 percent energy loss (140 Kev $-$ 14 $= 126$ KeV), $\Delta\lambda = 0.0099$ Å, cos $\phi = 0.5926$, and $\phi = 54°$ (Compton photon scatter angle). In a Compton interaction in which the incident photon may lose only 1 percent of its initial energy, these differences in the scatter angle of the Compton photons become even more significant for the low-energy photon emitters. It is apparent, therefore, that lower-energy photons, which lose relatively little energy in Compton interactions, are scattered at a much larger angle than higher energy photons, even for the same relative energy loss. This becomes extremely important in the clinical setting, where scattered photons degrade image quality, and the primary process of eliminating scatter is by energy discrimination (as will be discussed further in the section on radiation detection). Therefore, energy selection for low-energy photon emitters must be rather more precise than for higher-energy radionuclides, to achieve the same image quality relative to scatter radiation.

The third major type of interaction of photons with matter is known as *pair production* and may occur only when the incident photon has at least the mass/energy equivalent of two electrons. As the photon (of at least 1.02 MeV) enters the vicinity of a nucleus of the absorber, the photon is transformed into a negatron and a positron, each having as *kinetic* energy one-half the energy *in excess* of the 1.02 MeV, which was possessed by the incident photon. Both particles then expend their kinetic energy in excitation and/or ionization in the absorber, until the negatron comes to rest, and the positron annihilates with a "nearby" electron, with the typical release of two 511 KeV photons in opposite directions, just as in positron decay. The variables influencing the occurrence of the three major modes of interaction of nonparticulate radiation with matter are summarized in Table 12.3; the relationship of these three interactions to photon energy and Z number is illustrated in Figure 12.9.

The final important considerations regarding interactions of nonparticulate radiation in any medium are: (1) the mathematics of *attenuation* (defined as the decrement in the amount of radiation emerging from a medium, compared to the incident radiation, which is produced by one or more of the types of absorption or scatter described above); and (2) the definitions of *attenuation coefficient* (in general), and of *half-value layer*. In a manner similar to radioactive

decay, the number of photons passing through the medium may be expressed by the equation:

$$A = \mu N$$

where A is the attenuation or rate of removal of photons from an incident beam with N photons initially, while traversing and interacting with an absorbing medium; and $\mu$ is the coefficient of attenuation for the particular medium and photon beam of interest. It should be emphasized that $\mu$ is unique and specific to the type of medium *and* to the energy of the photons in the beam (analogous to the uniqueness of $\lambda$, the disintegration constant for each radionuclide, as discussed earlier). If the photon beam is monoenergetic, and is narrow and contains no scatter photons (i.e., attenuation occurring under conditions of good geometry), then the following equations pertain:

$$N = N_0 e^{-\mu X}$$

where N is the number of photons *penetrating* (or emerging from) the absorbing medium; $N_0$ is the original number of photons in the beam as it enters the medium; X is the thickness of the absorbing medium, in units of inches or centimeters, etc.; and $\mu$ is the attenuation coefficient for the beam in this medium, which implies that $\mu$ has units of in$^{-1}$, or cm$^{-1}$, and so on. Therefore, $\mu$ in this instance is defined as the *linear attenuation coefficient*. In general, $\mu$ varies with the energy of the incident X- or $\gamma$-ray beam, the atomic number of the absorber, and the density of the absorber. (In point of fact, there are also mass ($\mu_m$), atomic ($\mu_a$), and electronic ($\mu_e$) attenuation coefficients for each beam-absorber combination, the use of which require certain alterations in the above equa-

**Table 12.3. Variables that Influence the Principle Modes of Interaction of X and $\gamma$ Rays**

| Mode of Interaction | Dependence of Linear Attenuation Coefficient on: | | | |
| | Photon Energy hv | Atomic Number Z | Electron Density $\rho_e$ | Physical Density $\rho$ |
|---|---|---|---|---|
| Photoelectric | $1/(h\nu)^3$ | $Z^3$ | — | $\rho$ |
| Compton | $1/h\nu$ | — | $\rho_e$ | $\rho$ |
| Pair Production | $h\nu$ (above 1.02 MeV) | Z | — | $\rho$ |

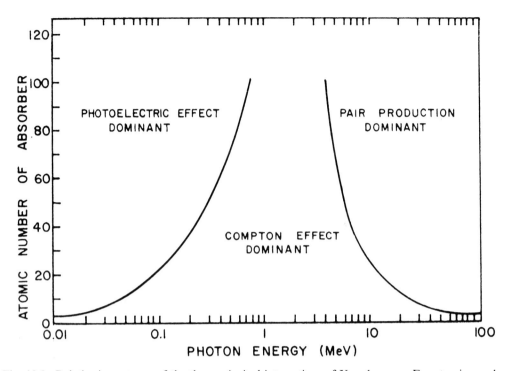

Fig. 12.9 Relative importance of the three principal interactions of X and γ rays. For atomic numbers and photon energies falling *on* the curves shown, the probability of occurrence of either of the two adjacent types of interactions is equal. (Hendee: Medical Radiation Physics, 2nd ed., 1979, by permission of Year Book Medical Publishers.)

tion, but which need not be further mentioned in this discussion.) The similarity between the above *attenuation equation* and the previously discussed *decay equation* is obvious. And logically, just as the *half-life* of a radionuclide may be defined in terms of λ, so we may define *half-value layer* in terms of μ as,

$$HVL = \frac{\ln 2}{\mu}$$

or                $HVL = 0.693/\mu$

where HVL, or half-value layer, is the thickness of a particular material required to reduce the intensity (or number of photons) of an X- or γ-ray beam to one half the initial or incident number of photons. The HVL of a beam describes its "quality" or penetrating ability. If we plot the relationships expressed in the attenuation equation, in terms of percent of photons transmitted versus thickness of the absorbing medium (for soft tissue and certain diagnostic-

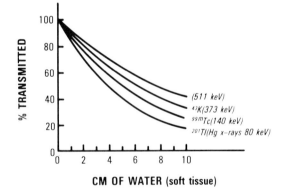

Fig. 12.10 Percent transmission of photons plotted as a function of tissue thickness through which the photons pass. Note that the half-value thickness of soft tissue (e.g., muscle) for ⁹⁹ᵐTc photons is about 4.6 cm and for ²⁰¹Tl photons is about 3.8 cm. Therefore, 50 percent of the photons emitted from ⁹⁹ᵐTc or ²⁰¹Tl localized in the heart would be attenuated by less than 2 inches of overlying soft tissue. Attenuation decreases with increasing photon energies. (Adapted from Budinger and Rollo: Principles of Cardiovascular Nuclear Medicine, 1978, by permission of Grune and Stratton.)

range photons), the resulting graph would appear as shown in Fig. 12.10. From this graph, we see that the HVL of soft tissue for ²⁰¹Tl is only about 3.8 cm and for ⁹⁹ᵐTc about 4.6 cm. The clinical importance of these values will be evident after we have discussed the constraints of radiation safety and dosimetry, and the requirements of radiation detection, counting statistics, and imaging instrumentation.

## RADIATION DETECTION AND COUNTING STATISTICS

Inasmuch as the process of nuclear medicine imaging is based on one type of radiation detection, it seems useful to briefly discuss the principles of detecting and counting radioactivity. The most common detection systems are based on the physical interaction of radiation with matter and are classified in one of the three following ways: (1) by the medium in which the interaction occurs, e.g., liquid, solid or gas detectors; (2) by the nature of the phenomenon produced, i.e., excitation or ionization; or (3) by the type of electronic pulse generated, i.e., amplitude that is constant, or proportional to the energy delivered in the interaction.[6] Of the above types of detectors, gas-filled ionization chambers are common in nuclear medicine and have important uses, such as for personnel dosimetry, dose calibrators, laboratory monitors, proportional counters for measuring charged particles, and Geiger-Müller tubes for measuring ambient radiation. All gas-filled detectors operate on the same principle: the ability of ionized gas within an electrically-charged enclosure to alter the voltage potential between two electrodes. Ionizing radiation entering the detector chamber produces negative and positive ion pairs, which are collected by the electrodes of the chamber, based on the direction of the electric field. A capacitor in the circuit between the two electrodes undergoes a change in charge proportional to the number of ions collected. The pulse height thus produced is shown as a function of the voltage applied across the electrodes, for α and β particles, in Figure 12.11. In the recombination region of these curves, the electric field is too weak to attract many ion pairs before they can reform into neutral

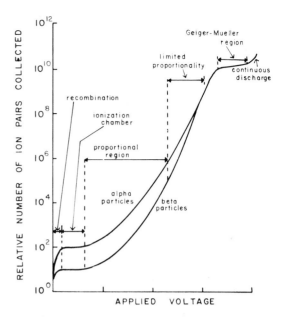

Fig. 12.11 Relationship of pulse height (or total number of ion pairs collected by the electrodes) in a gas-filled detector, to the high voltage between the electrodes. (Hendee: Medical Radiation Physics, 2nd ed., 1979, by permission of Year Book Medical Publishers.)

atoms. As the voltage increases, the fraction of ion pairs collected, and thus charge, increases. With further increases in voltage, all ion pairs produced are collected with no recombination. In this ionization plateau, the capacitor charge or pulse height remains relatively constant over a range of applied voltages. The saturation voltage is the charge necessary for operation in this region. As voltage is increased beyond saturation, the charge collected is increased by gas amplification, due to secondary ionization from the primary ions, which may even become an avalanche with tertiary ions, and so forth. The pulse height in this range depends on the initial energy of the ionizing radiation, and therefore, is called the proportional region. At the upper end of this region, the two curves come together, such that the pulse height becomes more dependent on the voltage applied than on the energy of the initial ionizing event. This is the range of limited proportionality. In the Geiger-Müller region, the pulse height becomes entirely independent of the energy of the original event, and a plateau is again reached. Above this region, *continuous* discharge occurs within the chamber.

The most useful of these curve regions are the *proportional* and *Geiger-Müller* ranges. Geiger-Müller tubes are highly sensitive for measuring all types of radiation, including weak X-rays and are, therefore, useful in low-level radiation surveying, such as is encountered in the majority of nuclear medicine usage. However, due to the independence of radiation energy and pulse height in these tubes, discrimination of one type of radiation from another is not possible.

## Scintillation Detectors

Compared to gas-filled detectors, scintillation detectors have two advantages that make them highly useful in nuclear medicine: (1) they are capable of much higher counting rates, and (2) they are much more efficient for γ-ray detection

(while maintaining pulse-height proportionality). The basic components of a solid scintillation detector system, with a thallium-activated NaI(Tl) crystal, are shown in Figure 12.12; this type of detector is the basis of the design for the Anger-type gamma camera used most commonly for nuclear medicine imaging. As gamma photons enter the crystal, they are absorbed by the three processes of photoelectric and Compton interactions and pair production, in proportion to the energy of the incident photon, as shown in Figure 12.13. It may be seen from this figure that most of the interactions of useful tracer photon energies involve photoelectric or Compton attenuations, due to the density of NaI(Tl), 3.67 g/cc, and the Z-number of iodide, which = 53. As the incident photon strikes the crystal, its energy is imparted to the electrons of the atoms of the crystal lattice. The excited electrons then give off light photons, or *scintillations,* as they return to ground state. The Tl

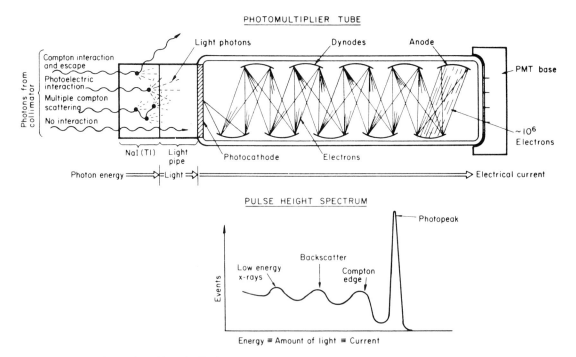

Fig. 12.12  The basic solid scintillation detector consisting of a NaI(Tl) crystal optically coupled to a photomultiplier tube. Photons absorbed in the crystal produce scintillations, the light intensity being proportional to the amount of energy absorbed. Light photons from the crystal striking the photocathode of the photomultiplier tube liberate photoelectrons which are multiplied many times by cascading through the series of metal grids (dynodes) shown. The pulse height spectrum shows the distribution of photon energies arriving at the detector. (Budinger and Rollo: Principles of Cardiovascular Nuclear Medicine, 1978, by permission of Grune and Stratton.)

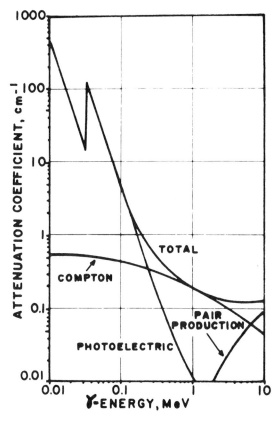

Fig. 12.13 Attenuation coefficients as a function of photon energy in NaI. (Rocha and Harbert: Textbook of Nuclear Medicine: Basic Science, 1978, by permission of Lea and Febiger.)

tillation crystal are detected by a photomultiplier (p.m.) tube (Fig. 12.12), or in the case of a gamma camera, many p.m. tubes arranged evenly across the crystal surface, as seen in Figure 12.14*B*. Because NaI crystals are hygroscopic and become discolored when they absorb moisture (which in turn causes more *internal* light absorption and less light emission), the

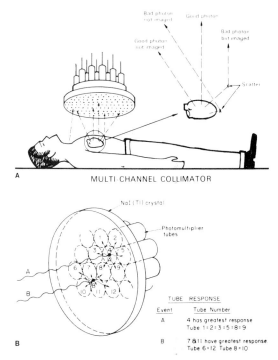

Fig. 12.14 The principle of the Anger-type gamma camera: *(A)* The relationships of the organ to be imaged to the face of the camera collimator, which acts as a multihole "lens." Only photons emitted in a direction parallel to the holes of the collimator will be allowed to reach the face of the camera crystal. Between the holes are lead septa which attenuate (or stop) the scattered photons entering at an unacceptable angle. Some "good photons" will also be attenuated, if they strike the face of the septa; conversely, some lower energy "bad" photons, if they are parallel to the holes, will be allowed to enter the crystal, but most of these should be screened out via pulse height analysis (see later text). *(B)* The position of the "good" photons (or "good" scintillation events) is deduced by the amount of light detected by the photomultiplier tubes relative to one another, as they are distributed over the surface of the camera crystal. (Adapted from Budinger and Rollo: Principles of Cardiovascular Nuclear Medicine, 1978, by permission of Grune and Stratton.)

impurities in the crystal greatly speed up this process by acting as electron acceptors. A single gamma photon may produce many ion pairs in the crystal and thus many photons. If the γ-ray energy is completely absorbed within the crystal, the number of light photons emitted is directly proportional to the energy of the incident photon. This would be true if 100 percent photoelectric interaction occurred, which is more nearly the case for photons of energy < 150 KeV. Above this energy, more Compton scatter occurs, and frequently part of the γ-energy escapes the crystal, with fewer light photons produced, and the resulting output is less than the input photon energy. This energy loss accounts for the Compton portion of the γ-ray spectrum *(pulse-height spectrum)* shown in Fig. 12.12.

The visible light photons emitted by the scin-

crystal is usually hermetically sealed and is coupled to the p.m. tubes via light pipes. When the light photons from the crystal strike the photocathodes of the p.m. tubes, the position of the incident photon in the crystal is deduced by the amount of light detected by the p.m. tubes relative to one another (Fig. 12.14). Each photon releases an electron from the photocathode, which is accelerated through a "high voltage" potential in multiple steps, like an energy amplifier. At each step, the electron strikes a metal plate, releasing secondary electrons, all of which are then accelerated to the next stage, and so on. The end result yields about $10^6$ electrons for each photon emitted from the crystal into a photocathode. This electron current from the p.m. tubes is proportional to the number of light photons emitted from the crystal, which is in turn proportional to the energy of the incident $\gamma$-photon. Therefore, the signal from the p.m. tubes is proportional to the photon energy absorbed in the crystal. (A typical pulse-height spectrum from the p.m. tubes, as noted earlier, is shown in Fig. 12.12.) This output pulse from the p.m. tubes is amplified and shaped by preamplifier and amplifier circuits prior to pulse-height analysis.

The pulse-height analyzer is the mechanism whereby the primary photoelectric events are differentiated from scattered or less energetic events, which may also interact with the detector crystal. If such "lesser" photons were accepted by the system as primary events, significant image degradation would result. Therefore, the primary photopeak is specifically selected by means of an "energy window" in the pulse-height analyzer, usually set at 20 percent around the primary photopeak energy. Thus, for a primary photon energy of 140 KeV, a 20 percent window would allow acceptance of output pulses resulting from photons of energies ranging from 126 to 154 KeV (10 percent of 140, on either side of 140 KeV). This energy discrimination in the pulse-height analyzer is accomplished by means of anticoincidence circuitry. This means that a *lower* discriminator produces an output pulse whenever an input pulse (in the above example) falls *above* 126 KeV; if the input pulse is also *less* than 154 KeV, the upper discriminator does

nothing, and the output pulse is passed on to the display device (see later). If the input pulse is *greater* than 154 KeV, the upper discriminator also produces a pulse, which blocks the pulse from the lower discriminator, so that no signal is passed on. If the input is < 126 KeV, also no output pulse appears. It is apparent from the pulse-height spectrum in Figure 12.12, that the most important discrimination function is to eliminate Compton scatter, as was alluded to earlier. The scintigraphic image produced by the accumulation of many such "discriminated" photons from many parts of the camera crystal, may be displayed by registering an X and Y pulse for each event (to discern location) and a Z pulse to quantify input energy of the event. The display device can be a persistence scope, or special cathode ray tube (CRT), which may be viewed directly, or used to produce images directly on X-ray or Polaroid film; or the signals may be routed to a single or multiple imaging device, such as a Matrix formatter; or the signals may be digitized and stored in computer matrices, as will be described in Chapter 28.

So, in summary, a scintigraphic image is produced when a specific radioactive tracer, localizing in a specific organ in the body, emits $\gamma$-photons. Of these photons, which may be emitted in any direction from the source organ, only those emitted straight toward the detector will be potentially useful. And while passing through the intervening soft tissue, 50 percent of these primary photons will be eliminated for each half-value-layer thickness of soft tissue encountered, prior to exiting the body. Of the exiting "good" photons approaching the detector face, some will be eliminated by the camera collimator, a special lead-septated focusing device used to improve images by screening out scatter photons from the body (see Fig. 12.14; this will be further discussed in Chapter 28). The number of good photons reaching the collimator face is also affected by the distance that must be traversed through air, from the body surface to the collimator. The further away the collimator is from the body surface, the fewer photons will reach it, according to the relationship $n = n_o/d^2$, where $n_o$ is the initial number of photons leaving the body surface, n is the number of photons arriving at the detector face, and d is the distance between the body and the detector (assuming the attenuation of air itself is negligible). This relationship is known as the *inverse square law.*

After photons have passed through the collimator, they may then interact in the crystal partially or totally, or may not interact at all. Of those "interacting," ultimately only those passing the "discrimination test" of pulse-height analysis will be used to produce the image. It is obvious then, that the more photons of ideal energy emitted from the source organ, the better and/or faster the image will be produced. Therefore, within the dead time count-rate limitations of the detector, for purposes of creating an image, the higher and more differential the concentration of radioisotope in the organ of interest, the better. However, we must also deal with the realities of radiation dosimetry and safety, both for radiation workers and for patients; and, therefore, appropriate limits must be set. These considerations spur the constant search for better and more efficient imaging technology, and more ideal radiopharmaceuticals, to be discussed briefly in the next section.

There are other types of radiation detection devices, such as liquid scintillation counters and semiconductor detectors. Discussion of these, however, is neither within the scope of this chapter, nor germane to the topic.

## Counting Statistics

It *is* necessary and pertinent to briefly mention certain aspects of counting statistics. Because radioactive decay is entirely a random behavior and, therefore, *not* equally distributed through time, the measurement of radioactivity becomes complex, since most such measurements are based on a determination of the rate of disintegration, by means of counting over a time period that is short relative to the half-life of the nuclide. What we really hope to determine by such a measurement is the true mean count rate, $\mu$. If a series of these interval measurements is taken, of N counts each time, the actual values of N will approximate a Poisson distribution centered about a mean value, $\mu$.

Each count, N, is an estimate of the true count rate, $\mu$. But a better estimate of $\mu$ is achieved by the mean of all Ns, or $\overline{N}$, the *average* N. In fact, the larger the number of counts sampled, regardless of the sampling or measurement time, the closer the approximation of $\overline{N}$ to $\mu$. However, all estimates involve some degree of error, which is important to determine. The percent error may be assessed by knowing the mean and standard deviation of the distribution of measurements, where the mean is defined as:

$$\overline{N} = \frac{\sum\limits_{i=1}^{i=x} N_i}{x}$$

and x is the *number of measurements* of N counts each. The *standard deviation* ($\sigma$) specifies the spread of the distribution about $\mu$, and is defined as:

$$\sigma = \sqrt{\mu}$$

Just as $\mu$ is approximated by $\overline{N}$, so $\sigma$ is approximated by s, the *sample standard deviation,* and the best measure of s is:

$$s = \sqrt{\frac{\sum (N - \overline{N})^2}{N - 1}}$$

where $N - \overline{N}$ is the *deviation* of any given value of N from $\overline{N}$ and $N - 1$ is called the number of *degrees of freedom.* The *sample standard deviation of the mean is Sm:*

$$Sm = \frac{s}{\sqrt{N}}$$

Therefore, the best estimate of sample activity becomes:

$$\overline{N} \pm Sm$$

In a Poisson distribution of counts as described above, as the number of counts, N, in each measurement, becomes large, the more closely the distribution begins to assume a *Gaussian* distribution, which may also be defined by the mean and standard deviation. In a Gaussian distribution, the values of N must be distributed symmetrically about the mean, such that 68.3 percent of the values of N will be within $\pm 1\sigma$ of the mean, 95.4 percent will be within $\pm 2\sigma$, and 99.7 percent will be within $\pm 3\sigma$. These limits express the probability that a given count rate is due only to random decay and *not* to some systematic error, and are called *confidence limits*. The value of $\sigma$ may be approximated by:

$$\sigma = \sqrt{N}$$

The primary way to reduce *random error* and, thus, make a measurement more sensitive to *systematic variations,* is to increase the number of counts in the sample. Thus, a total of *10,000 counts* is frequently chosen as an end point, since:

$$\sigma = \sqrt{N}$$

which is approximately equal to

$$\sigma = \sqrt{10,000} = 100$$

and    $100 = 1$ percent of 10,000

Therefore, with 10,000 counts in a sample, the random error should be $\pm 2$ percent for 95.4 percent of the times such a sample is taken. This discussion will assume major importance in the methodologic considerations to be presented in Chapter 28.

## A Brief Overview of Radiopharmaceuticals, Radiation Dosimetry and Radiation Safety

A *radiopharmaceutical,* or *radioactive drug,* is defined as a "radioactive element or labeled compound whose physical, chemical and biological properties render it both safe and useful for administration to humans."[7] The majority of these agents are classified for *diagnostic uses,* which implies that "the amount of drug that must be administered to provide useful information will produce no effects due to chemical toxicity, and that the resultant radiation dose

will be much smaller than the levels producing demonstrable somatic radiation damage."[7] A "radiopharmaceutical" is different from a "radiochemical" in that the radiopharmaceutical is considered a *drug* or *medicinal,* which is, therefore by law subject to biological control testing to avoid any adverse reaction that might result after it is administered (by the appropriate route) to patients. Since most of the current diagnostic radiopharmaceuticals are injected intravenously, these agents must meet the following criteria:

1. *Sterility.* Most agents are rendered sterile (free of all living microorganisms and their spores) either by *autoclaving* at 125°C at 20 pounds per square inch for 15 to 20 minutes or by *filtration* through fine cellulose ester membranes.[1]

2. *Apyrogenicity.* An intravenously injected agent must be free of *pyrogens,* which are particles having a diameter of 0.05 to 1.0 $\mu$ that do not decompose at elevated temperatures, and which produce elevated body temperature if present in an intravenous injection.[1] Meticulous attention to chemical preparation techniques is the only sure method to eliminate these particles.

Routine techniques for meeting these two criteria are carried out, either by culture or radiometric methods for sterility or by either rabbit or Limulus testing for apyrogenicity.[7]

Further major criteria, which should be applied regarding all such agents for human use, are as follows:[1,7]

1. *pH.* Should be within a range of 3.5 to 9.0 and *ideally* should be near 7.

2. *Injected volume of 10 ml or less.* Should contain the required amount of radioactivity and chemical form.

3. *Aqueous form.* Should be either a *solution* or a suspension of colloidal or larger particles.

4. *Radiochemical purity.* Defined as the percent of the desired radioisotope present in the desired chemical form (vs. any of the desired isotope present in some other chemical form).

5. *Radioisotopic purity.* Ratio of the amount of activity present as the desired radioisotope vs. the *total* activity in the sample.

6. *Carrier-free.* If possible, the radiopharmaceutical should contain only radioactive iso-

topes of the desired element (and little or *none* of the ground-state or nonradioactive form).

For the purposes of routine nuclear imaging techniques employing an Anger-type gamma camera, ideally the radioiosotope portion of the radiopharmaceutical should have a primary photon energy between 20 and 600 KeV (most ideally about 150 KeV) and a physical half-life between 1 hour and 1 year.[7] Nuclides with a physical $T_{1/2}$ longer than 1 year may potentially produce unwarranted radiation to the patient, because even though a short *biologic* $T_{1/2}$ may, in part, compensate, a small fraction of the administered dose is usually retained for a long period. (Exceptions to the rule are the noble gases, such as $^{133}Xe$ and $^{85}Kr$, which are readily eliminated via pulmonary excretion into expired air, and have a biologic $T_{1/2}$ of 4 to 5 minutes and no excessively long components.) Conversely, an isotope with a physical $T_{1/2}$ shorter than 1 hour is not practical for labeling and sterilization of appropriate chemical compounds. [The new positron emitters, such as $^{11}C$, $^{15}O$, and $^{13}N$, are currently being explored, particularly with applications to nuclear cardiology, by centers equipped with cyclotrons (for production of such ultrashort-lived isotopes— $T_{1/2}$ from 2 to 20 minutes), and with appropriate imaging devices, such as the positron emission transaxial tomographic camera. These agents appear to offer very exciting, new information in the areas of myocardial metabolism, blood flow, and oxygen consumption. However, general availability of the required production and imaging technology seems unlikely in the near future.]

Further "ideal" characteristics for radioisotope imaging are that the isotope be easily produced; readily available; inexpensive; have a high enough *specific activity* (defined as activity per unit mass of a sample, e.g., Ci/g) so as to produce *no* physiologic or toxic effects (when used in "tracer quantities" for imaging); decay by isomeric transition or electron capture without internal conversion (so that there is *no particulate* radiation produced, thus resulting in lower patient radiation dose); and be easily labeled to a variety of pharmaceuticals, which remain intact after administration to the patient and are readily and specifically localized in particular organ systems.

Technetium–99m, as mentioned previously, is the radionuclide that most nearly satisfies the above list of criteria. With the many available "instant" kits for producing a wide variety of $^{99m}Tc$-labeled radiopharmaceuticals, it is easy to see why $^{99m}Tc$ has become the "workhorse" of nuclear imaging. Technetium is produced either by neutron bombardment of $^{98}Mo$ or by fission from the neutron bombardment of $^{235}U$:

$$^{98}Mo(n,\gamma) \searrow$$
$$^{235}U \text{ (n, fission)} \nearrow \quad ^{99}Mo \xrightarrow[T_{1/2} = 67 \text{ hr}]{\beta^-} \, ^{99m}Tc \xrightarrow[T_{1/2} = 6 \text{ hr}]{140 \text{ KeV } \gamma} \, ^{99}Tc$$

The most efficient method of maintaining an abundant and readily available supply of $^{99m}Tc$ is by means of the *generator system,* in which the $^{99}Mo$ is adsorbed on an alumina column in a lead-shielded container. As $^{99}Mo$ decays to $^{99m}Tc$, a *transient equilibrium* is established in which the activity of $^{99}Mo$ and the activity of $^{99m}Tc$ (in an undisturbed system) become equal over time. Once equilibrium is established, the daughter ($^{99m}Tc$) activity thereafter decreases with an apparent $T_{1/2}$ equal to the physical $T_{1/2}$ of the parent ($^{99}Mo$). Then, at any point in time, the column may be eluted or "milked" with normal saline, bringing out the available $^{99m}Tc$, while leaving essentially all $^{99}Mo$ adsorbed to the column. Thereafter, transient equilibrium may be allowed to become reestablished, the column then "milked" again, and so on. These principles are illustrated graphically in Figure 12.15. $^{99m}$Technetium eluted from the generator is in the chemical form of Tc-pertechnetate, $^{99m}TcO_4^-$, which is Tc VII oxidation state. With few exceptions, this form must be reduced to allow labeling of the various pharmaceuticals with technetium. The reducing agent in most kits is stan-

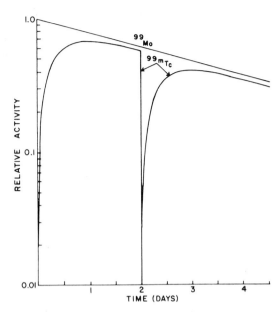

Fig. 12.15 The generator principle: After transient equilibrium has been established (at approximately 1 day on the X-axis), the daughter ($^{99m}$Tc) decays with an apparent half-life approximately equal to the half-life of the parent ($^{99}$Mo). Note that the $^{99m}$Tc activity remains less than that of $^{99}$Mo because about 14 percent of the parent nuclei decay promptly to $^{99}$Tc without passing first through the metastable state of $^{99m}$Tc. The sharp decline in $^{99m}$Tc activity shown at 2 days is due to "milking" of the generator, after which transient equilibrium is again gradually reestablished over about 24 hours. (Hendee: Medical Radiation Physics, 2nd ed., 1979, by permission of Year Book Medical Publishers.)

nous ion, a fact that has been serendipitously advantageous to nuclear cardiology, as will be further discussed in Chapter 28.

The theory of calculation of radiation doses to patients resulting from radioisotope imaging procedures is beyond the scope of this chapter; however, it should be noted that the majority of these procedures produce organ and whole-body doses of approximately one-half rad or less. (In most cases, the dose is about equivalent to a standard chest X-ray.) *Rad* is an acronym for *radiation absorbed dose* and is a measure of the amount of energy absorbed in a medium, such as soft tissue, as the result of exposure to ionizing radiation: *1 rad = 10⁻² joule/kg.* The unit of radiation exposure is the *roentgen (R)*, where *1 R = 2.58 × 10⁻⁴ coulomb/kg* of air.

A third commonly encountered term is the *rem,* which is a *dose equivalent* (DE) measurement, based on the fact that the chemical or biologic effect of a particular type of radiation is a function of the *linear energy transfer* (LET) of that radiation. This is reflected in the formula:

$$DE \text{ (rem)} = D \text{ (rad)} \times QF$$

where QF is a *quality factor* that varies with the LET of the radiation. The QF for $\gamma$-rays is *one.* Therefore, for $\gamma$-radiation, *rads = rems.* Dose limits for the general public and for occupationally-exposed persons have been set at 0.5 rem/yr and 5 rem/yr, respectively, excluding background environment radiation and medical diagnostic exposure; these are the *maximum permissible doses* (MPD) to the whole body. Such figures are based on concern for the genetic effects of radiation on the population and determination of the dose furnishing a genetic burden that is acceptably low in the population.[1] The radiation dosimetry of nuclear medicine, and the radiation wastes resulting from this medical subspecialty, are generally considered to be "low-level radiation." While standard procedures in handling any radioactive materials are observed by those who work in the field of nuclear medicine, no special precautions are considered necessary after a patient has undergone a nuclear imaging procedure.

From our introductory review of the fundamental principles of nuclear decay, radiopharmaceutical preparation, radiation safety, and knowledge of the instrumentation necessary for nuclear imaging, it is apparent that there is a great deal of technical proficiency needed to perform nuclear diagnostic procedures. Precisely because so much is involved in the performance of these tests, they are best considered to be an area for shared responsibility, involving experts in several clinical disciplines, e.g., a nuclear physician or radiologist who is usually more aware of the technical aspects of nuclear imaging, and a cardiologist who is sometimes better able to judge when a specific procedure is indicated and how the results may affect treatment. An integrated approach to the quality control of methods, materials, equipment, and personnel in such procedures is obviously of great importance. Further reference to quality control in these areas, as well as a discussion of computer applications and quality control, will be presented in Chapter 28.

## MYOCARDIAL IMAGING WITH THALLIUM-201

Since the early 1960s a number of radioactive agents have been proposed and shown to be suitable for direct myocardial imaging.[8-10] These include radioactive potassium and its analogues, cesium, rubidium, and thallium, several labeled fatty acids, and a variety of positron-labeled compounds, such as ammonia, various amino acids, and manganese. These agents have, in common, the propensity to concentrate in normally perfused myocardium, but accumulate in reduced amounts in ischemic, scarred, or infarcted tissue. Although the mechanisms of myocardial accumulation and clearance vary among these compounds, most investigators agree that within certain limits of coronary blood flow, initial concentration generally reflects the state of regional perfusion.[11,12]

For a variety of reasons thallium-201 ($^{201}$Tl) is currently the most commonly used myocardial imaging agent.[13-15] The radioactive decay of $^{201}$Tl is associated with the production of gamma and X-ray photons whose energies (80, 130, and 160 keV) are well suited for nuclear imaging. Its physical half-life of 73 hours allows scheduled shipments to be made from the source of production to virtually anywhere in the world. However, pharmaceutical grade $^{201}$Tl, available as the chloride, is produced at a limited number of cyclotron facilities in the U.S. and Europe, and is fairly expensive in comparison with most $^{99m}$Tc-labeled compounds used for routine nuclear imaging. For example, the average cost of a single administered dose of $^{201}$Tl in 1980 is approximately $100.

Virtually all modern 15-inch diameter, large field and 10-inch smaller field-of-view mobile scintillation cameras are capable of producing $^{201}$Tl images of high diagnostic quality. However, some older instruments manufactured prior to 1974 produce images of unacceptable quality. This can be determined by using appropriate test sources such as those supplied by the commercial producer of $^{201}$Tl. Some older cameras can be modified or upgraded at a lower cost than purchasing a new instrument.

When one views a $^{201}$Tl myocardial perfusion image, the picture observed is primarily that of the left ventricular, and, to a much lesser extent, the right ventricular myocardium. Whether presented as an image consisting of white dots on a black background, as with Polaroid print film, or black dots on a clear base, as with X-ray film, the density of dots on the image reflects two factors governing the distribution of the radiopharmaceutical. The most important factor is myocardial blood flow and the second is the distribution of myocardial muscle mass.

Following the intravenous administration of a typical dose of 1.5 to 2.0 mCi, peak concentration of $^{201}$Tl in normally perfused regions is usually reached within 2 to 5 minutes. The actual percent of the administered dose present within the myocardium may vary, depending on myocardial perfusion, but also depending on the physiologic state of the patient at the time of injection, e.g., rest vs. exercise. Generally, only 2 to 4 percent of the administered dose accumulates in the heart, the remainder being distributed throughout the skeletal muscles and organs, such as the liver and kidneys. Indeed, when $^{201}$Tl is administered at rest, considerable uptake may be noted beneath the diaphragm, primarily within the liver, and this may occasionally cause difficulty in evaluating the inferior left ventricular wall. Imaging is normally begun when the peak myocardial-to-blood ratio is reached, which usually occurs 10 minutes following injection.

An exact kinetic model that describes the mechanism of $^{201}$Tl extraction from the blood and initial concentration within the myocardium is not available, but would appear to be fairly similar to that associated with potassium accumulation.[12] Experimental evidence in animals suggest an almost linear relationship between blood flow and initial $^{201}$Tl concentration, although not in direct proportion. Thus, a reduction of approximately 70 percent of normal resting blood flow may be associated with only a 60 percent decrease in initial $^{201}$Tl tissue concentration.

The clearance rate of $^{201}$Tl from normally perfused myocardium appears to be significantly slower than for potassium, suggesting a different kinetic mechanism, again, one that is not well understood.[14] Nevertheless, myocardial clearance of $^{201}$Tl appears to be blood flow related in the sense that washout may be retarded in poorly perfused regions.[15] At the same time, clearance of $^{201}$Tl from skeletal muscles and its reappearance in the blood allows a small fraction to be extracted by the myocardium, presumably in proportion to perfusion.

The term "redistribution" has been used to describe the different rates of thallium accumulation and clearance from normal versus ischemic myocardium.[17-21] Whether more rapid washout from normal than from ischemic regions is the predominant factor, or whether peak accumulation in poorly perfused zones is reached more slowly than in normal regions, the net effect of redistribution is that the concentration of thallium tends to equalize over time. This frequently makes it more difficult to recognize focal deficits in $^{201}$Tl uptake in ischemic zones on images obtained beyond about 45 minutes. This stresses the need to complete the initial imaging procedure as quickly as possible.

Animal evidence suggests that early redistribution reflects the delayed active uptake of $^{201}$Tl by transiently ischemic tissue [21], while during the later stages, redistribution is primarily due to the more rapid loss of $^{201}$Tl from the normal myocardium.[19,20] Thus, it appears that the redistribution of thallium in the heart is a dynamic process. The various rate constants and factors that govern this process are unknown, and the phenomenon probably also depends to some extent on blood levels of $^{201}$Tl over time as well as on the physiologic state of the patient. The clinical implications of thallium redistribution will be discussed later.

The kidney is the primary organ for the excretion of $^{201}$Tl, which proceeds satisfactorily provided the patient is not in renal failure and renal perfusion is adequate.

As mentioned earlier, the distribution of myocardial tissue mass is a second factor governing radioactive count density on the scintillation camera images. The normally varying thickness of the left ventricular walls is often reflected by irregular shapes on the myocardial images. Frequently, one can observe increased count density (intensity) due to papillary muscle superimposition upon an adjacent wall when a tangential view is employed. Normal anatomic thinning at the apex may sometimes produce a slight reduction in count density, which may be difficult to distinguish from a true apical perfusion abnormality. Similarly, left ventricular dilatation may be associated with apparent thinning at the apex, a point to remember in the setting of suspected acute infarction.

The different projections used for image recording, i.e., the relationship between the scintillation camera detector and the heart, have a profound effect on which portions of the left ventricular anatomy are seen on any particular view (Fig. 12.16). Multiple views, therefore, are necessary to precisely localize most perfusion abnormalities. These focal reductions in uptake are generally best seen in the projection in which the deficit in counts is imaged tangentially. This provides maximum contrast between the focal area of reduced thallium concentration and the surrounding normal tissue. The angle of the long axis of the left ventricle with respect to the detector also affects image perspective. This is most pronounced in terms of the appearance of the base of the ventricle. Horizontal hearts are more frequently associated with a ring or "doughnut" pattern of uptake when viewed in the left anterior oblique projection. In more vertically oriented hearts the ventricular image may resemble a horseshoe, open at the top at the level of the mitral valve plane.

Right ventricular visualization is variable. While the right ventricle is routinely visualized when $^{201}$Tl is injected during exercise, identification of this chamber is much less frequent when the study is performed at rest. When the count density approaches that in the left ventricular wall, several possibilities should be considered, including right ventricular hypertrophy or increased right ventricular myocardial perfusion secondary to a greater workload of this

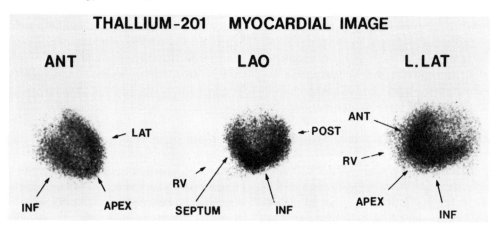

**THALLIUM-201   MYOCARDIAL IMAGE**

Fig. 12.16  [201]Tl images in a normal subject showing uniform uptake in the left ventricular myocardium plus slight accumulation in the right ventricular (RV) wall. Projections: ANT = anterior, LAO = left anterior oblique, L.LAT. = left lateral (decubitus, right side down). INF = inferior wall, LAT = lateral wall, POST = posterior wall, ANT = anterior wall.

chamber in response to increased pulmonary vascular resistance.

Lung background accumulation of [201]Tl is variable, but rarely exceeds approximately 50 percent of the left ventricular myocardial count density. Excessive pulmonary radioactivity is sometimes seen with left ventricular failure in association with a variety of causes, including acute infarction.[21]

Another feature that distinguishes rest from exercise images is the accumulation of [201]Tl beneath the diaphragm, which is due primarily to uptake in the liver. Imaging in multiple projections should serve to overcome any bothersome overlap of the liver and left ventricular accumulations. To minimize liver uptake, injecting the [201]Tl with the patient sitting, or while in the fasting condition is sometimes recommended.

Patterns of normal [201]Tl distribution in the heart are variable, depending on the various factors described above. Familiarity with the many variations of normal is important and can be gained with experience, as with any diagnostic method. Four views are usually needed to examine all aspects of the left ventricular wall. These views should include: anterior, 45° left anterior oblique (LAO), 60° LAO, and left lateral. Some laboratories omit the lateral view and substitute a more steeply angled LAO projection. To avoid a potential defect from diaphragmatic attenuation of the gamma ray pho-

tons, i.e., a spurious decrease in counts along the posterior and inferior walls, the left lateral image should be performed with the patient positioned with the right side dependent and the left chest upward beneath the detector.[22,23]

Proper and reproducible detector positioning are absolutely necessary for successful studies. Correct exposures are likewise essential. While scintillation techniques vary, the need to acquire sufficient counts to produce high quality images cannot be overemphasized. A convenient method to accomplish this is to begin with the anterior view and to record for the period of time necessary to acquire 2,000 counts/cm² over a normal region of myocardium. This is referred to as "information density" and an I.D. of 2,000 should not require more than 5 to 7 minutes per view when a general-purpose or all-purpose low energy, parallel hole collimator is used. During this period of time, a total of approximately 400,000 counts in the entire camera field of view will have been recorded, depending on liver and other soft tissue background activity. Once the time needed to achieve the desired I.D. or total counts has been determined for the initial image, the remaining views are then recorded for the same time.

Some laboratories simultaneously record all raw image data in a digital computer system to facilitate interpretation, thus permitting contrast to be adjusted and other manipulations to be made to provide images of more uniform quality. While this practice has certain advantages, including the potential for rough quantitation of regional activity, it is our recommendation that laboratories should first strive to achieve consistently good quality unprocessed images and gain experience in interpreting these whenever possible.

Scintillation camera recording is usually started 10 minutes following the injection of 1.5 to 2.0 mCi of [201]Tl. Images obtained at this time generally reflect the state of regional perfusion within the first 2 to 5 minutes following injection, during which time the maximum concentration of [201]Tl is reached in the normal zones. Reimaging, using the same initial dose (i.e., without reinjection), several hours later or even the next day constitutes redistribution imaging. As mentioned earlier, the mechanism of regional [201]Tl redistribution over time is poorly understood. Transiently ischemic regions, such as those associated with coronary artery spasm or, more typically, with exercise stress, may be expected to produce focal defects (reduced uptake) on the initial images, which may no longer be appreciated on the redistribution images.

The time needed to achieve this normalization or apparent obliteration of an initial regional deficit in counts is variable. It may be relatively rapid, as in transient ischemia secondary to coronary artery spasm, but more prolonged in unstable angina without infarction. Therefore, it may be helpful to characterize initial perfusion defects as to how quickly, if at all, they tend to "disappear." This can be accomplished by selecting one or more of the views during the initial study which best demonstrate the extent and location of the apparent perfusion abnormality for redistribution imaging 2 to 4 hours later. This may be repeated at 6 to 8 hours if normalization is not achieved or is indeterminate. Identical projections and comparable scintillation camera exposure parameters (i.e., I.D.) between the initial and delayed views are essential.

Redistribution imaging requires additional recording time due to the physical decay as well as the clearance of [201]Tl from the heart. A perfusion defect that seems to disappear or rapidly "fills in" is more likely to be associated with transient ischemia, while a regional deficit in counts that remains essentially unchanged with respect to adjacent areas over 6 to 8 hours tends to be more consistent with scar formation secondary to a previous acute infarction, i.e., reduced myocardial mass.[20,21]

The redistribution pattern in acute myocardial infarction is less well characterized. Although a defect corresponding to the site of infarction is usually identified on the initial [201]Tl images in the vast majority of cases early after the clinical onset of symptoms (Fig. 12.17), redistribution imaging may suggest some degree of apparent "reperfusion," perhaps as a reflection of the extent of transient or reversible ischemia, possibly surrounding or included within the region of irreversibly damaged myocardium. Similarly, repeat [201]Tl imaging over the succeeding days may show a surprising rate of apparent improvement in the infarcted zone.

Clearly, this is a complex issue that is not helped by the inability of even modern scintillation cameras using conventional planar imaging to isolate one volume of myocardial tissue from all others. On the other hand, it is possible to observe count changes over time by computer-assisted methods in which identical regions of the myocardium are compared during the redistribution period.[20,21] Thus, the dynamics of [201]Tl accumulation and clearance may be characterized and possibly used in the future to help differentiate between reversible and irreversible ischemia.

From the foregoing, it should be evident that a focal deficit in [201]Tl uptake, seen on the initial postinjection images in the clinical setting of suspected acute myocardial infarction, must be interpreted with the following in mind. While such defects may, in fact, represent acute infarction,[24,25] similar defects can be observed in chronic coronary artery disease with unstable angina,[26] coronary artery spasm associated with transient ischemia,[27,28] or scar formation resulting from a previous infarction. An entirely normal study, on the other hand, when performed within the first few hours following the onset of symptoms, provides reasonable evidence that acute infarction is unlikely.[29] Indeed a 96 percent sensitivity for detecting acute myocardial infarction within the first 6 to 12 hours follow-

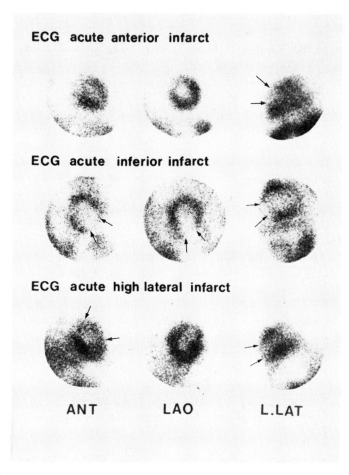

Fig. 12.17 ²⁰¹Tl images in three patients with proven acute myocardial infarctions as indicated. Focal reductions in uptake, (between the arrows), correspond to the site of infarction. The anterior infarct shown in the top panel also involves the intra-ventricular septum. The inferior and high lateral infarcts shown in the second and third panels also involve the apex of the left ventricle. Similar defects, however, may be seen with other causes of reduced perfusion or from scar formation following a previous infarction (see text).

ing the onset of symptoms has been reported.[30] However, in this and other reports, sensitivity tends to be somewhat lower when initial imaging is performed 24 to 48 hours following the onset of symptoms.[30,31] The explanation for this diminished sensitivity over time is not clear, but may reflect more extensive ischemia accompanying the onset of symptoms, which partially or totally recovers in some zones, though presumably not in the region of irreversible damage.

To summarize the above, normal ²⁰¹Tl images obtained within the early hours following a sus-

pected acute myocardial infarction can provide reasonable assurance that this diagnosis is unlikely. It does not, however, rule out coronary artery disease nor that transient ischemia may have occurred sometime prior to the imaging procedure with subsequent reestablishment of normal perfusion. An abnormal study, on the other hand, showing a clearly defined defect on at least two views, should alert the clinician to the high probability of myocardial ischemia, which has led or may lead to infarction. In any event, it strongly suggests the diagnosis of coronary artery disease, but differentiation may be impossible between acute infarction, unstable angina with transient reversible ischemia, or scar formation from a prior infarction whether apparent by history or not. Obviously, other methods to establish the specific diagnosis of acute infarction are available. Nevertheless, [201]Tl imaging can be useful in providing a graphic picture of the location and extent of acute or chronic ischemia. At the very least, the imaging procedure may provide the first laboratory evidence of acute infarction, even prior to the appearance of characteristic ECG changes or definitive elevation in cardiac related enzymes.

It is quite possible that in the future the primary role of [201]Tl myocardial imaging may be to help differentiate between the extent of reversible versus nonreversible ischemia by characterizing [201]Tl distribution over time and from these data perhaps provide some indication of short- and long-term prognosis. In this connection, Silverman et al. reported that [201]Tl scintigraphy—performed within 15 hours of the onset of symptoms in 42 class I and II patients with acute myocardial infarction and expressed as a summed perfusion defect score—was a highly accurate predictor of both in-hospital and late mortality.[31a]

## MYOCARDIAL IMAGING WITH "INFARCT-AVID" AGENTS

In the preceding section, the role of [201]Tl perfusion imaging to detect zones of ischemic myocardium associated with acute infarction was discussed. In this section, we will consider a second method to detect acute infarction using an agent that preferentially concentrates in injured myocardial tissue.

Direct visualization of the location and size of an infarcted zone would in many ways seem preferable to current methods used to detect myocardial infarction. With these methods the diagnosis is made indirectly by noting characteristic ECG changes or the appearance of enzymes in serum which are released from injured myocardial cells. Although a number of radioactive compounds have been suggested in the past as being suitable "infarct-avid" agents, the use of [99m]Tc-labeled stannous pyrophosphate

has become well established and is the current agent of choice.[32]

Credit must be given to Bonte et al. who, in 1974, hypothesized that since hydroxyappatite crystals can be detected within mitochondria of histologically damaged myocardial cells, [99m]Tc-pyrophosphate, an agent commonly used for bone scanning, might become incorporated within acutely infarcted tissue.[33,34]

Following the intravenous injection of [99m]Tc-pyrophosphate, approximately 40 percent of the radiopharmaceutical accumulates in the skeletal structures; the remainder is excreted by the kidneys. Blood clearance is facilitated in the well-hydrated patient with normal renal function. Within 90 to 120 minutes, blood concentration decreases to a level where the bone-to-background radioactivity ratio is maximum and suitable for imaging. Poor renal function or reduced renal perfusion associated with low cardiac output frequently delays excretion so that blood pool and soft tissue background may be excessive even 2 hours following injection, thus occasionally necessitating imaging at 3 to 4 hours.

The mechanism for pyrophosphate accumulation in infarcted myocardium is not entirely known.[35-41] While related to the histologic demonstration of calcium deposits in irreversibly damaged myocardial cells, the exact site of incorporation of the radiopharmaceutical in the injured cells and the role of calcium are not completely understood. Regardless of the precise mechanism, the preponderance of evidence suggests that pyrophosphate accumulation within the myocardium is an indication of the presence of irreversibly injured cells and the degree of uptake is roughly proportional to the extent of damage. On the other hand, some blood flow to the area of infarction must be preserved in order to deliver pyrophosphate to the region of damaged cells. It has been shown that while a reduction in normal perfusion by 20 to 40 percent results in maximum pyrophosphate accumulation, uptake actually decreases as blood flow is further reduced.[42] It is easy, therefore, to understand why, in very large infarcts, accumulation of this infarct-avid agent may occur only in the peripheral zones giving rise to the familiar "doughnut" pattern and why the amount of total uptake is not a good indicator per se of the quantity of infarcted tissue.

Imaging with the scintillation camera is normally begun approximately 2 hours following the intravenous injection of 10 to 15 mCi of stannous pyrophosphate labeled with $^{99m}$Tc. Three standard projections are ordinarily required to determine the presence and location of abnormal accumulations within the heart: anterior, left anterior oblique (LAO), and left lateral. The imaging technique should be standardized for consistent results and sufficient counts acquired to permit detection and localization of abnormal deposits in the heart, if present. The time required to record at least 500,000 counts rarely exceeds 2 minutes per view when a high resolution, parallel-hole collimator is used. As with $^{201}$Tl imaging (see above), a convenient method is to determine the time necessary to achieve the desired counting statistics on the anterior view and record each subsequent image for the same time. An information density of at least 2,000 counts per square centimeter over the sternum should result in images capable of demonstrating focal cardiac accumulations. Some experimentation with the degree of LAO angulation may be needed to assure that the "clear space" between the sternum and costochondral junction is positioned to allow viewing of the heart in an unobstructed manner.

Since pyrophosphate is a bone seeking agent, a good indicator of the quality of the study is the ability to clearly define skeletal structures such as the ribs and sternum. Indeed, in laboratories accustomed to obtaining high quality bone scans, imaging with this infarct-avid agent should present no problem. The degree of clarity of skeletal structures, or focal accumulations in the heart, if present, or both, depends to a large extent on minimizing soft tissue and blood pool background. As mentioned earlier, this can be accomplished by either increasing fluid intake or by delaying imaging for up to 3 to 4 hours postinjection.

Diffuse uptake in the cardiac area at 2 hours postinjection can result in an indeterminate study. Therefore, delayed imaging in one or more views should clarify whether excessive blood pool activity versus true myocardial uptake is present, since in the latter, focal areas should become more easily outlined with time. An additional clue to the presence of persistent cardiac blood pool activity is visualization of other vascular pools, such as the liver and spleen.

Another potential source of interpretative error is improper radiopharmaceutical preparation, sometimes manifested by excessive amounts of nonreduced, free $^{99m}$Tc-sodium pertechnetate, which can be recognized by noting accumulation in the thyroid gland or in the stomach beneath the heart. Again, the best biologic evidence of proper radiopharmaceutical preparation is clear visualization of the skeletal structures and minimal soft tissue and blood pool background activity.

Other bone imaging agents such as $^{99m}$Tc-labeled methylene diphosphonate, commonly used in clinical nuclear medicine, have not proved superior for infarct-avid imaging.[44] Stannous pyrophosphate, therefore, currently remains the agent of choice.

Precise localization of the site of infarction should not be difficult on properly exposed images obtained in multiple projections (Figs. 12.18 to 12.21). Overlying radioactivity in the ribs and sternum makes visualization of cardiac uptake more difficult, but does serve to help define the surrounding anatomy for orientation. Computer recording of the scintillation camera image data may be helpful in some cases by permitting the viewer to perform various degrees of background suppression and contrast enhancement. This, however, should not be a substitute for the practice of regularly obtaining high quality, original (unprocessed) scintigrams.

Various descriptive terms are sometimes used to characterize $^{99m}$Tc–pyrophosphate accumulation in zones of infarcted myocardium. It is important to differentiate between diffuse and focal uptake, and the accumulation may be described as being 1+ through 4+ (see Fig. 12.18). Grading schemes such as this can be useful in terms of establishing the degree of certainty with which the accumulation of pyrophosphate is present within the heart, but it can not always be relied on to estimate infarct size, since intensity of uptake also depends on the amount of

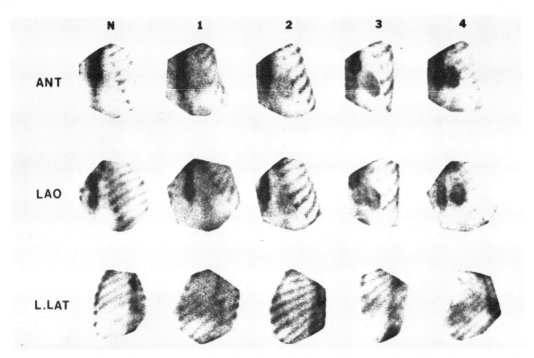

Fig. 12.18  $^{99m}$Tc labeled stannous pyrophosphate images in five subjects, (patients N and 1 are normal). Images were obtained between day 2 to 3 in the three other patients, all of whom had documented acute anterior or anterolateral transmural infarctions. A rough grading system is sometimes used: 4+ = uptake greater than rib uptake, 3+ = essentially equal to rib uptake, 2+ = less than rib uptake; a 1+ is usually considered equivocal and may result from delayed blood clearance of radioactivity (see text). Views: ANT = anterior, LAO = left anterior oblique, LAT = left lateral.

blood flow remaining in the infarcted region. Furthermore, the timing of the procedure with respect to the onset of clinical symptoms may have a profound effect on the intensity of accumulation, since pyrophosphate imaging within the initial 8 hours frequently fails to reveal uptake in an acutely infarcted region and maximum accumulation may not be achieved for 2 to 3 days. Thereafter, the intensity of uptake tends to decline in the period beyond approximately 7 days, but this is variable.

Methods for estimating the size of an acute infarction on infarct-avid scans have generally consisted of determining the largest area of $^{99m}$Tc-pyrophosphate accumulation as visualized in one of the three standard views.[38,43] In the case of an anterior wall infarct (see Fig. 12.19), the area of pyrophosphate accumulation can be determined by direct planimetry after correction is made for size. This can be done by enlarging the image to an appropriate 1:1 ratio and expressing the area in cm². For ante-

rior and anterolateral infarcts, this method generally yields size estimates that correlate well with those made by multiple serum creatine kinase (CK) sample techniques. Inferior wall infarcts are more difficult to assess by simple area measurement due to the lack of a suitable projection (e.g., an inferior view) to outline the extent of pyrophosphate uptake according to its largest area. This has led to the suggestion that a more complex geometric model might be used.[38]

Not all focal or diffuse accumulations of $^{99m}$Tc-pyrophosphate identified scintigraphically to be within the heart represent acute myocardial infarction. Some reports have indicated that patients with unstable or variant angina may demonstrate diffuse or even 2+ focal accumulations in the heart.[45-47] This has tended to confuse the issue of specificity of infarct-avid imaging with pyrophosphate for detecting acute myocardial infarction. Human biopsy and autopsy material obtained in such patients without clinical evidence of infarction has disclosed 99mTc-pyrophosphate accumulation in regions associated with histologic alterations characteristic of myocardial cell death using conventional as well as electron microscope techniques. This would suggest that identifiable accumulations of 99mTc-pyrophosphate in the heart on routine imaging are not normal and should at least raise

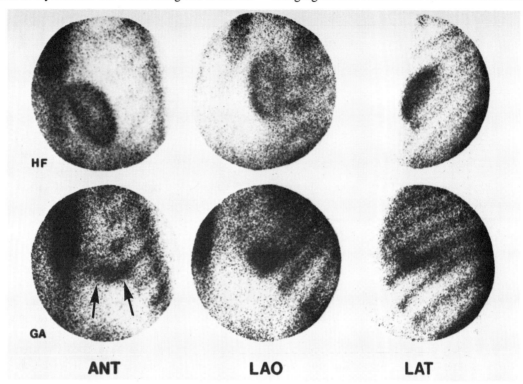

Fig. 12.19  Images in two patients with acute infarction studied 2 days after onset of symptoms. 99mTc pyrophosphate (PYP) images in patient HF (top row) show typical "doughnut" pattern seen in large anterior wall infarcts; location is confirmed on the lateral view. Patient GA (bottom row) shows PYP deposition in an inferior wall infarct (arrows). Views labeled as in Fig. 12.18.

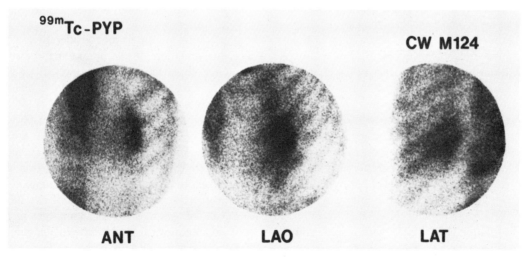

Fig. 12.20  Patient CW M124 demonstrates focal 99mTc pyrophosphate accumulation in the anterolateral wall consistent with the site of acute infarction suggested by ECG. Views labeled as in previous figures.

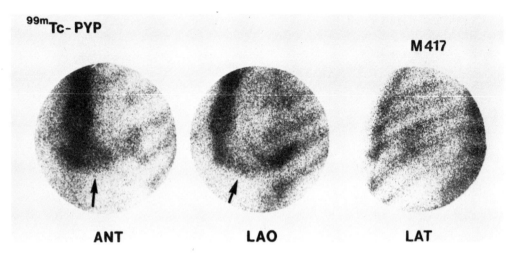

Fig. 12.21   Focal $^{99m}$Tc PYP uptake in the location of the inferior and right ventricular walls (arrows), consistent with right ventricular infarction. Views labeled as in previous figures.

the possibility of some degree of myocardial cell death, whether or not infarction is present by the usual clinical or laboratory criteria.

Other possible causes of $^{99m}$Tc-pyrophosphate uptake in the heart should be considered in the differential diagnosis of a positive study.[48-55] In addition to patients with unstable angina, the list should include: those patients with a documented prior myocardial infarction who have persistently positive accumulations over a several month period (to be discussed later); cases of traumatic cardiac contusion; ventricular aneurysms; calcified valves whether radiographically evident or not; various cardiac tumors; chronic pericarditis; and occasionally adriamycin cardiac toxicity. It is unclear whether to include acute pericarditis in the list of possible causes of a false positive study. As mentioned earlier, one must be careful not to confuse residual cardiac blood pool activity with true myocardial uptake.

Extracardiac accumulations of $^{99m}$Tc-pyrophosphate should also be considered among the possible causes for misinterpretation.[56-61] These include pyrophosphate uptake: in breast tumors; within rib or sternal fractures, which may persist up to a year or more following trauma; at the site of paddle placement for electrical defibrillation (Fig. 12.22); within some soft tissue tumors and at the site of various skin lesions. These extracardiac accumulations should not be the cause of interpretative error if atten-tion is given to their superficial location as identified in multiple projections.

Cardiac imaging with $^{99m}$Tc–pyrophosphate has been widely used for the detection of acute myocardial infarction and its sensitivity evaluated in many centers.[38,62-70] In transmural myocardial infarction, sensitivities generally exceeding 90 percent have been reported. In nontransmural infarction, some variation has been noted. Some reports indicate a sensitivity no better than 40 to 50 percent. Several investigators have suggested that at least 3 to 4 g of tissue must be infarcted before sufficient $^{99m}$Tc-pyrophosphate uptake can be detected by conventional imaging techniques.[38,43]

The time-course of $^{99m}$Tc-pyrophosphate accumulation is an important consideration in image interpretation. While uptake may be sufficient for visualization of an infarcted zone on images obtained as early as 8 to 10 hours following the onset of symptoms, sensitivity of the technique increases over time; indeed, its peak seems to be reached between 24 to 72 hours, at which time images obtained 2 to 3 hours following $^{99m}$Tc-pyrophosphate injection are most likely to be positive.[38] Peak accumulation, however, may not be reached until as late as 5 days. This emphasizes the point that in the case of an equivocal study early in the clinical course, repeating the procedure as late as the fifth day may be useful in helping to establish the diagnosis. On the other hand, it is not infre-

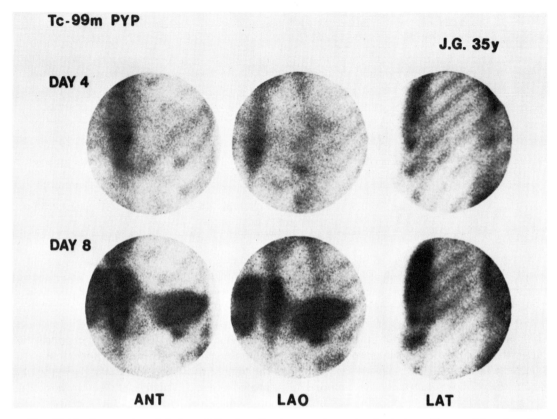

Fig. 12.22  Images 4 and 8 days following direct current countershock in a 35-year-old male with cardiac arrest from an electrical injury. There was no subsequent clinical or laboratory evidence of acute myocardial infarction. Day 4 images (top row) show 2+ focal uptake in a pattern similar to Figure 12.18 in the anterior (ANT) view, but poorly localized on the other projections. Day 8 images (bottom row) show typical soft tissue (muscle) burn injury at the paddle sites; their superficial location is confirmed on the lateral (LAT) view.

quent to find that a 4+ accumulation, observed within the first 24 to 48 hours, has become 3+ by the third day and only 2+ when repeated on the fifth day following the onset of symptoms (Fig. 12.23). It would seem important, therefore, to strive to perform [99m]Tc-pyrophosphate cardiac imaging within the initial 24 to 72 hour period. Failure to clearly identify abnormal [99m]Tc-pyrophosphate accumulation prior to this time is not sufficient to exclude acute infarction and repeat imaging at 3 to 5 days might be helpful in some cases. Similarly, an entirely negative study obtained 7 to 14 days following the onset of symptoms does not rule out acute infarction since it is not unusual for the image to become normal by this time.

In addition to the intensity of accumulation, various patterns of uptake have been described,

which would appear to relate to short- and long-term prognosis. The "doughnut" configuration, as described earlier, is frequently seen with large anterior or anterolateral infarcts and is more frequently associated with ventricular failure, presumably due to the extent and location of injury.[71,72]

Infarct size, as determined by the area of pyrophosphate uptake, also appears to relate to morbidity and mortality (see Fig. 12.23). For example, it has been reported that patients with planimetered areas of less than 16 cm² had no complications while in the hospital or during a mean follow-up period of 6 months, whereas a total complication rate of 68 percent (including a 12 percent mortality rate) was observed when the areas ranged between 16 and 40 cm².[73] Death from ventricular pump failure occurred

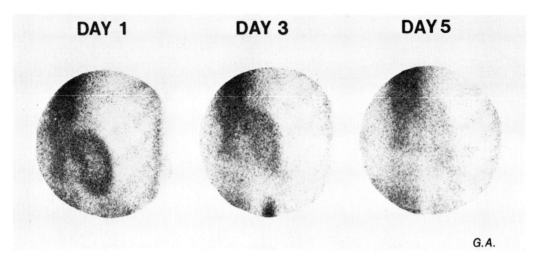

Fig. 12.23 Serial $^{99m}$Tc pyrophosphate images obtained on days 1, 3, and 5 following an acute anterior wall infarction. A planimetered area of 51 cm² and the "doughnut" pattern indicate a large infarct and would suggest a poorer prognosis. On the other hand, the reduction in extent of PYP uptake over the 5-day period may be an encouraging sign (see text).

in 6 out of 8 patients in whom the areas were larger than 40 cm². In the same report, intense (i.e., 4+) focal uptake was associated with a significantly higher mortality and morbidity compared with less intense or diffuse accumulations.

Patients with persistently positive $^{99m}$Tc-pyrophosphate studies, i.e., patients continuing to show uptake 3 or more weeks beyond the time of the original infarction, appear to exhibit a higher incidence of recurrent angina and left ventricular failure than do patients in whom the images quickly revert to normal within a 7- to 14-day period.[49,74,75] Persistently positive studies have been reported to occur in as high as 40 percent of patients with documented acute infarctions.[38] The degree of uptake, however, is rarely as intense at the time of late follow-up imaging as during the initial 24- to 72-hour postinfarction period. Thus, a positive image may represent a potential source of confusion, i.e., the possibility that a positive study in the clinical setting of suspected acute infarction is actually due to a prior acute episode. However, differentiation can usually be made by the history of a previous infarction, a discordance between the serum level of CK-MB isoenzyme and the intensity of uptake on the image, and by noting a change in the uptake pattern on serial imaging during the initial 5 to 7 days postinfarction.

In most cases of suspected acute myocardial infarction, traditional methods for establishing the diagnosis suffice. Thus, $^{99m}$Tc-pyrophosphate imaging is usually reserved for those situations in which either ECG or serum enzyme levels are equivocal, or indeed at odds with the history or clinical findings. For example, the ECG patterns in subendocardial, isolated right ventricular, and old myocardial infarction, as well as in the case of ventricular conduction defects, such as left bundle branch block, frequently make the diagnosis of acute infarction difficult or impossible. In such cases a positive pyrophosphate image may be helpful in establishing the diagnosis with greater certainty. Similarly, imaging with $^{99m}$Tc–pyrophosphate may provide confirmatory evidence of acute myocardial infarction in cases in which a spurious elevation in serum enzymes may have occurred or when an unexpectedly low level is obtained several days after the acute clinical event.

One particularly noteworthy application of $^{99m}$Tc-pyrophosphate is its use in the detection of perioperative myocardial infarction, particularly following coronary revascularization surgery.[78-81] It has been suggested that the imaging procedure may provide greater specificity for acute infarction during the immediate postoperative period than enzyme criteria, since elevation of CK-MB isoenzyme may result merely from cardiac manipulation or from other factors that occur during the time of surgery.

Perhaps the most valuable application of 99mTc-pyrophosphate imaging in the future may be in the early assessment of the extent, location, and uptake characteristics over time, and their use as predictors of clinical outcome. Understandably, it would be preferable if imaging with 99mTc-pyrophosphate could be counted on to detect acute infarction within the initial few hours following the onset of symptoms. In this regard several newer radioactive compounds are being currently investigated.[32,82-84] These

include labeled cardiac myosin antibody, indium-111 ([111]In)-labeled white blood cells, labeled heparin, and various iodinated fluorescein compounds.

Finally, we should consider the relationship between [201]Tl myocardial perfusion imaging (sometimes called "cold-spot" imaging) and 99mTc-pyrophosphate imaging (often called "hot-spot" imaging) and which (if either or both) procedure should be employed in the setting of a suspected acute infarction. In most cases there appears to be a close correspondence between the finding of a focal reduction in [201]Tl

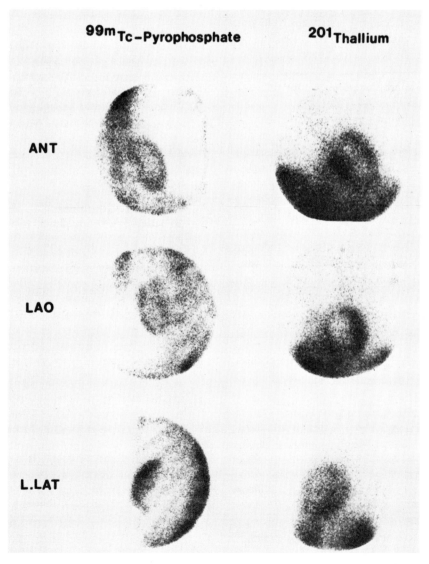

Fig. 12.24  Same patient as in Fig. 12.23 showing focal 99mTc pyrophosphate accumulation (left column) and corresponding reduction in [201]Tl uptake (right column). The anterior location of the site of acute infarction is best appreciated on the lateral views (L. LAT) below.

uptake in an infarcted zone and a comparable site of focal accumulation of $^{99m}$Tc-pyrophosphate (Fig. 12.24). Whereas "cold-spot" imaging primarily reflects the state of regional myocardial perfusion and provides a rough indication of the amount of viable myocardium, and "hot-spot" imaging defines the presence and extent of myocardial cell injury, it should not be surprising to find occasional discordant results, depending on the time following the onset of symptoms that each procedure is performed. If it is important to exclude the presence of an acute myocardial infarction within the initial 8 hours, then $^{201}$Tl imaging appears to be a reasonable confirmatory test, bearing in mind the relatively high cost of the procedure and the low specificity of an abnormal result. In general, the somewhat higher overall sensitivity of $^{99m}$Tc-pyrophosphate imaging for the detection of acute infarction during the 24 to 72 hour period following onset of the patient's symptoms would tend to favor its use in most clinical situations in which the results of cardiac imaging might be helpful in establishing the diagnosis of acute infarction, estimating the extent and location of myocardial injury, and as a possible predictor of short- and long-term morbidity and mortality. Under some circumstances, however, $^{201}$Tl myocardial imaging, when combined with exercise testing 3 weeks after myocardial infarction, may be useful in the identification of residual jeopardized myocardium.[85]

# REFERENCES

1. Hendee WR: Medical Radiation Physics: Roentgenology, Nuclear Medicine and Ultrasound. 2nd ed. Year Book Medical Publishers, Chicago, 1979.
2. Budinger TF: Physics and Physiology of Nuclear Cardiology. *In* Nuclear Cardiology, Willerson JT, editor, Cardiovascular Clinics. FA Davis, Philadelphia, 1979.
3. Lewis SE, Stokely EM, Bonte FJ: Physics and Instrumentation. *In* Clinical Nuclear Cardiology, Parkey RW, Bonte FJ, Buja LM, Willerson JT, editors. Appleton-Century-Crofts, New York, 1979.
4. Budinger TF, Rollo FD: Physics and Instrumentation. *In* Principles of Cardiovascular Nuclear Medicine, A Progress in Cardiovascular Disease Reprint, Holman BL, Sonnenblick EH, Lesch M, editors. Grune and Stratton, New York, 1978.
5. Radiological Health Handbook, Compiled and edited by the Bureau of Radiological Health and the Training Institute, Environmental Control Administration, U.S. Department of Health, Education, and Welfare, Public Health Service, Consumer Protection and Environmental Health Service, Rockville, Maryland, January, 1970, revised edition.
6. Rocha AFB, Harbert JC, editors: Textbook of Nuclear Medicine: Basic Science. Lea and Febiger, Philadelphia, 1978.
7. McAfee JG, Subramanian G: Radioactive Agents for Imaging. *In* Clinical Scintillation Imaging, 2nd ed, Freeman LM, Johnson PM, editors. Grune and Stratton, New York, 1975.
8. Zaret B: Myocardial imaging with radioactive potassium and its analogs. Prog Cardiovasc Dis 20:81–95, 1978.
9. Weiss ES, Siegel BA, Sobel BE, et al: Evaluation of myocardial metabolism and perfusion with positron emitting radionuclides. Prog Cardiovasc Dis 20:191–206, 1978.
10. Chauncey DM, Schelbert, HR, Halpern SE, et al: Tissue distribution studies with radioactive manganese. J Nucl Med 18:933–936, 1977.
11. Prokop E, Strauss HW, Shaw J, et al: Comparison of regional myocardial perfusion determination by ionic potassium-43 to that determined by microspheres. Circulation 50:978–984, 1974.
12. Strauss HW, Harrison K, Langer JK, et al: Thallium-201 for myocardial imaging. Relation of thallium-201 to regional myocardial perfusion. Circulation 51:641–645, 1975.
13. Lebowitz E, Green MV, Fairchild R, et al: $^{201}$Tl for medical use. J Nucl Med 16:151–155, 1975.
14. Schelbert HR, Henning H, Rigo P, et al: Consideration of thallium-201 as a myocardial radionuclide imaging agent in man. Invest Radiol 11: 163–171, 1976.
15. Welch H, Strauss HW, Pitt B: The extraction of thallium-201 by the myocardium. Circulation 56:188–198, 1977.
16. Gewirtz H, O'Keefe D, Pohost G, et al: The effect of ischemia on thallium-201 clearance from the myocardium. Circulation 58:215–219, 1978.
17. Pohost G, Zir L, Moore R, et al: Differentiation of transiently ischemic from infarcted myocardium by serial imaging after a single dose of thallium-201. Circulation 55:294–302, 1977.

18. Schwartz J, Ponto R, Carlyle P, et al: Early redistribution of thallium-201 after temporary ischemia. Circulation 57:332–340, 1978.

19. Schelbert HR, Schuler G, Ashburn WL, et al: Time-course of "redistribution" of thallium-201 administered during transient ischemia. Eur J Nucl Med 4:351–358, 1979.

20. Berger BC, Watson DD, Burwell LR, et al: Redistribution of thallium at rest in patients with stable and unstable angina and the effect of coronary artery bypass surgery. Circulation 60:1114–1125, 1979.

21. Pohost GM, Alpert NM, Ingwall JS, et al: Thallium redistribution: mechanisms and clinical utility. Sem Nucl Med 10:70–93, 1980.

22. Gordon D, Pfisterer W, Williams R, et al: The effect of diaphragmatic attenuation on thallium-201 images. Clin Nucl Med 4:150–151, 1979.

23. Johnstone DE, Wackers FJ, Berger HJ et al: Effect of patient positioning on left lateral thallium-201 myocardial images. J Nucl Med 20:183–188, 1979.

24. Wackers FJ, vd Schoot JB, Busemann Sokole E, et al: Non-invasive visualization of acute myocardial infarction in man with thallium-201. Br Heart J 37:741–749, 1975.

25. Wackers FJ, Becker A, Samson G, et al: Location and size of infarction estimated from thallium-201 scintigrams. Circulation 56:72–79, 1977.

26. Wackers FJ, Lie KI, Liem KL, et al: Thallium-201 scintigraphy in unstable angina pectoris. Circulation 57:738–742, 1978.

27. Maseri A, Parodi O, Severi S, et al: Transient transmural reduction of myocardial blood flow, demonstrated by thallium-201 scintigraphy as a cause of variant angina. Circulation 54:280–288, 1976.

28. Maseri A. Severi S, DeNes M, et al: "Variant" angina; one aspect of a continuous spectrum of vasospastic myocardial ischemia. Am J Cardiol 42:1019–1035, 1978.

29. Wackers FJ, Lie KI, Liem KL, Busemann Sokole E, et al: Potential value of thallium-201 scintigraphy as a means of selecting patients for the coronary care unit. Br Heart J 41:111–117, 1979.

30. Wackers FJ, Busemann Sokole E, Samson G, et al: Value and limitation of thallium-201 scintigraphy in the acute phase of myocardial infarction. N Engl J Med 295:1–5, 1976.

31. Ritchie J, Zaret B, Strauss H: Myocardial imaging with thallium-201: A multicenter study in patients with angina pectoris or acute myocardial infarction. Am J Cardiol 42:345–350, 1978.

31a. Silverman KJ, Becker LC, Bulkley BH et al:

Value of early thallium-201 scintigraphy for predicting mortality in patients with acute myocardial infarction. Circulation 61:996–1003, 1980.

32. Wynne J, Holman BL, Lesch M: Myocardial scintigraphy by infarct-avid radiotracers. Prog Cardiovasc Dis 20:245–267, 1978.

33. Bonte FJ, Parkey RW, Graham KD, et al: A new method for radionuclide imaging of myocardial infarcts. Radiology 110:473–474, 1974.

34. Parkey RW, Bonte FJ, Meyer SL, et al: A new method for radionuclide imaging of acute myocardial infarction in humans. Circulation 50:540–546, 1974.

35. Buja LM, et al: Morphologic correlations of technetium-99m stannous pyrophosphate imaging of acute myocardial infarcts in dogs. Circulation 52:576–607, 1975.

36. Stokely EM, Buja LM, Lewis SE, et al: Measurement of acute myocardial infarcts in dogs with technetium-99m stannous pyrophosphate scintigrams. J Nucl Med 17:1–5, 1976.

37. Holman BL, Ehrie M, Lesch M: Correlation of acute myocardial infarct scintigraphy with post-mortem studies. Am J Cardiol 37:311–313, 1976.

38. Willerson JT, Parkey RW, Bonte FJ, et al: Pathophysiologic considerations and clinico-pathological correlates of technetium-99m stannous pyrophosphate myocardial scintigraphy. Sem Nucl Med 10:54–69, 1980.

39. Buja LM, Tage AJ, Mukhergee A, et al: Role of elevated tissue calcium in myocardial infarct scintigraphy with technetium pyrophosphate radiopharmaceuticals. Circulation (suppl II) 54:219, 1976.

40. Dewanjee MK: Localization of skeletal-imaging Tc-99m chelates in dead cells in tissue culture. J Nucl Med 17:993–997, 1976.

41. Schelbert H, Ingwall J, Sybers H, et al: Uptake of infarct-imaging agents in reversibly and irreversibly injured myocardium in cultured fetal mouse hearts. Circ Res 39:860–868, 1976.

42. Zaret B, DeCola V, Donabedram R, et al: Dual radionuclide study of myocardial infarction. Circulation 53:422–429, 1976.

43. Henning H, Schelbert H, Righetti H, et al: Dual myocardial imaging with technetium-99m pyrophosphate and thallium-201 for detecting, localizing and sizing acute myocardial infarction. Am J Cardiol 40:147–154, 1977.

44. Kelly RJ, Chilton HM, Hackshaw BT, et al: Comparison of Tc-99m pyrophosphate and Tc-99m methylene diphosphonate in acute myocardial infarction. J Nucl Med 20:402–406, 1979.

45. Donsky MS, Curry GC, Parkey RW: Unstable

angina pectoris. Clinical, angiographic and myocardial scintigraphic observations. Br Heart J
38:257–263, 1976.

46. Abdulla AM, Canedo MI, Cortez BC, et al:
Detection of unstable angina by technetium-99m
pyrophosphate myocardial scintigraphy. Chest
69:168–173, 1976.

47. Prasquier R, Taradash MR, Botvinick E, et al:
The specificity of the diffuse pattern of cardiac
uptake in myocardial infarction imaging with
technetium-99m stannous pyrophosphate. Circulation 55:61–66, 1977.

48. Perez LA, Hoyt BB, Freeman LM: Localization
of myocardial disorders other than infarction
with Tc-99m labeled phosphate agents. J Nucl
Med 17:241–246, 1976.

49. Buja M, Poliner L, Parkey R, et al: Clinicopathologic study of persistently positive technetium-
99m stannous pyrophosphate myocardial scintigrams and myocytolytic degeneration after myocardial infarction. Circulation 56:1016–1023,
1977.

50. Go RT, Chiu CL, Doty DB, et al: Radionuclide
imaging of experimental myocardial contusion.
J Nucl Med 15:1174–1175, 1974.

51. Ahmmod M, Dubiel JP, Verdon TA Jr., et al:
Technetium-99m stannous pyrophosphate myocardial imaging in patients with and without left
ventricular aneurysm. Circulation 53:833–838,
1976.

52. Righetti A, O'Rourke RA, Schelbert H, et al:
Usefulness of preoperative and postoperative Tc-
99m (Sn) pyrophosphate scans in patients with
ischemic and valvular heart disease. Am J Cardiol 39:43–49, 1977.

53. Jengo JA, Mena I, Joe SH, et al: The significance
of calcified valvular heart disease in Tc-99m pyrophosphate myocardial infarction scanning: radiographic, scintigraphic and pathologic correlation. J Nucl Med 18:776–780, 1977.

54. Charko AK, Gordon DH, Bennett JM, et al:
Myocardial imaging with Tc-99m pyrophosphate in patients on adriamycin treatment for
neoplasm. J Nucl Med 18:680–683, 1977.

55. Klein MS, Coleman RE, Roberts R, et al: False
positive Tc-99m (Sn) pyrophosphate myocardial
infarct images related to delayed blood pool
clearance. Clin Nucl Med 1:45–47, 1976.

56. Serafini AN, Raskin MM, Zand LC, et al: Radionuclide breast scanning in carcinoma of the
breast. J Nucl Med 15:1149–1152, 1974.

57. Hisada K, Suzuki Y, Iimari M: Technetium-99m
pyrophosphate bone imaging in the evaluation
of trauma. Clin Nucl Med 1:18–25, 1976.

58. Kim E: Calcified costal cartilage as a cause of

false interpretation on myocardial imaging. Clin
Nucl Med 1:159–161, 1976.

59. Pugh BR, Buja LM, Parkey RM, et al: Cardioversion and "false positive" technetium-99m
stannous pyrophosphate myocardial scintigrams.
Circulation 54:399–403, 1976.

60. Davison R, Spies S, Przybylek J, et al: Techne-
tium-99m stannous pyrophosphate myocardial
scintigraphy after cardiopulmonary resuscitation
with cardioversion. Circulation 60:292–299,
1979.

61. Bassuyt A, Verberlen D: Accumulation of Tc-
99m pyrophosphate in the skin lesions of pseu-
doxanthoma elasticum. Clin Nucl Med 1:245,
1976.

62. Botvinick EH, Shames D, Lappin H, et al: Noninvasive quantitation of myocardial infarction
with technetium-99m pyrophosphate. Circulation 52:909–915, 1975.

63. Marcus M, Kerber R: Present status of the tech-
netium-99m pyrophosphate infarct scintigram.
Circulation 56:335–240, 1977.

64. Walsh WF, Karunaratne HB, Resnekov L, et
al: Assessment of diagnostic value of technetium-
99m pyrophosphate myocardial scintigraphy in
80 patients with possible acute myocardial infarction. Br Heart J 39:974–984, 1977.

65. Holman BL, Lesch M, Alpert J: Myocardial
scintigraphy with technetium-99m pyrophosphate during the early phase of acute infarction.
Am J Cardiol 41:39–41, 1978.

66. Poliner L, Buja LM, Parkey R, et al: Clinicopathologic findings in 52 patients studied by
technetium-99m stannous pyrophosphate myocardial scintigraphy. Circulation 59:257–267,
1979.

67. Willerson J, Parkey R, Buja LM, et al: Detection
of acute myocardial infarcts using myocardial
scintigraphic techniques. In Clinical Nuclear
Cardiology, Parkey R, Bonte F, Buja LM, Willerson J, editors. Appleton-Century-Crofts, New
York, 1979.

68. Cuaron A, Acero AP, Cardenas M, et al: Interobserver variability in the interpretation of myocardial images with Tc-99m labeled diphosphonate and pyrophosphate. J Nucl Med 21:1–9,
1980.

69. Willerson JT et al: Acute subendocardial myocardial infarction in patients; its detection by
technetium-99m stannous pyrophosphate myocardial scintigrams. Circulation 51:436–441,
1975.

70. Massie B. Botvinick E, Werner J, et al: Myocardial scintigraphy with technetium-99m stannous
pyrophosphate: an insensitive test for nontrans-

mural myocardial infarction. Am J Cardiol 43:186–193, 1979.

71. Rude RE, Parkey RW, Bonte FJ, et al: Clinical implications of the technetium-99m stannous pyrophosphate myocardial scintigraphic "doughnut" pattern in patients with acute myocardial infarcts. Circulation 59:721–730, 1979.

72. Ahmad M, Logan KW, Martin R: Doughnut pattern of technetium-99m pyrophosphate myocardial uptake in patients with acute myocardial infarction: a sign of poor longterm prognosis. Am J Cardiol 44:13–17, 1979.

73. Holman BL, Chisholm RJ, Braunwald E: The prognostic implications of acute myocardial infarct scintigraphy with technetium-99m pyrophosphate. Circulation 57:320–326, 1978.

74. Olson H, Lyons K, Aranow WS, et al: Followup technetium-99m stannous pyrophosphate myocardial scintigrams after acute myocardial infarction. Circulation 56:181–188, 1977.

75. Olson H, Lyons K, Aranow WS, et al: Prognostic value of a persistently positive technetium-99m stannous pyrophosphate myocardial scintigram after myocardial infarction. Am J Cardiol 43:889–898, 1979.

76. Sharpe DN, Botvinick EH, Shames DM, et al: The noninvasive diagnosis of right ventricular infarction. Circulation 57:483–490, 1978.

77. Tobinick E, Schelbert H, Henning H, et al: Right ventricular ejection fraction in patients with acute anterior and inferior myocardial infarction assessed by radionuclide angiography. Circulation 57:1084, 1978.

78. Platt MR, Parkey RW, Willerson JT, et al: Technetium-99m stannous pyrophosphate myocardial scintigrams in the recognition of myocardial infarction in patients undergoing coronary artery revascularization. Ann Thoracic Surg 21:311–317, 1976.

79. Righetti A, Crawford M, O'Rourke R, et al: Detection of perioperative myocardial infarction after coronary artery bypass graft surgery. Circulation 55:173–178, 1977.

80. Klausner S, Botvinick E, Shames D, et al: The application of radionuclide infarct scintigraphy to diagnose perioperative myocardial infarction following revascularization. Circulation 56:173–180, 1977.

81. Burdine J, DePuey EG, Drzan F, et al: Scintigraphic, electrocardiographic and enzymatic diagnosis of perioperative myocardial infarction in patients undergoing myocardial revascularization. J Nucl Med 20:711–714, 1979.

82. Alonso D, Jacobstein J, Apriano P, et al: Early quantification of experimental myocardial infarction with technetium-99m glucoheptonate. Scintigraphic and anatomic studies. Am J Cardiol 42:251–258, 1978.

83. Khaw B, Beller G, Haber E: Experimental myocardial infarct imaging following intravenous administration of iodine-131 labeled antibody (Fab')$_2$ fragments specific for cardiac myosin. Circulation 57:743–750, 1978.

84. Thakur ML, Gottschalk A, Zaret B: Imaging experimental myocardial infarction with indium-111 labeled autologous leukocytes: effects of infarct age and residual regional myocardial blood flow. Circulation 60:297–304, 1979.

85. Turner JD, Schwartz KM, Logic JR et al: Detection of residual jeopardized myocardium 3 weeks after myocardial infarction by exercise testing with thallium-201 myocardial scintigraphy. Circulation 61:729–737, 1980.

# Section 5
# COMPLICATIONS OF ACUTE MYOCARDIAL INFARCTION AND THEIR TREATMENT

# 13 | Pathophysiology of Arrhythmia

## Guy P. Curtis, M.D., Ph.D.

Normal synchronous mechanical activity of the heart depends upon a specific sequence of electrical activation for all myocardial cells during each beat, beginning first at the sinoatrial (SA) node and ending with depolarization of the ventricle. This normal activation sequence occurs during most cardiac cycles for several reasons:

1. A single pacemaker with the most rapid rate will trigger electrical activation of the heart, suppressing other pacemakers. The pacemaker cells with the most rapid rates are usually found within the SA node.

2. The specialized conduction system rapidly and uniformly conducts the impulse from the SA node to the atria and then to the ventricles so that these structures are synchronously activated.

3. Recovery of electrical excitability is delayed following myocardial activation resulting in a considerable distance and many inexcitable cells between activated fibers and those that have recovered and are thus capable of being reexcited. This barrier of inexcitable cells normally assures that a fiber will be activated one time only during each cardiac cycle.

Cardiac arrhythmias result when there are alterations in myocardial impulse formation (automaticity) and/or myocardial impulse propagation (conduction). These alterations in electrophysiologic properties of the myocardium are manifested by abnormalities in the heart rate, the heart rhythm, or both.

Even the normal heart possesses electrophysiologic properties that can produce arrhythmias. A variety of abnormal cardiac rhythms have been reported in subjects with no known cardiac disease.[1-5] Single as well as multiple ventricular and/or atrial premature beats have been observed in this population, with a few patients demonstrating paroxysmal atrial or ventricular tachycardia. The electrophysiologic alterations necessary to initiate and sustain these arrhythmias can apparently be elicited in the normal heart under special circumstances (i.e., during increases in autonomic tone). For instance, sustained atrial fibrillation can be initiated during maintained vagal stimulation, and sustained ventricular arrhythmia occurs in association with discharge of the cardiac adrenergic nerves which can be accomplished via stimulation of the left stellate ganglion.[6-9]

In the presence of coronary artery disease, premature beats, which are commonly well tolerated in the normal myocardium, may trigger a rapid sustained arrhythmia with its attendant hemodynamic embarrassment; such an arrhythmia may even result in sudden death.[10] Thus, the duration, characteristics, and frequency of an arrhythmia appear to depend upon both the electrophysiologic properties of the myocardial cells participating in the arrhythmia and the frequency with which suitable initiating events (i.e, premature beats) occur. Ischemic heart disease is known to result in conditions favorable to sustained rapid ventricular arrhythmia, which is presumably the mechanism for sudden death associated with coronary artery disease. Furthermore, the extent of ischemic disease may influence the incidence of single premature beats which can act as initiating stimuli for life-threatening arrhythmias.

In order to understand the pathophysiology of arrhythmia, it is necessary to go from the multicellular level where the summed vectors of cardiac electrical activation are monitored via the electrocardiogram to the cellular level where the behavior of individual cells and networks of cells can be monitored and understood. The reason for this is that very different electrophysiologic mechanisms can lead to the same electrocardiographic result.

To define the pathologic mechanisms of arrhythmia in man, a number of different types of electrophysiologic studies have been carried out:

1. In vitro studies of tissue obtained from patients with ischemic heart disease at the time of operation.[11]

2. Intraoperative conduction studies in areas of scar or aneurysm where arrhythmias are thought to originate.[12-14]

3. Studies in patients with arrhythmias employing electrically induced premature beats, overdrive suppression of arrhythmias, and His bundle studies to characterize abnormal rhythm.[15-18]

4. Classification of arrhythmia mechanism by therapeutic response to antiarrhythmic drugs.[19]

5. The study of experimental models of arrhythmia that behave like the clinical counterpart.[20]

The aim of all these studies is the acquisition of knowledge of the electrophysiologic mechanisms facilitating these arrhythmias so that these conditions can be effectively prevented with treatment.

In this chapter, basic electrophysiologic concepts that are important in normal and pathologic states will be reviewed and cellular mechanisms postulated for the production of arrhythmias will be outlined. In addition, the electrophysiologic alterations that accompany ischemia will be discussed in relation to these mechanisms for arrhythmia.

## NORMAL CARDIAC ELECTROPHYSIOLOGY

Myocardial fibers or cells are in some ways similar to electric wires. The cell membrane can be viewed as an insulator wrapped around the intracellular contents, the conducting core. There are low-resistance connections (tight junctions or nexus) between cells allowing intercellular current flow. The cell membrane demonstrates selective permeability and, when current is passed across it, demonstrates behavior best modeled electrically with a resistance and capacitance connected in parallel (see Fig. 13.1).

There is a voltage that can be measured across the cell membrane between cardiac cycles called the resting membrane potential (RMP). The inside of the cell is more negative than the outside. This RMP reflects an electrochemical equilibrium resulting from the selective permeability characteristics of the cell membrane (potassium crosses the cell membrane but other ions are much less permeable), and the relative concentrations of ions inside and outside the cell (see Table 13.1). The equilibrium potential for each ion (Eion) distributed across the cell membrane can be calculated from the Nernst equation:

$$E_{ion} = \frac{R\,T}{Z\,F} \ln \frac{C_2}{C_1}$$

where Z is the valence of the ion in question; $C_1$ and $C_2$ are the concentrations of ion inside

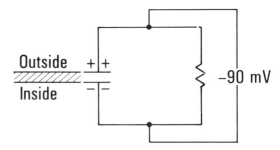

Fig. 13.1 Circuit diagram representing the myocardial cell membrane during diastole. The transmembrane potential is −90 mV with the inside of the membrane negative with respect to the outside. The cell membrane at rest is represented by a resistor and a capacitor connected in parallel.

Table 13.1. Approximate steady state ion concentrations across the cell membrane with their equilibrium potentials

| Ions | Intracellular | Extracellular | Nernst $E_{ion}$ (mV) |
|---|---|---|---|
| *Cations* | | | |
| Sodium | 10 mM | 140 mM | +42 |
| Potassium | 150 mM | 4 mM | −97 |
| Calcium | 0.0001 mM | 2 mM | +133 |
| *Anions* | | | |
| Chloride | 30 mM | 140 mM | −41 |
| Bicarbonate | 8 mM | 27 mM | −24 |

and outside of the cell membrane; R is the gas constant; T is the absolute temperature; and F is Faraday's constant. Rearranging for 37°C and $\log_{10}$, one obtains $E_{ion}$ millivolts = 61.5 $\log \frac{C_1}{C_2}$. The calculated equilbrium potential for potassium is −97 mV and for sodium +42 mV. The RMP for most cells in the heart is from −90 to −80 mV, approximating the potassium equilibrium potential. This value is not exactly the same as the potassium equilibrium potential because the cell membrane is permeable to other ions besides potassium, and a more exact approximation for the RMP ($V_r$) can be made using the Goldman equation[21,22] where membrane permeability is considered.

$$V_r = \frac{R\,T}{F} \log \frac{K_i\,P_K + Na_i\,P_{Na} + Cl_o\,P_{Cl}}{K_o\,P_K + Na_o\,P_{Na} + Cl_i\,P_{Cl}}$$

where $P_K$, $P_{Na}$ and $P_{Cl}$ refer to the relative permeability of potassium, sodium, and chloride ions, respectively, and o refers to ion concentration outside the cell and i refers to ion concentration inside the cell.

If the RMP is truly determined primarily by potassium, its value should vary with the concentration of potassium in the extracellular fluid. Figure 13.2 compares the potassium equilibrium potential, calculated from the Nernst equation, with the measured RMP as the concentrations of extracellular potassium changes. There is good agreement between the two values until extracellular potassium reaches low levels, reflecting the larger contribution of other ions to the RMP when $K_o$ is low. Changes in potassium permeability induced by decreasing the concentrations of extracellular potassium are

also involved. Thus, the RMP appears to be primarily determined by the potassium equilibrium potential because of the permeability characteristics of the cell membrane.

Local application of a small depolarizing current results in membrane depolarization at the site of current application which decreases exponentially with distance from the site of current application (see Fig. 13.3). The permeability characteristics of the membrane do not change, depolarization is not propagated, and this perturbation is called a "local response."

Application of larger amounts of depolarizing current will cause the cell membrane to reach threshold potential at the site of current

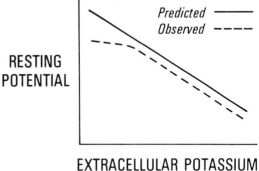

RESTING POTENTIAL

EXTRACELLULAR POTASSIUM CONCENTRATION

Fig. 13.2 The observed transmembrane potential (TMP) with variations in extracellular potassium ion concentration compared with the calculated equilibrium potential for potassium from the Nernst equation. Decreased correlation between predicted and observed values for TMP at low extracellular potassium ion concentrations reflects the influence of other ions on TMP under these conditions as well as the influence of extracellular potassium on potassium conductance.

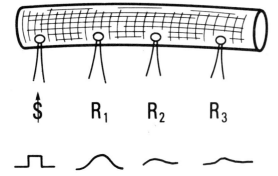

Fig. 13.3 The effects of a subthreshold stimulus on the transmembrane potential at recording sites $R_1$, $R_2$, and $R_3$. As distance from the stimulus site increases, the amplitude and rate of depolarization for the local response decreases.

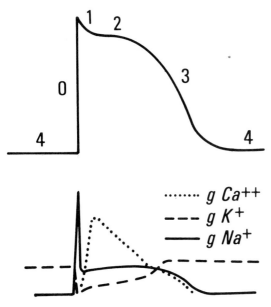

Fig. 13.4 An action potential *(top panel)* and the membrane conductances for potassium ($K^+$), sodium ($Na^+$), and calcium ($Ca^{++}$) *(lower panel)* during the different phases of the action potential. In the upper panel, Phase 0 represents rapid cellular depolarization secondary to a transient increase in sodium conductance while potassium conductance is simultaneously decreased. During Phase 1, the transmembrane potential achieved during the overshoot of the action potential rapidly returns to zero potential. Phase 2 of the action potential—the plateau phase—is associated with increased calcium movement. Phase 3 or repolarization of the action potential is associated with decreases in $Ca^{++}$ flux and increases in potassium conductance.

application. When the cell membrane reaches the threshold potential, a sudden, very transient change in permeability characteristics occurs resulting in the transmembrane potential alterations called the "action potential" (see Fig. 13.4).

### The Action Potential

The action potential has been divided into five phases, as Figure 13.4 shows. *Phase 0,* the *rapid-rising phase,* is known to be mediated by transient inward movement of sodium ion ("fast response"). Translocation of sodium ion occurs because the membrane permeability to sodium increases for a few msec, allowing sodium to approach its equilibrium potential of +42 mV.[23-26] There is also a slower developing, longer lasting inward movement of positive charges carried largely but not exclusively by calcium ion, as Figure 13.4 shows.[27] This slower movement of positive ions begins at membrane potentials less negative than threshold potential (−35 mV) and can be observed in cells where sodium currents are inactivated with tetrodotoxin or by slow depolarization. These resultant "slow response" action potentials are normally found in the atrioventricular (A-V) node area, in the SA node, and around the A-V valves. The slow current for slow response action potentials inactivates with a long time constant (100 msec).[27] How rapidly Phase 0 develops is a function of (1) the resting membrane potential (see Fig. 13.5) and (2) the equilibrium potential for sodium in "fast response" action potentials and calcium in "slow response" action potentials.[27,28]

*Phase 1* of the action potential is seen in the fast response action potential and results because the transmembrane potential reaches a value influenced by the sodium equilibrium potential where the inside of the cell is positive relative to the outside. This is called the *overshoot* and is not seen in slow response action potentials. Chloride ions seem to be involved in bringing the transmembrane potential to zero following the overshoot.[28]

During *Phase 2,* or the *plateau* of the action potential, the slowly developing inward movement of positive charge carried largely by cal-

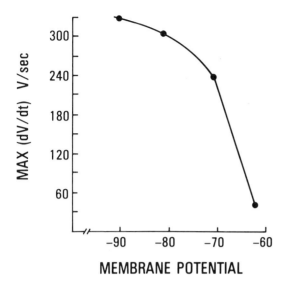

Fig. 13.5  The influence of membrane potential on the slope of Phase 0 of the action potential. As transmembrane potential is decreased, the upstroke velocity of the action potential also decreases.

cium ion peaks and begins to inactivate. Potassium permeability which falls with Phase 0 of the action potential begins to return. *Phase 3, repolarization,* results from inactivation of transmembrane calcium flux and a time- and voltage-dependent increase in potassium permeability[30-33] (see Fig. 13.4).

*Phase 4* of the action potential is not associated with any net current flow or ionic translocation in cells without automaticity. Purkinje fibers demonstrate automaticity and slow diastolic depolarization during Phase 4, a characteristic of all automatic cells (see Fig. 13.6). Phase 4 depolarization in Purkinje fibers is known to be related to the constant diastolic inward movement of sodium ion and a time-dependent decrease in potassium permeability, allowing the cell to gain net positive charge and to slowly depolarize to threshold potential.[34,35] Other pacemaker fibers may not share this mechanism for Phase 4 depolarization; rather, this change may be mediated by a time-dependent increase in the slow inward current carried largely by calcium.[36,37]

Once the membrane is depolarized, another action potential cannot be immediately elicited, and the membrane is refractory to stimulation. The absolute refractory period is defined as the

time period that this condition is present. There follows a voltage- and time-dependent recovery of excitability when the cell is relatively refractory to stimulation and increased current is required to elicit an action potential (see Fig. 13.7).[28] This relative refractory period ends when excitability reaches a stable value during Phase 4. The relation of voltage to time for excitability may be different in different fibers as refractoriness may outlast action potential duration in fibers where slow response action potentials are observed, while this would be most uncommon in fibers with fast response action potentials.[38]

The action potential serves as a source for potential difference and current flow within the myocardial fiber. Current flow between resting and depolarized membrane segments results in membrane depolarization of resting segments to threshold potential and action potential propagation. Impulse conduction, therefore, depends on the cable properties (current-conducting properties) of myocardial fibers as well as the action potential characteristics discussed above.

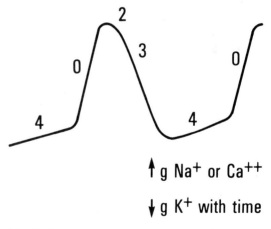

↑ g Na⁺ or Ca⁺⁺

↓ g K⁺ with time

Fig. 13.6  Action potential drawn from a pacemaker cell with action potential phases labeled. Pacemaker cells differ from other cells in that, during Phase 4, sodium and/or calcium membrane conductance is increased and there is a time-dependent decrease in outward current (represented here as gK⁺). These Phase 4 alterations lead to Phase 4 depolarization which reaches threshold potential, resulting in subsequent Phase 0 depolarization and spontaneous automaticity.

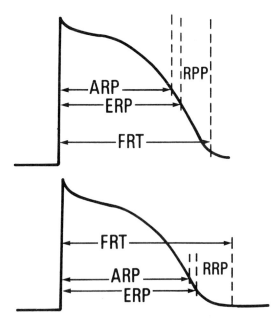

Fig. 13.7 Relationship between the action potential and the recovery of excitability in two different fibers. ARP = absolute refractory period; ERP = effective refractory period; RRP = relative refractory period; and FRT = full recovery time. Recovery of excitability is both time- and voltage-dependent. In the lower panel action potential duration is slightly abbreviated while ARP, ERP, and FRT are increased compared to the upper panel. Premature responses from the fiber in the lower panel would arise later, from more negative transmembrane potentials, and thus have greater amplitude and Phase 0 slope. This would lead to enhanced depolarizing current flow and enhanced conduction.

## CABLE PROPERTIES OF MYOCARDIAL FIBERS

Local application of a small depolarizing current results in membrane depolarization at the site of current application which does not reach the threshold potential. The steady state value for the effective decrease in membrane potential falls exponentially if the membrane potential is sampled further and further away from the site of current application. The decrease in effective membrane potential depolarization with distance occurs because cardiac cells demonstrate internal resistivity; therefore, current ($i_a$) flowing in the longitudinal direction along the fiber can be described as:

$$i_a = \frac{dV}{dx} \cdot \frac{1}{r_a}$$

where $r_a$ is internal resistance of the fiber, x is the distance from the site of current application, and V is the change in transmembrane potential from the resting state. The transmembrane current at any point along the fiber will be related to how rapidly current flow decreases as the distance from the current source is increased:

$$i_m = \frac{di_a}{dx}$$

where $i_m$ is the membrane current and $i_a$ is the axial current. Combining these two equations for determination of membrane current yields:

$$i_m = \frac{d^2V}{dx^2} \cdot \frac{1}{r_a}$$

Since the electrical behavior of the myocardial fiber can be represented by a resistance-capacitance circuit (see Fig. 13.1), membrane current flow must consist of two components: the ionic current ($i_e$) and the capacitance current ($i_c$). Thus, the membrane current can be represented as the sum of capacitance and ionic currents:

$$i_m = C_m \cdot \frac{dV}{dt} + i_e$$

Expressions for axial current flow and summed transmembrane currents can be combined, and the equation for conduction velocity $\theta$ for an action potential can be derived:

$$\theta = \sqrt{\frac{a \cdot K}{2 R_i C_m}}$$

where a is fiber radius; K is a constant proportional to current flow during excitation; $C_m$ is membrane capacitance; and $R_i$ is internal resistance of the fiber to current flow.[39-41] Once the initial large capacitance current ceases to flow as the capacity is charged up, dV/dt declines to zero, and the extent of spatial spread of current is related to the ratio between the membrane resistance and the internal resistance of the fiber. From these expressions, it is apparent that the relationship between internal resistance of the myocardial fiber to current flow compared with the membrane resistance to current flow, and the membrane capacitance are cable properties important in determining conduction velocity.[41] Changes in these parameters could importantly influence conduction in the absence of any change in the action potential characteristics. It is also apparent that the form of the action potential will influence the value for current flow during excitation and the value for the constant K in the expression above. If the action potential is of large amplitude, more current will flow than if the action potential amplitude is small.

The rate of rise of the action potential during Phase 0 is also an important determinant of conduction velocity. When current flows along the fiber, there is an initial large capacity current that results in an initial rapid change in voltage. However, as the membrane capacity

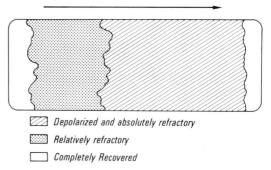

Depolarized and absolutely refractory
Relatively refractory
Completely Recovered

Fig. 13.9 Schematic representation of depolarization and recovery of excitability in an infinitely long strip of cardiac muscle. The arrow *(top)* represents the direction of movement for the depolarizing wavefront. The absolute refractory period represents a barrier to reexcitation of cells previously depolarized, as there are many inexcitable cells between the wavefront of depolarizing cells and cells capable of being reexcited.

becomes charged up, the capacity current will decline toward zero—as will the change in voltage with time—and an equilibrium state will be achieved. The more rapid the rise of Phase 0 of the action potential, the more rapid will be the approach to this equilibrium state at sites removed from the action potential; this directly influences the depolarization time to threshold potential and thus the conduction velocity (see Fig. 13.8). Depolarization initiated early in recovery is associated with low amplitude and slowly rising action potentials. It follows, then, that these abnormal action potentials result in slow conduction because they are associated with less effective depolarizing current distal to the action potential site and because the membrane being depolarized by current flow is relatively refractory to depolarization.

The absolute refractory period of the membrane and the plateau phase of the action potential result in an inexcitable barrier between depolarizing and recovered cells (see Fig. 13.9). This barrier tends to prevent retrograde excitation of previously depolarized membranes. Slowing the conduction velocity and/or decreasing the absolute refractory period and action potential duration brings depolarizing cells closer to recovered cells and increases the chances of retrograde excitation.

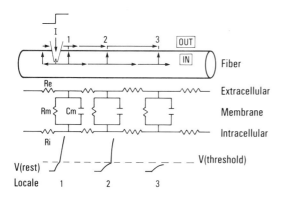

Fig. 13.8 Schematic representation of sequential myocardial fiber depolarization. Top panel represents myocardial fiber with current, I, applied as a square wave voltage across the membrane. Circuit diagrams and transmembrane potentials are presented in the middle and lower panels for recording sites 1, 2, and 3. In the circuit diagram, Rm = membrane resistance; Cm = membrane capacitance; Re = extracellular resistance to current flow; and Ri = intracellular resistance to current flow. Vrest = resting transmembrane potential and Vthreshold = threshold potential in the lower panel. (The effects of applied current on the membrane potential are discussed in the text.)

# CELLULAR MECHANISMS FOR ARRHYTHMIA

Mechanisms postulated to cause arrhythmias can be classified under three broad categories: (1) altered cellular automaticity, (2) reentry, and (3) altered excitability. Each of these mechanisms will be discussed separately below, but in ischemia and infarction they may coexist.

## Altered Cellular Automaticity

Cells that demonstrate Phase 4 diastolic depolarization have the potential for becoming pacemakers and thus a focus for ectopic beats. Increased focal activity will result when such a cell begins to fire independently at a faster rate than the sinus node or begins to compete with the normal sinus mechanism because of unidirectional block into the area where the automatic cell is located, protecting the automatic cell from sinus node initiated depolarization. (i.e., a parasystolic focus).

The rate of discharge for an automatic cell can be altered in several ways. Phase 4 diastolic depolarization will reach threshold potential more rapidly if: (1) there is a decrease in the maximum diastolic potential; (2) there is an increase in the threshold potential; or (3) there is an increase in the rate of Phase 4 depolarization (see Fig. 13.10). Pacemaker cells operating during Phase 4 in the range of normal resting potentials (from $-70$ to $-90$ mV) may demonstrate subthreshold oscillations before pace-

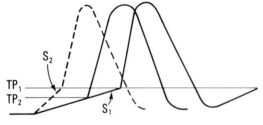

Fig. 13.10 Mechanisms for increasing spontaneous pacemaker fiber rate. $TP_1$ and $TP_2$ represent two different threshold potentials, while $S_1$ and $S_2$ represent two different slopes for Phase 4 diastolic depolarization. Mechanisms illustrated include decreasing the voltage between resting potential and TP, and increasing the slope for diastolic depolarization as in $S_2$ (i.e., catecholamine administration).

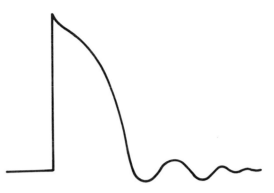

Fig. 13.11 Afterpotentials following an action potential. If positive afterpotentials reach threshold potential repetitive spontaneous activity can result.

maker discharge occurs, and Phase 4 depolarization may depend on transmembrane sodium flux as well as time-dependent decreases in potassium efflux ($iK_2$ current).[41,42] Drugs depressing transmembrane sodium flux (e.g., local anesthetics) or activating $iK_2$ will suppress these pacemakers. Automaticity initiated from less negative membrane potentials where fast sodium current is inactivated ($-40$ mV or less) depends on slow current that seems, at least in part, to be calcium mediated.

Low-voltage oscillations—in the form of positive afterpotentials following a normal action potential or in the form of prolonged Phase 2 depolarization with associated low-voltage oscillations—have been observed in Purkinje fibers and may be associated with focal activity (see Fig. 13.11).[43] Such low-voltage oscillations have been observed when extracellular potassium is low, in anoxia, in chloride-free solutions, and after treatment with ouabain, aconitine, and dinitrophenol.[41] The mechanism producing these oscillations is unclear. High extracellular calcium concentration, catecholamines, and hypokalemia tend to increase the amplitude of low-voltage oscillations, and they could be significant sites of focal activity in ischemia.

Automaticity has also been reported in depolarized fibers with slow response action potentials after these fibers have been driven for several cycles.[44-46] This type of automaticity is felt to be related to diastolic oscillatory activity similar to that discussed above. It also contrasts sharply with the behavior of normal pacemakers, where overdriving the spontaneous discharge rate results in diastolic hyperpolarization and overdrive suppression.

It has been appreciated that, in addition to time-dependent increases in inward current and decreases in outward current, changes in cell-to-cell coupling could produce changes in automaticity in cells with spontaneous Phase 4 activity. Pacemaker cells may demonstrate enhanced automaticity if they are freed from the electrotonic influences of cells with more negative transmembrane potentials which would tend to increase the diastolic membrane potential and slow Phase 4 depolarization rate; this sort of uncoupling may occur in areas of ischemia.[11]

Focal activity due to afterpotential oscillations may arise in adjacent cells that have different time courses for recovery of the resting membrane potential following depolarization. Recovered cells may hasten repolarization of adjacent cells with longer action potential durations, while depolarized cells would tend to depolarize cells that have achieved their resting membrane potentials. At the moment that repolarization is complete in all adjacent cells, current ceases to flow between cells; the aftereffects of current flow might theoretically produce positive afterpotentials reaching threshold potential, resulting in an action potential. Such a mechanism is similar to the redistribution of charge that is observed following termination of a low-intensity, long duration current pulse.[41]

## Reentry

Continuous conduction of an impulse will occur when conduction alterations are present that allow recovered tissue previously excited to be in close proximity to depolarizing cells so that reexcitation of cells occurs (the impulse reenters cells previously depolarized). The requirements for a reentrant loop have been summarized by Moe: (1) block of an impulse at some site within the conducting network; (2) slow conduction over an alternative pathway; (3) delayed activation of tissue beyond the block; and (4) reexcitation of tissue proximal to the block.[47] Given the normal conduction velocities for areas outside of the SA and A-V nodes, and the duration for refractory periods, very long pathways would be required for reentry and such a process would be unlikely in the intact heart. If conduction is slowed by low voltage or slow rising action potentials, however, conduction would be slow enough to support such a mechanism. Slow response action potentials in a localized area of a conduct-

Table 13.2. Comparison of characteristics of slow and fast response action potentials

| Property | Fast Response | Slow Response |
|---|---|---|
| 1. Resting membrane potential | $-80$ to $-90$ mV | $-40$ to $-60$ mV |
| 2. Ion carrying depolarizing current | Sodium | Calcium |
| 3. Depolarizing current blocker | Tetrodotoxin, depolarization | Verapamil, D-600 |
| 4. Threshold for depolarizing current activation | $-60$ to $-70$ mV | $-30$ to $-40$ mV |
| 5. Action potential amplitude | 100 to 130 mV | 35 to 75 mV |
| 6. Conduction velocity | 0.5 to 3.0 m/sec | 0.01 to 0.1 m/sec |
| 7. Safety factor for conduction | High | Low |
| 8. Recovery of full excitability | Complete with full repolarization | Often outlasts action potential duration |
| 9. Latent automaticity | Rarely demonstrated | Often demonstrated |
| 10. Catecholamines | Little effect | Enhancement |
| 11. Location | Normal atrial & ventricular muscle fibers & Purkinje fibers | SA node AV node Ischemic tissue |

ing pathway would increase the likelihood for reentry in the intact heart (see Table 13.2). Slow potentials normally are present in the SA node and the A-V node and are observed in depolarized myocardial cells where fast sodium current is inactivated.[48-50] Such potentials have also been recorded from ischemic tissues.[20]

What has been described as "circus movement" or, more recently, "macro-reentry" occurs when a wave of excitation travels around an anatomical obstacle, an anatomical loop, or along functional pathways (see Fig. 13.12). Macro-reentrant arrhythmias have been demonstrated in tissues with slow response action potentials (i.e., the A-V node, the SA node) as well as in those with clearly separate parallel pathways possessing different electrophysiologic characteristics (i.e., paroxysmal atrial tachycardia associated with Wolf-Parkinson-White preexcitation syndromes)[51-55] (see Figs. 13.13, 13.14).

Multiple wavelets have been proposed as a reentrant mechanism for atrial fibrillation by Moe[47] and represent the concept of micro-reentry with small wavelets and everchanging reentrant loops derived from functional tissue differences resulting from inhomogeneous electrical properties. Many wavelets encountering islands of tissue in different stages of recovery "change velocity, number, direction, and breadth" but continue to circulate because of random but adequate small reentry circuits. Obviously, a mixture of tissue with normal and slow response action potentials would best support such a mechanism; such a mixture has been docu-

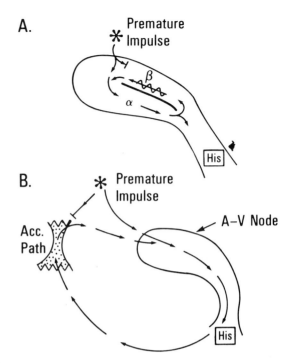

Fig. 13.13 Two examples of macroreentry. *(A)* The mechanism for nodal reentrant paroxysmal atrial tachycardia. A premature impulse is blocked because of incomplete recovery in the beta pathway and conducts over the alpha pathway. Beta pathway excitation occurs in a retrograde manner allowing reentry to occur. *(B)* Reentry in the Wolff-Parkinson-White syndrome. The premature impulse is blocked at the accessory pathway because of incomplete recovery, enters the ventricle via the A-V node and His-Purkinje system; it then reenters the atrium via retrograde conduction over the accessory pathway.

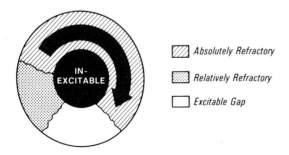

Fig. 13.12 Schematic representation of circus movement with arrow showing the direction of movement for fiber activation. As long as an "excitable gap" of recovered cells precedes the wavefront of depolarizing cells, this mechanism should be sustained.

mented in the infarct zone in dogs surviving experimentally induced myocardial infarction.[43,56,57]

Moe and coworkers have proposed another mechanism for continuous conduction termed "reflection."[58] In this model, electrotonic current flow across an inexcitable gap results in sufficient current flow to depolarize fibers distal to the gap to the threshold potential; after some delay, an action potential results. Enough time can elapse for excitation of cells distal to the gap such that reexcitation in the reverse direction of proximal cells occurs across the gap by electrotonic transmission leading to "reflection" of the impulse. Reflection may be a mechanism involved in extrasystoles and parasystole.

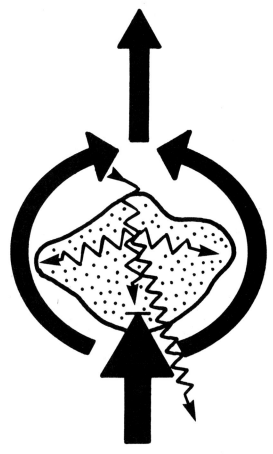

Fig. 13.14 Schematic representation of microreentry. The wavefront encounters an island of refractory tissue (stippled area), then fragments and coalesces with reentry via retrograde excitation through a previously refractory island. Slowed conduction is represented by wavy arrows.

## Altered Excitability

Changes in membrane capacity, membrane resistance, and internal myocardial fiber resistance can obviously have an effect on current flow that results from the action potential. Cell-to-cell coupling and intercellular resistance to current flow will also affect conduction velocity. These factors could slow conduction and produce effects similar to those that accompany slow response action potentials that would facilitate reentry. Standard microelectrode techniques do not assess these parameters, and only recently has their potential importance been appreciated. Recently, Spear and coworkers have de-

scribed abnormalities of cellular activation within infarcted tissue that could be explained, in large part, by alterations in tissue excitability.[11]

## ELECTROPHYSIOLOGIC ALTERATIONS ACCOMPANYING ISCHEMIA

Microelectrode studies and studies using suction microelectrodes on the epicardial surface have shown that acute ischemia is accompanied by a progressive decrease in action potential duration, amplitude, and upstroke velocity.[59-64] Cells in severely ischemic areas of the myocardium may eventually become and remain depolarized. Postrepolarization refractoriness develops with evidence for local block and decremental conduction. Inhomogeneity for electrophysiologic properties is evident between cells and from beat to beat within the same cell. Slow response action potentials have been noted, and the slope for Phase 4 depolarization is increased in ischemic Purkinje fibers.

Studies in tissue after chronic infarction have shown a variety of electrophysiologic findings.[56,57,65] There is usually a rim of surviving Purkinje fibers and myocardial cells on the endocardial surface with normal electrophysiologic characteristics. However, this area also contains slow response fibers that demonstrate spontaneous automaticity that can be suppressed by a "slow channel" [calcium] inhibitor (verapamil). In addition, there are cells with normal resting potentials and variable electrophysiologic properties as well as inexcitable cells. Deeper within the infarct is primarily scar tissue.

These known electrophysiologic alterations accompanying ischemia would support most of the mechanisms for arrhythmia proposed above. Through continued investigation of the electrophysiologic characteristics of ischemic myocardial fibers and a more complete knowledge of the effects of antiarrhythmic agents in ischemic tissue, both the effects of antiarrhythmic agents in ischemic tissue and the true pathophysiologic mechanisms of arrhythmia can be identified.

# REFERENCES

1. Brodsky M, et al: Arrhythmias documented by 24 hour continuous electrocardiographic monitoring in 50 male medical students without apparent heart disease. Am J Cardiol 39:390–394, 1977.
2. Hinkle LE, Carver ST, Stevens M: The frequency of asymptomatic disturbances of cardiac rhythm and conduction in middle-aged men. Am J Cardiol 24:629–650, 1969.
3. Raftery EB, Cashman PNM: Long-term recording of the electrocardiogram in a normal population. Postgrad Med J 52 (suppl 7):32–37, 1976.
4. Clarke JM, et al: The rhythm of the normal human heart. Lancet 2:508–512, 1977.
5. Glasser SP, Clark PI, Applebaum HJ: Occurrence of frequent complex arrhythmias detected by ambulatory monitoring. Chest 75:565–568, 1979.
6. Loomis TA, Krop S: Atrial fibrillation induced and maintained in animals by acetylcholine or vagal stimulation. Circ Res 3:390–396, 1955.
7. Kure K: Über die Pathogenese der heterotopen Reizbildung unter dem Einflusse der extracardialen Herznerven. Zeitschrift fur Experimentelle Pathologie und Therapie 12:389–459, 1913.
8. Han J, Garcia de Jalon P, Moe GK: Adrenergic effects on ventricular vulnerability. Circ Res 14:516–524, 1964.
9. Verrier RL, Thompson PL, Lown B: Ventricular vulnerability during sympathetic stimulation: Role of heart rate and blood pressure. Cardiovasc Res 8:602–610, 1974.
10. Lown B: Sudden cardiac death: The major challenge confronting contemporary cardiology. Am J Cardiol 43:313–328, 1979.
11. Spear JF, et al: Cellular electrophysiology of human myocardial infarction. I. Abnormalities of cellular activation. Circulation 59:247–256, 1979.
12. Gallagher JJ, et al: Ventricular aneurysm with ventricular tachycardia. Report of a case with epicardial mapping and successful resection. Am J Cardiol 35:696–700, 1975.
13. Josephson ME, et al: Comparison of endocardial catheter mapping with intraoperative mapping of ventricular tachycardia. Circulation 61:395–404, 1980.
14. Wittig JH, Boineau JP: Surgical treatment of ventricular arrhythmias using epicardial, transmural, and endocardial mapping. Ann Thor Surg 20:117–125, 1975.

15. Wellens HJJ, Lie KI, Durrer D: Further observations on ventricular tachycardia as studied by electrical stimulation of the heart. Chronic recurrent ventricular tachycardia and ventricular tachycardia during acute myocardial infarction. Circulation 49:647–653, 1974.
16. Wellens HJJ, Duren DR, Lie KI: Observations on mechanisms of ventricular tachycardia in man. Circulation 54:237–244, 1976.
17. Denes P, et al: Electrophysiological studies in patients with chronic recurrent ventricular tachycardia. Circulation 54:229–236, 1976.
18. Josephson ME, et al: Recurrent sustained ventricular tachycardia. I. Mechanisms. Circulation 57:431–440, 1978.
19. Elharar V, Gaum WE, Zipes DP: Effect of drugs on conduction delay in the incidence of ventricular arrhythmias induced by acute coronary occlusion in dogs. Am J Cardiol 39:544–549, 1977.
20. Elharar V, Zipes DP: Cardiac electrophysiologic alterations during myocardial ischemia. Am J Physiol 233:H329–H345, 1977.
21. Goldman DE: Potential, impedance, and rectification in membranes. J Gen Physiol 27:37–60, 1943.
22. Hodgkin AL, Katz B: The effect of sodium ions on the electrical activity of the giant axon of the squid. J Physiol (London) 108:37–77, 1949.
23. Hodgkin AL, Huxley AF: Currents carried by sodium and potassium ions through the membrane of the giant axon of loligo. J Physiol (London) 116:449–472, 1952.
24. Hodgkin AL, Huxley AF: The components of the membrane conductance in the giant axon of loligo. J Physiol (London) 116:473–496, 1952.
25. Hodgkin AL, Huxley AF: A quantitative description of membrane current and its application to conduction and excitation in nerve. J Physiol (London) 117:500–544, 1952.
26. Noble D: Application of Hodgkin-Huxley equations to excitable tissues. Physiol Rev 46:1–50, 1966.
27. Trautwein W: Membrane currents in cardiac muscle fibers. Physiol Rev 53:793–835, 1973.
28. Weidmann S: The effect of the cardiac membrane potential on the rapid availability of the sodium carrying system. J Physiol (London) 127:213–224, 1955.
29. Dudel J, et al: The dynamic chloride component of membrane current in Purkinje fibers. Pflugers Arch Ges Physiol Menschen Tiere 295:197–212, 1967.
30. McAllister RE, Noble D, Tsien RW: Reconstruction of the electrical activity of cardiac

Purkinje fibers. J Physiol (London) 251:1–59, 1975.

31. Noble D: The Initiation of the Heart Beat. Clarendon Press, Oxford, 1975.

32. Noble D, Tsien RW: The repolarization process of heart cells. In: Electrical Phenomena in Heart, Ed. by WC deMello, Academic Press, New York, 1972.

33. Trautwein W: The slow inward current in mammalian myocardium. Eur J Cardiol 1:169–175, 1973.

34. Noble D, Tsien RW: The kinetics and rectifier properties of the slow potassium current in cardiac Purkinje fibers. J Physiol (London) 195: 185–214, 1968.

35. Vassalle M: Analysis of cardiac pacemaker potential using a "voltage clamp" technique. Am J Physiol 210:1335–1341, 1966.

36. Brown HF, Clarke A, Noble SJ: Identification of pacemaker current in frog atrium. J Physiol (London) 258:521–530, 1976.

37. Strauss HC, Prystowsky EN, Scheinman MM: Sino-atrial and atrial electrogenesis. Prog Cardiovasc Dis 19:385–404, 1977.

38. Wit AL, Rosen MR, Hoffman BF: Electrophysiology and pharmacology of cardiac arrhythmias. II. Relationship of normal and abnormal electrical activity of cardiac fibers to the genesis of arrhythmias. A. Automaticity. Am Heart J 88:515–525, 1974.

39. Hodgkin AL: A note on conduction velocity. J Physiol (London) 125:221–224, 1954.

40. Jack JJB, Noble D, Tsien RW: Electric Current Flow in Excitable Cells. Clarendon Press, Oxford, 1975.

41. Hauswirth O, Singh BN: Ionic mechanisms in heart muscle in relation to the genesis and the pharmacological control of cardiac arrhythmias. Pharm Rev 30:5–63, 1979.

42. Hashimoto K, Moe GK: Transient depolarizations induced by acetylstrophanthidin in specialized tissue of dog atrium and ventricle. Circ Res 32:618–624, 1973.

43. Lazzara R, El-Sherif N, Scherlag BJ: Electrophysiological properties of canine Purkinje cells in one-day-old myocardial infarction. Circ Res 35:391–398, 1974.

44. Cranefield PF, Wit AL, Hoffman BF: Conduction of the cardiac impulse. III. Characteristics of very slow conduction. J Gen Physiol 59:227–246, 1972.

45. Imanishi S: Calcium-sensitive discharges in canine Purkinje fibers. Jpn J Physiol 21:443–463, 1971.

46. Surawicz B: Calcium responses ("calcium spikes"). Am J Cardiol 33:689–690, 1974.

47. Moe GK: Evidence for reentry as a mechanism of cardiac arrhythmias. Rev Physiol Biochem Exp Pharmacol 72:64–81, 1975.

48. Cranefield PF: The Conduction of the Cardiac Impulse. p.p. 1–315, Futura Publishing Company, Mt. Kisco, NY, 1975.

49. Wit AL, Cranefield PF: Triggered activity in cardiac muscle fibers of the simian mitral valve. Circ Res 38:85–94, 1976.

50. Zipes DP, Besch HR, Watanabe AM: Role of the slow current in cardiac electrophysiology. Circulation 51:761–768, 1975.

51. Goldreyer BN, Bigger JT Jr: Site of reentry in paroxysmal supraventricular tachycardia in man. Circulation 43:15–26, 1971.

52. Wellens HJJ, Durrer D: Effect of procainamide, quinidine and ajmaline in the Wolff-Parkinson-White syndrome. Circulation 50:114–120, 1974.

53. Wit AL, Goldreyer BN, Damato AN: An in vitro model of paroxysmal supraventricular tachycardia. Circulation 43:862–870, 1971.

54. Wit AL, Hoffman BF, Cranefield PF: Slow conduction and reentry in the ventricular conducting system. I. Return extrasystole in canine Purkinje fibers. Circ Res 30:1–10, 1972.

55. Wit AL, Hoffman BF, Cranefield PF: Slow conduction and reentry in the ventricular conducting system. II. Single and sustained circus movement in networks of canine and bovine Purkinje fibers. Circ Res 30:11–22, 1972.

56. Friedman PL, et al: Survival of subendocardial Purkinje fibers after extensive myocardial infarction in dogs; in vitro and in vivo correlations. Circ Res 33:597–611, 1973.

57. Friedman PL, Stewart JR, Wit AL: Spontaneous and induced cardiac arrhythmias in subendocardial Purkinje fibers surviving extensive myocardial infarction in dogs. Circ Res 33:612–626, 1973.

58. Antzelevitch C, Jalife J, Moe GK: Characteristics of reflection as a mechanism of reentrant arrhythmias and its relationship to parasystole. Circulation 61:182–191, 1980.

59. Brooks C McC, et al: Excitability and electrical response of the ischemic heart muscle. Am J Physiol 198:1143–1147, 1960.

60. Kupersmith JE, Antman EM, Hoffman BF: In vivo electrophysiologic effects of lidocaine in canine acute myocardial infarction. Circ Res 36:84–91, 1975.

61. Kupersmith J, Shiang H, Litwak RS, Herman

MV: Electrophysiological and antiarrhythmic effects of propranolol in canine acute myocardial ischemia. Circ Res 38:302–307, 1976.

62. Kardesch M, Hogancamp CE, Bing RJ: The effect of complete ischemia on the intracellular electrical activity of the whole mammalian heart. Circ Res 6:715–720, 1958.

63. Printzmetal M, et al.: Myocardial ischemia. Nature of ischemic electrocardiographic patterns in the mammalian ventricles as determined by in-

tracellular electrographic and metabolic changes. Am J Cardiol 8:493–503, 1961.

64. Downar E, Janse MJ, Durrer D: The effect of acute coronary artery occlusion on subepicardial transmembrane potentials in the intact porcine heart. Circulation 56:217–224, 1977.

65. Lazzara RN, El-Sherif N, Scherlag BJ: Early and late effects of coronary artery occlusion on canine Purkinje fibers. Circ Res 35:391–399, 1974.

# 14 | *Pharmacology of Antiarrhythmic Agents*

*Guy P. Curtis, M.D., Ph.D.*

The drugs discussed in this chapter are most frequently employed to suppress or control the abnormal heart rhythms or rapid heart rates discussed in the previous chapter. These agents are commonly used in patients with coronary artery disease because of the serious consequences of untreated arrhythmia in this patient population. Sudden death, presumably due to spontaneously occurring ventricular fibrillation, is associated with active myocardial ischemia and arrhythmia.[1] Klein and coworkers have shown that patients with coronary artery disease and supraventricular tachyarrhythmias with rapid ventricular response rates may be at increased risk for sudden death.[2] Furthermore, particular patterns of arrhythmia are associated with an increased risk of sudden death in the patient with active coronary artery disease.[1] These include:

1. Premature beats exhibiting the "R on T" phenomenon.
2. Frequent ventricular premature beats.
3. Multifocal ventricular premature beats.
4. Ventricular group beating (two or more ventricular premature beats in succession).

Suppression of these arrhythmias should decrease the risk of sudden death in patients with active coronary artery disease. Although such a positive relationship has yet to be convincingly demonstrated, it provides one of the prime reasons for instituting antiarrhythmic therapy in this patient population.

Arrhythmias compromise myocardial hemodynamic performance; deterioration in pump function is poorly tolerated in patients whose left ventricular performance is already diminished because of prior myocardial infarction or active ischemia. Dysrhythmia is frequently accompanied by a fall in cardiac output, an elevation in venous pressures, and a fall in arterial pressure. These hemodynamic alterations can precipitate congestive heart failure in patients with marked left ventricular dysfunction secondary to coronary artery disease and seriously limit functional exercise capacity in less severely afflicted patients. In addition, arrhythmia-associated elevation in intraventricular pressures, increases in heart chamber dimensions, and elevated heart rates are often associated with increases in myocardial oxygen consumption and work. These consequences of arrhythmia could be critical in ischemic areas of the myocardium where regional blood supply and available oxygen are limited. Resultant increases in regional oxygen consumption could be expected to lead to diminished regional shortening in ischemic myocardial segments, an increase in angina pectoris, and perhaps extension of myocardial necrosis in patients with acute myocardial infarction.

Symptoms associated with arrhythmia can also lead to attempts at arrhythmia suppression in patients with active coronary artery disease. Palpitations accompanying arrhythmia can be associated with considerable anxiety in a patient who knows he has coronary artery disease and may die suddenly. Paroxysmal tachyarrhythmia can also cause precipitous hypotension resulting in sudden loss of consciousness or lightheadedness and ataxia. These symptoms expose the patient to risk of serious injury if the patient is operating machinery or driving an automobile at the time of an attack.

## MECHANISMS FOR ARRHYTHMIA SUPPRESSION

Treatment of cardiac arrhythmias has been empiric in the past because the electrophysiologic mechanisms involved in the initiation and perpetuation of the majority of abnormal cardiac rhythms were unknown. Thus, it has not been possible to logically predict from each antiarrhythmic drug's known electrophysiologic properties whether or not it would be effective against a particular arrhythmia. A goal of electrophysiologists and pharmacologists has been to place antiarrhythmic drug therapy on a scientific base so that the therapeutic agent is chosen on electrophysiologic rather than on empiric data. This requires a knowledge of the complete pharmacology of the antiarrhythmic agents as well as complete electrophysiologic knowledge of arrhythmogenesis. While this goal has not yet been achieved, advances in the knowledge of pharmacology as well as electrophysiology in normal and pathologic states have occurred over the past decade that allow a shift away from a purely empiric to a more rational approach for antiarrhythmic therapy.

The therapeutic goal of suppressing abnormalities in heart rate and/or rhythm can theoretically be accomplished in several ways. Mechanisms responsible for arrhythmia initiation could be blocked without affecting myocardial electrophysiologic properties that sustain an arrhythmia once it is initiated. Thus, if a premature beat initiates continuous arrhythmia, effective arrhythmia suppression could be accomplished by suppressing all premature beats.

An antiarrhythmic drug that blocked mechanisms facilitating continuous arrhythmia but did not control the initiating event (i.e., premature beats) would also provide effective antiarrhythmic prophylaxis. Bretylium may some-

times demonstrate this mode of action because in some reported cases premature beats have not been suppressed with bretylium therapy at a time when ventricular tachycardia or ventricular fibrillation, previously associated with these beats, is controlled.[3]

Supraventricular tachyarrhythmias can be controlled or suppressed by regulating the electrophysiologic properties of the specialized conducting system of the heart through agents producing pharmacologic effects at the atrioventricular node. For example, digitalis glycosides are frequently employed in this manner to control the ventricular rate in the presence of atrial flutter or fibrillation. The same agent can suppress paroxysmal atrial tachycardia (PAT) by slowing A-V nodal conduction and blocking continuous conduction of a circulating waveform at this site.

An antiarrhythmic agent therefore can produce arrhythmia suppression or control through a combination of mechanisms or a single action. The agent may (1) suppress the initiating conditions facilitating the genesis of arrhythmia; (2) block electrophysiologic properties necessary for maintenance of arrhythmia; or (3) selectively depress A-V nodal conduction so that ventricular rate is controlled.

## ELECTROPHYSIOLOGIC PROPERTIES OF IMPORTANCE FOR ANTIARRHYTHMIC AGENTS

Electrophysiologic studies on antiarrhythmic agents in normal and diseased tissue have revealed effects on impulse formation (pacemaker activity), intramyocardial conduction, and/or recovery of electrical excitability. Since the cellular mechanisms for the various commonly encountered clinical arrhythmias are incompletely understood, it is often not possible to state which electrophysiologic property is of prime importance for the suppression of a particular arrhythmia. Useful information can be derived, however, from comparing empirically determined antiarrhythmic efficacy with known shared electrophysiologic properties of efficacious agents.

## Effects on Pacemaker Cells (Impulse Initiation)

Most antiarrhythmic agents suppress *abnormal* pacemaker activity but produce little effect on *normal* pacemaker activity until toxic concentrations are attained. Since many cardiac rhythm disorders may be initiated and/or maintained by spontaneously occurring ectopic automaticity, this property may be of key importance in arrhythmia suppression. Mechanisms responsible for ectopic automaticity and its suppression are not completely understood. Pacemaker cells demonstrate a time-dependent, net inward current (movement of positive charge). Two different mechanisms for the production of net inward current and automaticity have been elucidated in the normal heart.[4] Purkinje fiber automaticity has been demonstrated at membrane potentials between −90 and −60 mV. This automaticity is due to a time- and voltage-dependent decrease in outward potassium ion current while inward sodium ion movement continues. Another mechanism has been demonstrated in the sinoatrial (S-A) node and also in myocardial cells depolarized to less than −60 mV where sodium current is inactivated. Under these conditions a time- and voltage-dependent inward current carried largely by calcium ion has been demonstrated. Antiarrhythmic drugs can suppress abnormal automaticity occurring at membrane potentials between −90 and −60 mV at concentrations that do not affect normal S-A node function.[5] Thus, interference with transmembrane sodium flux and/or facilitation of potassium movement may be desirable electrophysiologic properties for drugs that suppress ectopic automaticity.

## Effects on Impulse Propagation

Many drugs used to control or suppress arrhythmias produce decreases in the conduction velocity of intramyocardial depolarization, block the propagation of early beats, and slow the recovery of full excitability. When these effects are focused on the A-V node, they result in a slowed ventricular response rate during supraventricular tachyarrhythmias or blockade of A-V nodal reentry in paroxysmal atrial tachycardia. Reentrant rhythms elsewhere in the heart may also be suppressed by these mechanisms via the conversion of areas of slowed conduction or unidirectional block to areas where impulses either are completely blocked or are conducted at a later time in recovery at near-normal velocities.

Antiarrhythmic agents can produce these effects on impulse propagation through several different electrophysiologic mechanisms.

1. *The rate of rise of the action potential* (dV/dt) may be reduced as well as the *magnitude* of voltage change during the upstroke (phase 0) of the action potential (see Fig. 14.1). The action potential serves as a voltage source for current flow—and it is current flow that depolarizes the membrane to threshold potential and is responsible for propagation of electrical depolarization (see Ch. 13). Decreasing dV/dt as well as decreasing the change in voltage during phase 0 will decrease the effective current flow responsible for bringing the myocardial cell membrane to threshold potential and thus alter impulse propagation.

2. *Membrane responsiveness* (change in membrane potential to applied depolarizing current) may be diminished and threshold potential may be decreased by antiarrhythmic agents. These alterations require that more current be supplied before threshold potential is attained and an action potential results. Such changes in

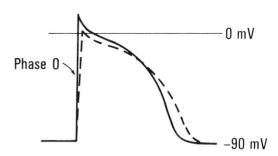

Fig. 14.1 Effects of quinidine on action potential upstroke velocity (Phase 0) and amplitude. The action potential drawn with the dashed line represents quinidine effect, while the solid line represents the control state. Upstroke velocity and amplitude of the action potential are reduced by quinidine without an effect on resting membrane potential. Action potential duration is increased after large doses of quinidine, as the figure shows.

membrane responsiveness and threshold potential would tend to slow conduction velocity, suppress conduction of early beats and suppress conduction in areas of unidirectional block where dV/dt for phase 0 and action potential amplitude are reduced.

3. Antiarrhythmic agents may *slow recovery of electrical excitability* and *alter the relationship between membrane potential during repolarization* and *recovery of excitability*. Recovery of electrical excitability is defined by measuring refractory periods in the myocardium (see Fig. 14.2). The effective refractory period (ERP) is that time following depolarization when a propagated response cannot be elicited by an applied stimulus. Propagated responses can be obtained during the relative refractory period (RRP), but the stimulus intensity necessary to evoke a response is greater than when full recovery is attained. If one could see electrical events in a long piece of cardiac muscle, there

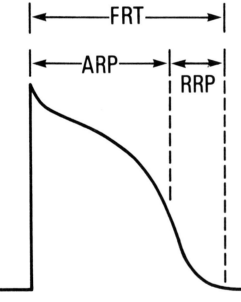

Fig. 14.2 Usual relationships between local refractory periods, representing recovery of excitability, and the action potential. FRT = full recovery time; ARP = absolute refractory period; RRP = relative refractory period. Refractoriness has time- and voltage-dependent characteristics. Usually, the ARP ends when the cell has repolarized to between −60 and −70 mV, and full recovery occurs with full repolarization. These relationships can be altered by antiarrhythmic drugs.

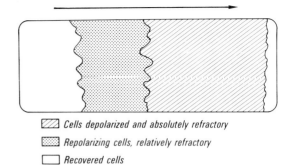

☐ Cells depolarized and absolutely refractory
☐ Repolarizing cells, relatively refractory
☐ Recovered cells

Fig. 14.3 Schematic representation of depolarization and recovery of excitability in an infinitely long strip of cardiac muscle. Arrow *(top)* represents the direction of movement for the depolarizing wavefront. The absolute refractory period represents a barrier to reexcitation of cells previously depolarized, as there are many inexcitable cells between the wavefront of depolarizing cells and cells capable of being reexcited.

should be recovered tissue ahead of a band of depolarizing cells. Behind the wave of depolarizing cells, there should be tissue that is refractory to stimulation, separating the depolarizing cells in phase 0 from cells that are either in their relative refractory periods or are completely recovered (see Fig. 14.3). The refractory period, then, is a barrier to reentry, separating recovered from depolarizing cells. Many antiarrhythmic agents (i.e., Class I agents) increase the duration of the ERP, thus increasing the distance between depolarizing and recovered cells. If reentry or continuous conduction depends in part on the recovery of cells along the conducting pathway so that areas previously depolarized can be "reentered," increasing the ERP could result in recirculating wavefronts of depolarization encountering refractory tissue in previously activated areas and being extinguished.

Drugs that alter the relationship between membrane potential and recovery of electrical excitability also can produce an antiarrhythmic effect by improving conduction of premature beats in areas of conduction depression. These agents produce electrophysiologic effects requiring that a more negative (greater) transmembrane potential be achieved before an action potential can be elicited (see Fig. 14.4). The resulting action potential exhibits an en-

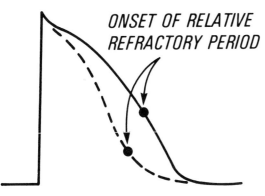

ONSET OF RELATIVE
REFRACTORY PERIOD

Fig. 14.4  Schematic representation of the effects of lidocaine and diphenylhydantoin on action potential duration and recovery of excitability. The action potential after drug is shown by the dashed line. Action potential duration is abbreviated more than the recovery of excitability in the normal myocardium so that early beats arise from more negative transmembrane potentials. This results in enhanced action potential amplitudes and rates of rise for Phase 0, resulting in more effective depolarizing current flow and improved conduction for early beats after drug (see text).

hanced amplitude and dV/dt during phase 0 when a premature response is elicited. Under these circumstances the action potential is more effective in eliciting depolarizing current flow, and an improved conduction velocity results. Drug-induced electrophysiologic changes of this type have been suggested as a mechanism to eliminate areas of unidirectional block and thus block reentrant rhythms.[6]

Studies in normal and ischemic tissues have revealed that drugs may have disparate effects under different circumstances.[7] An agent that abbreviates the refractory period and speeds the conduction of premature beats in normal myocardial cells may prolong refractoriness and slow conduction in ischemic tissue. These alterations could reduce electrophysiologic inhomogeneity at the cellular level, a condition postulated as a prime prerequisite for reentry. The effective refractory period decreases in the ischemic zone shortly after blood flow interruption and then increases as ischemia continues.[8] An agent that reduced the refractory period in normal tissue but increased refractory periods in the ischemic zone early after coronary flow interruption might reduce disparate re-

covery and inhomogeneity between normal and ischemic zones, removing a factor facilitating continuous conduction and reentrant rhythm.

## DRUG CLASSIFICATION

Antiarrhythmic agents can be divided into at least four groups based on what is known of their electrophysiologic actions, as originally suggested by Vaughn-Williams and coworkers: Class I, Local Anesthetics; Class II, $\beta$-Blocking Drugs; Class III, Drugs Sustaining Depolarization; and Class IV, Slow Channel Blocking Drugs.[9]

Many theoretical as well as practical benefits derive from such a classification system. Theoretically, antiarrhythmic drug selection for a particular arrhythmia should be facilitated by such a grouping if the electrophysiologic mechanism for arrhythmogenesis is known, since electrophysiologic properties required for arrhythmia suppression and drugs likely to successfully produce arrhythmia suppression should be available from such a drug classification. While this goal has almost been attained with a few selected arrhythmias, dysrhythmia suppression remains empiric in the majority of cases, particularly when ventricular arrhythmias are considered. This empiric approach reflects an incomplete understanding of arrhythmogenesis and electrophysiologic antiarrhythmic drug properties required for dysrhythmia suppression.

Classification schemes are helpful for the pharmacologist, as they allow comparison of structure-activity relationships between the antiarrhythmic agents and assist in the development and evaluation of new antiarrhythmic drugs. Potential toxicity of new compounds can also be predicted from previous knowledge of toxicity of drugs from a similar class.

The most practical use of the classification system for the clinician occurs when therapy with two antiarrhythmic agents is necessary. Unpleasant side effects accompanying large doses of a single drug can be avoided by utilizing lower doses of two drugs with the same electrophysiologic properties but different side effects. A satisfactory electrophysiologic result can be achieved with both drugs acting in concert while drug doses of the individual agents are low enough so that side effects are minimized.

Combination therapy for arrhythmia suppression is more likely to be successful if drugs with different electrophysiologic properties are employed. Thus, drugs from different classes may be successfully combined (e.g., quinidine and propranolol) or drugs within the same class that differ in some major electrophysiologic effects but have the same spectrum of activity may be successfully utilized (e.g., quinidine and lidocaine).

The fact that two drugs are in the same class does not mean they have identical electrophysiologic properties or side effects; it means only that the spectrum of major electrophysiologic effects is the same. Different subsidiary actions are possible and some drugs may possess extracardiac effects which alter the observed direct myocardial electrophysiologic effects.

## Class I: Local Anesthetic Drugs

Class I agents interfere with action potential generation and conduction of electrical activity within the myocardium. Quinidine is the prototype of antiarrhythmic drugs in this class. The major electrophysiologic effect of this class of drugs is a reduction in the maximum rate of myocardial cell depolarization during phase zero of the action potential without any effect on the resting membrane potential. Further, these agents suppress ectopic pacemaker activity at lower concentrations than those required to produce a decrease in the slope of phase zero of the action potential.[10] Since sodium movement into the cell is responsible for diastolic depolarization of some pacemaker fibers and for the rapid ascent of the action potential, an effect on a postulated sodium carrier to reduce the rate of entry of sodium into the cell has been proposed as the cellular mechanism by which these drugs act.[11] The result is a decrease in the effective depolarizing current associated with the action potential.

In the presence of these agents, conduction velocity is decreased and the threshold for excitability (current required for cellular depolarization) is increased. Repolarization and recovery of excitability must proceed to a greater extent

before another impulse can be initiated because of drug-induced decreases in depolarizing current. This results in an increase in the effective refractory period (ERP), and an altered relationship between the end of the ERP and the transmembrane potential (i.e., the ERP ends and impulse propagation occurs at more negative transmembrane potentials).

The resting membrane potential is related to the ratio of extra- to intracellular potassium ion concentration, and a reduction in extracellular potassium makes the transmembrane potential more negative (see Ch. 13). Increases in the transmembrane potential are known to increase the maximal rate of depolarization during the action potential and thus would tend to antagonize the effects of Class I agents. Thus, these drugs are less effective in hypokalemic states or following other interventions which tend to increase the transmembrane potential.[12]

Class I agents depress contractile force and produce local anesthetic actions on nerves at concentrations higher than those required for antiarrhythmic effects. However, conduction is affected in the specialized conducting system in the heart at much lower concentrations than those required to produce comparable effects on ventricular tissues.[13]

The major drugs with Class I actions are quinidine, procaineamide, lidocaine, diphenylhydantoin, and disopyramide.

## Class II: β-Adrenergic Blocking Agents

Drugs in Class II produce arrhythmia suppression by blocking the effects of catecholamine stimulation on the myocardial cell. Propranolol is the prototype drug for this group. Catecholamines are known to increase the rate of diastolic depolarization in cardiac cells that possess spontaneous automaticity. Local increases in catecholamine activity that accompany centrally mediated sympathetic nervous system discharge or myocardial ischemia can be associated with sufficient local enhancement in automaticity so that competing rhythms and ectopy emerge.[14,15] β-adrenergic blocking drugs can suppress this type of automaticity.

β-adrenergic blocking drugs also can produce direct effects on the myocardial cell membrane. Effects similar to those described for Class I agents have been described for some $\beta$-adrenergic blocking drugs at higher-than-therapeutic concentrations.[16] Impressive antiarrhythmic suppression has been demonstrated with a quaternary derivative of propranolol which may be present in very small amounts when propranolol is administered.[17] However, the role of direct membrane effects in arrhythmia suppression produced by propranolol and other $\beta$-adrenergic blockers is presently uncertain, and $\beta$-adrenergic blockade is probably the major mechanism for arrhythmia suppression in this class.

## Class III: Agents That Prolong the Action Potential Duration

Bretylium is the prototype for Class III drugs. These agents share the common property of prolonging both action potential duration and the effective refractory period. Unlike Class I drugs, they do not seem to affect resting membrane potential, rate of rise of phase 0 of the action potential, conduction velocity, or membrane responsiveness. Bretylium and amiodarone suppress cardiac catecholamine effects that result from sympathetic nerve stimulation; however, it is unlikely that the major antiarrhythmic effect for these drugs resides with adrenergic receptor blockade, since $\beta$-receptor blockade or blockade of neuronal release of catecholamines with guanethidine does not produce similar antiarrhythmic effects.[18,19]

The most impressive action of Class III drugs has been their ability to suppress ventricular tachycardia and/or ventricular fibrillation. Bretylium administration has been associated with the spontaneous reversion of ventricular fibrillation to normal sinus rhythm in the canine heart.[20] There are few drugs that are capable of chemical defibrillation of the cardiac ventricles; the existence of such drugs for chronic antiarrhythmic therapy might be important for the prevention of sudden death in many patients.

## Class IV: Slow Channel Blocking Drugs

Sodium entry into the myocardial cell during phase 0 of the action potential can be suppressed by the administration of tetrodotoxin or by de-polarizing the cell membrane to potentials less than $-60$ mV. These interventions are associated with a marked decrease in the slope for phase 0 of the action potential and the loss of that portion of the action potential where the inside of the cell membrane is more positive than the outside (overshoot). These slowly rising action potentials have been associated with marked reductions in conduction velocity, unidirectional block, reentry, and also with the appearance of spontaneous automaticity.[21,22] Voltage clamp studies have shown that calcium is responsible for cellular depolarization during these slow response action potentials and that selective calcium antagonists will suppress this type of electrical activity.[22]

Class IV drugs are such selective calcium antagonists; the prototype drug for this class is verapamil. Agents in this group produce their most profound effects in tissue where slow response action potentials are normally found—i.e., the A-V node and the A-V valve leaflets.[23] Catecholamines are known to induce automaticity in cells with slow response potentials, and Class IV agents can abolish these effects.[24] Clinical use of these drugs has shown them to be effective in controlling ventricular response rates to supraventricular arrhythmias, presumably via depressant effects on slow response potentials involved in A-V nodal conduction.[25] Reentrant rhythms within the A-V node, such as paroxysmal atrial tachycardia (PAT), are also suppressed, probably by similar mechanisms.[26] Ventricular arrhythmias have not been effectively suppressed by agents from this group, despite the demonstration in experimental models of ischemia that slow potentials are present in areas where arrhythmias arise.

## INDIVIDUAL DRUGS

### Quinidine

Quinidine has been the standard to which other antiarrhythmic drugs have been compared for many years. This drug is the dextrorotary optical isomer of quinine; its use as an antiarrhythmic agent stemmed from reports of dysrhythmia suppression in patients taking quinine for malaria.[27]

Quinidine administration is associated with all of the electrophysiologic myocardial effects normally associated with Class I agents,[28-30] namely:

(1) a depression of phase 4 depolarization in cells demonstrating automaticity, more marked for ectopic pacemakers with a resting membrane potential of less than 60 mV than for sinus node cells.

(2) a reduction in the rate of depolarization and the overshoot during phase 0 of the action potential.

(3) little effect on action potential duration and the duration of the absolute refractory period at therapeutic concentrations, but a prolongation of the effective refractory period.

(4) depression of the membrane-responsiveness curve. Effects (3) and (4) are probably in large part due to action number (2), a reduction in phase 0 dV/dt as explained above. The net effect of these cardiac actions is conduction depression or slowing most marked in the atrium, Purkinje, and ventricular muscle fibers; suppression of ectopic pacemakers; and an elevated threshold for excitability. As toxic concentrations of the drug are given, there is further conduction depression at all cardiac tissue sites. Decreases in mechanical shortening and a prolongation of action potential duration with refractory period prolongation are also noted. Clinically, increases in QRS duration of the electrocardiogram reflect conduction slowing, while increases in the Q-Tc interval reflect repolarization changes. Therapeutic quinidine plasma levels have been found to correlate best with QRS duration changes, while toxic effects are found most consistently with marked Q-Tc prolongation.[31]

Quinidine has other important effects. The drug has anticholinergic activity, and vagolytic effects can be demonstrated. These effects are of clinical importance at the A-V node. The ventricular response rate to atrial flutter and fibrillation can increase after quinidine administration. It is known that increased cholinergic (vagal) activity can increase the rate of atrial flutter and fibrillation, increase conduction block, and enhance decremental conduction at the A-V node. These cholinergic effects slow the ventricular response rate when atrial flutter

or fibrillation are present. Quinidine slows the atrial rate during flutter or fibrillation of these structures via its direct electrophysiologic effect and its atropine-like action. Quinidine also antagonizes vagal effects at the A-V node, reducing decremental conduction and conduction slowing of premature beats at this structure. The resulting more rapid A-V nodal transmission of impulses can produce marked increases in the ventricular response rate during these arrhythmias.

Nodal reentrant paroxysmal atrial tachycardia is suppressed by A-V node conduction depression that is vagally mediated; this arrhythmia, when established, is therefore not effectively treated with quinidine because of this agent's indirect anticholinergic drug effects.

Quinidine produces weak $\alpha$-receptor blockade and has a direct relaxant action on vascular smooth muscle. These effects in combination with the negative inotropic effect may explain why intravenous quinidine administration is often accompanied by substantial increases in reflex adrenergic tone and, on occasion, cardiovascular collapse. However, under ordinary circumstances quinidine when given orally is not a significant myocardial depressant;[32] recent experimental evidence indicates that the depressant effects of intravenous quinidine are usually masked by reflex adrenergic mechanisms.[33]

**Clinical Use.** Quinidine continues to be the standard against which other drugs are compared for the treatment of atrial and ventricular arrhythmias. It has been employed successfully to suppress atrial flutter, atrial fibrillation, premature atrial contractions, PAT associated with the Wolff-Parkinson-White (WPW) syndrome, and all forms of ventricular ectopic beats.

**Atrial Flutter and Fibrillation.** Drug therapy for patients with chronic atrial flutter and fibrillation is usually aimed at the control of the ventricular response rate. Quinidine administration in these patients may be associated with slowing of atrial rate during the arrhythmia but seldom results in the restoration of normal sinus rhythm even when therapeutic drug levels are achieved. Quinidine causes slowing of the atrial rate during arrhythmia, and its anticholinergic effects at the A-V node make the ventricular response rate more difficult to control. Thus, quinidine does not have a role in patients with sustained atrial flutter and fibrillation.

Quinidine therapy is effective in maintaining normal sinus rhythm in patients with paroxysmal atrial flutter or fibrillation and in patients undergoing cardioversion for these arrhythmias. Initiation of atrial flutter and fibrillation has been shown to be associated with critically timed atrial premature contractions.[34] Quinidine can suppress the premature atrial contractions triggering arrhythmia, resulting in maintained normal sinus rhythm after cardioversion or after the spontaneous appearance of sinus rhythm.

PAT associated with WPW syndrome usually involves sequential excitation of the specialized conducting system and then the accessory pathway, bypassing the A-V node.[35] The arrhythmia can be blocked via conduction suppression at the level of the A-V node or at the accessory pathway. Premature contractions are thought to trigger this arrhythmia.[36] Quinidine can suppress conduction in the accessory pathway and suppress premature atrial or ventricular contractions initiating arrhythmia. Prophylaxis with quinidine is particularly advantageous in patients with preexcitation and concomitant atrial fibrillation or flutter, since conduction slowing in the accessory bundle will limit the ventricular response rate during atrial fibrillation or flutter.

Nodal reentrant PAT can also be suppressed with quinidine therapy if premature atrial contractions initiating the arrhythmia are blocked. However, once the arrhythmia is initiated, therapy is focused on increasing A-V nodal vagal tone, and quinidine with its anticholinergic effects is not helpful in arrhythmia termination. Therefore this arrhythmia is usually treated prophylactically with agents increasing vagal tone (i.e., digoxin and/or propranolol).

Paroxysmal atrial tachycardia that results from a rapidly firing atrial ectopic focus is effectively suppressed with quinidine therapy.[37]

Ventricular ectopic beats and group beating can be suppressed with quinidine. This agent is still considered to be a first-line drug for chronic prophylaxis against ventricular arrhythmia. However, arrhythmia associated with Q-Tc prolongation or digitalis intoxication may be better treated with other agents. Digitalis toxicity can be associated with marked conduction depression within the specialized conducting system that can be exacerbated by quinidine resulting in A-V block and asystole.

**Administration, Fate, and Excretion.** Quinidine is almost completely absorbed from the gastrointestinal tract following oral administration. Peak plasma levels occur 1 to 2 hours later. A similar time course has been demonstrated after intramuscular administration, but the peak plasma levels are approximately 30 percent lower.[38] The intravenous administration of quinidine is not recommended except under unusual circumstances because of the potential adverse hemodynamic effects noted above.

Quinidine's therapeutic effects persist for 6 to 8 hours. The plasma half-life is 5 to 6 hours, and up to 95 percent of the drug is metabolized by the liver to less active hydroxylated compounds.[39] Virtually all of the administered drug can be recovered in the urine. Dose-related toxicity is seen in patients with congestive heart failure, liver, or renal failure. It has recently also been appreciated that concomitant administration of digoxin and quinidine can result in increases in serum digoxin levels through possible effects on digoxin absorption and renal clearance.[40,41]

Quinidine sulfate or quinidine gluconate is usually administered every 6 hours in the absence of impaired renal or hepatic function at doses of 200 or 300 mg and 324 mg, respectively. On this regime stable plasma levels are usually achieved in 48 to 72 hours. Loading doses have been used when chemical conversion of atrial fibrillation was attempted. Patients received drug every two hours for five doses (i.e., 200 mg every 2 hours) with increases in the dose of 200 mg/day until toxicity or the desired effect was achieved.

**Side Effects and Toxicity.** Chronic quinidine therapy is discontinued because of side effects in 20 to 30 percent of patients.[42] The most frequently troublesome side effects are directed against the gastrointestinal tract and manifest as loose stools, diarrhea, abdominal colic, nausea, vomiting, and anorexia. These gastrointes-

**Table 14.1  Clinical Pharmacology of Commonly Employed Antiarrhythmic Agents**

| *Drug* | QUINIDINE | PROCAINAMIDE | DISOPYRAMIDE |
|---|---|---|---|
| Route | Oral, IM; not IV | Oral, parenteral | Oral |
| Usual dose | $SO_4$ 200 mg po q6h<br>Gluconate 324 mg po q6h<br>Gluconate 200–400 mg q2-6h IM | 250 to 500 mg po q4-6h<br>100 mg IV over 1 min q5 min until arrhythmia is controlled or 1000 mg is given<br>Maintenance 2–3 mg/min | 100–300 mg po q6h |
| *Absorption* | Oral 90% or more<br>IM 80 to 90% | Oral 90–100% | 90–100% |
| *T½* | 6.3 hr; range 3–16 hr | $\alpha$ 5 min<br>$\beta$ 2.5–4.7 hr. | 4–7 hours |
| *Peak level* | Oral and IM 60–90 min | Oral 60–90 min | 2–3 hours |
| *Protein bound* | 60–80% | 15%–20% | 30% |
| *Metabolism*<br>  site<br>  mechanism | Liver<br>Hydroxylation (active) | Liver<br>N-acetylation (active)<br>Plasma hydrolysis | Liver<br>N-dealkylation (anti-cholinergic) metabolite |
| *Percent unchanged in urine* | 10–27% | 50–60% | 40–60% |
| *Renal failure* | Follow levels | Reduce dose | Reduce dose |
| *Hepatic failure* | Reduce dose | Follow levels | Reduce dose |
| *Effective plasma concentrations* | 3–6 µg/ml | 4–10 µg/ml | 3–8 µg/ml |
| *Common side effects* | 1) Gastrointestinal<br>2) Cinchonism with overdose<br>3) Q-Tc prolongation<br>4) Elevated digoxin levels | 1) Hypotension (IV)<br>2) ⊕ANA<br>3) Lupus-like syndrome (10–20%)<br>4) Q-Tc prolongation | 1) Anticholinergic<br>2) Depressed contractility in patients with CHF |

tinal side effects may be reduced in intensity when the polygalacturonate form of the drug is used (Cardioquin) but less active drug may be available in this dosage form.

Hypersensitivity reactions to quinidine manifest as fever, urticaria, rash, and hematologic abnormalities, with thrombocytopenia being the most frequently reported.[42] The most feared idiosyncratic response to the drug has been termed "quinidine syncope" and is not common;[43] there is usually Q-T prolongation out of proportion to the drug level with an associated increased incidence of complex ventricu-

lar arrhythmias in this syndrome. The hemodynamic effects of the drug-induced arrhythmias can cause lightheadedness, syncope, and sudden death.

Quinidine overdose produces a constellation of symptoms termed cinchonism. Mild cases of quinidine toxicity may be accompanied by headache, blurred vision, temporary deafness, and tinnitus. In more severe cases, diplopia, photophobia, vertigo, confusion, delirium, and psychosis are seen, and the skin may be hot and flushed, with concomitant abdominal pain, nausea, vomiting, and diarrhea. Respiratory ar-

| LIDOCAINE | PROPRANOLOL | BRETYLIUM |
|---|---|---|
| Parenteral only | Oral, parenteral | Parenteral |
| Load: 1–2 mg/kg IM or IV slowly. Repeat 3–5 min. to 300 mg total. Maintenance: 2–4 mg/min | 10 to 100 mg po q6h 1–2 mg q5 min IV until arryhthmia is controlled; a total dose usually not to exceed 0.1 mg/kg. | IV: Load: 5–10 mg/kg over 10–20 min. 5 mg/kg in emergency. Repeat 15 to 30 min. to total 30 mg/kg/24h Maintenance: 1–2 mg/kg/min. |
| — | Oral variable | — |
| $\alpha$ 8–20 min. $\beta$ 100 min. | 2-4½ hr | 10 hr (4–17 hr range) |
| 30 min after IM Immediate IV | 1–4 hr po | 90 min after IM |
| 50% | 4–9% | — |
| Liver Deethylation Hydrolysis | Liver Several metabolites | Insignificant |
| <10% | <1% | Virtually 100% |
| Maintain dose | Reduce dose | Reduce dose |
| Reduce dose | Reduce dose | No effect |
| 2–6 μg/ml | Variable | Variable |
| CNS | 1) CNS 2) Bronchospasm in asthma 3) Cardiac depression | 1) Postural hypotension 2) Enhanced pressor response to sympathomimetics 3) Nausea & vomiting after IV bolus |

IM = intramuscular; IV = intravenous; po = by mouth; T½ = time for the plasma concentration to reach one-half of its peak value; $\alpha$ = rapid redistribution phase of drug metabolism; $\beta$ = slow elimination by hepatic metabolism, renal excretion and fecal loss; ANA = antinuclear antibody; CHF = congestive heart failure; CNS = central nervous system.

rest may occur secondary to central nervous system effects of the drug. Cardiovascular collapse may occur if this agent is administered intravenously because of the hemodynamic effects outlined above. QRS duration and Q-Tc intervals are prolonged as toxic quinidine levels are approached. All ECG waveforms are broadened and flattened. Spontaneous ventricular arrhythmia and high-grade conduction block occur under these circumstances.

## Procainamide

The local anesthetic procaine was observed to raise the threshold of ventricular muscle to electrical stimulation when directly applied to the heart.[49] However, procaine could not be used as an antiarrhythmic agent because it was not suitable for systemic administration. Marked central nervous system side effects accompanied its administration, and the duration

**Table 14.2   Antiarrhythmic Therapy: Choice of Agents (USA) ***

| ARRHYTHMIA | THERAPY (In Order of Preference) |
|---|---|
| *Supraventricular* | |
| Atrial premature contractions | Quinidine, procainamide, disopyramide |
| Reentrant paroxysmal atrial tachycardia | Propranolol, digoxin |
| Paroxysmal atrial tachycardia with preexcitation | Quinidine, procainamide, propranolol; or digoxin if no atrial fibrillation |
| Atrial flutter | Cardioversion, digoxin |
| Atrial fibrillation | Cardioversion, quinidine, procainamide, disopyramide (to maintain sinus rhythm) Digoxin, propranolol (to control ventricular response) |
| *Ventricular* | |
| Ventricular premature contractions | |
|    Emergency | Lidocaine, procainamide, bretylium |
|    Chronic | Quinidine, procainamide, disopyramide, combinations (see below) |
| Tachycardia | Lidocaine, procainamide, bretylium, cardioversion |
| *Digitalis-Induced* | |
| Supraventricular or ventricular | Lidocaine, diphenylhydantoin |

*Combination Therapy for Suppression of Ventricular Ectopy*

1. Quinidine—procainamide (for maximal quinidine-like effect at a lower dose for each agent).

2. Quinidine or procainamide with propranolol in patients without congestive heart failure.

3. #1 above with lidocaine or diphenylhydantoin.

\* As new drugs become available—e.g., verapamil for supraventricular tachycardia—the order of preference may change.

of drug effect was extremely short because of rapid hydrolysis by plasma esterases leading to inactivation. Substitution of an amide for the ester linkage was associated with fewer central nervous system side effects, increased resistance to plasma hydrolysis, and retention of antiarrhythmic activity.

**Actions.** The cardiac actions of procainamide are the same as those described for quinidine. Automaticity and conduction are depressed while the effective refractory period is increased. As with quinidine, the ECG reflects drug induced cellular electrophysiologic alterations. QRS widening is associated with therapeutic effects and Q-T interval prolongation is associated with toxicity.

Anticholinergic activity, similar to that observed following quinidine administration, can be demonstrated leading to similar problems with control of ventricular response rate when atrial flutter or fibrillation is present. Negative inotropic effects accompany procainamide administration, but these may be less marked than after quinidine ingestion. Hypotension after procainamide is related to its negative inotropic effect and to peripheral vasodilatation due to a direct action on vascular smooth muscle. As with quinidine, these effects are negligible in most patients during oral administration of procainamide.

**Uses.** One of the primary therapies for emergency treatment and prophylaxis of paroxysmal atrial tachycardia associated with the Wolff-Parkinson-White syndrome involves suppression of bypass tract conduction so that ventricular activation occurs predominantly via the A-V node and His-Purkinje system. Procainamide is the drug of choice for *emergency intravenous* therapy to achieve accessory tract suppression.[45,46] Similar therapy is also used in patients with preexcitation and atrial fibrillation, since the high ventricular response rates to atrial tachyarrhythmia can be life-threatening under the circumstances. Chronic therapy is usually with quinidine.

Procainamide is not as effective as quinidine against atrial arrhythmias and is not usually the first choice for their therapy. If quinidine cannot be employed, however, procainamide may satisfactorily suppress these arrhythmias.

Single premature ventricular contractions and more complex ventricular arrhythmias often are suppressed with procainamide. Intravenous procainamide is a mainstay in the emergent therapy for ventricular arrhythmia and, until bretylium became available, was the only effective intravenous agent for emergency therapy of arrhythmia refractory to lidocaine. Oral procainamide chronic therapy for ventricular arrhythmia is certainly at least as effective as quinidine therapy for the same arrhythmias.

**Absorption, Fate, and Excretion.** Procainamide can be administered by the oral, intramuscular, or intravenous route, although absorption after intramuscular administration can be erratic.[47] Intravenous boluses are usually given over 2 to 5 minutes to avoid hypotension and reflex increases in sympathetic nervous system activity. The usual intravenous dose is 100 mg every 5 minutes until arrhythmia suppression has occurred or until a total of 1 g of drug has been administered. The antiarrhythmic effect is then maintained by instituting a continuous infusion of from 20 to 80 $\mu g/kg$ per minute. Oral therapy usually involves 2 to 4 g/day in divided doses at 6-hour or, more frequently, 4-hour intervals, as the drug half-life is between 2.2 and 4 hours.[48]

Peak plasma concentration after oral drug ingestion is 1 hour. Plasma levels decline thereafter at a rate between 10 to 20 percent per hour. Liver acetylation and plasma hydrolysis are responsible for drug disappearance, and 90 percent of the drug or its metabolites can be recovered in the urine.[48,49] Drug accumulation is associated with renal insufficiency or renal tubular acidosis but not with hepatic insufficiency, congestive heart failure, or states where plasma protein available for drug binding is altered, since plasma hydrolysis can be extensive.

N-acetyl procainamide (NAPA) is an active metabolite produced by acetylation of drug in the liver. This metabolite occurs in high concentration in rapid acetylators or in patients with renal insufficiency and may exert important antiarrhythmic effects.[50] Trials of NAPA as an antiarrhythmic agent have revealed several potential benefits for the metabolite over the parent drug:

(1) There is less individual variability in drug level after an administered dose, since elimination of drug depends only on renal excretion.

(2) The half-life of NAPA is about twice as long as that for procainamide, thus allowing less frequent oral administration.

(3) The potential for immunologic reactions to the drug may be less (see below).

**Side Effects and Toxicity.** Effective therapy with procainamide is frequently limited by the appearance of side effects and drug toxicity; these have been of sufficient magnitude to limit its use in long-term antiarrhythmic prophylaxis. The most serious problem involves the drug's ability to induce serologic abnormalities with chronic use and a syndrome that resembles systemic lupus erythematosus. Most patients receiving more than 2 g of procainamide per day develop a positive antinuclear antibody test. Migratory polyarthralgia, fever, and skin rashes may appear in at least one third of patients maintained on chronic procainamide therapy, in association with abnormal serology.[51] Initial symptoms of the lupus syndrome may appear within 10 to 14 days of drug administration, when drug fever is often first encountered. Myalgia, arthritis, pleuropericarditis, and hepatomegaly may also be found as symptoms of the lupus-like syndrome. Pulmonary manifestations are more prominent with drug-induced lupus than with the idiopathic form, but renal and cerebral involvement and false positive serologic tests for syphilis are not observed. Hematologic abnormalities are also uncommon. Symptoms generally clear rapidly following drug withdrawal.

Recently, it has been appreciated that the rate at which procainamide is acetylated may reflect the propensity for developing positive serology and the lupus-like syndrome.[52] Patients rapidly acetylating procainamide may take longer to develop positive antinuclear antibodies and the lupus syndrome. This finding suggests that a procainamide metabolite may be responsible for this type of toxicity, since acetylated drug is cleared by the kidneys, resulting in partial protection, leaving less parent compound to be converted to other metabolites that may be toxic. If N-acetyl-procainamide replaced procainamide as a therapeutic agent, significant reduction in drug toxicity might result.

Patients receiving chronic therapy should be followed closely for evidence of drug-induced lupus and for agranulocytosis, which also has been reported. Baseline studies should include complete blood count, erythrocyte sedimentation rate, antinuclear antibody test, and determination of acetylator phenotype. Hematologic studies should be repeated several times during each year that the patient is on drug therapy, and the drug should be withdrawn if lupus symptoms appear.

Procainamide can produce the same cardiac toxicity observed after quinidine administration (see Table 14.1). Doses of 4 gm or more per day are associated with anorexia, nausea, vomiting, or diarrhea.

## Disopyramide (Norpace)

Disopyramide phosphate was released in this country for treatment of ventricular arrhythmias in 1977, but the drug has been available in Europe for 10 years. Its spectrum of cardiac and noncardiac actions is very similar to those of quinidine and procainamide, although it resembles neither drug structurally.

**Actions.** Disopyramide has been shown to produce the cardiac electrophysiologic effects commonly associated with Class I agents.[53,54] Phase 4 diastolic depolarization is decreased in cells possessing automaticity, and upstroke velocity of the action potential (phase 0) and overshoot are decreased without a change in the resting membrane potential. The terminal phase of repolarization may be prolonged, and the effective refractory period is increased. These effects are associated with a depression in ectopic automaticity and fast fiber conduction velocity. There is a direct depressant effect of disopyramide on A-V nodal conduction.

Studies in Purkinje fibers from normal and infarcted myocardium have revealed that disopyramide decreases the disparity between refractory periods in these two zones and may reduce inhomogeneous recovery within the infarct zone.[55]

Like quinidine and procainamide, disopyramide has potent anticholinergic effects. Its major N-monodealkylated metabolite is about 20 times more potent than the parent compound in anticholinergic activity.[56] The direct and indirect effects of disopyramide lead to variable effects on A-V nodal transmission and the electrocardiographic intervals (see Table 14.1). However, if sinus node or conduction system disease is present, it can be exacerbated by disopyramide. Problems with control of ventricular response rate to atrial fibrillation and flutter are also encountered with disopyramide for the same reasons cited above for quinidine and procainamide. Like quinidine and procainamide, disopyramide also depresses accessory bypass tract conduction in the WPW syndrome.[57]

Negative inotropic effects have been demonstrated for disopyramide in animal preparations and in man in the presence of preexisting congestive heart failure.[58,59] The drug is not well tolerated in patients with cardiomyopathy. Podrid et al. have reported that disopyramide is far more potent as a negative inotropic agent when compared to quinidine; they observed that, if congestive heart failure has occurred at any time in the past, disopyramide may precipitate recurrence in as many as 50 percent of patients.[59a]

**Uses.** Disopyramide may occasionally be effective in arrhythmia suppression where quinidine and procainamide have failed. However, most frequently the drug is employed for chronic arrhythmia suppression for the same dysrhythmias as quinidine and procainamide. The claim that disopyramide treatment is as effective as quinidine therapy but associated with fewer side effects and toxicity has not been adequately documented.[60]

Many clinical studies document the efficacy of disopyramide for suppression of simple and complex ventricular arrhythmias.[61-63] The drug has been successfully employed to suppress atrial arrhythmias and appears to be as active as quinidine in this regard.[64] Control of ventricular response rate in the presence of ongoing atrial flutter or fibrillation may be a problem with disopyramide for the reasons cited above with quinidine and procainamide. Nodal reentrant PAT would likely not be suppressed by disopyramide once initiated, but the drug might block initiating premature atrial contractions. Disopyramide should also control the ventricular response rate in atrial flutter and fibrillation complicating preexcitation because, like quinidine and procainamide, it prolongs the refractory period of the accessory pathway.[57] Disopyramide is not used for emergency intravenous antiarrhythmic treatment, as only the oral preparation is available in the United States.

**Administration, Fate, and Excretion.** Disopyramide is absorbed slowly but almost completely following oral administration. In the United States, the drug is available in capsules containing either 100 mg or 150 mg of active base. Total daily dose ranges from 400 mg to 2.4 grams, usually given at 6-hour intervals because the plasma half-life is approximately 6 to 7 hours. Peak blood levels are attained 2 to 3 hours after drug ingestion.[65] A loading dose of 200 mg or 300 mg of disopyramide may be used to achieve more rapid therapeutic blood levels (2 to 5 $\mu$g/ml) but loading should be discouraged in patients with marked congestive heart failure, conduction system disease, hepatic or renal insufficiency, as marked depression in myocardial shortening, conduction block and other signs of drug toxicity may appear.

The major metabolite results from hepatic N-dealkylation of the parent compound and serum concentrations of this metabolite are usually approximately 10 percent that of disopyramide.[66] The N-monodealkylated metabolite is one quarter as potent as disopyramide in producing electrophysiologic Class I actions, 20 times as potent as a cholinergic antagonist, and has a positive inotropic effect.

Approximately 90 percent of the drug appears in the urine, with the remainder in the feces. Forty to sixty percent of an administered dose appears in the urine as unchanged drug, with 25 percent appearing in the urine as the N-monodealkylated metabolite. It follows that drug half life should increase with decreases in renal function or hepatic insufficiency. It is recommended that the interval between 100 mg doses be increased to 10 hours for creatinine clearance ($C_{cr}$) from 40 to 15 cc/min, to 20 hours for $C_{cr}$ 15 to 5 cc/min, and to 30 hours for $C_{cr}$ 5 to 1 cc/min.[67]

**Side Effects and Toxicity.** Disopyramide has been marketed as an antiarrhythmic agent that is as effective in arrhythmia suppression as quinidine or procainamide, with fewer side effects than either of these two agents. This claim is supported by several studies, but more clinical experience with the drug will be required before it is adequately proven.

The anticholinergic actions of the drug account for the majority of reported side effects. Dry mouth and urinary hesitancy are noted in from 10 to 40 percent of the patients; although they are seldom severe enough to occasion discontinuation of therapy, they can cause considerable patient discomfort. Urinary retention is one of the most serious anticholinergic effects; although it is relatively uncommon (2 percent of patients) disopyramide should be used with caution in patients with benign prostatic hypertrophy. The therapeutic indications for disopyramide treatment in patients with glaucoma should be carefully considered because of anticholinergic effects. Other adverse reactions due to anticholinergic drug effects appear in 3 to 9 percent of patients receiving disopyramide and include blurred vision, and constipation with pain, bloating, and gas.

Potentially harmful cardiac effects of disopyramide deserve special attention since further clinical experience with this medication has indicated that cardiac decompensation may be precipitated in as many as 50 percent of patients with a history of heart failure.[59a] Thus, the negative inotropic effects of disopyramide appear to be far more potent than those observed after quinidine or procainamide administration. Indeed, Podrid et al. remark that "There have been no reports of congestive heart failure precipitated by quinidine or procainamide, although both these agents have been extensively employed over many decades as the mainstay for treatment of cardiac arrhythmias." [59a] Patients with cardiomyopathy or severe congestive heart failure should not receive loading doses of disopyramide and should be observed closely for worsening heart failure. Similar precautions should be observed in patients with renal or hepatic failure. QRS widening or QT prolongation of 25 percent or greater are indications for drug discontinuation.[67] Cautious administration and frequent monitoring are indicated in patients with preexisting sinus node disease, high-degree A-V block, or bundle branch block. A syndrome similar to quinidine syncope has been reported for disopyramide, and therefore QT prolongation without arrhythmia suppression may be an indication for drug withdrawal.[68]

## Lidocaine

Lidocaine hydrochloride was developed by Lofgren, and has been used extensively as a local anesthetic agent.[69] It is the antiarrhythmic drug of choice for the emergency therapy of ventricular arrhythmias. Despite extensive investigation of the electrophysiologic actions of lidocaine in normal and ischemic myocardial fibers, its antiarrhythmic mechanism of action has not been definitely delineated.

**Cardiac Actions.** Lidocaine suppresses some types of spontaneous automaticity in experimental preparations. In this regard, lidocaine resembles quinidine and procainamide in affecting spontaneous automaticity occurring at membrane potentials greater than $-60$ mV, while automaticity occurring at less negative membrane potentials ($-50$ to $-40$ mV) is unaffected until toxic drug concentrations are achieved.[70,71,72] Spontaneous Phase 4 diastolic depolarization is suppressed in isolated, perfused stretched Purkinje fibers. In these same fibers exposed to low potassium concentrations, epinephrine- or ouabain-induced automaticity is also suppressed. Spontaneous discharge rates for the SA node or for ventricular pacemakers providing escape rhythms in patients with A-V block are little affected.

Conflicting data have been obtained in experi-

mental preparations when the effects on conduction velocity and the maximal rate of action potential depolarization are considered. Lidocaine does not affect upstroke velocity of the action potential in fibers with resting membrane potentials greater than $-80$ mV or in fibers bathed in perfusion solutions with potassium concentrations of 3 mM or less (these solutions are hypokalemic and tend to increase the resting membrane potential of myocardial fibers). [73-75] However, studies in blood-perfused preparations and preparations where the potassium is raised or in depolarized cardiac fibers revealed that lidocaine does slow upstroke velocity of the action potential.[76,77]

During recovery of excitability, lidocaine also alters the relationship between membrane potential and the upstroke velocity of the action potential; in this respect, it is like other Class I agents.[78,79] Following drug administration, recovery of maximum upstroke velocity occurs later after depolarization while action potential duration is either little affected or abbreviated. The effects on upstroke velocity of the action potential would be expected to prolong the effective refractory period and preferentially suppress the conduction of premature beats through partially depolarized tissue, while in normal fibers abbreviation of the refractory period should predominate and result in improved conduction of premature beats.

Lidocaine has no effects on A-V nodal, His, and Purkinje conduction in the absence of disease in these structures. However, infra-His A-V block has been described after lidocaine in the presence of preexisting conduction system disease.[80] Lidocaine is contraindicated in complete A-V block with a spontaneous escape rhythm, as are other Class I agents.

Negative inotropic effects are transient following bolus injections of lidocaine, and therapeutic concentrations are well tolerated by patients with significant congestive heart failure. However, hypotension and negative inotropic effects have been reported with lidocaine toxicity.[81]

**Clinical Uses.** Lidocaine is the drug of choice for the suppression of simple and complex ventricular arrhythmias in emergencies. Lidocaine prophylaxis during the peri-infarction period may reduce the incidence of spontaneous ventricular fibrillation.[82,83] Ventricular arrhythmia during digitalis intoxication can also be suppressed with lidocaine.[84] There are reports of suppression of paroxysmal atrial tachycardia associated with Wolff-Parkinson-White syndrome and conversion of atrial fibrillation to normal sinus rhythm after lidocaine therapy.[85,86] However, most often arrhythmias arising at or above the A-V junction do not respond to lidocaine.

**Absorption, Fate and Excretion.** Lidocaine is most commonly administered by the intravenous route, although intramuscular administration has been proposed as a prophylactic measure in patients with acute myocardial infarction.[83] Oral lidocaine administration is not practical because so much of the drug is metabolized on the first pass through the liver after it enters the circulation via the portal system.[87,88] Oral doses that produce therapeutic blood levels are associated with the central nervous system toxicity that is secondary to high blood levels of drug metabolites.[89,90] Recently, an oral analogue of lidocaine, tocainide, has become available for clinical investigation (see below).

Therapeutic blood levels of lidocaine can be achieved within 15 minutes following intramuscular administration of 200 to 300 mg of lidocaine with peak levels within 30 minutes after injection. Intramuscular drug absorption depends upon blood flow through the injection site, the surface area available for drug absorption, and the concentration of the injected solution.[91] The deltoid muscle injection site has been found to result in higher blood levels than the lateral thigh or the buttock. Therapeutic blood levels and effects have been observed for 45 to 60 minutes following intramuscular administration of lidocaine.[92] However, intramuscular injections are associated with a rise in serum creatine kinase from skeletal muscle, and this will tend to confuse the clinical picture in patients where the diagnosis of acute myocardial infarction has not been definitely made.

A single intravenous bolus of lidocaine produces an antiarrhythmic effect that lasts from 15 to 20 minutes. This correlates well with the study showing a 10- to 20-minute half-life for the rapid disappearance of drug from the blood following intravenous bolus administration, reflecting drug redistribution throughout the body.[93] A second, slower phase of drug elimination reflecting hepatic metabolism and renal excretion has a half-life of approximately 100 minutes. Administration by constant intravenous infusion alone would require 5 hours before stable blood levels are achieved. Therefore the drug is given in a bolus loading dose of 1 to 1.5 mg/kg followed by constant infusion of 1 to 4 mg/min. Plasma levels may dip below the therapeutic range with this regimen approximately 30 minutes after the initial bolus injection, so a second bolus of one half of the loading dose may be given at this time.[94]

Lidocaine is rapidly and almost completely metabolized in the liver, and only 10 percent of the parent compound is removed by renal excretion.[95-97] The major metabolites result from drug deethylation and hydrolysis. The deethylation product, ethylglycine xylidide, may contribute to antiarrhythmic effects.[98] Any condition reducing hepatic function or blood flow will result in slower elimination of drug and require dosage adjustment (e.g., congestive heart failure, hepatic disease, and hepatic failure.)[99]

**Side Effects and Toxicity.** Wide experience with lidocaine in a variety of patients has shown that the drug lacks significant cardiac toxicity. However, in patients with intramyocardial conduction block and other conducting system disease, lidocaine may transiently increase conduction disturbances, and A-V block has been reported.[100-101] Further, toxic concentrations are associated with bradycardia and hypotension due to myocardial depression and peripheral vasodilation that is mediated through a direct action of the drug on vascular smooth muscle.

The most common side effects and toxicity involve the central nervous system.[102,103] Dizziness, drowsiness, paresthesias, and euphoria are most frequently encountered at therapeutic lidocaine concentrations. Speech disturbances, confusion, excitement, and frank psychosis also occur, particularly in patients with previous central nervous system disease or in elderly individuals. Both petit and grand mal seizures with respiratory arrest and coma accompany toxic drug levels.

## Phenytoin (diphenylhydantoin, DPH, Dilantin)

DPH has electrophysiologic properties similar to those described for lidocaine. The drug has not been as effective as other available antiarrhythmic agents for the acute or chronic suppression of ventricular arrhythmias and soon may be of historical interest only. Currently, DPH is utilized as a drug of last resort, alone and in combination with quinidine or procainamide. In addition, arrhythmias associated with digitalis toxicity may be effectively treated with DPH, and this agent may antagonize digoxin-induced depression of atrioventricular conduction. In the future, DPH may be employed less and less as an antiarrhythmic agent as other, more effective drugs with similar electrophysiologic properties (e.g., tocainide) become available.

**Cardiac Actions.** Electrophysiologic effects described above for lidocaine are also shared by DPH.[104] Spontaneous depolarization at membrane potentials more negative than −60 mV are suppressed. Action potential upstroke is slowed most noticeably in partially depolarized fibers; this accounts for the conduction slowing observed after DPH action in depressed myocardial fibers.[105,106] DPH shortens the action potential duration more than the refractory period in *normal* myocardial fibers so that beats arriving during the relative refractory period begin at more negative potentials and have an improved rate of rise making them more effective generators of depolarizing current flow; improved conduction of premature beats in normal fibers would result from this electrophysiologic alteration.

DPH has important noncardiac effects. It accelerates conduction across the AV node perhaps via central extracardiac effects.[104] The direct effect of this agent can be documented in isolated tissues and results in depression of slow response action potentials similar to those normally found at the A-V node. Conduction slowing at the A-V node can be demonstrated in denervated or atropinized experimental preparations. However, the effects of DPH in man

without conduction system disease are to improve A-V nodal conduction velocity, probably through a centrally mediated withdrawal of vagal tone.

Chronic oral administration of DPH is not known to be associated with significant hemodynamic alterations, even in patients with depressed myocardial function. However, rapid intravenous administration of DPH has resulted in spontaneous ventricular fibrillation, negative inotropic effects, and hypotension, perhaps in part secondary to the diluent used in the commercially available preparation.[107-109] Following chronic administration, other drug effects primarily involve the central nervous system and the liver and will be covered below.

**Clinical Uses.** DPH may be the drug of choice for the control of digitalis-toxic ventricular arrhythmias. DPH is also used as a second-line drug in the treatment of refractory ventricular arrhythmia, often as a part of combination therapy with another Class I agent. Therapeutic trials with DPH as the primary agent for arrhythmia suppression have yielded conflicting results but generally have been disappointing;[110-115] blood levels must be used to guide administration, as the blood level after a given dose can vary considerably. Side effects are frequent and troublesome.

DPH has no role in the therapy of supraventricular arrhythmia.

**Administration, Fate, and Elimination.** The intravenous and oral routes are preferred for administration of DPH. Intravenous loading can be accomplished with 100 mg injections of DPH at 5-minute intervals until arrhythmia is controlled, toxicity ensues, or a total of 1,000 mg has been given.[116] Generally, patients are loaded with 1,000 mg in the first 24 hours in divided doses followed by 500 mg over the next 24 hours with maintenance doses ranging from 300 to 400 mg per day. This regimen may be used for the parenteral or the oral route. Intramuscular DPH administration leads to local tissue inflammation and erratic systemic absorption and is not recommended.[125]

There are several factors that importantly influence the plasma concentrations of DPH that are attained after a given dose in each patient; this leads to a variable dose-response relationship and therefore plasma levels must be determined to assure that adequate but not toxic concentrations of drug are present. DPH absorption occurs in the small bowel and so must await gastric emptying after oral ingestion.[117] The drug may then enter the enterohepatic cycle, be reintroduced into the small bowel, and be reabsorbed.[117,118] Peak plasma levels follow drug ingestion by 4 to 6 hours, and the plasma half-life for DPH is long. This is in part because of enterohepatic recycling of drug but also because the drug-metabolizing enzymes can be saturated (see below). DPH can be given once per day, and concentrations effective in maintaining arrhythmia suppression will result. DPH binding to plasma proteins is decreased in uremia, liver disease, hyperbilirubinemia, and in the presence of certain drugs.[119-123] The DPH dose should be adjusted downward in patients with these disorders.

DPH metabolism is via the hepatic microsomal system and consists primarily of hydroxylation of one of the phenyl rings followed by glucuronide conjugation. This enzyme system is saturated when therapeutic plasma concentrations of DPH are achieved (greater than 10 $\mu g/ml$), and DPH disappearance rate is constant and independent of plasma concentration under these circumstances (0 order kinetics).[124] Thus, the higher the plasma concentration, the longer the duration of action. Agents that induce hepatic microsomal activity, such as phenobarbital, hasten DPH metabolism, while concurrent isoniazid administration interferes with DPH degradation. Patients with hepatic failure or genetic absence of hepatic hydroxylating enzymes must have the drug dose reduced because of slow disposition.

**Side Effects and Toxicity.** Rapid intravenous treatment with DPH in elderly patients has resulted in respiratory arrest, bradycardia, heart block, and sinus arrest.[126-127] Also reported have been ventricular fibrillation, negative inotropic effects, and hypotension, perhaps in part due to the effects of the diluent used in the commercial preparation (see above). Chronic administration results in side effects and toxicity that exclude the heart.[128] Gingival hyperplasia may be the most frequent drug-associated side effect, present in up to 40 percent of pa-

tients receiving this agent. Central nervous system effects are often dose-related and include nystagmus, diplopia, visual blurring, dysarthria, ataxia, and dizziness. Drug allergy occurs in the form of toxic hepatitis, systemic lupus erythematosis, pseudolymphoma, and a variety of cutaneous problems including rash, depigmentation, and hirsutism. Megaloblastic anemia associated with low blood folate levels may be found in patients on DPH therapy.

## Propranolol

Inhibition of catecholamine effects on the heart through $\beta$-receptor blockade is thought to be the primary mechanism for arrhythmia suppression for Class II drugs. Until recently, propranolol was the only Class II agent available in the United States. Other agents—including metoprolol, timolol, altenolol, sotalol, and alprenolol—either are or will soon be available. These agents block cardiac $\beta$-receptors and can be used for antiarrhythmic actions similar to those described for propranolol. Their pharmacology will not be discussed in this chapter.

**Actions.** Propranolol blocks the effects of $\beta$-one and $\beta$-two receptorstimulation.[129,130] Catecholamine-induced stimulation of $\beta$-one receptors causes increases in cardiac automaticity both at the SA node and in the specialized conducting system. In addition, $\beta$-one receptor stimulation increases conduction velocity across the A-V node and shortens the effective refractory period of this structure. Stimulation of $\beta$-one receptors, both in the atria and in the ventricles, causes increased shortening in these areas. Cardiac effects of $\beta$-receptor blockade depend on the resting level of adrenergic tone, but generally the effects of $\beta$-blockade are diametrically opposed to those for $\beta$-one receptor catecholamine induced stimulation.

The effects of $\beta$-two receptor stimulation include dilatation of blood vessels in skeletal muscle, relaxation of bronchial smooth muscle, enhanced insulin release from the pancreas, and glycolysis in skeletal muscle. These catecholamine effects are also blocked by propranolol. In addition, propranolol decreases plasma renin activity, and this effect may be important in mediating the antihypertensive effects of this agent.

The basis for grouping agents which block catecholamine receptors into a separate class stems from the observation that hyperactivity of the sympathetic nervous system is important in the genesis of many cardiac arrhythmias, and that catecholamine depletion or blockade will lower the incidence of clinical and experimental arrhythmias associated with ischemia and other etiologies.[131-134] Propranolol and some other $\beta$-blockers also have potent local anesthetic properties, and controversy has existed concerning the relative contributions of $\beta$-adrenergic blockade and Class I effects to observed antiarrhythmic actions. It now appears that $\beta$-receptor antagonists in therapeutically relevant concentrations act largely and perhaps exclusively by adrenergic blockade and that their local anesthetic properties (which are apparent at high concentrations) are probably not usually important in the control of cardiac arrhythmias.[135,136] Propranolol-induced depression of Phase 4 depolarization in automatic cells, resulting in decreased automaticity, may be the principal electrophysiologic mechanism for arrhythmia suppression.[137,138] This action results from $\beta$-blockade. Further, propranolol suppresses supraventricular tachycardias due to atrioventricular nodal reentry and slows the ventricular response rate during atrial flutter or fibrillation. This action also is dependent on the inhibition of adrenergic tone to the atrioventricular node, resulting in a secondary increase in A-V nodal refractoriness and a slowing of conduction in the A-V nodal fibers. On the other hand, potent antiarrhythmic Class I effects have been demonstrated with quaternary propranolol derivatives, and these drugs may be the first in an important new group of antiarrhythmic agents.[139]

**Uses.** $\beta$-blockers are effective in treating arrhythmia from several different etiologies: [130,140]

1. Ventricular arrhythmias unresponsive to other antiarrhythmic agents, usually in combination with Class I agents.

2. Digitalis toxic arrhythmias.

3. Nodal reentrant supraventricular tachycardia.

4. Supraventricular tachycardia associated with the Wolff-Parkinson-White syndrome.

5. Ventricular rate control during atrial flutter and fibrillation.

6. Control of arrhythmias associated with increased adrenergic activity (see above).

7. Sudden death prophylaxis in ambulatory patients with coronary artery disease.

All of these uses involve the blockade of adrenergic effects on local automaticity or conduction.[130] Propranolol influences A-V nodal conduction by blocking the effects of catecholamines that facilitate conduction velocity at the A-V node, allowing the parasympathetic nervous system to act unopposed to slow conduction. This results in a slowed ventricular response to atrial flutter and fibrillation, and block of recirculating rhythms at the A-V node during paroxysmal atrial tachycardia. Other uses listed above probably reflect blockade of local catecholamine effects to enhance spontaneous automaticity.

Digitalis-induced arrhythmias are suppressed by propranolol. However, diphenylhydantoin and lidocaine are preferred because of the potential of propranolol to exacerbate bradycardia and conduction blocks.

Recent reports have stimulated interest in the role of $\beta$-receptor blocking agents during and after myocardial infarction, since three controlled trials using prophylactic $\beta$-blockers have shown a reduced incidence of sudden death in patients during the late postinfarction period.[140-142] However, until further confirmatory information is available, routine use of $\beta$-blockers for this purpose is not recommended.

**Absorption, Fate and Distribution.** Propranolol blood levels are quite variable following oral administration; the magnitude of $\beta$-blockade for any given plasma level is also variable.[143] These differences may reflect variations in hepatic first pass metabolism, as at least eight metabolites for propranolol have been identified in man and little unchanged drug is recovered from the urine.[144] Thus, hepatic blood flow and the status of hepatic binding sites are critically important in determining plasma concentrations during propranolol therapy.[145] Observed variations between drug plasma levels and the degree of $\beta$-blockade require that the decision as to what dose of propranolol to use for $\beta$-blockade be based on physiologic parameters such as resting heart rate and the response of heart rate to exercise or change in body position.

Following discontinuation of propranolol, $\beta$-blocking activity disappears in less than 48 hours.[146]

Several conditions have been noted to alter the disposition of propranolol usually requiring a downward adjustment in dosage.[147,148] These include: (1) uremia; (2) alcoholic cirrhosis; (3) chronic active hepatitis; (4) cardiac cirrhosis; and (5) portacaval shunting. In these conditions, altered hepatic metabolism, volume of drug distribution, and bioavailability are thought to be responsible for alterations in blood levels.

For acute therapy, propranolol may be administered in 1-mg increments at 1- to two-minute intervals while the ECG and blood pressure are monitored. A total dose between 7 and 10 mg may be administered in this manner if well tolerated. Oral dosage is usually between 80 and 320 mg daily, given in 2 to 4 divided doses—although total doses approaching 1,000 mg have rarely been employed.

**Side Effects and Toxicity.** The most commonly seen side effects of propranolol involve the central nervous system. These include generalized fatigue, depression, and nightmares. Other reported adverse effects include nausea, diarrhea, alopecia, impotence, increased peripheral vascular insufficiency, and hypo- or hyperglycemia.

Cardiac actions of propranolol can result in worsening of congestive heart failure in patients dependent upon sympathetic nervous system tone for adequate cardiac function; for this reason, propranolol must be employed with caution in such patients. Sinus bradycardia may also be associated with propranolol therapy but is usually well tolerated with rates above 44 per minute unless sinus node disease is present. Similarly, A-V block may be uncovered or exacerbated during propranolol therapy, and atropine and/or isoproterenol should be available when the drug is given intravenously. Sudden propranolol withdrawal in patients with angina has been associated with serious rebound phenomena including a marked increase in the frequency of chest pain and, on occasion, myocardial infarction.[149,150]

Asthma and chronic obstructive pulmonary disease can be exacerbated by propranolol, and the drug is relatively contraindicated in such patients. However, selective $\beta$-1 antagonists are becoming available in this country, and these agents can be employed in such patients with relative safety.

### Bretylium Tosylate

Bretylium, a bromobenzyl quaternary ammonium derivative, was first introduced as an antihypertensive agent in 1959.[151,152] After bretylium administration blockade of catecholamine release from adrenergic nerve endings was observed and was thought to be a mechanism for drug-induced hemodynamic effects. Subsequent experience with bretylium in the therapy of chronic hypertension was disappointing because of variable drug effects resulting from inconstant absorption and the rapid appearance of drug tolerance. Subsequently, the antiarrhythmic effects of bretylium were appreciated in the mid 1960s, and this agent is now generally available for the treatment of ventricular arrhythmias.[153,154]

**Actions.** Bretylium produces cardiac effects via effects on the adrenergic nervous system and via direct membrane effects on myocardial fibers. High concentrations of bretylium release norepinephrine from adrenergic nerve endings.[155] Subsequently, the drug inhibits the neuronal release of norepinephrine in response to nerve stimulation and blocks the uptake of norepinephrine into adrenergic nerve endings.[155,156] Blockade of neuronal uptake of norepinephrine produces higher concentrations of this substance at postjunctional receptor sites on the cell membrane, resulting in an enhanced response to circulating or locally released catecholamines. The relationship of these catecholamine effects to the observed antiarrhythmic activity of bretylium is uncertain, but the effects of both catecholamine release and subsequent inhibition on arrhythmias and hemodynamics will depend on electrophysiologic conditions in the area of drug action and on existing resting adrenergic tone.

The direct action of bretylium on cardiac fibers is to increase the action potential duration and prolong the effective refractory period in ventricular myocardial fibers without altering the relationship between effective refractory period and action potential duration.[157-159] Bretylium also decreases the disparity in action potential duration between normal and infarcted regions of the canine heart.[160] Since inhomogeneity is thought to be an important prerequisite for ectopic activity, this could be the basis for at least part of the antifibrillatory action of this agent. The most impressive effects of bretylium have been demonstrated in animal models of ventricular fibrillation, where the drug is effective in reversing fibrillation in the canine heart without electrical countershock.[161,162] Bretylium also increases the electrical threshold for ventricular fibrillation in normal hearts, hypothermic hearts, ischemic hearts, and hearts exposed to regional hyperkalemia.[161-167] Unlike other antiarrhythmic drugs, bretylium does not suppress automaticity. In fact, transient increases in automaticity have been noted following bretylium administration; this effect is probably related to the above-mentioned release of catecholamines.

The hemodynamic effects of bretylium are complex. The drug increases shortening in isolated papillary muscles with catecholamine stores intact. However, this is probably due largely to the release of endogenous catecholamines, as positive inotropic effects have not been observed at clinically achieved concentrations in the presence of $\beta$-blockade or catecholamine depletion following reserpine.[155] Bretylium may have direct positive inotropic effects at concentrations greater than those achieved in man.[168] Studies in man have demonstrated an initial significant increase in heart rate and systemic arterial pressure which lasts for 15 minutes, followed by a decrease in heart rate, systemic arterial pressure, systemic vascular resistance, and no change in cardiac index.[169] Thus, ventricular function may be maintained after bretylium-induced removal of sympathetic nervous system tone by a reduction of the "afterload" on the myocardium. However, this effect could be deleterious in patients with preexisting hypotension.

**Clinical Uses.** Bretylium is particularly effective in preventing recurrences of ventric-

ular tachycardia and fibrillation that are resistant to therapy with other antiarrhythmic agents.[3,170,171] In addition, chemical defibrillation has been reported in man following bretylium administration.[172] This phenomenon has not been reported for any other antiarrhythmic agent. On the other hand, the response of premature ventricular depolarizations to bretylium is inconsistent, and this agent may not be as effective as other antiarrhythmic drugs in suppression of these rhythms. Data obtained to date indicate that bretylium may be the drug of choice for the emergency treatment of truly resistant and recurrent ventricular tachycardia or ventricular fibrillation; an early trial of bretylium in patients with these arrhythmias appears justified based on the present experience with the drug.

Bretylium has been found to be ineffective in the treatment of supraventricular arrhythmias.

**Absorption, Fate, and Excretion.** In the past, bretylium has been administered by the oral, intravenous, and intramuscular routes, but currently it is approved for parenteral use only. Following oral ingestion, absorption is incomplete, and doses of 400 mg to 600 mg every 6 hours have been employed to achieve arrhythmia suppression.[171,173] Tolerance to the hypotensive effects of bretylium has been noted with chronic oral therapy while arrhythmia suppression appeared to be maintained.[173,174] After 2 to 4 months of oral therapy with bretylium, parotid pain—associated with salivation and mastication, but without inflammation of the parotid gland—has been reported.

The intravenous dose of bretylium for emergency arrhythmia suppression is 5 to 10 mg/kg. This dose can be given as a bolus from the ampule containing 500 mg of bretylium in 10 ml of water; in less urgent situations, the dose can be diluted in 50 ml or more of isotonic dextrose or sodium chloride and given over 10 minutes while the ECG and blood pressure are monitored. Boluses can be repeated at 15- to 30-minute intervals with a total dose not to exceed 30 mg/kg. Once effective arrhythmia suppression has been achieved, an antiarrhythmic effect can be maintained by repeating the 5 to 10 mg/kg dose intramuscularly or intravenously every 6 to 8 hours or with an intravenous infusion of one to 2 mg/min. The total daily dose of bretylium should not exceed 30 mg/kg for any 24-hour period.

Bretylium appears to be avidly taken up by the neuronal membranes of the adrenergic nervous system as well as by the myocardial membranes.[175] The onset of action is fastest after the intravenous route, and arrhythmia suppression can occur within minutes—although in some patients the onset of action may be delayed for from 20 minutes to one hour. In some patients full antiarrhythmic effects may not develop for several hours. Plasma levels peak following intramuscular administration at 1½ hours after injection.[176]

Bretylium does not appear to undergo significant hepatic metabolism; the majority of the administered dose in man and experimental animals has been recovered in the urine within the first 24 hours following administration.[177,178] Elimination has not been studied following the intravenous administration of bretylium, but following intramuscular administration the plasma half-life ranges from 4.2 to 16.9 hours (mean 9.8 hours).[176] Plasma bretylium concentrations have not correlated with arrhythmia suppression and cannot be used as a guide to therapy.

**Side Effects and Toxicity.** The most common undesirable effect associated with bretylium administration is hypotension which is due to blockade of the adrenergic nervous system and resultant decreases in peripheral vascular resistance. Significant postural hypotension can be found in most patients; decreases in mean arterial pressure, even in the supine position of 10 to 20 mm Hg, are not uncommon but often are not clinically detrimental. In some patients excessive hypotension has been observed and can be treated with the intravenous administration of fluids and vasopressor drugs.[171,179,180] Hypersensitivity to infused catecholamines occurs during bretylium therapy, presumably due to blockade of uptake of these catecholamines into nerve endings. Therefore, blood pressure must be monitored carefully when vasopressors are employed to reverse hypotension.

Release of norepinephrine, produced by initiation of bretylium therapy by bolus injections, can be associated with transient increases in blood pressure or arrhythmias or both. In cases of digitalis toxicity, bretylium is not recommended for arrhythmia suppression, since initial release of catecholamines can exacerbate digitalis induced arrhythmias.

Nausea and vomiting are not uncommon when bretylium is given very rapidly by bolus injections, but these rarely occur when the drug is administered over several minutes. Parotid swelling and pain have been associated with chronic oral therapy but have not been a problem with short-term parenteral administration.[171] Other major side effects have not been noted, and bretylium is generally well tolerated, with only 6 to 8 percent of patients demonstrating adverse effects that have required discontinuation of the drug.[171,179]

## NEW ANTIARRHYTHMIC DRUGS

The drugs that follow are in clinical trial in the United States, and some may become generally available. Each agent appears to possess potent antiarrhythmic properties. Aprindine, tocainide, and mexiletine are Class I agents. Amiodarone is a Class III agent, and verapamil is a Class IV drug.

### Aprindine

Aprindine hydrochloride is a tertiary amine with local anesthetic properties that was developed and initially used in Belgium. It most closely resembles quinidine or procainamide in its electrophysiologic action.[181]

**Actions.** Electrophysiologic studies reveal that aprindine produces changes in recovery of excitability and conduction depression in both atrial and ventricular muscle. Aprindine shortens Purkinje fiber action potential duration and, to a lesser extent, shortens effective refractory period.[182-184] In cardiac muscle fibers, however, action potential duration is only slightly reduced, but the duration of the effective refractory period is lengthened.[182,183] The rate of rise of phase zero of the action potential is depressed, with greater effects noted as the heart rate is increased or the resting membrane potential is decreased.[185] In normal Purkinje fibers, automaticity is decreased by aprindine; the same effect is seen in the presence of the digitalis glycoside acetylstrophanthidin.[181] Aprindine injections into the sinus node artery in intact dogs decrease the spontaneous sinus rate, and injections into the A-V nodal artery prolong the functional refractory period and conduction time through the A-V node. The drug also produces direct effects similar to quinidine when A-V nodal conduction is studied in that aprindine prolongs the A-H interval, H-V interval, transmural ventricular conduction time, and the effective refractory period of the ventricle.[181] Widespread conduction depression following aprindine is reflected by significant widening of the QRS complex (up to 15 to 20 percent) in patients receiving this agent.[186] Accessory pathway conduction in patients with the Wolff-Parkinson-White syndrome is also suppressed, more reliably in the antegrade than in the retrograde direction.[187,188]

Aprindine is effective in suppressing both atrial and experimental ventricular arrhythmias. The drug also suppresses ventricular arrhythmias occurring 24 hours after coronary artery occlusion as well as digitalis-induced arrhythmias.[187,189,190]

Hemodynamic studies reveal that at therapeutic doses aprindine is a mild depressant of myocardial function, the effects being similar to those noted after quinidine administration.[186,191]

**Clinical Uses.** Several studies have shown that aprindine is effective in suppressing a variety of supraventricular and ventricular arrhythmias in patients with different types of heart disease. Chronic stable ventricular arrhythmias have been totally suppressed in up to 67 percent of patients receiving this drug; many of these patients had been previously given procainamide, quinidine, or β-blocking agents with little or no therapeutic response.[192] In another study, arrhythmias following acute myocardial infarction appearing on the 4th through the 20th day were more effectively suppressed by aprindine than by disopyramide.[193] Recently, Zipes and Troup[194] have reported on a group of patients who were treated chronically with aprindine for frequent symptomatic premature ventricu-

lar complexes (2 patients), recurrent ventricular tachycardia (36 patients), or recurrent ventricular tachycardia and ventricular fibrillation (12 patients). The subjects were intolerant of or did not respond to quinidine, procainamide, propranolol, lidocaine, diphenylhydantoin, and overdrive pacemaker suppression. Mean serum concentrations of 1.8 μg/ml of aprindine were achieved. In 13 patients, aprindine was discontinued because it did not control arrhythmia, because it produced intolerable side effects, or because ventricular arrhythmias could no longer be demonstrated at the time of antiarrhythmic testing. Excluding an additional 3 patients who died, 30 of 34 remaining patients receiving aprindine at the time of the study had no episodes of ventricular fibrillation or ventricular tachycardia. In addition, it was found that these patients had achieved 80 percent suppression of premature ventricular complexes when the results of 24-hour Holter examinations during aprindine therapy were compared with those obtained before the drug was started. Thus, aprindine appears to be quite effective against complex ventricular arrhythmias which are resistant to treatment with more conventional antiarrhythmic drugs.

Aprindine successfully suppressed tachyarrhythmia secondary to the Wolff-Parkinson-White syndrome in 12 of 14 patients in the study reported by Zipes and Troup.[194] Electrophysiologic evaluation performed during this study and others has revealed that aprindine produces complete block or increased refractoriness of the accessory pathway that is greater for the antegrade than the retrograde direction. This makes it a particularly useful drug for ventricular response rate control in patients with an accessory pathway and atrial fibrillation or flutter.

**Absorption, Fate, and Excretion.** Aprindine is available only in the oral dosage form in the United States. It is almost completely absorbed following oral ingestion, and is 85 to 95 percent protein bound.[194] Hepatic metabolism accounts for elimination of the majority of the drug, and 95 percent appears as hydroxylated metabolites that undergo glucuronidation in the liver. Sixty-five percent of aprindine and its metabolites is found in the urine, with the remaining 35 percent in the feces.[191] Elimination half-life ranges from 12 to 60 hours, and the full antiarrhythmic effect of the drug may not appear for several days, even when the agent is administered with a loading dose. Dosage regimens usually include a loading dose ranging from 200 to 400 mg followed by maintenance doses of 100 to 200 mg daily, given in twice daily dosing as this is thought to yield a more uniform therapeutic effect.[186,191,192]

**Side Effects and Toxicity.** Side effects with aprindine are quite common, particularly during the initial loading period and adjustment of maintenance dose, since the ratio between toxic and therapeutic drug concentrations is rather narrow. Central nervous system side effects are most common and are most often dose related. Tremor is most common; as the serum concentration increases dizziness, intention tremor, ataxia, nervousness, hallucinations, diplopia, memory impairment, or seizures may occur.[194,195] Gastrointestinal side effects are seen less frequently, and nausea and diarrhea are most common among these. Central nervous system side effects can be controlled with concomitant administration of meclizine.[194] Cholestatic jaundice and agranulocytosis have recently been reported in association with aprindine therapy; it is thought that these are idiosyncratic reactions as opposed to dose-related toxicity.[196] Both of these complications appear to be reversible if the drug is discontinued. In addition, transient abnormalities of liver function tests have been noted in some studies but no abnormalities persisted or led to discontinuation of the drug. In a similar vein, QRS widening and prolongation are common but do not progress to advanced conduction system block unless serious underlying conduction system disease is present.

## Tocainide

Lidocaine is one of the more efficacious and less toxic antiarrhythmic agents but it has a major disadvantage that it must be given parenterally to be effective. Tocainide is a primary amine analog of lidocaine which differs from the parent drug in that it lacks two ethyl groups that contribute to lidocaine's first pass hepatic

degradation after oral administration. Tocainide is now undergoing clinical trials in the United States. The drug has already been shown to be effective in suppressing arrhythmias that are refractory to treatment with currently available antiarrhythmic preparations and may achieve its greatest use in combination therapy with other agents.

**Actions.** The electrophysiologic effects of tocainide are similar to those already described for lidocaine. At low doses in normal Purkinje fibers, tocainide increases the rate of rise of phase zero of the action potential and decreases it at higher doses. Action potential duration is decreased at 50 percent repolarization but not at 100 percent repolarization, while the effective refractory period is decreased.[197] When infused into patients, tocainide does not produce significant electrophysiologic effects at peak plasma concentrations averaging $11 \pm 1.7$ $\mu g/ml$ (range 3.7 to 22.7 $\mu g/ml$).[198] Anderson and coworkers [198] showed that the atrial, A-V nodal, and right ventricular effective refractory periods were slightly decreased while the sinus node recovery time and Wenckebach cycle length for the A-V node was unchanged. In addition the Q-Tc interval was slightly decreased during atrial pacing while the A-H interval was slightly increased under similar circumstances. H-V and QRS intervals were unchanged. Studies in animals have shown that the ventricular fibrillation threshold is elevated after tocainide and that the compound is effective against arrhythmias induced by coronary ischemia.[197,199]

Like lidocaine, tocainide is thought to produce minimal hemodynamic effects in therapeutic concentrations. Mean aortic and pulmonary pressures and vascular resistances exhibit a small but significant increase during a 15-minute infusion of drug, and these rises are accompanied by small increases in right and left ventricular end-diastolic pressures without significant changes in left ventricular shortening, heart rate, or cardiac index.[200]

**Arrhythmia Suppression—Clinical Studies.** Tocainide has been shown to be effective in suppressing premature ventricular complexes and ventricular tachycardia in patients with associated coronary artery disease, cardiomyopathy, mitral prolapse, and other disease states. Short-term studies in patients with stable chronic premature ventricular complexes have shown a 50 to 75 percent suppression of arrhythmia in the majority of individuals receiving the drug.[200,201,202] Ryan et al.[203] investigated tocainide efficacy for arrhythmia suppression in patients with ventricular arrhythmias refractory to quinidine, procainamide, and propranolol, and found 75 percent suppression of ventricular premature beats in 13 of 30 patients enrolled in the study. In this study, ventricular tachycardia was present in 21 of 30 patients and was completely abolished in 14 patients. Tocainide doses employed in these studies have ranged from 400 to 800 mg/day and have been given either as a single oral dose of drug or at 8- to 12-hour intervals. Peak tocainide blood levels in patients responding to the drug have ranged from 5 to 15 $\mu$g/ml.[203]

Recent studies indicate that tocainide is effective in the long-term suppression of refractory ventricular arrhythmias. Engler et al.[204] followed 18 patients for 3 to 10 months who had previously demonstrated greater than 70 percent suppression of average hourly ventricular premature complex counts on 24-hour electrocardiographic monitoring or conversion of grade 4B arrhythmias (Lown and Wolf classification) to a lower grade of arrhythmia. Effective chronic arrhythmia suppression subsequently was defined as an 80 percent or greater decrease in ventricular premature complexes in followup 24-hour ambulatory ECGs compared to the frequency in recordings obtained in the absence of tocainide. Significant arrhythmia suppression was observed in 17 of the 21 patients initially entered in the study, and in the remaining 4 patients ventricular tachycardia was abolished despite a less than 80 percent reduction in ventricular premature complexes. The mean peak blood level 30 minutes to 4 hours after dosing in these patients was 10.3 $\mu$g/ml with a range of from 6.6 to 13.9 $\mu$g/ml. These blood levels were obtained after an average of 7.4 months from the start of therapy. Three to ten months after entry into this study, 18 patients were readmitted to the hospital for tocainide withdrawal to retest drug efficacy and the need for continued antiarrhythmic therapy. Ventricular

tachycardia recurred in 9 of 15 patients who had this rhythm before starting tocainide therapy; thus, continued arrhythmia suppression could be demonstrated in these patients. Grade 2 or 3 arrhythmias without ventricular tachycardia were present in 3 of 18 patients in this withdrawal study, and arrhythmia recurred in all three patients, indicating continued suppression of arrhythmia with tocainide therapy. Thus, tocainide appears to be an effective oral agent in some patients for the therapy of potentially lethal ventricular arrhythmias refractory to other medication.

**Absorption, Fate, and Excretion.** Tocainide is rapidly absorbed following oral administration; peak serum levels occur 60 to 90 minutes after drug ingestion.[200,205] Plasma half-life ranges from 12 to 15 hours, and the drug is 50 percent protein bound. Forty percent of the drug is excreted unchanged in the urine, while the remainder is presumed to undergo hepatic degradation.[205,206] Therapeutic plasma concentrations range from 4 to 15 $\mu$g/ml and can be achieved by an oral dose regimen of from 400 to 800 mg every 8 to 12 hours.[200,201,204,207] Side effects appear to be dose related.

**Side Effects and Toxicity.** Minor central nervous system side effects are observed in virtually all patients maintained on chronic tocainide therapy. These include decreased recent memory, decreased mental alertness, difficulty concentrating, paresthesias, mild tremor, light-headedness, and incoordination. These symptoms tend to occur at doses of 600 mg every 8 hours or greater but not infrequently can be found in patients receiving 400 mg every 8 hours when such individuals are questioned closely. Paranoid delusions and thought impairment responding to discontinuation of tocainide have been observed on occasion in patients receiving higher doses of this drug.

Gastrointestinal complaints are frequent at the initiation of therapy but seldom persist during chronic administration. These include anorexia, nausea, abdominal pain, vomiting, and constipation. Chronic cervical muscle spasms have been exacerbated by this drug and have necessitated discontinuation of therapy.[204] In addition, drug allergy has been observed manifested by erythematous maculopapular rash.[204]

There have been no significant changes observed in indices of hepatic, renal, or hematologic function during long-term tocainide administration. The possibility that antinuclear antibody titers may become positive in some patients receiving tocainide has been raised, but lymphocytotoxicity has not been demonstrated in these patients when investigated.[204]

In summary, tocainide frequently causes mild to moderate side effects which do not require discontinuation of drug and which tend to be well tolerated by patients with serious arrhythmias. Severe toxicity appears to be unusual. The drug is promising because of demonstrated efficacy in arrhythmia suppression, high oral bioavailability, and convenient dosing interval.

## Mexiletine

Mexiletine, a primary amine analog of lidocaine, was developed in a search for a preparation which would replace phenmetrazine as an anorectic compound with minimal central nervous system effects. Investigation of this compound has revealed that it was a potent anticonvulsant and in addition had local anesthetic and antiarrhythmic activity.[208] The drug has been used an an antiarrhythmic agent in Europe and Great Britain since 1972, and its actions appear similar to those of lidocaine.[209]

**Actions.** Electrophysiologic studies of mexiletine in cardiac tissue demonstrate a decrease in the rate of rise of phase zero of the action potential.[210] In addition the ventricular fibrillation threshold is increased in experimental animals, and mexiletine is as effective as lidocaine in abolishing ventricular tachycardia and other experimentally induced ventricular arrhythmias following experimental coronary artery occlusion, digitalis intoxication or adrenaline and halothane administration.[211,212,213] In man, mexiletine produces no consistent effect on the frequency of sinus node discharge rate, intraatrial conduction, or atrial refractoriness.[214] Effects on the specialized conduction system have been variable and include: increase in refractoriness at the A-V node and His-Purkinje system; a prolonged H-V interval (noted in one study); and shortening of the relative refractory period of the His-Purkinje system (the only consistent effect noted in another study conducted in man).[214,215] As with lidocaine, the effects may depend on the presence or absence of disease in the specialized conducting system.

Studies in isolated cardiac tissue reveal that mexiletine has a mild negative inotropic effect similar to that seen with lidocaine.[216] Similar results have been obtained in clinical studies in several groups of patients with a variety of disorders including coronary artery disease and aortic valve disease with prosthetic valve replacement.[217-220] The drug has no activity as an antagonist of the autonomic nervous system and has anesthetic activity equipotent with lidocaine, procainamide, or propranolol.[216]

**Clinical Antiarrhythmic Activity.** Mexiletine is effective in suppressing both acute and chronic ventricular arrhythmias. Campbell et al.[221] treated 89 patients with acute and chronic ventricular arrhythmia with 200-mg injections of mexiletine followed first by intravenous infusions of 3 mg/min for one hour and subsequently by 1.5 mg/min steady state infusions. A greater than 75 percent reduction in the number of PVCs was noted in 51 of the 89 patients, and 4 additional patients had 50 percent or greater suppression of PVCs. These investigators also treated 57 patients with an oral dose of 400 mg of drug followed by 200 to 400 mg 2 hours later. It was found that two thirds of the patients had a 50 percent or greater suppression in the number of PVCs. It was noteworthy that mexiletine produced arrhythmia suppression in some cases where lidocaine had failed. Similar results have been noted by Talbot et al.,[222] who reported that 31 of 43 patients had a 95 percent or greater suppression of arrhythmia following mexiletine therapy; an additional 9 patients demonstrated a 75 percent or greater reduction in the number of VPCs with abolition of ventricular tachycardia or prolongation of the R-R interval so the VPCs no longer fell into the preceding T wave. Of 32 patients in this series treated with intravenous mexiletine, 26 had been refractory to lidocaine. An additional 13 patients had not responded to additional antiarrhythmic agents.

Mexiletine at a dose of 250 mg every 8 hours has been compared with oral procainamide, 500 mg every 4 hours in a double-blind, placebo control study conducted in the first 2 weeks following myocardial infarction.[223] After 36 hours of intravenous lidocaine therapy, 32 percent of patients treated with mexiletine and 35 percent of patients treated with procainamide experienced further arrhythmias, while the patients receiving placebo had a 77 percent incidence of further arrhythmias. In addition mexiletine was found to be a more acceptable antiarrhythmic drug than procainamide because it was administered less frequently, with lower associated toxicity and with better suppression of ventricular ectopic beats and complex ventricular arrhythmias. The results of this study are supported by other data which indicate that mexiletine administration within 48 hours of acute myocardial infarction reduces the incidence of spontaneously occurring ventricular tachycardia and R-on-T ventricular ectopic beats.[222]

There is no evidence that mexiletine is beneficial for the therapy of supraventricular arrhythmias.

**Absorption, Fate and Distribution.** Mexiletine is virtually completely absorbed following oral administration with peak plasma levels occurring between 2 to 4 hours following ingestion.[224] A parenteral preparation is available in Great Britain and Europe but is not yet available in this country. The mean plasma half-life in healthy subjects following intravenous administration has been reported to be 10.4 hours and after oral administration 9.3 hours. In patients stopping chronic oral therapy, a similar value of 12.1 hours for plasma half-life was obtained, but in patients with myocardial infarction mean half-life has been reported to be significantly longer, with an average of 16.7 hours.[224] Under normal circumstances mexiletine is eliminated primarily by metabolism which is presumed to occur predominately in the liver; thus, the prolonged half-life in patients with myocardial infarction may reflect reduced hepatic blood flow. Thus, the mexiletine dose must be adjusted in patients with congestive heart failure or hepatic disease, as only 5 to 10 percent of the drug appears unchanged in the urine. The drug is given at 8 to 12-hour intervals; total daily doses in the range of 600

to 1,000 mg are required to maintain therapeutic plasma levels of between 1 and 2 $\mu$g/ml.

**Side Effects and Toxicity.** Following oral administration, mild adverse reactions may be seen in up to 65 percent of patients treated with mexiletine with severe adverse effects occurring in up to 35 percent.[221] Mild side effects most often involve the central nervous system, with tremor and nystagmus being the most common. Other central nervous system side effects include lightheadedness, blurred vision, paresthesias, ataxia, confusion, and drowsiness. Indigestion, nausea, and vomiting have also been reported on initiation of drug therapy and on a chronic basis shortly after drug ingestion, but these side effects rarely require drug withdrawal. Severe side effects which have required either dosage reduction or drug withdrawal have included tremor, nystagmus, and nausea. Rarely, hypotension, bradycardia, and aggravation of rhythm disturbances have been associated with mexiletine therapy. There is one case where thrombocytopenia and a positive antinuclear antibody were associated with mexiletine therapy, but the relationship between drug ingestion and these findings may have been fortuitous.[221] Severity and frequency of side effects appear to be related to plasma concentrations, as side effects are more frequently seen at plasma levels between 1.5 and 3 $\mu$g/ml, although there is considerable overlap with therapeutic levels.

## Amiodarone

Amiodarone is a benzofuran derivative which has been employed as an antianginal agent.[225] It has recently been appreciated that this drug has potent antiarrhythmic effects.[226] Amiodarone, a Class III agent, produces increases in action potential duration as its major electrophysiologic effect. This compound has structural similarities to thyroxine, and it has been noted that increases in action potential duration are seen in hypothyroidism.[227] Further, atrial arrhythmias are rare in hypothyroidism but common in thyrotoxicosis, where atrial intracellular action potentials are markedly abbreviated. Currently, the relation of the thyroxine-like structure of this compound to its antiarrhythmic effects is unclear but represents an interesting area for further study.

**Actions.** Amiodarone prolongs the action potential duration in atrial and ventricular muscle as well as Purkinje fibers without altering resting membrane potential or automaticity.[226,228] The drug's effects on automatic cells in the SA node are to increase action potential duration and to decrease the slope of diastolic depolarization.[229] Amiodarone has no local anesthetic effects on nerve or cardiac membranes, but in experimental studies extremely weak Class I actions have been reported (decreases in the slope of phase zero of the action potential in Purkinje fibers, atrial, and ventricular muscle).[230] In intact hearts, the sinus node discharge rate is slowed following administration of amiodarone even after pharmacologic autonomic blockade.[231] Electrophysiologic studies in man have revealed that amiodarone slows sinus nodal discharge rate, lengthens A-V nodal conduction time, and increases the atrial and ventricular monophasic action potential duration and refractory period.[232-235] In patients with Wolff-Parkinson-White syndrome, the effective refractory period of the accessory pathway is prolonged by amiodarone, more in the antegrade than the retrograde direction.[232] Following amiodarone administration, electrocardiographic abnormalities have also been noted and have involved T-wave changes, U waves, and prolongation of the Q-T interval.[226] Experimental arrhythmias produced by administration of barium chloride, myocardial ischemia, acetylcholine, aconitine, or digitalis have been suppressed by amiodarone.[236]

In the coronary and systemic vascular beds, amiodarone is a potent smooth muscle relaxant. It increases coronary blood flow with a concomitant decrease in peripheral vascular resistance, cardiac work, and oxygen consumption.[231,237] A negative inotropic effect occurs, particularly at higher doses, but because of peripheral vasodilatation amiodarone is usually well tolerated by patients with congestive heart failure and severe left ventricular dysfunction.[226,238] Negative inotropic effects may be related in part to

decreased adrenergic tone which has been noted following amiodarone. The drug does not exhibit competitive $\beta$-receptor blocking activity but does have a mild noncompetitive inhibitory effect on sympathetic nerve stimulation.[236] Inotropic and chronotropic effects of glucagon are also antagonized by amiodarone.[240]

**Clinical Uses.** The reports of initial clinical trials with amiodarone against a variety of arrhythmias have been extremely favorable. Rosenbaum et al.[226] observed complete suppression of arrhythmia in all but one out of 30 patients who had recurrent atrial flutter and fibrillation, in 96 percent of 59 patients with repetitive supraventricular tachycardia, in all of the 27 patients who had Wolff-Parkinson-White syndrome and in the majority (77 percent) of 44 patients with recurrent ventricular tachycardia that had been resistant to other agents. Subsequent studies have confirmed these favorable results in a wide variety of arrhythmias, and the drug continues to show promise as a remarkably effective antiarrhythmic agent with a very broad spectrum.[194,232,238]

**Absorption, Fate, and Excretion.** Following oral ingestion about 50 percent of the drug is absorbed, resulting in low blood levels.[239] But the native compound and its metabolites are widely distributed, accounting in part for an exceedingly long duration of action. It has been estimated that the total concentration of drug in the body decreases by only 16 to 34 percent 30 days after amiodarone has been stopped. Antiarrhythmic effects have been noted for as long as 30 to 45 days after the drug has been discontinued.[226,239] Thus, this agent seems to accumulate slowly in tissues, and it has been estimated that several weeks may be required for its full antiarrhythmic effects to become manifest.[226] At this time drug half-life and fate in the body have not been determined.

Amiodarone has a wide margin of safety, and the median lethal dose of the drug is reported to be more than 10 times the therapeutic dose when the compound is given intravenously and even greater when the drug is given orally.[240] Amiodarone is usually given as a single daily dose of from 200 to 800 mg for antiarrhythmic effects.

**Side Effects and Toxicity.** The most consistent undesirable effect associated with amiodarone therapy is the occurrence of corneal microdeposits which appear as a yellow-brown granular pigmentation of the cornea.[241-245] These deposits tend to be reversible with cession of drug therapy, and irreversible damage has never been reported.[226] Eye drops containing methylcellulose or sodium iodide heparinate seem to prevent or diminish these deposits.[244,246]

Amiodarone appears otherwise to be very well tolerated. There is a small incidence of gastrointestinal complaints such as constipation, nausea, and vomiting. Amiodarone also may cause a slight gray-blue discoloration of the skin which may take months to disappear after the drug is stopped.[247,248] In addition, amiodarone may cause thyroid dysfunction; patients may exhibit hypo- or hyperthyroidism which is presumably due to the large iodine load. Therefore, thyroid function should be followed during therapy.[249,250]

Because of its depressant effects on the SA node and specialized conducting system, amiodarone is contraindicated in patients with significant conduction delays, and complete heart block has been precipitated during amiodarone therapy.[226]

## Verapamil

This agent is a papaverine derivative that produces its primary effects through antagonism of transmembrane calcium fluxes associated with the action potential through what has been termed the "slow channel." Verapamil is also a vasodilator and was originally introduced as an antianginal drug in the United States. It was withdrawn, however, when it appeared to induce cataracts in beagle dogs during early toxicology studies. Subsequently, it has become clear that this reaction was a species-specific verapamil effect. Verapamil is now in use at medical centers all over the world, and it is currently under clinical investigation in the United States.

**Actions.** The electrophysiologic effects of verapamil-induced decreases in calcium flux are most marked in areas of the heart where slow response action potentials are normally found. Thus the A-V node is particularly sensitive to verapamil's effects, and suppression of electrical activity in this area is associated with drug administration. Conduction suppression through the A-V node, reflected by A-H interval prolongation, can be demonstrated in the absence of atrial (P-A interval), His-Purkinje (H-V interval), or intraventricular (QRS interval) conduction time prolongation.[250-253] In addition to conduction slowing, recovery of full excitability within the A-V node is prolonged following depolarization and is reflected by increases in the A-V nodal functional and effective refractory periods.[254] The spontaneous discharge rate of the sinus node is also showed by verapamil. None of these effects appear to be mediated via alterations in autonomic tone to the heart.[254] The A-V nodal depressant effects of verapamil are clearly related to this agent's beneficial effects in suppressing A-V nodal reentrant rhythms—i.e., supraventricular tachycardia and controlling the ventricular response to atrial fibrillation—but in the presence of conduction system disease, $\beta$-blockade or digitalis therapy, heart block may occur.[255,256]

Verapamil has a local anesthetic potency 1.6 times that of procaine, but it does not share the electrophysiologic actions of the Class I agents at clinically relevant concentrations.[230] The drug does not affect resting membrane potential, maximum action potential rate of rise, or action potential amplitude, and accelerates only phase 2 of repolarization in atrial, ventricular, or Purkinje fibers.[230,257] However, slow channel dependent activity in these tissues can be suppressed by this agent in depolarized, diseased, or digitalis toxic myocardial fibers.[257-262]

Verapamil has a direct negative inotropic effect and causes peripheral vasodilitation. However, these effects are accompanied by a reflex-induced increase in sympathetic tone; thus, the net effect of verapamil administration will depend on the level of autonomic tone, prevailing myocardial contractility, and other factors such as the resistance of the systemic vascular bed, preload, etc.[263-269] In the absence of coronary artery disease, coronary blood flow is increased by verapamil and the drug is thought to act as a direct vasodilator of coronary arteries.[266,270,271] In most patients the hemodynamic effects of verapamil result in mild hypotension only.

**Clinical Uses.** Verapamil is particularly useful in the therapy of supraventricular arrhythmias. The drug effectively controls the ventricular response rate to atrial fibrillation and flutter and will occasionally cause spontaneous reversion of these ectopic rhythms to normal sinus rhythm following intravenous or oral administration.[263]

Verapamil is an effective antianginal agent and currently appears useful in the therapy of variant angina.[279] This agent may also prove useful in the treatment of hypertrophic cardiomyopathies.

**Absorption, Fate and Excretion.** Oral absorption of verapamil is rapid and almost complete.[272,273] The dose employed is usually 80 to 120 mg every 8 hours. The intravenous dose is about one tenth the oral dose (range 5 to 15 mg) since verapamil entering the body via the gastrointestinal tract and the portal circulation is rapidly metabolized in the liver to N or O-demethylated forms or both.[274]

The intravenous bolus administration of 10 mg is ideally carried out over a 60-second period while the ECG and blood pressure are monitored, although the entire dose can be given over 10 to 15 seconds if a rapid response is desired. Boluses can be repeated at 30-minute intervals with infusions of 0.005 mg/kg per minute to maintain the response.[275] If left ventricular dysfunction is present, the dose should be reduced.

Verapamil is 90 percent protein-bound in the serum. Following intravenous or oral administration, the agent disappears from the plasma in a biexponential fashion. There is an initial distribution phase lasting 18 to 35 minutes with the half-life for elimination thereafter ranging from 3 to 7 hours.[272] The majority of the administered dose is found in the urine as metabolized drug.

**Side Effects and Toxicity.** Verapamil is usually very well tolerated if conditions that will amplify its pharmacologic effects are avoided. Thus, the drug should not be administered to patients with sick sinus syndrome, high-degree

or unstable A-V block, overt congestive heart failure, or marked hypotension. The drug should not be used in presence of $\beta$-adrenergic blockade or in conjunction with quinidine-like drugs because shock and asystole have been reported under these conditions.[276-278] Catecholamines are recommended to reverse the negative inotropic effects of verapamil.

After oral administration, approximately 2 percent of patients will complain of gastrointestinal disturbances, with constipation and nausea being the most common; central nervous system symptoms, such as headache and dizziness, also occur. A variety of other miscellaneous side effects have been reported in a few patients receiving verapamil, including skin rashes and dyspnea.[255]

# REFERENCES

1. Lown B: Sudden cardiac death: The major challenge confronting contemporary cardiology. Am J Cardiol 43:313–328, 1979.
2. Klein GJ, et al: Ventricular fibrillation in the Wolff-Parkinson-White syndrome. N Engl J Med 301:1080–1085, 1979.
3. Dhurandhar RW, Teasdale SJ, Mahon WA: Bretylium tosylate in the management of refractory ventricular fibrillation. Can Med Assoc J 105:161–166, 1971.
4. Noble D: Potassium currents and pacemaker activity. In The Initiation of the Heartbeat. Oxford University Press, New York, 2nd ed., 1979, p. 85–102.
5. Hauswirth O, Singh BN: Ionic mechanisms in heart muscle in relation to the genesis and the pharmacological control of cardiac arrhythmias. Pharmacol Rev 30:5–63, 1979.
6. Bigger JT Jr, Mandel WJ: Effect of lidocaine on canine Purkinje fibers and at the ventricular muscle-Purkinje fiber junction. J Pharmacol Exp Ther 172:239–254, 1970.
7. Rosen MR, et al: Effects of therapeutic concentrations of diphenylhydantoin on transmembrane potentials of normal and depressed Purkinje fibers. J Pharmacol Exp Ther 197:594–604, 1976.
8. Han J, Goel BG, Hanson CS: Reentrant beats induced in the ventricle during coronary occlusion. Am Heart J 80:778–784, 1970.
9. Vaughan Williams EM: Classification of antiar-

rhythmic drugs. J Pharmacol Ther 1:115–138, 1975.

10. Singh BN: Rational basis for antiarrhythmic therapy: Clinical pharmacology of commonly used antiarrhythmic drugs. Angiology 29:206–242, 1978.

11. Ducouret P: The effect of quinidine on membrane electrical activity in frog auricular fibers studied by current and voltage clamp. Br J Pharmacol 57:163–184, 1976.

12. Watanabe Y, Dreifus LS: Interactions of quinidine and potassium on atrioventricular transmission. Circ Res 20:434–446, 1967.

13. Hoffman BF, Rosen MR, Wit AL: Electrophysiology and pharmacology of cardiac arrhythmias. VII. Cardiac effects of quinidine and procaineamide. Am Heart J 90:117–122, 1975.

14. Verrier RL, Thompson PL, Lown B: Ventricular vulnerability during sympathetic stimulation: Role of heart rate and blood pressure. Cardiovasc Res 8:602–610, 1974.

15. Corr PB, Witkowski FX, Sobel BE: Mechanisms contributing to malignant dysrhythmias induced by ischemia in the cat. J Clin Invest 61:109–119, 1978.

16. Davis LD, Temte JV: Effects of propranolol on transmembrane potentials of ventricular muscle and Purkinje fibers in the dog. Circ Res 22:661–677, 1968.

17. Schuster DP, Lucchesi BR, et al: The antiarrhythmic properties of UM-272, the dimethyl quaternary derivative of propranolol. J Pharmacol Exp Ther 184:213–227, 1973.

18. Boura ALA, Green AF: The actions of bretylium: Adrenergic neuron blocking and other effects. Br J Pharmacol 14:536–548, 1959.

19. Polster P, Broekhuysen J: The adrenergic antagonism of amiodarone. Biochem Pharmacol 25:131–134, 1976.

20. Bacaner M: Quantitative comparison of bretylium with other antifibrillatory drugs. Am J Cardiol 21:504–512, 1968.

21. Cranefield PF: The Conduction of the Cardiac Impulse. Futura Publishing, Mt. Kisco, New York, 1975.

22. Kohlhardt M, Bauer B, Krause H, Fleckenstein A: Selective inhibition of the transmembrane calcium conductivity of mammalian myocardial fibers. Pflugers Arch 338:115–123, 1973.

23. Trautwein W: Membrane currents in cardiac muscle fiber. Physiol Rev 53:793–835, 1973.

24. Rosen MR, Wit AL, Hoffman BF: Electrophysiology and pharmacology of cardiac arrhythmias. IV. Cardiac effects of verapamil. Am Heart J 89:665–673, 1975.

25. Singh BN, Ellrodt G, Peter PT: Verapamil: A review of its pharmacological properties and therapeutic uses. Drugs 15:159–197, 1978.

26. Heng MK, Singh BN, Roche AHC, Norris RM, Mercer CJ: Effects of intravenous verapamil on cardiac arrhythmias and on the electrocardiogram. Am Heart J 90:487–498, 1975.

27. Beckman H: Treatment in General Practice. W. B. Sanders, Philadelphia, 1934.

28. Vaughan Williams EM: The mode of action of quinidine on isolated rabbit atria interpreted from intracellular records. Br J Pharmacol 13:276–287, 1958.

29. Johnson EA, McKinnon MG: The differential effect of quinidine and pyrilamine on the myocardial action potential at various rates of stimulation. J Pharmacol Exp Ther 120:460–468, 1957.

30. Chen CN, Gettes LS, Katzung BG: Effect of quinidine and lidocaine on steady state and recovery kinetics of (dv/dt) max. Circ Res 37:20–29, 1975.

31. Heissenbuttel RH, Bigger JT Jr: The effect of oral quinidine on intraventricular conduction in man: Correlation of plasma quinidine with changes in QRS duration. Am Heart J 80:453–462, 1970.

32. Crawford MH, White BH, O'Rourke RA: Effects of oral quinidine on left ventricular performance in normal subjects and patients with congestive cardiomyopathy. Am J Cardiol 44:714–718, 1979.

33. Engler RL, Le Winter MM, Karliner JS: Depressant effects of quinidine gluconate on left ventricular function in conscious dogs with and without volume overload. Circulation 60:828–835, 1979.

34. Reynolds EW Jr, MacDonald WJ, Greenfield BM, Semion AA: Mechanisms of onset and termination of abnormal cardiac rhythm studied by constant monitoring. Am Heart J 74:473–481, 1967.

35. Gallagher JJ, Gilbert M, Svenson RH, Sealy WC, Cassel J, Wallace AG: Wolff-Parkinson-White syndrome. The problem, evaluation, and surgical correction. Circulation 51:767–785, 1975.

36. Gallagher JJ, Svenson RH, Sealy WC, Wallace AG: The Wolff-Parkinson-White syndrome and the preexcitation dysrhythmias. Med Clin North Am 60:101–123, 1976.

37. Goldreyer BN, Gallagher JJ, Damato AN: The electrophysiologic demonstration of atrial ectopic tachycardia in man. Am Heart J 85:205–215, 1973.

38. Greenblatt CJ, Pfeifer HJ, Ochs HR, Franke K, Smith TW, Koch-Weser J: Pharmacokinetics of parenteral quinidine in humans. Clin Pharmacol Ther 21:105, 1977.

39. Palmer KH, Martin B, Baggett B, Wall ME: The metabolic fate of orally administered quinidine gluconate in humans. Biochem Pharmacol 18:1845–1860, 1969.

40. Hooymans PM, Merkus FWHN: Effect of quinidine on plasma concentration of digoxin. Br Med J 2:1022, 1978.

41. Hager WD, Fenster P, Mayersohn M, Perrier D, Graves P, Marcus FI, Goldman S: Digoxin-quinidine interactions. Pharmacokinetic evaluation. N Engl J Med 300:1238–1241, 1979.

42. Lown B, Wolf M: Approaches to sudden death from coronary heart disease. Circulation 44:130–142, 1970.

43. Selzer A, Ray HW: Quinidine syncope: Paroxysmal ventricular fibrillation occurring during treatment of chronic atrial fibrillation. Circulation 30:17–26, 1964.

44. Mautz FR: Reduction of cardiac irritability by the epicardial and systemic administration of drugs as a protection in cardiac surgery. J Thorac Surg 5:612–628, 1936.

45. Wellens HJJ, Durrer D: Effect of procainamide, quinidine, and ajmaline in the Wolff-Parkinson-White syndrome. Circulation 50:114–120, 1974.

46. Mandel WJ, Laks MM, Obayashi K, Hayakawa H, Daley W: The Wolff-Parkinson-White syndrome: Pharmacologic effect of procainamide. Am Heart J 90:744–754, 1975.

47. Koch-Weser J: Antiarrhythmic prophylaxis in ambulatory patients with coronary artery disease. Arch Int Med 129:763–772, 1972.

48. Koch-Weser J: Pharmacokinetics of procainamide in man. Ann NY Acad Sci 179:370–382, 1971.

49. Weiley HS, Genton E: Pharmacokinetics of procainamide. Arch Intern Med 130:366–369, 1972.

50. Elson J, Strong JM, Lee WK, Atkinson AJ: Antiarrhythmic potency of N-acetylprocainamide. Clin Pharmacol Ther 17:134–140, 1975.

51. Henningsen NC, Cederberg A, Hanson A, Johansson BW: Effects of long term treatment with procainamide. A prospective study with special regard to ANF and SLE in fast and slow acetylators. Acta Med Scand 198:475–482, 1975.

52. Woosley RL, Drayer DE, Reidenberg MM, Nies AS, Carr K, Oates JA: Effect of acetylator phenotype on the rate at which procainamide induces antinuclear antibodies and the lupus syndrome. N Engl J Med 298:1157–1159, 1978.

53. Danilo P, Rosen MR: Cardiac effects of disopyramide. Am Heart J 92:532–536, 1976.

54. Koch-Weser J: Drug therapy. Disopyramide. N Engl J Med 300:957–962, 1979.

55. Sasyniuk BI, Kus T: Cellular electrophysiologic changes induced by disopyramide phosphate in normal and infarcted hearts. J Int Med Res 4(suppl I):20–25, 1976.

56. Baines MW, Davies JE, Kellett DN, et al: Some pharmacological effects of disopyramide and a metabolite. J Int Med Res 4(suppl. I):5–7, 1976.

57. Spurrell RAJ, Thorburn CW, Camm J, et al: Effects of disopyramide on electrophysiological properties of specialized conduction system in man and on accessory atrioventricular pathway in Wolff-Parkinson-White syndrome. Br Heart J 37:861–867, 1975.

58. Mathur P: Cardiovascular effects of a newer antiarrhythmic agent, disopyramide phosphate. Am Heart J 84:764–770, 1972.

59. Story JR, Abdulla AM, Frank MJ: Cardiogenic shock and disopyramide phosphate. JAMA 242:654–655, 1979.

59a. Podrid PJ, Schoeneberger A, Lown B: Congestive heart failure caused by oral disopyramide. N Engl J Med 302:614–617, 1980.

60. Koch-Weser J: Prevention of sudden coronary death by chronic antiarrhythmic therapy. Adv Cardiol 25:206–228, 1978.

61. Smith WS, Vismara L, Kalmansohn RV, et al: Clinical studies of Norpace. Angiology 26 (suppl. I):124–153, 1975.

62. Heel RC, Brogden RN, Speight TM, et al: Disopyramide: A review of its pharmacological properties and therapeutic use in treating cardiac arrhythmias. Drugs 15:331–368, 1978.

63. Vismara LA, Vera Z, Miller RR, et al: Efficacy of disopyramide phosphate in the treatment of refractory ventricular tachycardia. Am J Cardiol 39:1027–1034, 1977.

64. Hartel G, Louhija A, Konttinen A: Disopyramide in the prevention of recurrence of atrial fibrillation after electroconversion. Clin Pharmacol Ther 15:551–555, 1974.

65. Hinderling PH, Garrett ER: Pharmacokinetics of the antiarrhythmic disopyramide in healthy humans. J Pharmacokinet Biopharm 4:199–230, 1976.

66. Grant AM, Marshall RJ, Ankier SI: Some effects of disopyramide and its N-dealkylated metabolite on isolated nerve and cardiac muscle. Eur J Pharmacol 49:389–394, 1978.

67. Norpace. Searle Laboratories Product Information, Physicians Desk Reference, 1980.

68. Zipes DP, Troup PJ: New antiarrhythmic agents. J Cardiol 41:1005–1024, 1978.

69. Lofgren N: Xylocaine: A New Synthetic Drug. Hoeggstroms, Stockholm, 1948.

70. Weld FM, Bigger JT Jr: The effect of lidocaine on diastolic transmembrane currents determining pacemaker depolarization in cardiac Purkinje fibers. Circ Res 38:203–208, 1976.

71. Mandel WJ, Bigger JT Jr: Electrophysiologic effects of lidocaine on isolated canine and rabbit atrial tissue. J Pharmacol Exp Ther 178:81–93, 1971.

72. Imanishi S, Surawicz B: Lidocaine resistant automaticity in depolarized guinea pig ventricular myocardium. Circulation 50(suppl III):145A, 1974.

73. Davis LD, Temte JV: Electrophysiological actions of lidocaine on canine ventricular muscle and Purkinje fibers. Circ Res 24:639–655, 1969.

74. Bigger JT Jr, Mandel WJ: Effect of lidocaine on transmembrane potentials of ventricular muscle and Purkinje fibers. J Clin Invest 49:63–77, 1970.

75. Rosen MR, Hoffman BF, Wit AL: Electrophysiology and pharmacology of cardiac arrhythmias. V. Cardiac antiarrhythmic effects of lidocaine. Am Heart J 89:526–536, 1975.

76. Singh BN, Vaughan Williams EN: Effects of altering potassium concentration on the action of lidocaine and diphenylhydantoin on rabbit atrial and ventricular muscle. Circ Res 29:286–295, 1971.

77. Chen CM, Gettes LS: Comparison of antiarrhythmic drug effect on the determinants of (dv/dt) max. Fed Proc 34:775A, 1975.

78. Bigger JT Jr, Mandel WJ: Effect of lidocaine on conduction in canine Purkinje fibers and at the ventricular muscle-Purkinje fiber junction. J Pharmacol Exp Ther 172:239–254, 1970.

79. Singh BN: Explanation for the discrepancy in reported cardiac electrophysiological actions for diphenylhydantoin and lidocaine. Br J Pharmacol 41:385–386, 1971.

80. Gupta PK, Lichstein E, Dhadda KD: Lidocaine induced heart block in patients with bundle branch block. Am J Cardiol 33:487–497, 1974.

81. Jewitt DE, Kishon Y, Thomas N: Lidocaine in the management of arrhythmia after acute myocardial infarction. Lancet 1:266–270, 1958.

82. Lie JI, Wellens HJ, VanCapelle FJ, Durrer D: Lidocaine in the prevention of primary ventricular fibrillation. A double blind randomized study of 212 consecutive patients. N Eng J Med 291:1324–1326, 1974.

83. Valentine PA, Frew JL, Mashford ML, Sloman JG: Lidocaine in the prevention of sudden death in the prehospital phase of acute infarction. N Engl J Med 291:1327–1331, 1974.

84. Anderson JL, Harrison DC, Meffin BJ, Winkle RA: Antiarrhythmic drugs: Clinical pharmacology and therapeutic uses. Drugs 15:271–309, 1978.

85. Josephson ME, Kastor JA, Kitchen JG: Lidocaine in Wolff-Parkinson-White syndrome. Ann Intern Med 84:44–45, 1976.

86. Malach M, Kostis JB, Fischetti JL: Lidocaine for ventricular arrhythmias in acute myocardial infarction. Am J Med Sci 257:52–60, 1969.

87. Rowland M, Thomson PD, Guichard A, et al: Disposition kinetics of lidocaine in normal subjects. Ann NY Acad Sci 179:383–397, 1971.

88. Stenson RE, Constantino RI, Harrison DC: Interrelationships of hepatic blood flow, cardiac output, and blood levels of lidocaine in man. Circulation 43:205–211, 1971.

89. Smith ER, Duce BR: The acute antiarrhythmic and toxic effects in mice and dogs of 2-ethylamino-2′, 6′-acetoxylidine (L-86), a metabolite of lidocaine. J Pharmacol Exp Ther 179:580–585, 1971.

90. Blumer J, Strong JM, Atkinson AJ Jr: The convulsant potency of lidocaine and N-dealkylated metabolites. J Pharmacol Exp Ther 180:31–36, 1973.

91. Cohen LS, Rosenthal JE, Horner DW, Atkins JM, Matthews OA, Sarnoff SJ: Plasma levels of lidocaine after intramuscular administration. Am J Cardiol 29:520–523, 1972.

92. Bernstein V, Berstein B, Griffiths J, Peretz DI: Lidocaine intramuscularly in acute myocardial infarction. JAMA 219:1027–1031, 1972.

93. Benowitz NL: Clinical applications of the pharmacokinetics of lidocaine. Cardiovasc Clin 6:77–101, 1974.

94. Harrison DC, Meffin PJ, Winkle RA: Clinical pharmacokinetics of antiarrhythmic drugs. Prog Cardiovasc Dis 20:217–242, 1977.

95. Hollunger G: On the metabolism of lidocaine. II. The biotransformation of lidocaine. Acta Pharmacol Toxicol 17:365–373, 1960.

96. Becket AH, Boyes RN, Appleton PJ: The metabolism and excretion of lignocaine in man. J Pharm Pharmacol 18(suppl):76–81, 1966.

97. Stenson RE, Constantino RT, Harrison DC: Interrelationships of hepatic blood flow, cardiac output and blood levels of lidocaine in man. Circulation 43:205–211, 1971.

98. Singh BN: Rational basis of antiarrhythmic therapy: Clinical pharmacology of commonly

used antiarrhythmic drugs. Angiology 29:206–242, 1978.

99. Thomson PD, Melmon KL, Richardson JA, et al: Lidocaine pharmacokinetics in advanced heart failure, liver disease and renal failure in humans. Ann Intern Med 78:499–508, 1973.

100. Cheng TO, Wadhwa K: Sinus standstill following intravenous lidocaine administration. JAMA 223:790–792, 1973.

101. Gupta PK, Lichstein E, Chadda, KD: Lidocaine-induced heart block in patients with bundle branch block. Am J Cardiol 33:487–492, 1974.

102. Boston Collaborative Drug Surveillance Program: Drug induced convulsions. Lancet 2:677–679, 1972.

103. Wagman IH, deJong RH, Prince DA: Effects of lidocaine on the central nervous system. Anesthesiology 28:155–172, 1967.

104. Wit, AL, Rosen MR, Hoffman BF: Electrophysiology and pharmacology of cardiac arrhythmias. VIII. Cardiac effects of diphenylhydantoin. Am Heart J 90:397–404, 1975.

105. Rosen MR, Danilo P, Alonso MB, et al: Effects of therapeutic concentrations of diphenylhydantoin on transmembrane potentials of normal and depressed Purkinje fibers. J Pharmacol Exp Ther 197:594–604, 1976.

106. Jensen RA, Katzung BG: Electrophysiological actions of diphenylhydantoin on rabbit atria. Circ Res 26:17–27, 1970.

107. Louis S, Kutt H, McDowell F: The cardiocirculatory changes caused by intravenous dilantin and its solvent. Am Heart J 74:523–529, 1967.

108. Lieberson AD, Schumacher RR, Childress RH, Boyd DL, Williams JF: Effects of diphenylhydantoin on left ventricular function in patients with heart disease. Circulation 36:692–699, 1967.

109. Karliner JS: Intravenous diphenylhydantoin sodium (Dilantin) in cardiac arrhythmias. Dis Chest 51:256–269, 1967.

110. Collaborative Group: Phenytoin after myocardial infarction. Controlled trial in 568 patients. Lancet 2:1055–1057, 1971.

111. Bigger JT Jr, Schmidt DH, Kutt H: Relationship between the plasma level of diphenylhydantoin sodium and its cardiac antiarrhythmic effects. Circulation 38:363–374, 1968.

112. Lovell RRH: Antiarrhythmia prophylaxis: Long term suppressive medication. Circulation 52(suppl III):236–240, 1975.

113. Stone N, Klein MD, Lown B: Diphenylhydantoin in the prevention of recurrent ventricular tachycardia. Circulation 43:420–427, 1971.

114. Vajda FJE, Prineas RJ, Lovell RRH, Sloman JG: The possible effect of long term high plasma levels of phenytoin on mortality after acute myocardial infarction. Eur J Clin Pharmacol 5:138–144, 1973.

115. Atkinson AJ Jr, Davison R: Diphenylhydantoin as an antiarrhythmic drug. Ann Rev Med 25:99–113, 1974.

116. Bigger JT Jr, Schmidt DH, Kutt H: Method for estimation of plasma diphenylhydantoin concentration. Am Heart J 77:572–573, 1969.

117. Albert KS, Sakmar E, Hallmark MR, Weidler DJ, Wagner JG: Bioavailability of diphenylhydantoin. Clin Pharmacol Ther 16:727–735, 1974.

118. Glazko AJ: Diphenylhydantoin. Pharmacology 8:163–177, 1972.

119. Reidenberg MM, Odar-Cederlöf I, von Bahr C, Borga O, Sjöqvist F: Protein binding of diphenylhydantoin and desmethylimipramine in plasma from patients with poor renal function. N Engl J Med 285:264–267, 1971.

120. Odar-Cederlöf I, Borga O: Kinetics of diphenylhydantoin in uraemic patients: Consequences of decreased plasma protein binding. Eur J Clin Pharmacol 7:31–37, 1974.

121. Blaschke TF: Protein binding and kinetics of drugs in liver diseases. Clin Pharmacokinet 2:32–44, 1977.

122. Rane A, Lunde PJ, Jalling B, Yaffee SJ, Sjöqvist F: Plasma protein binding of diphenylhydantoin in normal and hyperbilirubinemic infants. Pediatr Pharmacol Ther 78:877–880, 1971.

123. Winkle, RA, Glantz SA, Harrison DC: Pharmacologic therapy of ventricular arrhythmias. Am J Cardiol 36:629–650, 1975.

124. Gerber N, Lynn R, Oates J: Acute intoxication with 5,5-diphenylhydantoin (Dilantin) associated with impairment of biotransformation. Ann Intern Med 77:765–771, 1972.

125. Serrano EE, Roye DB, Hammer RH, Wilder BJ: Plasma diphenylhydantoin values after oral and intramuscular administration of diphenylhydantoin. Neurology 23:311–317, 1973.

126. Mercer EN, Osborne JA: The current status of diphenylhydantoin in heart disease. Ann Intern Med 67:1084–1107, 1967.

127. Rosen M, Lisak R, Ruben IL: Diphenylhydantoin in cardiac arrhythmias. Am J Cardiol 20:674–678, 1967.

128. Yahr MD: Drugs in the treatment of convulsive disorders. In Drill's Pharmacology in Medicine, ed. DiPalma JR. 4th ed, McGraw-Hill, New York, 1971.

129. Lands AM, Arnold A, McAuliff JP, et al: Differentiation of receptor systems activated by sympathomimetic amines. Nature 214:597–598, 1967.

130. Conolly ME, Kerstig F, Dollery CT: The clinical pharmacology of beta-adrenoceptor-blocking drugs. Prog Cardiovasc Dis 19:203–234, 1977.

131. Singh BN, Jewitt DE: Beta-adrenergic receptor blocking drugs in cardiac arrhythmias. Drugs 7:426–461, 1974.

132. Webb SW, Adgey AAJ, Pantridge JF: Autonomic disturbance at the onset of acute myocardial infarction. Br Med J 3:89–92, 1972.

133. Katz RL, Epstein RA: The interaction of anesthetic agents and adrenergic drugs to produce cardiac arrhythmias. Anesthesiology 29:763–784, 1968.

134. Krasnow N, Babarosh H: Clinical experiences with beta-adrenergic blocking agents. Anesthesiology 29:814–827, 1968.

135. Parmley WW, Braunwald E: Comparative myocardial depressant and antiarrhythmic properties of d-propranolol, dl-propranolol and quinidine. J Pharmacol Exp Ther 158:11–21, 1967.

136. Lucchesi BR, Whitsitt LS, Brown NL: Propranolol (Inderal) in experimentally induced cardiac arrhythmias. Can J Physiol Pharmacol 44:543–547, 1966.

137. Coltart DJ, Gibson DG, Shand DG: Plasma propranolol levels associated with suppression of ventricular ectopic beats. Br Med J 1:490–491, 1971.

138. Jewitt DE, Singh BN: The role of beta-adrenergic blockade in myocardial infarction. Prog Cardiovasc Dis 16:421–438, 1974.

139. Schuster DP, Lucchesi BR, Nobel-Allen NL, et al: The antiarrhythmic properties of UM-272, the dimethylquaternary derivative of propranolol. J Pharmacol Exp Ther 184:213–227, 1973.

140. Green KG, Chamberlin DM, Fulton RN, et al: Multicentre international study: Improvement in prognosis of myocardial infarction by long-term beta-adrenoceptor blockage using practolol. Br Med J 3:735–740, 1975.

141. Ahlmark G, Seatrie H, and Korsgren M: Reduction of sudden death after myocardial infarction by treatment with alprenolol. Lancet 2:1563, 1974.

142. Wilhelmsen C, Vedin JA, Wilhelmsen L, Tibblin G, Werkö L: Reduction of sudden deaths after myocardial infarction by treatment with alprenolol. Lancet 2:1157–1159, 1974.

143. Shand DG: Individualization of propranolol therapy. Med Clin North Am 58:1063–1069, 1974.

144. Walle T, Gaffney TE: Propranolol metabolism in dog and man: Mass spectrometric identification of six new metabolites. J Pharmacol Exp Ther 182:83–92, 1972.

145. Evans GH, Shand DG: Disposition of propranolol. V. Drug accumulation and steady-state concentrations during chronic oral administration in man. Clin Pharmacol Ther 14:487–493, 1973.

146. Coltart DJ, Cayen MN, Stinson EB, Goldman RH, Davies RO, Harrison DC: Investigation of the safe withdrawal period for propranolol in patients scheduled for open heart surgery. Heart J 37:1228–1234, 1975.

147. Bianchetti G, Graziani G, Brancaccio D, et al: Pharmacokinetics and effects of propranolol in terminal uraemic patients and in patients undergoing regular dialysis treatment. Clin Pharmacokinet 1:373–384, 1976.

148. Branch RA, Shand DG: Propranolol disposition and chronic liver disease: A physiological approach. Clin Pharmacokinet 1:264–279, 1976.

149. Diaz RG, Somberg J, Freeman E, et al: Myocardial infarction after propranolol withdrawal. Am Heart J 88:257–258, 1974.

150. Alderman EL, Coltart J, Wettach GE, et al: Coronary artery syndromes after sudden propranolol withdrawal. Ann Intern Med 81:625–627, 1974.

151. Dollery CT, Emslie-Smith D, McMichael J: Bretylium tosylate in the treatment of hypertension. Lancet 1:296–299, 1960.

152. Boura ALA, Green AF, McCoubrey A, et al: Darenthin: Hypotensive agent of a new type. Lancet 2:17–21, 1951.

153. Leveque PE: Antiarrhythmic action of bretylium. Nature 207:203–204, 1965.

154. Bacaner MB: Bretylium tosylate for suppression of induced ventricular fibrillation. Am J Cardiol 17:528–534, 1966.

155. Markis JE, Koch-Weser J: Characteristics and mechanisms of inotropic and chronotropic actions of bretylium tosylate. J Pharmacol Exp Ther 178:94–102, 1971.

156. Kirpekar SM, Furchgott RF: The sympathomimetic action of bretylium on isolated atria and aortic smooth muscle. J Pharmacol Exp Ther 143:64–76, 1964.

157. Wit AL, Steiner C, Damato AN: Electrophysiologic effects of bretylium tosylate on single fibers of the canine specialized conducting system and

ventricle. J Pharmacol Exp Ther 173:344–356, 1970.

158. Bigger JT Jr, Jaffe CC: The effect of bretylium tosylate on the electrophysiologic properties of ventricular muscle and Purkinje fibers. Am J Cardiol 27:82–92, 1971.

159. Waxman MB, Wallace AG: Electrophysiologic effects of bretylium tosylate on the heart. J Pharmacol Exp Ther 183:264–274, 1972.

160. Cardinal R, Sasyniuk BI: Electrophysiological effects of bretylium tosylate on subendocardial Purkinje fibers from infarcted canine hearts. J Pharmacol Exp Ther 204:159–174, 1978.

161. Bacaner MB: Bretylium tosylate for suppression of induced ventricular fibrillation. Am J Cardiol 17:528–534, 1966.

162. Bacaner MB: Quantitative comparison of bretylium with other antifibrillatory drugs. Am J Cardiol 21:504–512, 1968.

163. Bacaner MB, Schrienemachers D: Bretylium tosylate for suppression of ventricular fibrillation after experimental myocardial infarction. Nature 220:494–496, 1968.

164. Kniffen FJ, Lomas TE, Counsell RE, Lucchesi BR: The antiarrhythmic and antifibrillatory actions of bretylium and its o-iodobenzyltrimethylammonium analog, UM360. J Pharmacol Exp Ther 192:120–128, 1975.

165. Cervoni P, Ellis, CH, Maxwell RA: The antiarrhythmic action of bretylium in normal, reserpine-pretreated and chronically denervated dog hearts. Arch Int Pharmacodyn Ther 190:91–102, 1971.

166. Nielsen KC, Owman C: Control of ventricular fibrillation during induced hypothermia in cats after blocking the adrenergic neurons with bretylium. Life Sci 7:159–168, 1968.

167. Buckley JJ, Bosch OK, Bacaner MB: Prevention of ventricular fibrillation during hypothermia with bretylium tosylate. Anesth Analg (Cleve) 50:587–593, 1971.

168. Hammermeister KE, Boerth RC, Warbasse JR: The comparative inotropic effects of six clinically used antiarrhythmic agents. Am Heart J 84:643–652, 1972.

169. Chatterjee K, Mandel WJ, Vyden JK, et al: Cardiovascular effects of bretylium tosylate in acute myocardial infarction. JAMA 223:757–760, 1973.

170. Terry G, Vellani CW, Higgins MR, et al: Bretylium tosylate in the treatment of refractory ventricular arrhythmias complicating myocardial infarction. Br Heart J 32:21–25, 1970.

171. Berstein JG, Koch-Weser J: Effectiveness of bretylium toyslate against refractory ventricular arrhythmias. Circulation 45:1024–1034, 1972.

172. Sanna G, Arcidiacono R: Chemical ventricular defibrillation of the human heart with bretylium tosylate. Am J Cardiol 32:982–987, 1973.

173. MacAlpin RN, Zalis, EG, Kivowitz GV: Prevention of recurrent ventricular tachycardia with oral bretylium tosylate. Ann Intern Med 72:909–912, 1972.

174. Evanson JM, Sears HTN: Bretylium tosylate in the treatment of hypertension. Lancet 1:544, 1960.

175. Namm DH, Wang CN, El-Sayad S, Copp FC, Maxwell RA: Effects of bretylium on rat cardiac muscle: The electrophysiologic effects and its uptake and binding in normal and immunosympathectomized rat hearts. J Pharmacol Exp Ther 193:194–208, 1975.

176. Romhilt DW, Bloomfield SS, Liticky, RJ, Welch RM, Fowler NO: Evaluation of bretylium toyslate for the treatment of premature ventricular contractions. Circulation 45:800–807, 1972.

177. Duncombe WG, McCoubrey A: The excretion and stability to metabolism of bretylium. Brit. J. Pharm. 15:260–264, 1960.

178. Kuntzman R, Tasi I, Chang R, and Conney AH: Disposition of bretylium in man and rat. Clin Pharmacol Ther 11:829–837, 1970.

179. Cohen HC, Gozo EG Jr, Langendorf R, et al: Response of resistant ventricular tachycardia to bretylium: Relation to site of ectopic focus and location of myocardial disease. Circulation 47:331–340, 1973.

180. Loumannaki K, Heikkila J, Hartel G: Bretylium tosylate: Adverse effects in acute myocardial infarction. Arch Intern Med 135:515–518, 1975.

181. Elharar V, Foster PR, Zipes DP: Effects of aprindine HCl on cardiac tissues. J Pharmacol Exp Ther 195:201–205, 1975.

182. Carmeliet E, Verdonck F: Effect of aprindine and lidocaine on transmembrane potentials and radioactive K efflux in different cardiac tissues. Acta Cardiol (Brux) Suppl 18:73–90, 1974.

183. Steinberg MI, Greenspan K: Intracellular electrophysiological alterations in canine cardiac conducting tissue induced by aprindine and lidocaine. Cardiovasc Res 10:236–244, 1976.

184. Verdonck F, Vereecke J, Velugels A: Electrophysiological effects of aprindine on isolated heart preparations. Eur J Pharmacol 26:338–347, 1974.

185. Elharrar B, Bailey JC, Lathrop DA, et al: Effects of aprindine HCl on slow channel action

potentials and transient depolarizations in canine Purkinje fibers. Fed Proc 36:416, 1977.

186. Kesteloot H: General aspects of antiarrhythmic treatment with aprindine. Acta Cardiol (Brux) Suppl 18:303–316, 1974.

187a. Zipes DP, Gaum WE, Foster PR, et al: Aprindine for treatment of supraventricular tachycardias with particular application of Wolff-Parkinson-White syndrome. Am J Cardiol 40:586–596, 1977.

187b. Zipes DP, Elharrar V, Noble RJ, et al: Effects of various drugs on ventricular conduction delay and ventricular arrhythmias during myocardial ischemia in the dog. In Reentrant Arrhythmias, ed. Kulburtus HE. NTP Press, London, 1977, pp. 312–326.

188. Neuss H, Schlepper M: Influence of various antiarrhythmic drugs (aprindine, ajmaline, verapamil, oxprenolol, or ciprenaline) on functional properties of accessory A-V pathways. Acta Cardiol (Brux) Suppl 18:279–288, 1974.

189. Kroll DA, Lucchesi BR: Antiarrhythmic and antifibrillatory properties of aprindine. J Pharmacol Exp Ther 194:427–434, 1975.

190. Ueda M, Kimoto S, Matsuda S, et al: Antiarrhythmic effect of aprindine on several types of ventricular arrhythmias. Jpn J Pharmacol 25:549–561, 1975.

191. Fasola AF, Carmichael R: The pharmacology and clinical evaluation of aprindine—a new antiarrhythmic agent. Acta Cardiol (Brux) Suppl 18:317–333, 1974.

192. VanDurme JP, Rousseau M, Mbuyamba P: Treatment of chronic ventricular dysrhythmias with a new drug aprindine (AC1802). Acta Cardiol (Brux) Suppl 18:335–340, 1974.

193. Pouleur H, Chaudron JM, Reyns P: Effects of disopyramide and aprindine on arrhythmias after acute myocardial infarction. Eur J Cardiol 5:397–404, 1977.

194. Zipes DP, Troup PJ: New antiarrhythmic agents. Am J Cardiol 41:1005–1024, 1978.

195. Fasola AF, Noble RJ, Zipes DP: Treatment of recurrent ventricular tachycardia and fibrillation with aprindine. Am J Cardiol 39:903–909, 1977.

196. VanLeeuwen R, Meyboom RHB: Agranulocytosis and aprindine. Lancet 2:1137, 1976.

197. Investigators brochure for tocainide HCl. Astra Pharmaceutical Products Inc, Jan 1977.

198. Anderson JL, Mason JW, Winkle RA, et al: Clinical electrophysiologic effects of tocainide. Circulation 57:685–691, 1978.

199. Coltart DJ, Brendt TB, Kernoff R, et al: Antiarrhythmic and circulatory effects of Astra

W36095, a new lidocaine-like agent. Am J Cardiol 34:35–41, 1974.

200. Winkle RA, Meffin PJ, Fitzgerald JW, et al: Clinical efficacy and pharmacokinetics of a new orally effective of antiarrhythmic, tocainide. Circulation 54:884–889, 1976.

201. McDevitt DG, Nies AS, Wilkinson GR, et al: Antiarrhythmic effects of a lidocaine congener, tocainide, 2-amino-2′,6′-proprionoxylidide, in man. Clin Pharmacol Ther 19:396–402, 1976.

202. Woosley RL, McDevitt DG, Nies AS, et al: Suppression of ventricular ectopic depolarization by tocainide. Circulation 56:980–985, 1977.

203. Ryan W, Engler R., LeWinter M, Karliner JS: Efficacy of a new oral agent (tocainide) in the acute treatment of refractory ventricular arrhythmias. Am J Cardiol 43:285–291, 1979.

204. Engler R, Ryan W, LeWinter M, Bluestein H, Karliner JS: Assessment of long-term antiarrhythmic therapy: Studies on the long-term efficacy and toxicity of tocainide. Am J Cardiol 43:612–618, 1979.

205. Lalka D, Meyer MB, Duce BR, et al: Kinetics of the oral antiarrhythmic lidocaine congener, tocainide. Clin Pharmacol Ther 19:757–766, 1976.

206. Harrison DC, Meffin PJ Winkle RA: Clinical pharmacokinetics of antiarrhythmic drugs. Prog Cardiovasc Dis 20:217–242, 1977.

207. Meffin PJ, Winkle RA, Blaschke TF, Fitzgerald JW, Harrison DC: Response optimization of drug dosage: Antiarrhythmic studies with tocainide. Clin Pharmacol Ther 22:42–57, 1977.

208. Koppe HG: The development of mexiletine. Postgrad Med J 53(Suppl I):22–25, 1977.

209. Singh BN, Vaughan Williams EM: Investigations of the mode of action of a new antidysrhythmic drug, KO1173. Br J Pharmacol 44:1–9, 1972.

210. Weld FM, Bigger JT Jr, Swistel D, Bordiuk J, Lau YH: Electrophysiological effects of mexiletine (KO1173) on bovine cardiac Purkinje fibers. J Pharmacol Exp Ther 210:222–228, 1979.

211. Okuma K, Sugiyama S, Wada M, et al: Experimental studies on the antiarrhythmic action of lidocaine analog. Cardiology 61:289–297, 1976.

212. Iwamura N, Shimizu T, Toyoshima H, et al: Electrophysiological actions of a new antiarrhythmic agent on isolated preparations of the canine Purkinje fiber and ventricular muscle. Cardiology 61:329–340, 1976.

213. Allen JD, Kofi A, Ekue JM, Shanks RG, et al: The effect of KO1173, a new anticonvulsant agent on experimental cardiac arrhythmias. Br J Pharm 45:561–573, 1972.

214. Roos JC, Paalman ACA, Dunning AJ: Electrophysiological effects of mexiletine in man. Br Heart J 38:62–72, 1976.

215. McComish M, Robinson C, Kitson D, et al: Clinical electrophysiological effects of mexiletine. Postgrad Med J 53(suppl I):85–91, 1977.

216. Dannenberg PB, Shelly JH: The pharmacology of mexiletine. Postgrad Med J 53(suppl I):26–29, 1977.

217. Banim SO, DaSilva A, Stone D, et al: Observations on the hemodynamics of mexiletine. Postgrad Med J 53(suppl I):74–76, 1977.

218. Shaw TRD: The effect of mexiletine on left ventricular ejection: A comparison with lignocaine and propranolol. Postgrad Med J 53(suppl I):69–73, 1977.

219. Pozenel H: Hemodynamic studies on mexiletine. A new antiarrhythmic agent. Postgrad Med J 53(suppl I):78–80, 1977.

220. Kuhm P, Klictera M, Kroiss A, et al: Antiarrhythmic and hemodynamic effects of mexiletine. Postgrad Med J 53(suppl I):81–83, 1977.

221. Campbell NPS, Shanks RG, Kelly JG, et al: Long-term oral antiarrhythmic therapy with mexiletine. Postgrad Med J 53(suppl I):143–145, 1977.

222. Talbot RG, Gulian JG, Prescott LF: Long-term treatment of ventricular arrhythmias with oral mexiletine. Am Heart J 91:58–65, 1976.

223. Campbell RWF, Dolder MA, Prescott DLF, Talbot RG, et al: Ventricular arrhythmias after acute myocardial infarction treated with procainamide or mexiletine. Postgrad Med J 53(suppl I):150–153, 1977.

224. Prescott LF, Pottage A, Clements JA: Absorption, distribution and elimination of mexiletine. Postgrad Med J 53(suppl I):50–55, 1977.

225. Vastesaeger M, Gillot P, Asson G: Etude clinique d'une nouvelle medication anti-angoreuse. Acta Cardiol (Brux) 22:483–500, 1967.

226. Rosenbaum NB, Chiale PA, Halpern MS, Nau GJ, et al: Clinical efficacy of amiodarone as an antiarrhythmic agent. Am J Cardiol 38:934–944, 1976.

227. Freedberg AS, Papp JG, Vaughn Williams EM: The effect of altered thyroid state on atrial intracellular potentials. J Physiol (Lond) 207:357–370, 1970.

228. Singh BN, Vaughn Williams EM: The effect of amiodarone, a new antianginal drug on cardiac muscle. Br J Pharmacol 39:657–667, 1970.

229. Goupil N, Lenfant J: The effects of amiodarone on the sinus node activity of the rabbit heart. Eur J Pharmacol 39:23–31, 1976.

230. Pritchard DA, Singh BN, Hurley PJ: Effects of amiodarone on thyroid function in patients with ischemic heart disease. Br Heart J 37:856–860, 1975.

231. Charlier R: Cardiac actions in the dog of a new antagonist of adrenergic excitation which does not produce competitive blockade of adrenoceptors. Br J Cardiol 39:668–679, 1970.

232. Wellens HJJ, Lie KI, Bar FW, et al: Effect of amiodarone in the Wolff-Parkinson-White syndrome. Am J Cardiol 38:189–194, 1976.

233. Touboul P, Huerta F, Porte J, et al: Bases electrophysiologiques de l'action antiarythmique de l'amiodarone chez l'homme. Arch Mal Coeur 69:845–853, 1976.

234. Coutte R, Fontaine G, Frank R, et al: Etude electrocardiologique des effets de l'amiodarone sur la conduction intracardiaque chez l'homme. Ann Cardiol Angeiol (Paris) 18:543–548, 1977.

235. Cabasson J, Puech P, Mellet JM, et al: Analyze des effets electrophysiologiques de l'amiodarone par l'enregistrement simultane des potentiels d'action monophasiques et du faisceau de His. Arch Mal Coeur 69:691–699, 1976.

236. Charlier R, Deltour G, Baudine A, et al: Pharmacology of amiodarone: An antianginal drug with a new biological profile. Arzneim Forsch 11:408–417, 1968.

237. Olsson SB, Brorson L, Varnauskas E: Class III antiarrhythmic action in man. Observations on monophasic action potential recordings in amiodarone treatment. Br Heart J 35:1255–1261, 1973.

238. Swan JH, Chisholm AW: Control of recurrent supraventricular tachycardia with amiodarone hydrochloride. Can Med Assoc J 144:43–44, 1976.

239. Broekhuysen J, Laruel R, Sion R: Etude comparee du transit et du metabolisme de l'amiodarone chez diverses especes animales et chez l'homme. Arch Int Pharmacodyn Ther 177:340–359, 1969.

240. Charlier R, Deltour G, Tondeur R, et al: Researches dans la serie des benzofurannes. VII. Etude pharmacologique preliminaire du butyl-2 (diodo-3',5'butyl-N-diethylaminoethoxy 4'benzoyl) -3 benzofuranne. Arch Int Pharmacodyn Ther 139:255–264, 1962.

241. Francios J: Cornea verticillata. Doc Ophthalmol 27:235–251, 1969.

242. Facquet J, Nivet M, Alhomme P, et al: Traitement de l'angine de poitrine par l'amiodarone. Presse Med 77:725–726, 1969.

243. Toussaint D, Pohl S: Aspect histologique et ultrastructure des depots corneens dus au

chlorhydrate d'amiodarone. Bull Soc Belge Ophthalmol 153:675–686, 1969.

244. Verin P, Gendre P, Barchewitz G, et al: Thesaurismose corneenne par amiodarone. Arch Ophthalmol 31:581–596, 1971.

245. Babel J, Stangos N: L'action de l'amiodarone sur les tissus occulaires. Schweiz Med Wochenschr 102:220–223, 1972.

246. Soussi A, Colonna D: Troubles du rythme auriculaire et amiodarone. J Agreges 7:43–55, 1974.

247. Wanet J, Achten G, Barchewitz G, et al: Amiodarone et depots cutanes. Etude clinicique et histologique. Ann Dermatol Syphil (Paris) 98:131–140, 1971.

248. Geerts ML: Amiodarone pigmentation. An electron microscopic study. Arch Belg Dermatol Syphil 27:339–349, 1971.

249. Grand A: Myxoedeme l'amiodarone. Coeur Med Interne 14:163–167, 1975.

250. Jonckheer MH, Block P, Kaivers R, et al: Hyperthyroidism as a possible complication of the treatment of ischemic heart disease with amiodarone. Acta Cardiol (Brux) 28:192–200, 1973.

251. Krikler D: Verapamil in cardiology. Eur J Cardiol 2:3–10, 1974.

252. Husaini MH, Kvasnicka J, Ryden L, et al: Action of verapamil on sinus node, atrioventricular and intraventricular conduction. Br Heart J 35:734–737, 1973.

253. Roy PR, Spurrell RAJ, Sowton E: The effect of verapamil on the cardiac conduction system in man. Postgrad Med J 50:270–275, 1974.

254. Wellens HJJ, Tan SL, Bar FWH, et al: The effect of verapamil studied by programmed electrical stimulation of the heart in patients with paroxysmal reentrant supraventricular tachycardia. Br Heart J 39:1058–1066, 1977.

255. Krikler DM, Spurrell RAJ: Verapamil in the treatment of paroxysmal supraventricular tachycardia. Postgrad Med J 50:447–453, 1974.

256. Sacks H, Kennelly BM: Verapamil in cardiac arrhythmias. Br Med J 2:716, 1972.

257. Rosen MR, Ilvento JP, Gelband H, et al: Effects of verapamil on electrophysiologic properties of canine cardiac Purkinje fibers. J Pharmacol Exp Ther 189:414–422, 1974.

258. Davis LD: Effects of changes in cycle length on diastolic depolarization produced by ouabain in canine Purkinje fibers. Circ Res 32:206–214, 1973.

259. Ferrier GR, Saunders JH, Mendez C: A cellular mechanism for the generation of ventricular arrhythmias by acetylstrophanthidin, Circ Res 32:600–609, 1973.

260. Hofdof AJ, Edie R, Malm JR, et al: Electrophysiologic properties in response to pharmacologic agents of fibers from diseased human atria. Circulation 54:774–779, 1977.

261. Spear JF, Horowitz LN, Moore EN, et al: Verapamil sensitive "slow response" activity in infarcted human ventricular myocardium. Circulation 53 & 54(suppl II):75, 1976.

262. Cranefield PF, Aronson RS, Wit AL: Effect of verapamil on the normal action potential and on a calcium-dependent slow response of canine cardiac Purkinje fibers. Circ Res 34:204–213, 1974.

263. Verapamil clinical information. Investigators brochure. Knoll Pharmaceutical. Feb 1977.

264. Wolf R, Habel F, Witt E, et al: Wirkung von Verapamil auf die Hamodynamik und Grosse des akuten Myokardinfarkts. Herz 2:110–119, 1977.

265. Angus JA, Richmond DR, Dhumma-Upakorn P, et al: Cardiovascular action of verapamil in the dog with particular reference to myocardial contractility and atrioventricular conduction. Cardiovasc Res 10:623–632, 1976.

266. Newman RK, Bishop VS, Peterson DF, et al: Effect of verapamil on left ventricular performance in conscious dogs. J Pharmacol Exp Ther 201:723–730, 1977.

267. Vincenzi M, Allegri P, Galbaldo S, et al: Hemodynamic effects caused by I.V. administration of verapamil in healthy subjects. Arzneim Forsch 6:1221–1223, 1976.

268. Lewis BS, Mitha AS, Gostman MS: Immediate hemodynamic effects of verapamil. Cardiology 60:366–376, 1975.

269. Singh BN, Phil D, Roche AH: Effects of intravenous verapamil on hemodynamics in patients with heart disease. Am Heart J 94:593–599, 1977.

270. Luebs ED, Cohen A, Zaleski E, et al: Effect of nitroglycerin, intensain, Isoptin, and papaverine on coronary blood flow in man. Am J Cardiol 17:535–541, 1966.

271. Rowe GG, Stenlund RR, Thomsen JH, et al: The systemic and coronary hemodynamic effects of iproveratril. Arch Int Pharmacodyn Ther 193:381–390, 1971.

272. Schomerus M, Spiegelhalder B, Stieren B, et al: The physiological disposition of verapamil in man. Cardiovasc Res 10:605–612, 1976.

273. Spiegelhalder B, Eichelbaum M: Determination of verapamil in human plasma by mass fragmentography using stable isotope-labeled verapamil as internal standard. Arzneim Forsch 27:1–7, 1977.

274. Belz GG, Bender F: Therapie der Herzrhythmusstorungen mit Verapamil. Gustav Fischer Verlag, Stuttgart, 1974.

275. Singh BN, Roche AHG: Effects of intravenous verapamil on hemodynamics in patients with heart disease. Am Heart J 94:593–599, 1975.

276. Spurrell RAJ, Krikler DM, Sowton GE: Concealed bypasses of the atrioventricular node in patients with paroxysmal supraventricular tachycardia revealed by intracardiac electrical stimulation and verapamil. Am J Cardiol 33:590–595, 1974.

277. Benaim ME: Asystole after verapamil. Br Med J 2:169–170, 1972.

278. Vaughn-Neil EF, Snell NJC, Bevan G: Hypotension after verapamil. Br Med J 2:529, 1972.

# 15 | Supraventricular Arrhythmias: Diagnosis, Treatment, and Prognosis

*William P. Nelson, M.D.*

Supraventricular arrhythmias are frequently encountered in the patient with ischemic heart disease—particularly in the setting of acute myocardial infarction. By arbitrary definition, "normal sinus rhythm" is a rate varying from 60 to 100 beats per minute. Although there are numerous ways to catalogue atrial arrhythmias, the major importance of changes in heart rate permits a useful and simple separation into two categories—"bradyarrhythmias" and "tachyarrhythmias" (Fig. 15.1). Specific varieties of each will be discussed, as well as the responsible mechanisms, the altered physiology which may occur, and the concepts of treatment for each. When known, prognosis of the arrhythmia will be reviewed.

Some preliminary generalizations about tachyarrhythmias and bradyarrhythmias are in order. The inherent rate of the sinoatrial node exceeds that of other potential pacemakers (and that, of course, is why the sinoatrial node normally remains the dominant pacemaker). Alterations in sinoatrial node automaticity or the appearance of ectopic supraventricular pacemakers can be due to a number of factors:

1. Autonomic nervous system effects can impose powerful influences, resulting in either a decrease in sinus node rate (excessive vagal "tone"), or in its acceleration (release of vagal suppression or excess sympathetic activity). Although autonomic nervous system reflexes may be responsible for such changes during cardiac ischemia, it is important to emphasize that psy-

chological factors associated with apprehension or continuing pain may exert important influences on heart rate.

2. Anatomic abnormalities may be present with either "ischemia" or actual infarction of the sinus node.

3. Biochemical derangements can be a potent stimulus for atrial arrhythmias. Particularly common ones are hypoxia, hyper- or hypocarbia, acidosis, and electrolyte derangements—especially hypokalemia.[1,2]

4. Drugs being taken at the time of the acute myocardial infarction may influence the genesis of atrial arrhythmias. Drugs commonly involved include digitalis, antihypertensive medications, diuretic agents, and "tranquilizers" (particularly "antidepressant" drugs).

It is important to emphasize these possible causative factors because their recognition may permit treatment aimed at the true cause, thereby preventing the use of potentially dangerous antiarrhythmic drugs. Decisions regarding treatment of supraventricular arrhythmias must stem from "bedside" appraisal of the patient's condition. It is impossible to provide a "recipe of therapy" for an arrhythmia without such knowledge. Similarly, it is impossible to suggest what might be the appropriate dosage of a given antiarrhythmic drug that could apply to *all* patients. Each judgment must include reflections on numerous variables: the patient's clinical condition, age, state of renal and hepatic function, presence or absence of electrolyte derangement, etc. Although specific drugs will be mentioned, I do not intend to dwell on dosage, since the concept of an "average dose" is largely meaningless until the time that every patient agrees to be an "average patient!" The duration of the arrhythmia is more important than the particular type. Obviously, a brief tachyarrhythmia or bradyarrhythmia has less impact than a lasting one. Accurate diagnosis and prompt therapy greatly influence prognosis. There is little meaning in efforts to assign "risk" of a given arrhythmia without considering the duration of time during which the rhythm disturbance is present.

## BRADYARRHYTHMIAS

Bradyarrhythmias represent a disturbance of impulse formation in the sinus node (or "exit block" of sinus node impulses) and can lead to undesirable consequences by the following mechanisms:

1. Slow heart rates may significantly compromise cardiac output. (Recall that cardiac output represents the product of stroke volume and heart rate). Myocardial infarction may decrease left ventricular (and possibly right ventricular) performance and thus reduce stroke volume, requiring an increase in heart rate to maintain adequate cardiac output to accomplish effective organ perfusion. Thus, bradycardia may be a decisive factor in the limitation of cardiac output.

2. Slow heart rates may enhance the appearance of ectopic pacemakers (in the atria, atrioventricular junction, or ventricles). Such stimuli, when ill-timed, may be ineffective in producing ventricular excitation (e.g., nonconducted premature atrial complexes); or, they may not result in an effective cardiac contraction (e.g., premature cardiac activation before adequate diastolic filling of the ventricles has occurred). Such foci may also precipitate additional dysrhythmias (to be discussed below).

3. Slow heart rates may permit the appearance of ectopic pacemakers as "escape pacemakers" (e.g., junctional escape complexes). Although this may be desirable, cardiac activation lacking the appropriate synchrony of atrial

and ventricular mechanical events may not result in an adequate stroke volume. Thus, their efficacy may be decreased by the absence of effective atrial contribution to ventricular filling, further compromising an already diminished cardiac output.

## TACHYARRHYTHMIAS

Supraventricular tachyarrhythmias impose a rate burden, which may be intolerable, in one of the following ways: (1) by diminishing the time needed for adequate ventricular filling; or (2) by decreasing the time available for diastolic coronary perfusion of ischemic myocardium.

With this brief background, specific examples of supraventricular bradycardia and tachycardia will be discussed.

## SINUS BRADYCARDIA

Although one would anticipate that the life-threatening insult of acute myocardial infarction would lead to sinus tachycardia, it is surprising how frequently slow atrial rates are encountered.

### Mechanism

Sinus node suppression is most frequently due to excess vagal tone, and less frequently due to anatomic destruction (infarction) or physiologic suppression from "ischemia." A particularly pernicious cause is the "Bezold-Jarisch reflex," in which there is the combination of a decrease in the sinoatrial node discharge rate and peripheral vasodilatation, leading to bradycardia and hypotension. Although the exact receptors initiating this reflex are in dispute, it is clear that the reflex may be initiated by myocardial stretch and perhaps by coronary artery distension.[3,4]

Occasionally, sinus node impulse formation continues normally, but the stimulus is unable to penetrate to the atria ("sinoatrial exit block"). An example is shown in Fig. 15.2. Exit block may represent "injury" or ischemia of

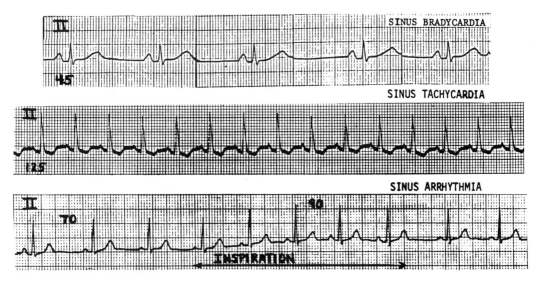

Fig. 15.1 Examples of sinus bradycardia of 45/min and sinus tachycardia of 125/min. These are so familiar that they require no additional comment. Respiratory variation in sinus rhythm (sinus arrhythmia) is shown in the bottom tracing with inspiratory acceleration and expiratory slowing of sinus node discharge. Sinus arrhythmia of this degree is rarely seen in adults with ischemic heart disease but is common in young, healthy patients. (Reprinted by permission of the publisher, from Davies, Hywel, and Nelson, William P., *Understanding Cardiology*. Woburn: Butterworth Publishers, Inc., 1978.)

the sinus node, but it is frequently due to excess digitalis effect (and this should be kept in mind if the drug is in use).

## Pathophysiology

The hemodynamic consequences of sinus bradycardia occur when the heart rate is sufficiently slow that inadequate cardiac output occurs. It is important to emphasize, however, that many patients may have heart rates less than 60/min and be completely stable, with adequate blood pressure and tissue perfusion. The axiom "one should always treat the *patient* rather than the electrocardiogram" is particularly applicable in this situation. Many patients tolerate a slow heart rate quite well and require careful observation rather than treatment with drugs. In such individuals, sinus node responsiveness can frequently be determined by having

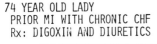

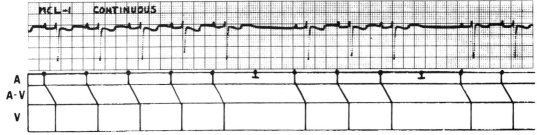

Fig. 15.2 Episodes of "sinoatrial exit block" in an elderly woman. The ladder diagram indicates that the "pause" in cardiac rhythm, without evidence of atrial activiation, is due to the block of the sinoatrial node stimulus. Despite the "missing P wave," there is no disruption of regular sinus discharge: the P-P interval remains constant and the recovery P wave after the pause appears at its anticipated time.

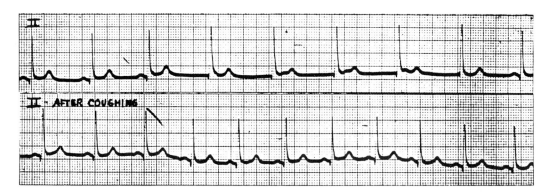

Fig. 15.3 Sinus node slowing permits the emergence of a junctional escape focus, with the SA node and junctional focus dissociated and competing for ventricular activation. Although the ventricular rate is adequate (averaging 60/min), the lack of an appropriately synchronized atrial contribution resulted in intermittent hypotension. In the lower strip, the simple expedient of having the patient cough increased the sinus rate, with resumption of normal sinus rhythm. Small doses of intravenous atropine were utilized to maintain the sinus rate above that of the junctional escape focus, and there was return of normal blood pressure with an uncomplicated subsequent convalescence.

the patient cough several times (Fig. 15.3) or by momentarily raising the legs to promote an increase in venous return to the heart. If such measures promote sinus acceleration, there can be reasonable assurance that sinus node responsiveness can be relied upon if needed later.

### Treatment and Prognosis

Therapy should be reserved for patients who are intolerant of the slow rate and show signs or symptoms of diminished cardiac output. In such cases, small intravenous doses of atropine (0.2 to 0.4 mg) can be given—repeatedly if necessary—until the sinus rate increases (Fig. 15.4). Although atropine has been reported to cause an abrupt shift in sinus bradycardia to sinus tachycardia, creating an undesirable increase in myocardial oxygen demand, this usually occurs if a single, large dose (1.5 to 2.0 mg) is administered, or if multiple smaller doses are given in a brief period of time. In such circumstances, it is usually the *dose* and not the *drug* which should be blamed.[5,6,7]

In general, the prognosis of patients with sinus bradycardia is good. Occasionally, however, symptomatic sinus bradycardia is unresponsive to atropine, even in full dosage (2 mg). In such a circumstance, it is futile to administer larger amounts of the drug, and a temporary

electronic transvenous pacemaker provides the most reliable control of the problem.

Isoproterenol has been used to increase the sinus node rate, but it is a potent and treacherous drug, with a very narrow margin separating its desirable and undesirable effects. Thus, isoproterenol may induce ventricular ectopy (or ventricular tachycardia) before sinus node acceleration is achieved. Additionally, it is a powerful myocardial stimulant and will increase myocardial oxygen requirements in a situation where the demands may not be met. A temporary electronic pacemaker appears to be a safer and more dependable form of therapy in the patient with unresponsive sinus bradycardia. However, in a patient who has been receiving β-adrenoceptor antagonists such as propranolol, careful titration of the heart rate with isoproterenol, a potent β-adrenergic agonist, may be warranted.

## SINUS TACHYCARDIA

### Mechanisms

During myocardial infarction, increase in sinus node discharge rate may be due to inhibition of vagal suppression or to sympathetic dis-

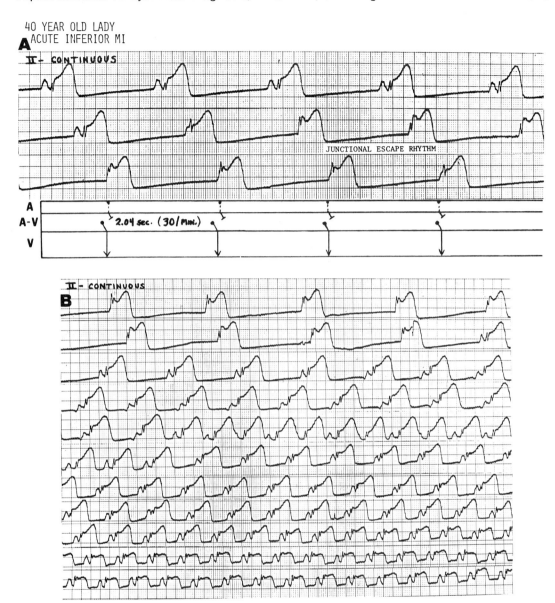

Fig. 15.4  *(A)* Acute inferior myocardial infarction has resulted in marked bradycardia (30/min). The "default" of sinus impulse formation promotes the appearance of a junctional escape focus with an escape interval of 2.04 sec (approximately 30/min). Dissociation of atrial and ventricular events occurs and is depicted in the ladder diagram. *(B)* Therapy with intravenous atropine results in sinus acceleration (accompanied by acceleration of the AV junctional "escape focus"). This continuous recording shows a gradual increase in rate until the sinus node resumes command. Note the decrease in the degree of ST segment elevation as heart rate increases. Prompt clinical improvement accompanied the increase in sinus rate, and her subsequent recovery was uneventful.

charge. As previously mentioned, this is commonly due to fright or continuing pain. It is mandatory that adequate relief of pain be obtained (with intravenous morphine), and that fear and apprehension be removed (by reas-

surance and, when necessary, sedation). It is a common experience that the relief of pain and anxiety results in sinus node slowing, removing the undesirable burden of sinus tachycardia.

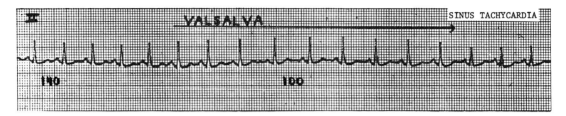

Fig. 15.5 Proof that supraventricular tachycardia in this patient is of sinus origin is provided by the Valsalva maneuver, which results in prompt but temporary deceleration from a rate of 140/min to an average rate of 100/min.

## Treatment and Prognosis

If sinus tachycardia persists despite such relief (e.g., when the patient is asleep), the continuing tachycardia should be an alert to possible "pump failure." Sinus tachycardia *alone* does not justify the diagnosis of "heart failure." The presence of tachypnea, dyspnea, basilar lung rales, and a third heart sound provides confirmatory bedside evidence. If such objective evidence is found, therapy with a diuretic drug is indicated. There remains disagreement regarding the efficacy of digitalis in this setting, and preplanned "digitalizing doses" may be hazardous. Small intravenous doses of digoxin, administered at intervals of not less than every two hours, can be tried and may be beneficial, without undue risk of digitalis intoxication. It should be emphasized that sinus node rate *cannot* be used as a predictable guide to digitalis dosage. The factors controlling sinus node discharge are complex, and attempts to effect its slowing, using the drug, may be unsuccessful and may lead to digitalis intoxication. Similarly, efforts to suppress sinus node rate by producing β-adrenergic blockade (propranolol) can lead to significant depression of myocardial contractility and is a potentially hazardous therapy which should be used with caution.

## PREMATURE SUPRAVENTRICULAR COMPLEXES

### Premature Atrial Complexes (PACs)

#### Mechanism

Present evidence indicates that PACs usually represent the *reentry* of a stimulus, arising in the sinoatrial node, which "echoes" back to the atrium, either at the atrioventricular junctional level or via intraatrial conduction pathways (see Paroxysmal Supraventricular Tachycardia, later in this chapter). Less frequently, ectopic foci may become enhanced and compete with the sinus node pacemaker. Often, it is difficult or impossible to distinguish the site of ectopic impulse formation (atrial vs. junctional premature origin); fortunately, the distinction is seldom important.

#### Pathophysiology

Premature supraventricular stimuli are frequently encountered during acute myocardial infarction. They may be single or multiple and may be conducted normally, aberrantly, or not at all. Although these stimuli are frequently of little consequence, they may have the following important effects:

1. PACs that occur early in the refractory period of the preceding cycle may be nonconducted; or, achieving conduction may not permit adequate time for ventricular diastolic filling, and may result in an ineffective mechanical contraction. When nonconducted, the PACs may "hide" in the T wave of the preceding beat, and, although not an effective stimulus for ventricular activation, they may repetitively cause resetting of the sinus node, delaying its discharge. The resulting slow rhythm may suggest to the unwary that "sinus bradycardia" is present.

2. PACs may encounter refractoriness in the intraventricular conduction pathways and be aberrantly conducted. (Such an example is shown in Fig. 15.6). Again, this can result in confusion and prompt the diagnosis of "ven-

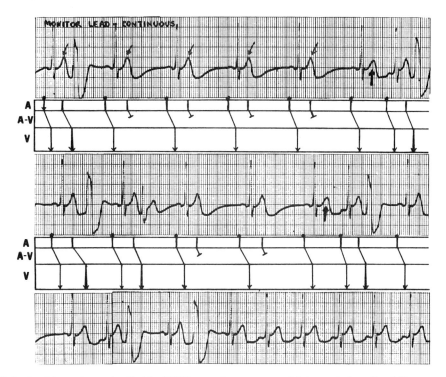

Fig. 15.6  In this patient, the "wide QRS" complexes were misinterpreted as "multiform ventricular ectopic beats," and the slow heart rate was misconstrued to be sinus bradycardia. The fact of the matter is shown in the bottom strip. Contrast the morphology of the T waves of the sinus beats which terminate the bottom strip, and compare them with the T waves of the impulses preceding the PVCs and the lengthy pauses. In doing so it becomes obvious that a premature P wave is hiding in the T wave (upper arrows). When nonconducted, PACs can "reset" the sinus node and trap the unwary into a diagnosis of "sinus bradycardia." When aberrantly conducted, they may be misinterpreted as "premature ventricular complexes." This patient needs neither lidocaine, nor a pacemaker! Since he was asymptomatic, no treatment was given. If therapy was required, oral quinidine would almost certainly have eradicated the multiple PACs.

tricular premature complexes," resulting in unnecessary concern and/or ineffective therapy. Lidocaine is frequently utilized for the latter diagnosis and is usually successful in suppression of ventricular ectopy, but seldom eliminates PACs.

3. When premature atrial stimuli occur during mechanical activation of the preceeding sinus impulse, atrial contraction cannot contribute to ventricular filling against the closed atrioventricular valve. The pressure generated may be dissipated retrogradely into the systemic and pulmonary venous circuits. Perhaps this contributes to the dyspnea frequently encountered in patients with such dysrhythmias.

4. The major threat of isolated supraventricular premature impulses is that, when crit-

ically timed, they may establish a continuing reentrant supraventricular tachycardia, imposing an undesirable rate burden on the ventricles (see Paroxysmal Supraventricular Tachycardia, later in this chapter).

## Treatment

When infrequent, PACs usually do not significantly compromise cardiac function and require no therapy. When PACs are frequent, or result in brief bursts of supraventricular tachycardia, or repetitively reset the sinus node (such as in nonconducted atrial bigeminy), they can result in an important decrease in effective cardiac output. As mentioned, atrial ectopic beats infrequently respond to lidocaine, but usually they are promptly responsive to quinidine or procainamide therapy. As a trial, one may administer procainamide in incremental, intravenous doses (no more than 50 mg/min) until the PACs are eliminated or until 500 mg of the drug has been given. If this initial therapeutic trial is successful, therapy with oral quinidine (0.2 to 0.3 gm q. 6 hr) usually results in continuing suppression of the dysrhythmia.

## ABERRANT VENTRICULAR CONDUCTION

An impulse arising in the atria may activate the ventricles in an abnormal manner, with a "wide QRS" complex resulting. Possible causes for this include:

1. Fixed intraventricular conduction disturbances, such as would be seen with established left or right bundle branch block (L- or RBBB).

2. Intermittent intraventricular conduction disturbance: "functional"; or "nonfuctionnal" —as can be seen in the patient who develops bundle branch block when the sinus node accelerates to a "critical rate."

3. Alternate atrioventricular pathways—the "preexcitation syndrome"—Wolff-Parkinson-White pattern.

In this discussion I will concentrate on aspects of 'functional" disturbances of the intraventricular conduction of supraventricular stimuli.

### Mechanism

A premature impulse arising in the atria or atrioventricular (AV) junction may be propagated to the ventricles while a portion of the intraventricular conduction network is completely (or partially) refractory. Thus, the impulse may be conducted either not at all or in

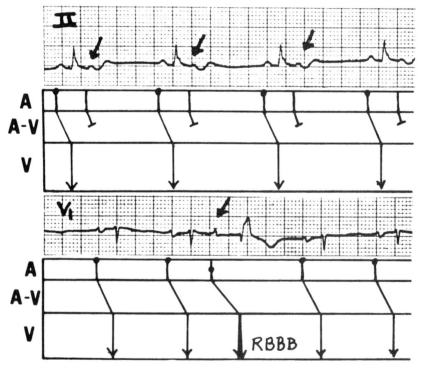

Fig. 15.7  In the top strip, coupled atrial premature complexes occur early in the recovery period of the preceding cycle and are not conducted ("nonconducted atrial bigeminy"). In the lower strip, a premature atrial stimulus (arrow) is conducted through the AV junction with a prolonged P-R interval, and with intraventricular conduction aberrancy of complete right bundle branch block. (Adapted and reprinted by permission of the publisher, from Davies, Hywel, and Nelson, William P., *Understanding Cardiology.* Woburn: Butterworth Publishers, Inc., 1978.)

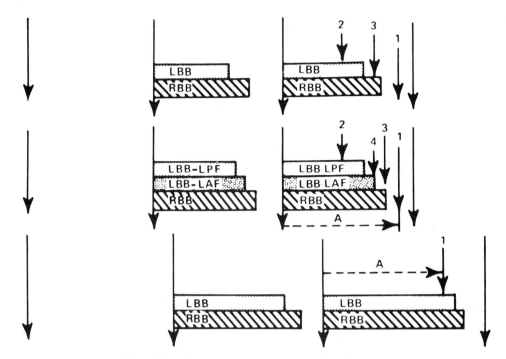

Fig. 15.8   Aberrant ventricular conduction (see text).

an abnormal fashion. An example of this is shown in Fig. 15.7, and the concept is illustrated in Fig. 15.8.

In Fig. 15.8, ventricular depolarization is indicated by the vertical arrows. The refractory period (recovery time) of the specialized intraventricular conduction pathways—left and right bundle branches—are depicted as horizontal bars. In the top portion of Fig. 15.8, the numbered arrows represent atrial stimuli which are premature in the previously established cycle. Stimulus #1, although premature, would find the conduction pathways "recovered" and would be conducted in a normal fashion. (The correct terminology for this is "atrial premature complex—normally conducted.") Stimulus #2 is sufficiently premature that neither bundle branch has "recovered" and it would not be conducted to the ventricles. (Terminology: "atrial premature complex—nonconducted.") In the normal individual, the right bundle branch has a somewhat longer refractory period than the left bundle branch. Stimulus #3 is critically timed to find the left bundle branch (LBB) responsive but the right bundle branch (RBB) still refractory. The stimulus is successfully conducted into the ventricle

via the left bundle branch (LBB), and is propagated as though RBBB were present. (Terminology: "atrial premature complex—aberrantly conducted—RBBB morphology.") This variety of aberrant ventricular conduction—typical RBBB—is frequently encountered with premature atrial stimuli. Although the premature P wave responsible for the aberrantly conducted complex may be obvious, it frequently is hidden in the T wave of the preceding beat and may not be apparent. Often there may be only a subtle distortion of the preceding T wave to reveal its presence (Figs. 15.6 and 15.10). Nonetheless, before deciding that a premature complex with a wide QRS is a ventricular premature beat (particularly if it shows typical RBBB morphology), the preceding T wave should be carefully scrutinized in multiple leads for a telltale P wave that may be causing the "wide QRS beat."

The middle portion of Fig. 15.8 is a further extension of this concept. In it, the left bundle branch is displayed to show the differing refractory periods of its divisions—the left anterior fascicle (LAF) and the left posterior fascicle (LPF). Normally, "recovery time" of the LAF is somewhat longer than that of the LPF. In

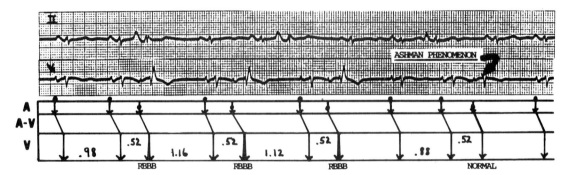

Fig. 15.9 Identically timed atrial premature complexes (see text). (Nelson WP: "The Ashman Phenomenon." Med Times 106:96, 1978.)

this portion of the illustration, premature stimuli #1, #2, and #3, as described above, would result in normal conduction, nonconduction, or aberrant ventricular conduction. The only additional element is premature stimulus #4. Note that its timing finds the LPF responsive while the LAF and RBB remain refractory. The stimulus, thus, would be conducted via the left posterior fascicle and distributed as though there were left anterior fascicular block (LAFB) and RBBB. (Terminology: "atrial premature complex—aberrantly conducted—left anterior fascicular and right bundle branch block morphology.") (An example of this is shown in Fig. 15.11.) Such a combination of LAFB and RBBB is frequently seen as a pattern of ventricular aberrancy, since a critically timed stimulus may find both fascicles partially or completely refractory.

The lower portion of Fig. 15.8 adds an additional concept and reflects the effect of a change in heart rate ("cycle length") on the recovery periods. In general, when the cycle length is prolonged, so is the refractory period. On the ECG, the total recovery time—the QT interval—depends on heart rate, shortening as the rate speeds and lengthening as the rate slows. The effect of this phenomenon is illustrated in the bottom portion of Fig. 15.8. The vertical arrows, representing ventricular depolarization, are further separated to depict slowing of the heart rate. As a result, the recovery period is prolonged. Note in the middle strip of Fig. 15.8 that premature stimulus #1 (separated from the preceding depolarization by interval A) is *normally* conducted. As the heart rate slows

and the recovery time prolongs, a premature stimulus with the same timing (interval A) finds neither the LBB nor the RBB "recovered" and thus would be *nonconducted*. This phenomenon is demonstrated in Fig. 15.9.

Figure 15.9 shows identically timed atrial premature complexes in which the same separation of the resulting ventricular depolarization and the preceding QRS complex (0.52 sec) are aberrantly conducted three times (with RBBB morphology). The fourth PAC is conducted normally. A little reflection will explain why this occurs. Note that the cycles preceding the first three PACs are relatively long (0.98, 1.16, 1.12 sec), whereas the cycle preceding the fourth PAC is significantly shorter (0.88 sec). The shortened cycle length results in a decrease in the refractory period of the conduction pathways, permitting the last PAC to be normally conducted, while the previous ones were aberrantly conducted. The concept that changing cycle lengths determines the recovery period of conducting pathways was described many years ago by Dr. Richard Ashman of Louisiana State University Medical School; the term "Ashman Phenomenon" is a valid and useful eponym to apply to the phenomenon.[8]

These concepts are readily understood and the presence of a preceding premature atrial stimulus serves as an alert that the "wide QRS" complex is supraventricular in origin. The same concepts can be applied to the patient with atrial flutter, atrial fibrillation, or junctional premature stimuli, but it is evident that the absence of discrete P waves (or uncertainty as to which atrial stimulus might have been conducted) makes the judgment more difficult. In such settings, the differential consideration of "wide QRS complexes" as being of ectopic ventricular origin vs. aberrant conduction of supraventricular stimuli may be difficult (and at times impossible). If the morphology is that of "typical RBBB," there is reasonable assurance that it represents aberrant conduction of a supraventricular stimulus.[9,10,11] This subject has been recently and extensively reviewed, and the reader is referred to this excellent reference for additional information and discussion.[12]

### Pathophysiology

As previously indicated, single nonconducted or aberrantly conducted impulses of supraventricular origin have little impact on cardiac function and, when they occur infrequently, have little importance. However, it is worthwhile to emphasize that repetitive supraventricular ectopic stimuli may result in recurrent "resetting" of the sinus node, leading to decrease in effective cardiac rate; or, because of their abnormal configuration, they may be misinterpreted as ventricular in origin.

### Treatment

When infrequent, aberrantly conducted PACs do not require specific therapy. When they recur often or lead to short bursts of aberrantly conducted supraventricular tachycardia, I believe that therapy should be attempted, and I have found that oral quinidine is usually an effective agent.

## PAROXYSMAL SUPRAVENTRICULAR TACHYCARDIA

### Mechanism

The AV junction is not a single electrical conduit but can be envisioned as being divided into parallel pathways (much like separate strands in a multicable electrical conduit). This is depicted in fig. 15.12. Normally, a penetrating impulse from the atrium enters the AV junction and travels with equal velocity through the parallel limbs, reaching the more distal pathways as a synchronized signal. The parallel AV junctional pathways may have dissimilar recovery times, and, if challenged by a premature atrial

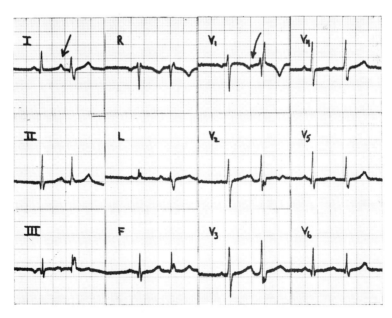

Fig. 15.10 Atrial premature complexes with aberrant ventricular conduction of RBBB morphology. Note how the PACs attempt to "hide" in the T waves of preceding beats (arrows). (Reprinted by permission of the publisher, from Davies, Hywel, and Nelson, William P., *Understanding Cardiology*. Woburn: Butterworth Publishers, Inc., 1978.)

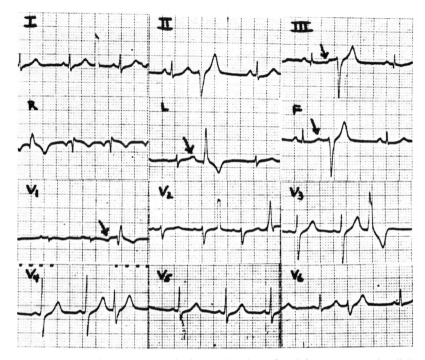

Fig. 15.11   An example of aberrant ventricular conduction of atrial premature stimuli (arrows). The limb leads show left axis deviation (due to left anterior fascicular block), and the precordial leads indicate the presence of RBBB. Thus, this is the combination of intraventricular aberrancy of LAFB and RBBB. (Nelson WP: Cherchez les P Waves Hiding in the T Waves. Med Times 106:97, 1978.)

stimulus, one limb may be accommodating and allow its transmission; the other may not be fully recovered and, as a result, the antegrade signal is blocked. The initial stimulus may then pass retrograde through the blocked limb and "reenter" in the AV junction, with each circular passage stimulating the ventricles (and usually the atria as well). The ladder diagram in Fig. 15.12 serves as an illustration of this mechanism.[13-21]

Current evidence indicates that the majority of regular supraventricular tachycardias are *not* due to the discharge of an ectopic focus,[22] but rather to reentry of a premature stimulus in

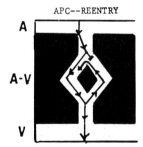

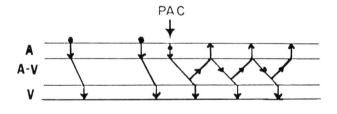

Fig. 15.12   The potential reentry of a supraventricular impulse, utilizing parallel pathways in the AV junction. In this schema, an PAC is blocked in one of the potential pathways but is transmitted through the alternate pathway, discharging the ventricles and "reappearing" through the limb that had not been utilized. Repetitive use of this "circular pathway" would result in a "reentrant supraventricular tachycardia." A ladder diagram demonstrating this mechanism is shown. (Adapted and reprinted by permission of the publisher, from Davies, Hywel, and Nelson, William P., *Understanding Cardiology*. Woburn: Butterworth Publishers, Inc., 1978.)

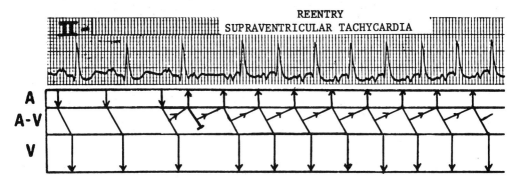

Fig. 15.13   Sinus rhythm is interrupted by retrograde passage of the penetrating impulse—with the first returning impulse transmitted to the atria but blocked in antegrade passage to the ventricle. In this example, retrograde activation of the atria is convincing because the sinus P waves are upright, but those due to the reentrant impulse are inverted. The ladder diagram depicts the dysrhythmic phenomenon. (Reprinted by permission of the publisher, from Davies, Hywel, and Nelson, William P., *Understanding Cardiology.* Woburn: Butterworth Publishers, Inc., 1978.)

the AV junction ("AV nodal reentry"). Thus, although these dysrhythmias are frequently due to a disturbance of impulse *formation* (the premature atrial complex), they are perpetuated by a disturbance of impulse *conduction* (reentry pathways in the AV junction).

There is increasing evidence that many individuals have, in addition to the AV junctional "bridge," accessory pathways that are available for transmission of stimuli from the atria to the ventricles. These paths may allow "preexcitation" and result in "WPW complexes." However, they may remain latent and not permit antegrade conduction to the ventricles, so that normal ventricular activation is consistently seen. Such accessory pathways may be present in the lateral aspect of the atrioventricular groove ("Kent bundles") or may connect the atrial septum with some part of the ventricle ("septal pathways"). Although these anatomic structures may not be utilized for impulse transmission, they constitute a potential "reentry pathway" from the ventricles to the atria. In such individuals, reentrant supraventricular tachycardias can occur, the impulse using the "concealed accessory pathway" to regain access to the atria and returning to the ventricles via the normal AV junctional tissue.[23]

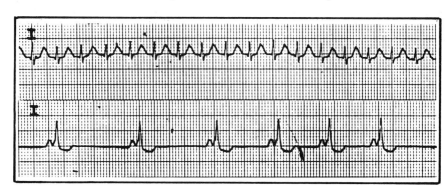

Fig. 15.14   Reentry supraventricular tachycardia in a patient with "preexcitation." Note that during the tachycardia the QRS morphology is normal, but after conversion typical "Wolff-Parkinson-White complexes" are seen. The postconversion tracing helps to clarify the mechanism responsible for the recurrent episodes of tachycardia. In many cases, however, the "accessory pathway" may not be utilized during normal rhythm but may be available for retrograde activation, establishing a reentry tachycardia. (Reprinted by permission of the publisher, from Davies, Hywel, and Nelson, William P., *Understanding Cardiology.* Woburn: Butterworth Publishers, Inc., 1978.)

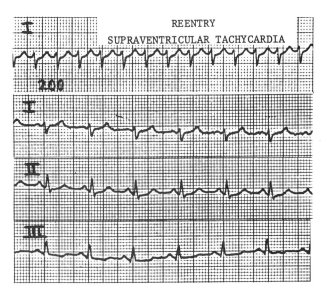

Fig. 15.15   During the tachycardia, despite the absence of discernible P waves, one can be confident that the dysrhythmia is supraventricular in origin because of the narrow QRS complexes (which, after conversion, have the same morphology as sinus-conducted beats). In such a circumstance, the exact reentrant pathway responsible cannot be determined; however, most frequently it represents "AV junctional reentry." (Reprinted by permission of the publisher, from Davies, Hywel, and Nelson, William P., *Understanding Cardiology.* Woburn: Butterworth Publishers, Inc., 1978.)

Thus, paroxysmal supraventricular tachycardia (SVT) may represent reentry, using the AV junction or these accessory pathways. It is impossible to determine, from the "surface" EKG, which anatomic structure is functioning during the dysrhythmia. Present evidence indicates the "AV junctional reentry" is the more common of the two possible mechanisms.

## Pathophysiology and Treatment

SVT is an infrequent rhythm disturbance during acute myocardial infarction, but, when it occurs, every circulating impulse may succeed in producing ventricular activation with a major rate burden (150 to 200/min). Such a tachycardia is rarely tolerated, and prompt therapy is essential. Once established, the circulating impulse can be extinguished by blocking a portion of its reentrant pathway.[24] Such block can be provided by a vagal stimulus (carotid sinus massage or Valsalva maneuver), by drugs (digitalis or propranolol), or by "overdrive" electrical pacing.[25] The commonly used vagal maneuvers, mentioned above, should be attempted but frequently are unsuccessful. In such a circum-

stance, and if the patient is intolerant of the tachycardia, prompt application of synchronized electrical shock (cardioversion) should be undertaken. After conversion to sinus rhythm, ectopic supraventricular premature complexes can usually be suppressed with orally administered quinidine.

## ATRIAL FLUTTER

### Mechanisms

Atrial flutter is characterized by regular deflections on the EKG, usually at a rate of 300/min. It is also regarded as a "reentry" dysrhythmia, rather than due to the repetitive discharge of a single ectopic focus. There is evidence that specialized conducting tracts (the internodal tracts) connecting the sinoatrial and AV nodes may serve as the reentrant pathway.[26-28]

### Pathophysiology

Usually, 2:1 AV conduction of the impulse occurs, but even at this "half-rate," the rapid

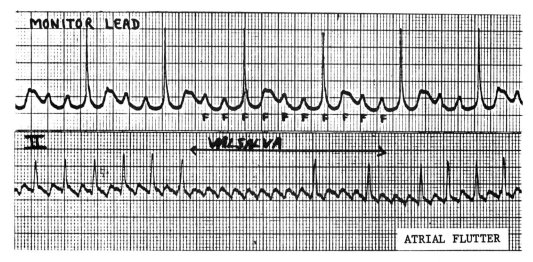

Fig. 15.16 In the lower portion of this figure, typical "saw-tooth" flutter waves are demonstrated during temporary vagal suppression provided by a Valsalva maneuver. Note how readily they might have been missed in the initial portion of the lead (during the period of 2:1 conduction). In the upper portion, atrial flutter is also present; but, instead of a distinctive "flutter pattern," atrial stimuli are seen as upright P waves. It is worthwhile to emphasize that, in monitor leads (as used in many intensive care units), the typical morphology of atrial flutter waves may not be seen; instead they may present as discrete upright deflections. (Reprinted by permission of the publisher, from Davies, Hywel, and Nelson, William P., *Understanding Cardiology*. Woburn: Butterworth Publishers, Inc., 1978.)

ventricular rate (150/min) results in an excessive burden and is often intolerable, with obvious evidence of impaired cardiac output.

## Treatment

Although an occasional patient may tolerate the tachycardia resulting from atrial flutter, the majority do not, and expedient therapy is required. Reversion of this dysrhythmia can be accomplished with synchronized precordial shock (usually at very low energy levels). Rapid atrial pacing will also result in conversion, but this is an "invasive" procedure and requires special equipment which is unavailable in many hospitals. If the situation is less urgent, therapy to decrease the number of penetrating impulses may be tried, using incremental intravenous doses of digoxin. In many patients, the dysrhythmia is short-lived and converts, either spontaneously or with small doses of digoxin. After reversion, normal sinus rhythm can be maintained with oral quinidine (0.2 to 0.3 gm every 6 hr). Subsequent convalescence may be uneventful; when transient, atrial flutter does not impair the prognosis for ultimate recovery.

## ATRIAL FIBRILLATION

### Mechanism

Atrial fibrillation is frequently initiated by a premature atrial stimulus but may arise from preexisting atrial flutter. Present evidence suggests that atrial fibrillation is due to "microreentry" circuits in the atria rather than multiple sites of ectopic discharge.[30,31] It is identified as irregular baseline activity in the EKG rather than a series of regular events, reflecting an atrial rate of 400 to 700/min.

### Pathophysiology

The important issue in the patient with atrial fibrillation is not the atrial rate, but the number of stimuli that penetrate to the ventricles per minute. Frequently, atrial fibrillation induces a rapid ventricular response, resulting in impaired cardiac function. Additionally, the lack of an effective atrial contraction to augment ventricular filling, and recurring short periods

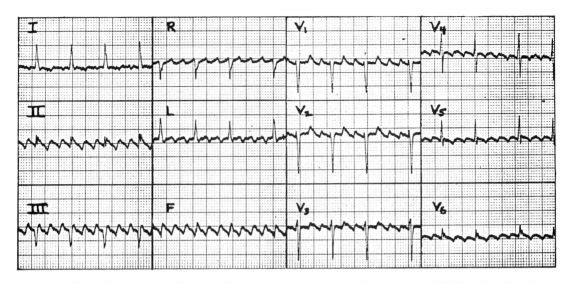

Fig. 15.17 Atrial flutter is evident in this patient with an acute inferior myocardial infarction. Variable AV conduction is present but the average ventricular rate exceeds 100/min, and the patient showed evidence of compromised cardiac output. Cardioversion was accomplished with return of normal rhythm and disappearance of signs and symptoms of the low cardiac output state.

for diastolic ventricular filling, further compromise cardiac output.[32,33]

## Treatment and Prognosis

During myocardial infarction, atrial fibrillation usually causes a decrease in cardiac output. This can result in hypotension, persistence of chest pain, and signs or symptoms of congestive heart failure, and may further jeopardize zones of ischemic myocardium surrounding the area of actual infarction.[34,35] In such individuals, prompt reversion utilizing synchronized precordial electrical shock is a simple and effective mode of therapy.[36] Subsequently, antiarrhythmic drugs (e.g., oral quinidine) may be

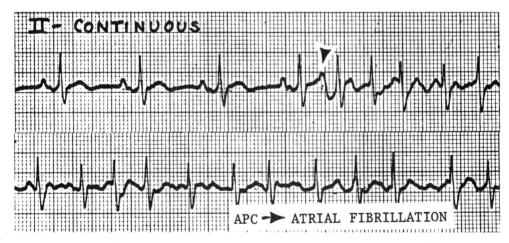

Fig. 15.18 Sinus rhythm is interrupted by an atrial premature complex (arrow) which "triggers" the patient into a sustained run of atrial fibrillation with a rapid ventricular response. In approximately 50 percent of patients, atrial fibrillation develops from such premature atrial stimuli; in the other 50 percent, it occurs as a "degeneration" of atrial flutter. (Reprinted by permission of the publisher, from Davies, Hywel, and Nelson, William P., *Understanding Cardiology*. Woburn: Butterworth Publishers, Inc., 1978.)

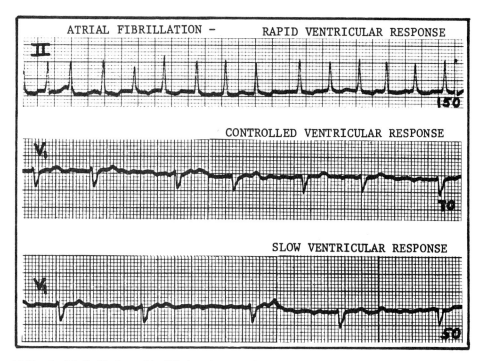

Fig. 15.19  Atrial fibrillation with differing degrees of AV conduction. In the top strip, many impulses penetrate the AV junction with an average ventricular response of 150/min. The middle strip shows a controlled ventricular response of 70/min. The bottom strip shows excessive AV junctional suppression with a slow ventricular response of 50/min. (Reprinted by permission of the publisher, from Davies, Hywel, and Nelson, William P., *Understanding Cardiology.* Woburn: Butterworth Publishers, Inc., 1978.)

utilized to suppress the atrial ectopy that initially caused the arrhythmia.[36] If the situation is less urgent, therapy with incremental intravenous doses of digoxin may decrease the number of penetrating stimuli, resulting in a slower ventricular rate and improved cardiac function. It is important to emphasize that the effect of digitalis in diminishing AV conductivity is, to an important degree, due to its autonomic action (vagal stimulation) rather than a *direct* effect of the drug. Thus, if there is excessive sympathetic activity, it may be difficult (or impossible) to achieve adequate AV junctional suppression, despite large doses of digitalis. In such a circumstance, partial $\beta$-adrenergic blockade with small intravenous doses of propranolol may decrease the number of conducted impulses. When the dysrhythmia lasts for only a brief period of time, or is promptly reverted (by electrical shock or drugs), there is little influence on prognosis. When protracted, especially when accompanied by a rapid ventricular rate, atrial

fibrillation may seriously jeopardize cardiac function. Prognosis for life or uncomplicated recovery decreases with each minute of the rapid cardiac rate; hence, prompt treatment is mandatory.

## MULTIFOCAL ATRIAL TACHYCARDIA (CHAOTIC ATRIAL RHYTHM)

### Mechanism

As implied by the name, this dysrhythmia represents the appearance of multiple ectopic foci within the atria. Usually, it occurs in the setting of significant hypoxemia or serious electrolyte derangement. During these situations, enhancement of other potential atrial pacemakers results and multiform PACs are seen. (An example is shown in Fig. 15.20.) The irregularity and changing P-wave morphology help to distinguish this dysrhythmia from paroxysmal

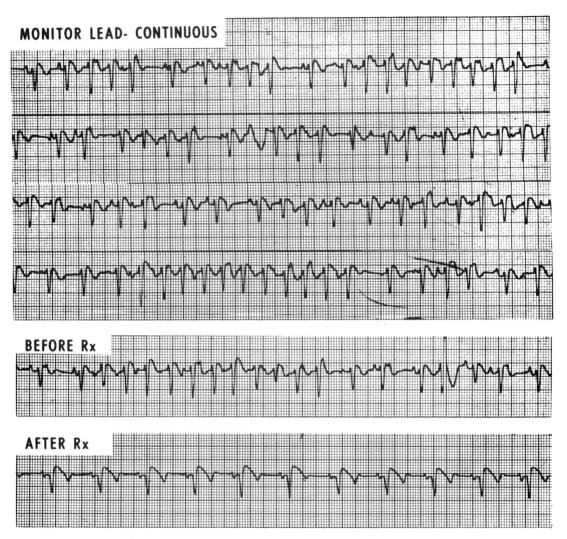

Fig. 15.20 Multifocal atrial tachycardia in a patient with serious lung disease. Note the multiform premature atrial complexes and their unpredictable occurrence. These features help distinguish this dysrhythmia from paroxysmal atrial tachycardia. The irregularity of R-R cycling could suggest atrial fibrillation, but the discrete P waves help in this important differentiation. The lower portion of the illustration demonstrates successful therapy—not with drugs, but with improved pulmonary function and removal of hypoxia. (Adapted and reprinted by permission of the publisher, from Davies, Hywel, and Nelson, William P., *Understanding Cardiology*. Woburn: Butterworth Publishers, Inc., 1978.)

supraventricular tachychycardia. However, the irregularity and changing P-wave morphology can be misdiagnosed as "coarse atrial fibrillation." It is important to distinguish between these two dysrhythmias, since multifocal atrial tachycardia, in general, does not respond to digitalis administration, whereas such therapy in the patient with atrial fibrillation may result either in rhythm conversion or in adequate AV block of the atrial stimuli.[37-40]

Treatment and Prognosis

In the setting in which this arrhythmia occurs (usually a desperately ill patient with myocardial infarction and serious hypoxic lung disease), therapy may be ineffectual and disappointing. Treatment should be aimed at eliminating the causative factors rather than attempting suppression of the ectopic impulse sites with antiarrhythmic drugs. Treatment is frequently unsuccessful unless the underlying cause can be remedied. Multifocal atrial tachycardia (with or without acute infarction) has a mortality rate approximating 50 percent.

## AV JUNCTIONAL RHYTHMS AND AV DISSOCIATION

### Mechanism

The appearance of AV junctional pacemakers is quite common during acute myocardial infarction.[41] Several varieties occur, and distinctions regarding them are important:

1. "Escape junctional pacemakers" may appear whenever the sinus rate slows sufficiently (Fig. 15.21).

2. "Accelerated junctional rhythm" occurs when an ectopic focus in the AV junction appears at a rate greater than that expected of an escape focus[42,43] (Figs. 15.22,23). This dysrhythmia has been called "nonparoxysmal junctional tachycardia," but this terminology has disadvantages because:

(a) It is confusing ("nonparoxysmal" indicates what the rhythm is *not* rather than what it is!); and

(b) It is misleading ("tachycardia" should be reserved for a rate of discharge greater than 100/min, and frequently the accelerated junctional focus has a lesser rate, usually 70 to 100/min).

3. "Paroxysmal junctional tachycardia" may be considered the same as paroxysmal atrial tachycardia, and differentiation cannot be made from the surface electrocardiogram.[44]

During the presence of either "escape junctional rhythm" or "accelerated junctional rhythm," it is common for the atria to continue to be discharged by the sinus node, while the ectopic junctional focus activates the ventricles. This, by definition, is AV dissociation.[45-49] It is important to emphasize that AV dissociation *is not synonomous with AV block;* and the terms and their meanings should be carefully distinguished. Although incomplete AV block may coexist, it need not be present.

### Junctional Escape Rhythm with AV Dissociation

When the sino-atrial node discharge slows to a critical degree, an escape focus may surface in the AV junction and assume responsibility for cardiac activation. The ectopic pacemaker will maintain its dominance until the sinus rate

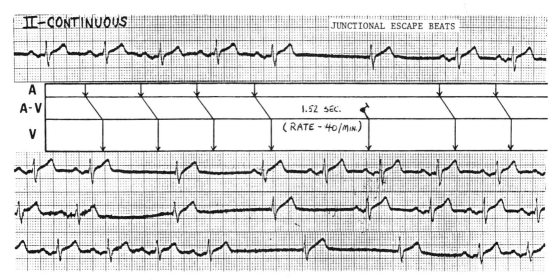

Fig. 15.21 The ladder diagram depicts the result of sinus node "default." After an escape interval of 1.52 sec (rate 40/min), a junctional focus surfaces to activate the heart. It reappears at the same interval whenever sinus node stimuli do not. (Reprinted by permission of the publisher, from Davies, Hywel, and Nelson, William P., *Understanding Cardiology.* Woburn: Butterworth Publishers, Inc., 1978.)

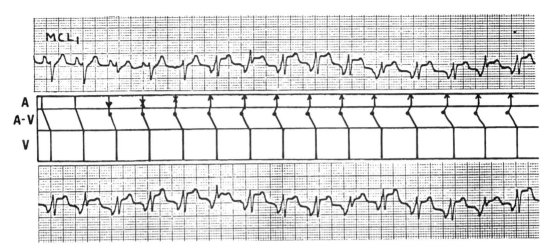

Fig. 15.22  Sinus rhythm is interrupted by the appearance of an accelerated junctional rhythm (low atrial rhythm?) with a discharge rate of 110/min. In the top strip, the ladder diagram demonstrates the interesting interplay of the sinus and ectopic foci. Two atrial fusion beats are seen before the ectopic focus succeeds in producing consistent retrograde atrial excitation, with inverted P waves preceding each QRS complex.

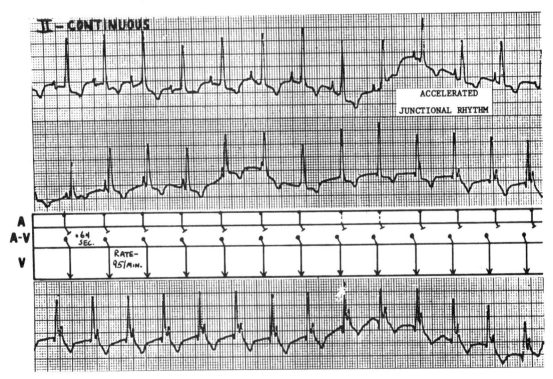

Fig. 15.23  An example of a junctional focus competing with sinus node stimuli for ventricular activation. The ectopic focus has been accelerated to a rate of 95/min and frequently succeeds in producing ventricular activation despite the presence of an adequate sinus rate. The ladder diagram depicts the dissociation of atrial and ventricular events, with the P waves gradually "marching through" the QRS complex until they appear in its wake. Although accelerated junctional rhythm can occur as a result of myocardial infarction, it frequently is due to excess digitalis effect. (Reprinted by permission of the publisher, from Davies, Hywel, and Nelson, William P., *Understanding Cardiology*. Woburn: Butterworth Publishers, Inc., 1978.)

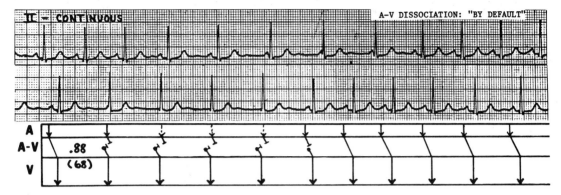

Fig. 15.24  Sinus node slowing permits the appearance of an escape junctional pacemaker at a cycle length of 0.88 sec (rate 68/min). The "default" of the sinus node allows the ectopic pacemaker to continue to function until the sinus rate increases. The interplay of the two pacemakers is illustrated in the ladder diagram. (Reprinted by permission of the publisher, from Davies, Hywel, and Nelson, William P., *Understanding Cardiology*. Woburn: Butterworth Publishers, Inc., 1978.)

increases to exceed the "escape interval" of the junctional focus. Such a dysrhythmia represents the emergence of a "passive" auxilliary pacemaker because of the "default" of the sinus node (see Fig. 15.24). Therapy, if any, should be to increase the rate of the sinus node discharge (e.g., atropine); or, if sinus node activity cannot be accelerated, to provide a predictable electrical stimulus (e.g., an electronic pacemaker). It is obvious that therapy to suppress the escape focus would be illogical and potentially disastrous.

### Accelerated Junctional Rhythm with AV Dissociation

In the course of myocardial infarction, and despite an adequate rate of sinus node, a focus in the AV junction may become enhanced and compete with the sinus node pacemaker. The ectopic pacemaker thus "usurps" the role of the sinus node and provides ventricular activation, leaving the sinus impulse to activate the atria—resulting in AV dissociation, as shown in Fig. 15.25.

Accelerated junctional rhythm is commonly due to digitalis intoxication; if the drug has been used, this possibility should always be considered. When the dysrhythmia occurs during the myocardial infarction and is not due to digitalis excess, it is commonly well tolerated and usually does not need therapy. Occasionally, however, the dissociation of atrial and ventricular

events, with resulting loss of an appropriately timed atrial contribution to ventricular filling, may lead to serious cardiac impairment. If the accelerated focus has a relatively rapid rate of discharge (90 to 100 min or greater), it can usually be suppressed with antiarrhythmic drugs, allowing the sinus node to resume control of ventricular activation. If the discharge rate of the ectopic focus is slower (60 to 70/ min), small intravenous doses of atropine may increase sinus node discharge to a level slightly above that of the ectopic pacemaker, permitting the sinus node to resume its dominance.

### AV Dissociation Due to AV Block

Note that, in the two varieties of AV dissociation discussed above, the disturbance is that of *impulse formation;* the two pacemakers may coexist while *AV conduction* remains unimpaired. If incomplete AV block is present, the number of effective stimuli may be less than the discharge rate of an ectopic auxiliary focus, and AV dissociation may result, as shown in Fig. 15.26. As suggested above, therapy should be directed to diminish the AV block, rather than to suppress the ectopic pacemaker. Therapy with intravenous atropine is often successful in increasing the transmission of atrial stimuli. If such therapy is not successful, a temporary transvenous pacemaker may be required to insure predictable activation of the ventricles. (This subject is discussed further in Chapter 18.)

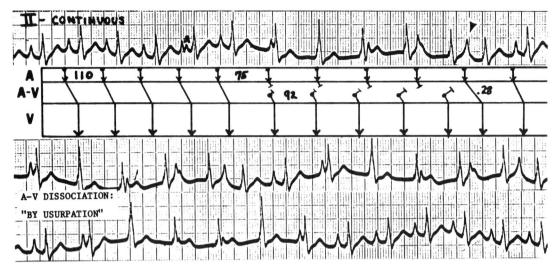

Fig. 15.25   The ladder diagram illustrates what is occurring in this patient with AV dissociation due to "usurpation" by an accelerated junctional focus. (In the top strip one of the P waves contains an artifact and is marked with an "A"). Initial sinus tachycardia of 110/min slows to a rate of 75/min, permitting the appearance of an accelerated AV junctional focus at a rate of 92/min and allowing dissociation of atrial and ventricular events by the usurpation of the enhanced AV junctional pacemaker. The lower sinus pacemaker follows in the wake of the junctional focus. At a given point, it finds the AV junction responsive, and penetrates to capture the ventricle (arrow), temporarily disrupting the discharge of the junctional focus. This phenomenon occurs repetitively in the second and third strips. (Nelson WP: Is There a Smart Aleck in the A-V Junction? Med Times 107:83, 1979.)

## DIGITALIS-INDUCED ATRIAL ARRHYTHMIAS

### Mechanisms

Excess digitalis suppresses the rate of sino-atrial node discharge and enhances the automaticity of ectopic atrial or AV junctional pacemaker sites. Simultaneously, it can decrease AV conductivity. The most common digitoxic atrial arrhythmias result from these effects and include:

1. atrial tachycardia (with either 1:1 AV conduction or with variable degrees of AV block) (Figs. 15.26,27).

2. accelerated junctional rhythm ("nonparoxysmal junctional tachycardia") (Fig. 15.28).

3. excessive AV block (e.g., atrial fibrillation or atrial flutter with a slow ventricular response) (Fig. 15.29).

Since any of these arrhythmias can result from myocardial infarction and could be legitimately ascribed to it, it is of the utmost impor-tance to ensure that digitalis is not the true cause. In many cases, the only solution is to stop the drug. Plasma assays of digitalis can be helpful if the result is either a significant elevation or a low level—but it is foolhardy to presume that a "therapeutic blood level" re-moves the possibility that an arrhythmia is due to digitalis excess!

### Treatment

The treatment of digitoxic arrhythmias con-sists of withdrawal of the drug. In my experi-ence, usually little else is required. Occasionally, however, AV block may be excessive, resulting in a symptomatic bradycardia that requires treatment. Frequently, incremental small doses of intravenous atropine are successful in dimin-ishing the degree of AV block and increasing cardiac rate to an effective level. In rare circum-stances, a temporary transvenous pacemaker may be required to permit appropriate increase in heart rate while the excess digitalis effect is eliminated by renal excretion of the drug.

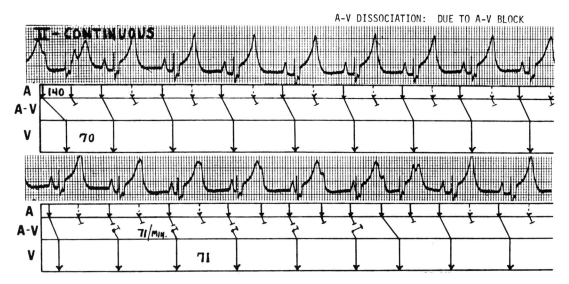

Fig. 15.26 The ladder diagram illustrates what is occurring in this patient with AV dissociation due to AV block. Note that there is atrial tachycardia at a rate of 140/min, but AV block permits the passage of only alternate stimuli (2:1 AV block). Note also that the alternate, nonconducted P waves attempt to hide in the T wave of the conducted beat and are convincingly seen only in the lower tracing. The effective *conductible rate* is, therefore, 70/min. In the lower strip a junctional focus at a rate of 71/minute appears. This ectopic pacemaker succeeds in producing ventricular activation until one of the (potential) penetrating atrial stimuli succeeds in crossing the AV-junctional bridge, reestablishing atrial tachycardia with 2:1 AV block. Although the disturbance in AV-junctional transmission may be due to myocardial infarction, it is frequently seen as a manifestation of digitalis excess (and such was the case in this patient). It is obvious that therapy should be to decrease the AV block and *not* to suppress the ectopic pacemaker, which has appeared due to the diminished number of effective atrial stimuli. (Nelson WP: AV Disassociation Due to AV Block. Med Times 107:145, 1979.)

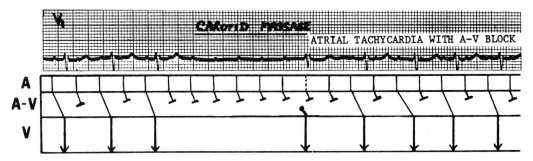

Fig. 15.27 At first glance, this patient's rhythm appears to be normal sinus rhythm with a somewhat prolonged P-R interval. The suspicion of atrial tachycardia was raised by the small deflections in the interval between the QRS and T waves. Carotid sinus massage confirmed the presence of atrial tachycardia by exaggerating the degree of AV block. The ladder diagram indicates the conduction sequence. There is atrial tachycardia with 2:1 AV conduction; the block increased during brief carotid sinus massage. After a lengthy interlude, an escape junctional focus surfaces before resumption of 2:1 conduction of the supraventricular stimuli. This tracing demonstrates the need for careful attention to "routine rhythm strips" in the patient receiving digitalis. Had the dysrhythmia not been recognized and digitalis continued, more serious dysrhythmias would certainly have occurred. (Nelson WP: Digitalis Effects and Excesses. Med Times 107:48, 1979.)

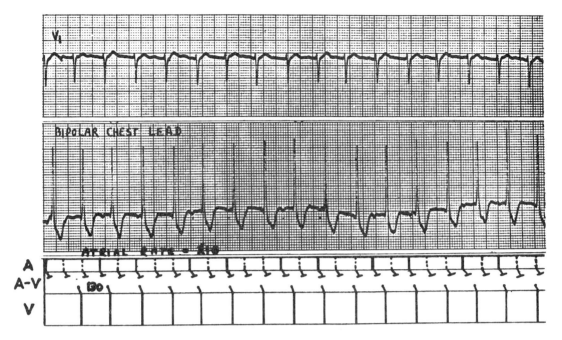

Fig. 15.28 This figure emphasizes several important points in a patient with digitalis intoxication. Note that, although discrete P waves are not seen in Lead V1, they are evident in the bipolar chest lead. When they are carefully plotted, there is found to be an atrial tachycardia at a rate of 210/min. The P waves, however, "march through" the QRS complexes, and it is evident that they are dissociated from them. There is an independent, enhanced focus in the AV junction which stimulates the heart at a rate of 130/min. Digitalis, in addition to prompting atrial and junctional tachycardia, has also resulted in AV block; if the atrial stimuli could penetrate antegrade, and if the junctional stimuli could pass retrograde, the two pacemakers could not coexist. This is an example of "double supraventricular tachycardia." With the recognition of atrial tachycardia with AV block, digitalis intoxication must lead the list of causes, and the drug must be stopped before more serious dysrhythmias occur.

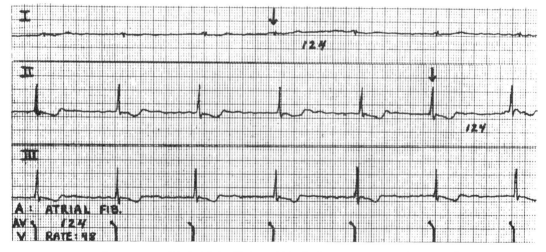

Fig. 15.29 In this patient with atrial fibrillation, digitalis has caused excessive AV block, permitting the appearance of a junctional "escape" pacemaker at a rate of 48/min. Note the regularity of the majority of the R-R cycles. Occasionally, an earlier QRS complex occurs (arrows), indicating that AV block is not complete and that an occasional stimulus of atrial origin can penetrate the AV junction and activate the ventricles. Since the patient was stable, the offending drug was withheld, and no other therapy was given. Had there been need for increased ventricular rate, small doses of intravenous atropine would almost certainly have lessened the degree of AV block and increased the number of conducted atrial stimuli.

362

## ARTIFACTS

There are a variety of artifacts that can appear on both the monitors and ECG recordings of patients, even in the best of coronary care units. The majority are due to muscle potentials, motion, loose electrodes, and, less commonly, to electrical signals from other equipment in use (respirators, suction devices, etc.). At times, they can closely resemble atrial arrhythmias—particularly atrial fibrillation or atrial flutter—and evoke concern, prompting

55 YEAR OLD MAN
4TH DAY AFTER ANTERIOR MI

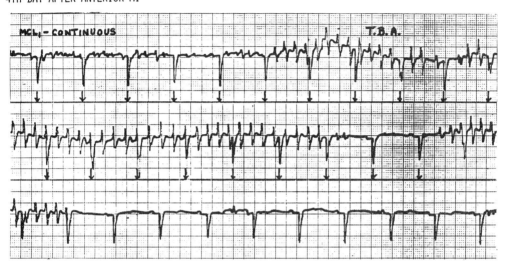

Fig. 15.30 Imagine the concern of the ICU personnel when the rhythm shown appeared in this patient during convalescence from acute myocardial infarction! The initial reaction was that he was having "bursts of atrial fibrillation or coarse atrial flutter," but, in point of fact, the irregular baseline is due to muscle motion. The artifact was due to the patient's brushing his teeth! (TBA-tooth brush artifact!)

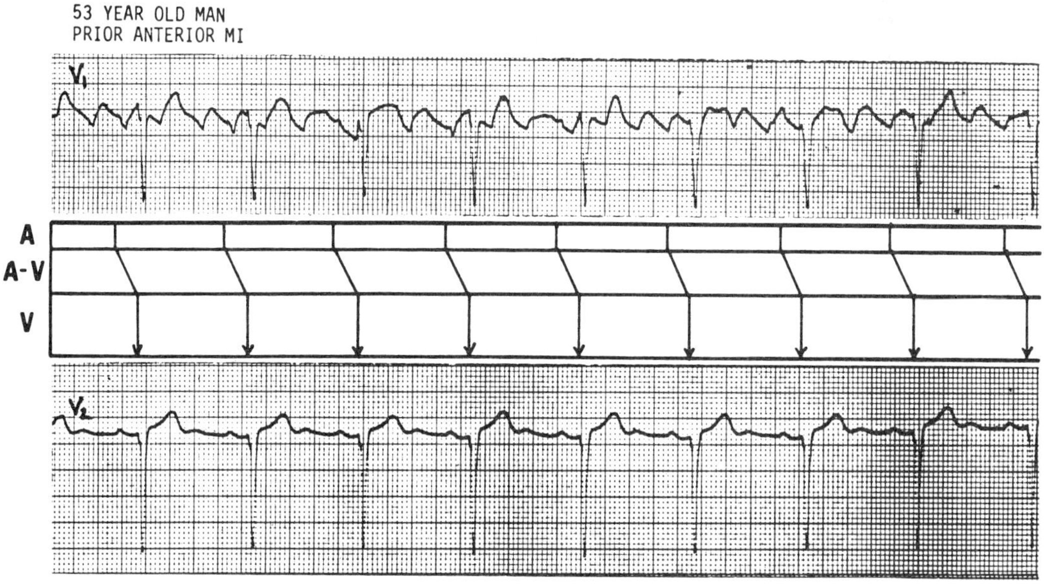

53 YEAR OLD MAN
PRIOR ANTERIOR MI

Fig. 15.31 Another example of an artifact simulating an atrial dysrhythmia. In Lead V1, the deflections simulate atrial flutter, but, in the simultaneously recorded lead V2, it is obvious that the patient has normal sinus rhythm. This artifact was presumably due to a loose recording electrode.

antiarrhythmic drug therapy when none is required. Even experienced CCU personnel can be fooled (the reader is invited to recall the last occasion when such an event occurred!) Examples are shown in Figs. 15.30 and 15.31.

## SUGGESTED READINGS

Hoffman BF, Cranefield PF, Wallace AG: Physiological basis of cardiac arrhythmias. Mod Concepts Cardiovasc Dis 35:103, 1966, 35:107, 1966.

Watanabe Y, Dreifus LS: Newer concepts in the genesis of cardiac arrhythmias. Am Heart J 76:114, 1968.

Cranefield PF, Wit AL, Hoffman BF: Genesis of cardiac arrhythmias. Circulation 47:190, 1973.

De Sanctis RW, Block P, Hutter AM: Tachyarrhythmias in myocardial infarction. Circulation 45:681, 1972.

Hoffman BF, Rosen M, Wit AL: Electrophysiology and pharmacology of cardiac arrhythmias III: The causes and treatment of cardiac arrhythmias. Am Heart J Part A 89:115, 1975, Part B 89:253, 1975.

Cristal N, Szwarcberg J, Gueron M: Supraventricular arrhythmias in acute myocardial infarction: Prognostic importance of clinical setting: Mechanism of production. Ann Intern Med 82:35, 1975.

Liberthson RR, Salisburg KW, Hutter AM, De Sanctis RW: Atrial tachyarrhythmias in acute myocardial infarction. Am J Med 60:956, 1976.

## REFERENCES

1. Ayres SM, Grace WJ: Inappropriate ventilation and hypoxemia as causes of cardiac arrhythmias. Am J Med 46:495, 1969.
2. Dreifus LS, de Azevedo IM, Watanabe Y: Electrolyte and antiarrhythmic drug interaction. Am Heart J 88:95, 1974.
3. Kezdi PM, Korenat RK, Misra SN: Reflex inhibitory effects of vagal afferents in experimental myocardial infarction. Am J Cardiol 33:853, 1974.
4. Chadda KD, Lichstein E, Gupta PM, Choy R: Bradycardia hypotension syndrome in acute myocardial infarction: Reappraisal of the overdrive effects of atropine. Am J Med 59:158, 1975.
5. Scheinman MM, Thorburn D, Abbott JA: Use of atropine in patients with acute myocardial infarction and sinus bradycardia. Circulation 52:627, 1975.
6. Das G, Talmers FN, Weissler AM: New observations on the effects of atropine on the sinoatrial and atrioventricular nodes in man. Am J Cardiol 36:281, 1975.
7. Dhingia R, Amat-y-Leon F, Wyndham C, Denes P, Wir D, Pouget JM, Rosen KM: Electrophysiologic effects of atropine on human sinus node and atrium. Am J Med 38:429, 1976.
8. Denes P, Wu D, Dhingia RC, Pietras RJ, Rosen KM: Effects of cycle length on cardiac refractory periods in man. Circulation 49:32, 1974.
9. Sandler IA, Marriott HJ: Differential morphology of anomalous ventricular complexes of RBBB type in lead V$_1$. Circulation 31:551, 1965.
10. Marriott HJ, Sandler IA: Criteria old and new for differentiating between ectopic ventricular beats and aberrant ventricular conduction in the presence of atrial fibrillation. Prog Cardiovasc Dis 9:18, 1966.
11. Marriott HJ: Differential diagnosis of supraventricular and ventricular tachycardia. Geriatrics 25:91, 1970.
12. Wellens HJ, Bar FW, Lie KI: Value of the electrocardiogram in the differential diagnosis of tachycardia with a widened QRS complex. Am J Med 64:27, 1978.
13. Bigger JT, Goldreyer BN: The mechanism of supraventricular tachycardia. Circulation 42:673, 1970.
14. Goldreyer BN, Damato AN: Essential role of atrioventricular conduction delay in the initiation of paroxysmal supraventricular tachycardia. Circulation 43:679, 1971.
15. Janse MJ, van Capelle FJ, Freud G, Durrer D: Circus movement within the AV node as a basis for supraventricular tachycardia as shown by multiple microelectrode recording in the isolated rabbit heart. Circ Res 28:403, 1971.
16. Rosen KM, Mehta A, Miller RA: Demonstration of dual atrioventricular nodal pthways in man. Am J Cardiol 33:291, 1974.
17. Wu D, Amat-y-Leon F, Denes P, Dhingra RC, Pietras RJ, Rosen KM: Demonstration of sustained sinus and atrial reentry as a mechanism of paroxysmal supraventricular tachycardia. Circulation 51:234, 1975.
18. Denes P, Wu D, Dhingra RC, Chuquimia R, Rosen KM: Demonstration of dual AV nodal pathways in patients with paroxysmal supraventricular tachycardia. Circulation 48:549, 1973.
19. Wu D, Denes P: Mechanisms of paroxysmal supraventricular tachycardia. Arch Intern Med 135:473, 1975.
20. Schuilenburg RM, Durrer D: Further observa-

tions on the ventricular echo phenomenon elicited in the human heart: Is the atrium part of the echo pathway? Circulation 45:629, 1972.

21. Josephson ME, Kastor JA: Paroxysmal supraventricular tachycardia: Is the a atrium a necessary link? Circulation 54:430, 1976.

22. Goldreyer BN, Gallagher JJ, Damato AN: Electrophysiologic demonstration of atrial ectopic tachycardia in man. Am Heart J 85:205, 1973.

23. Barold SS, Coumel P: Mechanisms of atrioventricular junctional tachycardia: Role of reentry and concealed accessory bypass tracts. Am J Cardiol 39:97, 1977.

24. Klein HO, Hoffman BF: Cessation of paroxysmal supraventricular tachycardias by parasympathomimetic interventions. Ann Intern Med 81:48, 1974.

25. Vergara GS, Hildner FJ, Schoenfeld CB, Javier RP, Cohen LS, Samet P: Conversion of supraventricular tachycardias with rapid atrial stimulation. Circulation 46:788, 1972.

26. Rytand DA: The circus movement (entrapped circuit wave) hypothesis and atrial flutter. Ann Intern Med 65:125, 1966.

27. Gavrilescu S, Luca C: Right atrium monophasic action potentials during atrial flutter and fibrillation in man. Am Heart J 90:199, 1975.

28. Waldo AL, Mac Lean WA, Karp RB, Kouchoukos NT, James TN: Entrainment and interruption of atrial flutter with atrial pacing. Circulation 56:737, 1977.

29. Das G, Kamanahally MA, Ancinudu K, Chinnavaso T, Talmers FN, Weissler AM: Atrial pacing for cardioversion of atrial flutter in digitalized patients. Am J Cardiol 41:308, 1978.

30. Abildskov JA, Millar K, Burgess MJ: Atrial fibrillation. Am J Cardiol 28:263, 1971.

31. Bennett MA, Pentecost BL: The pattern of onset and spontaneous cessation of atrial fibrillation in man. Circulation 41:981, 1970.

32. Orndahl G, Thulesuis O, Hood B: Incidence of persistent atrial fibrillation and conduction defects in coronary heart disease. Am Heart J 84:120, 1972.

33. Klass M, Haywood LJ: Atrial fibrillation associated with acute myocardial infarction: A study of 32 cases. Am Heart J 79:752, 1970.

34. Harrison DC: Editorial: Atrial fibrillation in acute myocardial infarction: Significance and therapeutic implications. Chest 70:3, 1976.

35. Cristal N, Petersburg, I, Szwarcberg J: Atrial fibrillation developing in the acute phase of myo-

cardial infarction: Prognostic implications. Chest 70:8, 1976.

36. Sodemark J, Jonsson B, Olsson A, Oro L, Wallin H, Edhag O, Sjogren A, Danielsson M, Rosenhamer G: Effects of quinidine on maintaining sinus rhythym after conversion of atrial fibrillation or flutter. Br Heart J 37:986, 1975.

37. De Maria AN, Lies JE, King JF, Miller RM, Amsterdam EA, Mason DT: Echographic assessment of atrial transport mitral movement and ventricular performance following electroversion of supraventricular arrhythmias. Circulation 51:273, 1975.

38. Shine KI, Kastor JA, Yurchak PM: Multifocal atrial tachycardia. N Engl J Med 279:344, 1968.

39. Phillips J, Spano J, Burch G: Chaotic atrial mechanism. Am Heart J 78:171, 1969.

40. Berlinerblau R, Feder W: Chaotic atrial rhythm. J Electrocardiol 5:135, 1972.

41. Lipson MJ, Shapur N: Multifocal atrial tachycardia. Circulation 42:397, 1970.

42. Fisch C, Knoebel SB: Junctional rhythms. Prog Cardiovasc Dis 13:141, 1970.

43. Konecke LL, Knoebel SB: Nonparoxysmal junctional tachycardia complicating acute myocardial infarction. Circulation 45:367, 1972.

44. Knoebel SB, Fisch C: Accelerated junctional escape: A clinical and electrocardiographic study. Circulation 50:151, 1974.

45. Rosen KM: Junctional tachycardia: Mechanisms diagnosis differential diagnosis and management. Circulation 47:654, 1973.

46. Pick A: AV dissociation: A proposal for a comprehensive classification and consistent terminology. Am Heart J 66:147, 1963.

47. Marriott HJL, Menendez MM: AV dissociation revisited. Prog Cardiovasc Dis 8:522, 1966.

48. Zipes DP, Fisch C: ECG analysis No. 12: Atrioventricular dissociation Arch Intern Med 131:593, 1973.

49. Zipes DP, Fisch C: ECG analysis No. 13: Atrioventricular dissociation. Arch Intern Med 132:130, 1973.

50. Zipes DP, Fisch C: ECG analysis No. 14: Atrioventricular dissociation. Arch Intern Med 132:612, 1973.

51. Lown B, Marcus F, Levine HD: Digitalis and atrial tachycardia with block. N Engl J Med 260:301, 1959.

52. Bernstein RB, Stanzler RM: Paroxysmal atrial tachycardia with latent block. Arch Intern Med 118:154, 1966.

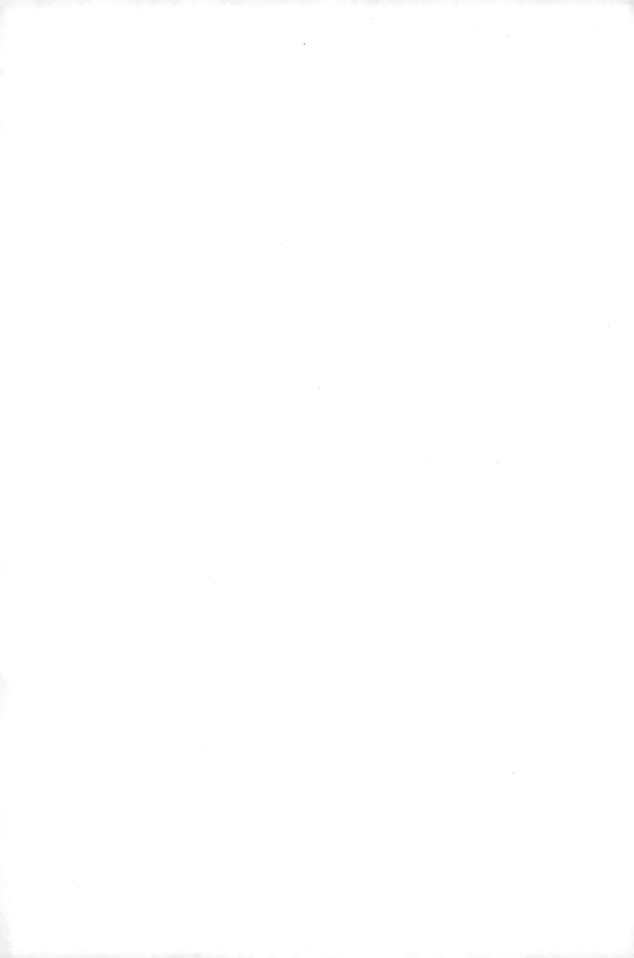

# 16 | Ventricular Arrhythmias: Diagnosis, Treatment, and Prognosis

*Robert L. Engler, M.D.*
*Martin M. LeWinter, M.D.*

The major impact of the coronary care unit on the mortality rate of acute myocardial infarction is on arrhythmia detection and treatment. Arrhythmia detection has two levels of significance: (1) immediate recognition of any arrhythmias likely to have hemodynamic consequences; and (2) recognition of "warning" arrhythmias. We will discuss the value of arrhythmia detection in these two areas in the next section. We will then review the rationale for prophylactic administration of antiarrhythmic drugs, the diagnosis and therapy of ventricular tachycardia, and the current evidence regarding the prognostic implications of ventricular arrhythmias.

## MONITOR LEADS

The most convenient monitor lead is MCL-1, in which the negative electrode is on the left shoulder; the positive electrode is at the right sternal edge in the fourth intercostal space, and the ground is on the right shoulder (Fig. 16.1). This lead configuration generally demonstrates good amplitude p waves and allows detection of left and right bundle branch block and distinction of left ventricular premature complexes from supraventricular impulses conducted with right bundle branch aberration.[1,2] Aberrantly conducted beats occur when a supraventricular impulse (usually a premature atrial or junctional depolarization) arrives at

the His bundle when part of the conducting system is refractory. For example, if the left bundle branch (LBB) is refractory, the impulse would be conducted down the right bundle branch (RBB) only and a left bundle branch block (LBBB) pattern would be recorded on the electrocardiogram. Because the refractory period of the RRB is longer than the refractory period of the LBB in the majority of patients, right bundle branch block (RBBB) aberrancy

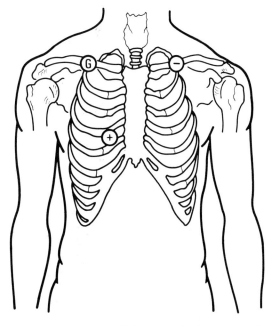

Fig. 16.1 Placement of electrodes for MCL-1 monitor lead.

367

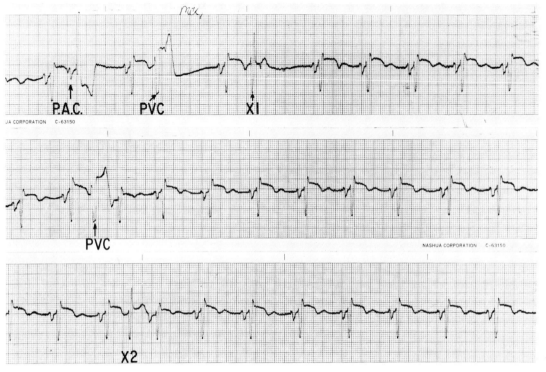

Fig. 16.2   A premature atrial beat (PAC) conducted with right bundle branch block (rSR′) and a premature ventricular complex (PVC) are demonstrated on this MCL-1 rhythm strip. The complex labeled "X-1" has the rSR′ configuration of right bundle branch block suggesting supraventricular origin. The complex labeled "X-2" is identical to X-1 has an rSR′ form but is clearly an interpolated PVC.

is more common. For this reason, a typical RBBB pattern in MCL-1 is more likely to represent a supraventricular depolarization conducted with aberrancy. The RBBB pattern in MCL-1 is of the general form RSR′, with the R′ generally longer than the initial R. However, there are exceptions to this principle; thus, it is necessary to apply other criteria (Fig. 16.2).

## ARRHYTHMIA DETECTION

The monitor watcher is the original arrhythmia detector; continuous visual oscilloscope observation by trained observers is used in many coronary care units. This method allows detection of some dysrhythmias, but many are missed. Romhilt and coworkers, in a study of 31 patients monitored for up to 5 days, found that only 54.5 percent of patients with ventricular premature complexes (VPCs), 6.5 percent

with multifocal VPCs, and 13 percent with coupling were detected by monitor observation alone.[3] These data indicate that warning arrhythmias are not reliably detected by trained personnel. The individual who must watch the monitor should be changed at least every hour. Detection can be aided by the use of a storage oscilloscope which displays the most recent 10 to 15 seconds of rhythm. A continuously recording memory loop is also helpful; the value of this device is that electrical events preceding dysrhythmias can be identified. When a patient is suddenly noted to have dysrhythmia, activation of the memory playback loop causes the several minutes immediately preceding the arrhythmia (usually three) of ECG to be written or stored for later playback. By this means, the presence or absence of warning arrhythmias and the initiation of the arrhythmia can be reviewed. Some memory devices provide automatic sampling at pre-set intervals.

Automated or computer-assisted detection of arrhythmias is a mixed blessing. The simplest example is the "rate alarm." Low and high limits for heart rate are set, and a QRS detection device counts complexes and continuously averages the heart rate; when the prescribed limits are exceeded, an alarm sounds. There are several drawbacks to this still widely used system. First, it takes several beats of a changing average heart rate to detect an arrhythmia; therefore, the initiation of the arrhythmia may be lost unless an automated memory loop is used. Second, movement artifact may trigger the "heart rate too high" alarm, causing the coronary care unit staff to respond by inactivating the alarm. Third, in patients with electronic pacemakers, arrhythmias may be missed. For example, a patient with primary ventricular fibrillation (VF) might not trigger the alarm because his pacemaker continues to generate impulses which are falsely detected as QRS complexes.

Computer recognition of ventricular premature complexes is currently in the developmental stage. The hardware systems (the computer itself) are available from almost every manufacturer of monitoring equipment, and the variety is overwhelming to the uninitiated. Display of premature beats, trend analysis, and 24-hour memory (storage of all detected dysrhythmias) are available options. However, very few of the computer programs for ventricular premature complex detection used in these systems have been rigorously tested and subjected to peer review. A few reports indicate false-positive detection rates between 2 and 13 percent and false-negative detection rates of 2 to 5 percent [4-6] for ventricular premature complexes. These rates are slightly higher for atrial arrhythmias and higher still in patients with atrial fibrillation. The main problems are false-positive detection of ventricular premature complexes due to electrical noise and false classification of aberrantly conducted premature atrial beats as ventricular. The goal of automated detection of all warning arrhythmias has not yet been achieved. Nonetheless, when automated detection is compared to monitor watching in real time, the computer has a much higher percent detection rate—probably greater than 95 percent detection in programs now being tested. So far, no significant impact of automated arrhythmia detection has been demonstrated. However, it seems to us that the more precise data regarding arrhythmia frequency available from a computer would be desirable. Exactly how (and if) this information should be used is so far unknown.

## WARNING ARRHYTHMIAS

Lown and others proposed the concept that the occurrence of primary ventricular fibrillation (VF) in the absence of severe myocardial failure or cardiogenic shock is more common in patients with ventricular premature complexes which have certain characteristics.[7-16] These characteristics are: (1) greater than 5 beats per minute; (2) more than 2 beats in succession; (3) multiform configuration (Fig. 16.3); or (4) prematurity index of less than 0.85. The prematurity index is based on the vulnerable period during late repolarization when the electrical threshold for ventricular fibrillation is at a minimum. It is calculated as follows: The coupling interval between the normally conducted ventricular depolarization and the premature complex (RQ) is divided by the QT interval of a normally conducted complex. While premature ventricular complexes possessing these characteristics may precede ventricular fibrillation, 40 to 83 percent of patients who develop primary VF have no preceding arrhythmia.[11,12,16,17]

## PRIMARY VENTRICULAR FIBRILLATION

Primary ventricular fibrillation occurs in the absence of cardiogenic shock, severe left ventricular failure, or specific metabolic or toxic causes (Fig. 16.4). Ventricular fibrillation associated with shock is multifactorial and is called secondary ventricular fibrillation. It is thus called because the major associated factors include low perfusion pressure, high left ventricular diastolic pressure, increasing ischemia, acidosis, and electrolyte abnormalities.

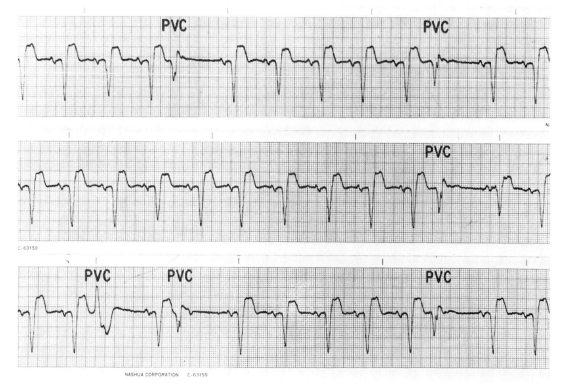

Fig. 16.3  Multiform premature ventricular complexes. Five complexes with one form and a single complex of different form are present.

A major goal of coronary care in patients with acute infarction is prevention and therapy of primary ventricular fibrillation. Primary VF occurs in up to 11 percent of acute infarction patients when prophylactic antiarrhythmic agents are not used.[18] One approach to prevention is to treat all warning dysrhythmias. This approach is limited by the previously mentioned data that 40 to 83 percent of primary ventricular fibrillation is not preceded by warning arrhythmias. The rationale for the prophylactic administration of antiarrhythmic agents to patients

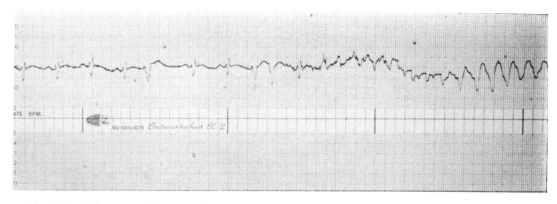

Fig. 16.4  Primary ventricular fibrillation or ventricular flutter. Only one PVC was noted during the previous hour.

with acute myocardial infarction is to suppress VPCs which may trigger VF. If such an agent can reduce the incidence of primary VF without significant side effects or other risks, it would be highly desirable to use it prophylactically.

One approach might be to administer a prophylactic antiarrhythmic agent to all patients with possible acute myocardial infarction. A second approach is to select patients who are at high risk for developing primary ventricular fibrillation. In selecting patients for arrhythmia prophylaxis, it is necessary to identify predictive criteria for primary ventricular fibrillation other than the type of VPC. The incidence of primary VF with acute myocardial infarction decreases with increasing age;[14,15] however, this criterion is not of itself sufficient for patient selection. After 24 to 48 hours have elapsed from the onset of infarction, the incidence of primary ventricular fibrillation is low,[19] and prophylaxis is not warranted. The site of infarction does not correlate with the incidence of primary VF.[16,18] Although it is unclear whether "infarct size" is related to the incidence of primary VF, congestive heart failure and shock are associated with a high incidence of secondary ventricular fibrillation.[14,20-21]

## Prophylactic Use of Lidocaine

The classification of VPCs suggested by Lown can be used as a basis for arrhythmia prophylaxis. Greater than 5 VPCs per minute, more than 2 VPCs in a row, or multiform VPCs are reasonable indications for administration of prophylactic antiarrhythmic agents, but the prematurity index (RQ/QT) is a less reliable predictor of primary ventricular fibrillation.[22] However, we prefer to use arrhythmia prophylaxis for all patients within the first 24 to 48 hours of onset of acute myocardial infarction who do not have specific contraindications to such therapy. Prophylaxis with intravenous lidocaine has been shown to be efficacious in reducing the incidence of primary ventricular fibrillation. However, there is not complete unanimity on this point.[9-12,16,23-35,45-47,50]

The rationale for prophylactic lidocaine administration was summarized by Harrison.[31] The absence of preceding warning arrhythmias in 20[33] to 83 percent of patients[15] and the mean incidence (from several reports) of primary VF of 6 percent argue in favor of prophylaxis for patients without specific contraindications. Electronically controlled intravenous delivery devices which accurately regulate the dose and knowledge of the pharmacokinetics of lidocaine have been important in reducing the number of adverse reactions. However, the toxic effects of lidocaine (and other antiarrhythmic drugs) can be significant and occasionally fatal. Frequent checks of mental status for lethargy which may indicate lidocaine toxicity are necessary. Seizures are the major toxic manifestation of lidocaine. Avoidance of toxicity by appropriate reductions in dose when congestive heart failure or underlying liver disease is present is discussed in the next section.

Patients who have primary VF in the first 48 hours of acute myocardial infarction may have a worse prognosis. Thompson and Sloman reported 23 patients who had sudden death in the hospital after leaving the CCU and 250 control patients without progressive congestive heart failure or shock.[34] Six of those who died had primary VF in the CCU, whereas 12 of the 250 controls had primary VF. Of interest was the formulation of a prognostic index for late sudden death in hospital and confirmation by Graboys.[35] Patients with three of the following five criteria were at increased risk: anterior infarction, supraventricular or sinus tachycardia persisting after the second day, ventricular tachycardia, primary VF, and a new conduction disorder. In Graboys' series, of nine patients who died unexpectedly in the hospital, three had had primary VF in the CCU.[35] By using prophylaxis, the predictive value of primary VF is lost.

In hospitals where physicians are not readily available in the CCU, arrhythmia prophylaxis would be important. Selection of patients could be based on length of time after probable infarction and perhaps on age. To prevent primary VF during transport to the CCU, arrhythmia prophylaxis should begin in the admitting area or emergency room. We also recommend that a portable monitor be used during transport to the CCU and that a physician accompany the patient. The concept of warning arrhyth-

**Table 16.1**   Intravenous Administration of Antiarrhythmic Drugs (see also Table 14.1, pp. 306–307)

| Agent | Loading Dose | Infusion Rate | Toxicity | Contraindications |
|---|---|---|---|---|
| Lidocaine | 2.3 mg/kg in two divided doses 5 min apart | 20 to 55 μg/kg/min (for congestive heart failure or known liver disease, use half this dose) | Central nervous system: lethargy, confusion, tinnitus, visual changes, nausea | Allergy, high-grade heart block, severe bradycardia |
| Procainamide | 10 mg/kg: initially 100 mg over 5 min, then 20 mg/min | 1 to 5 mg/min | Hypotension, myocardial depression, QRS prolongation, psychosis, nausea | Allergy, high-grade heart block |
| Propranolol | 1 to 2 mg q. 5 min until arrhythmia is controlled; total dose usually not to exceed 0.1 mg/kg | Oral maintenance | Hypotension, bronchospasm in asthma, myocardial depression | Asthma, high-grade heart block |
| Bretylium tosylate | 5 to 10 mg/kg infused over 10 minutes | Repeated | Catecholamine release followed by adrenergic blockade, nausea, vomiting | Digitalis toxicity, concomitant digitalis administration |
| Disopyramide phosphate (not approved for i.v. use in U.S.A.) | 2 mg/kg infused over 8 min; 2 mg/kg infused over 52 min | 20 to 40 mg/min | Nausea, vomiting, myocardial depression, urinary retention | Allergy, high-grade heart block, left ventricular failure |

mias seems less reliable. Our current practice is to give antiarrhythmic prophylaxis to patients in the first 48 hours of acute infarction who do not have heart block or new conduction disturbances and who are not allergic to lidocaine.

## Selection of Antiarrhythmic Agents for the Treatment of Primary VF

Many agents have been subjected to small clinical trials for prevention of primary VF. However, there are some difficulties which arise in analyzing small clinical trials. When the efficacy of a therapeutic intervention is being tested against a therapy or placebo, patients must be randomly assigned to therapy or no therapy, and all potentially significant patient characteristics must be the same in both groups. Further, the sample size should not be too small to detect therapeutic efficacy. (See discussion of Type 2 error, Ch. 42.)

Lidocaine is the most widely used prophylactic agent that reduces the incidence of primary VF acute myocardial infarction (MI). Because lidocaine suppresses warning arrhythmias[18,23,36-38] in acute MI, numerous clinical trials of prophylaxis for primary ventricular fibrillation have been carried out. The data have been well reviewed by Bigger et al.[11] Many studies using infusion rates less than 2 mg/min demonstrated suppression of warning arrhythmias but not of ventricular fibrillation.[18,27,38-40] When higher doses were employed, efficacy in the suppression of ventricular fibrillation or ventricular tachycardia was demonstrated in some studies.[12,27,41] When effective suppression of ventricular fibrillation has not been found, it can be ascribed to too small a frequency of VF relative to sample size. (The pharmacokinetics of this agent are discussed in Ch. 14.)

As indicated in Table 16.1, we routinely use a dose of 20 to 55 mcg/kg/min in a patient without left ventricular failure after a bolus injection of 2.3 mg/kg in two doses. The importance of the multiple bolus technique and reaching a therapeutic level deserves emphasis.[42-43] This is illustrated schematically in Fig. 16.5. Congestive heart failure and decreased hepatic function result in a low clearance rate, and dosages should be reduced.[44] Renal failure does not alter the pharmacokinetics of lidocaine.

There has been some interest in administering intramuscular lidocaine before transport to the hospital in patients with acute MI. Singh[29] demonstrated suppression of VPCs at serum lidocaine levels below the usual therapeutic range. Valentine et al.[28] conducted a double-blind, randomized trial using 300 mg of intramuscular lidocaine. The mortality in the placebo group (8/113) was greater than the lidocaine group (3/256). However, studies by Lie et al.[45] and Zener et al.[46] have suggested that larger doses (450 mg) are necessary to achieve effective blood levels, but peak levels then approach the toxic range. It is therefore preferable to use intravenous lidocaine in the prehospital phase of acute MI, but intramuscular administration is a reasonable alternative when the support personnel for transport with intravenous therapy are not available.

Clinical trials of quinidine have been inconclusive. Two clinical studies demonstrated that quinidine suppressed ventricular premature complexes.[25,26] However, no conclusions can be reached regarding efficacy in preventing primary VF because of the low incidence of primary VF in these trials.

The same type of clinical trial data are available for procainamide. Koch-Weser et al. reported effective suppression of ventricular premature complexes and ventricular tachycardia.[24] Primary VF occurred in 2/33 control patients and 0/37 treated patients (inconclusive). Thus, procainamide has been shown to reduce VPCs and ventricular tachycardia, but prevention of primary ventricular fibrillation was not demonstrated.

Based on the above evidence, we routinely administer prophylactic lidocaine to patients who arrive at the CCU within 48 hours of symptoms suggestive of acute myocardial infarction, provided there is no history of allergy to lidocaine or atrioventricular conduction disturbance. Until temporary standby ventricular pacing is available, contraindications to lidocaine or procainamide include: (1) second or third degree heart block; and (2) first degree heart block with evidence of bifascicular block in the setting of anterior infarction. Utilizing automated delivery systems to avoid accidental increases in the delivered dose, minor toxicity has been reported in up to 39 percent of patients,[18] but the incidence is less than 10 percent in most of the previously cited studies. Major toxicity (seizures, coma) has been reported, especially in patients with impaired hepatic function or reduced hepatic blood flow.[41,47,57,70] Reduced doses should be used in these patients.[44,48,49] In patients with severe congestive heart failure or in whom hepatic function is likely to be abnormal, we administer one-half the usual dose.

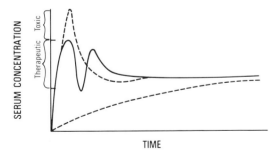

TIME

Fig. 16.5 Typical pharmacokinetic data for a drug such as lidocaine with a short plasma half-life. The solid line represents administration with two boluses and an intravenous drip. A single bolus followed by an intravenous drip and an intravenous drip alone are shown by the upper and lower dashed lines, respectively.

## USE OF ATROPINE IN ACUTE MYOCARDIAL INFARCTION

Vagal stimulation has been reported to reduce the ventricular fibrillation threshold and the frequency of ventricular premature complexes in experimental myocardial infarction.[50-54] The ventricular fibrillation threshold is the minimal current delivered during the vulnerable period necessary to induce ventricular fibrillation. The mechanism of reduction of this threshold in dogs is mediated through cholinergic innervation of the ventricular septum in proximity to the Purkinje system.[50] Kolman et al. demonstrated that the beneficial effects of vagal tone were exerted only when $\beta$-adrenergic stimulation was enhanced.[56] Atropine administration may induce VF by blocking vagal impulses; thus, Goldstein et al. demonstrated an increase in spontaneous VF in dogs treated with atropine.[55] However, two other canine studies failed to demonstrate any vagal effect on ventricular fibrillation.[57-58] The data are difficult to apply to patients with acute myocardial infarction because the existence of ventricular cholinergic nerves in man has not been shown. Furthermore, the relation between ventricular fibrillation threshold in the dog and ventricular fibrillation in man is unknown.

In spite of conflicting experimental data on the use of atropine, interest in its use continues because of the problem of bradycardia after acute MI. In this context, the findings of Grauer et al. of frequent bradycardia and associated hypotension during transport to the hospital of patients with acute MI stimulated interest in the level of vagal tone and the potential benefits of atropine.[59] Two clinical studies support the use of atropine in specific circumstances. Warren and Lewis reported 70 patients with bradycardia shortly after acute myocardial infarction.[60] The incidence of ventricular fibrillation was 1/45 in those who received atropine and 2/25 in those who did not. Thirty-nine of the 45 patients who received atropine had significant hemodynamic improvement. Scheinman et al. reviewed 56 patients with bradycardia.[61] Atropine resulted in improvement of hypotension in 88 percent, of A-V block in 85 percent, and of ventricular ectopy in 87 percent.

However, three patients developed ventricular tachycardia or ventricular fibrillation, and three patients had sustained sinus tachycardia. Adverse reactions were more common in patients receiving an initial dose of 1 mg or greater or more than 2.5 mg in 2.5 hours.

Thus, under some circumstances, atropine may enhance the likelihood of ventricular tachycardia or ventricular fibrillation. However, atropine should be used when symptomatic bradycardia or heart block are present. The initial dose should be 0.4 to 0.6 mg because adverse reactions are less common than with a dose of 1.0 mg or more. However, routine use of atropine in asymptomatic patients with relative bradycardia for overdrive suppression of VPCs is not indicated.

## CONTINUED THERAPY OF WARNING ARRHYTHMIAS

When warning arrhythmias are present, how vigorous should one be in suppression? When lidocaine is ineffective or contraindicated, we administer procainamide. The dose and safety of procainamide administration are discussed in the next section. If neither of these drugs suppresses the warning dysrhythmias, we continue drug administration and continue monitoring. If VPCs continue after 2 or 3 days, an oral agent for chronic suppression is selected. The indications for therapy of VPCs in the post-CCU setting are discussed in a subsequent section.

## VENTRICULAR TACHYCARDIA

Ventricular tachycardia (VT) is a regular or slightly irregular rhythm of ventricular origin with QRS complexes wider than 120 ms, often greater than 160 ms (Figs. 16.6–16.8). In the setting of acute myocardial infarction, VT is usually of left ventricular origin, and the mechanism is probably reentry (see Ch. 13). Another feature which is helpful in recognizing VT is the absence of retrograde (ventricular-atrial) nodal conduction in about one-half of the in-

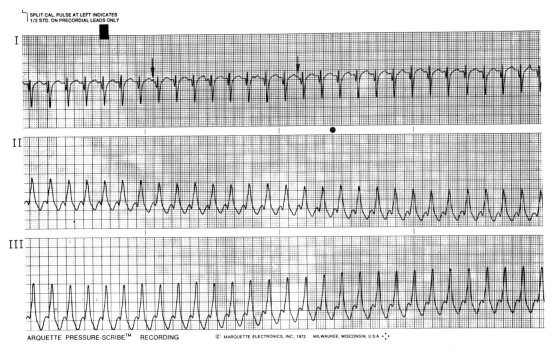

Fig. 16.6  Rhythm strips from leads I, II, and III show continuous ventricular tachycardia. Independent atrial activity is visible in lead I (arrows).

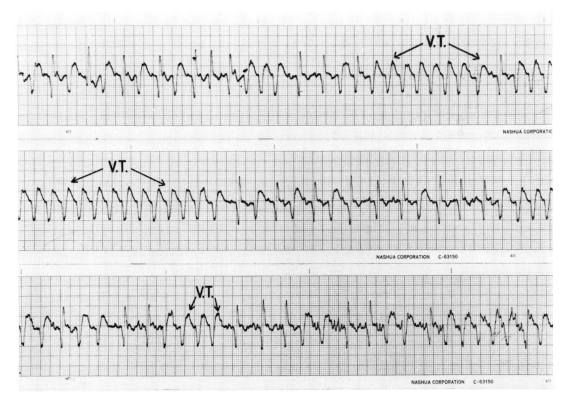

Fig. 16.7  Intermittent ventricular tachycardia (VT), MCL-1 rhythm strip. Atrial fibrillation results in irregular supraventricular beats with frequent PVCs. Episodes of regular ventricular tachycardia (VT) are present.

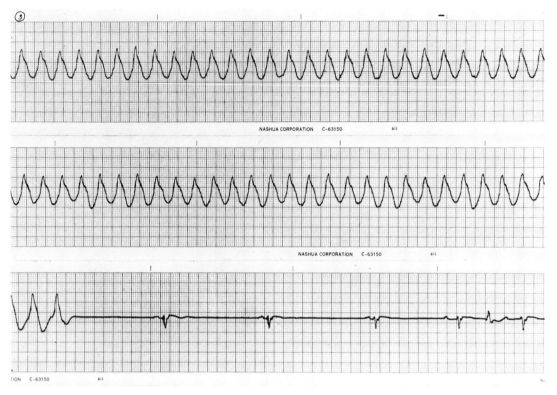

Fig. 16.8  Rapid ventricular tachycardia (150/min) converted to sinus brachycardia. Lead is MCL-1.

stances. This results in independent atrial activity and occasional antegrade AV nodal conduction with partial ventricular capture and fusion beats (Fig. 16.9).

The ventricular rate is important in prognosis and treatment. Ventricular tachycardia is said to exist when the rate is greater than 100/min. Ventricular rhythms with a rate of 60 to 100/min are defined as accelerated idioventricular rhythm (AIVR). Ventricular rhythm at a rate

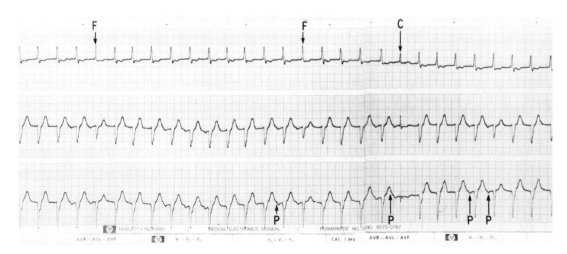

Fig. 16.9  Continuous ventricular tachycardia interrupted by a single supraventricular capture beat (C) and several fusion beats (F). Independent atrial activity is visible, and several P waves are labeled (P). Rhythm strip is not continuous.

of less than 60/min is defined as idioventricular rhythm (IVR) (Figs. 16.10–16.11).

Ventricular tachycardia can occur within the first few days of acute infarction or may not appear until later. As noted in Chapter 13, there is some experimental evidence supporting different pathophysiologic mechanisms at these times. The first task of the clinician is to differentiate ventricular tachycardia from supraventricular tachycardia with aberrant conduction (Table 16.2).

There are several diagnostic points to consider. First is the presence of atrioventricular dissociation. Atrial activity at a rate different from ventricular activity may be visible. One clue may be the appearance of a regular variation in the ST-T segment or QRS morphology due to p waves which vary in relation to the QRS complex (Figs. 16.6, 16.9).

However, retrograde atrial activation does occur in 50 percent of episodes of VT.[62] In addition, junctional tachycardia may occasionally occur with retrograde block and atrioventricular (A-V) dissociation.[63]

The opportunity to observe the onset of the dysrhythmia may clarify the mechanism. Initiation by a premature atrial beat favors supraventricular origin whereas initiation by a VPC favors VT. (In the presence of accessory pathways, reentrant tachycardia may be initiated by either atrial or ventricular premature complexes). Atrioventricular dissociation may also be confirmed on physical examination by: (1) appearance of irregular cannon (giant a) waves in the jugular venous pulse, caused by contraction of the atrium against a closed tricuspid valve; or (2) variation in intensity of the first heart sound.

Thus, the presence of A-V dissociation suggests VT but does not exclude an unusual case of junctional tachycardia. The presence of one-to-one atrial and ventricular activity is not very

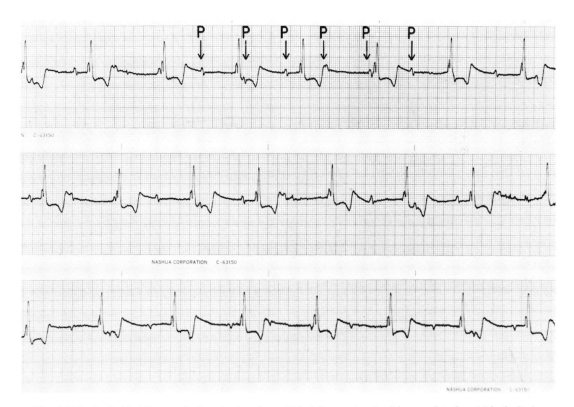

Fig. 16.10 Probable idioventricular rhythm (rate 40/min) associated with complete heart block. Independent atrial activity (P) is present at 70/min. The QRS width of 120 ms and right bundle branch block pattern in lead MCL-1 suggest the possibility of a low junctional or His bundle location of the escape pacemaker.

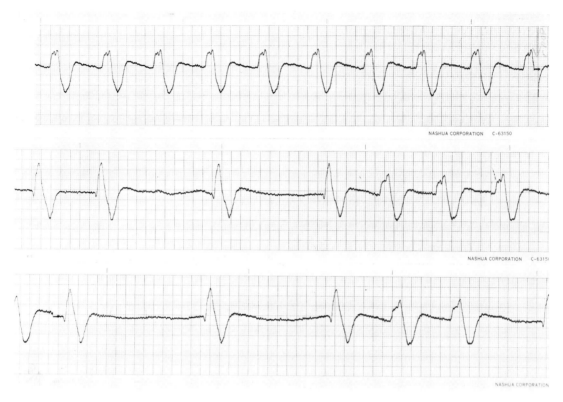

Fig. 16.11  Idioventricular rhythm at a rate of 50 to 60/min. No atrial activity is present. There is variation in rate, and two different ventricular complexes are present.

helpful, since retrograde ventriculoatrial conduction is seen in one-half the instances of VT. One may also observe the presence of fusion beats (Figs. 16.7, 16.9). A fusion beat is generated when part of the QRS is formed by ventricular depolarization from a conducted supraventricular impulse and part is formed from the ventricular ectopic or reentrant depolarization wave. It usually has different form (shape) from the underlying VT and is narrower. A capture beat is a normal supraventricular complex interrupting the tachycardia (Fig. 16.9).

Table 16.2  Use of the ECG to Differentiate Ventricular Tachycardia from Supraventricular Tachycardia

|  | Supraventricular Tachycardia | Ventricular Tachycardia |
|---|---|---|
| QRS duration | ≤ .14 ms | > .14 ms |
| Configuration of QRS | Right bundle branch block | Left axis in frontal plane |
| Atrioventricular dissociation | Very rare | Occurs in about one-half of patients |
| Capture and fusion beats | Do not occur | Diagnostic when they occur |
| Lead MCL-1 configuration | rSR′ | Monophasic R or qR |

Since this beat must arrive before the next expected ventricular depolarization and is narrow, it makes aberrancy as a mechanism of tachycardia unlikely. While there are rare exceptions, observation of ventricular-atrial dissociation and fusion or capture beats is strongly suggestive of VT.[64] A less specific criterion is the QRS width which is usually greater with VT than with supraventricular tachycardia. Thus, a QRS duration greater than 140 ms favors a ventricular origin.[64] Wellens found the QRS width greater than 140 ms in 48/70 instances of ventricular tachycardia.[64] However, none of these patients had acute infarction or bundle branch block or were receiving antiarrhythmic agents. In the presence of depressed conduction due to ischemia, drugs, or conduction system disease, the QRS duration during supraventricular tachycardia with aberrancy might be as wide as 140 ms. A QRS width of 120 ms favored aberrancy in 53/63 patients in Wellens' series.[64]

Most VT in the setting of acute MI will have the configuration of a monophasic R or a QR complex in a right precordial lead such as MCL-1.[1,2,63-66,70,71,74-76] This suggests left ventricular origin of the tachycardia. However, in patients with precordial Q waves in $V_1$–$V_2$ due to anteroseptal infarction, a RBBB aberrancy pattern in lead $V_1$ or MCL-I will resemble the qR configuration suggestive of left ventricular origin (Table 16.2).

Identical configuration of the tachycardia QRS to isolated premature ventricular complexes previously recorded can be an important clue to ventricular origin.

It is of critical importance to assess the hemodynamic consequences of an arrhythmia immediately. If a tachycardia with widened QRS is present and perfusion is not adequate, immediate DC cardioversion should be performed. The proper procedures to follow when cardioversion is not successful will be considered below. If the apparent ventricular tachycardia results in adequate systemic perfusion, there is time to review the rhythm and confirm whether ventricular tachycardia is present. The bedside clues should not be overlooked. The appearance of cannon waves in the jugular venous pulse suggesting atrioventricular dissociation, or variation in intensity of the first heart sound also suggesting atrioventricular dissociation, will help confirm the ventricular origin of the tachycardia. It should be kept in mind, however, that about one-half of patients with ventricular tachycardia will have 1-to-1 retrograde atrial conduction and, thus, the signs of AV dissociation will not be found.[64]

## Treatment of Ventricular Tachycardia: Initial Drug Therapy

Sustained ventricular tachycardia with inadequate perfusion should be treated with immediate electrical cardioversion. Injection of a bolus of lidocaine (usually 100 mg) should be tried if the defibrillator is not immediately ready. In patients who maintain adequate blood pressure despite VT, pharmacologic therapy can be initiated. However, one should keep in mind that perfusion is seldom adequate and acidosis and other effects of tissue hypoxia may accumulate rapidly. The best drug to start with is lidocaine in a dose of 100 mg intravenously. If the patient is already receiving lidocaine but the dose is inadequate, a second bolus of one-half the usual loading amount and an increase in the intravenous infusion rate to a maximum of 55 mcg/kg/min can be tried.

Procainamide is the second best drug. Pharmacokinetic data indicate that the intravenous loading dose to give a therapeutic level of 5 mg/l is 10 mg/kg.[4,6,24,36,43,67-69,77] The maximum rate at which procainamide should be administered, however, is 50 to 100 mg given as an infusion over 5 minutes. This dose may be repeated every 5 minutes until the tachycardia is abolished or until a maximum dose of 1 gr has been given. However, in situations where VT is refractory to lidocaine, this dose rate can be cautiously exceeded. Careful monitoring of blood pressure for hypotension and the ECG are necessary. Maintenance intravenous administration at a dosage of 1 to 5 mg/min can be begun after the initial loading dose to prevent recurrent VT. It is apparent that, for the average 75 kg patient, it will take 35 minutes to administer the loading dose, clearly much too long for acute therapy of VT. It is the impression in most CCUs that ventricular arrhythmias responding to procainamide will respond to the initial 100 mg bolus. Therefore, when ventricular tachycardia resistant to lidocaine recurs, one can usually decide if procainamide is going to be effective after the first dose or after the first two doses. Occasionally, patients will require the full loading dose before a therapeutic response is seen. For initial therapy of ventricular tachycardia in patients with acute infarction who maintain an adequate blood pressure, we use electrical cardioversion if lidocaine or procainamide are not successful within about 5 minutes.

Diphenylhydantoin (Dilantin) has been found to be effective in digitalis toxicity.[70] For the emergency therapy of ventricular arrhythmias in acute infarction, only one clinical study has reported marginal success.[71] It seems unlikely that diphenylhydantoin will ever be an important agent for the treatment of ventricular arrhythmias in acute MI.

However, diphenylhydantoin may be tried when other agents have failed. The intravenous dosage should not exceed 50 mg/min during administration of a 500 to 600 mg loading dose. The total dose given during the first 24 hours is 1 g. Maintenance therapy requires 300 to 500 mg daily. Intravenous therapy may cause hypotension due to vasodilatation and diphenylhydantoin should not be given with dextrose in the infusion line.

## Treatment of Ventricular Tachycardia: Secondary Drug Therapy

Quinidine has marginal efficacy in the suppression of VPCs and VT in acute myocardial infarction.[75-76] Quinidine has not been widely used for the suppression of acute VT, largely because of administration problems. The oral route acts too slowly, and intramuscular quinidine requires large volumes and is painful. Recently, quinidine has been administered by slow intravenous infusion (experimentally) to five cardiac transplant recipients.[74] However, intravenous quinidine is a vasodilator resulting in reflex augmentation of sympathetic tone to the myocardium, and is a direct myocardial depressant of possibly significant magnitude.[75] Therefore, the use of intravenous quinidine is not currently accepted practice in coronary care units, but it may be tried under unusual circumstances when other approaches have failed. The dose used in the experimental study cited [74] was 10 mg/kg infused over a 20-minute period.

Bretylium tosylate is a second-line drug for treatment of ventricular fibrillation (see Ch. 31) and tachycardia.[76,77] A dosage of 5 mg/kg has been used with good results in patients with VT.[7,8,76-78,91] Bretylium tosylate may also be effective as prophylaxis for ventricular fibrillation in acute MI.[79] The usual dosage is 5 to 10 mg/kg given by intravenous infusion over 8 to 10 minutes for the treatment or suppression of ventricular tachycardia. Bretylium must be used with caution for several reasons. First, there is a release of catecholamines with the onset of adrenergic blockade (see Ch. 14), which leads to an increase in blood pressure and inotropic stimulation. Second, after adrenergic blockade, moderate or severe hypotension is a fairly constant finding, and postural hypotension is almost always present. Nausea and vomiting occur after rapid intravenous administration. Since catecholamine stimulation may be involved in digitalis-induced ventricular arrhythmias, it seems prudent to avoid using bretylium in patients receiving digitalis until more substantial data are available. In addition, the release of catecholamines is undesirable in the setting of acute MI.

Disopyramide may also be effective in the treatment of VPCs and ventricular tachycardia.[29,30,80,81] Disopyramide was administered in a double-blind placebo trial to patients with acute MI beginning at the time of arrival at the hospital and continuing for seven days.[122] Mortality and the presence of warning dysrhythmias were reduced in the disopyramide group. The reduced mortality was presumably due to prevention of primary ventricular fibrillation. The dosage used was 100 mg every 6 hours.

In patients with acute MI and ventricular tachycardia refractory to other agents, disopyramide has been effective in preventing recurrences.[123] Disopyramide is not approved for intravenous use in the U.S.A. The dosage used was 2 mg/kg infused over 8 min followed by mg/kg infused over 52 min. The maintenance infusion rate is then 20 to 40 mg/min.[123] Other side effects of disopyramide include nausea, vomiting, myocardial depression, and urinary retention due to its anticholinergic properties.

### Therapy of Ventricular Tachycardia: Overdrive

Occasionally, sinus bradycardia will be the atrial mechanism in patients with recurrent VT, and increasing the sinus rate with atropine or electrical pacing will suppress VT by overdrive. The shorter cycle length does not permit the ectopic or reentrant pathway to capture the ventricle. However, if the ventricular rate is slow (in the range of AIVR, see below), there is considerable debate over the necessity of any therapy. Paradoxically, an increased vagal tone produced by $\alpha$-adrenergic agonists[72] or edrophonium[73] has been reported to convert ventricular tachycardia to sinus rhythm.

In patients refractory to electrical cardioversion and pharmacologic therapy, overdrive atrial or ventricular pacing is the next treatment to try.

## PRECAUTIONS IN THE USE OF ANTIARRHYTHMIC AGENTS

Most antiarrhythmic agents depress ventricular performance—e.g., quinidine by direct myocardial depression,[75] propranolol or bretylium by adrenergic blockade.[78-79,92-93] However, the hemodynamic influence of ventricular arrhythmias and the risk of progression to ventricular fibrillation are usually more important than the depression of ventricular performance in the clinical situation. With quinidine and procainamide, depression of left ventricular performance has occurred primarily with intravenous administration. There is little evidence to suggest that oral therapy with these agents is associated with a significant reduction in left ventricular function except in the most marginal of circumstances. Thus, depending on the agent or agents required, one might elect not to suppress occasional VPCs in a patient with left ventricular failure. In fact, improvement of myocardial performance may improve pH and electrolyte disturbances or favorably alter the balance between myocardial oxygen demand and delivery and thus ameliorate the underlying pathologic mechanism of arrhythmia.

A second area of concern is the effect of these agents on atrioventricular conduction. During lidocaine infusion, impulse formation and atrioventricular node conduction are generally not affected, but there is a slight enhancement of AV nodal conduction in patients with supraventricular tachycardia.[82-83] However, lidocaine can lead to decremental intraventricular conduction, and peak blood levels after an intravenous bolus can cause transient heart block.[82-85] Therefore, in patients with impaired distal conduction such as new bundle branch block, or new bifascicular block, lidocaine should be infused with full cognizance of its potential adverse effects, and consideration should be given to the prophilactic insertion of a temporary transvenous pacemaker. In patients with complete heart block and ventricular escape rhythm, lidocaine should not be administered; in patients with both narrow QRS complexes (<.08 sec) and wide QRS complexes, lidocaine may induce exit block, causing sudden slowing of the ventricular rate.[86] Patients are also at risk for other clinical toxicity (Ch. 14).

Procainamide prolongs conduction time in the His-Purkinje system.[17-19,87-89] Several studies have not demonstrated progressive heart block even in patients with intraventricular conduction delay.[88,89] However, patients with acute ischemia have not been studied, and it would seem prudent to take the same precaution as is taken with lidocaine of prophylactic pacing in patients at high risk for complete heart block. Quinidine can also lead to progressive conduction block in the His-Purkinje system and should be used with stand-by ventricular pacing in patients with impaired distal AV conduction in the setting of acute MI. Both quinidine[75] and procainamide[67] are vasodilators and may cause hypotension. As indicated above, intravenous administration should be accompanied by careful monitoring of the blood pressure.

## USE OF PROPRANOLOL AS AN ANTIDYSRHYTHMIC AGENT

The use of propranolol in acute MI for therapy of excessive $\beta$-adrenergic discharge or recurrent chest pain, or for possible "infarct size" limitation, is discussed elsewhere. When used as an antiarrhythmic agent, propranolol may be effective by two mechanisms. One mechanism is by reduction in $\beta$-adrenergic stimulation to the myocardium. The second mechanism involves direct membrane effects (quinidine-like properties). In man, conventional doses of propranolol yield serum levels that are well below the concentration which produces membrane effects in vitro. Thus, with the possible exception of digitalis toxicity (which remains controversial) the antiarrhythmic effects of propranolol are mediated by $\beta$-adrenergic blockade.

The rationale for using $\beta$-adrenergic blockade for therapy of arrhythmias in acute myocardial infarction is based on increased $\beta$-sympathetic and adrenal discharge which occurs in some patients. The role of sympathetic tone in arrhythmias resulting from acute coronary occlusion has been summarized by Corr and Gillis.[115] Studies of sympathetic nerve traffic in animals indicate simultaneous increases and decreases in neural activity to different areas of the myocardium during acute ischemia. This may induce inhomogeneity in refractory periods and conduction velocity and predispose to reentrant dysrhythmias. Studies of circulating catecholamines in man have been inconclusive. It is also known that local hyperkalemia associated with acute ischemia sensitizes the myocardium to the arrhythmogenic action of $\beta$-adrenergic stimulation.[113]

In dogs, sympathectomy protects against ventricular arrhythmias associated with acute coronary occlusion.[114] However, primary VF in dogs is not prevented by stellate ganglionectomy. Nevertheless, depletion of endogenous catecholamines in the myocardium by chronic neural ablation does decrease the incidence of VF. These findings suggest that either asymmetric spinal reflexes or inhomogeneous $\beta$-sympathetic tone predispose to VF at least in dogs and provides a rationale for pharmacologic alterations of sympathetic tone as an antiarrhythmic therapy. $\beta$-adrenergic receptor blockade decreased the incidence of VF in dogs subjected to acute coronary occlusion in some studies[116,117] but failed in others.[118] In one study, practolol decreased the mortality of acute coronary occlusion in dogs, but propranolol did not; practolol does not have direct membrane effects, but propranolol does.[119] Therefore, the question of whether $\beta$-adrenergic blockade prevents primary ventricular fibrillation in man has no general answer at this time. It seems likely that intrinsic differences between $\beta$-adrenergic blocking agents will require that they be tested individually until further data are available.[115] Because there have been no definitive clinical trials, $\beta$-adrenergic blockade should not be used for prophylaxis against primary VF. The question of long-term post-MI antiarrhythmic therapy with $\beta$-blockade in order to prevent sudden death is discussed at the end of this chapter.

### Propranolol in the Therapy of Other Ventricular Dysrhythmias

Lemberg et al. reported successful suppression of recurrent ventricular tachycardia resistant to conventional antiarrhythmic agents in patients with acute MI.[112] The total dose used was 2 to 4.5 mg intravenously. We have used propranolol in patients with recurrent VT that is resistant to lidocaine and procainamide. A total dose of up to 0.1 mg/kg in increments of 0.5 to 1.0 mg intravenously may be given with monitoring of blood pressure and the ECG. Propranolol may be used as a first-line drug for ventricular arrhythmias in patients with clinical evidence of inappropriately high sympathetic tone only after determination of the pulmonary capillary wedge pressure to exclude congestive heart failure. (We feel that, until more clinical experience with the use of beta-adrenergic blockade in acute MI is available, monitoring of the pulmonary capillary wedge pressure is desirable in these patients). Signs of inappropriate sympathetic tone after pain has been relieved include sinus tachycardia in the absence of congestive left ventricular failure, diaphoresis, and hypertension. If continued therapy is necessary, oral propranolol 20 to 40 mg every 6 hours should be started immediately because of the short effective half-life of intravenous propranolol. $\beta$-adrenergic blockade should not be used when impaired atrioventricular conduction is present without a standby electronic pacemaker in place.

## REFRACTORY VENTRICULAR TACHYCARDIA

True "refractory" ventricular tachycardia implies that insufficient energy is being delivered to the myocardium by the direct current cardioverter. Following direct current cardioversion, a majority of the myocardium is depolarized simultaneously and, thus, VT or VF is interrupted. Immediate reappearance of VT or VF is really "recurrent." Causes of insufficient energy delivery include inadequate capacitor charge, poor paddle position, and poor paddle-skin electrical contact. These should be checked when electrical cardioversion is unsuccessful.

If recurrent ventricular tachycardia still proves to be the problem, the following should be checked: serum pH, arterial oxygen content, and plasma electrolyte levels. The period of asystole following DC cardioversion should be inspected to determine the initial escape rhythm. Atropine may be useful if the sinus mechanism is not the first to emerge. If a supraventricular rhythm is interrupted by ventricular tachycardia, administration of an antiarrhythmic agent prior to cardioversion is indicted (lidocaine, procainamide, bretylium, or disopyramide). If the initial escape rhythm following DC cardioversion is ventricular despite atropine and despite adequate antiarrhythmic therapy, ventricular pacing should be considered as a last resort to try to suppress the ventricular tachycardia by overdrive pacing.

## ACCELERATED IDIOVENTRICULAR RHYTHM

Accelerated idioventricular rhythm (AIVR) is defined as three or more ventricular com-

plexes in sequence at a rate faster than 60/min but less than ventricular tachycardia. AIVR is distinguished from parasystole by lack of entrance block—i.e., the ventricular focus is capable of being captured by an occasional supraventricular conducted impulses. AIVR is usually seen with relative sinus bradycardia, as the AIVR rate is often similar to the sinus rate and, thus, competition and fusion beats are common. AIVR can easily be overdriven by increasing the sinus rate; however, this is often not necessary.

Idioventricular rhythm (IVR) is analogous to AIVR, except that the rate is less than 60/min. IVR is usually seen only with complete heart block and infarction which usually is anterior.

Harris described AIVR in dogs after coronary artery ligation.[7] AIVR occurs when an enhanced idioventricular pacemaker rate competes with a relatively slow sinus rate.[8,23–25,90–92] The relationship of AIVR to sinus rhythm is analogous to that of an electronic demand ventricular pacemaker to sinus rhythm. The AIVR rate is usually constant. However, Castellanos et al. have described some acute MI patients in whom the rate was variable and exit block occurred.[8]

The experience of Norris and Mercer is that the AIVR rate is usually very close to the sinus rate and AIVR captures the ventricle during the slow phase of sinus arrhythmia.[93] The incidence of AIVR in acute MI is 9 to 23 percent.[90,93] AIVR is more commonly associated with inferior than with anterior infarction and generally has a benign prognosis.[9,93] Primary VF occurs in up to 12 percent of patients with AIVR, an incidence which is not significantly different from the incidence in all patients with acute infarction. Thus, the presence of AIVR is not associated with higher mortality or an increased incidence of VF.[90,92,93] However, Talbott and Greaves found an association of AIVR at rates between 75 and 100 per min with ventricular tachycardia.[9] They also noted that AIVR was irregular (greater than 10 percent variation in cycle length) in patients who later developed VT. DeSoyza et al. reprorted frequent VT in patients with accelerated idioventricular rhythm, defining AIVR as rates of up to 120/min in 52 patients.[10] However, their patient population did not demonstrate slow sinus rates with AIVR, nor strong association with inferior infarction. Thus, their series is not typical of other series in the literature. AIVR at slow rates in association with inferior infarction and sinus bradycardia is benign, and patients are not at increased risk to develop VT or VF. At "faster" rates (perhaps greater than 75/min), in the setting of acute anterior MI, or when the rate is variable, the prognosis is not benign and VT may ensue.[9,10]

Treatment of AIVR in the setting of inferior infarction and sinus bradycardia usually is not necessary. However, atropine should be used to accelerate the sinus rate in patients with symptomatic bradycardia associated with AIVR. In asymptomatic patients, we do not administer antiarrhythmic agents. Therapy is indicated when the rate approaches 100 per min or, in anterior infarction, when the rate is variable. Lidocaine is the drug of choice.

AIVR usually disappears within 24 hours. Talbott and Greaves noted that the incidence decreased from 35/224 in the first 24 hours to 9/192 in the second 24 hours after acute MI.[9]

## IDIOVENTRICULAR RHYTHM

Idioventricular rhythm (IVR) is defined as the presence of ventricular complexes at rates less than 60/min. It is almost exclusively seen in myocardial infarction associated with complete heart block. In inferior infarction, the conduction block is usually at the AV node and usually responds to atropine.[94] Only occasionally in our experience has ventricular pacing been required in inferior infarction. However, in anterior infarction, IVR is usually the escape rhythm when complete heart block ensues.[95-97] The indicated treatment is demand ventricular pacing (see Ch. 18). In this setting, it is generally not wise to suppress idioventricular rhythm and in fact, stimulation with isoproterenol is often necessary to maintain an adequate cardiac output while an electronic ventricular pacemaker is inserted.

## VENTRICULAR FIBRILLATION

The treatment of ventricular fibrillation is discussed in detail Chapter 31. Factors to consider when DC cardioversion is not successful are the same as with recurrent ventricular tachycardia. The important clue to the mechanism of recurrent ventricular fibrillation may be found by attention to the rhythm that emerges immediately after direct current countershock.

## PARASYSTOLE

Parasystole is an independent ectopic rhythm occurring alongside the native dominant pacemaker. The focus which initiates the parasystolic depolarization is protected: it is not depolarized by the native depolarization. The parasystolic focus usually demonstrates exit block, which is a variable multiple of its intrinsic rate. In the case of ventricular parasystole, this results in PVCs that are not coupled in a fixed fashion to accompanying "native" sinus or other beats, and occur at intervals which are multiples of the underlying parasystolic cycle length (Fig. 16.12).

Baxter et al. found an incidence of ventricular parasystole of 4 percent in patients with acute MI.[98] Ventricular parasystole was not associated with VT or VF. Parasystole is a benign rhythm in acute MI and may not be related to the acute infarction.

## VENTRICULAR ARRHYTHMIAS IN THE POST-CCU PHASE

Ventricular ectopy early in the course of acute MI (CCU) does not correlate with the occurrence of late arrhythmias.[99-103] The incidence of ventricular premature complexes in the late postinfarction setting is not markedly different than in asymptomatic subjects.[99,101,104] However, Moss et al. demonstrated an increased mortality in MI patients who have frequent ventricular premature complexes compared to similar individuals with infrequent

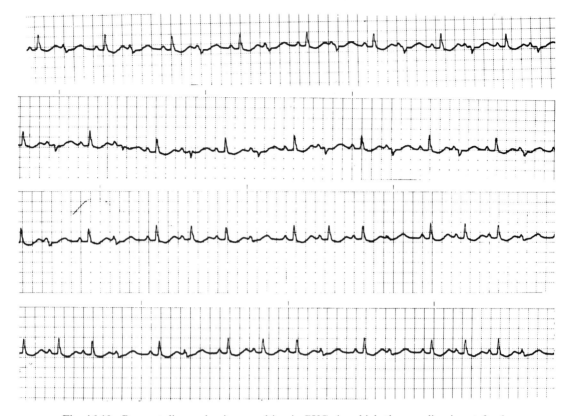

Fig. 16.12  Parasystolic mechanism resulting in PVCs in which the coupling is not fixed.

VPCs [100,105,106] studied 2 to 4 weeks after infarction. This might seem to offer a rationale for chronic antiarrhythmic prophylaxis. However, over 51 percent of patients exhibit VPCs in the two months after acute infarction.[99,100,101,103] Furthermore, those patients with frequent VPCs and ventricular tachycardia have markedly reduced ejection fractions.[102] Thus it is unclear whether VPCs in patients after acute infarction are associated with more severe myocardial damage, or if they represent electrical instabiliy and increased risk of sudden death from ventricular fibrillation or both.

Several small clinical trials of antiarrhythmic agents in patients several months to one year after acute infarction have been inconclusive due to small sample size.[107-109] The results of a multicenter double-blind trial of practolol administered for 12 to 36 months after MI in 3,038 patients are encouraging.[110] There was a significant decrease in overall death rate when practolol was compared to placebo, which appeared to be due entirely to the anterior infarction subgroup, and the mortality was due to sudden death (5 deaths in the treated subgroup compared to 18 in the corresponding control subgroup). The implication is that the antiarrhythmic effect was directly responsible for the reduced mortality. However, the large numbers of patients treated for such a small improvement in mortality is discouraging. Practolol is no longer used in patients because of ocular and other toxicity.

A multicenter (USA) trial of propranolol vs. placebo is currently underway in patients after MI. Until further information is available, there is no sound rationale for antiarrhythmic prophylaxis except in the first 48 hours after MI. One exception is the patient with ventricular tachycardia who, although asymptomatic, should be given antiarrhythmic treatment. In patients with infrequent, unifocal VPCs two or more weeks after acute infarction, we generally do not recommend arrhythmia prophylaxis if the patients are asymptomatic. However, the clinician should be alert to the results of ongoing trials.

Despite the lack of conclusive clinical trials, however, it is the practice in some hospitals to obtain ambulatory ECG recordings prior to hospital discharge and to modify, discontinue, or initiate antiarrhythmic therapy on the basis of the findings. Followup ambulatory recordings to assess the efficacy of therapy should be interpreted with due regard to the marked variability of VPC frequency.[111,112] Thus, for a 24-hour ECG recording, an 80 percent decrease in VPC count is necessary to assure drug effect at the 95 percent confidence level.[111,112] More complex methods of assessing the effectiveness of single and combination antiarrhythmic drug therapy, involving amubulatory monitoring and exercise testing, may be necessary in certain patients.

## REFERENCES

1. Marriott HJL, Sandler, JA: Criteria old and new for differentiating between extopic ventricular beats and aberrant ventricular conduction in the presence of atrial fibrillation. Prog in Cardiovasc Dis 9:18–28, 1966.
2. Sandler JA, Marriott HJL: The differential morphology of anomalous ventricular complexes of RBBB type in V1: Ventricular ectopy vs. aberration. Circ 31:551–555, 1965.
3. Romhilt DW, Bloomfield SS. Chou TC, Fowler NO: Unreliability of conventional electrocardiographic monitoring for arrhythmia detection in coronary care units. Am J Cardiol 31:457–461, 1973.
4. Shah, PM, Arnold JM, Haberern NA, Bliss DT, McClelland KM, Clarke WB: Automatic real time arrythmia monitoring in the intensive coronary care unit. Am J Cardiol 39:701–708, 1977.
5. Yanowitz F, Kinias P, Rawling D, Fozzard HA: Accuracy of a continuous real time ECG arrhythmia monitoring system. Circ 50:65–72, 1974.
6. Knoebel SB, Lovelace DE, Rasmussen S, Wash SE: Computer detection of premature ventricular complexes: A modified approach. Am J Cardiol 38:440–447, 1976.
7. Harris AS: Delayed development of ventricular ectopic rhythms following experimental coronary occlusion. Circ 1:1318–1328, 1950.
8. Castellanos A, Lemberg L, Arcebal AG: Mechanisms of slow ventricular tachycardias in acute myocardial infarction. Dis of the Chest 56:470–476, 1969.
9. Talbot S, Greaves M: Association of ventricular extrasystoles and ventricular tachycardia with idioventricular rhythm. Brit Heart J 38:457–464, 1976.
10. deSoyza N, Bissett JK, Kane JJ, Murphy ML, Doherty JE: Association of accelerated idioventricular rhythm and paroxysmal ventricular tachycardia in acute myocardial infarction. Am J Cardiol 34:667–670, 1974.
11. Bigger JT, Dresdale FJ, Heissenbuttel RH, Weld M. Wit AL: Ventricular arrhythmias in ischemic heart disease: Mechanism, prevalence, significance and management. Prog in Cardiovasc Dis 19:255–300, 1977.
12. Wyman MG, Hammersmith L: Comprehensive treatment plan for the prevention of primary ventricular fibrillation in acute myocardial infarction. Am J Cardiol 33:661–666, 1974.
13. Lown B, Sakhro AM, Hood WB: The coronary care unit. New perspectives and directions. J Am Med Assoc 199:188–198, 1967.
14. Lawrie DM, Higgins MR, Godman MJ, et al: Ventricular fibrillation complicating acute myocardial infarction. Lancet 2:523–528, 1968.
15. Julian DT, Valentine PA, Miller GG: Disturbances of rate, rhythm and conduction in acute myocardial infarction. A prospective study of 100 consecutive unselected patients with the aid of electrocardiographic monitoring. Am J Med 37:915–927, 1964.
16. Dhurandhar RW, MacMillan RL, Brown KWG: Primary ventricular fibrillation complicating acute myocardial infarction. Am J Cardiol 27:347–351, 1971.
17. Lie KI, Wellens HJJ, Downar E, Durrer D: Observations on patients with primary ventricular fibrillation complicating acute myocardial infarction. Circ 52:755–759, 1975.
18. Morgensen L: Ventricular tachyarrhythmias and lignocaine prophylaxis in acute myocardial infarction. Acta Med Scand 513:1–80, 1971.
19. Adgey AAJ, Allen JD, Geddes JS, et al: Acute phase of myocardial infarction. Lancet 2:501–504, 1971.
20. Killip T, Kimball JT: Treatment of myocardial infarction in a coronary care unit. Am J Cardiol 20:457–464, 1967.

21. Goble AJ, Sloman G, Robinson JS: Mortality reduction in a coronary care unit. Brit Med J 1:1005–1009, 1966.

22. DeSoyza M, Bissett JK, Kane JJ, Murphy ML, Doherty JE: Ectopic ventricular prematurity and its relationship to ventricular tachycardia in acute myocardial infarction in man. Circ 50:529–532, 1974.

23. Gianelly R, VonderGroeben JO, Spivack AP, Harrison DC: Effect of lidocaine on ventricular arrhythmias in patients with coronary artery disease. N Eng J Med 277:1215–1219, 1967.

24. Koch-Weser J, Klein SW, Foo-Canto LL, Kastor JA, DeSanctis RW: Antiarrhythmic prophylaxis with procainamide in acute myocardial infarction. N Eng J Med 281:1253–1260, 1969.

25. Bloomfield SS, Romhilt DW, Chou TC, et al: Quinidine for prophylaxis of arrhythmias in acute myocardial infarction. N Eng J Med 285:979–986, 1971.

26. Jones DT, Kostuk WJ, Gunton RW: Prophylactic quinidine for the prevention of arrhythmias after acute myocardial infarction. Am J Cardiol 33:655–660, 1974.

27. Lie KI, Wellens HJ, VanCapelle FJ, Durrer D: Lidocaine in the prevention of primary ventricular fibrillation. N Eng J Med 292:1324–1326, 1974.

28. Valentine PA, Frew JL, Mashford ML, Sloman JG: Lidocaine in the prevention of sudden deaths in the prehospital phase of acute infarction. N Eng J Med 291:1327–1330, 1974.

29. Singh JB, Kocot SL: A controlled trial of intramuscular lidocaine in the prevention of premature ventricular contractions associated with acute myocardial infarction. Am Heart J 91:430–436, 1976.

30. Noneman JW, Rogers JF: Lidocaine prophylaxis in acute myocardial infarction. Medicine 57:501–516, 1978.

31. Harrison DC: Should lidocaine be administered routinely to all patients after acute myocardial infarction? Circ 58:581–584, 1978.

32. Borer JS, Harrison LA, Kent KM, Levy R, Goldstein RE, Epstein SE: Beneficial effect of lidocaine on ventricular electrical stability and spontaneous ventricular fibrillation during experiment myocardial infarction. Am J Cardiol 37:860–864, 1976.

33. Lown B, Klein MD, Hirshberg PI: Coronary and pre-coronary care. Am J Med 46:705–724, 1969.

34. Thompson P, Sloman G: Sudden death in hospital after discharge from coronary care unit. Brit Med J 4:136–139, 1971.

35. Graboys TB: In hospital sudden death after coronary care unit discharge. A high risk profile. Archives of Int Med 135:512–514, 1975.

36. Bigger JT Jr, Heissenbuttel RH: The use of procainamide and lidocaine in the treatment of cardiac arrhythmias. Prog Cardiovasc Dis 11:515–533, 1969.

37. Jewitt DE, Kishon Y, Thomas M: Lignocaine in the management of arrhythmias after acute myocardial infarction. Lancet 1:266–270, 1968.

38. Chopra MP, Thadani U, Portal RW, et al: Lignocaine therapy for ventricular ectopic activity after acute myocardial infarction: A double-blind trial. Brit Med J 3:668–670, 1972.

39. Bennett MA, Wilner JM, Pentecost BL: Controlled trial of lignocaine in prophylaxis of ventricular arrhythmias complicating acute myocardial infarction. Lancet 2:909–911, 1970.

40. Bleifeld, W, Merx W, Heinrich KW, et al: Controlled trial of prophylactic treatment with lidocaine in acute myocardial infarction. Eur J Clinical Pharm 6:119–126, 1973.

41. Pitt A, Lipp H, Anderson ST: Lignocaine given prophylactically to patients with acute myocardial infarction. Lancet 1:612–616, 1971.

42. Wyman MG, Lalka D, Hammersmith L, Cannom DS, Goldreyer BN: Multiple bolus technique for lidocaine administration during the first hours of acute myocardial infarction. Am J Cardiol 41:313–316, 1978.

43. Collinsworth KA, Kalman SM, Harrison DC: The clinical pharmacology of lidocaine as an anti-arrhythmic drug. Circ 50:1217–1230, 1974.

44. Thompson PD, Melmon KL, Richardson JA, Cohn K, Steinbrunn W, Cudihee R, Rowland M: Lidocaine pharmacokinetics in advanced heart failure, liver disease and renal failure in humans. Annals Int Med 78:499–508, 1973.

45. Lie KI, Liem KL, Louridtz WJ: Janse MJ, Willebrands AF, Durrer D: Efficacy of lidocaine in preventing primary ventricular fibrillation within 1 hour after a 300 mg intramuscular injection. Am J Cardiol 42:486–488, 1978.

46. Zener JC, Kerbert RE, Spivack AP, Harrison DC: Blood lidocaine levels and kinetics following high dose intramuscular administration. Circ 47:984–988, 1973.

47. O'Brien KP, Taylor PM, Croxson RS: Prophylactic lignocaine in hospitalized patients with acute myocardial infarction. Med J Aust 2 (suppl):36–37, 1973.

48. Stenson RE, Constantino RT, Harrison DC:

The interrelationships of hepatic blood flow, cardiac output and blood levels of lidocaine in man. Circulation 43:205–211, 1971.

49. Pfeifer HJ, Greenblatt DJ, Koch-Weser J: Clinical use and toxicity of intravenous lidocaine. Am Heart J 92:168–173, 1976.

50. Harrison LA, Harrison LH, Kent KM, Epstein SE: Enhancement of electrical stability of acutely ischemic myocardium by edrophonium. Circ 50:99–102, 1974.

51. Kent KM, Smith ER, Redwood DR, Epstein SE: Electrical stability of acutely ischemic myocardium. Circulation 47:291–298, 1973.

52. Corr PB, Gillis RA: Role of the vagus nerves in the cardiovascular changes induced by coronary occlusion. Circulation 49:86–97, 1974.

53. Myers RW, Pearlman AS, Hyman RM, Goldstein RA, Kent KM, Goldstein RE, Epstein SE: Beneficial effects of vagal stimulation and bradycardia during experimental acute myocardial infarction. Circ 49:943–947, 1974.

54. Yoon MS, Han JC, Tse WW, Rogers R: Effects of vagal stimulation, atropine and propranolol on fibrillation threshold of normal and ischemic ventricles. Am Heart J 93:60–65, 1977.

55. Goldstein RE, Karsh, RB, Smith, ER, Orlando M, Norman D, Farnham G, Redwood DR, Epstein SE: Influence of atropine and of vagally mediated bradycardia on the occurrence of ventricular arrhythmias following acute coronary occlusion in closed chest dogs. Circ 47:1180–1190, 1973.

56. Kolman, BS, Verrier RL, Lown B: The effect of vagus nerve stimulation on vulnerability of the canine ventricle. Circ 52:578–584, 1975.

57. James RGG, Arnold JMO, Allen JD, Pantridge JF, Shanks RG: The effects of heart rate, myocardial ischemia, and vagal stimulation on the threshold for ventricular fibrillation. Circ 55:311–317, 1977.

58. Kerzner J, Wolf M, Kosowsky BD, Lown B: Ventricular ectopic rhythms following vagal stimulation in dogs with acute myocardial infarction. Circ 47:44–50, 1973.

59. Grauer LE, Gershen BJ, Orlando MM, Epstein SE: Bradycardia and its complications in the pre-hospital phase of acute myocardial infarction. Am J Cardiol 32:607–611, 1973.

60. Warren JV, Lewis RP: Beneficial effects of atropine in the pre-hospital phase of coronary care. Am J Cardiol 37:68–72, 1976.

61. Scheinman, MM, Thorburn D, Abbott JA: Use of atropine in patients with acute myocardial infarction and bradycardia. Circ 52:627–632, 1975.

62. Lister JW, Delman AJ, Stein E, Grunwald R, Robinson G: Dominant pacemaker of human heart: Antegrade and retrograde activation of the heart. Circulation 35:22–31, 1967.

63. Rosen KM: Junctional tachycardia. Circulation 47:654–664, 1973.

64. Wellens HJ, Bar FW, Lie KI: The value of the electrocardiogram in the differential diagnosis of a tachycardia with a widened QRS complex. Am J Med 64:27–33, 1978.

65. Lown B, Temte JV, Arter WJ: Ventricular tachyarrhythmias. Circ 47:1364–1380, 1973.

66. Schamroth L: How to approach an arrhythmia. Circ 47:420–426, 1973.

67. Cote P, Harrison DC, Basile J, Schroeder JS: Hemodynamic interaction of procainamide and lidocaine after experimental myocardial infarction. Am J Cardiol 32:937–942, 1973.

68. Giardina EGV, Heissenbuttel RH, Bigger JT: Intermittent intravenous procainamide to treat ventricular arrhythmias. Ann Int Med 78:183–193, 1973.

69. Lima JJ, Goldfarb AJ, Conti RD, Golden LH, Bascomb BL, Benedetti GM, Jusko WJ: Safety and efficacy of procainamide infusions. Am J Cardiol 43:98–105, 1979.

70. Mercer EN, Osborne JA: The current status of diphenylhydantoin in heart disease. Ann of Int Med 67:1084–1107, 1967.

71. Bashour FA, Jones RE, Edmundson R: Ventricular tachycardia in acute myocardial infarction. Preliminary report on the prophylactic use of Dilantin. Clin Res 13:399, 1966.

72. Waxman MB, Downar E, Berman ND, Felderhof CH: Phenylephrine (neosynephrine) terminated ventricular tachycardia. Circ 50:656–663, 1974.

73. Waxman MB, Wald RW: Termination of ventricular tachycardia by an increase in cardiac vagal drive. Circ 56:385–390, 1977.

74. Mason JW, Winkle RA, Ingles MB, Daughters GT, Harrison DC, Stinson EB: Hemodynamic effects of intravenously administered quinidine on the transplanted human heart. Am J Cardiol 40:99–104, 1977.

75. Engler RL, LeWinter MM, Karliner JS: Depressant effects of quinidine gluconate on left ventricular function in conscious dogs with and without volume overload. Circ 60:828–835, 1979.

76. Bacaner MB: Quanitative comparison of bretylium with other antifibrillatory drugs. Am J Cardiol 21:504, 1968.

77. Bacaner MB: Treatment of ventricular fibrillation and other acute arrhythmias with bre-

tylium tosylate. Am J Cardiol 21:530–543, 1968.

78. Bernstein JG, Koch-Weser J: Effectiveness of bretylium tosylate against refractory ventricular arrhythmias. Circ 45:1024–1034, 1972.

79. Taylor SH, Saxton C, Davies PS, et al: Bretylium tosylate in prevention of cardiac dysrhythmia after myocardial infarction. Brit Heart J 32:326–329, 1970.

80. Vismara LA, Vera Z, Miller RR, Mason DT: Efficacy of disopyramide phosphate in the treatment of refractory ventricular tachycardia. Am J Cardiol 39:1027–1034, 1977.

81. Befeler B, Castellanos A, Wells DE, Vagueiro MC, Yeh BK: Electrophysiologic effects of the antiarrhythmic agent disopyramide phosphate. Am J Cardiol 35:282–287, 1975.

82. Roos JC, Dunning AJ: Effects of lidocaine on impulse formation and conduction defects in man. Am Heart J 89:686–699, 1975.

83. Kunkel F, Rowland M, Scheinman MM: The electrophysiologic effects of lidocaine in patients with intraventricular conduction defects. Circ 49:894–899, 1974.

84. Gupta PK, Lichstein E, Chadda KD: Lidocaine-induced heart block in patients with bundle branch blocks. Am J Cardiol 33:487–492, 1974.

85. Gerstenblith G, Scherlag BJ, Hope RR, Lazzara R: Effects of lidocaine on conduction in the ischemic His-Purkinje system of dogs. Am J Cardiol 42:587–591, 1978.

86. Aravindakshan V, Kuo C, Gettes LS: Effect of lidocaine on escape rate in patients with complete atrioventricular block. Am J Cardiol 40:177–182, 1977.

87. Ogunkelu JB, Damato AN, Akhtar M, Reddy CP, Caracta AR, Lau SH: Electrophysiologic effects of procainamide in subtherapeutic to therapeutic doses on human atrioventricular conduction system. Am J Cardiol 37:724–731, 1976.

88. Scheinman MM, Weiss AN, Shafton E, et al: Electrophysiologic effects of procainamide in patients with intraventricular conduction delay. Circ 49:522–528, 1974.

89. Josephson ME, Caracta AR, Ricciutti MA, et al: Electrophysiologic properties of procainamide in man. Am J Cardiol 33:596–603, 1974.

90. Rothfeld EL, Zucker IR, Leff WA, Parsonnet V: Idioventricular rhythm in acute myocardial infarction. Circ 42:111–193, 1970.

91. Rothfeld, EL, Zucker IR, Parsonnet V, et al: Idioventricular rhythm in acute myocardial infarction. Circulation 37:203–209, 1968.

92. Schamroth L: Idioventricular tachycardia. J Electrocardiology 1:205–212, 1968.

93. Norris RM, Mercer CJ: Significance of idioventricular rhythms in acute myocardial infarction. Prog in Cardiovasc Dis 16:455–468, 1974.

94. Zipes DP: The clinical significance of bradycardic rhythms in acute myocardial infarction. Am J Cardiol 24:814–826, 1969.

95. Norris RM: Heart block in posterior and anterior myocardial infarction. Brit Heart J 31:352–356, 1969.

96. Kimball JT, Killip T: Aggressive treatment of arrhythmias in acute myocardial infarction: Proceedures and results. Prog Cardiovasc Dis 10:483–503, 1968.

97. Norris RM, Mercer CJ: Significance of idioventricular rhythms in acute myocardial infarction. Prog Cardiovasc Dis 16:455–468, 1974.

98. Baxter RH, McGuinnes JB: Comparison of ventricular parasystole with other dysrhythmias after acute myocardial infarction. Am Heart J 88:443–448, 1974.

99. Wenger TL, Bigger JL Jr, Merrill GS: Ventricular arrhythmias in the late hospital phase of acute myocardial infarction. Circulation 51–52 (suppl)2:110, 1975.

100. Moss AJ, Schnitzler R, Green R, et al: Ventricular arrhythmias three weeks after acute myocardial infarction. Ann of Int Med 75:837–941, 1971.

101. deSoyza N, Kane JJ, Bissett JK, et al: Correlation of ventricular arrhythmias during acute and late phase of myocardial infarction. Circ 49–50 (suppl III):223, 1974.

102. Schulze RA, Roleau J, Rigo P, et al: Ventricular arrhythmias in the late hospital phase of acute myocardial infarction: Relation to left ventricular function detected by gated cardiac blood pool scanning. Circ 52:1006–1011, 1975.

103. Vismara LA, Amsterdam EA, Mason DT: Relation of ventricular arrhythmias in the late hospital phase of acute myocardial infarction to sudden death after hospital discharge. Am J Med 59:6–12, 1975.

104. Hinkle LE, Carver ST, Stevens M: The frequency of asymptomatic disturbances of cardiac rhythm and conduction in middle aged men. Am J Cardiol: 24:629–650, 1969.

105. Moss AJ, DeCamilla JJ, Davis HP, Boyer L: Clinical significance of ventricular ectopic beats in the early post-hospital phase of myocardial infarction. Am J Cardiol 39:635–640, 1977.

106. Moss AJ, DeCamilla JJ, Mietlowski W, et al: Prognostic grading and significance of ventricular premature beats after recovery from myo-

cardial infarction. Circ (suppl III) 51:204–210, 1975.

107. Collaborative Group. Phenytoin after recovery from myocardial infarction, controlled trial in 568 patients. Lancet 2:1055–1057, 1971.

108. Kosowsky BD, Taylor J, Lown B, et al: Long-term use of procainamide following acute myocardial infarction. Circ 47:1204–1210, 1973.

109. Wilhelmsson C, Vedin JA, Wilhelmsen L, et al: Reduction of sudden death after myocardial infarction by treatment with alprenolol. Lancet 2:1157–1160, 1974.

110. Improvement in prognosis of myocardial infarction by long-term beta-adrenergic receptor blockade using practolol. A multicenter internation study. Brit Med J 3:735–740, 1975.

111. Morganroth J, Michelson EL, Horowitz LN, Josephson ME, Pearlman AS, Dunkman WB: Limitations of routine long term abulatory electrocardiographic monitoring to assess ectopic frequency. Circ 58:408–414, 1978.

112. Engler RL, Ryan W, LeWinter M, Bluestein H, Karliner JS: Assessment of long term antiarrhythmic therapy: Studies on the long term efficacy and toxicity of tocainide. Am J Cardiol 43:612–618, 1979.

113. Wit AL, Hoffman BF, Rosen MR: Electrophysiology and pharmacology of cardiac arrhythmias IX. Cardiac Electrophysiologic effects of beta-adrenergic receptor stimulation and blockade. Am Heart J 90:795–803, 1975.

114. Schaal AF, Wallace AG, Sealy WC: Protective influence of cardiac denervation against arrhythmias of myocardial infarction. Cardiovasc Res 3:241–244, 1969.

115. Corr PB, Gillis RA: Autonomic neuro-influ-

ences on the dysrrhythmias resulting from myocardial infarction. Circ Res 43:2–9, 1978.

116. Fearon RE: Propranolol in the prevention of ventricular fibrillation due to experimental coronary occlusion. Am J Cardiol 20:222–228, 1967.

117. Pentecost BL, Austen WG: Beta-adrenergic blockade in experimental myocardial infarction. Am Heart J 72:790–796, 1966.

118. Khan MI, Hamilton JT, Manning GW: Early arrhythmias following experimental coronary occlusion in conscious dogs and their modification by beta-adrenoreceptor blocking drugs. Am Heart J 86:347–358, 1973.

119. Pearle DL, Williford D, Gillis RA: Superiority of practolol versus propranolol in protection against ventricular fibrillation induced by coronary occlusion Am J Card 42:960–964, 1978.

120. Skinner JE, Lie JT, Entman ML: Modification of ventricular fibrillation latency following coronary artery occlusion in the conscious pig. Circ 51:656–657, 1975.

121. Lemberg L, Castellanos A, Arcebal AG: The use of propranolol in arrhythmias complicating acute myocardial infarction. Am Heart J 80:479–487, 1970.

122. Zainal N, Carmichael DJS, Griffiths JW, Besterman EMM, Kidner PH, Gillham AD, Summers GD: Oral disopyramide for the prevention of arrhythmias in patients with acute myocardial infarction admitted to open wards. Lancet 2:887–889, 1977.

123. Vismara LA, Vera Z, Miller RR, Mason DT: Efficacy of disopyramide phosphate in the treatment of refractory ventricular tachycardia. Am J Cardiol 39:1027–1034, 1977.

# 17 | *The Use of the Defibrillator*

## *L. A. Geddes, M.E., Ph.D.*

A cardiac defibrillator may be defined as an electrical device that stores energy in a capacitor and delivers this energy to the heart as a short-duration pulse of current. In this role, the defibrillator sees three different types of service; each is associated with different shock strengths and different degrees of urgency. First, the defibrillator is used in cardiac surgery when the ventricles are often intentionally fibrillated to obtain a tranquil operating field. In this situation, the patient's circulation is supported by cardiopulmonary bypass. For this reason, ventricular defibrillation can be accomplished when the surgeon desires by placing electrodes across the ventricles and delivering the shock. This type of defibrillation requires the least shock strength, expressed in joules or watt-seconds. Typically, 5 to 10 joules of damped sine wave current are used to defibrillate the adult human heart.

The second use for the defibrillator is to arrest ventricular fibrillation in the closed-chest subject. This situation is one of circulatory collapse and constitues an emergency of the highest order. Cardiopulmonary resuscitation must be applied immediately, and defibrillation must be achieved as soon as possible. Electrodes are placed on the chest, and a relatively strong shock is delivered to achieve defibrillation. In the adult subject, typically a 200 to 350-joule shock is delivered from a damped sine wave defibrillator.

Termination of tachyarrhythmias, other than ventricular fibrillation, is the third use for the defibrillator. The urgency for correcting the dysrhythmia is related to the cardiac chamber (atria or ventricles) and the severity of the dysrhythmia. In this situation, thoracic electrodes are used, and often the procedure can be scheduled—except in the coronary-care unit, where such dysrhythmias often progress to an emergency situation of severe circulatory impairment or collapse. Ventricular tachycardia can be terminated with a low-energy shock, as can atrial dysrhythmias. Atrial defibrillation requires a shock strength much less than for ventricular defibrillation, but above that required to terminate ventricular tachyarrhythmias.

In using a defibrillator to terminate tachyarrhythmias, two techniques are used: synchronized and unsynchronized. Delivery of the shock so that it does not fall in the vulnerable period of the ventricles, which occurs during the T wave of the ECG, is called synchronized countershock. If the shock is delivered randomly, there is the risk of precipitating ventricular fibrillation. Synchronization requires providing the defibrillator with an ECG signal, which may be obtained either from a separate pair of electrodes or directly from the defibrillating electrodes. A delay circuit in the defibrillator causes delivery of the shock late in the QRS complex when the ventricles are refractory to electrical stimulation.

Before presenting the requirements for terminating the various cardiac dysrhythmias, it is

391

important to understand how the strength of a shock is specified. In all defibrillators, the shock strength is expressed in joules (J) or watt-seconds, which are units of energy. The dial on a defibrillator identifies the energy that will be delivered into a 50-ohm test resistor. Older defibrillators have output controls calibrated in terms of stored energy, which is more than is delivered because of internal resistance in the defibrillator. Modern defibrillators deliver between 75 and 95 percent of the stored energy.

In clinical practice, the delivered energy is rarely known because it depends on the resistance of the subject. With transventricular electrodes, the resistance ranges from 15 to about 50 ohms. With precordial electrodes, the resistance varies between 25 and 125 ohms.[1]

Notwithstanding these facts, the output control, calibrated in joules, is what is used to select the shock strength. Most damped sine wave defibrillators indicate a maximum of 400 J.

Low-tilt trapezoidal (square) wave defibrillators provide 250 J. A commercially available, high-tilt, trapezoidal-wave defibrillator provides 400 J. With some of these defibrillators, an override control will allow the defibrillator to provide a higher output.

## CHARACTERISTICS OF VENTRICULAR FIBRILLATION

Prior to discussing ventricular defibrillation, it is of value to have a clear understanding of its true significance. Ventricular fibrillation can be defined as a condition in which all of the fibers of the ventricles are contracting and relaxing randomly, the net result being a loss of the pumping action and therefore a precipitous fall in blood pressure and consequently circulatory arrest. Electrophysiologically, the R and T waves of the electrocardiogram are replaced by

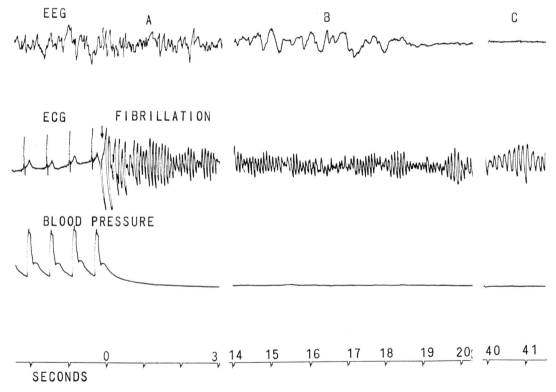

Fig. 17.1  The electroencephalogram (EEG), electrocardiogram (ECG), and femoral artery blood pressure of a dog prior to, during, and following the induction of ventricular fibrillation by direct-heart stimulation. Note that with about 19 seconds of circulatory arrest the EEG became isoelectric. (Br J Clin Eqpt 2:13–18, 1977.)

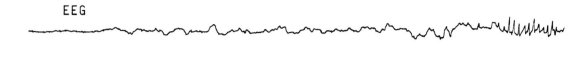

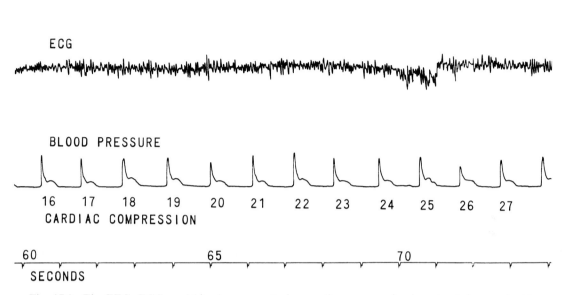

Fig. 17.2   The EEG, ECG, and blood pressure during cardiac compression in a dog being respired by intermittent positive-pressure respiration. Note that with about 25 cardiac compressions the EEG was restored. (Br J Clin Eqpt 2:13–18, 1977.)

a high-frequency, spindling type of activity. Unless circulatory support is provided within a few minutes, irreversible changes start to take place in the brain, heart, and other organs. In addition, it is generally found that the myocardial hypoxia, resulting from circulatory arrest, makes the ventricles more difficult to defibrillate. Moreover, when defibrillated, hypoxic ventricles are very slow to resume their normal pumping.

In ventricular fibrillation, the enemy is time. Just how rapidly the situation deteriorates without circulatory support is demonstrated by Figure 17.1, which illustrates the electroencephalogram (EEG), electrocardiogram (ECG), and femoral artery blood pressure of an anesthetized dog. The chest was open and the animal was supported by intermittent positive-pressure respiration. At the arrow on the record, 60-Hz current was applied to the ventricles, producing a rapid tachycardia that progressed to ventricular fibrillation. Note the immediate fall in blood pressure. After about 20 seconds of untreated

fibrillation, the EEG has become isoelectric, indicating that the cortex has become hypoxic. At this point, rhythmic cardiac compression was applied, as shown in Figure 17.2. Note that after about 25 compressions the EEG returned, indicating the effectiveness of the cardiac compression in perfusing the cortex with oxygenated blood.

The route to restoration of ventricular pumping is via cardiac standstill. The fibrillatory process must be abolished by rendering all of the excitable cells refractory and by prolongation of the refractory period of those cells that are excited. The only safe and effective method of attaining this goal is by the passage of a pulse of electric current (of adequate strength) through the ventricles. In Figure 17.3, electrodes were placed across the ventricles, and a pulse of defibrillating current (5 J) was delivered. Following the shock, there was a brief period of asystole, after which sinus rhythm and ventricular pumping resumed.

Thus, the two cardinal signs of ventricular

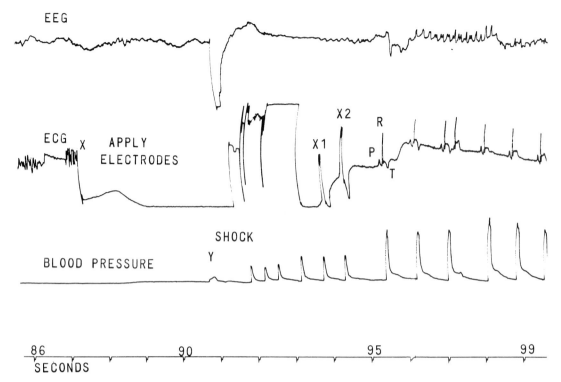

Fig. 17.3 Electrical ventricular defibrillation. The shock was delivered as indicated and the ventricles started beating while the EEG and ECG amplifiers were blocked. The first few ECG complexes (X1,2) indicated ectopic beats, following which sinus rhythm was restored. (Br J Clin Eqpt 2:13–18, 1977.)

fibrillation are a loss of the pulsatile pumping of the ventricles and replacement of the R and T waves of the ECG by high-frequency random (fibrillation) waves. Ventricular defibrillation rarely occurs spontaneously in warm-blooded animals larger than the rat, cat, rabbit, and monkey. Therefore, restoration of the circulation by cardiopulmonary resuscitation (CPR) is mandatory, unless defibrillation can be effected within minutes of its onset.

## HISTORICAL BACKGROUND

The fact that the ventricles could be thrown into a state of fibrillation has been known since 1850, when Hoffa and Ludwig[2] precipitated fibrillation in the dog heart by direct repetitive (faradic) stimulation. The loss of blood pressure indicated that all ventricular pumping had ceased. Direct observation of the ventricles revealed that they were far from quiescent; all ventricular fibers were contracting and relaxing

independently and had a shimmering appearance. Ludwig and Hoffa were impressed with the fact that the ventricles were dilated and full of blood.

A few years earlier in 1842, Ericksen[3] had unknowingly produced fibrillation in the dog heart by ligating the coronary arteries. In each animal, he carefully observed the result. Ericksen wrote: "At twenty one minutes (after ligation) the (pumping) action of the ventricles had ceased, with the exception of a slight tremulous motion." The nature of this tremulous motion was, of course, not known at that time. The terms used then to describe what we now know as ventricular fibrillation were mouvement fibrillaire, fibrillary motion, and tremulous motion. Fibrillation in the atria was called delirium cordis. At that time, the electrophysiological consequences were not known because the electrical activity of the heart had not been recorded.

Ventricular defibrillation was not achieved for almost one-half century and was discovered only tangentially. At the dawn of the twentieth century, there was considerable interest in determining whether direct or alternating current would be the safest for electric power distribution. Studies of the effect of each type of current on the heart were conducted in 1899 by Prevost and Battelli in Switzerland.[4,5,6] In these papers, which lay dormant for three decades, they reported that low-intensity alternating and direct current could cause fibrillation; higher intensity current of both types arrested ventricular fibrillation when applied directly to dog hearts. It may have been that because their papers were in the French language, their message was not received by those studying methods for arresting fibrillation.

The first concerted research on ventricular defibrillation started in 1930. At that time, Hooker et al.[7,8] and Wiggers et al.[9] reported that perfusion of the canine coronary arteries with potassium chloride solution would arrest ventricular fibrillation. If followed by a perfusate of calcium chloride, contractile force was restored rapidly. Thus, the chemical method of ventricular defibrillation was born. This method was employed experimentally for a few years; its use required left-ventricular injection, cross-clamping of the aorta, and rhythmic cardiac compression to flush the intracardiac solutions through the coronary arteries.

In 1933, just as the chemical defibrillation technique was being perfected, Hooker et al. discovered the Prevost and Battelli papers. Immediately, Hooker and Kouwenhoven set themselves the task of determining the feasibility of achieving ventricular defibrillation with 60-Hz domestic power-line current (Figure 17.4). Hooker et al.[10] and Kouwenhoven et al.[11] reported the successful defibrillation of dog hearts using 60-Hz applied to transventricular electrodes. The first human heart to be defibrillated electrically was reported in 1947 by Beck et al.,[12] who applied 120 volts from the 60-Hz power line to transventricular electrodes for a fraction of a second. Successful closed-chest defibrillation in man was reported in 1956 by Zoll et al.,[13] who used up to 720 volts of 60-Hz current applied to precordial electrodes for a fraction of a second.

Despite its life-saving value, the 60-Hz defi-

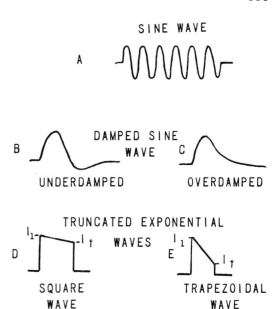

Fig. 17.4  Current waveforms used for cardiac defibrillation.

brillator had many defects; it was bulky, heavy, and drew an extremely high current from the power line. To achieve defibrillation, 6 to 12 cycles of 60 Hz were delivered. In addition, atrial fibrillation was sometimes a complication. Finally, the shock hazard to the operator was not negligible. Notwithstanding, use of the 60-Hz defibrillator was the therapy of choice for ventricular fibrillation. Such defibrillators are in use in only a few hospitals today and they are being replaced by single-pulse defibrillators.

The modern era of defibrillation had its beginnings long before its clinical application. Gurvich and Yuniev[14] in Russia had shown that defibrillation could be achieved in animals by a single pulse of current delivered to transchest electrodes from a charged capacitor. In the following year, Gurvich and Yuniev[15] found that, by placing an inductor in series with the capacitor and transthoracic electrodes, the duration of the current pulse was prolonged and defibrillation could be achieved with less current. Thus, the DC or damped sine wave defibrillator was born. (Fig. 17.4B, C illustrates the damped sine wave.) Again, this discovery was relatively unnoticed. Mackay and Leeds[16] verified the study by Gurvich and Yuniev, and the discovery became available to the English-speaking world. The study by MacKay and

Leeds recommended that energy be used as a measure of shock strength required for defibrillation; this measure is still in use.

The first successful defibrillations of human hearts with damped sine wave current were reported by Lown et al.[17,18] and Edmark et al.[19,20] Lown et al. used thoracic electrodes to terminate atrial fibrillation, and Edmark et al. used transventricular electrodes to terminate ventricular fibrillation. From the mid-1960s, damped sine wave defibrillation has been in clinical use. Sometimes this waveform is called the Gurvich-Lown-Edmark waveform, in recognition of the research carried out to establish its efficacy.

More recently, Schuder et al.[21] reported that square and trapezoidal waveforms are effective in defibrillating dog hearts; Figures 17.4D,E illustrate these waveforms. Soon, such defibrillators providing these waveforms were scaled up in size to permit defibrillation of human hearts with precordial electrodes.

As it stands now, there are really only two waveforms used for defibrillation: the damped sine wave, and the trapezoidal wave. The damped sine wave may be underdamped (Fig. 17.4B) or overdamped (Fig. 17.4C). The trapezoidal wave may be nearly square (Fig. 17.4D), or 'the current may decrease considerably during the pulse (Fig. 17.4E). Tilt is a term used to describe the percent decrease in current during the pulse. A square wave is really a low-tilt trapezoidal wave.

In this chapter the energy levels required to achieve defibrillation with the damped sine and trapezoidal waveforms will be presented. It will be seen that the various waveforms have different efficacies—i.e., different energy levels are required for defibrillation. As yet, there has been no study designed to identify which waveform achieves defibrillation and leaves the ventricles with the maximum ability to contract and pump blood.

## FIBRILLATION: THEORETICAL CONSIDERATIONS

Several overlapping theories have been proposed to account for fibrillation. One theory states that fibrillation results from "circus motion" or reentrant excitation; another holds that it originates from multiple ectopic pacemakers. Although different mainly in the genesis of fibrillation, both theories admit that, in fibrillation, excitation travels randomly and incessantly through excitable myocardium. It will not be the objective of the following discussion to uphold either theory; instead, each will be presented to illustrate that there are two possible mechanisms for precipitating fibrillation. Evidence can be adduced to uphold both theories.

The circus-motion theory was proposed and verified by Mines[22] (1913) and Garrey (1914).[23] The specimen that both used was a ring of cardiac muscle. The former made the ring from excised ray-fish atrium; the latter used turtle ventricle. Figure 17.5 illustrates an idealized ring of cardiac muscle. Suppose that a single stimulus is delivered, as shown in Figure 17.5A. Excitation will travel up both sides of the ring, as shown in Figure 17.5B, followed by a tail of recovering tissue. The two waves of excitation will ultimately run into each other's refractory period and be extinguished at the top of the ring, as shown in Figure 17.5C.

Now, suppose the ring of tissue is not uniform in its ability to recover. For example, in Figure 17.6A, suppose that the left side of the ring is slower to recover than the right side. A single stimulus delivered, as in Figure 17.6A, will cause excitation to proceed up the left and right sides of the ring equally well. However, since recovery in the left side is longer, more of the left side of the ring will be depolarized longer;

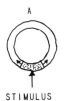  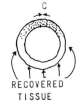

STIMULUS        EXCITED TISSUE        RECOVERED TISSUE

Fig. 17.5  A single stimulus delivered to a uniform ring of irritable tissues (A) will result in waves of excitation traveling up both sides of the ring (B). When the waves of excitation reach the top of the ring (C), they are extinguished because they run into each other's refractory period.

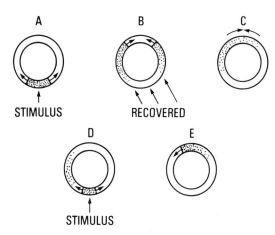

Fig. 17.6 A ring of irritable tissue with delayed recovery on the left. A stimulus will cause excitation to travel up both sides of the ring (A, B). The two waves of excitation will run into each other's refractory period (C). The recovery in the left side of the ring is slower; if a second stimulus is delivered during this time (D), excitation to the left will be blocked and will travel up the right side of the ring. If, when excitation reaches the top of the ring (E), recovery has occurred in the left side, excitation will continue around the ring (E). This is the basis for the circus-motion theory for fibrillation.

recovery will therefore occur on the right before the left, as shown in Figure 17.6B, C. If a second stimulus is delivered at this instant, the ring to the left has not recovered—i.e., it is refractory—but the right side of the ring is excitable (Figure 17.6D). Therefore, excitation will proceed only up the right side of the ring. If, when it reaches the top of the ring, the left side has recovered, the excitation wave will find recovered tissue in front of it and continue around the ring (Fig. 17.6E). If the ring is big enough, the propagation velocity is slow enough and the refractory period is short enough, the wave of excitation will continue to circle the ring. With Mines' excised ray atrial ring, 50 trips were made before excitation died out. With Garrey's turtle ventricular ring, excitation continued to circle for 7 hours.

The circus-motion model provides a self-sustained excitation because of (1) a nonuniformity of recovery in the myocardium; and (2) the delivery of a second stimulus at the appropriate point and time. Of course, for the circus motion to be sustained, there needs to be a critical rela-

tionship between the velocity of propagation of excitation, the duration of the refractory period, and the size of the excitable ring.

From the foregoing, it can be seen that sustained excitation can occur in cardiac muscle if the mass of tissue is large enough and repetitive stimuli are provided, as in the case of an irritable ectopic focus which increases its firing rate. Self-sustaining excitation can also occur if ectopic beats arise at different sites at different times. In either case, a wave of excitation could be blocked in one direction, travel in another, and return later to excite the area that was previously blocked but has since recovered.

As stated earlier, it makes little difference whether the precipitating factor is repetitive firing from one site or firing from multiple pacemakers. The essential requirement for sustaining fibrillation is a critical relationship between propagation velocity, refractory period, and mass of irritable tissue. The critical-mass theory for sustaining excitation is supported by the inability of small, warm-blooded hearts to remain in fibrillation when stimulated repetitively. MacWilliam et al.[24] found that ventricular fibrillation does not persist in the cat, rabbit, rat, mouse, hedgehog, and fowl. Studies by the author have shown that the ventricles of the cat, rat, rabbit, monkey, and very small dog do not remain in fibrillation. Interestingly enough, if the persistence of ventricular fibrillation is tested in the dog as it grows, ventricular fibrillation is found to persist in the puppy only after it increases in size. In addition, rabbit and monkey ventricles can be made to remain in fibrillation if the body temperature is increased slightly. An increase in temperature increases propagation velocity and decreases the refractory period. Increasing propagation velocity does not favor the persistence of fibrillation (because excitation would return too soon). However, decreasing the refractory period (i.e., by shortening the recovery period, which is strongly affected by an increase in temperature) favors the genesis of reentrant excitation.

Additional evidence for the critical-mass theory for supporting fibrillation comes from atrial fibrillation studies. Atrial fibrillation is sustained in very large horses. It is only sustained in dogs with hypertrophied atria. There is strong evidence that atrial fibrillation is sustained in man with atrial hypertrophy.

As just described, the maintenance of fibrillation requires that the mass of cardiac muscle be in excess of a critical minimum, and that there exist an appropriate relationship between the propagation velocity for excitation and the refractory period. It is obvious that fibrillation can be abolished by manipulating any of these three properties of cardiac muscle. Fibrillation has been abolished experimentally by decreasing the mass of cardiac muscle by surgical excision. For example, Garrey [23] precipitated ventricular fibrillation in the dog heart; then he reduced the ventricular mass surgically. Ventricular fibrillation ceased when about three quarters of the ventricles had been removed. In addition to demonstrating the need for a critical mass, Garrey found that the shape of the remaining myocardial tissue influenced the ability to sustain fibrillation. Long, thin strips would not maintain fibrillation; shorter strips with a greater cross-section could sustain fibrillation.

Additional studies supporting the concept of a critical mass of myocardium for the maintenance of fibrillation were offered by Zipes et al.[25] Using fibrillating canine ventricles supported by cardiopulmonary bypass, potassium chloride solution was injected into selected coronary artery branches. Such a solution depolarizes myocardial cells, rendering them inexcitable. Zipes et al. found that fibrillation was abolished when about 70 percent of the ventricular myocardium was depolarized.

The evidence presented thus far clearly demonstrates that there is a critical mass necessary for the maintenance of fibrillation. Reducing the excitable mass by surgical excision or by selective chemical depolarization arrests the self-sustaining excitation that characterizes fibrillation.

Hypothermia reduces cellular metabolism and hence delays recovery—i.e., lengthens the refractory period. In human cardiac surgery, hypothermia is used, and the ventricles are fibrillated intentionally to obtain a tranquil operating field. Often the hypothermia increases the refractory period to such an extent that fibrillation sometimes ceases spontaneously.

The most controllable method for arresting fibrillation employs a pulse of electric current which is strong enough to depolarize most of the excitable myocardial cells, thereby rendering them simultaneously refractory. On recovery, the cells will be able to accept a stimulus, contract, and pump blood.

From this discussion, it should be obvious that, if electric current is used to achieve defibrillation, the intensity required will be related to heart size. To defibrillate large hearts, more myocardial cells must be rendered inexcitable, which will require more current. This argument forms the basis of the dose concept—namely, that the shock strength required for defibrillation is related to heart and is therefore related to body weight. There is ample evidence from animal studies and from pediatric and adult defibrillation to provide support for the dose concept.

Since a defibrillator delivers a therapeutic agent, it is appropriate to equate a defibrillating shock to a drug; this analogy can be carried quite far. For example, the required drug dose is related to subject size; so it is with defibrillator shocks. Because a child requires a weaker shock than an adult, single or multiple smaller doses of a drug are used; the same is true with defibrillating shocks. Moreover, there are subject variables—that is, the same dose produces a lesser or greater effect in different subjects, and the same is true with defibrillating shocks. Some subjects require less or more shock strength than others of the same weight, due to such factors as metabolic status, the underlying cardiac disease, and the presence of drugs, all of which affect the shock strength required. The synergistic and antagonistic effects of drugs are well recognized; the same is true with defibrillation shocks. These facts should be borne in mind when examining the data on shock strength required for ventricular defibrillation.

For a given electrode size and placement, the most important factors to consider are subject size and the type of waveform provided by the defibrillator. As stated previously, there are two waveforms used clinically: the damped sine (Gurvich, Lown, or Edmark) wave and the trapezoidal wave. The damped sine wave can be underdamped or overdamped. The trapezoidal wave can be low-tilt (square) or high-tilt. As indicated earlier, tilt refers to the decrease in current during the shock. A high-tilt wave exhibits a considerable decrease in current during the pulse. Such a waveform behaves like a damped sine wave of a similar duration in that a similar energy is required. The shock strengths required will be discussed elsewhere in this chapter.

## DIRECT VENTRICULAR (SURGICAL) DEFIBRILLATION

Defibrillation with transventricular electrodes has been possible in the experimental animal since 1933, when Kouwenhoven and his associates first accomplished it using 60-Hz power-line alternating current. As stated previously, the first human heart was defibrillated in 1947 by Beck et al., who also applied 60-Hz alternating current to transventricular electrodes. In 1963 and 1966, Edmark et al. reported successful ventricular defibrillation of the human heart using damped sinusoidal current. In these studies, which included children and adults, Edmark recommended the use of 15 J to defibrillate the ventricles of children and 50 J for adult human hearts (although he did defibrillate the heart of a 61-year-old man with 10 J). Until recently, a level of 20 to 50 J has been used more or less routinely.

In a 1974 study involving animal hearts ranging in weight from 60 to 3800 g, Geddes et al.[26] reported the threshold energy levels required using damped sine wave current applied to electrodes which were adequately large to encompass the ventricles. Figure 17.7 illustrates the threshold energy-versus-body-weight relationship. To achieve defibrillation, the 300-g animal heart required about 6 J, and the 500-g heart, required 15 J. Tacker et al.[27] noted that these values were less than the 20 to 50 J used clinically. He therefore initiated a study in human subjects to determine the minimum (threshold) energy required for defibrillation with transventricular electrodes.

The study conducted by Tacker et al.[27] involved nine adult surgical patients on cardiopulmonary bypass and under hypothermia (34.6

to 26.1°C core temperature). Ventricular fibrillation was induced or occurred spontaneously. Prior to defibrillation, 100 mg of lidocaine were given. Defibrillation was attempted with 1 or 5 J; if unsuccessful, higher energies were used. In seven of the nine patients, defibrillation was accomplished with 5 J or less. In one subject, 10 J were required, and in another, 20 J were necessary. These latter two patients had higher estimated heart weights (550 gm) and higher body temperatures (34.6 and 36.3°C). Figure 17.8 illustrates the energy-versus-heart-weight data obtained in this study and subsequent data obtained by these investigators.

Tacker et al.[27] pointed out that the ventricles of human patients require slightly less energy than is required for normal animal ventricles; Figure 17.8 makes this comparison. Tacker et al. stated that defibrillation with the least energy impairs contractility the least and proposed that 5 J be used for the first shock applied to the adult human heart. If this shock fails, shocks of increasing intensity should be used. If fibrillation recurs after successful defibrillation, the same shock strength should be used for subsequent trials.

To date there is no comparable ventricular defibrillation study on human hearts with the low- and high-tilt trapezoidal waves. However, animal studies by Koning et al.,[28] who used 5-msec, low-tilt trapezoidal (square) waves, indicate that slightly less energy is required than with the damped sine wave. Animal studies with damped sine waves and high-tilt trapezoidal waves indicate that the energy levels required are similar.

## CLOSED-CHEST VENTRICULAR DEFIBRILLATION

The important factors to be considered in achieving ventricular defibrillation with thoracic electrodes are body size, defibrillator waveform, electrode size and placement, metabolic status of the subject, and underlying cardiac disease. In addition, the manner by which the energy is delivered (e.g., single or multiple shocks), may affect the shock strength required. These factors will be discussed, and the energy

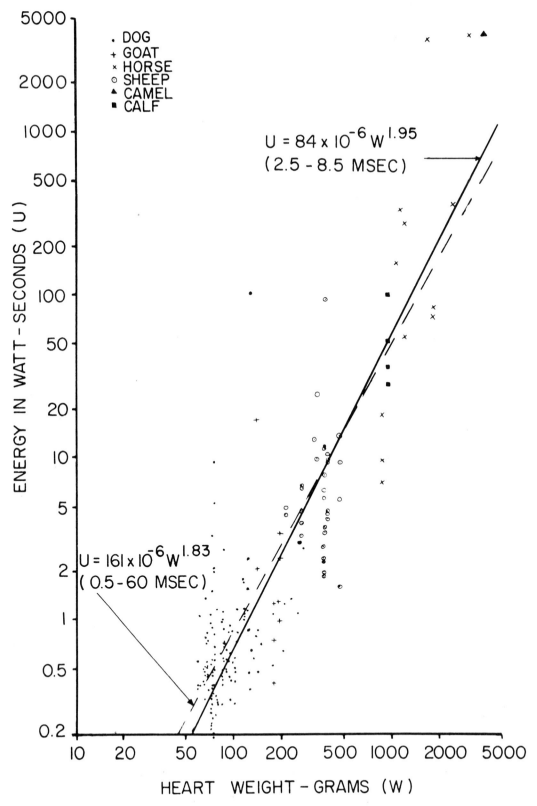

Fig. 17.7 Threshold delivered energy vs. heart weight for defibrillating animals with damped sine wave current. (Redrawn from Geddes et al: J Thorac Cardiovasc Surg 68:593–602, 1974.)

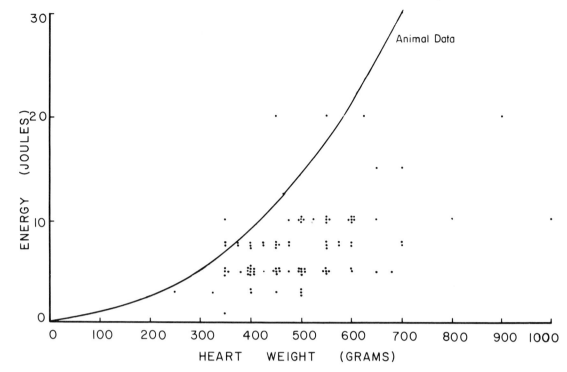

Fig. 17.8 Energy vs. heart weight for defibrillating human hearts with damped sine wave current (dots). The curve is for animal data from Fig. 17.7. (Courtesy of W. A. Tacker.)

levels required for defibrillation will be presented.

Despite the fact that the importance of body weight among adults does not seem to be a major factor in fine-tuning the shock strength, there is undeniable evidence from animal studies (Geddes et al.,[29,30] Gold et al.[31,32]) that the minimum energy required increases with body weight. The studies by Geddes et al. demonstrated, in a series of animals ranging from 2 to 340 kg, that the energy and current required increased with body weight. Figure 17.9 illustrates the threshold energy body-weight relationship. A similar relationship holds for low- and high-tilt trapezoidal waves. In a study by Gold et al.,[31] which employed square waves, the increase in energy needed to defibrillate calves was clearly demonstrated as they grew from 50 to 150 kg. In addition, it is well known that children require much less shock strength than adults.

As stated previously, there are two different current waveforms used for defibrillation: the damped sine wave and the trapezoidal wave.

Figure 17.4 illustrates these waveforms. The damped sine wave, 4 to 8 msec in duration, is the most popular. Obviously, the square wave is a low-tilt trapezoid. Low-tilt trapezoidal waves (10 to 50 percent) and high-tilt (above 70 percent) trapezoidal waves are delivered from commercially available defibrillators. The damped sine wave and high-tilt trapezoidal wave defibrillators store 400 J. The low-tilt trapezoidal wave stores 250 J. The defibrillating efficacies of these waveforms have been shown to be different by animal studies (Bourland et al.[33,34]). It is for this reason that the defibrillators have different stored energies.

## Electrode Location and Technique

There is considerable controversy over the optimum size and placement of the electrodes for ventricular defibrillation in man. At present, most electrodes for precordial placement are about 9 cm in diameter. The American Heart Association has recommended the two electrode locations shown in Figures 17.10 and

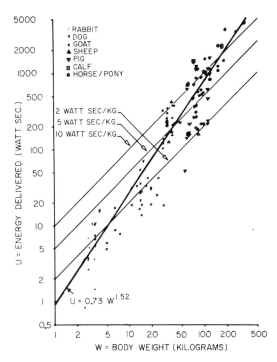

Fig. 17.9 Threshold energy-body weight relationship for defibrillating animals ranging from 5 to 340 kg in body weight using damped sinusoidal current. (Redrawn from Geddes, et al.: J Clin Invest 53:310–319, 1974.)

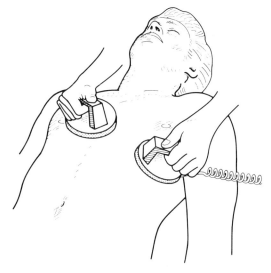

Fig. 17.10 Precordial or antero-anterior placement of electrodes. (Redrawn from Advanced Life Support, Am Heart Assoc, 1975.)

17.11. The precordial placement (Fig. 17.10) is preferred because it is easy to apply in an emergency situation. The chest-to-back placement derives from atrial defibrillation studies by Lown.[35] Often a larger electrode is used on the back. To date there is no definitive clinical study that documents the superiority of one electrode placement over the other for ventricular defibrillation. Animal studies by the author[36] have shown that the lowest energy and current are required when one electrode is over the apex-beat area. There was an insignificant difference in threshold when this electrode was paired against one on the right chest or back.

At present, two techniques are used for ventricular defibrillation. One employs multiple low-energy shocks, delivered in a rapid-fire sequence. Sometimes the shocks are alternated with cardiopulmonary resuscitation. After several shocks the strength is increased if defibrillation is not achieved. The other technique employs a single higher intensity shock with a desire to achieve defibrillation with the first shock. Although it appears that defibrillation can be achieved with a slightly lower energy setting using multiple shocks, it has not been shown that one technique causes less impairment to the ventricles than the other.

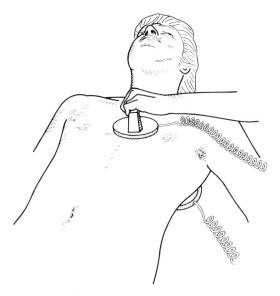

Fig. 17.11 Chest-back or antero-posterior placement of electrodes. (Redrawn from Advanced Life Support. Am Heart Assoc, 1975.)

## Pediatric Defibrillation

Using damped sinusoidal current, Gutgesell et al.[37] determined the shock strength required to defibrillate children ranging in weight from 2.1 to 50 kg. Figure 17.12 is a plot of their energy vs. body-weight data. In this study of 27 children, most of whom had congenital heart disease, there were 71 defibrillation attempts. It was found that an energy dose of 2 J/kg was 91 percent successful. For children less than 10 kg in body weight, the electrodes were 1.75 inches in diameter. For children above 10 kg, electrodes with a diameter of 3.5 inches were used. The electrodes were placed on the anterior chest wall. One electrode was placed over the apex beat area and the other was on the right chest, over the base of the heart. Gutgesell pointed out that, although an energy dose of 2 J/kg was applicable, there was a tendency for the heavier subjects to require a disproportionately higher energy when compared with lighter subjects. However, Gutgesell pointed out that, if fibrillation occurs again after successful defibrillation, there is no justification for increasing the energy to achieve subsequent defibrillation.

To date there have been no comparable pediatric data for the energy required with the low- and high-tilt trapezoidal waves. However, from animal and human studies on adults, it can be anticipated that the energy required with the high-tilt trapezoid is similar to that required with the damped sine wave. The energy required with the low-tilt trapezoid (square) wave is expected to be somewhat less.

### Adult Defibrillation

**Damped Sine Wave.** Since introduction of the damped sine wave defibrillator, considerable data have been accumulated which identify the

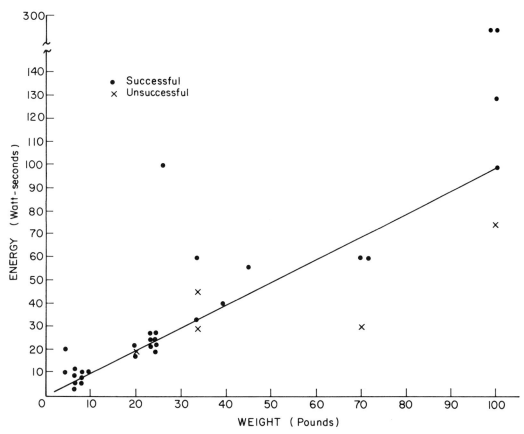

Fig. 17.12 Energy-body weight relationship for defibrillating children with damped sine wave current. (Redrawn from Gutgesell et al: Pediatrics, 58:898–901, 1976.)

energy levels used for defibrillating adult human subjects. Despite this fact, the data are not altogether consistent—probably because of the many variables, which include patient population, underlying cardiac disease, and electrode size and placement, as well as technique—i.e. single or multiple shocks. Technique probably is the area where the most controversy exists. For example, two techniques are used, and the energy levels are different. One group of clinicians believes that defibrillation should be achieved with the first shock; therefore, a slightly higher energy level is used. The other group believes that multiple lower-energy shocks delivered in a rapid sequence (sometimes alternated with cardiopulmonary resuscitation) is more effective. Which method is better has not been established. The data to be presented will identify the technique used.

Since their introduction, damped sine wave defibrillators have been available with output dials calibrated to 400 J. In the early defibrillators, the internal resistance was high; in order to achieve defibrillation in adults, it was necessary to turn the output control to the maximum setting. With the passage of time, defibrillators have improved and a larger fraction of the selected output is delivered to the subject. Unfortunately, the practice of turning the output to a maximum for all patients has not disappeared entirely.

Tacker et al.[38] and Collins et al.[39] conducted a retrospective study involving 178 patients in which a higher energy, single-shock (400 J, stored) was delivered to arrest ventricular fibrillation. The energy delivered by these defibrillators was 300 J into a 50-ohm resistor. Similar studies using multiple shocks were reported by Pantridge et al.[40,41] Figure 17.13 presents the result of these studies. This illustration demonstrates a decrease in percent success with increasing body weight.

The technique of multiple, low-energy shock defibrillation is advocated by Pantridge et al.,[40,41] Adgey et al.,[42] and Crampton et al.[43,44] Adgey et al.[42] reported two clinical studies with adult patients; in one, single and multiple 200-J shocks were delivered. In the other, single and multiple 100-J shocks were delivered. These values represent stored energy; the delivered

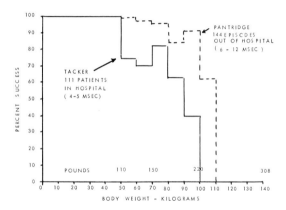

Fig. 17.13 Percent successful defibrillation of human subjects vs. body weight using 400 J (stored energy) defibrillators. (Redrawn from Tacker et al., 1974 and Pantridge et al., 1978.)

energy into a 50-ohm resistor was 83 percent of the stored energy. From the data presented in Adgey's study, which involved patients ranging in weight from 30 to 100 kg, it is possible to examine the percent success-versus-body-

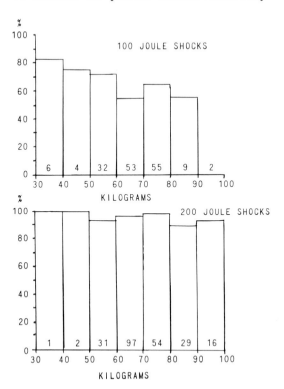

Fig. 17.14 Percent successful defibrillation of human subjects vs. body weight using single and multiple 100- and 200-J damped sine wave shocks. (Composed from data reported by Adgey et al., 1978.)

weight relationship. The percent success versus body weight histograms for the two energy levels are shown in Fig. 17.14.

The study by Adgey et al. merits comment. Clearly, the percent success is higher with the 200-J shocks. In 10 of the 120 patients, 200-J shocks failed to defibrillate. In 8 percent of the population, a 400-J shock was needed for defibrillation. Of particular significance was the fact that the percent successful defibrillation decreased after 2 minutes of circulatory arrest. For example, the average success rate with 100-J shocks in one group of patients was 69 percent for less than 2 minutes of fibrillation. For over 2 minutes of fibrillation, the average success was 50 percent. These findings clearly call attention to the importance of time. A similar observation was made by Schuder et al.,[45] who used animals.

The data reported by Adgey et al.[42] can be presented in terms of percent successful defibrillation vs. energy dose in J/kg. Figure 17.15 presents this relationship for the 100- and 200-J shocks. It is clear that there is a dose-response relationship and that the lowest energy dose for 100 percent successful defibrillation was about 4 J/kg.

Strong advocates for the rapid-fire serial defibrillation, using from 1 to 5 shocks, are Crampton et al.[43,44] In their human studies, the energy levels varied between 2.9 and 4.3 J per kg of body weight.

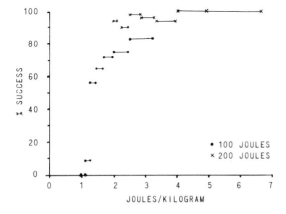

Fig. 17.15 Percent successful defibrillation of human subjects using various energy doses of damped sine wave current. (Composed from data reported by Adgey et al., 1978.)

From the foregoing, several important conclusions can be drawn. Perhaps the most obvious is that there is a difference in experience among those who report defibrillation data. The basic facts of biologic variability, underlying cardiac disease, and the circumstances under which defibrillation is carried out, may account for some of the difference. It would appear that an increased success attends multiple-shock defibrillation. An explanation for this situation is far from clear. One very important point to recognize is that it is current flow through the ventricles that achieves defibrillation, not delivered energy. With successive shocks, it has been shown in man by Chambers et al.[46] and in animals by Geddes et al.[47] and by Dahl et al.[48] that the thoracic resistance decreases with successive shocks. This means that, for the same energy setting, slightly higher current will flow through the thorax with successive shocks. Whether this is a major or minor contributor to the increased success with multiple shocks is not known. Due to biologic variability, it is very likely that there will be a small percentage of subjects who will require a stronger shock than expected. In Adgey's study, the number amounted to 8 percent.

Finally, the metabolic status of the myocardium plays an important role in determining the shock strength required for ventricular defibrillation. It is a common experience that prolonged circulatory arrest makes it more difficult to achieve defibrillation. This fact manifests itself in two ways: as a decrease in percent success with the same shock strength or as the need for a stronger shock to defibrillate. More important, however, is the fact that defibrillated hypoxic ventricles are very slow to resume their pumping load.

From the data presented thus far, it would appear that, with well-applied precordial electrodes, the energy dose used for children up to 50 kg is in the vicinity of 2 J/kg. For adults ranging in weight from 40 to 100 kg, single or multiple 100- to 200-J shocks are used. It would appear that the typical 70-kg adult can be defibrillated with about 2 to 4 J/kg, delivered in single multiple shocks. A small percentage of adults will require a higher dose. Very heavy adults (over 100 kg) may require more energy.

Because of the difficulty in defibrillating some heavy subjects, several manufacturers have developed experimental defibrillators that have a reserve energy. In such units there is a lock on the output control which requires a special maneuver to make the additional energy available. Some such defibrillators are capable of providing up to 500 or 600 J if needed. It is, however, too soon to report on the number of times when this reserve energy is needed.

**Low-Tilt Trapezoidal Wave.** A few commercially available defibrillators provide a low-tilt trapezoidal waveform; a typical example is shown in Figure 17.4D. It is important to note that the maximum energy provided by such defibrillators is lower than that provided by damped sine wave units. Because of the difference in waveform efficacy, low-tilt trapezoidal wave defibrillators are effective at a slightly lower energy level. This statement can be made from comparative studies on animals by Bourland et al.,[33,34] and by Geddes et al.[29,30] Using such a defibrillator, Anderson and Suelzer [49] reported efficacy data on 108 human subjects ranging in weight from 30 to 140 kg. The defibrillator was capable of delivering 250 J to a 50-ohm resistor at a voltage of 1200 and current of 24 amps. The maximum duration of the pulse was about 25 msec. In this defibrillator, the energy was controlled by varying the pulse duration. Internal circuitry adjusted the duration of the pulse of current to deliver the energy selected. Using 12-cm electrodes on the precordium, the percent success vs. body weight data obtained is shown in Figure 17.16. Aside from successful defibrillation of the 4 percent of subjects above 100 kg, the percent success-versus-body-weight histogram is similar to those presented by others who used the damped sine wave. Assuming that 250 J were used to defibrillate the subjects weighing from 60 to 140 kg, the average energy dose varied from 1.85 to 3.8 J/kg.

**High-Tilt Trapezoidal Wave.** There is at least one high-tilt trapezoidal wave defibrillator available; it provides a 10-msec constant duration pulse of current, has a 73 percent tilt and delivers 350 J into a 50-ohm load. Additional output is available from this defibrillator by releasing a lock on the output control. The output

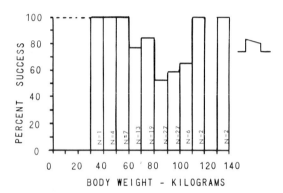

Fig. 17.16 Percent successful defibrillation of human subjects versus body weight for defibrillation using a low-tilt trapezoidal wave defibrillator. (Redrawn from Anderson and Suelzer: Chest 70:298–300, 1976.)

is regulated by controlling the voltage, which ranges from 0 to 2600. Using such a defibrillator equipped with 8.9-cm precordial electrodes, Tacker et al.[50] reported an efficacy study on eight adult human subjects ranging in weight from 50 to 77 kg. Using full output, an average of 63 percent successful defibrillation was achieved in the patients with an average weight of 66.8 kg. The average energy dose was 5.98 J/kg of body weight.

## Summary

From the foregoing, it is quite obvious that children require less energy for arresting ventricular fibrillation than adults. Experience indicates that among adult human subjects there does not appear to be a strong relationship between the energy required and body weight. However, for all waveforms currently in use, studies with normal animals have shown a clear relationship between energy and body weight. Why this relationship is not so evident among human subjects is not known. Part of the explanation must be attributed to the underlying cardiac disease, metabolic status of the patient, and the technique used for defibrillation.

To provide a guide for selecting the energy required, figure 17.17 is presented. In viewing this illustration, which merely calls attention to the energy requirement for an increase in body weight, it is necessary to remember that the amount of energy required depends on elec-

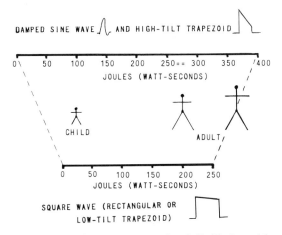

Fig. 17.17 The dose concept for defibrillation with damped sine, high-tilt, and low-tilt trapezoidal waves.

trode size, placement, type of electrolytic paste used, type of defibrillating waveform, technique used (single or multiple shocks), the underlying cardiac disease, and the metabolic status of the patient at the time when defibrillation is attempted. From the data summarized here, the reader can adopt a reasonable shock strength to achieve defibrillation.

## METABOLIC AND DRUG EFFECTS

The patient who is a candidate for ventricular defibrillation presents with rapidly advancing hypoxia and acidosis. In addition, the patient may or may not be on medication. All of these factors alter the threshold energy required for defibrillation. It will be the object of this section to identify those situations which make defibrillation easier or more difficult to achieve.

### Metabolic Effects

The metabolic status of the candidate for defibrillation merits some consideration. It is a common experience that hypoxic ventricles are difficult to defibrillate (i.e., more energy is required). This fact has been demonstrated by Schuder et al.[45] in animals and by Adgey et al.[42] in humans. The effect has shown up as a decreased percentage successful defibrillation following a prolonged period of fibrillation. In

Adgey's study, which employed 100-J shocks, the average percent successful defibrillation with less than 2 minutes of fibrillation was 67 percent. With more than 2 minutes of fibrillation, the success fell to 50 percent.

In a dog study by Yakaitis et al.,[51] metabolic and respiratory alkalosis and acidosis and hypoxia were induced selectively. In this study, it was not possible to demonstrate a clear effect of metabolic acidosis and hypoxemia on the energy required for defibrillation. They did note that, following defibrillation with metabolic acidosis and hypoxemia, restoration of the circulation was slow.

### Drug Effects

**Cardiac Glycosides.** Digitalis and digitalis-like drugs reduce the threshold energy for ventricular defibrillation. Lown et al.[52] showed in dogs that toxic doses of acetylstrophanthidin and ouabain decreased the defibrillation threshold by about 27 percent. A similar dog study by Tacker et al.[53] demonstrated a 25 percent reduction in defibrillation threshold.

Digitalis is not without its difficulties. High doses produce dangerous dysrhythmias. Lown[52] reported that, often when ventricular fibrillation was produced by digitalis, the heart could not be restored to a functional rhythm by multiple, high-energy shocks.

**Antidysrhythmic Drugs.** *Quinidine.* Following injection of a high dose of quinidine gluconate to dogs, Babbs et al.[54] measured the threshold energy for defibrillation over a period of three and one-half hours. It was found that the maximum increase in threshold energy was 172 percent. The energy threshold returned almost to the control value after 4 hours.

*Lidocaine.* Babbs et al.[54] determined the threshold energy required to defibrillate dog hearts following a single injection and continuous infusion of lidocaine. They found that in both instances the threshold energy increased 50 to 199 percent.

*Diphenylhydantoin.* In a dog study, Babbs et al.[54] measured the threshold energy for defibrillation before and after the continuous infusion of diphenylhydantoin. They found that the threshold energy increase was 85 percent.

## Summary

In the foregoing drug studies, the experimental animal was the dog. Therefore, the doses given are not comparable to those given in human subjects, although they were typical for the dog. However, the important point in each case is the direction of change in the threshold energy required for defibrillation. With more research in this area, it may be possible to identify a trend for inotropic drugs to reduce the threshold and antidysrhythmic drugs to increase the threshold energy for defibrillation.

## MYOCARDIAL INFARCTION

Animal studies by Tacker et al.[55] showed that the energy required for defibrillation rises and falls during the first two hours following coronary artery occlusion. Although this phenomenon was well demonstrated in the dog, caution must be used in applying this observation to man. Because of the critical mass theory for sustaining defibrillation, it may be that the energy required for defibrillation could conceivably be less if the infarct is very extensive.

When ventricular fibrillation (or its frequent precursor, ventricular tachycardia) is heralded by a warning signal or observed on the ECG monitor, it is the practice in many CCUs for the nurse to initiate resuscitative efforts—the first of which is the use of unsynchronized countershock.

## TACHYARRHYTHMIAS OTHER THAN VENTRICULAR FIBRILLATION

Cardioversion is the name usually applied to the use of a defibrillator to arrest tachyarrhythmias other than ventricular fibrillation. Use of the technique was pioneered by Lown in 1962. When using cardioversion, care must be exercised to avoid precipitating ventricular fibrillation by delivery of the countershock during the ventricular vulnerable period which occurs during the early to middle part of the T wave. Figure 17.18 illustrates the extent of the vulnerable period. During this time, a single threshold

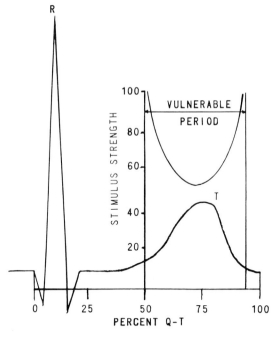

Fig. 17.18  The extent of the vulnerable period of the ventricles in relation to the ECG. The minimum stimulus strength to evoke ventricular fibrillation occurs just before the apex of the T wave.

stimulus will merely evoke an ectopic beat. However, if the strength of the shock is increased, the single shock will precipitate fibrillation. Figure 17.19 illustrates ventricular fibrillation by vulnerable-period stimulation. The ratio of shock strength for fibrillation to the strength for excitation may be 20 or more in the normal heart. In the ischemic heart, a shock only

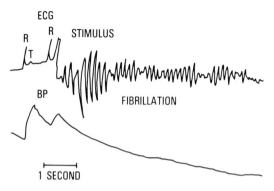

Fig. 17.19  The ECG and blood pressure before and after delivery of a single stimulus during the T wave of the ECG. Note the instant occurrence of ventricular fibrillation.

slightly in excess of threshold can precipitate fibrillation by vulnerable period stimulation.

The method used to avoid delivery of the countershock during the vulnerable period of the ventricles is called synchronized cardioversion. Such synchronization is achieved by the defibrillator and requires the ECG as a controlling signal. Some defibrillators require feeding in the ECG from an external electrocardiograph. Many defibrillators contain an ECG amplifier, and it is only necessary to apply the leads to the subject and connect them to defibrillator. An increasing number of defibrillators acquire the ECG from the defibrillating electrodes. Irrespective of how the ECG information is acquired, the defibrillator senses the QRS wave and delivers the countershock 20 to 50 msec after it. Thus, the countershock falls in the refractory period of the ventricles.

A few clinicians who use cardioversion feel that synchronization is not necessary. From experience they have noted that ventricular fibrillation has not been precipitated with unsynchronized cardioversion, due to the statistically low chance of hitting the vulnerable period, which occupies only about 75 msec. Resnekov[56] reported that the incidence of ventricular fibrillation due to random delivery of the countershock is 2 percent. Notwithstanding, it is unwise to use unsynchronized cardioversion if synchronization is available.

The type of complications following cardioversion are the same as those following ventricular defibrillation attempts. These have been outlined in the forthcoming section entitled "Myocardial Damage." However, it is to be noted that the energy level used for cardioversion is substantially less than is required for ventricular defibrillation. The side effects with cardioversion are therefore less.

## Atrial Fibrillation

The use of countershock to arrest atrial fibrillation has changed little since Lown[57] summarized his experience with 100 patients in whom high doses of quinidine could not abolish the dysrhythmia. The technique employed damped sinusoidal current. In order to prevent return of atrial fibrillation following the countershock, quinidine was given. In order to prevent the production of ventricular dysrhythmias, digitalis was withheld for at least 24 hours. Finally, a sedative was given to produce a short-duration amnesia so that the countershock was not perceived by the patient. More recently, a high dose of a tranquilizer has been used instead of a short-acting anesthetic to achieve the same goal.

Lown[57] found that the chest-to-back electrode location decreased the energy requirements for atrial defibrillation. The shock strength used varied among patients. Although the mean energy for adult subjects was 100 J, 40 percent of the patients were cardioverted with 50 J or less. Ninety-five percent were cardioverted with 200 J or less. The energy required was directly dependent on the duration of atrial fibrillation, being 87 J for less than one year and 240 J for more than ten years of atrial fibrillation. Lown also noted that the percentage of patients who remained in sinus rhythm was higher when the duration of fibrillation was shorter.

Interestingly enough, Lown also noted a correlation between the amplitude of the f waves in lead I of the ECG and the energy required for cardioversion and the percentage of patients remaining in sinus rhythm. For example, when the f waves were less than 0.1 mV, 140 J were required and 20 percent of the patients failed to remain in sinus rhythm. If the f waves were 0.2 mV or larger, 92 J sufficed, and only 4 percent failed to remain in sinus rhythm. According to Lown[57] and Resnekov,[58] certain subjects are unsuitable candidates for cardioversion. Included in this category are: patients who have recurrent atrial fibrillation while on high doses of quinidine; patients with enlarged atria; elderly patients with coronary artery disease with a slow ventricular rate in the absence of digitalis therapy; patients with lone or idiopathic atrial fibrillation; patients with small hearts and slow ventricular rates; patients with atrial fibrillation for longer than five years; and patients before and during valve replacement. Following cardioversion in many of these patients, intractable cardiac failure and/or atrial fibrillation recur.

## Atrial Flutter

Atrial flutter is easier to arrest than atrial fibrillation. A single, low-energy shock of about 50 J is usually adequate in the adult subject. The medication is the same as for atrial defibrillation. The danger of attempting cardioversion in a digitalized patient is the precipitation of ventricular dysrhythmias, including fibrillation.[52]

In acute myocardial infarction, however, it may not be possible to withhold digitalis for 24 hours if this drug has already been given for treatment of atrial dysrhythmias or if the patient had already been receiving this agent prior to hospital admission. If atrial fibrillation or flutter is the cause of progressive left ventricular failure or pulmonary edema, synchronized electrical conversion at low energy levels should be employed without hesitation. Prophylactic lidocaine (50 to 100 mg intravenously) may be given to prevent ventricular dysrhythmias after conversion to sinus rhythm. Two to 5 mg of diazepam IV may be used for tranquillization and muscle relaxation, but the blood pressure should be carefully monitored after this medication, and appropriate equipment for endotracheal intubation should always be available. Administration of 100 percent oxygen by mask after intravenous sedation and just before and after cardioversion is also indicated.

## Ventricular Tachycardia

Because of its variability, ventricular tachycardia is one of the most difficult arrhythmias to terminate. Although drugs can often control this arrhythmia, increasing numbers of patients with drug-resistant tachycardia are being identified. Various therapies have been used—ranging from ventricular pacing with complex trains of pulses, local sympathetic denervation, or surgical excision of irritable foci (documented electrophysiologically) to the application of synchronized countershock via precordial electrodes. Due to the different etiologies for ventricular tachycardia, it is difficult to recommend energy levels for countershock. Some forms of ventricular tachycardia (e.g., ventricular "flutter") can be converted with relatively low energy (e.g., 10 J of damped sinusoidal current). Other types of ventricular tachycardia may require up to the full 400-J setting of the defibrillator. However, only the lowest energy should be used. When an effective energy has been identified, it is probably unwise to raise the energy to convert subsequent episodes of tachycardia. To date there is little evidence that the use of higher energy will extinguish an irritable ventricular focus.

In the setting of acute myocardial infarction treated in the CCU, there is often little time for drug therapy for life-threatening ventricular tachycardia—other than the rapid intravenous administration of lidocaine or other antidysrhythmic agents. Thus, persistent ventricular tachycardia unresponsive to emergency drug therapy (or even in many instances before drug therapy is initiated) is an indication for immediate electrical conversion using the lowest possible energy level. Under these circumstances, the potential inciting role of hypokalemia should be recognized, and a serum potassium determination should be obtained routinely, especially in patients receiving diuretic therapy.

## MYOCARDIAL DAMAGE

There is no doubt that an excessively strong shock can impair contractility and cause damage to the myocardium. In normal animals, a shock that is 320 times the threshold energy required for defibrillation renders the ventricles of 50 percent of the animals incapable of contracting,[59] although QRS and T waves often persist. Obviously, shocks of this intensity are not used in clinical defibrillation. However, it is obvious that if the shock strength is made too low, defibrillation will not occur, and the patient will die. Therefore, it is useful to establish whether there is a margin of safety for defibrillating shocks. It would be comforting to know that myocardial impairment and damage do not occur until the shock strength is increased considerably above threshold. At present, some studies on this important topic have been reported, and many are now in progress. There is useful information from animal studies and some evidence from human atrial defibrillation which can aid in estimating the safety of electrical defibrillation.

Myocardial damage is a term that is used very loosely. Some identify myocardial damage as changes in the ECG (dysrhythmias, conduction disturbances, and S-T segment changes); others use microscopic evidence as an indicator, and still others use an elevation in serum enzymes (notably CK-MB fraction). Myocardial damage is also judged by scintigraphy. Changes can occur in the S-T segment of the ECG with little or no myocardial damage. Likewise, the presence of injured myocardial cells and elevated serum enzymes do not, by themselves, indicate the degree of functional impairment. In using scintigraphy, care must be taken to assure that abnormalities in structures between the heart and the electrodes are not interpreted as myocardial damage. Nonetheless, all of these indicators are useful to identify the response to defibrillating shocks.

## Animal Studies

Several energy overdose studies using defibrillating current have been carried out in dogs; Table 17.1 summarizes the results. In preparing this table, the threshold energies for defibrillation for damped sine waves were calculated from the weight of the animals and the data presented by Babbs et al.,[59] who reported that an energy dose of 3 J/kg defibrillated 95 percent of the animals. The energy levels for trapezoidal-wave defibrillation depend on the pulse duration and tilt. The thresholds were calculated for each study using the data of Bourland et al.[33,34]

The first study of myocardial impairment due to strong defibrillating shocks was presented by Peleska,[60] who applied damped sinusoidal current to thoracic electrodes on dogs ranging in weight from 20 to 25 kg. Peleska recorded the ECG and blood pressure following delivery of the shocks to normally beating hearts. He reported no dysrhythmias for shocks less than 120 J. Slight dysrhythmias were produced with 120- to 150-J shocks, and moderate dysrhythmias resulted from 150- to 340-J shocks. Very severe dysrhythmias were encountered with shocks greater than 340 J.

The threshold energy for defibrillating 20- to 25-kg dogs is about 67 J, and it would appear that the dysrhythmia threshold from Peleska's study is about 1.8 times the defibrillation threshold energy. Only slight dysrhythmias were encountered with 1.8 to 2.2 times defibrillation threshold, and moderate dysrhythmias were encountered with shock strengths of 2.2 to 5.1 times threshold. Very severe dysrhythmias were obtained with shocks 5 to 6 times threshold energy.

Lown[57] reported that 70 J of damped sine wave current was the threshold energy for defibrillation in the typical dog. The threshold for dysrhythmias (other than ventricular fibrillation) was given as 400 J. Lown stated that DC countershock provides "a five- to sixfold factor of safety."

Dahl et al.[61,62] undertook an extensive animal study designed to reveal gross and microscopic myocardial damage and ECG changes in response to suprathreshold damped sinusoidal current. The study involved 42 dogs ranging in weight from 14.2 to 27 kg. Three sizes of precordial electrodes (4.5 cm, 8 cm, and 12.8 cm) were used, and ten 400-J (stored) shocks were delivered with different spacing (15 sec, 1 min, and 3 min). Microscopic examination of the heart was carried out four days postshock. It was found that the S-T segment changes in the ECG were not a sensitive indicator of myocardial damage. Although 62 percent of the animals with myocardial damage showed S-T segment changes, 38 percent of the animals with myocardial damage did not exhibit S-T segment shifts.

Interesting observations were made relative to electrode size and temporal spacing between the shocks. Dahl et al. used a damage index to identify the severity of the shock-induced lesions. The index was defined by multiplying the damage (grades 1 to 3) by the area of the lesion in sq cm. Grade 1 identified patchy damage with many intact myocardial fibers. Grade 3 designated regions where all fibers had degenerated, and the lesion involved the full thickness of the wall. Grade 2 lesions were intermediate in severity between 1 and 3. Table 17.1 presents the data on myocardial damage and S-T segment deviation obtained by Dahl et al. It is

Table 17.1 Response to Defibrillating Shocks in Animals

| Investigator | Waveform* | Energy Ratio Used/Threshold | Observations |
|---|---|---|---|
| Peleska (1965) | DSW | 1.8 ×<br>1.8 to 2.2 ×<br>2.2 to 5.1 ×<br>More than 5.1 × | Threshold for dysrhythmias<br>Slight dysrhythmias<br>Moderate dysrhythmias<br>Very severe dysrhythmias |
| Lown (1967) | DSW | 5 to 6 × | Threshold for dysrhythmias |
| Dahl et al. (1974) | DSW | 10 shocks of 4 × delivered at 1.5 sec 1 min and 3 min to 4.5, 8, and 12.8 cm electrodes | *(see Damage Index / S-T Segment Change table below)* |
| Warner et al. (1975) | DSW | 10 shocks 2.7 to 5.3 × | Subepicardial lesions with 8 and 4.5 cm electrodes.<br>Minimal damage with 12.8 cm electrodes |
| Davis et al. (1976) | DSW | Multiple shocks 2 ×<br>Multiple shocks 5 × to 25 × | Mild to no damage<br>Focal to transmural damage |
| Tacker et al. (1978) | DSW | 1 shock 1.0 ×<br>6 shocks 9 to 23 × | No myocardial damage, transient dysrhythmias<br>Focal subepicardial to transmural damage; ECG changes persisting beyond the first day postshock. |

Dahl et al. (1974) — Observations:

| Electrode Diameter | Damage Index (average) | | | S-T Segment Change (mm) | | |
|---|---|---|---|---|---|---|
| | 15 sec | 1 min | 3 min | 15 sec | 1 min | 3 min |
| 4.5 cm | 60.2 | — | 4.0 | 8.6 | — | 0.2 |
| 8.0 cm | 4.4 | 15.0 | 1.1 | 2.5 | 1.2 | 0.0 |
| 12.8 cm | 3.0 | — | 0.5 | 0.1 | — | 0.0 |

| Reference | Waveform | Dose | Result |
|---|---|---|---|
| VanVleet et al. (1978) | DSW | 1 shock 400 ×<br>1 shock 225 ×<br>1 shock 144 ×<br>1 shock 36 ×<br>1 shock 9 ×<br>1 shock 1 × | Marked macroscopic damage in 80% of animals<br>20% of these animals receiving 400 ×, 225 × and 144 × died<br>Turgid areas in ventricular walls<br>Mild gross damage in 40% of animals<br>Mild microscopic damage in 20% of animals<br>No detectable macroscopic or microscopic damage |
| VanVleet et al. (1977) | Trap. | 6 shocks 135 ×<br><br>6 shocks 73 ×<br><br>1 shock 5.3 ×<br><br>3 shocks 11.6 × | 14% of animals died<br>70% had myocardial damage<br>70% had S-T segment changes, A-V block, and tachycardia<br>No microscopic damage<br>66% had S-T segment changes and ventricular tachycardia<br>No myocardial damage<br>50% with S-T segment changes<br>25% with tachycardia<br>25% with ventricular tachycardia |
| Ehsani et al. (1976) | DSW | 10 shocks 3.2 ×<br>to 4.8 × | 50% of animals showed S-T changes in the ECG<br>Serum enzymes (MB-CK) elevated<br>Gross and microscopic damage evident |
| DiCola et al. (1976) | DSW | 1 shock 2.9 ×<br>1 shock 5.9 ×<br>2 shocks 5.9 ×<br>3 shocks 5.9 × | 0.15% of heart damaged<br>1.11% of heart damaged<br>4.6% of heart damaged<br>6.4% of heart damaged |
| Schneider et al. (1977) | DSW | 2 shocks about 6 × | 8% of the heart damaged |
| Babbs et al. (1978) | DSW | 1 shock 1.0 ×<br>1 shock 20 ×<br>1 shock 313 × | No damage<br>Threshold for myocardial damage in 50% of animals<br>Threshold for death in 50% of animals<br>90% effective dose produced damage in 2% of animals<br>99% effective dose produced damage in 10% of animals |

* DSW = Damped Sine Wave.
* Trap. = Trapezoidal wave.
× = times threshold energy.

apparent that the myocardial response depends on both the electrode size and temporal spacing of the ten 4 times threshold energy shocks. The least myocardial damage was encountered with the largest (12.8 cm) electrodes and the most widely spaced shocks (3 min). In viewing these data, it must be recognized that ten shocks of 4 times threshold energy is a considerable overdose; yet, the damage was only moderate with standard-sized electrodes.

Another dog study was reported by Warner et al.,[63] who delivered ten 400-J shocks to the chests of dogs ranging in weight from about 15 to 30 kg. Three electrode sizes (12.8 cm, 8 cm, and 4.5 cm) were used. With the two smaller electrode sizes, gross and microscopic damage was seen in the ventricles. The lesions were confined to the subepicardium and along an imaginary line between the chest electrodes. There was minimal myocardial damage with the 12.8-cm electrodes.

The study by Warner et al. shows clearly that ten shocks of about 2.7 to 5.3 times threshold energy are damaging with standard and small electrodes. It also shows that myocardial damage is minimal when the current is spread by the use of larger electrodes.

Davis et al.[64] presented an extensive pathologic study on the hearts of dogs, examined 2 hours and 4 days after delivery of damped sine wave shocks to beating hearts. Among the animals receiving a shock of less than twice the threshold energy for defibrillation, minimal to no microscopic myocardial damage was found. Localized focal to transmural damage occurred in animals receiving shocks of 5 to 25 times threshold energy. The animals that received the lower-intensity shocks had less severe lesions, usually localized and subepicardial in extent.

A study by Tacker et al.[65] showed that there was no gross or microscopic damage when the nonfibrillating hearts of dogs ranging in weight from 12 to 19.5 kg were given one threshold energy shock of damped sine wave current. In some animals, transient ECG changes were seen. When six 400-J (stored) shocks were delivered, ECG changes were observed that lasted for more than a day. The animals were sacrificed 3 to 5 days postshock, and the hearts were examined grossly and microscopically. The

gross changes included pale yellow-tan to mottled reddish-tan areas, ranging from $1 \times 1$ cm to $4 \times 3$ cm over the anterior surface of the left ventricle. Similar lesions were seen high on the posterior wall of the right ventricle and adjacent right atrium. The lesions were transmural in one dog and almost transmural in another.

Clearly, in Tacker's study, threshold shocks produced no myocardial damage. The six 400-J shocks that produced myocardial damage were between 9 and 23 times the threshold energy required for defibrillation. It is interesting that these animals survived until they were sacrificed for the postmortem studies which were carried out three-and-one-half days after the shocks.

A study by VanVleet et al.[66] quantitated the myocardial damage in response to graded single damped sinusoidal shocks of threshold energy and overdose levels of 9, 36, 81, 144, 225, and 400 times threshold energy delivered to a large series of dogs with normally beating hearts. Interestingly enough, only 20 percent of the animals receiving 144, 225, and 400 times threshold intensity died following the shock. The lowest intensity shock for gross myocardial damage was 36 times threshold energy. The lowest intensity shock for microscopic damage occurred with 9 times threshold energy. The myocardial damage was found to be proportional to the shock strength. The animals were sacrificed at 2 hours, 1, 2, 4, 14, and 56 days postshock. At 2, 4, and 14 days, the lesions were yellow or white in appearance. After 2 days, calcification of necrotic cardiac muscle fibers occurred. At 4 days, macrophage invasion, early myocardial fibrosis, and epicardial thickening by fibrosis were evident. After 2 weeks, loss of cardiac muscle cells, or atrophy, and myocardial fibrosis were evident. At 56 days postshock, the sites of the myocardial damage had regressed to small, pale, firm, shrunken areas seen only in the left ventricle.

A study by VanVleet et al.[67] employed suprathreshold trapezoidal-wave shocks delivered to dogs with normally beating hearts. Arrhythmias and myocardial damage were sought in response to single and multiple shocks. It is possible to calculate the energy overdose given to these animals, and Table 17.1 presents the results which indicate that only with 6 shocks of 135 times threshold intensity did 14 percent of the animals die. Particularly interesting is the fact that the single shock at 5.3 times threshold intensity resulted in no microscopic myocardial damage, but did produce S-T segment changes in 50 percent of the animals and ventricular tachycardia in 25 percent of the animals.

Serum enzyme studies were carried out by Ehsani et al.[68] following delivery of suprathreshold defibrillating shocks to normally beating dog hearts. In this study, ten 240-J, damped sine wave shocks were applied to 8-cm diameter electrodes applied to the chests of dogs ranging in weight from 16.5 to 25 kg. These shocks were about 3.2 to 4.8 times the threshold for defibrillation. Changes in the S-T segment of the ECG were seen in about one-half of the dogs. In these animals, serum enzymes (MB CK) peaked at four hours postshock. At postmortem examination on the fourth day postshock, gross and microscopic damage was evident.

Scintigraphic studies on dogs have been reported by DiCola et al.[69] and Schneider et al.[70] to determine the intensity of defibrillating shocks required to produce myocardial damage. In the study of DiCola et al., 27 dogs ranging in weight from 11 to 29 kg (18.1 kg average) were used. Single and multiple 200- and 400-J (stored energy) damped sine wave shocks were delivered to precordial electrodes while the heart was beating. Myocardial imaging with Tc-99m stannous pyrophosphate was carried out four hours postshock. The data reported permits calculation of the energy overdose and the percentage of the heart that was damaged; Table 17.1 presents the results. With a single shock of 2.9 times threshold strength, 0.15 percent of the heart showed damage. The percentage of myocardium damaged increased to 6.4 percent following 3 shocks of 5.9 times threshold intensity. Table 17.1 presents the data for the other shocks and reveals that the damage increases with the number of shocks.

The study by Schneider et al.[70] employed 13 dogs with an average weight of 17.5 kg. Two 400-J (stored energy) damped sine wave shocks

were delivered 1 minute apart. From the scintigrams, the weight of the damaged region was estimated. From the data presented, the animals received 2 shocks at about 6 times threshold energy, which resulted in damage to 8 percent of the heart.

A most illuminating study of myocardial damage was presented by Babbs et al.,[71] in which the threshold energy dose in J/kg was determined in 36 dogs using damped sinusoidal current. The percent successful defibrillation vs. energy dose is shown in Figure 17.20. In another group of dogs, a single overdose shock of damped sine wave shock was given. These animals were sacrificed, and the hearts were examined grossly. Twenty-two blocks were then cut from each heart, and specimens were prepared for microscopic examination. The criterion for damage was any gross or microscopic evidence of damage in any heart or in any specimen derived from the myocardial blocks. The percentage of animals showing damage at the various energy doses and the percent of animals killed by the single high-energy shock are also shown in Figure 17.20.

The study by Babbs et al.[71] presents very interesting data. For example, if the 50 percent effectiveness point is taken, then it is seen that the threshold energy dose for defibrillation was 1.5 J/kg; the threshold for detecting myocardial damage (gross or microscopically) was 30 J/kg, and the lethal dose was 470 J/kg. Thus, the margin of safety between threshold defibril-

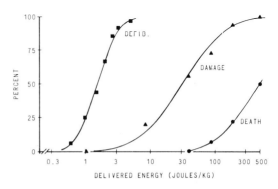

Fig. 17.20 Percent of animals versus energy dose for threshold defibrillation (DEFIB), for threshold myocardial damage (DAMAGE), and for death (DEATH). (Babbs et al: Cardiovasc Tech 20:88–98, 1978.)

lation and detectable myocardial damage in 50 percent of the animals was 20. The ratio of lethal energy dose to threshold defibrillation dose was 313 for 50 percent of the animals.

The data in Figure 17.20 may be examined in another way. Note that, for 90 percent successful defibrillation, 2 percent of the animals showed detectable gross or microscopic myocardial damage. Likewise, for 99 percent effectiveness, 10 percent of the animals showed detectable myocardial changes—either on gross inspection or in specimens from one or more of the 22 blocks of myocardium studied.

## Human Studies

The level of energy required to produce myocardial damage in the human is obviously of high importance. Because defibrillation is performed only in patients who have underlying cardiac disease, it is difficult to separate myocardial damage due to defibrillating shocks from damage due to the underlying cardiac disease. Although the normal dog studies just presented indicate that there is a fairly wide margin of safety—i.e., the lowest energy required to produce damage is much higher than the lowest energy required to achieve defibrillation—the same safety margin may not apply when cardiac disease is present.

Ehsani et al.[69] carried out enzyme studies (CK-MB fraction) in 35 normal subjects, 17 patients with myocardial infarction, and 30 patients with tachyarrhythmias without myocardial infarction who received countershocks of various strengths. Damped sinusoidal current was applied to chest-to-back electrodes. Shocks ranging in strength from 40 to 400 J were delivered. Multiple shocks were administered to 70 percent of the subjects. The total cumulative energy range was 40 to 700 J.

In the 35 normal subjects who did not receive a shock, the CK-MB level was 5 mIU. The average CK-MB level for the 17 patients with myocardial infarction was $39 \pm 6$ mIU. Among the 30 patients with tachyarrhythmias who received countershocks, the CK-MB fraction was normal in 28 patients. In two patients, the CK-MB levels were 13 and 11 mIU. One of

these patients received three shocks of 250 J (stored); the other received two shocks of 243 J (stored). It is noteworthy that the maximum CK-MB level in these two patients was only about twice the normal value. Many patients in the series had higher-energy shocks, yet failed to exhibit elevated CK-MB enzyme levels.

Resnekov[72] summarized his experience with 200 patients who had been shocked with damped sine wave and square wave current for terminating atrial tachyarrhythmias. Among the complications that he reported were elevated serum enzymes, hypotension, ECG changes, emboli, ventricular tachycardia, and cardiac failure. Among those patients who received 150 J, 6 percent had complications. When the energy level was raised to 400 J, 30 percent had complications. For these reasons, Resnekov was reluctant to use more than 400 J.

## Nature of Defibrillator-Induced Lesions

**Skin.** It is common to observe erythematous rings on the skin of humans and animals following the delivery of defibrillating current. A report by Corbitt et al.[73] described damage to the pectoral muscles in three human subjects following delivery of more than ten damped sine wave shocks designed to achieve defibrillation. The muscle changes included fragmentation, a loss of striations, and accumulation of lymphocytes and phagocytes. At that time, serum enzyme studies were being used to identify myocardial damage, and Corbitt et al suggested that skeletal muscle damage could be the cause of elevated serum enzymes, since the hearts of the three patients showed no lesions attributable to the defibrillating current.

The study by Corbitt et al. provided two interesting pieces of information: (1) the damage to the skin was not like that of a burn; and (2) a suggestion that the muscle cell damage was probably due to intense contraction of the muscle fibers and rupture of the sarcolemmal sheaths.

The concept that the erythematous rings on the skin are not thermally induced fits with measurements of skin-temperature rise. Unpublished studies in the author's laboratories (using high-speed thermography) reveal that extremely high-energy shocks (kJ) are needed to raise the skin temperature of dog skin one degree Celsius.

**Muscle.** The type of skeletal muscle-cell damage seen following multiple shocks may well be due to strong contraction due to the shock's acting as a stimulus. Pathologic examination does not indicate that a thermal process was present—although, at present, there is no explanation for the type of damage.

It has been assumed by many that the type of myocardial lesion due to high-energy countershock is thermally induced. A simple calculation can serve to provide information on this point. It is known that about one-fourth of the thoracic current traverses the heart to achieve defibrillation. This means that one-sixteenth of the energy delivered to the thorax reaches the heart. For a 320-J shock, about 20 J reaches the heart. In a typical adult, the heart may weigh 350 g. The caloric equivalent of electrical energy is 4.18 J for one calorie. Assuming a specific heat of 0.85 for the heart, the average myocardial temperature rise will be 0.016°C. This calculation assumes uniform current distribution throughout the heart. Therefore, to obtain a temperature rise large enough to produce thermal damage, multiple, extremely high-energy shocks would be required, or the current density distribution would have to be extremely nonuniform.

Lie et al.[74] described the type of myocardial damage due to multiple, high-energy shocks as follows:

> The cellular injury was characterized by disrupted myofilaments, and Z-lines that were malaligned or compressed, forming transverse contractile bands. The mitochondria showed disrupted cristae and contained electron-dense particles and lipid droplets. Irreparably damaged myocardium was replaced by fibrous granulation tissue seen as early as 4 days after EDS (electrical defibrillator shock).
>
> These changes were nonspecific and resembled myofibrillar degeneration described in a wide variety of both ischemic and nonischemic myocardial injuries seen in humans and experimental animals.

# DEFIBRILLATOR CHARACTERISTICS

Whether used to terminate an atrial or ventricular tachyrhythmia or ventricular fibrillation, the function of a defibrillator is to deliver a pulse of current having an intensity that corresponds to the setting of the output control. Thus, the requirements for a functional test are obvious: Discharge the defibrillator into a standard resistor (50 ohms) and measure the delivered energy or current. Before discussing the various tests for a defibrillator, several important items should be considered relative to defibrillators and their maintenance, especially if purchase is contemplated.

## Defibrillator Selection

Irrespective of the waveform produced, defibrillators are either portable or mobile. Portable defibrillators operate from rechargeable batteries; mobile defibrillators operate from the domestic power line. Whether a portable or mobile defibrillator is used depends on the type of service. For emergency or out-of-hospital service, or in cases of distance from power lines or failure of domestic power, battery-operated units are necessary. Size and weight may not be an important consideration for in-hospital use; however, for emergency service, size and weight are important considerations.

Defibrillators are available with and without an ECG monitor. Although a monitor is essential to identify ventricular fibrillation, some advocate "blind defibrillation" if an ECG monitor is not available and the patient is pulseless and cyanotic. Obviously, a defibrillator without an ECG monitor can be smaller than one with a monitor. However, advancing technology is rapidly removing the small weight and size penalty for the inclusion of a monitor which can be an oscilloscope or a stripchart recorder.

A defibrillator is a life-saving device and therefore must be ever ready to deliver the desired output. All defibrillators must have an indicator to identify when the selected output is available—i.e., when the energy-storage capacitor is charged.

If the defibrillator is battery operated, the

charge condition of the batteries must be indicated. Surprisingly, some battery-powered defibrillators cannot be operated while the batteries are charging. With dead batteries, such a defibrillator is useless. Other defibrillators permit operation while the batteries are charging and therefore can be used with dead batteries.

Another important consideration relates to the electrodes, which are the most vulnerable part of a defibrillator. Cables become frayed or broken, causing a short or open circuit, preventing delivery of the current, and constituting a hazard to the operating personnel. Electrodes usually cannot be interchanged among defibrillators. Often, electrodes provided by one manufacturer will not operate with all defibrillators provided by the same manufacturer. The availability of spare electrodes, or the rewiring of all defibrillators in the institution so that they can employ the same electrodes, could prevent a disaster.

Because a substantial current pulse must be delivered to the patient, the electrodes must be coupled to the skin with low-resistance electrode paste. Electrode creams and gels used for electrocardiography should not be used. Often, 0.9 percent saline-soaked pads can be employed with success. However, in all cases, the electrolyte must not be allowed to spread between the electrodes, because this will create a shunt path for the current and could cause a skin burn and prevent delivery of the full current to the heart.

## Defibrillator Testing

With all but one type of defibrillator, the delivered energy is always less than the stored energy. One low-tilt trapezoidal wave defibrillator electronically increases the pulse duration until the selected energy is delivered. In all damped sine wave and high-tilt trapezoidal wave defibrillators, the energy delivered to the standard 50-ohm load resistor is less than the energy stored in the capacitor. With newer defibrillators, the energy indicated is that which will be delivered into a 50-ohm load. Some defibrilators have two energy scales; one indicates stored energy and the other indicates the energy

that will be delivered into a 50-ohm load. If the load is other than 50 ohms, the indicated energy will not be delivered.

Routine testing of the output of all defibrillators is mandatory. There are many commercially available testers that contain a 50-ohm power resistor and straightforward electronic circuitry that performs the calculation of energy ($\int i^2 R dt$), where i is the current, R is 50 ohms, and t is time. Usually, the delivered energy is displayed on a scale. There are simpler output testers that contain some type of display that indicates that current was delivered to the internal resistor. Such types do not provide an accurate indication of the output capability of a defibrillator, although they are useful for spot-checking an instrument. Most hospitals have an electrical equipment maintenance department, and the appropriate CCU personnel should discuss the concepts presented in this section with those responsible for equipment maintenance.

Two tests which should not be performed by unauthorized personnel consist of discharging the defibrillator with no circuit between the electrodes—i.e., they are held apart in the air. The high voltage that appears across the electrodes is dangerous to the person holding the electrodes. In addition, this practice places undue stress on the insulation. Discharging the defibrillator with the electrodes joined together will cause extremely high current to be delivered and will pit the electrodes. It may also damage the output relay by spot-welding the contacts or damage the solid-state device that controls delivery of the output.

A convenient method of testing the output of a defibrillator consists of discharging it into a 50-ohm power resistor (usually 100 watts or so). The voltage across the resistor can be measured with a storage oscilloscope, which will display the current waveform. A typical damped sine wave defibrillator will deliver a peak voltage of about 2500; therefore, the peak current flowing through the resistor is about 50 amps. It is not easy to calculate the delivered energy using this method because the calculation depends on whether this waveform is underdamped, critically damped, or overdamped.

Nonetheless, this technique will permit checking the ability of the defibrillator to deliver current, which should be the same each time the test is performed. Therefore, by keeping a log of the peak voltage for each test, any deterioration of the defibrillator can be identified as an inability to deliver the same peak voltage. This type of test is applicable to all defibrillators, and it is of value to log the duration of the current pulse.

Babbs et al.[75] presented an excellent method of determining the magnitude of the inductance, capacitance, and internal resistance of damped sine wave defibrillators without gaining access to the internal circuitry. By knowing the internal resistance ($R_t$), the percent energy delivered into a standard resistor (R) can be calculated as $100R/(R_t + R)$. The method is illustrated in Figure 17.21 and consists of measuring the output of the defibrillator as it is discharged into any two resistors that result in producing an underdamped sine wave. The measurements consist of determining the time (in sec) from the onset of the wave to the peak ($t_1$) and to the first zero-crossing ($t_2$), as illustrated. From these two times, two parameters â and ĉ are calculated for each value of resistance (R). Plots of â and ĉ versus R are constructed as shown in Figure 17.22. From the slope and intercept of the â versus R curve, the internal resistance

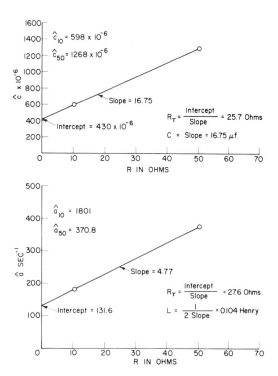

Fig. 17.22 The calculations for a typical defibrillator to which a 10- and 50-ohm resistor were connected; $t_1$ and $t_2$ were measured for each resistive load.

($R_t$) and inductance (L) can be calculated. From the slope and intercept of the ĉ versus R curve, the internal resistance ($R_t$) and capacitance (C) can be calculated. It is noteworthy that $R_t$ can be calculated from either plot.

Figure 17.22 illustrates the calculations for a typical defibrillator to which a 10- and 50-ohm resistor were connected, and $t_1$ and $t_2$ were measured for each resistive load. (In calculating â, the value obtained for the tangent is in radians.) For the defibrillator tested, the internal resistance was between 25.7 and 27.6 ohms; the inductance was 104 millihenries, and the capacitance was 16.75 microfarads. The plots of â and ĉ were obtained by measuring the time-to-peak and time-to-first-zero crossing using 50- and 10-ohm resistive loads connected to a damped sine wave defibrillator. From the plots of â and ĉ versus R, the slopes and intercepts are calculated, thereby providing the quantities for calculating the internal resistance, inductance, and capacitance. As shown from the test using a 10- and 50-ohm resistor, values for $t_1$

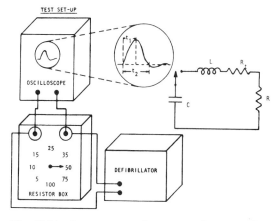

Fig. 17.21 Arrangement of apparatus for determining the internal resistance, inductance, and capacitance of a damped sine wave defibrillator. (Redrawn from Babbs et al: Med Instrum 1978, 12:34–37, 1978.)

and $t_2$ were obtained. From these, values for â and ĉ were calculated as follows:

$$\hat{a} = \frac{\pi}{t_2 \tan (\pi t_1 / t_2)}$$

$$\hat{c} = \frac{2\hat{a}}{\hat{a}^2 + (\pi / t_2)^2}$$

Performing these calculations provided the following:

| Test Resistor Ohms | Measured | | Calculated | |
|---|---|---|---|---|
| | $t_1$ ms. | $t_2$ ms. | â sec$^{-1}$ | ĉ $\times 10^{-6}$ |
| 10 | 1.77 | 4.16 | 180.1 | 598 |
| 50 | 1.58 | 4.64 | 370.8 | 1268 |

Figure 17.23 illustrates the circuit diagram of a typical trapezoidal-wave defibrillator. The energy-storage capacitor (C) is discharged by SCR 1, causing current to flow through the subject ($R_L$). Current flow is arrested by triggering SCR 2, which short-circuits the subject. Because of wiring, etc., the defibrillator has an internal series resistance ($R_s$). In order to provide effective operation of the SCR switches, a parallel resistance ($R_p$) is included. Thus, there are three important internal components in the trapezoidal-wave defibrillator: the energy-storage capacitor (C), the series ($R_s$), and parallel ($R_p$) resistances.

Babbs et al.[76] described a simple method for determining the internal components of trapezoidal-wave defibrillators. The method consists of discharging the defibrillator into various load resistors ($R_L$) and measuring the initial ($E_i$) and final ($E_f$) voltage and the duration (d) of the waveform. From the ratio of the initial ($E_i$) to final ($E_f$) voltage, the time constant ($\tau$) is calculated for each load resistor. The time constant

for open-circuit discharge ($\tau_\infty$) is also obtained. A plot of $\tau/(\tau_\infty - \tau)$ versus $R_L$ provides the information to calculate the internal series resistance ($R_s$) and the internal parallel ($R_p$) resistance. A second plot of time constant ($\tau$) versus the total equivalent internal resistance ($R_{eq}$) permits calculating the internal capacitance (C).

The method of testing a trapezoidal-wave defibrillator is best illustrated by the following example, in which the test just described was performed.

**Step 1.** The defibrillator is discharged into various load resistors $R_L$. The initial ($E_i$), final ($E_f$) voltages, and pulse duration (d) are measured on a storage oscilloscope. One trial is made with an open circuit, i.e. $R_L = \infty$. Table 17.2 illustrates the measured data.

**Step 2.** The time constant $\tau$ is calculated for each load resistance as follows: $\tau = d/\log E_i/E_f$. Then the magnitude of $\tau/(\tau_\infty - \tau)$ is calculated as shown in Table 17.2.

**Step 3.** A plot is made of $\tau/(\tau_\infty - \tau)$ versus $R_L$ as shown in Figure 17.24. From this plot, the slope and intercept are calculated as shown

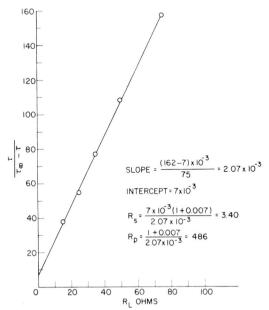

$$\text{SLOPE} = \frac{(162-7) \times 10^{-3}}{75} = 2.07 \times 10^{-3}$$

$$\text{INTERCEPT} = 7 \times 10^{-3}$$

$$R_s = \frac{7 \times 10^{-3}(1+0.007)}{2.07 \times 10^{-3}} = 3.40$$

$$R_p = \frac{1+0.007}{2.07 \times 10^{-3}} = 486$$

Fig. 17.24   Plot of $\tau/(\tau_\infty - \tau)$ versus different load resistors ($R_L$) used with a trapezoidal-wave defibrillator. From the slope and intercept, the internal series ($R_s$) and parallel ($R_p$) resistances can be calculated as shown.

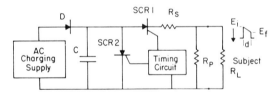

Fig. 17.23   The trapezoidal-wave defibrillator.

Table 17.2  Data for Calculating $R_p$ and $R_s$

| Measured Data | | | | | | Calculated Data | | |
|---|---|---|---|---|---|---|---|---|
| $R_L$ ohms | $E_1$ volts | $E_f$ volts | d msec | $\dfrac{E_i}{E_f}$ | $\ln \dfrac{E_i}{E_f}$ | $\tau$ msec | $\tau_\infty - \tau$ msec | $\dfrac{\tau}{\tau_\infty - \tau}$ |
| $\infty$ | 251 | 226 | 10 | 1.111 | 0.1053 | 94.970 | — | — |
| 75 | 240 | 113 | 10 | 2.124 | 0.7533 | 13.270 | 81.70 | 0.1620 |
| 50 | 236 | 81 | 10 | 2.914 | 1.0690 | 9.354 | 85.62 | 0.1090 |
| 35 | 230 | 55 | 10 | 4.182 | 1.4310 | 6.988 | 87.98 | 0.0794 |
| 25 | 221 | 32 | 10 | 6.906 | 1.9320 | 5.176 | 89.79 | 0.0576 |
| 15 | 210 | 12 | 10 | 17.500 | 2.8620 | 3.494 | 91.48 | 0.0382 |

in Figure 17.24. The internal series resistance ($R_s$) is calculated as follows:

$$R_s = \frac{\text{Intercept } (1 + \text{Intercept})}{\text{slope}} = 3.40 \text{ ohms}$$

Then the parallel resistance ($R_p$) is calculated as follows:

$$R_p = \frac{1 + \text{Intercept}}{\text{slope}} = 486 \text{ ohms}$$

**Step 4.** To determine C, the value of $R_{eq}$, the total effective resistance is calculated first as follows:

$$R_{eq} = R_s + (R_p R_L)/(R_p + R_L).$$

Table 17.3 presents the results of a typical calculation. A plot of $\tau$ versus $R_{eq}$ (Fig. 17.25) provides a line with a slope that is C, i.e.

$$C = \frac{\tau}{R_{eq}} = 194 \text{ microfarads.}$$

Note that this line passes through zero. In the example chosen, the capacitor in the defi-

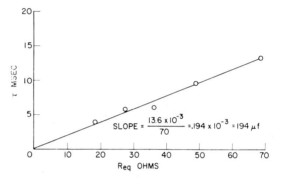

Fig. 17.25  Plot of $\tau$ versus the equivalent resistance ($R_{eq}$), from which its internal capacitance (C) is calculated as shown.

brillator was 200 $\mu f$, and the parallel resistor was 500 ohms.

## REFERENCES

1. Machin JW: Thoracic impedance of human subjects. Med Biol Eng & Comput 16:169–178, 1978.
2. Hoffa M, Ludwig C: Einige neue Versuche über Herzbewegung. Ztschr rat Med 9:107–144, 1850.
3. Ericksen JE: On the influence of the coronary circulation on the action of the heart. London Med Gazette 2:561–564, 1842.
4. Prevost JL, Battelli F: Death due to electric currents. Comptes Rendus Acad Sci 128:668–670, 1899.
5. Prevost JL, Battelli F: Some effects of electric discharge on the hearts of mammals. Comptes Rendus Acad de Sci 129:1267–1268, 1899.
6. Prevost JL, Battelli F: Some effects of electric discharge on the hearts of animals. Comptes Rendus Acad de Sci 129:1267–1268, 1899.
7. Hooker DR: On the recovery of the heart in electric shock. Am J Physiol 91:305–320, 1929.

Table 17.3  Data for Calculating C*

| $R_L$ | $R_{eq}$ | $\tau$ |
|---|---|---|
| ohms | ohms | msec |
| $\infty$ | — | — |
| 75 | 68.4 | 13.280 |
| 50 | 48.7 | 9.354 |
| 35 | 36.0 | 6.988 |
| 25 | 27.0 | 5.176 |
| 15 | 17.9 | 3.494 |

* $R_s = 3.40$, $R_p = 486$

8. Hooker DR: Chemical factors in ventricular fibrillation. Am J Physiol 92:639–647, 1930.

9. Wiggers CJ: Studies on ventricular fibrillation caused by electric shock. Revival of the heart from ventricular fibrillation by successive use of potassium and calcium salts. Am J Physiol 92:223, 1930.

10. Hooker DR, Kouwenhoven WB, Langworthy OR: The effect of alternating electrical current on the heart. Am J Physiol 102:444–454, 1933.

11. Kouwenhoven WB, Hooker RD: Resuscitation by countershock. Elect Engng 52:475–477, 1933.

12. Beck CS, Prilchard WH, Feil HS: Ventricular fibrillation of long duration abolished by electric shock. JAMA 135:985–986, 1947.

13. Zoll PM, Linenthal AJ, Gibson W, Paul M, Norman L: Termination of ventricular fibrillation in man by externally applied electric countershock. N Engl J Med 254:727–732, 1956.

14. Gurvich NL, Yuniev GS: Restoration of regular rhythm in the mammalian fibrillating heart. Amer Rev Soviet Med 3:236–239, 1946.

15. Gurvich, NL and Yuniev, GS: Restoration of heart rhythm during fibrillation by a condenser discharge. Am Rev Soviet Med 4:252–256, 1947.

16. MacKay RS, Leeds SE: Physiological effects of condenser discharge with application to tissue stimulation and ventricular defibrillation. J Appl Physiol 6(1):67–75, 1953.

17. Lown B, Amarasingham R, Newman J: New method for terminating cardiac arrhythmias. JAMA 182:548–555, 1962.

18. Lown B: A new method for terminating cardiac arrhythmias: the use of synchronized capacitor discharge. JAMA 182:566, 1962.

19. Edmark KW: Simultaneous voltage and current waveforms generated during internal and external direct current pulse defibrillation. Surgical Forum 14:262–264, 1963.

20. Edmark KW, Thomas GP, Jones TW: DC pulse defibrillation. J Thoracic and Cardiovasc Surg 51:326–333, 1966.

21. Schuder JC, Rahmoeller GA, Stoeckle H: Transthoracic ventricular defibrillation with triangular and trapezoidal waveforms. Circ Res 19:689–694, 1966.

22. Mines R: On dynamic equilibrium in the heart. J Physiol 46:344–383, 1913.

23. Garrey WE: The nature of fibrillary contractions of the heart—its relation to tissue mass and form. Am J Physiol 33:397–413, 1914.

24. MacWilliam JA: Fibrillar contractions of the heart. J Physiol 8:296–310, 1887.

25. Zipes D, Fischer J, King RM, Nicol AB, Jolly WW: Termination of ventricular fibrillation in dogs by depolarizing a critical mass of myocardium. Am J Cardiol 36:37–44, 1975.

26. Geddes LA, Tacker WA, Rosborough J, Moore AG, Cabler P, Bailey M, McCrady JD, Witzel D: The electrical dose for ventricular defibrillation with electrodes applied directly to the heart. J Thoracic Cardiovasc Surg 68:593–602, 1974.

27. Tacker WA, Rubio PA, Reeves LH, Korompai FL, Guinn GA: Low energy electrical defibrillation of human hearts during cardiac surgery. J Thor Cardiovasc Surg 68:603–605, 1974.

28. Koning G, Schneider H, Hoelen AJ, Reneman RS: Amplitude-duration relation for direct ventricular defibrillation with rectangular current pulses. Med Biol Engng (May):388–395, 1975.

29. Geddes LA, Tacker WA, Rosborough JP, Moore AG, Cabler P: Electrical dose for ventricular defibrillation of large and small animals with precordial electrodes. J Clin Invest 53:310–319, 1974.

30. Geddes LA, Bourland JD, Tacker WA: Energy and current requirements for ventricular defibrillation of dogs and ponies using trapezoidal waves. Am J Physiol Heart and Circulation, 238:231–236, 1980.

31. Gold JH, Schuder JC, Stoeckle H, Granberg TA, Dettmer JC, Schmidt DE: Scaling current and energy with body weight for the transthoracic ventricular defibrillation of calves as they grow from 50 to 150 kg. Circulation, 60:187–195, 1979.

32. Gold J, Schuder JC, Stoeckle H, Granberg TA, Hamdani SZ, and Rychlewski JM: Transthoracic ventricular defibrillation of the 100 kg calf with unidirectional rectangular pulses. Circulation 56:345–350, 1977.

33. Bourland JD, Tacker WA, Geddes LA: Strength-duration curves for trapezoidal waveforms of various tilts for transchest defibrillation in animals. Med Instrum 12:38–41, 1978.

34. Bourland JD, Tacker WA, Geddes LA, Chafee V: Comparative efficacy of damped sine wave and square wave current for transchest ventricular defibrillation in animals. Med Instrum 12:42–45, 1978.

35. Lown B: Cardioversion of arrhythmias. Mod Concepts Cardiovasc Dis 33:863–868, 1964.

36. Geddes LA, Grubbs SS, Wilcox P, Tacker WA: The thoracic windows for electrical ventricular defibrillation. Am Heart J 94:67–72, 1977.

37. Gutgesell H, Tacker WA, Geddes LA, Davis JS, Lie JT and McNamara D. Energy dose for ventricular defibrillation of children. Pediatrics 58(6):898–901, 1976.

38. Tacker WA, Galioto FM, Guiliani E, Geddes

LA, McNamara DG: Energy dosage for human transchest electrical ventricular defibrillation. N Engl J Med 290:214–215, 1974.

39. Collins RE, Guiliani ER, Tacker WA, Geddes LA: Transthoracic ventricular defibrillation: Success and body weight. Med Instrum 12:53, 1978.

40. Pantridge JF, Adgey AAJ, Geddes JS, Webb SW: The Acute Coronary Attack. New York, Grune and Stratton, 1975.

41. Pantridge JF, Adgey AAJ, Webb SW, Anderson J: Electrical requirements for ventricular defibrillation. Brit Med J 2:313–315, 1975.

42. Adgey AAJ, Campbell NPS, Webb SW, Kennedy AL, Pantridge JF: Transthoracic ventricular defibrillation in the adult. Med Instrum 12:17–19, 1978.

43. Crampton RS, Gascho JA, Cherwek ML, Sipes JN, Hunter FP: Low energy and fast serial dc shock ventricular defibrillation in man. Med Instrum 12:53, 1978.

44. Crampton RS, Cherwek ML, Gascho FA, Hunter FP: Efficacy of low energy and rapid sequency dc shock in human transthoracic ventricular defibrillation. Proc 12th AAMI Conf paper WAM-VI, 1977.

45. Schuder JC, Stoeckle H, Keskar PY, West J: Relationship between duration of ventricular fibrillation and effectiveness of therapeutic shock. Proc 25th AEMB 1972, paper 28.8.

46. Chambers W, Miles R, Stratbucker R: Human chest resistance during successive countershocks. Med Instrum 12:53, 1978.

47. Geddes LA, Tacker WA, Cabler P, Chapman R, Rivera R, Kidder H: The decrease in transthoracic impedance during successive ventricular defibrillation trials. Med Instrum 9:179–180, 1975.

48. Dahl CF, Ewy GA, Ewy MD, Thomas ED: Transthoracic impedance to direct current discharge: effect of repeated countershocks. Med Instrum 10:151–154, 1976.

49. Anderson GJ, Suelzer J: The efficacy of trapezoidal waveforms for ventricular defibrillation. Chest 70:298–300, 1976.

50. Tacker WA, Cole JS, Geddes LA: Clinical efficacy of a truncated exponential decay defibrillator. J Electrocardiol 9:273–274, 1976.

51. Yakaitis RW, Thomas JD, Mahaffey JE: Influence of pH and hypoxia on the successful defibrillation. Crit Care Med 3:139–142, 1975.

52. Lown B, Kleiger R, Williams J: Cardioversion and digitalis drugs; changed threshold to electric shock in digitalized animals. Circ Res 17:519–531, 1965.

53. Tacker WA, Geddes LA, Kline B, Burton C: Alteration of electrical defibrillation threshold by the cardiac glycoside, ouabain. Proc. 1st Purdue Cardiac Defib. Conf. 1975, Purdue University, Eng. Exp. Sta. Doc. #00147, Purdue University, West Lafayette, Indiana.

54. Babbs CF, Yim GKU, Whistler SJ, Tacker, WA, and Geddes LA: Elevation of ventricular defibrillation threshold in dogs by antiarrhythmic drugs. Am Heart J 98:345–350, 1979.

55. Tacker WA, Geddes LA, Cabler PS, Moore AG: Electrical threshold for defibrillation of canine ventricles following myocardial infarction. Am Heart J 88:476–481, 1974.

56. Resnekov L: Atrial defibrillation. Proc. 1st Purdue Cardiac Defibrillation Conf., 1975. Eng Exp Document No. 147, Purdue University, W. Lafayette, Indiana, 1975.

57. Lown B: Electrical reversal of cardiac arrhythmias. Brit Heart J 29:469–487, 1967.

58. Resnekov L: Direct current shock. In Cardiac Emergency Care. E. K. Chung, Ed., Philadelphia, Lea and Febiger, 1975.

59. Babbs CF, Tacker WA: Fundamental aspects of electrical ventricular defibrillation. J Cardiovasc Technol 20:88–98, 1978.

60. Peleska B: Cardiac arrhythmias following condenser discharge led through an inductance. Circ Res 16:11–18, 1965.

61. Dahl CF, Ewy GA, Warner ED, Thomas ED: Myocardial necrosis from direct current countershock. Circulation 50:956–961, 1974.

62. Dahl CF, Ewy GA, Warner ED, Thomas ED: Myocardial necrosis from direct current countershock. Circulation 50:956–961, 1974.

63. Warner ED, Dahl C, Ewy GA: Myocardial injury from transthoracic defibrillator countershock. Arch Pathol 99:55–59, 1975.

64. Davis JS, Lie JT, Bentinck DC, Titus JL, Tacker WA, Geddes LA: Cardiac damage due to electric current and energy. Proc Purdue 1st Cardiac Defibrillation Conference 1975, Eng. Exp. Sta. Document 147, Purdue University, West Lafayette, Indiana.

65. Tacker WA, Davis JS, Lie JT, Titus JL, Geddes LA: Cardiac damage produced by transchest damped sine wave shocks. Med Instrum 12:27–30, 1978.

66. Van Vleet JF, Tacker WA, Geddes LA, Ferrans VJ: Sequential cardiac morphologic alterations induced in dogs by single transthoracic damped sinusoidal waveform defibrillator shocks. Am J Vet Res 39:271–278, 1978.

67. Van Vleet JF, Tacker WA, Geddes LA, Farrans VJ: Acute cardiac damage in dogs given multiple

transthoracic shocks with a trapezoidal wave-form defibrillator. Am J Vet Res 38:617–626, 1977.

68. Ehsani A, Ewy GA, Sobel BE: Effects of electrical countershock on serum creatine phosphokinase isoenzyme activity. Am J Cardiol 37:12–18, 1976.

69. DiCola VC, Freedman GS, Downing SE, Zaret BL: Myocardial uptake of technetium-99m stannous pyrophosphate following direct current transthoracic shock. Circulation 54:980–986, 1976.

70. Schneider RM, Hayslett JP, Downing SE, Berger HJ, Donabedian RK, Zaret BL: Effect of methylprednisolone upon technetium pyrophosphate assessment of myocardiac necrosis in the canine countershock model. Circulation 56:1029–1034, 1977.

71. Babbs CF, Tacker WA, VanVleet JF, Bourland JD, and Geddes LA: Therapeutic index for defi-

brillation shocks. Effective, damaging, lethal electrical doses. Am Heart J, 99:734–738, 1980.

72. Resnekov L: High energy electrical current and myocardial damage. Med Instrum 12:24–26, 1978.

73. Corbitt JD, Sybers J, Levin JM: Muscle changes of the external chest wall secondary to electrical countershock. Am J Clin Path 51:107–112, 1969.

74. Lie JT, Davis JS, Tacker WA, Geddes LA: Histopathology and ultrastructure of myocardial injury caused by overdosed electrical defibrillation shocks. Am J Pathol 82:25a, 1976.

75. Babbs CF, Whistler SJ: Evaluation of the operating internal resistance, inductance and capacitance of intact damped sine wave defibrillators. Med Instrum 12:34–37, 1978.

76. Babbs CF, Whistler SJ, Geddes LA: Evaluation of the operating internal resistance and capacitance of intact trapezoidal waveform defibrillators. Med Instrum 14:67–69, 1980.

# 18 | Atrioventricular and Intraventricular Block in Patients with Acute Myocardial Infarction

*Melvin Scheinman, M.D.*
*Nora Goldschlager, M.D.*
*Robert Peters, M.D.*

A rational approach to the management of patients with acute myocardial infarction and atrioventricular or intraventricular block depends on an understanding of the blood supply to the specialized cardiac conduction system.

## THE ATRIOVENTRICULAR NODE

The atrioventricular node is an intra-atrial structure, located in the posteromedial area of the right atrium just anterior to the coronary sinus [1] (Fig. 18.1). Electrical impulses are relayed into the atrioventricular node via three internodal tracts, with the major electrical input proceeding via the anterior and middle internodal tracts; fibers [2] from the posterior internodal tract appear to end in "blind sacs" within the atrioventricular node.[3]

The atrioventricular node itself consists of interlacing whorls of fibers without apparent organization.[4] It is divided into three regions on the basis of both anatomic and electrophysiologic differences: the "AN" region is a transitional zone between working atrial muscle and atrioventricular nodal cells; the "N" region is the compact central compartment of the node; and the "NH" region is another transitional zone between atrioventricular nodal and His bundle cells.[5,6] The atrioventricular node is densely innervated by both sympathetic and parasympathetic fibers. Its blood supply is derived from the right coronary artery in approxi-

mately 85 to 90 percent of human hearts; in the remainder, it is derived from branches of the left circumflex coronary artery (Fig. 18.2).[7] Under normal circumstances, the atrioventricular node is seldom, if ever, supplied by the left anterior descending coronary artery. However, marked variations in atrioventricular nodal

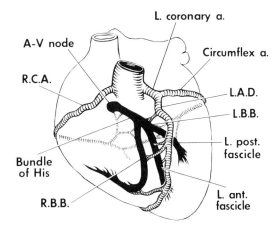

Fig. 18.1 The coronary blood supply to the specialized cardiac conduction system is detailed. The right coronary artery (RCA) travels in the right atrioventricular groove and carries the major blood supply to the atrioventricular node. Arterial branches from the RCA also supply the His bundle and proximal portion of the right bundle branch (RBB). The left anterior descending coronary artery (LAD) supplies the proximal bundle branches (RBBB, left anterior and posterior fascicles) while additional flow to the left posterior fascicle is derived from the left circumflex coronary artery.

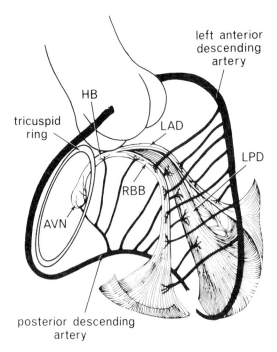

Fig. 18.2  More detailed view of the anatomic relationship of blood supply to the specialized cardiac
conduction system. The left anterior descending coronary artery is the major source of supply to proximal right bundle branch (RBB) and left anterior division (LAD) as well as the left posterior division
(LPD) of the left bundle branch.

blood supply may be present in patients with
coronary arterial occlusion, and collateral blood
supply may become the dominant source of
atrioventricular nodal blood flow. For example,
in a patient with proximal occlusion of the right
coronary artery, the posterior descending
branch of the right coronary artery system (and
thus also the atrioventricular node) may be fed
by collateral vessels derived from the left anterior descending coronary artery that course
around the apex of the heart.

## VENTRICULAR SPECIALIZED
## CONDUCTION SYSTEM

The ventricular specialized conduction system is comprised of the common and branching
portions of the bundle of His, the right and
left bundle branches, and the fascicular radia-

tions (or "divisions") of these bundle branches
(Fig. 18.1).

The His bundle serves to connect the atrial
and ventricular conduction systems and is the
continuation of the atrioventricular node. Although the atrioventricular node and His bundle are not clearly separable from each other
grossly, the fibers of the His bundle are generally orderly and parallel, in contrast to the interlacing network of the atrioventricular nodal
cells. The more distal portion of the His bundle
is organized into longitudinal columns (fascicles) separated by collagen septa.[8] The His
bundle consists of three portions: prepenetrat-
ing, penetrating, and branching. The penetrating portion of the His bundle passes through
the fibrous atrioventricular ring at the level of
the central fibrous body, at which point it lies
at the posteroinferior border of the membranous portion of the interventricular septum in
proximity to the noncoronary cusp of the aortic
valve; it then continues anteriorly just below
the membranous septum. In most instances, the
His bundle courses down the left side of the
interventricular septum, although it is occasionally found on the right side of the septum.[9]
"Branching" of the His bundle into the "divisions" or "fascicles" of the left bundle branch
occurs in this area of the membranous septum.
After the fibers of the left bundle branch have
been given off, the His bundle continues as the
right bundle branch. The length of the His bundle ranges from approximately 10 to 20 mm,
and its width from 1 to 2 mm,[10] if it is considered to begin at the central fibrous body and
end at the distal point of division of the bundle
branches.

Blood supply to the His bundle is almost always dual, arising from the atrioventricular nodal branch of the right coronary artery and
the septal perforator branch of the left anterior
descending coronary artery (Fig. 18.2). It is unusual for the left anterior descending coronary
artery alone to supply the bundle of His. Extensive intercoronary and intracoronary collateral
networks are present within the His bundle,
an important anatomical consideration in the
assessment of infranodal conduction blocks developing in the course of myocardial infarction.

## THE RIGHT BUNDLE BRANCH

The right bundle branch is the continuation of the His bundle (Fig. 18.1). It arises distal to the septal leaflet of the tricuspid valve and is about 40 to 50 mm in length and 1 to 2 mm in width. The right bundle branch resembles a nonpartitioned cylindrical conduit of fibers.[11] Three portions of the right bundle branch have been recognized: the first, located proximal to the area of origin of the fibers of the left bundle branch, is subendocardial and is related to the membranous portion of the interventricular septum; the second is intramyocardial, coursing within the interventricular septum; and the third is again subendocardial, coursing anteriorly from the interventricular septum toward the base of anterior papillary muscle of the right ventricle. The fascicles of the right bundle branch originate distally, near the anterior right ventricular papillary muscle, in contrast to those of the left bundle branch which have a much more proximal origination.

Blood supply to the right bundle branch is dual (Fig. 18.2). Branches of the atrioventricular nodal artery of the right coronary artery supply the first portion, and septal perforator branches of the left anterior descending coronary artery supply the second and third portions. Recognition of right coronary arterial blood supply to the proximal portion of the right bundle branch is extremely important, as patients who develop right bundle branch block in the course of inferior wall myocardial infarction would not be expected to have the same prognosis as those developing right bundle branch block with anterior myocardial infarction (see below).

## THE LEFT BUNDLE BRANCH

The left bundle branch is not, strictly speaking, a branch at all, but is a fan-like structure that extends from the common bundle of His in almost perpendicular fashion for 5 to 15 mm (Fig 18.2). Its fibers resemble those of the distal bundle of His.[11] Recent studies suggest that fibers destined for the left bundle branch may

in fact originate within the His bundle, as lesions experimentally produced in the non-branching (penetrating) portion of the common bundle of His result in conduction disturbances electrocardiographically indistinguishable from left bundle branch block.[12]

The wide left bundle branch radiates from the left side of the interventricular septum. At its area of origin, the left bundle branch lies in relation to the right and noncoronary cusps of the aortic valve. Calcification involving the aortic valve cusps and/or annulus may extend into this area of the interventricular septum producing conduction delay or block in the His bundle and left bundle branch (Lev's disease).[13]

The existence of discrete fascicles or divisions of the left bundle branch (anterior, posterior, and medial or septal), originally put forth in the late 1960s and early 1970s,[14-17] is a clinically and electrophysiologically useful concept, although its morphologic validation is controversial.[9] Within this conceptual framework, the fibers of the shorter, broader fascicle arise from the proximal portion of the left bundle branch; this fascicle appears to be the continuation of the left bundle branch. The posterior radiation courses away from the subaortic valve area and interventricular septum, posteriorly and inferiorly toward the posterior papillary muscle of the left ventricle, where branching into the peripheral Purkinje network occurs. The fibers of the longer, thinner anterior fascicle leave the left bundle branch more distally and course across the left ventricular outflow tract toward the anterior papillary muscle of the left ventricle. The septal, or medial, fascicle of the left bundle branch may originate from the left bundle branch as a discrete fascicle like the posterior and anterior divisions, or from either one of these fascicles; in some instances, a discrete septal fascicle is not readily demonstrable, and numerous rami resembling a plexus serve to connect the posterior and anterior fascicles.[15-17] The fibers of the left bundle branch all interlace peripherally, whether or not a discrete septal fascicle is present. As the left bundle branch consists of three fascicles, and not two, it is more accurate to consider the ventricular specialized conduction system as quadrifascicular rather than trifascicular in nature. As the radiations of the left bundle branch vary substantially with regard to size, shape, and area of origin, precise clinicopathologic correlations are precluded.

The blood supply to the predivisional portion and the posterior fascicle of the left bundle branch is usually derived from vessels arising from both anterior and posterior descending coronary arteries; however, blood supply from the atrioventricular nodal branch of the right coronary artery alone, and from the septal perforator branch of the left anterior descending coronary artery alone, has been demonstrated (Fig. 18.2). Blood supply to the anterior fascicle is usually derived from septal perforator branches of the left anterior descending coronary artery.

## ELECTROCARDIOGRAPHIC RECOGNITION OF FASCICULAR BLOCK

In the setting of acute myocardial infarction, consideration of the site of infarction, pattern of atrioventricular conduction disturbance, and QRS morphology usually allow for accurate localization of the site of atrioventricular block as well as the involved coronary artery. Electrocardiographic criteria for the identification of divisional or fascicular block in the ventricular specialized conduction system have recently been proposed,[18] and their recognition is of considerable importance in the evaluation of patients with acute myocardial infarction. Such recognition of fascicular block patterns depends on an understanding of the normal sequence of ventricular activation.

Ventricular activation normally begins in the area of left septal surface and proceeds rightward, anteriorly and inferiorly, toward the anterior papillary muscle of the right ventricle. Depolarization of the free walls of the ventricles then occurs; the right ventricle, being of smaller mass and thus generating smaller forces, contributes little to the mean QRS vector. Finally, the base of the heart is activated.

It is now recognized that conduction delay or block produced experimentally in the right bundle branch and in the anterior and posterior fascicles of the left bundle branch may result in rather specific and often reproducible electrocardiographic patterns.[19-22] Electrocardiographic patterns that resemble those resulting from section of fascicles in the experimental setting but that occur in the clinical setting have been accepted as reflecting fascicular "block." Less certain, and still largely unexplored experimentally, are the possible electrocardiographic patterns resulting from conduction delay or block in the left septal fascicle of the left bundle branch; observations based on clinical electrocardiograms are therefore theoretical and conjectural. The following discussion of the electrocardiographic recognition of fascicular block assumes that intraventricular conduction system is quadrifascicular in nature.

The electrocardiographic pattern of conduction delay in the right bundle branch consists of QRS duration prolonged to or beyond 0.12 seconds, a wide s wave in leads I, aVL, and $V_5$–$V_6$ and a late r' or R' in leads aVR and $V_1$ (Fig. 18.3). Abnormal deviation of the frontal plane QRS vector is not a feature of isolated right bundle branch block, and the calculation of mean frontal plane QRS axis should discount the terminal conduction delay. The electrocardiographic pattern of right bundle branch block does not necessarily reflect disease of the proximal ventricular specialized conduction system, but may be a manifestation of myocardial disease and/or disease of the distal right ventricular Purkinje network, or right ventriculotomy.[23]

Conduction delay in the predivisional portion of the left bundle branch (or equal delay in both anterior and posterior fascicles of the left bundle branch) produces a QRS complex of duration equal to or exceeding 0.12 seconds, and delayed intrinsicoid deflections in leads I, aVL, and $V_4$–$V_6$[24] (Fig. 18.4). It does not by itself result in abnormal deviation of the frontal plane QRS axis, although some leftward axis deviation may occur.[14] As normal left-to-right activation of the interventricular septum does not occur in left bundle branch block, the small q wave in the anterolateral leads, reflecting normal left-to-right septal depolarization, is not present in left bundle branch block (Fig. 18.4);

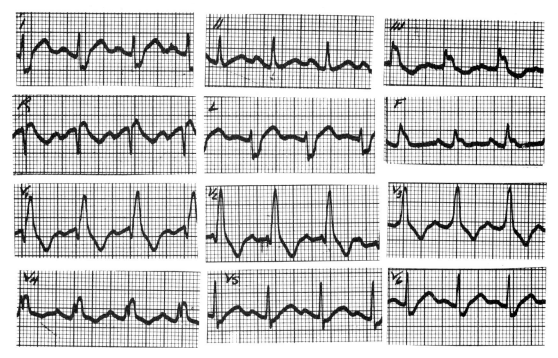

Fig. 18.3 The rhythm is sinus at a rate of 100/min and the PR interval is within the limits of normal (0.19 sec). An intraventricular conduction delay is present, indicated by the wide QRS duration of 0.13 sec. The mean frontal plane QRS axis is about +75°. The electrocardiographic diagnosis of right bundle branch block is established by the delayed R′ wave in Leads aVR, $V_1$, and $V_2$ and by the wide s wave in leads I, aVL, and $V_6$.

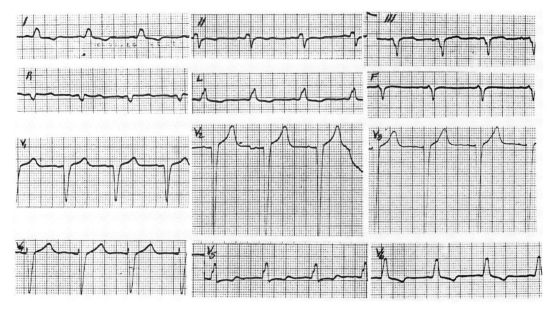

Fig. 18.4 Sinus rhythm is present at a rate of 65/min, and the PR interval is normal. The QRS duration is prolonged at 0.12 sec, and the QRS configuration indicates left bundle branch block, manifested by broad notched complexes over the left ventricular leads I, aVL, $V_5$, and $V_6$. The mean frontal plane QRS axis is about −30°. Because ventricular depolarization is abnormal, ventricular repolarization is also abnormal, and the ST-T wave abnormalities seen in this figure are secondary to the intraventricular conduction defect. The large QRS voltages may also reflect abnormal ventricular depolarization, although left ventricular hypertrophy cannot be excluded with certainty.

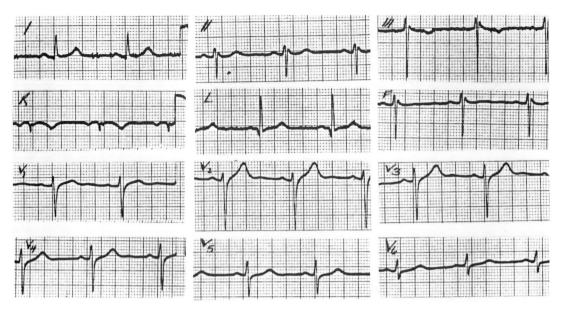

Fig. 18.5 Sinus rhythm is present at a rate of about 59/min, and the PR interval is 0.16 sec. The QRS duration is normal (0.08 sec). The mean frontal plane QRS axis is markedly superior and leftward at about −75°, reflecting left anterior fascicular block. The small q wave in leads I and aVL reflect early ventricular activation occurring in a rightward and inferior direction. The s wave seen in leads $V_5$ and $V_6$ and the abnormal R:S ratio in the lateral precordial leads reflect late leftward and superior ventricular activation rather than lateral wall myocardial infarction.

its existence has been considered to indicate infarction of the interventricular septum.

Conduction delay or block involving the anterior fascicle or the left bundle branch results in early ventricular activation proceeding inferiorly and posteriorly, and late ventricular activation proceeding anteriorly and superiorly (Fig. 18.5). This sequence of ventricular activation results in the inscription of an r wave in leads II, III, and aVF, and a q wave in leads I and aVL, although the latter finding is variable and not essential to the diagnosis.[25] The early infero-posterior activation of the left ventricle may mask Q waves of recent or remote inferior myocardial infarction and may suggest the presence of lateral infarction. Late leftward and superior ventricular activation produces leftward axis deviation (≥ 30 degrees) in the frontal plane and tall QRS voltage in leads I and aVL; in the horizontal plane, a small q wave (but not a QS wave) in leads $V_1$–$V_3$ and a narrow s wave in leads $V_5$ and $V_6$ may be inscribed due to inferiorly and posteriorly directed forces (Fig. 18.5).[26] As left anterior fascicular block per se may produce large QRS voltage in the limb

leads, the electrocardiographic diagnosis of left ventricular hypertrophy using standard limb lead criteria alone is precluded. The q waves produced in the anterolateral leads by left anterior fascicular block do not meet electrocardiographic criteria for infarction Q waves (≥ 0.04 seconds in duration or 25 percent of the height of the R wave). The small q waves in Leads $V_1$–$V_3$, being due to inferiorly and posteriorly directed forces,[27] will not be seen if these leads are recorded one interspace lower. Left anterior fascicular block does not prolong the QRS duration by more than about 20 msec; therefore, if abnormal left axis deviation is the only electrocardiographic abnormality, the QRS complex should be normal in duration or only minimally prolonged. If, in addition to superior axis deviation, wide QRS complexes are present, conditions such as left ventricular hypertrophy, myocardial disease, or additional conduction delay in the left bundle branch may be present.

The acute development of left anterior fascicular block almost always occurs in the setting of acute anterior wall myocardial infarction, with ischemia in the areas supplied by the left anterior descending coronary artery. The occurrence of left anterior fascicular block requires no specific therapy, but as its development may presage further necrosis of the proximal bundle branches and development of atrioventricular block, careful observation is warranted.

Conduction delay or block in the posterior fascicle of the left bundle branch results in initial ventricular activation proceeding leftward, anteriorly and superiorly, and late ventricular activation proceeding inferiorly and posteriorly, resulting in the inscription of an rS wave in leads I and aVL, and a tall R wave in leads II, III, and aVF (Fig. 18.6). The rS configuration in the lateral leads may mask the Q wave of recent or remote infarction, and the inscription of the q wave in the inferior leads may suggest inferior myocardial infarction, although neither its magnitude nor its duration meet criteria for Q waves of infarction. Because later ventricular activation proceeds inferiorly and posteriorly, the mean QRS axis in the frontal plane is rightward ($\geq$ 90 degrees) (Fig. 18.6). Although rightward axis deviation is an electro-

cardiographic requirement of left posterior fascicular block, more common causes—such as right ventricular hypertrophy of any etiology, chronic obstructive pulmonary disease, and lateral wall myocardial infarction—must be excluded before the diagnosis of left posterior fascicular block may be entertained.

The uncommon general occurrence of isolated conduction delay in the posterior fascicle of the left bundle branch reflects the relationship of this fascicle to the low pressure inflow tract of the left ventricle and its dual blood supply. Similarly, left posterior fascicular block is a relatively rare complication in patients with acute myocardial infarction.

The electrocardiographic pattern reflecting conduction delay in the septal fascicle of the left bundle branch is not well defined, although prominent anterior forces, absence of septal q waves, and appearance of q waves in the right precordial leads have all been described as being theoretically compatible with this diagnosis.[25,28,29] The usual underlying cardiac conditions in patients with the proposed electro-

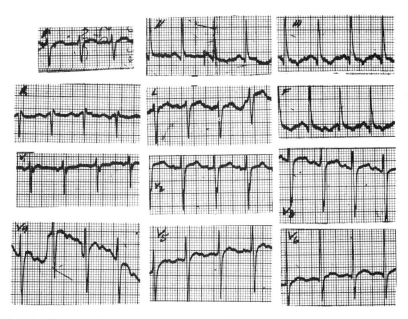

Fig. 18.6 In this 62-year-old man admitted to the CCU, sinus rhythm is present at a rate of 110/min and the PR interval is normal. The QRS duration is normal at 0.10 sec. The mean frontal plane QRS axis is abnormally rightward at about +110°. The rightward axis deviation and the qR pattern in leads II, III, and aVF may be attributed to left posterior fascicular block. Note that a slight right ventricular conduction delay is also present (r' in Leads aVR and V$_1$ with slurring of the s wave in leads I, aVL, and V$_6$).

cardiographic abnormalities in left septal fascicular block include ischemic heart disease, papillary muscle dysfunction, and hypertrophic cardiomyopathy, conditions no different from those in patients with conduction abnormalities in other fascicles.

Equal conduction delay in both anterior and posterior fascicles of the left bundle branch is manifested in the electrocardiogram as a left bundle branch block pattern and is indistinguishable from conduction delay in the predivisional portion of the left bundle branch. On the other hand, concomitant conduction delays in the right bundle branch and either fascicle of the left bundle branch have specific associated electrocardiographic patterns in which the general configuration of right bundle branch is preserved. When left anterior fascicular block is superimposed upon right bundle branch block, a leftward axis deviation and rS wave in Leads II, III and aVF will be present (Fig. 18.7); when left posterior fascicular block is su-

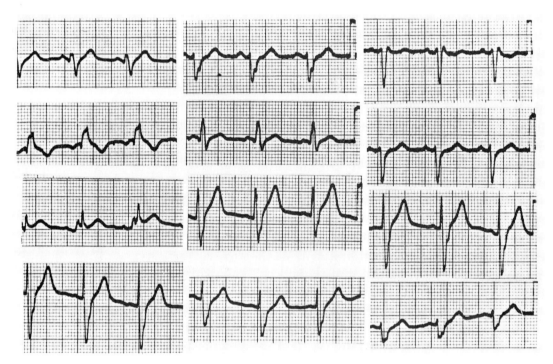

Fig. 18.7   Sinus rhythm is present at a rate of 84/min, and the PR interval is normal. The QRS duration is prolonged at 0.13 sec. The "unblocked" (reflecting left ventricular events and ignoring the terminal right ventricular conduction delay) mean frontal plane QRS axis is leftward at about −65°, indicating left anterior fascicular block. Small q waves are present in Leads I and aVL. Right bundle branch block is indicated by the wide R' wave in leads aVR and $V_1$, and by the wide S wave in leads I, aVL, $V_5$, and $V_6$. Note that the terminal conduction delay may be seen in lead II as a broad S wave; failure to recognize the contribution of the terminal conduction delay to the QRS morphology in lead II may result in improper calculation of the mean frontal plane QRS axis.

Fig. 18.8   This 79-year-old man was admitted to the CCU with severe chest pain and cardiogenic shock associated with anterior wall myocardial infarction. The admission electrocardiogram (A) shows an intraventricular conduction delay involving both the left anterior fascicle and the right bundle branch. The markedly prolonged duration of the QRS complex of about 0.16 sec suggests additional myocardial disease. The ECG recorded two days later (B), when the patient had improved somewhat, shows virtual disappearance of the right bundle branch block pattern and persistence of the left fascicular block. The mean frontal plane QRS axis is somewhat less leftward, and the QRS duration has shortened to about 0.13 sec with a left bundle branch block pattern. This sequence of events is compatible with involvement of both bundle branches. The PR interval remained normal.

A

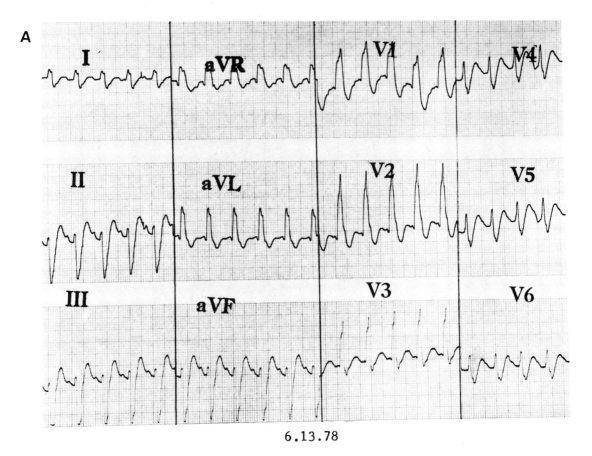

6.13.78

B

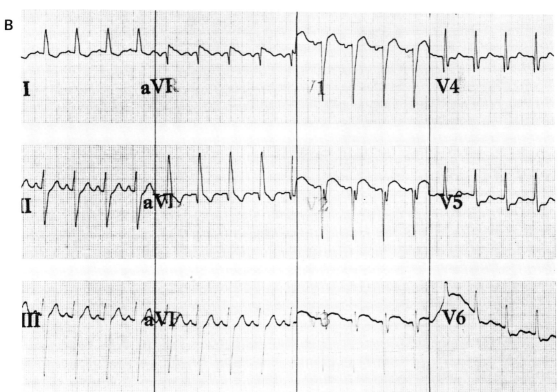

6.15.78

perimposed, rightward axis deviation and a qR wave in leads II, III and aVF occur. The presence of right bundle branch block, representing terminal intraventricular conduction delay, does not interfere with the early vectors of ventricular depolarization and thus does not mask left ventricular events, including conduction abnormalities and infarction patterns.

Because of anatomic relationships and specific blood supplies, bifascicular block most commonly involves the right bundle branch and the anterior fascicle of the left bundle branch, with less common involvement of the right and left posterior fascicles. It should be emphasized that conduction delay or block may occur in the proximal portion of a fascicle or may result from a more widespread process affecting many fibers of the more distal Purkinje network (Figs. 18.8A, B). The actual site of conduction delay, therefore, cannot be determined with certainty from the surface electrocardiogram.

Knowledge of both the relationship of blood supply to the ventricular specialized conduction system and the electrocardiographic diagnosis of fascicular block patterns aids the clinician in understanding the natural history of atrioventricular block occurring in the setting of acute infarction, and in the construction of a rational treatment plan.

## NATURAL HISTORY AND TREATMENT OF ATRIOVENTRICULAR AND INTRAVENTRICULAR CONDUCTION DISTURBANCES IN PATIENTS WITH ACUTE MYOCARDIAL INFARCTION

### Atrioventricular Nodal Block

**Pathogenesis.** The right coronary artery supplies the diaphragmatic surface of the left ventricle and most of the right ventricle. The atrioventricular node is nourished by the right coronary artery in the majority of subjects. Occlusion of the right coronary artery is associated with inferior wall myocardial infarction, and the atrioventricular block occurring in these patients is almost always localized to the atrioventricular node.[30] Atrioventricular nodal

block may be due to the effects of ischemia per se rather than necrosis, as postmortem studies in these subjects often show no evidence of atrioventricular nodal necrosis.[31,32] Another cause of atrioventricular block is an increase in vagal tone, which may be mediated by cholinergic ganglia near the atrioventricular node.[33] This type of atrioventricular block is occasionally seen during the course of inferior myocardial infarction, and intravenous atropine results in normalization of atrioventricular conduction.[34] Still another possible cause of atrioventricular block in patients with inferior myocardial infarction is regional atrioventricular nodal hyperkalemia; recent observations during experimental myocardial infarction suggest that an increased concentration of potassium in the lymphatic system draining the inferior left ventricular wall after occlusion of the right coronary artery may lead to impaired atrioventricular nodal conduction as the lymphatic channels travel in close proximity to the atrioventricular node.[35]

### Clinical Manifestations of Atrioventricular Block in Patients with Inferior Myocardial Infarction

Patients with atrioventricular nodal block may present with simple prolongation of the PR interval, Type I (Wenckebach) second-degree atrioventricular block, or complete atrioventricular block. Atrioventricular block is an early complication of inferior infarction, generally occurring within the first 72 hours and seldom after the first week.[36] The atrioventricular block is transient and almost always disappears within one week of onset.[37,38] In exceptional instances, the atrioventricular block may persist for up to three weeks, and in very rare instances chronic complete atrioventricular block may occur. Although some patients with inferior myocardial infarction may present with complete atrioventricular block, the sequence of events usually observed is serial development of first degree, Type I second degree, and finally third degree atrioventricular block. Type I (Wenckebach) second degree atrioventricular

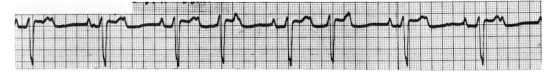

Fig. 18.9 MCL1 rhythm strip recorded in a patient with acute myocardial infarction. Sinus rhythm at a rate of 92/min is present. Type I (Wenckebach) second-degree AV block is present with atrioventricular conduction ratios of 2:1 and 3:2. The QRS complex has a duration of 0.13 sec, and its configuration suggests a left bundle branch block pattern. In patients with atrioventricular Wenckebach conduction and narrow QRS the site of conduction delay is almost always at the level of the atrioventricular node. In contrast, atrioventricular Wenckebach conduction in patients with bundle branch block may be occurring in the atrioventricular node, within the His bundle, or within the fascicles. Precise localization of the site of block cannot be determined from the surface electrocardiogram alone, and His bundle electrography is required.

block (Fig. 18.9) is characterized by gradual prolongation of the PR interval proximate to the nonconducted sinus impulse. The occurrence of this pattern of atrioventricular conduction in patients with inferior wall myocardial infarction and normal QRS duration strongly suggests that the site of atrioventricular block is within the atrioventricular node.[39] Similarly, complete atrioventricular block in this clinical setting is expected to be manifested by a ventricular pacemaker with normal QRS duration and with a discharge rate of 50 to 60 per minute.[40] The overall mortality rate for patients with inferior myocardial infarction and atrioventricular conduction disturbances is similar to that in patients with inferior myocardial infarction and normal atrioventricular conduction.[41]

## Treatment of Atrioventricular Block in Patients with Inferior Myocardial Infarction

Treatment of atrioventricular block in the setting of acute myocardial infarction depends primarily on the patient's hemodynamic status. First-degree atrioventricular block requires no specific therapy. If Type I second-degree atrioventricular block or even complete atrioventricular block are associated with a reasonable ventricular rate and no evidence of hemodynamic deterioration or serious ventricular arrhythmias, no specific treatment is required.

Pharmacologic therapy is indicated, however, in the presence of congestive heart failure and/or ventricular arrhythmias. The initial approach to the bradycardia-related impairment in hemodynamic function is use of an intravenous bolus injection of 0.5 mg of atropine, with repeat injection of 0.5 mg if no response is observed. Adverse effects of intravenous atropine, including sinus tachycardia, ventricular tachycardia, and other toxic manifestations of vagolysis are more common if doses exceeding 2.5 mg are administered within the first two to three hours.[34] If intravenous atropine is not effective in increasing the ventricular rate, low-dose isoproterenol (1–2 μg/min) may be used.[39] Isoproterenol is not recommended in patients with ventricular irritability. If augmentation of heart rate is deemed advisable and cannot be safely achieved by pharmacologic means, temporary transvenous pacing is indicated (see below).

## Atrioventricular and Intraventricular Block in Patients with Acute Anterior Myocardial Infarction

Atrioventricular block complicating acute anterior wall myocardial infarction represents a very different problem from inferior wall myocardial infarction. Most of the anterior wall of the left ventricle, interventricular septum, and proximal bundle branches receive their blood supply from the left anterior descending coronary artery system.[7] Thus, atrioventricular block occurring in this clinical setting reflects substantial necrosis of ventricular myocardium together with fibers of the ventricular specialized conduction system. Atrioventricular block developing during anterior wall infarction is often sudden and occurs without warning. It is associated with dire consequences, as the emerging subjunctional pacemaker is frequently unstable, has a very slow automatic rate, and is usually unresponsive to vagal influences.

First degree atrioventricular block with a narrow QRS complex occurring during anterior myocardial infarction warrants only close observation. Second degree atrioventricular block

in this setting is usually manifested by abrupt failure of atrioventricular conduction in which the nonconducted sinus impulse is preceded by a constant PR interval (Type II [Mobitz II] block). Type II second-degree atrioventricular block, even if it occurs only rarely during the course of anterior wall myocardial infarction, should be considered sufficient indication for immediate temporary transvenous pacing. Care should be taken not to mistake nonconducted premature atrial impulses or vagally induced nonconducted sinus impulses (characterized by simultaneous slowing of sinus rate and atrioventricular block) for true Type II second-degree atrioventricular block, since these rhythm dis-

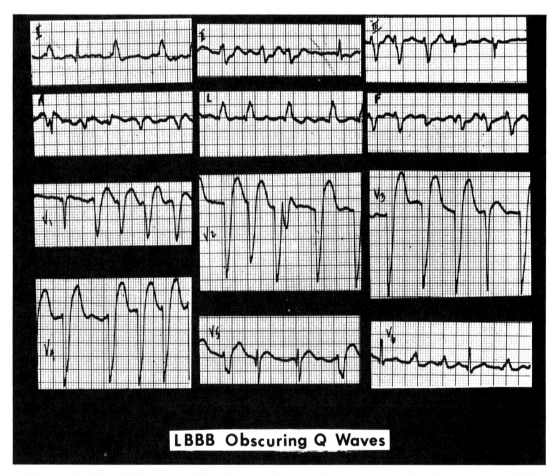

LBBB Obscuring Q Waves

Fig. 18.10   12-lead ECG recorded in a 70-year-old man with severe chest pain admitted to the CCU. The rhythm is atrial fibrillation with a moderately rapid ventricular response. Some QRS complexes are of normal duration and some show a left bundle branch block pattern. The q waves seen in the QRS complexes of normal duration are diagnostic of anterolateral infarction (in leads I, $V_5$, and $V_6$); they are completely masked in those QRS complexes showing left bundle branch block.

Atrioventricular and Intraventricular Block

turbances have a benign prognosis and usually warrant no specific therapy.[42] Patients with anterior myocardial infarction who develop complete atrioventricular block should also undergo prompt temporary transvenous cardiac pacing. In this emergency situation, it is appropriate to use an intravenous isoproterenol infusion in order to maintain an adequate heart rate while preparing for the pacemaker insertion.

It has long been appreciated that atrioventricular block occurring during anterior myocardial infarction is associated with a marked increase in mortality with the majority of deaths being due to severe pump failure rather than to ventricular arrhythmias; nevertheless, recent multicenter cooperative studies have suggested that an improvement in survival may eventuate with the use of a pacemaker.[43,44] While the site of atrioventricular block can usually be predicted on the basis of the site of infarction, the pattern of atrioventricular block, and the duration of the emerging QRS complex, at times the correct localization of the site of block (and hence appropriate therapy) may be uncertain on the basis of the surface electrocardiographic recordings. For example, the site of atrioventricular block that occurs in patients with left bundle branch block, in whom the area of infarction may be obscured by the conduction disturbance, may not be correctly ascertained (Fig. 18.10); and Type I (Wenckebach) second degree atrioventricular block developing in patients with bundle branch block may be occurring in the His-Purkinje system thus indicating severe infranodal pathology (Fig. 18.9). In the latter example, His bundle recordings may be of value in precisely localizing the site of the atrioventricular conduction disturbance and dictating the most appropriate mode of therapy.[45]

## Bundle Branch Block and Acute Myocardial Infarction

The role of pacemaker therapy in patients developing bundle branch block during acute myocardial infarction is still somewhat controversial.[46-48] As the proximal bundle branches receive much of their blood supply

from the left anterior descending coronary artery system, the majority of patients developing acute bundle branch block have *anterior* wall infarction. However, as the right coronary artery system often supplies the proximal portion of the right bundle branch as well as the diaphragmatic surface of the heart, acute right bundle branch block may develop during inferior wall myocardial infarction; in this circumstance, atrioventricular conduction defects may be associated with a more benign prognosis, similar to that observed in patients with inferior myocardial infarction without conduction disturbances.

Patients developing unifascicular block may also have a benign course. In one recent report, only three of 75 patients with isolated left anterior fascicular block and none of 14 with isolated left posterior fascicular block progressed to high grade atrioventricular block.[46]

A recently completed multicenter study has helped clarify the role of temporary pacing in patients with acute myocardial infarction and intraventricular conduction defects.[43,44] Of 432 patients with acute myocardial infarction and bundle branch block, 22 percent developed high-degree atrioventricular block (Type II second- or third-degree atrioventricular block progressing from a Type II conduction disturbance)(Table 18.1). Among the factors which predisposed the development of high degree atrioventricular block were bifascicular block, first degree atrioventricular block, or a new or indeterminate onset of the intraventricular conduction defect (Table 18.1). Thus, prophylactic pacemaker insertion seems justified in these circumstances. Of particular note was the occurrence or progression of atrioventricular block in the absence of significant left ventricular failure in 37 percent of 95 patients; 15 of these patients died due to the abruptness of the onset of high-grade atrioventricular block.

The role of intracardiac electrophysiologic studies in the evaluation of patients with acute myocardial infarction and intraventricular conduction defects, although promising, has not yet been fully established. Good correlation between abnormalities in infranodal conduction time and subsequent progression to high-grade atrioventricular block and overall mortality in

Table 18.1    Incidence and Risk of In-Hospital Progression to High-Grade Atrioventricular Block in 432 Patients with
Acute Myocardial Infarction and Bundle Branch Block*

| Type of Block | No. Patients | Progression to High Degree Block** |
|---|---|---|
| Left bundle branch block | 163 | 13% |
| Right bundle branch block | 48 | 14% |
| Right bundle branch block + left anterior fascicular block | 149 | 27% |
| Right bundle branch block + left posterior fascicular block | 45 | 29% |
| Alternating bundle branch block | 27 | 44% |
| New bifascicular block | 36 | 31% |
| New bundle branch block + first degree atrioventricular block | 12 | 19% |
| First degree atrioventricular block + new bilateral bundle branch block | 26 | 38% |

\* Adapted from Hindman et al.[43,44]
\*\* Type II second degree or third degree atrioventricular block progressing from a Type II conduction disturbance.

patients with right bundle branch block has been found,[49] suggesting that systematic study of such patients may be prognostically useful.

In this connection, it has been found that the commonly used antiarrhythmic drugs (lidocaine and/or quinidine, procainamide, digoxin, propranolol, or disopyramide) do not adversely affect atrioventricular conduction in patients with acute infarction who have a normal QRS and either normal, first-degree or Mobitz I atrioventricular block. Moreover, no subset of patients grouped by infarct location, specific antiarrhythmic agent used, or bundle branch block (except perhaps those with newly acquired bundle branch block) appear to be at risk of developing atrioventricular block during antiarrhythmic therapy.[49a]

## TECHNIQUE OF TEMPORARY PACEMAKER INSERTION

### Equipment

**Pacing Catheters.** There are two general types of bipolar pacing catheters available: floating and nonfloating. The floating (or flow-directed) type of electrode catheter is very thin and flexible and has a small inflatable balloon near the tip to facilitate its advancement into the right ventricle. The nonfloating pacing catheter is thicker and more rigid; it is best inserted with fluoroscopic guidance using an image intensifier.

**Pulse Generators.** Several types of pulse generators are available for temporary pacing. All have similar design, consisting of electrode terminals that connect to the pacing catheter wires and mechanisms or control switches by which pacing rate, current output, and sensing of intracardiac electrical signals may be adjusted.

**Defibrillator.** A standard defibrillator should be available at the time of pacemaker insertion because of the possibility of initiating ventricular dysrhythmias. Such dysrhythmias may result from premature ventricular complexes due to mechanical contact of the pacing catheter or from delivery of a pacing stimulus during the vulnerable period of the ventricle (Fig. 18.11).

### Means of Electrode Catheter Insertion

Transvenous pacemakers may be inserted from almost any vein, although antecubital, femoral, internal jugular or subclavian veins are used most frequently. Each of these approaches has advantages and disadvantages, and it is advisable to use the route with which one is most familiar.

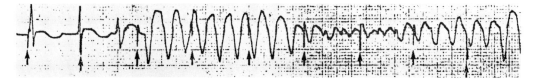

Fig. 18.11 A potential danger of fixed-rate ventricular pacing in the setting of acute myocardial infarction is illustrated. The pacing stimuli are indicated by the *arrows*. The first QRS complex is paced, and the second appears to be a pseudofusion complex, in which the pacing artifact occurs within the QRS complex but does not contribute to ventricular activation. The third QRS complex is premature and of uncertain origin, and is not sensed by the pacemaker. A pacing stimulus occurs on the downslope of the T wave of this premature complex, and initiates ventricular flutter-fibrillation. Pacing stimuli continue to be emitted at regular intervals but fail to capture the ventricles. The patient was successfully defibrillated.

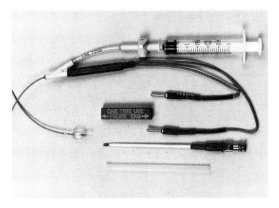

Fig. 18.12 Equipment for inserting an electrode catheter at the bedside, without fluoroscopic guidance, consists of a balloon-tipped catheter (the balloon is inflated by means of a syringe), an introducer, and an adaptor. The wire from the distal (tip) electrode is connected to the "probe" end of the adapter and the "ECG" end of the adaptor is connected to the V lead of the ECG machine in order to record the intracardiac electrogram as the catheter is advanced.

**Nonfluoroscopic Method.** A floating electrode catheter can usually be positioned in the apex of the right ventricle fairly easily at the bedside. Most balloon-tipped electrode catheters are available in disposable kits. In addition to the pacing catheter, these kits contain a means of introducing the catheter into the vein and an adapter to connect the catheter to an electrocardiographic lead and then to an ECG machine (Fig. 18.12). When the catheter has been advanced to the central venous system, the balloon is inflated, and the distal (tip) electrode is connected by means of the adapter to the V lead of the ECG machine. The unipolar electrogram which is then recorded may be utilized in the proper positioning of the catheter (Fig. 18.13). When the pacing catheter is in the right ventricle, the balloon should be deflated. A "pattern of injury" signifies contact with the endocardium (Fig. 18.13), and right ventricular pacing should be initiated at this time.

**Fluoroscopic Method.** It is usually preferable to position the more rigid nonfloating catheters with the aid of an image intensifier (fluoroscope) because of the danger of perforation of the myocardium. While the technique of pacemaker insertion is relatively simple, the patient must be moved to the cardiac catheterization laboratory if a portable image intensifier and radiolucent bed are not available.

**Transthoracic Method.** Transthoracic pacing should be utilized only in extremely emergent situations when it is not feasible to use either of the other two methods of pacemaker insertion (as, for example, in a patient with asystole). Prepackaged kits are available which include a long needle that serves as an introducer for the electrode catheter and a means of connecting the electrode catheter to the pulse generator. The transthoracic method is relatively simple and involves advancing the catheter into the right ventricle via a needle puncture from either the left parasternal or subxiphoid approach. It is often difficult to establish consistent pacing, and potential complications of this technique include myocardial laceration and cardiac tamponade; the technique should therefore be used only as a last resort. Once consistent ventricular pacing is achieved, electrode catheter insertion using the more conventional transvenous routes should be performed.

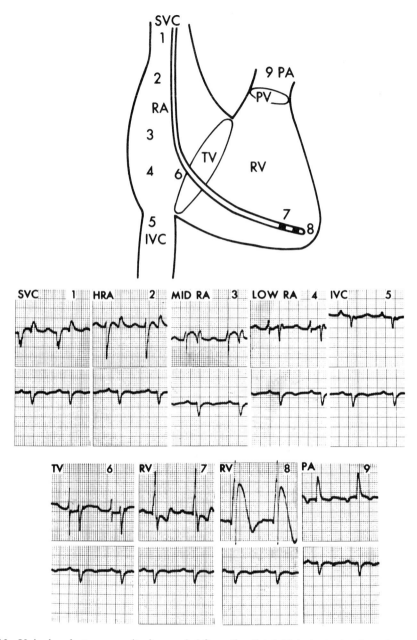

Fig. 18.13 Unipolar electrograms (top) recorded from the distal (tip) electrode of an electrode catheter are shown together with simultaneously recorded surface $V_3$ (bottom). The numbers in the schematic drawing of the right side of the heart represent the locations from which the unipolar electrograms were obtained during positioning of the pacing catheter. Note the change in size and polarity of atrial and ventricular deflections as the electrode catheter is advanced toward the right ventricle and into the pulmonary artery. At Position 8, the injury current signifies contact of the tip electrode with endocardium. SVC = superior vena cava, HRA = high right atrium, mid RA = mid right atrium, low RA = low right atrium, IVC = inferior vena cava, TV = tricuspid valve, RV = right ventricle, PV = pulmonary valve, and PA = pulmonary artery.

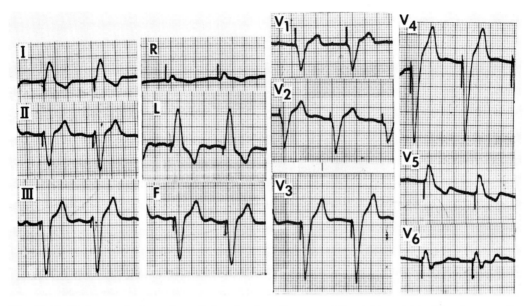

Fig. 18.14  Right ventricular endocardial pacing from the apex of the right ventricle. The electrocardiographic diagnosis of electrode catheter location may be made from the following observations: (1) the right ventricle is the chamber being paced, thus producing QRS complexes with a left bundle branch block configuration; (2) the mean frontal plane axis of the paced ventricular complexes is superior, indicating that the apex of the heart is being activated before the base; and (3) the frontal plane axis of the pacing artifacts is superior, compatible with the tip (cathodal, stimulating) electrode being inferior to the ring (anodal) electrode, with electrical current traveling in an inferior-to-superior direction.

### Initiation of Pacing

Ventricular pacing should be initiated when the electrode catheter is positioned in the apex of the right ventricle. The pacing rate should be set above the patient's intrinsic heart rate, and the current output should be gradually increased until consistent ventricular capture is achieved. Capture should be achieved at current outputs of less than 1.5 ma if the catheter is properly positioned. The current output is then set to two to three times the myocardial stimulation threshold (higher levels of current may predispose patients to ventricular dysrhythmias), and the input sensitivity control is adjusted to achieve maximal sensing of ventricular deflections. Fixed rate ventricular pacing is not advisable in the setting of acute infarction, as competitive rhythms may predispose these patients to serious ventricular dysrhythmias. Sensing of ventricular deflections is determined both by the rate of rise (slew rate) and the amplitude of the endocardial electrical signal. The intracardiac bipolar electrogram should be recorded to ensure that sufficient amplitude of intracar-

diac deflections for proper sensing are present. This is accomplished by connecting the wires from the two electrodes of the pacing catheter to the right and left arm electrocardiographic leads and recording lead I from a standard ECG machine. A minimum of 2.5 mV is generally required for proper sensing, but electrical signals exceeding 5 mV are desirable. The electrode catheter should then be sutured in place and covered with an antibacterial ointment and dry dressing. A 12-lead electrocardiogram and chest x-ray (PA and lateral, if possible) should be obtained to serve as a reference should problems develop later (Figs. 18.14 and 18.15).

## COMPLICATIONS OF TEMPORARY PACEMAKERS

### Failure to Pace and/or Sense

Failure to pace and/or sense appropriately is the most common complication encountered during temporary transvenous pacing and is most often due to dislodgement of the pacing

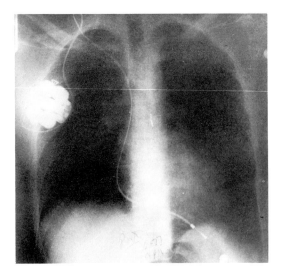

Fig. 18.15A  PA chest radiograph illustrating right ventricular apical position of a bipolar electrode catheter. Note that the catheter tip lies well to the left of the spine and is directed slightly inferiorly.

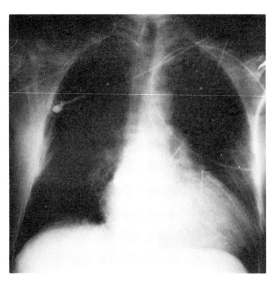

Fig. 18.16  The tip of the bipolar electrode catheter is seen to lie to the left of the spine, directed superiorly. This position is compatible with a location in either the coronary sinus (the corresponding 12-lead ECG would show atrial pacing or a *right* bundle branch block pattern) or the outflow tract of the right ventricle. That the latter was correct is established by the corresponding ECG shown in Fig. 18.17.

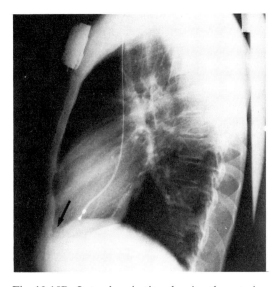

Fig. 18.15B  Lateral projection showing the anterior orientation of the electrode catheter. The arrow points to the right ventricular apex.

catheter from the apex of the right ventricle— an event which may be identified by means of a chest radiograph (Fig. 18.16) and/or by a change in frontal plane axis of both the pacing artifact and the paced QRS complexes (Fig. 18.17). Pacing and/or sensing may become intermittent before failing completely, and, although increasing the current output may temporarily restore normal function, increase in

myocardial stimulation threshold is a clue to electrode catheter displacement. Although the myocardial stimulation threshold is usually lower when the distal (tip) electrode serves as the cathode, a change in catheter position may alter this situation such that reversing the electrode polarity (so that the proximal [ring] electrode serves as cathode) may allow for more effective capture. Selective failure of sensing function may also occur in patients with right ventricular infarction, with consequent suboptimal electrical signals reaching the catheter electrodes. In this situation, converting the pacing system from a bipolar to a unipolar system may considerably amplify the electrical signal, thus allowing proper sensing to occur. Unipolarization is accomplished by substituting a surface (or subcutaneous) electrode for the positive pole of the electrode catheter (Fig. 18.18). Rectifiable problems that may occur with unipolarized temporary pacing systems include "oversensing" (sensing of P waves and T waves, for example) and loss of proper contact with the surface electrode.

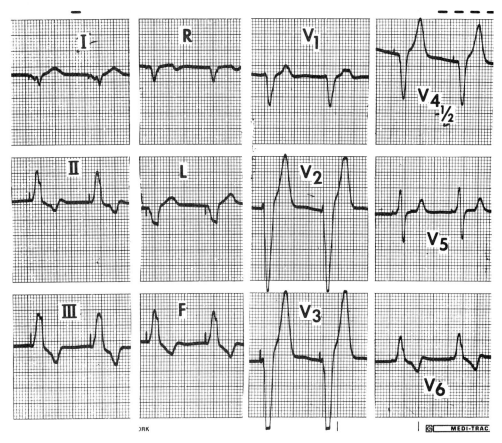

Fig. 18.17 Temporary transvenous pacing with the bipolar electrode catheter located in the outflow tract of the right ventricle. The electrocardiographic diagnosis of catheter location may be made from the following observations: (1) the right ventricle is the chamber being paced, as the QRS complexes have a left bundle branch configuration; (2) the axis of the pacemaker artifacts is inferior, indicating that electrical current is traveling in a superior-to-inferior direction, compatible with the location of the tip (cathodal) electrode being superior to the ring (anodal) electrode; and (3) the mean frontal plane axis of the paced ventricular complexes is inferior, indicating that the base of the heart is being activated before the apex.

## Perforation of the Myocardium

Perforation of the right ventricle is not a rare problem with some of the stiffer electrode catheters, but is very unusual with the more flexible "floating" pacing catheters. Myocardial perforation may be manifested clinically by an increase in myocardial stimulation threshold, failure of appropriate sensing, and a change in axis of the pacing artifact and paced QRS complexes. This is because in these circumstances the pacemaker may be initiating ventricular activation from the epicardium or the left ventricle. The onset of chest pain, pericardial friction rub, or stimulation of the chest wall musculature or diaphragmatic musculature should suggest the possibility of myocardial perforation. Catheter repositioning is usually required in this situation in order for proper pacing and sensing functions to be achieved, and the patient should be observed for signs of pericardial tamponade.

## Infection

Careful attention to sterile technique can limit pacemaker-related infections. The insertion site should be inspected daily; if signs of local inflammation or unexplained fever develop, appropriate cultures should be obtained. Catheter replacement using another insertion

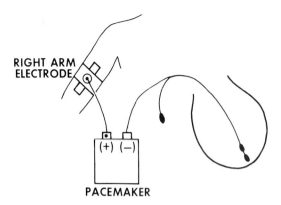

Fig. 18.18 The technique of "unipolarization" of a bipolar electrode catheter in an attempt to enhance the endocardial signal. The electrode connected to the positive terminal of the generator is detached. The positive terminal is then connected using an alligator clamp to a surface or subcutaneous electrode (needle). The subcutaneous electrode avoids the electrical resistance generated by the skin and allows for a lower myocardial stimulation threshold.

site should be promptly executed if there is continued need for cardiac pacing.

### Electrical Hazards

The presence of an indwelling temporary electrode catheter provides a potential low-resistance conduit for stray electrical current to be transmitted directly to the myocardium. Relatively small currents have been shown to be capable of producing ventricular fibrillation in man.[50,51] This problem is of special importance in the patient with acute myocardial infarction, as the ventricular fibrillation threshold may already be reduced. Improperly grounded or de-

fective electrical equipment in the critical care facility are potentially important sources of current leaks. It is imperative for equipment to be checked regularly for proper grounding and for all personnel to be aware of the danger of simultaneous manipulation of the electrode catheter and other electrical equipment. Therefore, it is a good idea to enclose the electrodes and the pulse generator in a well-insulated shield such as a surgical rubber glove.

### Dysrhythmias

Causes of pacemaker-related dysrhythmias should be sought out. For example, improper sensing can result in pacing stimuli being delivered in the vulnerable period of ventricular tissue. Similarly, mechanical irritation of the ventricle can cause ventricular dysrhythmias. Careful attention to catheter position and avoidance of "catheter whip" will help to limit these problems, but a defibrillator should be available at all times.

"Pacemaker runaway" (Fig. 18.19) is a very rare and potentially lethal complication in that ventricular rates of up to 300 pulses per minute have been recorded.[52] The cause of this pacemaker malfunction is a component problem, and it is readily treated by prompt replacement of the faulty pulse generator.

### Thromboemboli

Clinically apparent thromboemboli due to temporary pacemakers are sufficiently uncommon that prophylactic anticoagulation is not recommended; in addition, should myocardial perforation occur, the risk of hemorrhagic peri-

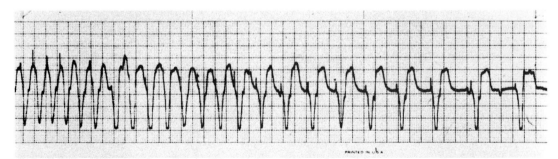

Fig. 18.19 Example of "runaway pacing" in a patient who underwent temporary transvenous pacing. The pacemaker generator spontaneously increased its discharge rate to a maximum of 300 beats/min and then spontaneously decreased its rate. The situation is rectified by changing the pulse generator.

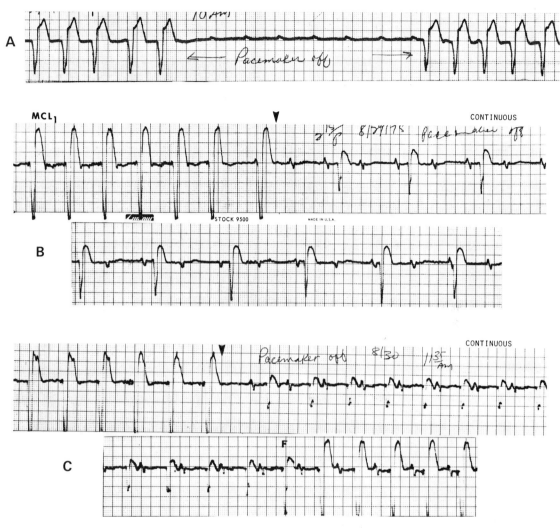

Fig. 18.20 *(A)* MCL1 rhythm strip recorded from a patient with acute inferior wall myocardial infarction who had developed complete AV block on the second hospital day, necessitating placement of a temporary transvenous right ventricular endocardial pacemaker. All QRS complexes are paced. After the fifth QRS complex, the pacemaker is abruptly turned off. No QRS rhythm emerges for over five seconds although sinus rhythm at a rate of about 75/min is present. The pause in QRS rhythm is terminated by the turning on of the pacemaker, and a paced QRS rhythm resumes. With a temporary transvenous endocardial pacemaker in place, follow-up of a patient's spontaneous cardiac rhythm, as well as changes in pacing and sensing thresholds in the setting of myocardial infarction, can be readily accomplished.

*(B)* A temporary transvenous right ventricular endocardial pacemaker is turned off at the *arrow.* Sinus rhythm at a rate of about 78/min, and a dissociated, slow ventricular rhythm at a rate of about 37/min are present. The ventricular rhythm, having a QRS contour similar to that of the paced complexes, and bearing no relationship to the P waves, is apparently originating in an area near the site of the pacemaker electrode.

*(C)* In these two continuous lead MCL1 rhythm strips recorded one day later from the same patient as in Fig. 18.2B, turning off the pacemaker reveals that sinus rhythm with marked first degree AV block is now the underlying spontaneous cardiac rhythm. The fifth QRS complex in the bottom strip, labeled "F," is a fusion complex between the sinus-stimulated and pacemaker-initiated impulses.

carditis might be increased. If an embolic episode does occur, the pacing catheter should be promptly replaced; if insertion has been accomplished via the femoral vein, signs of deep vein thrombophlebitis should be carefully sought.

## SUMMARY

Recent advances in our understanding of the relationship of the coronary blood supply to the cardiac conduction system and the ability to recognize fascicular block patterns allow for better prediction of the site of atrioventricular block occurring during acute myocardial infarction. Treatment is dependent on both the presumed site of atrioventricular block and the clinical status of the patient. In our view, most patients with inferior myocardial infarction and atrioventricular block may be successfully treated by atropine or low-dose isoproterenol infusion. Temporary transvenous pacemaker insertion is indicated in patients with acute inferior myocardial infarction and complete AV block if the dysrhythmia remains refractory to drug therapy and if evidence of power failure or ventricular irritability is present. The natural history of AV block in patients with inferior myocardial infarction is for resolution of the AV conduction disturbance; hence, permanent pacing is almost never required (Fig. 18.20). In contrast, patients with acute anterior myocardial infarction with evidence of second- or third-degree AV block should undergo temporary pacemaker insertion. Similarly, prophylactic pacemaker insertion is indicated for those with new or indeterminate bundle branch block associated with either first degree AV block or a bifascicular bundle branch block pattern. Permanent ventricular pacing is indicated for those with anterior myocardial infarction and fixed complete AV block. The role of permanent pacemaker insertion for patients with bundle branch block who transiently progress to high-grade AV block in the course of acute myocardial infarction still remains controversial. While the incidence of sudden death is higher for unpaced patients in this subgroup,[44,46] no control studies are available proving that transient progression to high-grade or complete AV block is an independent risk factor for sudden death.

## ACKNOWLEDGMENT

Supported in part by the National Institutes of Health grant HL-20238.

## REFERENCES

1. Becker AE, Anderson RH: Morphology of the human atrioventricular junctional area, in Wellens HJJ, Lie KI, Janse MJ (eds): The Conduction System of the Heart. Philadelphia, Lea & Febiger, 1976, pp 263–286.
2. James TN: The connecting pathways between the sinus node and the A-V node and between the right and left atrium in the human heart. Am Heart J 66:498, 1963.
3. Truex, RC: Anatomical considerations of the human atrioventricular junction, in Mechanisms and Therapy of Cardiac Arrhythmias, Dreifus LS, Likoff W (eds), Grune and Stratton, New York, 1966, pp 333–340.
4. Anderson RH, Janse MJ, van Capelle JL, et al: A combined morphological and electrophysiological study of the atrioventricular node of the rabbit heart. Circ Res 35:909, 1974.
5. Paes de Carvalho A, de Almeide DF: Spread of activity through the atrioventicular node. Circ Res 8:801, 1960.
6. Anderson RH: Histologic and histochemical evidence concerning the presence of morphologically distinct cellular zones within the rabbit atrioventricular node. Anat Rec 173, 1972.
7. James TN: Anatomy of the coronary arteries and veins, in Hurst JW, Logue RB (eds): The Heart: Arteries and Veins, New York, McGraw-Hill, 1966, pp 32–46.
8. James TN, Sherf L: Fine structure of the His bundle. Circulation 44:9, 1971.
9. Massing GK, James TN: Anatomical configuration of the His bundle and proximal bundle branches in the human heart. Circulation 44(Suppl. II):II–64, 1971.
10. Titus JL: Normal anatomy of the human cardiac conduction system. Mayo Clin Proc 48:24, 1973.
11. James TN, Sherf L, Urthaler F: Fine structure of the bundle branches. Br Heart J 36:1, 1974.
12. Fabregas RA, Tse WW, Han J: Conduction disturbances of the bundle branches produced by lesions in the nonbranching portion of the His bundle. Am Heart J 92:356, 1976.
13. Lev M: The pathology of complete atrioventricular block. Prog Cardiovasc Dis 6:317, 1964.

14. Rosenbaum MD, Elizari MV, Lazzari JO: The Hemiblocks. Tampa Tracings. Tampa, Florida, 1970.

15. Hecht HH, Kossman, CE: Atrioventricular and intraventricular conduction. Revised nomenclature and concepts. Am J Cardiol 31:232, 1973.

16. Demoulin JC, Kulbertus HE: Histopathological examination of concept of left hemiblock. Br Heart J 34:807, 1972.

17. Uhley HN: Some controversy regarding the peripheral distribution of the conduction system. Am J Cardiol 30:919, 1972.

18. Rosenbaum MB: The Hemiblocks: Diagnostic criteria and clinical significance. Mod Concepts Cardiovasc Dis 39:141–146, 1970.

19. Myerburg RJ, Nilsson K, Gelband H: Physiology of canine intraventricular conduction and endocardial excitation. Circ Res 30:217, 1972.

20. Durrer D, Van Dam RT, Freud GE, et al: Total excitation of the isolated human heart. Circulation 41:899, 1970.

21. Lazzara R, Yeh BK, Samet P: Functional transverse interconnections within the His bundle and the bundle branches. Circ Res 32:509, 1973.

22. Myerburg RJ, Nilsson K, Gelband H, et al: Comparison of anatomy and physiology of canine and primate left ventricular conduction systems. Clin Res 21:83, 1973.

23. Krongrad E, Hefler SE, Bowman FO Jr, et al: Further observations on the etiology of right bundle branch block pattern following right ventriculotomy. Circulation 50:1105, 1974.

24. The Criteria Committee of the New York Heart Association: Nomenclature and Criteria for Diagnosis of Diseases of the Heart and Great Vessels. Little, Brown and Co., Boston, 1969.

25. Jacobson LB, LaFollette L, Cohn K: An appraisal of initial QRS forces in left anterior fascicular block. Am Heart J 94:407, 1977.

26. Mihalick MJ, Fisch C: Electrocardiographic findings in the aged. Am Heart J 87:117, 1974.

27. McHenry PL, Phillips JF, Fisch C, et al: Right precordial QRS pattern due to left anterior hemiblock. Am Heart J 81:498, 1971.

28. Nakaya Y, Hiasa Y, Murayama Y. et al: Prominent anterior QRS force as a manifestation of left septal fascicular block. J Electrocardiol 11:39, 1978.

29. Gambetta M, Childers RW: Rate-dependent right precordial Q waves: "septal focal block." Am J Cardiol 32:196, 1973.

30. James TN: The coronary circulation and conduction system in acute myocardial infarction. Prog Cardiovasc Dis 10:410, 1968.

31. Sutton R, Davies M: The conduction system in acute myocardial infarction complicated by heart block. Circulation 38:987, 1968.

32. Blondeau M, Rizzon P, Lenegre J: Les trouble de la conduction auriculoventriculaire dans l'infarctus myocardique recent: II. Etude anatomique. Arch Mal Coeur 54:1104, 1961.

33. Paes de Carvalho A: Excitation of the atrioventricular node during normal rhythm. Effects of acetylcholine, in Dreifus LS, Likoff W (eds), Mechanisms and Therapy of Cardiac Arrhythmias. New York, Grune and Stratton, 1966, pp 341–352.

34. Scheinman MM, Thorburn D, Abbott JA: Use of atropine in patients with acute myocardial infarction and sinus bradycardia. Circulation 52:627–633, 1975.

35. Cohen HC, Gozo EG Jr, Pick A: The nature and type of arrhythmias in acute experimental hyperkalemia in the intact dog. Am Heart J 82:777–785, 1971.

36. Fontaine G, Guiraudon G, Frank R, Coutte R, Dragodanne C: Epicardial mapping and surgical treatment in six cases of resistant ventricular tachycardia not related to coronary artery disease, in The Conduction System of the Heart: Structure, Function and Clinical Implications, Wellens HJJ, Lie KI, Janse MJ (eds), Lea and Febiger, Philadelphia, 1976, pp 545–563.

37. Rotman M, Wagner GS, Wallace AG: Bradyarrhythmias in acute myocardial infarction. Circulation 45:703, 1972.

38. Brown RW, Hunt D, Sloman JG: The natural history of atrioventricular conduction defects in myocardial infarction. Am Heart J 78:460, 1969.

39. Rotman M, Wagner GS, Waugh RA: Significance of high degree atrioventricular block in acute posterior myocardial infarction. Circulation 47:257, 1973.

40. Jacobson LB, Lester RM, Scheinman MM: Management of acute bundle branch block and bradyarrhythmias. Med Clin N Am 63:93, 1979.

41. Rotman M, Wagner GS, Wallace AG: Bradyarrhythmias in acute myocardial infarction. Circulation 45:703, 1972.

42. Massie B, Scheinman MM, Peters R, Desai J, Hirschfeld D, O'Young J: Clinical and electrophysiologic findings in patients with paroxysmal slowing of the sinus rate and apparent Mobitz type II AV block. Circulation 58:305–314, 1978.

43. Hindman MC, Wagner GS, JaRo M, et al: The clinical significance of bundle branch block complicating acute myocardial infarction. 1. Clinical characteristics, hospital mortality, and one-year follow-up. Circulation 58:679, 1978.

44. Hindman MC, Wagner GS, JaRo M, et al: The

clinical significance of bundle branch block complicating acute myocardial infarction. 2. Indications for temporary and permanent pacemaker
insertion. Circulation 58:689, 1978.

45. Dhingra RC, Denes P, Wu D, Chuquimia R,
Rosen K: The significance of second degree AV
block and bundle branch block—observations regarding site and type of block. Circulation
49:638, 1974.

46. Mullins CB, Atkins JM: Prognosis and management of ventricular conduction blocks in acute
myocardial infarction. Mod Concepts Cardiovasc Dis 45:125, 1976.

47. Nimetz AA, Shabrooks ST, Hutter AM Jr, et
al: The significance of bundle branch block during acute myocardial infarction. Am Heart J
90:439, 1975.

48. Scheinman MM, Brenman B: Clinical and anatomic implications of intraventricular conduction blocks in acute myocardial infarction. Circulation 46:753, 1972.

49. Lie KI, Wellens HJ, Schuilenburg RM, et al:
Factors influencing prognosis of bundle branch
block complicating acute anteroseptal infarction.
The value of His bundle recordings. Circulation
50:935, 1974.

49a. Scheinman MM, Remedios P, Cheitlin MD et
al: Effects of antiarrhythmic drugs on atrioventricular conduction in patients with acute myocardial infarction. Circulation 62:20–28, 1980.

50. Geddes LA, Baker LE: Response to passage of
electric current through the body. Med Instrum
5:13, 1971.

51. Raftery EB, Green H, Gregory I: Electrical
safety: fibrillation threshold with 50 Hz leakage
currents in man and animals. Br Heart J 35:864,
1973.

52. Kallenbach J, Scott Millar RN, Obel IWP: Runaway temporary pacemaker. Heart & Lung
6:517, 1977.

# 19 | *Congestive Heart Failure: Pathophysiology and Treatment*

*Joel S. Karliner, M.D.*

## DEFINITION OF HEART FAILURE

Congestive cardiac failure is an abnormal physiologic state caused by the inability of the heart to deliver sufficient blood to satisfy the metabolic requirements of the tissues. Under ordinary circumstances, the diagnosis of congestive cardiac failure in the patient with acute myocardial infarction is not difficult; the usual criteria are not different in patients with acute infarction, and such patients exhibit typical findings on physical examination (see Ch. 9). These may include cardiomegaly, although one of the major causes of acute left ventricular failure in the presence of a normal heart size is acute myocardial infarction. This presumably occurs because of a marked increase in left ventricular end-diastolic pressure before there are any alterations in chamber volume (see below). The left ventricular impulse is frequently displaced, and gallop rhythm with prominent third and fourth heart sounds and signs of pulmonary congestion may be present. The murmur of papillary muscle dysfunction is not uncommon. Evidence of vascular blurring, dilatation of pulmonary arteries, or parenchymal clouding on a chest radiograph are frequent but not invariable associated findings (see Ch. 26). Based on the above criteria, mild-to-moderate left ventricular failure was found on physical examination in approximately half (range 23 to 71 percent) of 1800 hospitalized patients evaluated clinically prior to development of the Coronary Care Unit.[1] Wolk et al. noted approximately the same incidence in studies reported since 1967. Severe heart failure or pulmonary edema is less common, occurring in approximately 12 percent of patients with acute myocardial infarction.[1] Of 490 consecutive patients with acute myocardial infarction admitted to the Coronary Care Unit of University Hospital, San Diego, and studied in the Myocardial Infarction Research Unit, 228 (46 percent) had mild-to-moderate left ventricular failure, while 39 (8 percent) developed pulmonary edema and 34 (7 percent) were in cardiogenic shock. One hundred eighty-nine (39 percent) had no clinical evidence of heart failure whatever.

## PHYSIOLOGIC CONSIDERATIONS

### Determinants of Myocardial Oxygen Demand

Before discussing the treatment of congestive cardiac failure in patients with acute myocardial infarction, it is useful to consider the physiologic factors that determine the heart's demands for oxygen. Among the most important of these are the heart size, the left ventricular systolic pressure, the heart rate and the level of myocardial inotropic state (Fig. 1). Both heart size and left ventricular pressure are important determinants of myocardial wall tension, which in turn is probably the major influence on myocardial oxygen demands. Although resting cardiac size has been conventionally related to "preload" and left ventricular pressure to "afterload" on the myocardium, these two measures, according to the law of La Place, are directly related to left ventricular wall tension and hence to myocardial oxygen demand. The law of Laplace, a formula for thin-walled shells, states that wall force, or stress, is directly related to the product of intracavitary pressure (P) and radius (r); in addition, myocardial wall tension (T) usually is considered to be inversely related to ventricular wall thickness (h): $T = (P \times r)/h$. Thus, an increased "preload" at a given level of ventricular systolic pressure will augment wall tension, and vice versa, while an increase in "afterload" at any level of end-diastolic dimension or volume will also tend to increase wall stress. These considerations become particularly important when assessing the value of vasodilator agents in patients with congestive cardiac failure (see Ch. 22).

The heart rate exerts an independent influence on myocardial oxygen requirements: tachycardia causes an increase and bradycardia causes a decrease. Drugs which alter the inotropic state of the left ventricle also alter myocardial oxygen demands: agents that increase the inotropic state augment demand and drugs that decrease it diminish demand. According to these considerations, any therapeutic intervention that diminishes heart size, left ventricular pressure, heart rate, and inotropic state will tend to decrease myocardial oxygen demand. However, a depression of inotropic state may be harmful in patients with congestive cardiac failure. Therefore, combinations of drugs may be used either to maintain or augment inotropic state, while at the same time other agents may be used to counteract the increased myocardial oxygen demand resulting from a raised inotropic state. A clinical example is the combined use of digoxin and propranolol in patients with cardiomegaly and/or left ventricular dysfunction.[2]

Since virtually all patients with acute ischemic heart disease and congestive cardiac failure have abnormal left ventricular wall motion, the effects of therapeutic interventions on such areas of asynergy deserve consideration. It has been shown that the extent and severity of seg-mental wall motion abnormalities after myocardial infarction tend to correlate with reduced left ventricular performance.[3] Thus, amelioration of left ventricular asynergy produced by agents affecting congestive cardiac failure should have appropriate beneficial effects on left ventricular performance. Currently, it is uncertain whether improvement or reversal of asynergy by pharmacologic means is the result of enhanced inward motion of adjacent normally contracting segments or whether there is direct enhancement of performance in areas of resting or exercise-induced left ventricular asynergy.

## Determinants of Myocardial Oxygen Supply

Under ordinary circumstances, increases in myocardial oxygen demand, influenced by the factors discussed above, are met by an appropriate increase in myocardial oxygen supply (Fig. 19.1). However, in patients with acute coronary insufficiency this is frequently not the case, and myocardial damage ensues. The amount of oxygen utilized by the heart is directly related to coronary blood flow, the oxygen content of arterial blood, and the amount of oxygen extracted from the blood by the heart. Of these three considerations, the first is of the most practical importance, since the oxygen-carrying capacity of the blood cannot be significantly increased unless considerable hypoxemia is present. Further, the heart extracts a high and relatively fixed amount of oxygen from the blood flowing through the coronary circulation.

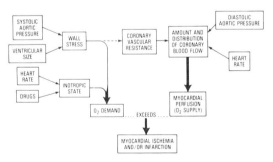

Fig. 19.1  The major determinants of myocardial oxygen supply and demand. The treatment of congestive heart failure in acute myocardial infarction depends on a favorable balance of the factors shown above.

Therefore, augmentation of coronary flow is the major practical mechanism by which increased metabolic demands can be met.

It should be recognized that coronary blood flow is markedly diminished during systole because the vascular tree is compressed by the myocardium. However, this phenomenon is not of major significance in the epicardial arteries, which extend primarily over the surface of the heart, as compared with the subendocardial vessels, which are compressed during systole. As a result of this compression, systolic flow is markedly diminished through these vessels and aortic diastolic pressure becomes a major influence on coronary blood flow. Indeed, in the presence of hypotension and frank cardiogenic shock, aortic diastolic pressure is probably the major determinant of coronary flow. However, under ordinary circumstances the absolute level of aortic diastolic pressure is not the sole hemodynamic determinant responsible for driving blood through the coronary circulation.[4] Because the coronary vessels are exposed to intramyocardial pressure during diastole as well as systole, it is clear that the net driving force responsible for maintaining coronary flow during diastole must be the difference between aortic diastolic pressure and intramyocardial diastolic pressure. The latter is related to left ventricular diastolic pressure. When this measure is elevated, as it often is in congestive cardiac failure, there may be significant diminution of subendocardial blood flow. This may be one of the reasons that vigorous treatment of congestive cardiac failure (see below) may prevent further ischemia. It is also clear that reduction in cardiac size will also reduce myocardial wall tension, thereby reducing myocardial oxygen demand. Thus, appropriate treatment of congestive cardiac failure should reduce demand while at the same time increasing supply.

## HEMODYNAMIC OBSERVATIONS

### Cardiac Output

In patients with acute myocardial infarction, the cardiac output, the cardiac index, and stroke volume often are diminished—and sometimes remarkably so in hypotensive patients. However, care must be exercised in the interpretation of values obtained by the indicator dilution technique, since undetected recirculation can occur throughout most of the inscription of an apparently exponential downslope.[5] Techniques in which recirculation is minimal, such as the thermodilution method,[6] appear to be more reliable in patients with a reduced cardiac output and now represent a standard approach for the measurement of cardiac output in acutely ill patients. Most thermodilution catheters are constructed as part of a balloon float catheter system (see below) so that both pulmonary wedge pressure and cardiac output can be measured simultaneously. The orifice of the additional lumen is approximately 30 cm proximal to the catheter tip, while the thermistor is immediately proximal to the end of the catheter. A known quantity of cold solution is injected into the right atrium, and the resultant change in pulmonary artery blood temperature is measured by the thermistor. Thus, this method measures the output of the right ventricle, which in the absence of intracardiac shunts is equal to left ventricular output.

A number of studies have documented that, in patients with uncomplicated myocardial infarction, the cardiac index, the stroke volume, and stroke work tend to be within normal limits; in patients with congestive cardiac failure, the cardiac index, although technically still within normal range, is at the lower limits of normal and stroke volume and stroke work both tend to be reduced.[7-9] Presumably, the maintenance of cardiac index in a marginally normal range is the result of an increased heart rate, which frequently complicates congestive cardiac failure in patients with acute myocardial infarction.[7] As with all the measures described below, the cardiac index and cardiac output tend to be depressed more in patients with anterior infarction as compared with those who have inferior wall myocardial infarction.[10] (The specific techniques for measuring cardiac output as well as for measuring intracardiac pressures in patients with acute myocardial infarction are discussed in more detail in Ch. 27.)

## Intracardiac Pressures

With increasing congestive cardiac failure and especially in the presence of a marginal blood pressure, it may be desirable to monitor intracardiac pressures continuously. For this purpose, a small balloon-tipped "float" catheter which is flow-directed was developed by Swan, Ganz, and their coworkers.[11] The Swan-Ganz catheter has come into routine use for this purpose in Intensive Care Units. The catheter allows rapid cannulation of the pulmonary artery with minimal irritation of the right ventricle; by intermittent inflation of the balloon, it is possible to monitor pulmonary arterial wedge or capillary pressure.

## Central Venous Pressure

While useful as a reflection of the right ventricular filling pressure, the central venous pressure has provided a relatively unreliable index of left ventricular filling pressure. For example, in patients with associated pulmonary disease, the venous pressure may be distinctly abnormal when the left ventricular diastolic pressure is normal or nearly so, and the left ventricular pressure may be substantially elevated in the face of a normal central venous pressure.[12] Furthermore, the central venous pressure may not be an accurate indicator of directional changes in the pulmonary wedge pressure during therapy with intravenous fluids.[13] One clinical condition in which the central venous pressure may be elevated is that of right ventricular infarction, with or without associated tricuspid regurgitation.[14] Indeed, jugular venous distension may not be present in the usual patient with left ventricular failure due to acute myocardial infarction, since, despite elevated left-sided pressures, the right ventricular and right atrial pressures usually remain within the normal range. Conversely, an elevated right atrial or right ventricular pressure in the presence of a normal or nearly normal pulmonary wedge pressure suggests the possibility of right ventricular infarction. Recent scintigraphic studies have documented the common occurrence of right ventricular infarction in patients with infe-

rior wall myocardial infarction [15,16] (see Ch. 12).

## Pulmonary Artery Pressure

Both the pulmonary artery pressure and the pulmonary capillary or wedge pressure tend to be elevated in the presence of congestive cardiac failure; with pulmonary edema, these pressures are even further elevated. Forrester and his colleagues reported that, in patients with x-ray evidence of pulmonary vascular congestion, the pulmonary capillary pressure usually exceeded a mean value of 18 mmHg.[8] It is sometimes not possible to obtain an accurate pulmonary wedge pressure; under these circumstances, measurement of the pulmonary artery end-diastolic pressure has been advocated as an indirect measure of left ventricular filling pressure. However, it should be recognized that, after acute myocardial infarction, pulmonary arterial pressures may not accurately reflect left ventricular end-diastolic pressure because atrial contraction makes a large contribution to ventricular filling pressure.[17,18] In addition, the pulmonary artery end-diastolic pressure may not be the same as the mean pulmonary arterial wedge pressure because of some increase of pulmonary vascular resistance in many patients. Nevertheless, measuring the pulmonary arterial end-diastolic pressure is often useful in following serial changes in patient status. It is actually more desirable to measure the pulmonary capillary pressure; however, failing this, the pulmonary artery end-diastolic pressure is an acceptable substitute if its limitations are recognized.

## Left Ventricular Pressures

In the early 1970s, a number of investigators reported on bedside retrograde catheterization of the left ventricle, using percutaneous femoral arterial cannulation. These techniques yielded considerable useful information, but it should be recognized that they have been employed in only a few studies and remain a highly specialized investigative method. Hamosh and Cohn reported that left ventricular end-diastolic pressure was elevated in 85 percent of 40 patients studied by retrograde catheterization of the left ventricle. In 14 patients with apparently uncomplicated infarcts, the left ventricular end-diastolic pressure averaged 15 mmHg, while in 12 patients with clinical signs of left ventricular failure, the average value was 30 mmHg. As indicated above, a large presystolic atrial "kick" (with an average amplitude of 9.5 mmHg) was an important factor in the high left ventricular end-diastolic pressure in patients with heart failure. Wolk et al. made similar observations and also indicated that there was a considerable range of left ventricular end-diastolic pressures.[1] Thus, seven of 13 patients without clinical evidence of left ventricular failure had an abnormal left ventricular end-diastolic pressure, while, in patients with congestive cardiac failure, the range of left ventricular end-diastolic pressures was between 16 and 43 mmHg. However, no patient with clinical evidence of heart failure had a normal left ventricular end-diastolic pressure, and, in about half the patients, the level was in the range where pulmonary interstitial fluid accumulation should occur (greater than 25 mmHg). In three patients with pulmonary edema, left ventricular end-diastolic pressure was markedly elevated and ranged from 32 to 42 mmHg. Even in patients with a normal heart size and adequate forward cardiac output, an inappropriate rise in left ventricular end-diastolic pressure may lead to a rise in pulmonary venous pressure and to signs and symptoms of pulmonary congestion. Presumably, such as increase in left ventricular "filling pressure" results from decreased diastolic compliance of ischemic and/or infarcted myocardium.

Measurements of the left ventricular "filling pressure," either as left ventricular end-diastolic pressure, pulmonary arterial end-diastolic pressure, or pulmonary capillary pressure, have been used in conjunction with measurements of cardiac output and systemic arterial pressure to plot left ventricular function curves in patients with acute myocardial infarction. It was reported by Russell et al. that a left ventricular filling pressure in the range of 20 to 24 mmHg was associated with the peak of such a curve and that, when the filling pressure exceeded this range, the curves became flattened or decreased.[19] Scheidt et al. reported that a left ventricular work index of less than 1.75 kg-m/minute/m² was associated with a very high mortality.[20] Based on this type of study, Crexelles et al. suggested that the optimal level of filling pressure on the left side of the heart in acute myocardial infarction was in the neighborhood of 18 mmHg.[21] Such a filling pressure appeared to provide an optimal relationship between filling pressure and cardiac output, but it is clear that the filling pressure in any given patient must be individualized. Recently, Shell et al. reported that the level of left ventricular filling pressure measured at any time during the first few days after myocardial infarction could be related to mortality and that, in patients with initial or subsequent values exceeding 18 mmHg, mortality ranged between 25 and 60 percent.[22]

When determinations of cardiac output are not readily available, a rather good clinical assessment can be made by observation of urine volume and systemic arterial pressure in relation to the pulmonary wedge pressure or pulmonary artery end-diastolic pressure. An excessive decrease in mean pulmonary capillary pressure due to vigorous diuretic therapy will be associated with a reduction in both urine volume and systemic arterial pressure as well as increasing hypoxemia, while a pressure that is too high will produce hypoxemia and other clinical signs of congestive cardiac failure, including persistent pulmonary rales, gallop rhythm, and tachycardia.

## Peripheral Vascular Resistance

Although systemic hypotension after acute myocardial infarction usually is associated with a low cardiac output and some compensatory elevation of systemic vascular resistance, the systemic arterial pressure alone may not be an adequate reflection of the cardiac output.[23] Occasionally, a fall in peripheral resistance occurs but is accompanied by no change or rise in cardiac output. It should be recognized that the peripheral vascular resistance is a measure derived from the relation between cardiac output and mean arterial pressure and thus is subject to the clinical limitations of these measurements.

## Serial Measurements of Cardiac Output and Left Ventricular "Filling Pressures"

In several studies, serial measurements of these parameters have been made. After initial acute measurements, repeat measurements were made several weeks later. In some patients, it has been found that left ventricular end-diastolic pressure returns to normal, but in others it remains persistently elevated.[24] During the first few days after acute myocardial infarction, Franciosa et al. reported that induced or spontaneous alterations in arterial pressure were probably the most important determinants of left ventricular filling pressure.[25] In 26 patients, these pressures averaged 147 (systolic) and 21 (diastolic) mmHg, respectively, on day one and decreased to 107 and 12.7 mmHg, respectively, by day five after acute infarction. In addition, the left ventricular function curve also may remain abnormal in these patients in response to a fluid challenge.[26] Thus, there appears to be considerable heterogeneity in left ventricular function as evaluated serially,[27] and this is consistent with observations that have been made by using radionuclide studies.[28,29] In most patients, the major changes in left ventricular hemodynamics occurred within the first four to six weeks after acute myocardial infarction; in the study of Kupper et al. there was almost no further alteration in left ventricular function during the following nine months.[30] Such alterations in left ventricular hemodynamics may be the basis for the abnormal physical findings (third heart sound, fourth heart sound, car-

diomegaly, abnormal apical impulse) often found in patients with chronic coronary artery disease.[31]

## SUMMARY OF USUAL AND UNUSUAL HEMODYNAMIC PATTERNS

Various hemodynamic patterns after acute myocardial infarction are summarized in Figure 19.2 and Table 19.1. An analogous classification has been presented by Forrester et al.[32] In patients with uncomplicated transmural myocar-

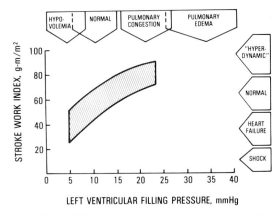

Fig. 19.2 The hemodynamic spectrum of cardiac function in acute myocardial infarction. In any given patient, the hemodynamic status can be assessed by using the function curve coordinates of filling pressure and left ventricular work depicted here. It should be recognized that the designations are only approximate and that considerable overlap probably occurs. (Modified after Heikkilä.[42])

Table 19.1 Summary of Hemodynamic Patterns Following Acute Myocardial Infarction

| Classification | Systemic Arterial Pressure | Cardiac Output | Peripheral Vascular Resistance | Left Ventricular End-Diastolic Pressure or Pulmonary Artery Wedge Pressure |
|---|---|---|---|---|
| Uncomplicated | Normal or ↓ | Normal or ↑ | Normal | Usually ↑ |
| Mild Congestive Heart Failure | Usually normal | ↓ | ↑ | ↑↑ |
| Severe Congestive Heart Failure | ↓ | ↓↓ | ↑↑ | ↑↑ or ↑↑↑ |
| Shock Cardiogenic (usual) | ↓↓↓ | ↓↓↓ | ↑↑↑ | ↑↑↑ |
| Cardiogenic (unusual) | ↓↓↓ | ↓↓ | ↑ | ↑↑ |
| Hypovolemic | ↓↓↓ | ↓↓↓ | ↑↑↑ | May be normal |

dial infarction, the left ventricular end-diastolic pressure usually is elevated. However, patients with nontransmural infarction and patients with hypovolemia may have a normal left ventricular end-diastolic pressure or mean pulmonary capillary pressure.[33] In uncomplicated patients, the cardiac output remains normal, the blood pressure is normal or only slightly diminished, and peripheral vascular resistance and central venous pressure tend to be normal. With congestive heart failure, the left ventricular end-diastolic pressure tends to be substantially elevated, but the degree of elevation does not necessarily coincide with the severity of the complication, nor does it necessarily parallel the alterations in chest radiograph. In general, however, the more severe the congestive heart failure, the lower the systemic arterial pressure and cardiac output, and the higher the peripheral vascular resistance. While an elevated output may occur occasionally in the face of acute myocardial infarction, its presence in a patient in whom the diagnosis is not definite may be a clue to another process, such as sepsis.

## DIURETIC THERAPY

As indicated earlier, pulmonary vascular congestion is commonly the result of an elevated left ventricular mean diastolic and end-diastolic pressure associated with acute myocardial infarction, and may occur in the presence of normal heart size by chest radiograph. Initially, fluid tends to accumulate in the perialveolar lymphatic spaces, and this accumulation may by itself lead to increased pulmonary vascular resistance. As congestion progresses, the hydrostatic pressure in the pulmonary vascular bed exceeds the plasma oncotic pressure and fluid may then accumulate in the alveolar spaces as well. Although there tends to be a reasonably good correlation between the levels of pulmonary arterial wedge pressure and congestive cardiac failure, exceptions occasionally occur where the pulmonary arterial wedge pressure is markedly elevated in the absence of clinical signs of congestive cardiac failure and vice versa.

There is considerable evidence that the pre-

ferred initial approach to the therapy of congestive cardiac failure in the setting of acute myocardial infarction involves the use of intravenous or oral diuretics rather than the use of digitalis glycosides. The common occurrence of atrial, ventricular, and junctional dysrhythmias during acute myocardial infarction may lead to confusion in a patient who is receiving digitalis. By contrast, diuretics act rapidly and are exceedingly effective in reducing dyspnea, which is the major symptom of congestive cardiac failure. The counterpart of this reduction from the hemodynamic standpoint can be seen in the reduction in pulmonary arterial wedge pressures and pulmonary arterial pressure that has been documented in a number of studies.[34-36] It should also be recognized that the acute use of intravenous diuretic therapy, specifically furosemide, may lead to a rapid amelioration in congestive signs and symptoms by the mechanism of venous pooling due to acute venous dilatation, as reflected by a 50 percent increase in venous capacitance within 5 minutes of drug administration, well before any diretic effect can be documented.[34]

Both furosemide and ethacrynic acid are known as "loop diuretics." Although unrelated chemically, both of these agents are potent diuretics which interfere with sodium reabsorption through the nephron, but especially in the ascending limb of the loop of Henle (Fig. 19.3). They may be used both orally and intravenously; however, for intravenous use furosemide is the preferred agent because of occasional reports of deafness after intravenous ethacrynic acid.[37] Occasionally, patients with advanced heart failure may respond only to the intravenous preparation, but, after initial diuresis, oral therapy may achieve satisfactory results. The usual initial dose of furosemide should be 20 or 40 mg given intravenously, depending on the level of pulmonary arterial wedge pressure or signs or symptoms of pulmonary congestion, or 40 mg given orally. It is recommended that the initial dose of furosemide not exceed 240 mg and the initial dosage of ethacrynic acid not exceed 250 mg, since higher doses are rarely more effective, and adverse reactions may be more common [38] (see below). Once the patient has responded to the initial dose of diuretic,

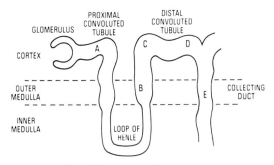

Fig. 19.3  The important sites for fluid and electrolyte transport within the nephron. In this simplified,
schematic diagram, they are:

*(A)* The proximal convoluted tubule. Ordinarily, 65
to 70 percent of sodium, chloride, and bicarbonate
reabsorption occurs here. This ionic movement occurs with an equivalent transfer of water.

*(B)* The ascending limb of the loop of Henle. Another
15 to 20 percent of filtered sodium chloride is reabsorbed here. Water is generally not reabsorbed at
this site, thus producing urinary dilution and accounting for the production of solute-free or "free"
water.

*(C)* In this segment of the distal convoluted tubule,
another 5 to 10 percent of filtered sodium is reabsorbed. Antidiuretic hormone (ADH) may act here.

*(D)* (and possibly *E*). Here, sodium not exceeding
3 percent of the filtered load is reabsorbed. In exchange, hydrogen and potassium ions are secreted
from the renal tubular cells into the tubular lumen.
Although this ionic transfer occurs independent of
aldosterone, the exchange process is in general sensitive to and regulated by this hormone.

*(E)* The collecting duct is also sensitive to antidiuretic
hormone, and water absorption occurs when this substance is present. (Modified after Puschett.[38])

subsequent doses may be given based on the
presence or absence of dyspnea, tachycardia,
and pulmonary rales—or on the level of the
pulmonary capillary pressure and/or cardiac
output, if these are being measured. Often, patients will require a maintenance dose of anywhere between 20 and 40 mg of furosemide
daily or subsequent therapy with one of the
benzothiadiazine ("thiazide") diuretics. These
inhibit sodium reabsorption primarily in the
proximal portion of the distal tubule and are
effective compounds for oral therapy as well.
Chlorothiazide and hydrochlorothiazide are
similar in action and differ only in dosage. The
dose for hydrochlorothiazide is between 50 and

100 mg daily, and for chlorothiazide between
500 and 1000 mg daily. Chlorthalidone is a
longer acting agent, and the usual dose is 100
mg/day. All the "thiazide" diuretics cause a
modest increase in renal vascular resistance and
depression of glomerular filtration rate, and are
relatively ineffective in patients with impaired
renal function. The sites of action and relative
potencies of the diuretics are summarized in
Table 19.2.

In the presence of acute myocardial infarction, spironolactone, which is an antagonist of
the salt-retaining hormone aldosterone and
which causes a reduction in the distal tubular
exchange of sodium and potassium, is rarely
indicated. Another diuretic which tends to
cause potassium retention is triamterene—
which is not, however, an aldosterone antagonist. Because of its tendency to produce hyperkalemia, triamterene is not recommended in the
treatment of acute myocardial infarction.

### Adverse Reactions to Diuretics

**Hypovolemia.** The locus of the major action
of ethacrynic and furosemide is also the locus
of the countercurrent multiplier apparatus that
is the basic mechanism responsible for urinary
concentration and dilution—i.e., the ascending
limb of the loop of Henle (Fig. 19.3). Normally,
this area is responsible for reabsorption of some
25 percent of the filtered load of sodium as
compared to the residual 10 percent on which
all the more distal reabsorptive mechanisms
operate. Thus, when the filtered load of sodium
is adequate, diuresis may be so massive as to
produce a marked fall in pulmonary arterial
pressure and left ventricular filling pressure and
a reduction in cardiac output. Subsequent to
the diuresis, the kidney may then exhibit an
appropriate response to the physiological stimulus of volume depletion, resulting in high osmolality and specific gravity of urine, a very high
concentration of creatinine and other nonreab-
sorbable solutes, and a low concentration of
sodium.[39] Renal blood flow and glomerular filtration rate are reduced, mediated in part by
sympathetic nervous system activity and possibly, in part, by activation of the renin-angioten-
sion system. With a severe deficit, renal blood

Table 19.2 Sites of Action and Relative Potency of Diuretics*

| Agent | Major Site of Action within the Nephron | Additional Site | Maximal Natriuretic Effect (% of Filtered Load Excreted) |
|---|---|---|---|
| Thiazides | Distal tubule | Proximal tubule | 5–8% |
| Furosemide | Ascending loop of Henle | Proximal tubule | 20–25% |
| Ethacrynic acid | Ascending loop of Henle | Proximal tubule | 20–25% |
| Spironolactone | Distal tubule | | 2–3% |
| Triamterene | Distal tubule | | 2–3% |
| Amiloride | Distal tubule | | 2–3% |

* Adapted from Puschett, J. B.: Physiologic basis for the use of new and older diuretics in congestive heart failure. Cardiovasc Med 2:255–261, 1976.

flow may be reduced to one-third of normal, despite an adequately maintained arterial pressure. Afferent arteriolar constriction then occurs so that glomerular capillary hydrostatic pressure is inadequate to maintain filtration at normal levels. Thus, depressed renal function under these circumstances ("prerenal azotemia") is a form of iatrogenic "renal ischemia," which results from a reduction in renal blood flow but is not due to an inadequacy of metabolic function of the renal parenchymal cells. It should be recognized that the combination of increased myocardial oxygen demand (tachycardia) and decreased coronary perfusion pressure (hypotension) resulting from excessive diuretic therapy may potentially produce extension of myocardial ischemia. It should also be recognized that a carefully controlled diuresis resulting in a reduction in left ventricular filling pressure may have little effect on cardiac output.[34] Nevertheless, when cardiac output is plotted against pulmonary arterial wedge pressure, yielding a "ventricular function curve," it can be shown that the response to the diuresis, if it is well-controlled, tends to be along the ascending limb of the function curve, suggesting a beneficial effect on left ventricular performance.[36]

**Hypokalemia and Hypomagnesemia.** The large amounts of sodium presented to aldosterone-sensitive sites of cation exchange in the distal nephron may induce large losses of potassium, with potentially serious consequences for inducing dysrhythmias in the patient with acute myocardial infarction, especially in the presence of digitalis. Potassium deficits should be corrected as rapidly as possible, but intravenous potassium chloride should not be given at a rate exceeding 15 meq/hr, and the concentration of potassium in the infusate should not exceed 40 meq/l. For oral replacement therapy, between 20 and 80 meq of $K^+$ are usually necessary, depending on renal function. Serum potassium levels should be monitored as the clinical situation indicates. Occasionally, magnesium deficits may result from diuretic therapy. For intravenous magnesium replacement, a 10 percent solution should be used: 40 ml of this preparation (3.25 meq) may be given at a rate not exceeding 1.5 ml/min.

When patients are changed to oral diuretic therapy, administration of the agent 5 days per week or on alternate days tends to help protect against serious potassium deficiency. Intake of food high in potassium and periodic monitoring of the serum potassium level are also indicated.

**Additional Side Effects.** Other adverse reactions which can occur following intravenous or oral diuretic therapy include excessive hyponatremia (reduction in serum sodium). Should this become a problem, water intake must be restricted to equal the estimated insensible loss (400 to 600 ml/day); diuretics are usually not effective until the electrolyte imbalance is corrected. Hypertonic saline should never be used in such a situation, except when the serum sodium is exceedingly low—i.e., less than 100 meq/l—and there are associated severe central nervous system disturbances and/or serious hypotension. Hyponatremia in nonedematous patients is usually the consequence of excessive diuretic therapy and salt restriction, both of

**Table 19.3    Adverse Reactions to Commonly Used Diuretics\***

| Reaction | Consequence in Acute Myocardial Infarction |
|---|---|
| 1. Hypovolemia | Tachycardia and hypotension with possible increase in ischemia |
| 2. Hypokalemia | ↑ in severity and duration of ventricular arrhythmias; precipitation of atrial, junctional or ventricular arrhythmias in digitalized patients |
| 3. Hypomagnesemia | Same |
| 4. Hyponatremia | Central nervous system disturbances; possible adverse effect on ventricular arrhythmias |
| 5. Metabolic alkalosis | Possible adverse effect on hypoxic myocardium; usually accompanied by hypokalemia, hypovolemia and hyponatremia |
| 6. Worsening of carbohydrate tolerance | May cause fluid and electrolyte disturbances; nonketotic hyperosmolar coma rare |
| 7. Hyperuricemia | Acute gout |
| 8. Deafness (ethacrynic acid, rare; furosemide, exceedingly rare) | |

\* These reactions may occur as a result of all of the commonly employed diuretics except where indicated. For details, see text.

which may have been used overenthusiastically. A less stringent diuretic regimen, with or without liberalization of dietary salt, is often sufficient to correct this imbalance.

Other adverse reactions which are seen occasionally include a metabolic alkalosis which occurs in previously edematous patients who have received diuretic therapy. This is usually accompanied by the hyponatremia mentioned above and has been called a "contraction alkalosis" because of the volume depletion and potassium loss required to produce the alkalosis.[40] Other, less common, adverse reactions include worsening of carbohydrate tolerance produced by furosemide and the rare occurrence of nonketotic diabetic coma.[41] Because of a fall in urea clearance caused by extracellular fluid volume depletion, hyperuricemia is common and acute gout can be precipitated in susceptible individuals. It should also be recognized that hyperuricemia in the absence of marked changes in volume may be the result of previous therapy or new therapy with the thiazide diuretics. The latter also may diminish carbohydrate tolerance as well.

Adverse reactions to the diuretics are summarized in Table 19.3.

## MANAGEMENT OF ACUTE PULMONARY EDEMA

From a technical standpoint, pulmonary edema occurs as soon as there is excessive fluid in the lungs, whether it be in the perialveolar lymphatic spaces or actually in the alveoli themselves. From a clinical standpoint, however, it seems appropriate to divide congestive cardiac failure into mild, moderate, and severe, with pulmonary edema being reserved as a term for the more severe cases of lung congestion usually, but not always, associated with severe left ventricular pump failure.[42] Under normal circumstances, the plasma oncotic pressure prevents the diffusion of fluids across the capillary membrane into the interstitial space. However, as congestive cardiac failure worsens in acute myocardial infarction, the capillary hydrostatic pressure increases, and the plasma oncotic pressure is exceeded with resulting transudation of fluid into the interstitial tissues, and, subsequently, into the pulmonary alveoli themselves. In the most severe instances, this can be seen as bubbling pink froth in the severely dyspneic patient.

The proper management of pulmonary edema, which can occur even in the absence of cardiomegaly,[43] involves several of the modalities of therapy already discussed. Intravenous furosemide, 20 to 240 mgm, is certainly a mainstay of treatment. In addition, morphine sulfate in doses of 5 to 15 mg intravenously may be exceedingly useful under these circumstances. It is advisable to begin with 5 mg intravenously, with increments of 2 mg every 5 to 15 minutes depending on the patient's response, to a maximum dose of 15 mg intravenously. It should be recognized that with severe pulmonary edema the usual circumstance is for the arterial carbon dioxide tension to be reduced, but some patients tend to retain carbon dioxide.[44] Although morphine in excessive amounts may cause hypercapnia, especially in patients with underlying chronic obstructive lung disease, hypercapnia under these circumstances does not appear to be a contraindication to morphine therapy, but may well be an indication for intubation.

It has previously been taught that morphine produces a "pharmacologic phlebotomy," and that its major mechanism of action in reducing acute pulmonary edema resides in its ability to produce venous pooling resulting from acute venodilatation. However, in recent studies of both normal volunteers and patients with congestive cardiac failure, no evidence of venodilatation could be shown.[45,46] In addition, in patients with chronic coronary artery disease, it could not be demonstrated that morphine had any effect on left ventricular end-diastolic dimension measured echocardiographically.[47] It is likely, therefore, that morphine exerts its major action by inhibiting central sympathetic outflow, thereby reducing both peripheral vascular resistance and left ventricular contractility, with a resulting decrease of myocardial oxygen demand. Definite proof of this hypothesis must await further investigation.

Other traditional treatment for pulmonary edema includes oxygen therapy (30 to 40 percent $O_2$ at a flow rate of 5 l/min); when rotating tourniquets are used, the blood pressure cuff is blown up to 50 to 80 mmHg systolic on three limbs and rotated every 5 to 10 minutes. An alternative is to use a rubber tourniquet fastened tightly about the upper arms and thighs in three of the four extremities. In patients with prior congestive cardiac failure, it has been shown that such rotating tourniquets produce little change in pulmonary arterial wedge pressure because of the decrease in venous distensibility that is characteristic of chronic heart failure.[48] Whether these results can be extrapolated to patients with acute pulmonary edema is problematical. Another neglected but often exceedingly useful measure in the treatment of acute pulmonary edema is direct removal of blood from the circulation. Such phlebotomy of 250 to 500 ml of blood with monitoring of pulmonary arterial wedge and systemic arterial pressures can often produce a dramatic relief in the acute congestive state.

With severe pulmonary edema, metabolic acidosis may be profound with an arterial pH of 7.1 or less.[44] Under these circumstances, there is a base deficit, and the diagnosis of lactic acidosis may be made with confidence. The major goal of therapy is to improve left ventricular performance; therapy with intravenous bicarbonate is not indicated, in part because the available solutions of bicarbonate are hyperosmolar. Such solutions may cause acute and undesirable increases in plasma volume as well as a hyperosmolar state.[49] Rapid change in blood pH to alkaline levels also may trigger cardiac dysrhythmias, perhaps because of changes in serum potassium. Patients who develop such severe acidosis tend to hypoventilate rather than hyperventilate in the face of pulmonary edema.

The presence of hypoxemia indicates serious disturbances in alveolar-capillary gas exchange; such a finding is, of course, common in acute myocardial infarction even in the absence of overt pulmonary edema. It has been shown that the alveolar-arterial oxygen difference in patients with acute myocardial infarction increases as pulmonary arterial wedge or left atrial pressure increases.[50] At some point, alveolar edema develops and a few rales may be apparent. Occasionally, bronchospasm reflecting peribronchial edema or subsequently florid pulmonary edema may develop. This can result in premature airway closure with resultant atelectasis leading to venoarterial shunting even in the absence of alveolar edema. Ayres has shown that the calculated venoarterial shunt in a group of patients with acute myocardial infarction decreased markedly after several deep breaths, suggesting recruitment of previously closed lung units.[50] The same author has also proposed that most patients with myocardial infarction and pulmonary edema lasting for more than several hours should be intubated. However, endotracheal intubation increases the risk of a complicating pneumonia and positive pressure ventilation may impair cardiac output by decreasing systemic venous return. Thus, the decision to intubate should not be made on the basis of blood gas data alone, but should be reserved for the patient who is obtunded or is not responding to conventional management.[49] (Techniques of intubation, the management of the ventilator, and arterial blood gas management are outlined in Chs. 32 and 35.)

It is known that extracellular lung water increases in proportion to the left atrial pressure even in the absence of major abnormalities in pulmonary blood volume,[51] and that a decline in colloid osmotic pressure in such patients, resulting in a decreased colloid osmotic-hydrostatic capillary pressure gradient, tends to favor transudation of fluid into the lungs.[56] These factors may in part account for discrepancies between the chest radiograph and clinical and hemodynamic measures,[53] and estimations of pulmonary extravascular water.[54] (Radiographic methods for detecting acute pulmonary edema and pulmonary vascular congestion are described in Ch. 26.)

As indicated earlier, the use of diuretics involves a reduction of "preload" on the myocardium. Additional methods of producing such a reduction fall into the realm of vasodilator therapy, discussed in Chapter 22. Such therapy may involve preload and/or afterload reduction. In this connection, the use of orally active

organic nitrates deserves comment. It was formerly thought that nitroglycerin should not be used in patients with acute myocardial infarction, but this is no longer the case. Indeed, intravenous nitroglycerin has been used experimentally to effect changes in the extent of myocardial ischemia,[55] and sublingual nitroglycerin is commonly employed in patients with acute myocardial infarction to treat chest pain. Severe hypotension and bradycardia can occasionally occur after the use of either intravenous or sublingual nitroglycerin.[56] The mechanism of this effect is uncertain, but it may involve a vagal discharge similar to that observed in dogs with volume overload acutely subjected to hemorrhage.[57] Bussmann and coworkers have demonstrated that, in patients with an initial elevation of left ventricular filling pressure, cardiac output rose and left ventricular filling pressure declined in response to oral isosorbide dinitrate,[58] while Miller et al. have stressed the importance of alterations in systemic arterial pressure on changes in coronary blood flow induced by nitroglycerin in patients with acute myocardial infarction.[59]

## DIGITALIS IN ACUTE MYOCARDIAL INFARCTION

### Experimental Considerations

Digitalis therapy in patients with acute myocardial infarction was first advocated by James B. Herrick, who in 1912 described for the first time in the American literature the "clinical features of sudden obstruction of the coronary arteries." [60] In the conclusion of his article, Herrick wrote as follows: "It would also seem to be far wiser to use digitalis, strophanthus or their congeners than to follow the routine practice of giving nitroglycerin or allied drugs. The hope for the damaged myocardium lies in the direction of securing a supply of blood through friendly, neighboring vessels so as to restore as far as possible its functional integrity. Digitalis or strophanthus, by increasing the force of the heart's beat, would tend to help in this direction more than the nitrites." Herrick, of course, wrote primarily by inference and had no clinical data to support his observations. Since his time, considerable controversy concerning the indications and usefulness of digitalis in such patients continues to exist.

It is now generally accepted that the beneficial effects of digitalis in patients with congestive cardiac failure result from direct stimulation of the contractile state of the myocardium. Thus, in hemodynamic studies of patients exhibiting chronic heart failure of the low-output type, it has been shown that digitalis augments the cardiac output and lowers the abnormally high left ventricular end-diastolic pressure.[61] It should be recognized that these studies largely employed intravenous digitalis preparations. More recently, it has been shown in the normal conscious dog [62] as well as in normal man [63] that either chronic intramuscular or oral digoxin experts a positive inotropic effect on the myocardium which can be shown especially when a stress is placed on the heart, such as raising the blood pressure with the α-adrenergic agonist phenylephrine. By contrast, some have proposed that there is little evidence to substantiate the effects of chronic digoxin therapy in patients with congestive cardiac failure and have advocated abandoning its use under these circumstances entirely because of the high incidence of toxicity that results from the use of this drug.[64,65] This will remain a matter of controversy until appropriate, prospective, well-controlled studies can be performed to further substantiate the time-honored use of digoxin in patients with chronic congestive cardiac failure. Indeed, it has recently been observed that, in nine patients with well-documented congestive heart failure and abnormal left ventricular function, there was definite hemodynamic deterioration (increased pulmonary artery wedge pressure and decreased left ventricular stroke work index) 2 to 7 weeks after stopping maintenance oral digoxin. These changes were reversed when the patients were redigitalized.[65a]

In patients in whom myocardial infarction has eliminated significant quantities of myocardium from contributing to the contractile process, cardiac output can be sustained only by an increase of shortening of the surviving myocardium—some of which may be ischemic but

much of which is adequately perfused and may, in fact, be normal. It is essential, therefore, to consider the effects of cardiac glycosides on hypoxic myocardium. Hypoxia of surviving myocardium occurs for a number of reasons in patients with acute myocardial infarction. First of all, systemic hypoxia is common in these patients, and it is presumably related to impaired pulmonary gas exchange as a consequence of elevated pulmonary capillary pressure resulting, as noted above, from impairment of left ventricular performance. The second important mechanism responsible for myocardial hypoxia is related to the relatively large amount of heart muscle surrounding an infarct which receives a portion of its blood supply from the occluded coronary vessel. The oxygen available to this portion of myocardium, which Edwards has aptly termed "the twilight zone," [66] is reduced to a varying extent, although not totally eliminated. The third cause of myocardial hypoxia in these patients is atherosclerotic narrowing in the unoccluded coronary vessels. Coronary arteriosclerosis is a diffuse disease, and segments of myocardium quite remote from the acute infarct may also suffer from an impairment of oxygen delivery, particularly during hypotensive episodes. A number of experimental studies have indicated that acutely administered intravenous digitalis glycosides may enhance contraction in the normal and border zones, but that the direct effect on the ischemic zone may be variable.[67,68] It should also be recognized, however, that enhancement of contractility under these circumstances may exert a deleterious effect. Thus, the effects of hypoxia may be of importance in the genesis of dysrhythmias associated with digitalis therapy. For example, hypoxic, hypercapnic patients with chronic obstructive pulmonary disease tend to develop dysrhythmias after bolus injections of acetylstrophanthin.[69]

The potentially beneficial effects of digitalis may also in part depend on initial heart size before administration. In the presence of cardiomegaly and left ventricular failure, digitalis may reduce myocardial oxygen demands, particularly due to a fall in end-diastolic volume, resulting in a decline in systolic wall tension (see Laplace relationship, above). Thus, the increase in contractility produced by digitalis tends to increase myocardial oxygen demand; however, in the dilated, failing heart which becomes smaller after glycoside administration, the concurrent reduction in wall tension presumably counteracts the oxygen cost of augmented contractility. Thus, the effects of digitalis on myocardial oxygen demands are conditioned importantly by the state of compensation existing at the time the drug is administered.[70] Extrapolating from these observations, it would be expected that digitalis might be of little benefit to the patient with a normal heart size, an elevated left ventricular end-diastolic pressure, and pulmonary congestion in whom the residual normal myocardium is functioning maximally. On the other hand, digitalis could conceivably be of use to the patient with cardiomegaly and congestive cardiac failure due to acute myocardial infarction.

Digitalis, when acutely administered, may have varying effects on different vascular beds, including the coronary vasculature. There is little information regarding the effects of cardiac glycosides on the human coronary arterial bed, but animal studies imply that a bolus intravenous injection of a rapid-acting glycoside might constrict the coronary bed, and, therefore, this may not be an advisable method of administration in patients with acute myocardial infarction.[70] Of course, the extent to which the results of studies in dogs are applicable to patients with coronary vascular disease remains to be demonstrated. Both generalized systemic and regional arteriolar constrictor and venoconstrictor effects of cardiac glycosides have been demonstrated in conscious, intact human subjects without heart failure, with opposite effects occurring in patients with heart failure.[71] In both animal and human conscious subjects, regardless of the state of compensation, large doses of cardiac glycosides administered intravenously produce a rise in systemic arterial pressure. Transient elevation of systemic arterial pressure resulting from rapidly acting glycosides might, therefore, be undesirable in patients with acute myocardial infarction, and it has been demonstrated that the early pressor effect of intravenously administered digitalis

may be harmful in some patients with cardiogenic shock.[72]

The propensity of patients with acute myocardial infarction to develop ventricular instability has led to the fear that such individuals may be more sensitive to the arrhythmogenic properties of the glycosides. However, clinical evidence that patients with acute myocardial infarction are particularly prone to develop digitalis-induced dysrhythmias is lacking. The role of the drug in the production of primary ventricular fibrillation complicating acute myocardial infarction is not known because many other factors in such patients—including bradycardia, increased sympathetic activity, hypoxia, and hypokalemia—may contribute to the genesis of serious dysrhythmias. Metabolic half-times and excretion rates of short, intermediate and long-acting glycosides have been well characterized.[73] It has been demonstrated that both renal insufficiency and advanced age are associated with impaired excretion of these agents. Since alterations in renal hemodynamics commonly occur after acute myocardial infarction, it is likely that digitalis dosage should be modified appropriately in such patients. When questions arise under these circumstances, blood should be obtained for analysis of the amount of digitalis in the serum.

### Clinical Observations

Recommendations concerning the use of digitalis glycosides in acute myocardial infarction reflect the somewhat controversial state of the experimental literature. As indicated above, Herrick in 1912 [60] and, subsequently, Hamman in 1926 [74] advocated the use of digitalis in all patients with acute myocardial infarction. In contrast, Friedberg recommended digitalis only when heart failure was not controlled by bedrest, opiates, or oxygen therapy.[75] Unless they persist after the first week, basilar rales alone, according to Friedberg, are insufficient indication for digitalis. The criteria for digitalis therapy after acute myocardial infarction proposed by Logue and Hurst are somewhat broader and include the presence of gallop sounds, pulmonary rales, radiographic evidence of interstitial pulmonary edema, and a sinus rate exceeding

110/min.[76] The same authors continue to recommend the use of digoxin in patients who have heart failure resulting from myocardial infarction.[77] Earlier, Lown and coworkers reported that 22 percent of patients with congestive symptoms demonstrated an inadequate response to digitalis, and diuretic measures were required.[78] A somewhat different approach was advocated by Swan and associates, who recommended administration of digoxin to patients with congestive heart failure who do not respond adequately to an initial trial of diuretic therapy,[79] and this indeed appears to be the optimal therapeutic sequence to follow.

The specific digitalis preparation recommended differs according to the circumstances. For urgent situations such as acute pulmonary edema complicating myocardial infarction, ouabain, because of its rapidity of onset and the ease of dosage adjustment, has been advocated as the preparation of choice by some.[78] Others have indicated that switching to other preparations for maintenance therapy may pose a problem, and, hence, the use of digoxin is favored.[76,77] The potential hazard of bolus intravenous injections of rapidly acting glycosides has already been commented upon. On the other hand, oral absorption may be variable in these patients, and the same is true for intramuscular absorption; therefore, the intravenous route may be the safest, provided it is used judiciously and the glycoside is administered over a period of 10 to 15 minutes with careful observation of heart rate and blood pressure.[78a]

While the glycosides may exert arrhythmogenic effects in profoundly ill patients, digitalis is frequently used in the treatment of certain dysrhythmias complicating acute myocardial infarction. Atrial fibrillation with a rapid ventricular rate occurring during a course of acute infarction appears to be a clear indication for the use of digitalis. Atrial and nodal tachycardia are frequently transient, and it has been suggested that digitalis may provide effective prophylaxis against their recurrence. Persistent atrial tachycardia causing hypotension should be treated with electrocardioversion followed by digitalis. Atrial flutter should be treated in a similar fashion, with the addition of both digitalis and quinidine as prophylactic measures.

Since the glycosides increase the contractile force developed by the myocardium, earlier concern had been expressed that digitalis might lead to rupture of the heart in patients with acute myocardial infarction, but clinical studies have concluded that there is little evidence that digitalis contributes to such rupture.

As indicated above, transmural myocardial infarction is almost always accompanied by an elevated left ventricular end-diastolic pressure.[7] In uncomplicated patients, the cardiac output remains normal. The systemic arterial pressure is normal or only mildly reduced, and peripheral vascular resistance and central venous pressure tend to be normal. A fourth heart sound is almost always present and does not necessarily indicate cardiac failure. It is unlikely that such patients would benefit from digitalis therapy. Measurements of cardiac output after intravenous administration of digitalis in patients with uncomplicated acute transmural infarction have revealed either no change or an actual fall in cardiac output.[80] Indeed, intravenous administration of glycosides in such patients has been reported to be associated occasionally with a sudden development of ischemic chest pain.[80]

With congestive cardiac failure, the left ventricular end-diastolic pressure tends to be substantially elevated. In general, the more severe the congestive heart failure or hypotension, the lower the systemic arterial pressure and cardiac output, and the higher the peripheral vascular resistance. Although numerous authors have advocated digitalis therapy for congestive cardiac failure complicating acute myocardial infarction, there are few studies in man which document benefit from the cardiac glycosides in this setting,[81-83] and others which have shown only marginal[84] or no benefit.[85] If digitalis is to be employed under these circumstances, the dosage regimen must be adjusted to the level of the blood urea nitrogen and serum creatinine, and hypokalemia must be scrupulously avoided.

It is necessary that the physician be thoroughly familiar with the specific digitalis preparation he or she tends to use. As indicated earlier, under most circumstances in acute myocardial infarction, this preparation will be digoxin. The dosage of the drug depends on many factors—among the most important of which is renal function, since digoxin is cleared primarily by the kidneys. Glomerular filtration rate declines with age, and older patients may be more susceptible to digitalis intoxication. Although the estimation of serum digoxin level may be of great help in the management of such patients, there is often insufficient time in the acute coronary care setting for the results of such a determination to be of much use. On the other hand, in a patient who is exhibiting ventricular dysrhythmias after several days of treatment, the availability of a serum digoxin level within a few hours may be of considerable aid. Nevertheless, complete reliance should not be placed on measurement of the serum digoxin level, since serious dysrhythmias due to digitalis intoxication may be present at levels below the usual "therapeutic range" which is considered in most laboratories to be in the neighborhood of 2 ng/ml. Digoxin dosage is easiest to manage in patients with atrial fibrillation, since reduction of the ventricular response to 60 to 80 beats per minute at rest is the ideal goal.

Recognition of digitalis toxicity is of the utmost importance. Nausea and vomiting are common symptoms and should not routinely be attributed to other causes in patients receiving the drug. Visual changes are uncommon but are a useful clue when present. Frequently, the diagnosis of digitalis intoxication is an electrocardiographic one, but this is much more difficult in the acute Coronary Care Unit setting than it is in an outpatient clinic. A commonly missed sign of digitalis intoxication is the appearance of an atrioventricular junctional rhythm in patients with atrial fibrillation. It cannot be overemphasized that regularization of the cardiac rhythm in patients with atrial fibrillation should not be attributed to the reappearance of sinus rhythm, unless this can be proved by an electrocardiogram. The presence of a regular rhythm ranging between 40 and 100 beats per minute in patients who have previously been in atrial fibrillation usually represents a junctional rhythm and indicates atrioventricular dissociation. Although this rhythm in itself is usually not a dangerous one, the continued administration of digoxin may lead to more serious and even fatal dysrhythmias.

Other arrhythmias that can be due to digitalis intoxication include paroxysmal atrial tachycardia with or without block; junctional and ventricular ectopic beats; ventricular tachycardia; and ventricular fibrillation. However, all these dysrhythmias, especially the ventricular ones, are common in patients with acute myocardial infarction and complicate the problem of the administration of digitalis in this setting. In addition, it has been claimed that patients with acute myocardial infarction may be more sensitive to the arrhythmogenic properties of the drug—especially in the presence of hypokalemia and/or hypoxia, both of which are also common during acute myocardial infarction. Other rhythms that can result from digitalis excess include sinus bradycardia and first-, second-, and third-degree atrioventricular block. Again, all of these rhythms may occur as a result of myocardial infarction alone. Repolarization abnormalities are common after digitalis administration and do not indicate the presence of intoxication; of course, such abnormalities also result from acute and chronic ischemic heart disease.

The method of digitalization will be dictated by the clinical situation. For example, in patients with rapid atrial fibrillation, digitalization within 12 hours may occasionally be indicated. For severe congestive cardiac failure, digitalization within 24 to 36 hours is usually the rule. Only in a monitored patient with sinus rhythm is more rapid digitalization indicated. As indicated earlier, for mild or borderline congestive cardiac failure, initial therapy with diuretics will usually be the treatment of choice, and digitalization over a period of several days is usually adequate. Experimental evidence indicates that even small amounts of digitalis may have a beneficial effect on a failing heart and, thus, "full digitalization" is not prerequisite for hemodynamic improvement.

**Digitalization by the Intravenous or Intramuscular Route.** The onset of action of intravenous digoxin is between 10 and 20 minutes; peak action occurs within 2 to 3 hours. The time required for disappearance of one-half of physiologic activity as well as the biologic half time are approximately equivalent in this preparation; in a patient without renal insufficiency, the half-life averages 33 hours. In the presence of renal insufficiency, the half-life is, of course, increased accordingly. In the patient who has not received a glycoside in recent past, the initial intravenous dose is 0.75 mg followed by 0.25 mg every 2 to 4 hours. Ordinarily, 1.5 mg intravenously should not be exceeded during the first 24 hours. Complete excretion of the drug takes anywhere from 3 to 6 days and is delayed, as indicated above, in patients with renal insufficiency. When renal failure, hypokalemia, or hypothyroidism is present, the initial dose should be reduced by 25 to 50 percent. In a study of the use of digoxin in patients with acute myocardial infarction, Sharpe, Norris, and White recommended that 1.5 mg be given in the first 36 hours.[86] They recommended that 0.5 mg be given intramuscularly and then the remainder in divided doses orally. It should be recognized that, if the diagnosis of myocardial infarction is in doubt, intramuscular digoxin may lead to elevation of serum creatine kinase (CK). Unless the determination of the specific isoenzyme of creatine kinase (MB-CK) is available (See Ch. 11), intramuscular digoxin as well as other intramuscular medications should be avoided in the patient with acute myocardial infarction.

**Moderately Rapid Oral Digitalization Within 24 to 36 Hours.** This method is appropriate for use in patients with rapid atrial fibrillation, when the situation is not urgent but when it is necessary to control the ventricular response within a relatively brief period of time. In addition, this method is appropriate for patients with acute congestive cardiac failure in whom reasonably rapid digitalization is desirable. In undigitalized patients, an initial dose of between 0.5 and 1.0 mg of digoxin may be given orally, followed by 0.25 mg orally every 6 hours until a clinical response is achieved. The average range for the total oral "digitalizing" dose is between 1.5 to 3.0 mg given over several days.

**Slow or Oral Digitalization.** When digitalization over a 2 to 4-day period is desirable, a starting dose of 1.0 mg of digoxin followed by 0.25 to 0.5 mg every 12 hours for 6 doses may be given. It should also be recognized that, in patients in whom digitalization over a period

of 5 to 8 days is desirable, it is possible to begin with a maintenance dose of digoxin of 0.25 mg daily or, more rarely, 0.5 mg daily. After one week, an adequate level of digitalis in the serum will be achieved even though a "digitalizing dose" was not given initially. Therefore, a loading dose is not necessary in patients in whom slow oral digitalization is the preferred method.[87]

**Maintenance Dosage.** In general, a maintenance dose of 0.25 mg orally daily for digoxin is adequate for adults. Some patients may require a larger amount, especially those with atrial fibrillation in whom the ventricular response is the guide to therapy. Other patients may exhibit symptoms or signs of digoxin intoxication on a daily dose of 0.25 mg and a smaller dose such as 0.125 mg daily may be adequate in some individuals. Other patients may require a combination of these doses on alternate days. It has recently been suggested that, in patients receiving oral quinidine, the level of serum digoxin may be higher than would be the case in the absence of quinidine.[88] Since the latter drug is often employed in patients with acute myocardial infarction, special care should be taken to observe patients for signs of digitalis intoxication who are receiving quinidine; also, under these circumstances, measurements of serum digoxin levels appear to be indicated. Further, in older patients the renal clearance of quinidine itself may be reduced.[89]

**Management of Digitalis Intoxication.** Digitalis intoxication may present in a variety of ways. Gastrointestinal symptoms such as nausea and vomiting are frequent. Occasionally, occular difficulties such as yellow vision have been reported. The most serious manifestations of digitalis intoxication are the cardiac dysrhythmias which have been described above. In some patients, the margin between the dose of glycoside required for an optimum therapeutic effect and for the development of toxicity is small. Hypokalemia, hypothyroidism, renal insufficiency, and old age all lower the threshold for digitalis intoxication. As emphasized earlier, evidence that patients with acute myocardial infarction are more sensitive to digitalis is not firm, but the fact that these patients are prone to develop serious dysrhythmias in any case suggests that digitalis should be used with caution in the presence of acute infarction.

The first step in the treatment of digitalis intoxication is discontinuation of the drug. The blood urea nitrogen, serum creatinine, serum potassium and, if possible, the serum digoxin levels should be measured. Occasionally, all of the measurements are normal, but hypomagnesemia is responsible for digitalis intoxication. Deficits of potassium and/or magnesium should be corrected. However, as indicated earlier, potassium should not be given intravenously at a rate exceeding 15 meq/hr, and the concentration of potassium should not exceed 40 meq/l. Magnesium should be administered intravenously as a 10 percent solution; 40 ml of this preparation (3.25 meq) may be given at a rate not exceeding 1.5 ml/min.

The mild arrhythmias, including first-degree A-V block, second-degree block of the Wenckebach type, atrioventricular junctional rhythm with a ventricular response of 60 to 100 beats per minute, sinus bradycardia, occasional premature ventricular or junctional contractions, and paroxysmal atrial tachycardia with block with a ventricular response of less than 100 beats per minute require little therapy other than discontinuation of the drug. On the other hand, two or more premature ventricular contractions occurring in a row, brief bouts of ventricular tachycardia, and higher degrees of atrioventricular block require more vigorous treatment.

In the setting of acute myocardial infarction, premature ventricular contractions occurring in the presence of a normal serum potassium level are a definite indication for treatment with intravenous lidocaine or intravenous procainamide. If these agents are unsuccessful, propranolol, quinidine, or diphenylhydantoin (Dilantin) may be used, but these drugs must be employed under appropriate hemodynamic monitoring.

Intractable supraventricular and ventricular dysrhythmias with ventricular rates exceeding 130/min may lead to circulatory collapse and/or pulmonary edema. When such dysrhythmias are thought to be caused by digitalis intoxication, D-C cardioversion may be utilized as a last resort if other measures such as the cautious administration of intravenous propranolol have failed, provided that the serum potassium is within normal limits. Low energies (10 to 15 joules) may be tried initially. Although such treatment is potentially hazardous, it may be indicated in desperate situations because of the ever-present danger of ventricular fibrillation. A temporary demand pacemaker is indicated for digitalis-induced bradyarrhythmias responsible for a low output state, if a trial of atropine has been unsuccessful. It cannot be emphasized too strongly that the diagnosis of these dysrhythmias as a result of digitalis intoxication in the presence of acute myocardial infarction must be a presumptive one, unless it can be shown that the digoxin level is indeed elevated, since all these dysrhythmias may be the result of infarction alone in the absence of therapy with digoxin.

## ADDITIONAL MEASURES FOR THE TREATMENT OF CONGESTIVE CARDIAC FAILURE

These measures are outlined under general patient care in Chapter 7; however, a number of points should be emphasized. With respect to diet, clinical experience indicates that it is quite difficult for patients to adhere to very low-sodium diets. Even with the availability of the newer diuretics, however, dietary control remains an important adjunct to the therapy of congestive heart failure. From the standpoint of patient education, it is useful to begin dietary control as treatment in the Coronary Care Unit. In many patients, dietary indiscretion precipitates recurrent bouts of heart failure and can also precipitate acute myocardial infarction, despite faithful adherence to medications such as digitalis and diuretics. Salt restriction to below 4 gm daily, which can be achieved by adding no extra salt to the meal, is usually advisable. Occasionally, patients with advanced heart failure require a 1 gm/day salt regimen, which necessitates limitation of salt in food preparation as well as elimination of many foods (for example, preprocessed meat and fish), but this is difficult for most patients to follow over prolonged periods of time. Another exceedingly important point in the control of congestive cardiac failure is the control of systemic arterial pressure. This, of course, is the goal of "afterload reduction," and it is a good idea to begin to educate the patient as soon as possible on the importance of controlling his or her arterial blood pressure.

# REFERENCES

1. Wolk MJ, Scheidt S, Killip T: Heart failure complicating acute myocardial infarction. Circulation 45:1125–1138, 1972.
2. Crawford MH, LeWinter MM, O'Rourke RA, Karliner JS, Ross J Jr: Combined propranolol and digoxin therapy in angina pectoris. Ann Intern Med 83:449–455, 1975.
3. Field BJ, Russell RO, Dowling JT, Rackley CE: Regional left ventricular performance in the year following myocardial infarction. Circulation 40:679–684, 1972.
4. Lesch M, Gorlin R: Pharmacological therapy of angina pectoris. Mod Concepts Cardiovasc Dis 43:5–10, 1973.
5. Oriol A, McGregor M: Indicator-dilution methods in the estimation of cardiac output in clinical shock. Am J Cardiol 20:826–830, 1967.
6. Forrester JS, Ganz W, Diamond G, McHugh T, Chonette DW, Swan HJC: Thermodilution cardiac output determination with a single flow-directed catheter. Am Heart J 83:306–311, 1972.
7. Hamosh P, Cohn JN: Left ventricular function in acute myocardial infarction. J Clin Invest 50:523–533, 1971.
8. Forrester JS, Diamond G, Chatterjee K, Swan, HJC: Medical therapy of acute myocardial infarction by application of hemodynamic subsets. New Engl J Med 295:1356–1362, 1976.
9. Weber KT, Janicki JS, Russell RO, Rackley CE: Identification of high risk subsets of acute myocardial infarction: derived from the myocardial infarction research units cooperative study data bank. Am J Cardiol 41:197–203, 1978.
10. Russell RO Jr, Hunt D, Rackley CE: Left ventricular hemodynamics in anterior and inferior myocardial infarction. Am J Cardiol 32:8–16, 1973.
11. Swan HJC, Ganz W, Forrester J, Marcus H, Diamond G, Chonette DW: Cardiac catheterization with a flow-directed balloon-tipped catheter. New Engl J Med 283:447–451, 1970.
12. Cohn JN, Tristani FE, Khatri IM: Studies in clinical shock and hypertension. VI. Relationship between left and right ventricular function. J Clin Invest 48:2008–2018, 1969.
13. Forrester JS, Diamond G, McHugh TJ, Swan, HJC: Filling pressures in the right and left sides of the heart in acute myocardial infarction. New Engl J Med 285:190–193, 1971.
14. McAllister RG Jr, Friesinger GC, Sinclair-Smith BC: Tricuspid regurgitation following inferior myocardial infarction. Arch Intern Med 136:95–99, 1976.
15. Rigo P, Murray M, Taylor DR, Weisfeldt ML, Kelly DT, Strauss HW, Pitt B: Right ventricular dysfunction detected by gated scintiphotography in patient with acute inferior myocardial infarction. Circulation 52:268–274, 1975.
16. Tobinick E, Schelbert HR, Henning H, LeWinter M, Taylor A, Ashburn WL, Karliner JS: Right ventricular ejection fraction in patients with acute anterior and inferior myocardial infarction assessed by radionuclide angiography. Circulation 57:1078–1084, 1978.
17. Rahimtoola SH, Loeb, HS, Ehsani A, Zinno MZ, Chuquimia R, Lai R, Rosen KM, Gunnar RM: Relationship of pulmonary artery to left ventricular diastolic pressures in acute myocardial infarction. Circulation 46:283–290, 1972.
18. Rahimtoola SH, Ehsani A, Sinno MA, Loeb HS, Rosen KM, Gunnar RM: Left atrial transport function in myocardial infarction: importance of its booster pump function. Am J Med 59:686–694, 1975.
19. Russell RO Jr, Rackley CE, Pombo J, Hunt D, Potanin C, Dodge HT: Effects of increasing left ventricular filling pressure in patients with acute myocardial infarction. J Clin Invest 49:1539–1550, 1970.
20. Scheidt S, Wilner G, Fillmore S, Shapiro M, Killip T: Objective haemodynamic assessment after acute myocardial infarction. Br Heart J 35:908–916, 1973.
21. Crexells C, Chatterjee K, Forrester JS, Dikshit K, Swan HJC: Optimal level of filling pressure in the left side of the heart in acute myocardial infarction. N Engl J Med 289:1263–1266, 1973.
22. Shell WE, Stankus K, Mickle D, Swan HJC: Early assessment and alteration of left ventricular filling pressure following myocardial infarction. Am J Cardiol 43:394 (abst) 1979.
23. Karliner JS, Ross J Jr: Left ventricular performance after acute myocardial infarction. Prog Cardiovasc Dis 13:374–391, 1971.
24. Broder MI, Cohn JN: Evolution of abnormalities in left ventricular function after acute myocardial infarction. Circulation 46:731–743, 1972.
25. Franciosa JA, Guiha NH, Limas CJ, Paz S, Cohn JN: Arterial pressure as a determinant of

left ventricular filling pressure after acute myocardial infarction. Am J Cardiol 34:506–512, 1974.

26. Rackley CE, Russell RO Jr: Left ventricular function in acute myocardial infarction and its clinical significance. Circulation 45:231–244, 1972.

27. Rahimtoola SH, DiGilio MM, Sinno MZ, Loeb HS, Rósen KM, Gunnar RM: Cardiac performance three to eight weeks after acute myocardial infarction. Arch Intern Med 128:220–228, 1971.

28. Rigo P, Murray M, Strauss HW, Taylor D, Kelly D, Weisfeldt M, Pitt B: Left ventricular function in acute myocardial infarction evaluated by gated scintiphotography. Circulation 50:678–684, 1974.

29. Schelbert HR, Henning H, Ashburn WL, Verba JW, Karliner JS, O'Rourke RA: Serial measurements of left ventricular ejection fraction by radionuclide angiography early and late after myocardial infarction. Am J Cardiol 38:407–415, 1976.

30. Kupper W, Bleifeld W, Hanrath P, Mathey D, Effert S: Left ventricular hemodynamics and function in acute myocardial infarction: studies during the acute phase, convalescence and late recovery. Am J Cardiol 40:900–905, 1977.

31. Karliner JS: Noninvasive evaluation of the patient with suspected coronary artery disease. Curr Probl Cardiol 3(4):18–22, 1978.

32. Forrester JS, Diamond G, Swan HJC: Correlative classification of clinical and hemodynamic function after acute myocardial infarction. Am J Cardiol 39:137–145, 1977.

33. Rigo P, Murray M, Taylor DR, Weisfeldt ML, Strauss HW, Pitt B: Hemodynamic and prognostic findings in patients with transmural and nontransmural infarction. Circulation 51:1064–1070, 1975.

34. Dikshit K, Vyden JK, Forrester JS, Chatterjee K, Prakush R, Swan HJC: Renal and extrarenal hemodynamic effects of furosemide in congestive heart failure after acute myocardial infarction. N Engl J Med 288:1087–1090, 1973.

35. Kiely J, Kelly DT, Taylor DR, Pitt B: The role of furosemide in the treatment of left ventricular dysfunction associated with acute myocardial infarction. Circulation 48:581–587, 1973.

36. Mond H, Hunt D, Sloman G: Haemodynamic effects of frusemide in patients suspected of having acute myocardial infarction. Br Heart J 36:44–53, 1974.

37. Meriwether WD, Mangi RJ, Serpick AA: Deafness following standard intravenous dose of ethacrynic acid. JAMA 216:795–798, 1971.

38. Puschett JB: Physiologic basis for the use of new and older diuretics in congestive heart failure. Cardiovasc Med 2:119–134, 1977.

39. Hollenberg NK, Adams DF: The renal blood supply in oliguric states: when is a kidney ischemic? A fundamental in cardiology. Am Heart J 91:255–261, 1976.

40. DeRobertis FR, Michelis MF, Beck H, Davis BB: Complications of diuretic therapy: severe alkalosis and syndrome resembling inappropriate secretion of antidiuretic hormone. Metabolism 19:709–719, 1970.

41. Lavender S, McGill RJ: Nonketotic hyperosmolar coma and furosemide therapy. Diabetes 23:247–248, 1974.

42. Heikkilä J: Pump failure and haemodynamic subsets in acute myocardial infarction. Ann Clin Res 9:112–123, 1977.

43. Dodek A, Kassebaum DG, Bristow JD: Pulmonary edema in coronary-artery disease without cardiomegaly. Paradox of the stiff heart. N Engl J Med 286:1347–1350, 1972.

44. Aberman A, Fulop M: The metabolic and respiratory acidosis of acute pulmonary edema. Ann Intern Med 76:173–184, 1972.

45. Zelis R, Mansour EJ, Capone RJ, Mason DT: The cardiovascular effects of morphine. The peripheral capacitance and resistance vessels in human subjects. J Clin Invest 54:1247–1258, 1974.

46. Vismara LA, Leaman DM, Zelis R: The effects of morphine on venous tone in patients with acute pulmonary edema. Circulation 54:335–337, 1976.

47. Ryan WF, Henning H, Karliner JS: Effects of morphine on left ventricular dimensions and function in patients with previous myocardial infarction. Clinical Cardiology 2:417–423, 1979.

48. Habak PA, Mark AL, Kioschos JM, McRaven DR, Abboud FM: Effectiveness of congesting cuffs ("rotating tourniquets") in patients with left heart failure. Circulation 50:366–371, 1974.

49. Grossman RF, Aberman A: Emergency management of acute pulmonary edema. Ann Intern Med 84:488, 1976.

50. Ayres SM: Ventilatory management in acute pulmonary edema. Am J Med 54:558–562, 1973.

51. Yu PN: Lung water in congestive heart failure. Mod Concepts Cardiovasc Dis 50:27, 1971.

52. daLuz PL, Shubin H, Weil MH, Jacobson E, Stein L: Pulmonary edema related to changes in colloid osmotic and pulmonary artery wedge pressure in patients after acute myocardial infarction. Circulation 51:350–357, 1975.

53. Kostuk W, Barr JW, Simar AL, Ross J Jr: Correlations between the chest film and hemodynamics in acute myocardial infarction. Circulation 48:629–632, 1973.

54. Luepker RV, Caralis DG, Voigt GC, Burns RF, Murphy LW, Warbasse JR: Detection of pulmonary edema in acute myocardial infarction. Am J Cardiol 39:146–152, 1977.

55. Epstein SF, Kent KM, Goldstein RE, Borer JS, Redwood DR: Reduction of ischemic injury by nitroglycerin during acute myocardial infarction. N Engl J Med 292:29–35, 1975.

56. Come PC, Pitt B: Nitroglycerin-induced severe hypotension and bradycardia in patients with acute myocardial infarction. Circulation 54:624–628, 1976.

57. LeWinter MM, Karliner JS, Covell JW: Alteration in heart rate response to hemorrhage in conscious dogs with volume overload. Am J Physiol 235 (4):H422–H428, 1978.

58. Bussmann W-D, Löhner J, Kaltenbach M: Orally adminstered isosorbide dinitrate in patients with and without left ventricular failure due to acute myocardial infarction. Cardiology 39:91–96, 1977.

59. Miller RR, Awan NA, DeMaria AN, Amsterdam EA, Mason DT: Importance of maintaining systemic blood pressure during nitroglycerin administration for reducing ischemic injury in patients with coronary disease. Effects on coronary blood flow, myocardial energetics and left ventricular function. Circulation 40:504–508, 1977.

60. Herrick JB: Clinical features of sudden obstruction of the coronary arteries. JAMA 49:2015–2020, 1912.

61. Bloomfield RA, Rapaport B, Milnor JP, Long WK, Mebane JG, Ellis LB: Effects of cardiac glycosides upon dynamics of circulation in congestive heart failure: ouabain. J Clin Invest 27:588–599, 1948.

62. Mahler F, Karliner JS, O'Rourke RA: Effects of chronic digoxin administration on left ventricular performance in the normal conscious dog. Circulation 50:720–727, 1974.

63. Crawford MH, Karliner JS, O'Rourke RA: Favorable effects of oral maintenance digoxin therapy on left ventricular performance in normal subjects: echocardiographic study. Am J Cardiol 58:843–847, 1976.

64. Johnston JD, McDevitt DG: Is maintenance digoxin necessary in patients with sinus rhythm? The Lancet I:567–570, 1979.

65. Guz A, McHaffie D: The use of digitalis glycosides in sinus rhythm. Clin Sci Mol Med 55:417–421, 1978.

65a. Byrd R, Arnold S, Meister S, Cheitlin M, Bristow D, Chatterjee K: Hemodynamic improvement at rest and exercise with chronic digoxin in heart failure. Circulation 59 and 60 (suppl II):75, 1979.

66. Edwards JE: What is myocardial infarction? Circulation 39–40 (Suppl IV):5–11, 1969.

67. Banka VS, Chadda KD, Bodenheimer MM, Helfant RH: Digitalis in experimental acute myocardial infarction. Differential effects on contractile performance of ischemic, border and nonischemic ventricular zones in the dog. Am J Cardiol 35:801–808, 1975.

68. Vatner SF, Baig H: Comparison of the effects of ouabain and isoproterenol on ischemic myocardium of conscious dogs. Circulation 58:654–662, 1978.

69. Baum GL, Dick MM, Blum A, Kaupe A, Carballo J: Factors involved in digitalis sensitivity in chronic pulmonary insufficiency. Am Heart J 57:460–462, 1959.

70. Karliner JS, Braunwald E: Present status of digitalis treatment of acute myocardial infarction. Circulation 45:891–902, 1972.

71. Mason DT, Braunwald E: Studies on digitalis: X. Effects of ouabain on forearm vascular resistance and venous tone in normal subjects and in patients in heart failure. J Clin Invest 43:532–543, 1964.

72. Cohn JN, Tristani FE, Khatri IM: Cardiac and peripheral vascular effects of digitalis in clinical cardiogenic shock. Am Heart J 78:318–330, 1969.

73. Karliner, JS, Braunwald E: Congestive heart failure. In Current Therapy 1973, edited by Conn HF, WB Saunders Co, Philadelphia, 1973, 25:189–197.

74. Hamman L: The symptoms of coronary occlusion. Johns Hopkins Med J 38:273–319, 1926.

75. Friedberg CK: Acute coronary occlusion and myocardial infarction. In Diseases of the Heart, 3rd ed, WB Saunders Co, Philadelphia, 1966, p 911.

76. Logue RB, Hurst JW: Management of patients with coronary atherosclerotic disease and its complications. In The Heart, 2nd ed, edited Hurst JW, Logue RB, New York, McGraw Hill Book Co, 1970, p 1017.

77. Hurst JW, Logue RB, Walter PF: The clinical recognition and medical management of coronary atherosclerotic heart disease. In The Heart, 4th ed, edited Hurst JW, Logue RB, Schlant RC, Wenger NK, New York, McGraw Hill Book Co, 1978, p 1239.

78. Lown B, Vassaux C, Hood WB Jr, Fakhro AM,

Kaplinsky E, Roberge G: Unresolved problems in coronary care. Am J Cardiol 20:494–508, 1967.

78a. Marcus FI: Editorial: Use of digitalis in acute myocardial infarction. Circulation 62:17–19, 1980.

79. Swan HJC, Danzig R, Sukumalchantra Y, Allen H: Current status of treatment of power failure of the heart in acute myocardial infarction with drugs and blood volume replacement. Circulation 39–40 (Suppl IV):277–284, 1969.

80. Balcon R, Hoy J, Sowton E: Haemodynamic effects of rapid digitalization following acute myocardial infarction. Br Heart J 30:373–376, 1968.

81. Sjögren A: Left heart failure in acute myocardial infarction. III. The early hemodynamic effects of ouabain and furosemide in patients with acute myocardial infarction and raised pulmonary artery diastolic pressures. Acta Med Scand (Suppl 510):53–62, 1970.

82. Mason DT, Amsterdam EA, Miller RR, Williams DO: What is the role of positive inotropic agents in the treatment of acute myocardial infarction? Cardiovasc Clin 8:113–122, 1977.

83. Morrison J, Coromilas J, Robbins M et al: Digitalis and myocardial infarction in man. Circulation 62:8–16, 1980.

84. Lipp H, Denes P, Gambetta M, Resnikov L: Hemodynamic response to acute intravenous digoxin in patients with recent myocardial infarction and coronary insufficiency with and without heart failure. Chest 63:862–867, 1973.

85. Goldstein RA, Bowen WG, Branconi JM et al: Comparison of the hemodynamic effects of digoxin and dobutamine in patients with cardiac failure and acute myocardial infarction. (Abstr.) Circulation 60 (Suppl II):II-70, 1979.

86. Sharpe DN, Norris RM, White B McL: Treatment with digoxin and measurement of serum digoxin levels after myocardial infarction. Br Heart J 37:530–533, 1975.

87. Marcus FI, Burkhalter L, Cuccia C, Pavlovich J, Kapadra GG: Administration of tritrated digoxin with and without a loading dose. A metabolic study. Circulation 34:865–874, 1966.

88. Rieffel JA, Leahey EB Jr, Drusin RE, Heissenbuttel RH, Lovejoy W, Bigger JT Jr: A previously unrecognized drug interaction between quinidine and digoxin. Clin Cardiol 2:40–42, 1979.

89. Ochs HR, Greenblat DJ, Woo E, Smith TW: Reduced quinidine clearance in elderly persons. Am J Cardiol 42:481–495, 1978.

# 20 | Cardiogenic Shock: Pathophysiology and Pharmacologic Therapy

## Joel S. Karliner, M.D.

Over the past few years much has been learned concerning the pathophysiology of cardiogenic shock in acute myocardial infarction. Several newer pharmacologic agents have been tried both experimentally and clinically in the treatment of this disorder, with modest claims for success. Over the last decade, mechanical ventricular assistance has also received considerable study; the use of this approach combined with surgical therapy is outlined in the following chapter. It should be recognized that shock due to acute myocardial infarction is, in general, the result of severe pump failure of the left ventricular myocardium. Thus, in pathologic studies it has been reported that over 40 percent of the left ventricular myocardium is generally involved.[1,2] Where angiographic studies have been performed under these circumstances, it has been noted that the residual myocardium appears to be contracting maximally, thereby raising the issue of whether inotropic support could even be of benefit (see below). The clinician should be aware, however, that the following may also have some of the clinical signs of cardiogenic shock: (1) a few patients suffering from hypovolemia resulting from either blood loss or diuretic therapy; and (2) other patients with pure right ventricular infarction. Although these two groups are small, recognition that such subsets exist may increase the salvage rate of such patients. These are described in more detail below.

## DEFINITION OF CARDIOGENIC SHOCK

Before proceeding to a discussion of the treatment of cardiogenic shock, it is necessary to have a reasonably rigid definition of the syndrome, since otherwise apparent therapeutic success may occur when true cardiogenic shock is, in fact, not present. This may lead to discouraging results when the true syndrome is encountered. In many units, the definition of shock utilized by the Myocardial Infarction Research Units of the National Heart, Lung and Blood Institute has been employed. While this represents a "committee approach," it nevertheless describes most features of cardiogenic shock and permits the discussion of results in a logical and cohesive manner. Thus, the criteria for cardiogenic shock are as follows:

1. A systolic arterial pressure less than 90 mmHg or 60 mmHg below the previous basal level.
2. Evidence of reduced blood flow as shown by the presence of all of the following:
   a. urine output less than 20 ml/hr, preferably with a low sodium content
   b. impaired mental function
   c. peripheral vasoconstriction associated with cold, clammy skin

Additional criteria are that urinary flow should be measured without the aid of diuretic therapy

471

and that hypovolemia, as judged by left-sided filling pressures, should be corrected. In addition, significant dysrhythmias such as rapid supraventricular and ventricular tachycardia should not be present. All efforts to correct systemic hypoxia should be made. With respect to blood pressure measurement, it is important to note that this should preferably be an intra-arterial pressure, since it has been shown that, in patients with shock syndrome of any etiology, the blood pressure measured by cuff sphygmomanometry may be 10 to 20 mmHg lower than that measured by intra-arterial needle due to intense vasoconstriction and the inability of the auscultator to hear the Korotkoff sounds properly.[3]

The presence of myocardial infarction should, of course, be confirmed by the appropriate electrocardiographic and enzymatic determinations. In this connection, it seems apparent that, in patients with acute myocardial infarction and cardiogenic shock, the nature of the myocardial injury appears to be a progressive one. Thus, Gutovitz et al. measured peak plasma cardiospecific creatine kinase (MB-CK) activity and found that it was significantly higher in seven patients with cardiogenic shock associated with an initial infarction than in pa-

tients with shock who had previous infarction or in patients with uncomplicated myocardial infarction.[4] A prolonged time to the peak level of MB-CK activity, averaging 26 hours, and a plateau of the elevated MB-CK activity were seen in patients with shock associated with initial infarction. The results reported by these investigators suggest that cardiogenic shock associated with initial infarction results from progressive myocardial damage causing continuous release of MB-CK into the circulation. These observations reflect a vicious cycle of spreading myocardial injury, progressive compromise of cardiac function and exacerbation of ischemia and perpetuation of myocardial damage.

## HEMODYNAMIC CHARACTERIZATION OF CARDIOGENIC SHOCK DUE TO ACUTE MYOCARDIAL INFARCTION

In a number of studies, it has been demonstrated that cardiogenic shock may be viewed as an extreme form of left ventricular failure. Thus, utilizing the concepts presented in Chapter 19, it can be seen that, in patients with cardiogenic shock, the relation between left ventricular stroke work and left ventricular end-diastolic pressure (the left ventricular function curve) is severely depressed and that, despite very high left ventricular filling pressures, the cardiac output remains markedly reduced (Fig. 20.1). Thus, Ratshin et al. reported that, despite intensive medical treatment, a 100 percent mortality rate occurred in patients who had: a pulmonary arterial end-diastolic pressure or left ventricular end-diastolic pressure greater than 28 mmHg; or a pulmonary artery end-diastolic pressure or left ventricular end-diastolic pressure of greater than 15 mmHg in association with a cardiac index of less than 2.3 1/min/m².[5] Forrester et al. have proposed that patients with acute myocardial infarction can be divided into various hemodynamic subsets and that those who exhibit evidence of both pulmonary congestion and hypoperfusion on clinical grounds (hypotension, tachycardia, confusion,

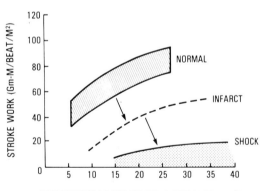

Fig. 20.1  Relation of stroke work to left ventricular end-diastolic pressure. The shaded area above depicts the normal range of this modified Frank-Starling relation. The broken line shows depression of left ventricular function. (This occurs in many patients with acute myocardial infarction, but most of these do not succumb.) The solid line shows the upper limits of ventricular function in patients dying of myocardial infarction shock. (Modified after Swan et al.[39])

cyanosis, oliguria) have a cardiac index averaging 1.6 1/min/m² and a pulmonary capillary pressure averaging 27 mmHg.[6] Over half of patients in this subgroup died. Bleifeld et al. reported that patients with a left ventricular end-diastolic pressure exceeding 17 mmHg in the presence of a cardiac index below 1.8 1/min/m² had a mortality rate of about 70 percent.[7] When the ratio of left ventricular stroke work index to left ventricular end-diastolic pressure declined below 1.2 gm-m/m²/mmHg, 80 percent of 42 patients had an immediate poor prognosis. It should be recognized that, where the definition of cardiogenic shock described above is rigidly adhered to, the mortality rate in most series has been between 80 and 90 percent. Additional metabolic features of cardiogenic shock that portend a poor prognosis include elevation in blood lactate and persistent marked depression of the arterial oxygen tension despite adequate oxygenation delivered by mask or even by endotracheal intubation.[8]

Among the additional mechanical complications of acute myocardial infarction leading to cardiogenic shock are papillary muscle rupture and ventricular septal defect (see Ch. 24). In both instances, the diagnosis may be made by bedside cardiac catheterization using a balloon-tipped catheter. In the presence of papillary muscle rupture, a large "V" wave may be recorded in the pulmonary wedge tracing. With a ventricular septal defect, there will be an increase in oxygen content between the superior vena cava and the right ventricle and, in addition, evidence of elevated right atrial and right ventricular pressures. These syndromes should be sought in any patient with cardiogenic shock, since they are potentially amenable to surgical correction. This is especially important because silent mitral insufficiency may occur in acute myocardial infarction. Thus, Forrester et al. described severe mitral regurgitation in the absence of an audible murmur in three patients with power failure secondary to acute myocardial infarction.[9] In each instance microscopic examination of all papillary muscles revealed evidence of extensive necrosis.

Because of the necessity of assessing intracardiac pressures in monitoring patients with cardiogenic shock, it is important to recognize that there is a good relationship between the pulmonary artery end-diastolic pressure and left ventricular filling pressure in such patients. Because of technical difficulties and balloon breakage, it may be difficult to obtain an adequate pulmonary capillary or wedge pressure in all circumstances; under these conditions, the pulmonary arterial end-diastolic pressure (PAEDP) can be utilized. Scheinman et al. reported that the PAEDP can be used over a wide range of heart rates (60 to 160 beats per minute) and a wide spectrum of aterial oxygen tensions ranging from 33 to 562 mmHg.[10] They reported that a PAEDP in excess of 15 mmHg nearly always reflected an increased left ventricular end-diastolic pressure, while a PAEDP of less than 10 mmHg was always associated with a normal left ventricular end-diastolic pressure. At least two cautionary notes are in order, however; Scheinman et al. pointed out that: (1) in 16 percent of their studies, the PAEDP suggested left ventricular failure in the presence of a normal left ventricular EDP, and (2) in an additional 3 percent of their studies, the PAEDP failed to reflect apparent left ventricular decompensation.[10] These false-positive and false-negative results almost always occurred with PAEDP levels in the borderline area (10 to 15 mmHg). Recent experimental work has emphasized that, in patients who require endotracheal intubation and positive end-expiratory pressure (PEEP), pulmonary capillary pressure (and hence PAEDP) may exceed the simultaneously measured left atrial pressure despite a decline in cardiac output.[11] In such patients, it seems best to discontinue PEEP for 30 to 40 secs before measuring PAEDP or pulmonary capillary pressure.

As the left ventricular end-diastolic pressure and the intrapulmonary pressures increase in patients with cardiogenic shock, pulmonary function may be further affected. How often the syndrome known as "shock lung" occurs in patients with cardiogenic shock is uncertain, but this syndrome has been characterized by progressive respiratory failure, falling $PO_2$ levels, increasing tachypnea, dyspnea and cough, cyanosis, respiratory acidosis and physical signs of pulmonary edema and pneumonia.[12] All of these may occur in patients with cardiogenic shock, and undoubtedly some lung damage does occur to complicate this syndrome.

Additional important hemodynamic features include the recognition of normal pulmonary arterial wedge pressure or pulmonary end-diastolic pressure in a patient with evidence of peripheral hypoperfusion. Under these circumstances, hypovolemia can be diagnosed, and the diagnosis of cardiogenic shock should not be made until an adequate left ventricular filling pressure (mean pulmonary capillary pressure averaging 18 mmHg) is achieved. The hypovolemia may be iatrogenic from previous or current diuretic therapy, may be the result of occult or overt gastrointestinal hemorrhage, or may reflect vomiting or diarrhea from any cause. The recent observation that right ventricular infarction occurs commonly in patients with inferior myocardial infarction [13] confirms observations made previously that occasional patients with acute inferior myocardial infarction may exhibit features compatible with severe congestive cardiac failure or even with cardiogenic shock.[14] Under these circumstances, the jugular venous pressure may be elevated, and increased right ventricular pressures may be noted in the presence of normal or near normal pulmonary arterial and pulmonary capillary pressures. Such combinations of hypovolemia and right ventricular infarction can lead to the erroneous diagnosis of cardiogenic shock.

## TREATMENT OF CARDIOGENIC SHOCK

Once a diagnosis has been made, the therapy of cardiogenic shock should be aimed toward the detection and correction of all possible hemodynamic and metabolic abnormalities. In patients with overt hypovolemia and/or significant dysrhythmias, these should obviously be corrected as rapidly as possible. In the vast majority of patients, however, the left ventricular filling pressure is elevated, and a sinus tachycardia is almost always present. The latter reflects the attempt of the cardiovascular system to maintain adequate cardiac output in the face of a marked reduction in pump function. Among the general measures which should be

employed toward the treatment of cardiogenic shock are the following:

1. Place the patient in a head-down position (unless the patient is in pulmonary edema).
2. Administer morphine sulfate 5 to 10 mg intravenously as necessary to control pain and agitation.
3. Administer 100 percent oxygen by nasal catheter or mask at a rate of 4 to 5 liters per minute.
4. Proceed with tracheal intubation in those patients who may require it (see Chs. 31 and 32).

Based on the level of the left ventricular filling pressure, a diuretic such as furosemide at a dose of 40 to 80 mg intravenously, may be given.

The use of digitalis in acute myocardial infarction is controversial. In recent experimental work, Vatner and Baig compared the effects of isoproterenol and ouabain at equi-inotropic doses on the mechanical function, electrograms, and blood flow of severely ischemic tissue in conscious dogs. The experiment showed that these agents had opposite effects.[15] Ouabain produced a favorable action as evidenced by improved flow and reduction in ST-segment elevation, while isoproterenol intensified ischemia, as reflected in augmented paradoxical bulging, further ST-segment increases, and a fall in blood flow, particularly to endocardial layers. Kirk et al. have emphasized that collateral coronary blood flow to the ischemic region is highly dependent on physical factors, primarily diastolic time, for coronary perfusion and the gradient for perfusion which is created by the diastolic aortic pressure and the left ventricular diastolic pressure.[16] When the left ventricular diastolic pressure is reduced after administration of a digitalis glycoside in an experimental preparation, the coronary diastolic flow in ischemic regions derived from collateral sources is increased, and this increased blood flow delivery may outweight any increase in oxygen requirements that might occur due to an increase in contractility.

Intravenous administration of either digoxin or ouabain has been recommended, but a number of years ago Cohn et al. observed that the intravenous administration of cardiac glycosides in patients with cardiogenic shock produced a prompt pressor effect that was characterized by increases in systemic vascular resistance and no change in left ventricular end-diastolic pressure.[17] Acute pulmonary edema developed during this period in one patient. Fifty to 60 minutes after infusion of digitalis, the left ventricular end-diastolic pressure tended to decrease, but, despite other evidence of improved myocardial function, cardiac output was not significantly increased and was always lower than that attained during infusion of isoproterenol. Thus, digitalis did not appear to be very effective by itself in restoring blood flow in cardiogenic shock, and the early peripheral vasoconstrictor effect following intravenous administration could be deleterious in some patients. Nevertheless, on the presumption that cardiogenic shock is an extreme form of left ventricular failure, its judicious use may be considered in most patients.[18] The drug of choice is digoxin, which, when given intravenously, has an onset of action between 10 and 30 minutes and a maximum effect between 2 and 3 hours after administration. In a patient who has not received a glycoside in the recent past, the intravenous dose of digoxin should be 0.75 mg, followed by 0.25 mg every 4 to 6 hours. Ordinarily, 1.5 mg of digoxin intravenously should not be exceeded during the first 24 hours. Complete excretion of the drug will be impaired in patients with cardiogenic shock and reduced renal blood flow. This suggests that either the initial or the subsequent doses should be reduced by 25 to 50 percent. However, no objective data regarding either the efficacy or the dose of digitalis in patients with acute myocardial infarction in cardiogenic shock have been published to date.

As indicated above, the major problem in cardiogenic shock is reduced pump function of the acutely ischemic and/or necrotic left ventricle. Because coronary flow is pressure-dependent and because most of this flow occurs during the diastolic period of the cardiac cycle, it is necessary to attempt to achieve an increase in aortic diastolic pressure to at least 60 mmHg. It is not, however, necessary to "normalize" the blood pressure in all patients. Thus, a general goal might be to bring the systemic arterial pressure to the level of 90/60 to 100/70 mmHg. Augmentation of blood pressure beyond this level may, in fact, increase myocardial oxygen demand, since the heart's ability to contract is in part dependent on the resistance to ejection (aortic pressure) as well as on the adequacy of coronary blood flow generated by that same aortic pressure. Thus, the goal is to elevate the systemic arterial pressure but not to produce too high a pressure, which would cause further deterioration of cardiac function. This emphasizes the importance of serial measurements of cardiac output in patients who are being treated for either extreme left ventricular failure or cardiogenic shock. A variety of pharmacologic means have been employed to raise the systemic arterial pressure under these circumstances and to achieve an increase in cardiac output. In addition, mechanical ventricular assistance has been used in combination with surgical therapy; in some centers, this is the treatment of choice for cardiogenic shock (see Ch. 21).

Before consideration of pharmacologic therapy, it is useful to review the basis for such treatment. The catecholamines are a group of chemical substances normally synthesized by the adrenal glands, the sympathetic nervous system, and the central nervous system (Fig. 20.2). These compounds have the function of chemical messengers in the central and peripheral autonomic nervous systems; their release at junctions between the nerve cell and its immediately adjacent muscle, mediated by receptors on the cell surface, causes muscular contraction or relaxation, usually in the skeletal muscle and mesenteric vascular beds. When a catecholamine causes contraction of arterial or smooth muscle, an $\alpha$-adrenergic agonist effect is said to occur, while relaxation of that same muscle is termed a $\beta$-adrenergic agonist action, mediated by $\beta$-adrenoceptors (see Table 20.1). A pure $\alpha$-adrenergic agonist is the synthetic substance methoxamine, which causes peripheral (arteriolar) smooth muscle vasoconstriction. A pure $\beta$-adrenergic agonist is isoproterenol, which causes peripheral arteriolar vasodilation (see Table 20.1 and Fig. 20.3). The naturally occurring catecholamines, norepinephrine and epinephrine, have mixed $\alpha$- and $\beta$-agonist functions in the periphery which are

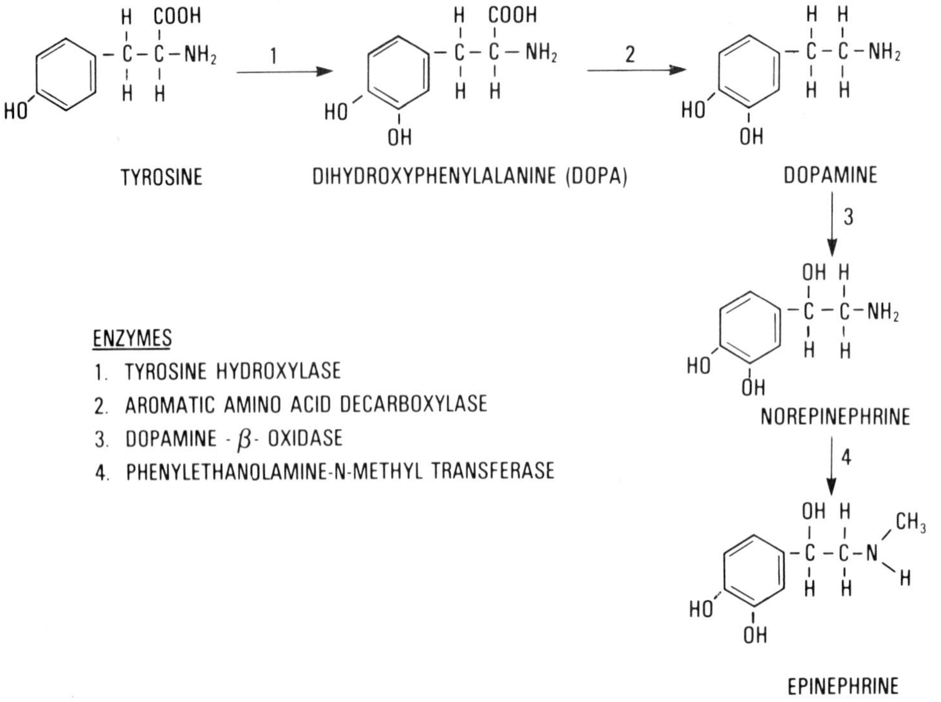

Fig. 20.2 The major natural biosynthetic pathways of catecholamines. Each of the numbers corresponds to the enzyme catalyzing each reaction.

to some degree dose dependent. Thus, in small doses, epinephrine may cause vasodilation, while in larger doses vasoconstriction may occur. Norepinephrine, on the other hand, always causes vasoconstriction. With respect to their effects on the heart, the catecholamines, when they are active, tend to exert a $\beta$-adrenergic agonist effect alone ($\beta_1$ effect). In the heart, this effect consists largely of an increase in the rate and force of cardiac action, and administration of a pure $\beta$-adrenergic agonist such as isoproterenol will increase the heart rate and increase the force of myocardial contraction. Norepinephrine and epinephrine are somewhat less potent $\beta$-adrenergic agonists with respect to their action on cardiac muscle; phenylephrine has little $\beta$-adrenergic agonist effect on the heart, and methoxamine has none at all. While the heart has the capacity to respond to $\alpha$-adrenergic stimulation by an increase in the force of contraction, the clinical importance of this response has yet to be determined.

The classification of catecholamines into $\alpha$- and $\beta$-adrenergic agonists was first described by Ahlquist.[19] As indicated above, it has be-

come evident that these drugs exert their actions in part by combining with receptors thought to be located on cell surfaces, the $\alpha$- and $\beta$-adrenoceptors respectively. Dopamine is a naturally occurring catecholamine that is an intermediate in the biosynthesis of noradrenaline and functions as an important neurotransmitter in the central nervous system (Fig. 20.2). Dopamine stimulates both $\alpha$- and $\beta$-adrenoceptors as well as specific dopamine receptors.[20] Which receptors are stimulated depends mainly on the dose of dopamine given. In healthy subjects, the effect of a low infusion rate (0.5 to 2.0 $\mu$gm/kg per minute) is to stimulate dopamine receptors in the renal artery, causing dilatation and an increased renal blood flow, and a rise in glomerular filtration rate and sodium excretion.[21] These effects occur with little or no change in cardiac output and are inhibited by dopamine receptor blocking agents such as haloperidol. In animals, the equivalent dose of dopamine also increases mesenteric arterial blood flow, but this effect has yet to be demonstrated in man. Infusion of dopamine in the range of 3 to 10 $\mu$gm/kg per minute stimulates

$\beta$-adrenoceptors in the heart with an increase in myocardial contractility, stroke volume, and cardiac output. Usually, total peripheral resistance falls, and heart rate and mean arterial pressure change little. These effects are prevented by $\beta$-adrenergic blockade, which will also prevent $\beta$-adrenergic effects produced by isoproterenol and norepinephrine. A commonly used $\beta$-blocker is, of course, propranolol. Higher doses of dopamine stimulate $\alpha$-adrenoceptors, causing an increase in vascular resistance and eventually a fall in renal blood flow. At the same time, cardiac dysrhythmias may develop as a result of excessive $\beta$-adrenergic stimulation, and this is true of all catecholamines.

Experimental studies in conscious dogs with regional myocardial ischemia induced by complete occlusion of one major coronary vessel have demonstrated that catecholamines elicit a spectrum of actions in tissues which are undergoing varying degrees of ischemia.[22] In severely ischemic zones, myocardial function tended to deteriorate, whereas almost all segments in moderately ischemic and border zones as well as in the normal zones displayed improved function. These results regarding mechanical function correlated well with regional flow determinations, which indicated enhanced perfusion along with improved function on the one hand and no change or reduced perfusion in those segments that deteriorated on the other. In patients with cardiogenic shock, it is likely that coronary perfusion of the myocardium is fixed and cannot increase; therefore, increases in myocardial oxygen demand induced by the systemic administration of catecholamines may not be met by an appropriate increase in oxygen delivery. Accordingly, the myocardium may

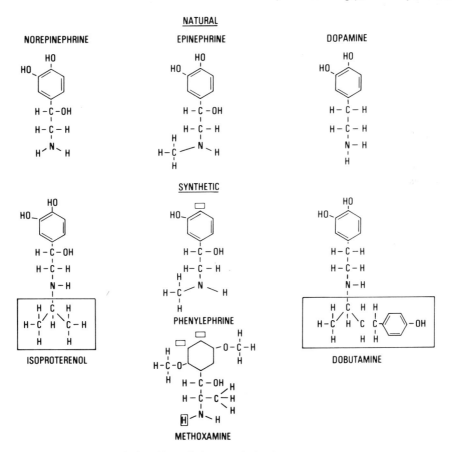

Fig. 20.3 Some structural relationships of the catecholamines used in the treatment of cardiogenic shock. Each large and small boxed area in the synthetic compounds shows a major structural alteration when compared to the natural compound.

rapidly exceed its nutrient blood supply, resulting in deterioration of left ventricular performance, especially if aortic pressure is excessively augmented. In patients with cardiogenic shock, the extent of coronary artery disease as well as the extent of collateral circulation may vary, and the balance of myocardial oxygen supply and demand produced by administration of catecholamines will depend on the extent to which coronary blood flow can be increased to ischemic and border zones.

Early studies by Gunnar et al. indicated that, when norepinephrine was compared with a pure $\alpha$-adrenergic agonist such as methoxamine, infusion of the former drug resulted in an increased cardiac output in patients with shock due to myocardial infarction.[23] Thus, it appears necessary to utilize a drug or combination of drugs which exhibit both an $\alpha$-adrenergic agonist action in the periphery (vasoconstriction) and $\beta$-adrenergic agonist action on the myocardium (increased contractility).

Mueller and her colleagues demonstrated that, during norepinephrine infusion to patients with cardiogenic shock, the cardiac index increased insignificantly but increased arterial pressure was associated in all patients with increases in coronary blood flow, averaging 28 percent.[24] Myocardial metabolism also improved. By contrast, during isoproterenol perfusion, the cardiac index increased uniformly, averaging 61 percent. Mean arterial pressure remained unchanged, but diastolic pressure fell. Coronary blood flow increased in three patients secondary to the decrease in coronary vascular resistance, but myocardial lactate metabolism deteriorated uniformly, lactate production increasing or extraction shifting to production. These investigators concluded that, since forward and collateral flow through the severely diseased coronary bed depends mainly on perfusion pressure, norepinephrine appears to be superior to isoproterenol. A subsequent study, again by Mueller and her colleagues, demonstrated that, during dopamine administration to eight patients with cardiogenic shock in doses averaging 17.2 $\mu$gm/kg per minute, myocardial contractility was increased as manifested by an augmentation of cardiac index and systolic ejection rate with a moderate decrease in systemic

vascular resistance.[25] Pulmonary arterial wedge pressure and right atrial pressure both decreased, but this improvement in hemodynamic status produced by dopamine was associated with deterioration of myocardial metabolism. Thus, myocardial oxygen extraction and arterial-coronary sinus oxygen differences both increased, as did myocardial lactate production. Although norepinephrine would seem to be the drug of choice when compared with isoproterenol and dopamine, on the basis of metabolic studies alone, Abrams et al. concluded that the usefulness of norepinephrine in patients with acute myocardial infarction is limited, as individuals most likely to receive this agent would be expected to respond with a small increase in cardiac output and a significant increase in afterload.[26] It should be pointed out that only small groups of patients were involved in each of these studies, but the results obtained serve to emphasize the point that improvement in hemodynamics may occur at the expense of potential deterioration in myocardial metabolism.

Recently, substantial clinical experience has been accumulated with dopamine in the treatment of cardiogenic shock. Thus, among 30 patients treated for shock due to acute myocardial infarction at the University of California, San Diego, 10 survived the shock episode and eight (27 percent) actually left the hospital.[27] In each patient, ventilatory assistance, antibiotics, digitalis, and other supportive measures were used as indicated. Other pressor or positive inotropic agents, including isoproterenol, norepinephrine and epinephrine were employed singly and in combination in these patients before administration of dopamine. For intravenous administration, dopamine was diluted in 5 percent dextrose and water to a concentration of 800 $\mu$gm/ml. Infusion usually began at the rate of 2 $\mu$gm/kg per minute, and this dose was then increased 1 to 4 $\mu$gm/kg per minute every 15 to 30 minutes until an optimal effect was obtained as judged by urinary flow and systemic arterial pressure. In a number of patients, either isoproterenol, norepinephrine, or both of these agents were discontinued after starting dopamine. In several instances, it was possible to discontinue the isoproterenol or norepinephrine and to utilize dopamine as the sole pressor agent. During the administration of dopamine, an intravenous diuretic agent, usually furosemide, was employed to aid in augmentation of urinary flow. In 24 selected patients, urinary volume was measured hourly and the maximum hourly flow rate was chosen as the primary indicator of the peak response to dopamine. The data in the 12 survivors of the shock episodes, among the 24 patients studied hemodynamically, revealed significant differences when compared with the nonsurvivors. Before dopamine infusion, the average heart rate of survivors averaged $113 \pm 7$ (SE) beats per minute and did not differ significantly from the mean heart rate of the nonsurvivors ($112 \pm 5$ beats per minute). During the peak urinary response of dopamine therapy, the heart rate of the survivors decreased significantly to $104 \pm 6$ beats per minute ($p < .05$, paired t-test), while in nonsurvivors mean heart rate was unchanged (Fig. 20.4). Similarly, alterations in mean arterial pressure demonstrated significant differences between the two groups. Before dopamine, mean arterial pressure averaged $58.6 \pm 9.3$ mmHg in survivors and $63 \pm 2.2$ mmHg in nonsurvivors, a difference which was not significant. During the peak renal response to dopamine, however,

mean arterial pressure increased in survivors to $82 \pm 3.6$ mmHg ($p < .05$), while in nonsurvivors the increment of mean arterial pressure to $72.4 \pm 4.3$ mmHg was not significant (Fig. 20.4).

Urinary flow in nonsurvivors before dopamine averaged $9.6 \pm 2.3$ ml/hr and was not different from survivors ($15.4 \pm 5$ ml/hr). During the optimal response to dopamine treatment, mean urinary flow in survivors increased to $250.4 \pm 59$ ml/hr ($p < .01$), while in nonsurvivors the increase to $100.9 \pm 55$ ml/hr was nonsignificant (Fig. 20.4). Although four nonsurvivors had large (greater than 100 ml/hr) increments of urinary flow, the other eight had either no change or a minimal change in urinary flow. By contrast, only one patient who survived had an increase of urinary flow of less than 35 ml/hr; the average increment was $224.7 \pm 59$ ml/hr. In four of six patients receiving intraaortic balloon counterpulsation (three of whom survived), dopamine augmented urinary flow from an average of 20 to 207 ml/hr.

Before dopamine, left ventricular filling pressure in eight survivors averaged $26.9 \pm 2.4$ mmHg and did not differ from that of ten nonsurvivors ($27 \pm 4$ mmHg). During the peak re-

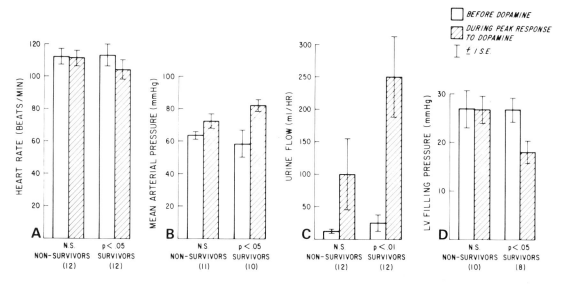

Fig. 20.4  Comparison of survivors and nonsurvivors with respect to alterations in heart rate *(A)*, mean arterial pressure *(B)*, urinary flow *(C)*, and left ventricular filling pressure *(D)*, before and during the peak response to dopamine. In each instance, the changes were statistically significant (paired t-test) only in the survivors. N.S. = not significant; p = probability; S.E. = standard error. (Holzer et al.: Effectiveness of dopamine in patients with cardiogenic shock. Am J Cardiol 32:79–84, 1973.)

nal response to dopamine, left ventricular filling pressure in survivors declined to $18.3 \pm 2.3$ mmHg ($p < .05$), while the average left ventricular filling pressure in nonsurvivors did not change ($26.8 \pm 3.4$ mmHg) (Fig. 20.4).

The dose of dopamine employed ranged from a starting dose of 0.2 $\mu$gm/kg per minute in one patient to a maximum of 53 $\mu$gm/kg/minute in another. The average duration of drug therapy for all patients was approximately 40 hours.

Dopamine was also evaluated in a larger group of 68 patients, among whom were included a subset of 30 patients with acute myocardial infarction.[28] Side effects among these 68 patients probably attributable to dopamine therapy were noted in 12 (18 percent). In one patient, a sinus tachycardia of 140 beats per minute was observed. Eight patients had ventricular ectopic beats during dopamine administration. Therapy with intravenous lidocaine controlled the ectopic beats in three patients, while in one other patient dopamine was discontinued. Two patients had ventricular tachycardia during dopamine therapy, and in one of these the drug was discontinued. Other side effects noted in patients with ventricular ectopic beats were nausea and vomiting (one patient) and angina pectoris (one patient). Another patient developed peripheral gangrene after 89 hours of dopamine therapy, but he was the only patient in whom we have observed this complication, which has subsequently been reported by others.[29-31] This patient had a persistently reduced cardiac index for 13 days after mitral valve replacement for a ruptured papillary muscle resulting from acute myocardial infarction. Whether there was a relation between dopamine therapy and the development of gangrene in this patient could not be definitely established, and it should be emphasized that this is an exceedingly rare complication of dopamine therapy. For treatment of this complication, either intravenous phentolamine (5 to 10 mg) or local phentolamine infiltration has been recommended.[21,29] Intravenous chlorpromazine (7 $\mu$g/kg per min) has also been used successfully.[31]

Of the 12 patients who exhibited adverse re-

sponse to therapy with dopamine, only two were receiving another pressor agent (norepinephrine) at the time the side effect was observed. Four of these 12 patients survived the shock episode (three with acute myocardial infarction and one who had a mitral valve replacement). Adverse reactions occurred predominantly in patients with acute myocardial infarction (eight of 12 patients), but were unrelated to the dose of dopamine employed (average maximum dose of 6.5 $\mu$gm/kg per min, range 1 to 16). One patient who died 21 days after pericardiectomy for constrictive pericarditis required dopamine treatment for the entire three-week postoperative period. No lesions in the heart or other organs attributable to dopamine were found. In addition, 19 other patients showed no evidence of cardiac, renal, or other lesions that could be attributed to dopamine therapy at postmortem examination.

Other potential adverse effects include rebound hypotension, which can occur after prolonged treatment with any catecholamine.[32] In part, this phenomenon may be due to depletion of intravascular volume; the status of the latter should, therefore, be periodically monitored, preferably by measurements of pulmonary capillary or pulmonary artery end-diastolic pressure. In any case, the infusion rate of dopamine (or any other catecholamine) should be reduced slowly. One suggested regimen for dopamine is a reduction of 1 $\mu$cg/kg per min every 30 to 60 minutes.

It should also be recognized that a number of drugs may block various receptors referred to above (also see Table 20.1). Thus, propranolol blocks $\beta$-adrenergic receptors, while phenothiazines and butyrophenones such as haloperidol block $\alpha$-adrenergic receptors. Under these circumstances, dopamine could produce excessive cardiac stimulation without raising blood pressure. It is also possible (but not proved in man) that large doses of phenothiazines or butyrophenones may also block dopamine receptors, thereby preventing the expected increase in renal blood flow.[32] Thus, when the dose of dopamine or other sympathomimetic agents is larger than expected or when the response appears to be inadequate, a drug interaction should be considered. The inactivation pathway of dopamine involves the enzyme monoamine oxidase, and prior use of monoamine oxidase inhibitors could result in an augmented hemodynamic effect from a given infusion of dopamine.[32]

It should also be emphasized that all catecholamines may be inactivated by alkaline solutions, and, therefore, these agents should never be mixed with solutions containing sodium bicarbonate or other basic compounds.

In comparative studies between isoproterenol and dopamine, Thompson has reported that optimal isoproterenol doses of 7 μgm/min maintained systemic arterial pressure at an average of 68 mmHg in patients with severe shock, whereas dopamine at an average dose of 1320 μgm/min promptly increased mean arterial pressure to 80 mmHg with improved perfusion.[33] These patients were relatively refractory to norepinephrine, requiring 26 μgm/min to maintain a mean arterial pressure of 75 mmHg with severe hypoperfusion. When dopamine was instituted in such patients, mean arterial pressure increased to an average of 80 mmHg at an average dopamine dose of 850 μgm/min. Dopamine caused minimal changes in heart rate, left ventricular end-diastolic pressure, or pulmonary arterial wedge pressure. The cardiac index was unchanged when dopamine was compared with an equivalent dose of isoproterenol, while dopamine caused a doubling of the cardiac index when compared with isoproterenol and norepinephrine. Despite these encouraging hemodynamic observations, the survival of patients was poor, reflecting the serious prognosis of shock which is refractory to volume expansion and initial treatment with isoproterenol and/or norepinephrine. Of 156 patients with cardiogenic shock, 29 left the hospital alive, 23 died more than two days after resolution of shock, and 80 died in shock. As observed by others, the prognosis of patients with shock due to acute myocardial infarction is considerably worse than that due to hypotension and myocardial depression associated with open-heart surgery.[28,34] Under the latter circumstances, dopamine seems to be an effective drug which may enhance survival. As Mueller

and her colleagues have indicated, an additional reason for the poor prognosis, aside from extensive myocardial necrosis, is that myocardial metabolism may in fact be worsened despite improvement in hemodynamics.[25]

A more recent approach that requires further study in patients with cardiogenic shock is the combination of α- and β-adrenergic agonists such as dopamine with afterload reduction therapy using nitroprusside. In patients with congestive cardiac failure, Stemple et al. reported that dopamine in average doses of 3 and 7μgm/kg per min produced increases in cardiac output and reductions in peripheral resistance.[35] At a dosage of 15 μgm/kg per min, dopamine increased heart rate, peripheral arterial pressure as well as side effects. Nitroprusside alone decreased left-sided filling pressures and increased cardiac output. When the agents were administered together, the increases in cardiac output were significantly greater than when either agent was used alone. Whether the combination of α- and β-adrenergic agonist and vasodilator therapy will produce metabolic improvement in acutely ischemic myocardium remains to be proved.

Despite apparent abnormalities in myocardial metabolism induced by dopamine, the clinical ease with which the drug can be administered, its relative lack of side effects, its potential for prolonged administration, and its beneficial effect on renal blood flow currently make it the drug of choice for the treatment of cardiogenic shock. If the shock is due to myocardial infarction and dopamine therapy alone is inadequate at the doses mentioned above, norepinephrine at a dose of 0.01 to 0.07 μg/kg per min should be added and isoproterenol avoided because of the effects of isoproterenol on myocardial oxygen demand. Following cardiopulmonary bypass, however, a combination of isoproterenol and dopamine often seems to be useful, especially when the former agent is ineffective alone. In this connection, Talley et al. have noted that the combination of isoproterenol and dopamine may be useful in selected patients by minimizing the danger of excessive vasoconstriction produced by dopamine and excessive vasodilatation produced by isopro-

Table 20.1 Relative Actions of Catecholamines on Adrenergic and Dopaminergic Receptors and Their Use in Cardiogenic Shock

| Receptor Site | Response to Stimulation | Isoproterenol | Norepinephrine | Epinephrine* | Phenylephrine | Methoxamine | Dopamine | Dobutamine** |
|---|---|---|---|---|---|---|---|---|
| Alpha | Vasoconstriction of cutaneous, skeletal muscle, mucosal, intestinal and renal vascular beds | None | Marked | Low doses: Small or none; Larger doses: Moderate | Marked | Marked | Low doses: Small or none; Larger doses: Small or none*** | Small or none |
| Beta$_1$ | Increase in force and rate of cardiac contraction | Marked | Small | Marked | Minimal | None | Moderate | Marked |
| Beta$_2$ | Vasodilatation of skeletal muscle and mesenteric vascular beds; bronchodilatation | Marked | None | Low doses: Moderate; Larger doses: Small or none | None | None | None | Small or none |
| Dopaminergic | Vasodilatation of mesenteric and renal vascular beds | None | None | None | None | None | Moderate | None |
| Dose in treatment of cardiogenic shock (μcg/kg/min) | | 0.02–0.18 | 0.01–0.07 | 0.06–0.18 | 0.5–1.0 | 7–20 | 1–30 | 2–40 |

* In small doses beta-adrenergic effects predominate, but alpha-adrenergic effects (i.e., vasoconstriction) occur in kidney. In larger doses, alpha-adrenergic effects predominate.

** Use in cardiogenic shock not yet established.

*** In many vascular beds, alpha-adrenergic effects may become more marked as the dose is increased.

terenol.[36] They have also demonstrated that in occasional cases this combination may augment cardiac output and urinary flow beyond that produced by either drug alone. Adverse reactions to dopamine are not frequent; ventricular irritability occasionally necessitates either a decrease in dose or discontinuation of the drug.

The doses and pharmacologic effects of other agents used to treat cardiogenic shock are shown in Table 20.1, and their structural interrelations are shown in Figures 20.2 and 20.3. In all instances, it is preferable to administer these agents using an infusion pump with a drop counter.

In some instances, parenteral diuretic therapy may be successful only after the administration of dopamine. Thus, the combination of dopamine and parenteral diuretic therapy, like combined administration of dopamine and isoproterenol, may increase urinary flow in some patients beyond that produced by either agent alone. Under these circumstances, furosemide at an initial dose of 20 mg intravenously should be employed. This dose should be increased by 20 mg if there is no augmentation of urine flow within 30 minutes. The dose may again be doubled after another 30 minutes if there is still no increase in urine flow.

As indicated above, isoproterenol should be used with great caution, if at all, in the treatment of cardiogenic shock because of its adverse effects on myocardial oxygen demand. There is one clinical situation, however, in which this agent may be of considerable clinical use: Patients receiving $\beta$-adrenergic blocking agents such as propranolol may on occasion be unable to maintain blood pressure and heart rate at adequate levels because of an inadequate sympathetic nervous system response to acute myocardial infarction. Under these circumstances, isoproterenol may be used cautiously to "titrate" the heart rate and blood pressure to acceptable levels.

Continued clinical pharmacological research appears to be indicated in this area. Newer agents such as dobutamine seem to hold some promise in patients with acute myocardial infarction,[37] although data are sparse with respect to the treatment of cardiogenic shock. Use of $\alpha$-adrenergic blockade with drugs such as

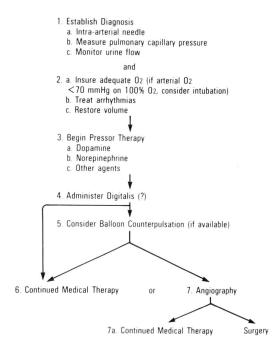

Fig. 20.5  An outline summary for a suggested approach to the treatment of cardiogenic shock.

phentolamine [38] (and, in the past, with chlorpromazine) seems in a few studies to have been useful. However, the relative ease with which the vasodilating agents can now be used has probably superseded the use of $\alpha$-adrenergic receptor blockade with phentolamine in this regard.

A summary of the current therapeutic approach to the treatment of cardiogenic shock is outlined in Figure 20.5.

## REFERENCES

1. Page DL, Caulfield JB, Kastor JA, DeSanctis RW, Sanders CA: Myocardial changes associated with cardiogenic shock. N Engl J Med 285:133–137, 1971.
2. Alonso DR, Scheidt S, Post M, Killip T: Pathophysiology of cardiogenic shock: quantification of myocardial necrosis, clinical, pathologic and electrocardiographic correlations. Circulation 43:588–596, 1973.
3. Cohn JN: Blood pressure measurement in shock: mechanism of inaccuracy in auscultatory and palpatory methods. JAMA 199:972–976, 1967.
4. Gutovitz AL, Sobel BE, Roberts R: Progressive

nature of myocardial injury in selected patients with cardiogenic shock. Am J Cardiol 41:469–475, 1978.

5. Ratshin RA, Rackley CE, Russell RO Jr: Hemodynamic evaluation of left ventricular function in shock complicating myocardial infarction. Circulation 45:127–139, 1972.

6. Forrester JS, Diamond GA, Swan HJC: Correlative classification of clinical and hemodynamic function after acute myocardial infarction. Am J Cardiol 39:137–145, 1977.

7. Bleifeld W, Hanrath P, Mathey D, Merx W: Acute myocardial infarction. V: left and right ventricular haemodynamics in cardiogenic shock. Br Heart J 36:822–834, 1974.

8. Afifi AA, Chang PC, Liu VY, da Luz PL, Weil MH, Shubin H: Prognostic indexes in acute myocardial infarction complicated by shock. Am J Cardiol 33:826–832, 1974.

9. Forrester JS, Diamond G, Freedman S, Allen HN, Parmley WW, Matloff J, Swan, HJC: Silent mitral insufficiency in acute myocardial infarction. Circulation 44: 877–883, 1971.

10. Scheinman M, Evans GT, Weiss A, Rapaport E: Relationship between pulmonary artery end-diastolic pressure and left ventricular filling pressure in patients in shock. Circulation 47:317–324, 1973.

11. Zarins CK, Virgilio RW, Smith DE, Peters RM: The effect of vascular volume on positive end-expiratory pressure-induced cardiac output depression and wedge-left atrial pressure discrepancy. J Surg Res 23:348–360, 1973.

12. Kamada RO, Smith JR: The phenomenon of respiratory failure in shock: the genesis of "shock lung." Am Heart J 83:1–4, 1972.

13. Tobinick E, Schelbert HR, Henning H, LeWinter M, Taylor A, Ashburn WL, Karliner JS: Right ventricular ejection fraction in patients with acute anterior and inferior myocardial infarction assessed by radionuclide angiography. Circulation 57:1078–1084, 1978.

14. Cohn JN, Guiha NH, Broden MI, Limas CJ: Right ventricular infarction: clinical and hemodynamic features. Am J Cardiol 33:209–214, 1974.

15. Vatner SF, Bary H: Comparison of the effects of ouabain and isoproterenol on ischemic myocardium of conscious dogs. Circulation 58:654–662, 1978.

16. Kirk ES, LeJemtel TH, Nelson GR, Sonnenblick EH: Mechanisms of beneficial effects of vasodilators and inotropic stimulation in the experimental failing ischemic heart. Am J Med 65:189–196, 1978.

17. Cohn JN, Tristani FE, Khatri IM: Cardiac and peripheral vascular effects of digitalis in clinical cardiogenic shock. Am Heart J 78:318–330, 1969.

18. Karliner JS, Braunwald E: Present status of digitalis treatment of acute myocardial infarction. Circulation 45:891–902, 1972.

19. Ahlquist RP: A study of adrenotropic receptors. Am J Physiol 153:586–599, 1948.

20. Goldberg LI: Cardiovascular and renal actions of dopamine: potential clinical applications. Pharmacol Rev 24:1–29, 1972.

21. Goldberg LI: Recent advances in the pharmacology of catecholamines. Intensive Care Medicine 3:233–236, 1977.

22. Vatner SF: Effects of sympathomimetic amines on myocardial function, electrograms and blood flow in conscious dogs with myocardial ischemia, in Proceedings of a Symposium, "Use of Dopamine in Shock III. Myocardial Infarction." Boston, Mass, August 5, 1976. Exerpta Medica pp 9–10.

23. Gunnar RM, Cruz A, Boswell J, Co BS, Pietras RJ, Tobin JR Jr: Myocardial infarction with shock: hemodynamic studies and results of therapy. Circulation 33:753–762, 1966.

24. Mueller H, Ayres SM, Gregory JJ, Giannelli S Jr, Grace WJ: Hemodynamics, coronary blood flow, and myocardial metabolism in coronary shock; response to ⅼ-norepinephrine and isoproterenol. J Clin Invest 49:1885–1902, 1970.

25. Mueller HS, Evans R, Ayres SM: Effect of dopamine on hemodynamics and myocardial metabolism in shock following acute myocardial infarction in man. Circulation 57:361–365, 1978.

26. Abrams E, Forrester JS, Chatterjee K, Danzig R, Swan HJC: Variability in response to norepinephrine in acute myocardial infarction. Am J Cardiol 32:919–923, 1973.

27. Holzer J, Karliner JS, O'Rourke RA, Ross J Jr: Effectiveness of dopamine in patients with cardiogenic shock. Am J Cardiol 32:79–84, 1973.

28. Karliner JS: Usefulness and limitations of dopamine in the therapy of cardiogenic shock. In Dopamin, Arbeitstagung über die klinische Anwendung. Berlin, Juli, 1974, R. Schroder, editor. F.K. Schattauer Verlag, Stuttgart-New York, 1975, pp 13–22.

29. Alexander CS, Sako Y, Mikulic E: Pedal gangrene associated with the use of dopamine. New Engl J of Med 293:591, 1975.

30. Greene SA, Smith JW: Dopamine gangrene. Ibid 294:114, 1976.

31. Valdez ME: Post-dopamine gangrene treated with chlorpromazine. Ibid 295:1081–1082, 1976.

32. Latts JR, Goldberg LI: Dopamine in the management of shock. Drug Therapy (Hosp) pp 25–30 (Jan) 1979.

33. Thompson WL: Dopamine in the management of shock. Proc R Soc Med 70 (Suppl 2):25–35, 1977.

34. Filner BE, Karliner JS, Dailey PO: Favorable influence of dopamine on left ventricular performance in patients refractory to discontinuation of cardiopulmonary bypass. Circulatory Shock 4:223–230, 1977.

35. Stemple DR, Kleiman JH, Harrison DC: Combined nitroprusside-dopamine therapy in severe chronic congestive heart failure: dose-related hemodynamic advantages over single drug infusions. Am J Cardiol 42:267–275, 1978.

36. Talley RC, Goldberg LI, Johnson CE, McNay JL: A hemodynamic comparison of dopamine and isoproterenol in patients in shock. Circulation 39:361–378, 1969.

37. Gillespie TA, Ambos HD, Sobel BE, Roberts R: Effects of dobutamine in patients with acute myocardial infarction. Am J Cardiol 39:588–594, 1977.

38. Gould L, Ramana Reddy CV: Appraisal and reappraisal of cardiac therapy. Phentolamine. Am Heart J 92:397–402, 1976.

39. Swan HJC, Forrester JS, Diamond G, Chatterjee, Parmley WW: Hemodynamic spectrum of myocardial infarction and cardiogenic shock: a conceptual model. Circulation 45:1097–1110, 1972.

# 21 | Intraaortic Balloon Pumping: Use in the Treatment of Cardiogenic Shock and Acute Myocardial Ischemia

*Robert C. Leinbach, M.D.*
*Herman K. Gold, M.D.*

Since the initial conception of balloon counterpulsation by Mouloupoulos et al. in 1962,[1] the intraaortic balloon pump (IABP) has become the most widely used form of mechanical circulatory assistance throughout the world. The IABP has been quickly adopted because it duplicates all the beneficial physiologic effects of more complicated counterpulsing circulatory assist devices.

The goal of counterpulsation is to simultaneously increase coronary perfusion pressure and reduce left ventricular pressure work. The IABP accomplishes this by displacing a volume of blood from the descending thoracic aorta equal to the volume of the balloon. If this blood displacement is made to occur once in each cardiac cycle and is timed appropriately, the goals of counterpulsation can be met.

## TIMING OF IABP

In order to insure a maximal increment in coronary perfusion pressure, the timing of IABP inflation should be adjusted so that the positive intraaortic pressure pulse reaches the aortic valve at the moment of valve closure. To accomplish this, the pump must be inflated slightly early to allow for pulse wave transmission around the aortic arch. Each balloon pulse is triggered by the QRS complex of the electrocardiogram. Inflation timing presents no problem if pressures are monitored from the aortic root. Here, the positive pulse from the IABP can be superimposed on the dicrotic notch (Fig. 21.1).

In most cases, arterial pressure is monitored from the radial artery. Timing adjustments must therefore take into account the fact that the radial artery pressures are slightly delayed; when the dicrotic notch is seen in the radial artery pressure pulse, the aortic valve has already been closed for a fraction of a second. Therefore, the positive balloon pulse should be advanced ahead of the radial dicrotic notch by 20 to 30 msec (Fig. 21.1).

In order to decrease left ventricular systolic work, the negative phase of the balloon pulse should be timed to arrive at the aortic valve just before valve opening. Again, timing delays from waveform transmission must be considered, and the deflation pulse must be set slightly ahead in the radial artery tracing. The general rule of thumb for deflation timing is to set deflation so that the minimal diastolic pressure measurement at the radial artery is about 10 mmHg below the off-balloon diastolic pressure (Fig. 21.1). These timing adjustments with a 40-cc IABP will generally induce a rise in mean diastolic arterial pressure of 10 to 15 mmHg and a fall in peak systolic pressure of about 15 mmHg. The effect of systolic unloading is to reduce left ventricular filling pressure by 5 to 10 mmHg (Fig. 21.2).

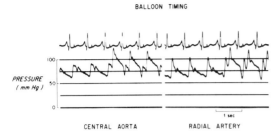

Fig. 21.1 Arterial pressure recorded from the central aorta (left panel) and from the radial artery (right panel) in the same patient during initiation of intraaortic balloon pumping (IABP). The electrocardiogram is shown above. The artifacts in the ST and PR segments are balloon timing markers. In the left panel the upstroke of the balloon pulse is precisely timed to coincide with the dicrotic notch as recorded from the central aorta. This timing requires slightly early balloon inflation as judged from the radial artery pressure measurements. Note the balloon pumping upstroke prior to the dicrotic notch in the right panel. Also, the minimal diastolic arterial pressure in the radial artery during balloon pumping is approximately 5 to 10 mmHg below diastolic radial artery pressure prior to pumping.

## CORONARY FLOW

Initiation of counterpulsation induces an immediate rise in coronary flow. At the same time, however, left ventricular systolic work has diminished. Therefore, autoregulation occurs, and coronary flow returns toward control. However, when coronary flow is pressure-dependent (as seen with coronary stenosis or shock), counterpulsation can cause an augmentation of coronary flow which is maintained (Fig. 21.3).

## CARDIAC OUTPUT

The effects of IABP on cardiac output vary with the condition of the patient. When cardiac output is not depressed, IABP (as with coronary flow) will produce a transient increase with autoregulation. When cardiac output is severely depressed by left ventricular failure, IABP will augment output primarily by reduction in afterload. When cardiac output is depressed by

ischemia, the IABP induces an improvement both by afterload reduction and by reversal of ischemic dysfunction.

## CLINICAL APPLICATION OF IABP

### Shock

Cardiogenic shock accompanying myocardial infarction (MI) is a result of cumulative myocardial dysfunction or dysfunction combined with a mechanical load such as mitral regurgitation or ventricular septal rupture. For this discussion, we exclude patients with shock from volume depletion, tamponade, or dysrhythmias. With these exclusions, patients presenting with clinical signs of shock can be classified hemodynamically by relating systolic left ventricular function to left ventricular filling pressure. Shock is generally associated with a depressed arterial pressure and cardiac output in association with an elevated pulmonary artery wedge pressure. The values most commonly accepted for initiation of IABP have been a cardiac index of less than 2.0 l/min/m², a systolic pressure less than 90 mmHg, and a mean pulmonary artery wedge pressure greater than 18 mmHg. There are two principal values to these criteria. First, at this level of hemodynamic depression, patients with acute myocardial infarction are unlikely to survive if circulatory assistance is withheld. Second, the results from trials of IABP can be compared only if hemodynamic patient classification is used.

Several groups have now reported the results of IABP support in patients with cardiogenic shock accompanying acute myocardial infarction.[2-4] Survival has ranged from 15 to 40 percent, with the majority of patients in recent series requiring surgical intervention. The most consistent success has been IABP support of patients presenting with shock complicated by a mechanical lesion. Late revascularization of infarcted myocardium has been disappointing.[5] Failure to observe a more consistent response pattern and the persistence of a high mortality in such patients treated with IABP are best explained by: (1) overly conservative attitudes

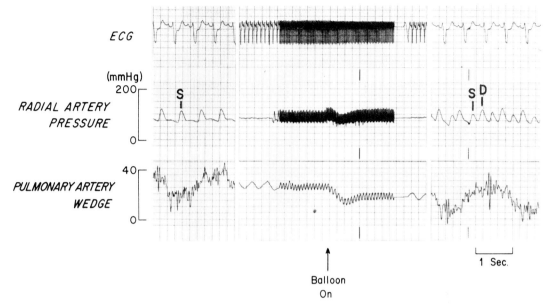

Fig. 21.2  Hemodynamic effects of initiation of IABP. Systolic arterial pressure (S) falls 15 mmHg. Mean diastolic arterial pressure rises 12 mmHg, and the mean pulmonary artery wedge pressure falls 7 mmHg. D = peak diastolic pressure. (Dunkman WB, Leinbach RC et al: Clinical and hemodynamic results of intraaortic balloon pumping and surgery for cardiogenic shock. Circulation 46:465–477, 1972.)

on the part of some physicians, leading to delays in instituting IABP, and (2) requirements for excessive myocardial depression before institution of IABP.[3] As a consequence of such delays, shock that was due to a large ischemic zone progresses to shock that is due to extensive (more than 40 percent) left ventricular infarction—and, hence, to unsalvageability of the myocardium.[6]

In the patient with cardiogenic shock, the critical factor in the use of IABP is speed. The physician is racing against progression of myocardial injury and, in the presence of mechanical lesions, against renal failure and refractory pulmonary edema that requires intubation. In general, patients with cardiogenic shock present in three patterns. The first is rapid onset of shock that reaches the full-blown syndrome within 6 hours of the onset of infarction.[7] This group requires the most rapid institution of

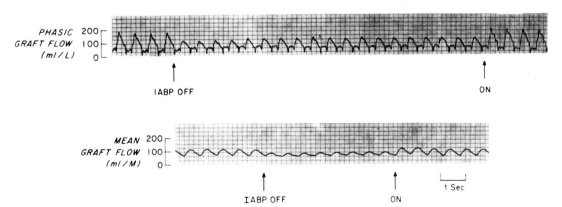

Fig. 21.3  Coronary flow in an aortocoronary venous bypass graft measured at operation with a flow probe. The effect of interruption of IABP is a sharp diminution in peak diastolic coronary flow. The mean regional coronary flow is reduced when the intraaortic balloon pump is off.

IABP. These patients should undergo rapid rhythm and blood gas analysis and hemodynamic categorization by a flow-directed thermodilution pulmonary artery catheter. If the combination of low left ventricular systolic work and high filling pressure is observed in the absence of dysrhythmia, acidosis, severe hypoxemia, or contraindication to the insertion of a balloon pump, then IABP should be started without a prolonged medical trial of various pharmacologic agents. During categorization, mean arterial pressure is maintained at a level greater than 60 mmHg with an infusion of norepinephrine.

The second pattern is a slower onset of shock, which is produced by the piecemeal progression of left ventricular ischemia and necrosis. In these patients, IABP should be started before a specific low hemodynamic level is reached. It is enough to isolate the problem to progressive injury refractory to standard medical therapy. This condition must be a result of inadequate regional coronary flow which is below the level necessary to prevent irreversible myocardial loss. Regional coronary flow in these cases is pressure dependent and can be boosted by IABP, halting the progression to necrosis.

The third pattern is the sudden development of shock and a systolic murmur days after the onset of a relatively uncomplicated myocardial infarction. This is caused either by rupture of papillary musculature or perforation of the interventricular septum. The diagnosis can be confirmed by passage of a Swan-Ganz catheter recording pulmonary wedge "V" waves and sampling for an oxygen step-up at the level of the right ventricle. Acute mitral regurgitation is associated with extreme elevation of pulmonary wedge pressure and pulmonary edema and ventricular septal rupture with extreme depression of systemic cardiac output. Failure to rapidly correct these abnormalities by pharmacologic means, including vasodilator therapy, is an indication for IABP.

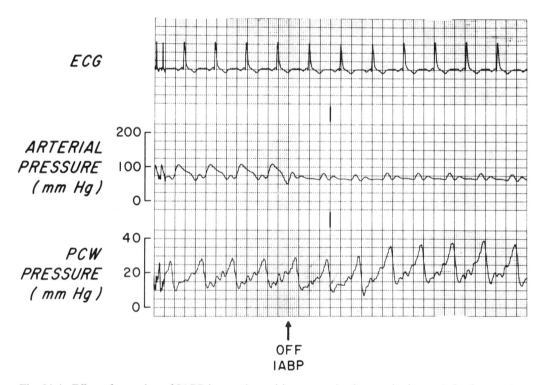

Fig. 21.4  Effect of cessation of IABP in a patient with severe mitral regurgitation and shock secondary to ruptured papillary muscle. Despite the large regurgitant waves in the pulmonary wedge pressure pulse (PCW pressure), the mean wedge pressure on the balloon pump is 19 mmHg. Off balloon pumping, arterial pressure is markedly reduced and the mean wedge pressure rises to 25 mmHg.

The hemodynamic effects of IABP in acute mitral regurgitation and ventricular septal rupture are, in most cases, just adequate to provide a temporary improvement in hemodynamic stability during angiographic evaluation and subsequent surgical correction. In acute mitral regurgitation, mean pulmonary wedge pressure can be reduced to a level below the pulmonary edema range (Fig. 21.4). In ventricular septal rupture, the systemic output can be augmented while the pulmonary flow remains essentially unchanged, thereby decreasing the pulmonary-to-systemic flow ratio and preventing acute renal failure [8,9] (Fig. 21.5).

Most patients in cardiogenic shock who receive IABP support without excessive delay will show hemodynamic stability within 12 to 24 hours. By this is meant a cardiac index greater than 2 l/min/m² without a rising BUN, maintenance of oxygenation without intubation, and a mean arterial pressure on minimal pressor

support of approximately 70 mmHg. However, the majority of these patients remain balloon dependent, with recurrence of ischemia or signs of shock when IABP is withdrawn on a trial basis for 15 to 30 minutes or is operated at a reduced frequency for several hours. There is no good alternative for these patients except angiography and consideration for cardiac surgery.

It is our practice to perform coronary and left ventricular cineangiography at the time of hemodynamic stabilization in all patients treated with IABP. This study is to delineate the mechanical defects and associated coronary artery pathology in patients with a new systolic murmur and to demonstrate areas of reversible ischemic dysfunction in patients with "pure" cardiogenic shock. Multiple-vessel disease is the rule with the left anterior descending coronary artery stenotic or occluded in nearly every case.[10] An irreversibly infarcted myocardial

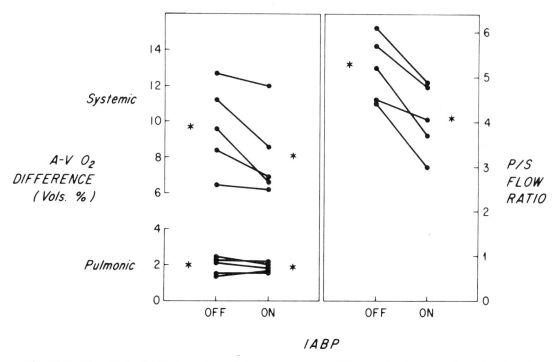

Fig. 21.5   The effect of IABP on the arteriovenous oxygen difference in the systemic and pulmonic circuits in a series of patients with ventricular septal rupture secondary to acute myocardial infarction. Onset of balloon pumping was associated with a decrease in the systemic AVO₂ difference (left panel above) and no significant change in the pulmonic AVO₂ difference (left panel below). There was a resultant fall in the pulmonic to systemic flow ratio from approximately 5:1 to 4:1. (Gold HK, Leinbach RC et al: Intraaortic balloon pumping for ventricular septal defect or mitral regurgitation complicating acute myocardial infarction. Circulation 47:1191–1196, 1973.)

zone is defined as one to which coronary flow cannot be identified either directly or by collateral circulation. When this involves the major territory of the left anterior descending coronary artery (Fig. 21.6), postmortem infarct size will often exceed 40 percent. Identification of large zones of necrosis by angiography can help to define inoperability. Wall motion abnormalities taken alone do not define irreversible necrosis.

Patients in whom cardiogenic shock is reversed by IABP and who become balloon independent may be weaned from IABP in about 4 to 5 days. The majority of such individuals will show multiple-vessel coronary disease. Reversal of shock therefore results from reversal of ischemia. We have most often discharged these patients without acute revascularization surgery. On follow-up, a higher percentage have experienced a subsequent ischemic event resulting in recurrent shock or death. It is uncertain whether prophylactic bypass surgery will prevent this outcome.

Patients in whom cardiogenic shock is reversed by IABP and who remain balloon dependent are evaluated for surgery. In "pure" shock without a systolic murmur, the best surgical outcome is seen when revascularization is performed early and flow is restored to major noninfarcted myocardial segments. Survival of 50 percent of such individuals can be achieved when patients with major avascular segments are excluded, when shock is a result of a single transmural myocardial infarction, and when shock is perpetuated by ischemic segments remote from the infarct zone.

Patients in whom cardiogenic shock is induced by the superimposed effects of marked mitral regurgitation and/or ventricular septal rupture must undergo urgent surgical correction, since stabilization with IABP is often marginal. Results are best when mechanical repair alone is all that is required; the risk is higher when revascularization is also necessary; and the yield is lowest when infarct size is large and mechanical dysfunction severe. Therefore, an important part of the preoperative assessment is the ventriculogram to quantitate the extent of mitral regurgitation and the magnitude of the residual ejection fraction.[12] Greater than 50 percent survival can be expected if the mechanical burden has been shown to be large and reparative surgery is not delayed.

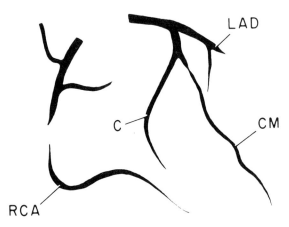

Fig. 21.6 An outline of the typical angiographic pattern in patients with cardiogenic shock and massive anterior myocardial infarction. The left anterior descending coronary artery is occluded without collateral flow to its distal portions. The circumflex marginal or other lateral left ventricular coronary arteries are small and posterior in position. (Leinbach RC et al: The role of angiography in cardiogenic shock. Circulation 47, 48 (suppl III):95–98, 1973.)

## THE CONTROL OF MYOCARDIAL ISCHEMIA

The IABP is highly effective in the control of recurrent myocardial ischemia at rest. This unstable myocardial ischemia is associated with either ST segment depression (subendocardial ischemia) or acute ST segment elevation which may be caused or aggravated by coronary spasm. Subendocardial ischemia is particularly responsive to IABP because it is induced by a regional inadequacy of flow that can be caused either by an increased demand, a decrease in coronary perfusion pressure, or an elevated end-diastolic (endocardial) left ventricular pressure. The IABP reverses each of these abnormalities; as a result, nearly every patient improves and greater than 90 percent become symptom free (Fig. 21.7).

Ten percent of patients will show recurrent subendocardial ischemia despite IABP. Most of these patients will show a specific angio-

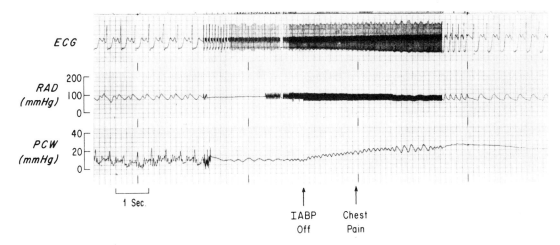

Fig. 21.7    Effect of the intraaortic balloon pump on a patient with severe subendocardial ischemia. In the center of the panel, the balloon pump is turned off. Within seconds, chest pain recurs and ST segment depression in the electrocardiographic lead (ECG) becomes more severe. There is an associated rise in the pulmonary wedge pressure to greater than 20 mmHg. RAD = radial artery pressure. PCW = pulmonary capillary wedge pressure.

graphic pattern: main left coronary stenosis, and right coronary occlusion. These patients represent the highest risk and may die during coronary angiography if IABP support has not been initiated.[13] Fifty percent of patients in whom pain has been completely relieved will show recurrence of pain during temporary cessation of IABP.[14]

Pharmacologic advances in the last few years have led to an improved control of subendocardial ischemia prior to and during coronary angi-

ography. There remains, however, a role for IABP in this condition in the most severe cases. The problem is patient identification before angiography. Presently, this differentiation is inexact, but the high-risk patients can sometimes be identified by a significant fall in arterial pressure during spontaneous ischemia or by a breakthrough of angina during β-blockade and continuous intravenous coronary vasodilator treatment.[15]

The therapy for recurrent angina with ST

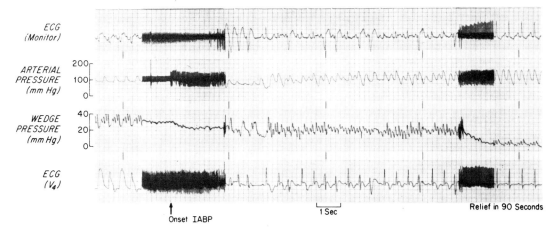

Fig. 21.8    Effect of balloon pumping on severe anterior transmural ischemia with ST segment elevation. The duration of this ischemic attack was 14 minutes. Within 90 seconds of the onset of balloon pumping, pulmonary wedge pressure falls from 35 to 4 mmHg and the ST segments are normalized. (Gold HK, Leinbach RC et al: Refractory angina pectoris: follow-up after intraaortic balloon pumping and surgery. Circulation 54 (suppl III):41–46, 1976.)

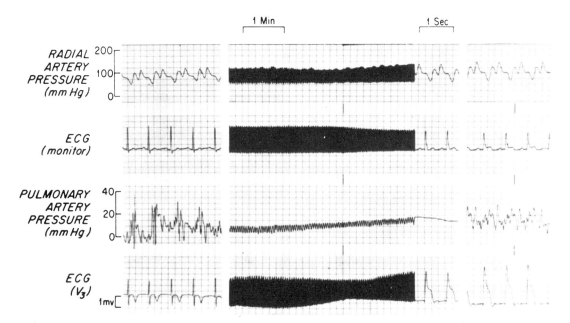

Fig. 21.9 Spontaneous occurrence of anterior transmural ischemia during properly timed IABP. In the center panel at the slow paper speed ST segment elevation develops in association with a slight rise in radial arterial pressure and in pulmonary artery mean pressure.

segment elevation at rest is changing. More potent coronary vasodilators specifically directed at coronary spasm such as "slow channel" (calcium) antagonists are undergoing clinical trials. Thus, it can be predicted that the number of patients resisting therapy will diminish. Introduction of IABP to patients with recurrent ischemic ST segment elevation is effective but less consistent than in patients with subendocardial ischemia (Fig. 21.8). Coronary spasm can induce ST segment elevation and pain even during optimally timed counterpulsation (Fig. 21.9). Therefore, the IABP may be best reserved for patients after angiographic identification of high-grade fixed coronary stenosis. In these cases, a small residual lumen in the coronary artery is adequate to allow prevention of ischemia if diastolic coronary perfusion pressure can be boosted.

Recurrence of myocardial ischemia during temporary cessation of IABP does not occur in half of the patients. Nevertheless, we have tended to recommend semiurgent coronary bypass surgery in all patients requiring IABP for control of ischemia. We have elected not to remove the balloon pump from those patients who remain pain-free during a trial period without counterpulsation. This decision is based on the observations that: (1) an aggressive medical program had failed; (2) postmortem examinations on patients who died of unstable ischemia demonstrated high-grade fixed stenoses complicated by plaque hemorrhage and rupture;[16] and (3) the mortality and morbidity of revascularization surgery under these conditions is low.[17]

## REDUCTION OF INFARCT SIZE BY IABP

Counterpulsation was suggested as treatment for early acute coronary occlusion in 1962.[18] We have applied balloon pumping to 11 patients without shock presenting with anterior myocardial infarction less than six hours after the onset of pain.[19] It was possible to produce a remarkable reduction in electrocardiographic injury current and in pain within minutes of induction of pumping (Fig. 21.10). However, certain criteria had to be met. The IABP had to be instituted within 4 hours of the onset of persistent pain and before irreversible left anterior descending occlusion occurred. Complete resolution of injury current was seen only in

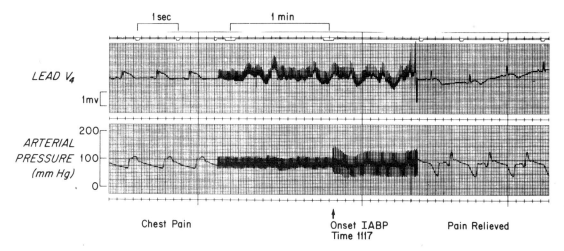

Fig. 21.10   Effect of IABP on injury current during acute anterior myocardial infarction. The pain had been present for 60 minutes. Immediately after the onset of balloon pumping, ST segments are nearly normalized. Systolic arterial pressure is dropped 20 mmHg and mean diastolic arterial pressure is increased 10 mmHg.

patients in whom the counterpulsation could be combined with a residual left anterior descending lumen. The rate of response strongly indicated restoration of coronary flow.

Preservation of ventricular function was seen only when this resolution of injury current was produced before precordial Q wave development. The patients with complete left anterior descending occlusion showed minor changes in injury current and progressed to R wave loss and left ventricular dysfunction. The importance of the IABP specifically for infarct size reduction has not been defined. Nevertheless, it is important to understand that myocardial injury can be controlled with subtotal coronary stenosis if counterpulsation is employed.

## COMPLICATIONS

The primary complications of balloon pumping are encountered at the time of balloon introduction. Arterial injury at the site of insertion or in the distal aortoiliac territory predominates.[20] Local or extensive aortic dissection and iliac perforations with death from retroperitoneal hemorrhage have been seen. These complications relate to tortuosity of the iliac vessels and aortoiliac atherosclerosis. The frequency of major dissections or arterial trauma is approximately 4 percent. A rare complication is cholesterol embolization with resultant peripheral gangrene.

Additional complications relate to duration of pumping. These include wound infection, local arterial thrombosis, mesenteric embolism, and peripheral arterial embolism during balloon withdrawal.[21] Platelet depression is seen in about 50 percent of patients, but the platelet count rarely falls to hemorrhagic levels.

We have attempted to reduce the frequency of complications during insertion by distal aortic cineangiography. This is not practical in cardiogenic shock. Severe distal aortoiliac stenosis can be identified, which will contraindicate use of the balloon. The site of balloon insertion can be selected by evaluation of vascular tortuosity. Local complications after insertion may be reduced by shortening the period of balloon pumping.

Experience with IABP has led to a growth in confidence and a more precise definition of the role of counterpulsation in all forms of ischemic myocardial disease.

## REFERENCES

1. Moulopoulos SD, Topaz S, Kolff WL: Diastolic balloon pump (with carbon dioxide) in the aorta:

Medical assistance to the failing circulation. Am Heart J 63:669, 1962.

2. Dunkman WB, Leinbach RC, Buckley MJ, Mundth ED, Kantrowitz AR, Austen WG, Sanders CA: Clinical and hemodynamic results of intra-aortic balloon pumping and surgery for cardiogenic shock. Circulation 46:465, 1972.

3. Scheidt S, Wilner G, Mueller H, Summers D, Lesch M, Wolff G, Krakauer J, Rubenfire M, Fleming P, Noon G, Oldham N, Killip T, Kantrowitz A: Intra-aortic balloon counterpulsation in cardiogenic shock. N Engl J Med 288:979, 1973.

4. Kantrowitz A, Tjenneland S, Krakauer JS, Phillips SJ, Freed PS, Butner AN: Mechanical intraaortic cardiac assistance in cardiogenic shock. Arch Surg 97:1000, 1968.

5. Willerson JT, Curry GC, Watson JT, Leskin SJ, Ecker RR, Mullins CB, Platt MR, Sugg WL: Intraaortic balloon counterpulsation in patients in cardiogenic shock, medically refractory left ventricular failure and/or recurrent ventricular tachycardia. Am J Med 58:183, 1975.

6. Page DL, Caulfield JB, Kastor JA, DeSanctis RW, Sanders CA: Myocardial changes associated with cardiogenic shock. N Engl J Med 285:133, 1971.

7. Caulfield JB, Leinbach RC, Gold HK: The relationship of myocardial infarct size and prognosis. Circulation 53 (Suppl I):141, 1976.

8. Gold HK, Leinbach RC, Sanders CA, Buckley MJ, Mundth ED, Austen WG: Intra-aortic balloon pumping for ventricular septal defect or mitral regurgitation complicating acute myocardial infarction. Circulation, 47:1191, 1973.

9. Daggett WM, Guyton RA, Mundth ED, Buckley MJ, McEnany MT, Gold HK, Leinbach RC, Austen WG: Surgery for post-myocardial infarct ventricular septal defect. Ann Surg 186:260, 1977.

10. Leinbach RC, Gold HK, Dinsmore RE, Mundth ED, Buckley MJ, Austen WG, Sanders CA: The role of angiography in cardiogenic shock. Circulation 48 (Suppl III):95, 1973.

11. Leinbach RC, Dinsmore RE, Mundth ED, Buckley MJ, Dunkman WB, Austen WG, Sanders CA: Selective coronary and left ventricular cineangiography during intra-aortic balloon pumping for cardiogenic shock. Circulation 45:845, 1972.

12. Radford MJ, Johnson RA, Buckley MJ, Daggett WM, Leinbach RC, Gold HK: Survival following mitral valve replacement for mitral regurgitation due to coronary artery disease. Circulation 60 (No. 2) (Suppl I):39, 1979.

13. Cohen MV, Cohn PF, Herman MV, Gorlin R: Diagnosis and prognosis of main left coronary occlusion. Circulation, 45 (Suppl I):57, 1972.

14. Gold HK, Leinbach RC, Sanders CA, Buckley MJ, Mundth ED, Austen WG: Intra-aortic balloon pumping for control of recurrent myocardial ischemia. Circulation 47:1197, 1973.

15. Johnson RA, Zir LM, Harper RW, Leinbach RC, Hutter AM, Pohost GM, Block PC, Gold HK: Patterns of haemodynamic alteration during left ventricular ischaemia in man: Relationship to the angiographic extent of coronary artery disease. Br Heart J 41:441, 1979.

16. Caulfield JB, Gold HK, Leinbach RC: Coronary artery lesions associated with unstable angina (abstr). Am J Cardiol 35:126, 1975.

17. Levine FH, Gold HK, Leinbach RC, Daggett WM, Austen WG, Buckley MJ: Management of acute myocardial ischemia with intraaortic balloon pumping and coronary bypass surgery. Circulation, 58 (No. 3) (Suppl I):69, 1978.

18. Jacobey JA, Taylor WJ, Smith GT, Gorlin R, Harken DE: A new therapeutic approach to coronary occlusion. Am J Cardiol 9:60, 1962.

19. Leinbach RC, Gold HK, Harper RW, Buckley MJ, Austen WG: Early intraaortic balloon pumping for anterior myocardial infarction without shock. Circulation 58:204, 1978.

20. McCabe JC, Abel RM, Subramanian VA, Gay WA Jr: Complications of intra-aortic balloon insertion and counterpulsation. Circulation 57:769, 1978.

21. McEnany MT, Kay HR, Buckley MJ, Daggett WM, Erdmann AJ, Mundth ED, Rao RS, deToeuf J, Austen WG: Clinical experience with intraaortic balloon pump support in 728 patients. Circulation 58 (Suppl I):124, 1978.

# 22 | *Role of Vasodilator Therapy*

## *John Ross, Jr., M.D.*

One of the most significant advances, during the past few years, in our understanding of the factors that regulate cardiac performance has been appreciation of the importance of the afterload on the myocardial fibers during ventricular ejection as an independent determinant of ventricular function.[1,2] This conceptual advance, coupled with a better understanding of the role of inotropic state or contractility, the preload (diastolic stretch on the myocardial fibers), and the various factors that affect the venous return,[3] has led to substantial improvements in the management of some patients with acute or chronic cardiac failure. Indeed, in certain forms of acute left ventricular failure the use of afterload and preload reduction alone, or in combination with other therapy, has now become the treatment of choice,[4,5] and in refractory chronic heart failure due to myocardial disease, valvular, and coronary heart disease, orally administered vasodilators are finding increasing application.[6] In the present chapter, we will focus primarily on the physiologic bases for vasodilator therapy, and its usefulness in the setting of acute myocardial infarction.

The earliest therapeutic use of afterload reduction occurred about 1960 when arterial counterpulsation by means of direct aortic cannulation was employed in the management of cardiogenic shock after myocardial infarction.[7] A reciprocating pump aspirated blood from the aorta during ventricular ejection, thereby lowering the systolic aortic pressure, and hence the afterload; the blood was then reinjected during diastole to augment the coronary artery perfusion pressure. Experimental studies showed that this intervention promoted increased shortening of the ventricular walls, while at the same time lowering myocardial oxygen requirements and improving coronary blood flow.[8] By 1970, the counterpulsation principle had evolved to intraaortic balloon counterpulsation, which also reduced the afterload and raised the diastolic aortic pressure.[9] In the presence of left ventricular "power failure," these effects were shown to improve cardiac output, and reduce left ventricular end-diastolic or mean filling pressure.[9] As discussed in Chapter 21, afterload reduction by balloon counterpulsation has constituted an important step in the management of some patients with acute myocardial ischemia or infarction. Thus, the importance of manipulating left ventricular afterload in the management of cardiogenic shock became evident,[10] and the stage was set for the introduction of pharmacologic vasodilators.

## PHYSIOLOGIC BASIS FOR THE ACTION OF VASODILATORS

The effects of various vasodilator drugs on the heart and circulation in the presence or absence of heart failure are complex, and our current understanding of mechanisms involved remains limited. A key observation, now securely

497

established, was the finding that when heart failure was absent vasodilator therapy usually resulted in a drop in cardiac output, whereas in the presence of left ventricular failure cardiac output improved (Fig. 22.1).[11] This response relates not only to more favorable afterloading conditions on the failing left ventricle but, as we shall see, to the highly important circulatory actions of vasodilators on the venous bed as well. The effects of vasodilator therapy in the setting of acute myocardial infarction also can be influenced by lowered coronary perfusion pressure, with associated effects on blood flow through stenotic coronary vessels, while at the same time reducing myocardial $O_2$ requirements. In addition, the marked drop in intracardiac filling pressures, particularly the left ventricular diastolic pressure, which usually accompanies the use of a vasodilator can have favorable effects on coronary perfusion, but, on occasion, the fall in filling pressure can affect ventricular function adversely. Such complex effects of vasodilators make it desirable to consider each of these potential actions in more detail in attempting to place the use of vasodilators in acute myocardial infarction on a rational basis.

## Definitions of Afterload and Impedance

We have preferred to define afterload as the force, or stress, developed in the ventricular wall during cardiac ejection; this load may be identified at a single point in time, or as the mean wall stress throughout ejection.[12] Aortic input impedance as a measure of the total afterload on the ventricle also has been advocated [13] and will be discussed further below. Although stress in the ventricular wall is closely related to systolic pressure in the left ventricle and

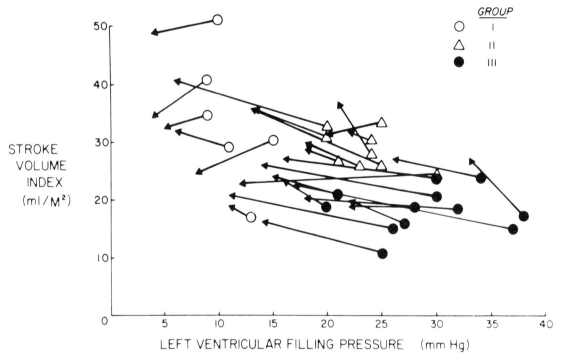

Fig. 22.1 Hemodynamic responses to nitroprusside infusion in patients with acute myocardial infarction. Patients in Groups II and III with elevated left ventricular filling pressures (20 mmHg or more) tend to respond to the vasodilator with an increase in the stroke volume and a marked drop in the filling pressure, whereas patients with left ventricular filling pressures below 15 mmHg (Group I) show a reduction in the stroke volume and tend to have less marked decreases in filling pressures during nitroprusside infusion. Group III patients had stroke work indices below 20 g-m/m². (Chatterjee K, Parmley WW: The role of vasodilator therapy in heart failure. Prog Cardiovasc Dis 19:301–325, 1977.)

aorta during ventricular ejection, the two values are not equivalent. Thus, according to a simplified Laplace formulation, the stress is directly related to the product of systolic pressure and diameter of the ventricular chamber, and inversely related to the thickness of the ventricular wall. In simplest terms, stress = P·r/2h (where P = systolic pressure, r = ventricular radius, and h = wall thickness), and a dilated heart with a thinned wall carrying the same systolic pressure as a normal heart must, therefore, develop a higher afterload or wall stress (force per unit area of muscle) than the normal ventricle.

As mentioned, the afterload also can be defined as impedance, a term that can include all factors that oppose active shortening of the ventricular fibers. Impedance is expressed as the ratio of pressure to flow within the vascular bed and is determined by peripheral vascular resistance, the properties of the blood vessel walls, and of the blood itself.[13] The aortic input impedance spectrum reflects those forces external to the heart that place a load on the left ventricle during ejection, but its calculation requires simultaneous high fidelity measurements of pressure and instantaneous blood flow in the ascending aorta, together with the use of Fourier analysis to describe the various harmonics of these waveforms in terms of amplitude and phase angle. The aortic input resistance (ratio of mean pressure to mean flow, which is equivalent to the total "peripheral or systemic vascular resistance") represents the impedance at zero frequency, and the characteristic impedance (which reflects primarily vascular wall characteristics), represents the average of the ratios of pressure to flow moduli at higher frequencies (2 to 12 Hz).[13]

Although afterload, defined either as wall stress or input impedance, can be calculated in man in the cardiac catheterization laboratory using appropriate instrumentation, such calculations are not available at the bedside. Moreover, even though changes in aortic stiffness without a change in mean arterial pressure can alter the characteristic impedance and produce changes in the stroke-volume,[14] recent studies in our laboratory have indicated that changes in the characteristic impedance are also accom-panied by alterations in wall stress and in the extent of wall shortening;[15] in fact, calculation of the relation between wall stress and wall shortening provided a better description of the afterload than the more complex calculations of characteristic impedance.[15]

In measuring the acute effects of vasodilator therapy at the bedside, we must rely primarily on measurements of the arterial or left ventricular systolic pressure and, if a measurement of the cardiac output is available, on the systemic vascular resistance (SVR) to reflect changes in the afterload on the left ventricle. The normal systemic vascular resistance * lies between 770 and 1500 dynes-sec cm$^{-5}$, or 10 to 19 units. Thus, an increase in afterload is generally manifested by an increase in systemic vascular resistance, as well as in the systolic and/or mean arterial pressures, whereas a reduction in afterload is reflected by a fall in these variables. In making such clinical assessments, however, it should be recalled that the systemic arterial pressure (AP) is equal to the product of the cardiac output and the systemic vascular resistance (AP = CO × SVR); hence, the response to a moderate dose of a vasodilator drug may consist of a sizeable increase in cardiac output without a change in systemic arterial pressure, which indicates that a substantial decrease in systemic vascular resistance must have occurred (no change in AP = CO ↑ × SVR ↓). In this setting, left ventricular filling pressure falls and heart size is reduced, so that the afterload must be lower despite a constant systemic arterial pressure; under such circumstances the fall in systemic vascular resistance would provide the best clinical measure of the decrease in afterload.[5] In the future, determination of ventricular chamber diameter and wall thickness by echocardiography may add to the clinical assessment of afterload changes by allowing

---

* In simplified terms the systemic vascular resistance or

$$SVR = \frac{MAP - MRAP \text{ mmHg}}{CO \text{ l/min}}, \text{ expressed in dimensionless}$$

"resistance units." The conversion factor of 80 converts these units to the commonly employed units of dynes-sec. cm$^{-5}$. MAP = mean arterial pressure (or diastolic arterial pressure plus ⅓ of the difference between systolic and diastolic pressures), MRAP = mean right atrial pressure, and CO = cardiac output. The right atrial pressure is often neglected.

estimates of heart size and wall stress at the bedside.

## Effects of Changing Afterload

The weight lifted by an isolated cardiac muscle during active shortening (the afterload) is well known to affect the muscle's performance. [1,16] If the resting muscle length (preload) is held constant, increasing the afterload (weight) will decrease both the extent and velocity of muscle shortening, whereas reducing the afterload will increase the extent and speed of muscle shortening. When cardiac muscle performance is studied over a range of afterloads with preload held constant, these experimental findings are responsible for the inverse relations between afterload and velocity (force = velocity curve) and between afterload (force) and the extent of myocardial fiber shortening. The relation between muscle length and the force developed at the end of active shortening in isolated muscle tends to fall on a single relation at any level of inotropic state, regardless of the level of preload and afterload, [16] a property of the muscle which is responsible for the usefulness of ventricular pressure-volume loops discussed below.

Similar effects of changing the afterload have been demonstrated in the intact heart. If the preload and inotropic state are held constant, increasing the afterload will decrease both the speed and the extent of left ventricular wall shortening, whereas reducing the afterload will increase both of these variables. [12] Although such responses are obtained experimentally, with the preload (diastolic stretch) of the heart held constant, comparable effects of increased and decreased afterload also occur in the heart when the preload reserve is fully utilized [17] and are manifested by the sharp decrease in stroke volume observed in the dilated human heart when the aortic pressure is elevated by administration of a vasopressor. [18]

Responses to afterload changes can be described most simply in diagrammatic form by using the pressure-volume loop in conjunction with the left ventricular function curve. As in isolated muscle, left ventricular tension-volume points at the end of ejection in individual beats tend to form a linear relation at any level of

inotropic state, [19] and during acute changes in ventricular performance, the pressure-volume relations at the end of ventricular ejection in individual pressure-volume loops also describe

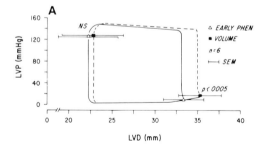

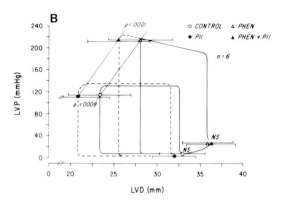

Fig. 22.2   Relations between left ventricular pressure (LVP) and left ventricular internal diameter (LVD) measured with ultrasonic crystals, producing pressure-volume loops in the conscious dog. Left ventricular systolic pressure was controlled by infusion of the vasopressor phenylephrine, and in some experiments a positive inotropic intervention (PII) was administered alone, or in combination with phenylephrine (PHEN + PII). *(A)* Response to acute volume overload by means of infusion, with systolic arterial pressure held constant. It can be noted that despite a larger end-diastolic dimension, the relation between ventricular diameter and pressure at the end of ejection is unchanged from control conditions (open symbols, solid lines). *(B)* The relations between left ventricular diameter and pressure at the end of ejection are dependent upon the left ventricular pressure, and when altered by phenylephrine infusion together with the control beats they form a straight line *(open symbols)*. Infusion of a positive inotropic agent shifts the entire end-systolic pressure-diameter relationship to the left *(closed symbols, dashed lines)*. (Mahler F, Covell JW, Ross J, Jr: Systolic pressure-diameter relations in the normal conscious dog. Cardiovasc Res 9:447–455, 1975.)

a linear relation at any level of contractility, regardless of the acute changes in preload and afterload [20,21] (Fig. 22.2). Thus an increase in systolic pressure alone will decrease the stroke volume, and vice versa, whereas an increase in preload alone will increase the stroke volume (Fig. 22.2).

This framework allows a description of the concept of "afterload mismatch" in describing the function of the normal and failing left ventricle.[2] The nonfailing heart, in the resting state, exhibits levels of preload and contractility which allow it to develop sufficient force and shortening to deliver an adequate stroke volume (normal ejection fraction) against a normal aortic pressure (Fig. 22.3); it also receives a normal

venous return and has a substantial preload reserve. In contrast, the failing heart with depressed contractility, despite maximal use of its preload reserve, exhibits a "mismatch" in the intrinsic ability of its muscle fibers to shorten against a load (Fig. 22.3). Often the afterload under these conditions is somewhat elevated due to increased vascular resistance and heart size; and if the inotropic state is severely depressed, it may be impossible for the ventricle to deliver an adequate stroke volume against even a normal or reduced aortic pressure (as in cardiogenic shock). Thus, in heart failure these factors set the stage for a highly beneficial effect of afterload reduction. Finally, in some clinical situations, e.g., acute systemic arterial hypertension or acute severe valvular regurgitation, when the left ventricle must acutely face a greatly elevated preload and afterload, an afterload mismatch with reduced stroke volume can occur even if contractility is normal or only mildly depressed. Again, such conditions are highly favorable for afterload reduction to produce an improved cardiac output.

Under conditions of severe acute left ventricular "power failure," with or without associated mechanical overload, the ventricle is operating on a "descending limb" of function [2] (Fig. 22.4). However, this descending limb is not due to diastolic overstretch of the sarcomeres, which would constitute a true descending limb of Starling's curve; [17] in fact, the failing heart responds to a reduction in preload alone with no change or a fall in cardiac output.[1] Rather, the descending limb is related to an acute afterload mismatch in the face of absent preload reserve (Fig. 22.4), similar to the marked drop in stroke volume observed a number of years ago in chronic heart failure during steady-state infusion of a vasopressor.[18] Thus, as shown in Figure 22.5, relief of such a mismatch by a vasodilator can be viewed as moving upward on a descending limb that was due to excessive afterload.[2]

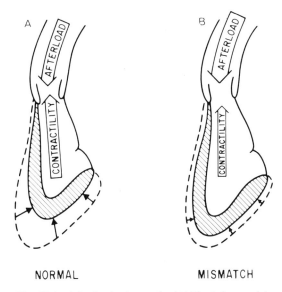

Fig. 22.3  Afterload mismatch. *(A)* The left ventricle is in the normal state; diastolic filling (preload), the basal level of contractility and afterload (reflected by the aortic pressure and impedance, but measured as the wall force or stress) are perfectly matched; thus ventricular ejection against a normal afterload leads to normal wall shortening and stroke volume (large arrows at bottom) and a normal percentage of ejection (ejection fraction). *(B)* In afterload mismatch, the preload reserve is fully utilized, myocardial contractility is depressed, and the impedance to ejection (afterload) is slightly increased because of elevation peripheral vascular resistance. Afterload mismatch leads to reduced shortening of the wall (small arrows at bottom) and reductions in the stroke volume and ejection fraction.

## The Role of Venous Return

Recent experiments in our laboratory have provided some insight into other mechanisms involved in acute adaptations to vasodilator

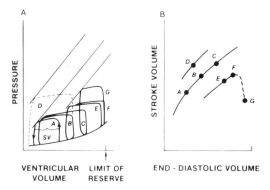

Fig. 22.4  *(A)* Pressure-volume loops of the normal and failing ventricle. The diagonal straight lines represent the relations between volume and pressure at the end of ejection at three levels of inotropic state: Normal *(middle line),* augmented contractility *(upper line),* heart failure (line shifted downward and to the right). The excursion of the pressure-volume loop on the x-axis, indicated by the brackets in loop A, represents the stroke volume (SV) for the normal heart, which is progressively increased by volume loading (loops B and C) but without significant change in the pressure-volume relationships at the end of ejection. If a positive inotropic intervention such as isoproterenol is administered while the ventricle is operating under conditions shown by loop B, despite an elevated systolic pressure during ejection, the ventricle can increase the stroke volume (loop D, dashed lines). In heart failure, (loop E) the stroke volume may be maintained compared to

that in loop B by increased use of the Frank-Starling mechanism, diastolic volume and pressure being markedly increased. The limited preload reserve is indicated by the vertical arrow and little increase in stroke volume is available with volume infusion (loop F). Under these conditions, pressure loading of the ventricle by infusion of a vasopressor such as phenylephrine in the absence of preload reserve will produce an afterload mismatch, and the stroke volume will drop as the systolic pressure rises (loop G). If the failing ventricle is initially operating at loop G, because of elevated peripheral vascular resistance and increased wall stress, administration of a vasodilator such as nitroprusside will cause the ventricle to move from loop G to loop E, producing an increase in the stroke volume.

*(B)* Relations between left ventricular end-diastolic volume and the stroke volume, based on the stroke volume generated by the pressure-volume loops shown in the left hand panel. The normal curve indicates a positive relation, and as the end-diastolic volume is progressively increased the stroke volume increases (points A, B, and C). A positive inotropic intervention moves the ventricle to point D. In heart failure, little preload reserve is available (point E to F) and acute pressure loading produces a descending limb of function (point F to G). If the ventricle is initially operating at point G, afterload reduction will move the ventricle to point F. See also Figure 22.5 for similar curves but using left ventricular end-diastolic pressure instead of diastolic volume.

treatment in the normal and failing circulations, and how opposite effects on the cardiac output can occur in the normal and failure states.[22] In these experiments, in which the venous return to the heart was assessed independently of the output of the ventricles, shifts in the volume of blood contained in peripheral and central (pulmonary) circulations, concomitant effects on venous return, and effects on performance of the left ventricle were found to play equally important parts in the observed responses of cardiac output.

In the normal circulation, intravenous infusion of the vasodilator nitroprusside led to a reduced left ventricular wall stress, a reduction in systemic vascular resistance, and a somewhat variable response of the characteristic input impedance. The normal left ventricle was sub-

jected to favorable loading conditions; however, there was concomitant peripheral vascular dilatation (predominantly in the venous bed) which was only partly compensated for by a small shift in blood volume from the central to the peripheral circulation. This effect, in turn, led to a striking decrease in the venous return to the heart, the venous return curve being displaced downward and to the left due to a reduced mean systemic pressure and effective systemic blood volume. This reduction in the venous return to the right heart was responsible for a reduction in cardiac output, despite the more favorable loading conditions on the left ventricle during systole (Fig. 22.6).[22]

In the presence of acute experimental left ventricular failure produced by coronary occlusion, in which the left ventricular end-diastolic

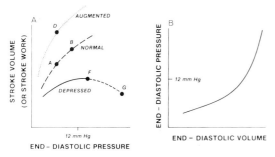

Fig. 22.5 *(A)* Left ventricular function curves similar to those shown in Figure 22.4 but plotted against left ventricular end-diastolic pressure. *(B)* The curvilinear relation between left ventricular end-diastolic volume and end-diastolic pressure is shown; it should be recalled that this relation is nearly exponential and that the pressure rises sharply with small changes in volume above an end-diastolic pressure of about 12 mmHg. Thus, in comparing the descending limb of function shown in the right hand panel of Figure 22.4 to that in the left hand panel of this figure, when the ventricle moves from point F to G or from point G to F, large changes in left ventricular end-diastolic pressure occur with only minimal changes in left ventricular diastolic volume.

pressures were elevated to over 20 mmHg, an opposite effect on cardiac output occurred during nitroprusside infusion. Again, venodilatation took place in the peripheral circulation; however, in the presence of left heart failure a large shift of blood volume from the central to the peripheral circulation occurred, which exactly counterbalanced the tendency for nitroprusside to lower the mean systemic pressure. Therefore, the venous return curve was not shifted downward, and a marked shift upward of the cardiac output curve due to correction of an afterload mismatch on the failing ventricle could be expressed as an increase in the cardiac output (Fig. 22.7).[22]

Thus, it is clear that effects of vasodilator drugs on the peripheral circulation are highly important in determining the overall hemodynamic responses to acute vasodilator therapy. Moreover, as discussed subsequently, different degrees of activity of these drugs on the resistance and capacitance vessels may lead to varying responses of the cardiac output in a given clinical setting, depending upon the drug employed.

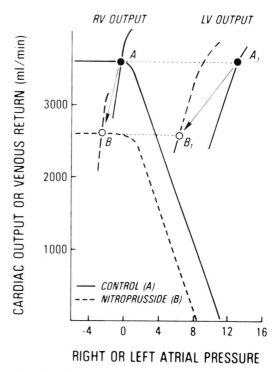

Fig. 22.6 Relation between cardiac output and venous return in the normal heart and circulation. The inverse relations between right atrial pressure and venous return are shown under control conditions *(solid lines)* and during nitroprusside infusion *(dashed lines)*. Segments of cardiac output curves relating right ventricular output to right atrial pressure (RV output) and left ventricular output to left atrial pressure (LV output) are also shown under these two conditions. Under control conditions, the cardiac output is limited by the venous return, and the equilibrium (Point A) where the venous return and cardiac output curves intersect is on the plateau of the venous return curve. In the steady-state, the right ventricular and left ventricular outputs are in equilibrium *(dashed horizontal line* and Point A₁). During nitroprusside infusion, venodilation produces a drop in mean systemic pressure and a shift downward of the venous return curve, the right ventricle reaching a new equilibrium point at a lower cardiac output (Point B) which, in turn, is in equilibrium with a lower left ventricular output at a lower mean left atrial pressure (Point B₁). Thus, despite upward shifts of the right and left ventricular function curves due to reduced afterload and lowered impedance to ejection, the cardiac output is lower. (Modified from Pouleur H, Covell JW, Ross J, Jr: Effects of nitroprusside on venous return and central blood volume in the absence and presence of acute heart failure. Circulation 61:328–337, 1980.)

## HEART FAILURE

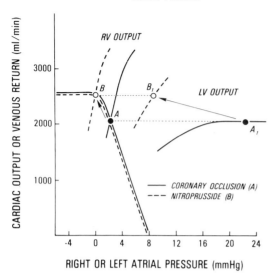

RIGHT OR LEFT ATRIAL PRESSURE (mmHg)

Fig. 22.7  Relations between cardiac output and venous return in acute heart failure produced by experimental coronary occlusion. Symbols same as in Figure 22.5. Under control failing conditions *(solid lines)*, the intersect between right ventricular output and venous return (Point A) is on the ascending limb of the venous return curve, cardiac output being limited by the failing left ventricle which is operating on a flat and depressed cardiac output curve (Point A). Following nitroprusside infusion *(dashed lines)* there is no shift downard of the venous return curve, this being prevented by a redistribution of the central blood volume to the periphery (see text). There is now a marked shift upward of the function curve of the left ventricle due to reduced afterload with correction of afterload mismatch, and a marked drop in left ventricular filling pressure occurs. The shift upward of the right ventricular output curve is now accompanied by an increase in the cardiac output (Point B), and at equilibrium both right and left ventricles (Point $B_1$) are now operating at lower filling pressures and with improved cardiac output (Modified from Pouleur H, Covell JW, Ross J, Jr: Effects of nitroprusside on venous return and central blood volume in the absence and presence of acute heart failure. Circulation 61:328–337, 1980.

## Effects on Ventricular Filling Pressures

During vasodilator therapy, reductions in the left and right ventricular end-diastolic pressures and in the pulmonary artery wedge pressure occur in both the normal and the failing heart,

an effect that is most marked when these pressures are high.[4,11] This fall has been equated with a reduction in diastolic fiber length, or preload, of the left ventricle. Reduction of the systemic vascular resistance in the setting of left ventricular failure results in enhanced left ventricular emptying with augmented stroke volume, the smaller residual volume moving the ventricle downward on its diastolic pressure-volume curve and leading to reduced intracardiac filling pressures (Fig. 22.5). An additional factor appears to be involved as well, however. Large downward shifts of the entire left ventricular diastolic pressure-volume curve have been described in patients with heart failure during treatment with nitroprusside; these shifts constituted small reductions or little change in the left ventricular diastolic volumes but striking reductions in left ventricular diastolic pressures.[23,24] That such shifts in the pressure-volume curve reflect an effect of the pericardium, rather than an alteration in left ventricular diastolic compliance, has been indicated by recent studies in our laboratory in acutely distended hearts of conscious dogs.[25,26] Following circulatory distension, the pressure-volume curve was displaced upward; under these conditions there was a downward shift of the diastolic volume-length curve with nitroprusside infusion when the pericardium was intact (Fig. 22.8). When the experiment was repeated after the pericardium was removed, the fall in the apparent filling pressure of the volume-loaded heart was less after nitroprusside, the left ventricle now moving downward on a single, undisplaced diastolic pressure-length curve (Fig. 22.8).[25] This finding suggests that decreases in intrapericardial pressure may contribute substantially to the dramatic reductions in left ventricular filling pressure observed during vasodilator therapy in some patients with acute or subacute heart failure. Such an additional component to the fall in filling pressures, relating to changes in the intrapericardial pressure, would imply a less marked fall in *transmural* left ventricular diastolic pressure and hence in heart size (preload) than would be estimated from the cardiac filling pressure alone. Thus, the true preload may not be so

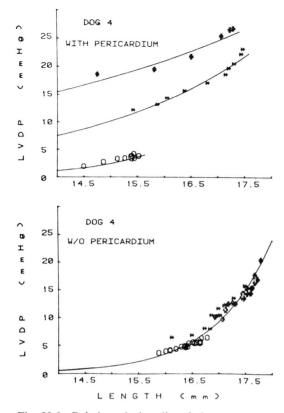

Fig. 22.8 Relations during diastole between a segment of the left ventricular wall and the left ventricular diastolic pressure (LVDP). Diastolic pressure-dimension relations were obtained during slow cardiac filling (diastasis). The upper panel shows this relation with the pericardium intact before *(open symbols)* and after the intravenous infusion of dextran to produce acute cardiac dilatation *(upper curve);* the middle curve shows the effects of an intravenous infusion of nitroprusside in the presence of such acute cardiac dilatation. In the lower panel the same dog is later studied again, but without (W/O) the pericardium. The same interventions, volume loading and nitroprusside, are produced. The ventricle now appears to be operating on a single diastolic pressure-length relation. (Shirato K, Shabetai R, Bhargava V, et al: Alteration of the left ventricular diastolic pressure-segment length relation produced by the pericardium: Effects of cardiac distension and afterload reduction in conscious dogs. Circulation 57:1191–1198, 1978.)

markedly reduced; indeed, if too great a reduction in preload does occur during vasodilator use, the effect on cardiac output will be detrimental.[11]

## Coronary Perfusion and Myocardial Oxygen Consumption

Vasodilator therapy following acute myocardial infarction can alter the balance between myocardial oxygen demand and supply[1] and can lead to improvement of the coronary perfusion pressure gradient to the subendocardium.[27] It is well to recall, however, that if mean coronary perfusion pressure is dropped below approximately 60 mmHg, autoregulation of the coronary vascular bed ceases[28] and the intravascular pressure distal to coronary stenosis, or in the coronary collateral circulation, then becomes the primary determinant of regional coronary blood flow. Therefore, lowering of mean systemic arterial pressure below 60 mmHg, particularly in the presence of coronary heart disease, should be avoided. Recent studies indicate that systolic as well as diastolic coronary perfusion pressure is important, since flow beyond a severe stenosis occurs primarily during systole in the outer myocardial layers,[29,30] whereas perfusion to the subendocardium occurs almost exclusively during diastole.[31] Therefore, a substantial fall in either systolic or diastolic arterial pressures may be detrimental. In addition, it is imperative to avoid substantial increases in heart rate, which may occur reflexly due to excessive reductions in arterial pressure, particularly with the use of vasodilators in the absence of significant heart failure. An increase in heart rate increases myocardial oxygen consumption in a nearly linear manner,[32] in addition to reducing the diastolic time available for subendocardial perfusion.[31]

Most experimental studies comparing the effects of various vasodilators on measures of ischemia and on coronary blood flow have been carried out in experimental animals subjected to coronary occlusion in the absence of heart failure. In the ensuing discussion this point should be kept in mind, since current indications for the use of vasodilators concern the treatment of heart failure rather than the reduction of ischemic injury, which is still in the experimental stage. Nevertheless, it is useful to review these effects and to assess their clinical relevance. Differing actions of nitroprusside and nitroglycerin on regional coronary blood flow and epicardial ST segment changes have been reported, and variations have also been observed in responses, depending on the animal species under study.

In dogs without heart failure, nitroprusside produces an increase in ST segment elevation together with reduced regional myocardial blood flow (measured by microspheres) in ischemic zones, whereas nitroglycerin causes a reduction of ST segment elevation and improved blood flow to ischemic zones.[33] Such effects of nitroglycerin were shown to result predominantly from increased subendocardial flow.[34] The addition of phenylephrine to maintain systemic arterial pressure during nitroglycerin administration to dogs results in a further increase in regional blood flow through collateral channels to the ischemic zones,[34,35] phenylephrine per se dominantly augmenting flow to the epicardium.[34] In contrast, use of nitroglycerin alone following acute coronary artery occlusion in the pig, a species in which there are relatively few coronary collateral channels, fails to show improved regional blood flow to ischemic regions,[36] and the addition of phenylephrine also did not improve coronary perfusion.[36] Nitroglycerin acts predominantly on larger conductance vessels, with relatively minor effects on the small resistance vessels,[37] and it may substantially improve coronary collateral blood flow by this mechanism in the dog. Nitroprusside, on the other hand, predominantly affects the small resistance vessels, and it might diminish flow through collateral channels by reducing the coronary perfusion from relatively normal adjacent vessels.[38] Despite findings with nitroprusside in the normal dog, when experiments are carried out in dogs with dilated failing hearts, nitroprusside has a favorable effect on coronary perfusion to the subendocardium, and it also decreases myocardial oxygen consumption.[39] These effects may relate to relief of both high ventricular filling pressure and reduced afterload on the left ventricle.[39] Such experiments appear more relevant to the usual clinical setting.

No studies in man have been concerned with the effects of vasodilators on acute ischemic in-

jury and coronary blood flow after coronary occlusion. In a small number of patients with chronic coronary artery disease, in whom pulmonary artery wedge pressures were not reported, the [133]xenon washout technique was used before and during either nitroprusside or nitroglycerin administration.[40] Recognizing the limitations of this method, the findings indicated that nitroprusside lowered regional myocardial blood flow about 15 percent in most patients, both in the presence and absence of coronary collateral vessels. Nitroglycerin, 0.4 mg sublingually, when given to patients with well-developed collateral vessels resulted in a 10 percent increase in regional myocardial flow; both drugs similarly reduced regional myocardial flow when there were no collaterals.[40] In these studies, left ventricular end-diastolic pressures were not measured and the average decrease in systemic arterial pressure was approximately 14 percent; therefore, it is likely that these responses resemble those in dogs without heart failure. In patients with congestive heart failure complicating myocardial infarction who are receiving nitroprusside, intravenous digoxin produced a further modest increase in cardiac output but did not produce any further decrease in pulmonary arterial wedge pressure.[41] Nitroprusside infusion (25 to 150 μg/min) has also been reported to increase ST segment elevations,[33] whereas sublingual nitroglycerin reduced the ST segment elevation in patients with acute myocardial infarction,[33,42] but more information is needed concerning the responses of coronary blood flow and cardiac oxygen consumption to vasodilator therapy, particularly in the presence of acute heart failure.

From the above considerations, it is evident that the potential effects of vasodilators on myocardial oxygen supply and demand should always be considered in relation to the hemodynamic status of the patient before undertaking vasodilator treatment in acute myocardial infarction.

The net effect on the left ventricular function curve of all factors discussed above (relief of afterload mismatch, increased venous return, improvement of subendocardial blood flow,

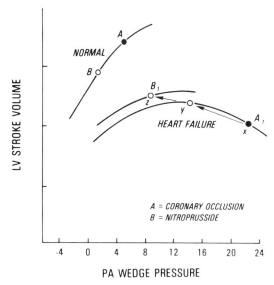

Fig. 22.9 Hemodynamic responses of the left ventricle (LV) diagrammed as changes in the stroke volume and the pulmonary artery (PA) wedge pressure in patients with coronary occlusion before and during nitroprusside infusion (compare to Fig. 22.1). The normal response of the left ventricle to the vasodilator is a modest fall in the pulmonary artery wedge pressure together with a drop in the stroke volume (Point A to Point B). In heart failure, there is a more marked decrease in the wedge pressure accompanied by a rise in the stroke volume (Point $A_1$ to $B_1$). The response in the normal heart is influenced dominantly by changes in venous capacitance and venous return (see text). In the failing heart, the marked improvement in left ventricular function produced by afterload reduction can be now expressed as an increased cardiac output because of the shift in central blood volume peripherally, which serves to prevent the normal fall in venous return produced by nitroprusside. At least two components of the left ventricular functional response seem likely. First, the ventricle moves upward on an apparent descending limb of function (Point X to Point Y); this response does not indicate operation of the ventricle on a true descending limb of the Starling curve, but rather relief by the vasodilator of an excessive afterload. Second, other factors including lowering of systolic wall stress, improvement of subendocardial blood flow by relief of cardiac distension, and lowering of intrapericardial pressure all may serve to shift the entire function curve upward and to the left (Point Y to Point Z).

lowering of intrapericardial pressure) is summarized in Figure 22.9.

## PHARMACOLOGIC AGENTS USED FOR AFTERLOAD REDUCTION

Several parenteral agents have been used for afterload reduction in the treatment of heart failure, and it seems likely that improved agents will become available for oral use. The drugs most commonly employed are listed in Table 22.1 along with their dominant sites of action and major hemodynamic effects. These drugs tend to have little or no direct effect on myocardial contractility.[11] Various vasodilators exert different degrees of activity on the arteriolar bed (the resistance vessels) and on the venous bed (the capacitance vessels). For example, a dominant action to dilate arterioles without appreciable venodilation (as produced by hydralazine) will lower systemic vascular resistance and thereby have a pronounced effect on left ventricular afterload but will be accompanied by only a small shift of blood from the central to peripheral circulations; hence, such a drug will tend to produce a substantial increase in cardiac output without much effect on left heart filling pressure. A dominant action to dilate the venous bed with less effect on arterioles (as produced by nitroglycerin) will tend to pool blood in the peripheral circulation by causing a shift of blood from the central circulation; therefore, such a drug will produce less increase in the cardiac output and a marked reduction of the left heart filling pressure, particularly when that pressure is elevated. Although mean arterial pressure may fall to some degree in response to most of these agents, there is usually little increase in heart rate in the presence of left ventricular dysfunction, which may reflect the blunting of cardiovascular reflexes accompanying heart failure.[1]

Intravenous sodium nitroprusside has been most commonly used in the treatment of acute heart failure; its action is to relax vascular smooth muscle [43] and it tends to have a balanced action on arteriolar and venous beds, resulting in both a substantial fall in pulmonary

**Table 22.1   Major Actions of Vasodilating Agents Used in Afterload Reduction Therapy**

| | Major Sites of Action | Chief Hemodynamic Effects | | | |
|---|---|---|---|---|---|
| | | ↓ *PAW* | ↑ *CO* | ↑ *HR* | ↓ *BP* |
| **Intravenous** | | | | | |
| Sodium nitroprusside | A + V | ++ | ++ | 0 | + |
| Phentolamine | A + V | ++ | +++ | ↑ | + |
| Nitroglycerin | V | +++ | + | 0 | + |
| **Oral** | | | | | |
| Isosorbide dinitrate (ISO) | V | +++ | + | 0 | + |
| Hydralazine (H) | A | ± | +++ | 0 | ± |
| Prazosin | A + V | ++ | ++ | 0 | + |
| ISO + H | A + V | ++ | ++ | 0 | + |

A = arterioles; V = veins; PAW = pulmonary artery wedge pressure; CO = cardiac output; HR = heart rate; BP = systemic blood pressure

artery wedge pressure and a rise in cardiac output (Table 22.1). It has been shown, in patients with chronic congestive heart failure, that nitroprusside infusion lowers the forearm vascular resistance and venous tone to approximately equal degrees.[44] No change, or a slight decrease, in heart rate ordinarily is observed in patients with congestive heart failure during nitroprusside infusion. This drug also produces a fall in pulmonary vascular resistance.[43] Other clinical aspects of concern during the use of nitroprusside are discussed in the ensuing section on clinical indications for therapy.

Nitroglycerin tends to act predominantly on the venous bed,[45] with a less marked arteriolar dilating action (Table 22.1) and, as mentioned, it has a more pronounced affect on pulmonary artery wedge pressure than cardiac output.[44,46] The action of this agent, administered sublingually, is probably too short to permit effective, sustained afterload reduction; in paste form its effect lasts up to 4 hours.[46] Intravenous administration of nitroglycerin in acute myocardial infarction has been shown to produce a less marked increase in cardiac output than does nitroprusside in patients with high left heart filling pressures.[47]

Phentolamine, one of the earliest drugs employed,[48] has a direct vasodilator action and also exerts an alpha-adrenergic blocking effect; it may have a small direct positive inotropic action as well.[5] Phentolamine appears to exhibit a somewhat more potent effect on arteries than on veins and appears to cause a somewhat greater increase in cardiac output and heart rate than does nitroprusside (Table 22.1).

The clinical use of oral vasodilators (Table 22.1) in subacute heart failure after myocardial infarction is discussed in the ensuing section. Isosorbide dinitrate, in chewable form, has been found to have an effect for 2 to 4 hours, whereas the oral form may be effective for 4 to 6 hours.[46] Its most prominent effect is on the pulmonary artery wedge pressure, only a small increase in cardiac output being produced in the presence of heart failure. Hydralazine tends to exert its most marked effect on arteriolar resistance, increasing cardiac output substantially with almost no effect on pulmonary artery wedge pressure in patients with heart failure.[15] It also may have a direct chronotropic effect,[49] but in patients with heart failure the effect on heart rate generally is minor. In addition, the combination of oral hydralazine with isosorbide dinitrate has been reported to lower pulmonary artery wedge pressure while maintaining the increase in cardiac output produced by hydralazine.[50] Prazosin, given orally, has a balanced action on the arteries and veins, resembling that of nitroprusside. This quinazoline derivative may act through direct arteriolar dilatation, together with a considerable degree of alpha-adrenergic blocking activity [51] and has been shown to have approximately equal actions on forearm vascular resistance and venous tone.[52] It has little effect on heart rate in patients with congestive heart failure.[51]

## CLINICAL INDICATIONS AND RESULTS OF VASODILATOR THERAPY IN ACUTE MYOCARDIAL INFARCTION

Current major indications for vasodilator therapy (Table 22.2) are severe left ventricular failure, which blends into the power failure or cardiogenic shock syndrome discussed in Chapter 20; systemic hypertension accompanying acute myocardial infarction; temporary support of patients with certain complications of myocardial infarction (ventricular septal rupture, acute mitral regurgitation, see Ch. 39); and refractory and persistent subacute left ventricular failure after acute myocardial infarction. The role of nitroglycerin in treating severe myocardial ischemia (intermediate coronary syndrome) and unstable angina pectoris is discussed elsewhere (Ch. 25).

### Acute Left Ventricular Failure

Afterload reduction has found increasing use in the management of severe, acute left ventricular failure. Mild to moderate degrees of heart failure after acute myocardial infarction often respond well to diuretics, with or without digitalis, but such measures may be ineffective when the failure is severe. In this setting, there may be a downward trend in blood pressure without frank hypotension, one or more signs of low

**Table 22.2   Indications for Vasodilator Therapy in Acute Ischemic Heart Disease**

---

1. Acute refractory left ventricular failure after myocardial infarction
2. Cardiogenic shock (milder forms) after myocardial infarction
3. Hypertension associated with acute myocardial infarction
4. Acute mitral regurgitation
5. Ventricular septal rupture
6. Subacute left ventricular failure
? 7. Reduction of ischemic injury after acute myocardial infarction

---

cardiac output (such as mental confusion, mild oliguria, cool and moist extremities), and marked pulmonary congestion on the chest roentgenogram.[53]

In such patients, a balloon-tipped catheter should be placed in the pulmonary artery to monitor pulmonary artery wedge pressure before any attempt is made to reduce afterload. Patients who will respond favorably to afterload reduction therapy generally show an elevated wedge pressure,[11] some reduction in cardiac index, and an elevated systemic vascular resistance. Beneficial effects of vasodilator therapy have been substantial *only* when there has been considerable elevation of the pulmonary artery wedge pressure (generally in excess of 15 mmHg) (Fig. 22.1); when the filling pressure is below 15 mmHg, the stroke volume often falls, sometimes with associated hypotension and an increase in heart rate.[11] Often, as systemic vascular resistance falls, it is possible to achieve a substantial increase in cardiac output with little or no reduction in systemic arterial pressure. If a significant fall in blood pressure occurs (mean systemic arterial pressure below 60 mmHg or systolic pressure below 80 mmHg), there may be adverse effects on both coronary perfusion pressure and blood flow.[28] Any reflex increase in heart rate stimulated by hypotension may unfavorably affect the ventricle by stimulating myocardial oxygen consumption in marginally perfused regions, which could even lead to extension of the infarction. Thus, use of vasodilator therapy should be limited to patients with an elevated pulmonary artery wedge pressure, and blood pressure should be carefully monitored by cuff or indwelling catheter with a view to lowering arterial pressure by no more than 10 to 20 mmHg (10 to 15 percent).

Nitroprusside has been the drug most commonly used in patients with heart failure arising after acute myocardial infarction. It is advisable to begin with a very small dose of nitroprusside (15 $\mu$g/min) to avoid sudden hypotension and tachycardia, and to increase the dosage every 10 to 15 minutes (average 75 $\mu$g/min; maximum 425 $\mu$g/min) to achieve a substantial reduction in pulmonary artery wedge pressure (to 10 or 12 mmHg) without a marked fall in systemic arterial pressure. Should wedge pressure fall below this level and/or signs of further lowering of cardiac output develop, it may be assumed that too much vasodilation, with consequent excessive reduction of left ventricular preload, has occurred. Infusion of fluid or colloid should be commenced to increase filling pressure to a more optimum level, usually about 12 to 13 mmHg during continued nitroprusside infusion. In some patients, even higher levels of filling pressure (15 to 20 mmHg) may be necessary to optimize the use of the Frank-Starling mechanism.[54] Although it is desirable to monitor the rise in cardiac output during nitroprusside administration for severe left ventricular failure, it is perhaps not essential if the patient is not in shock; improvement in the character of the pulse, decreased pulmonary congestion, warming of the extremities, and enhanced urine output are clinical signs that cardiac output has improved. Furosemide, given intravenously in small doses (20 mg), may be employed, if necessary, to further lower left heart filling pressure and improve urine flow.

Intravenous nitroprusside for the treatment of severe left ventricular failure after myocardial infarction has been reported to reduce hospital mortality from about 75 percent to 40 to 50 percent.[55] In those studies, the vasodilator was infused continuously for several hours up to 3 weeks. When prolonged nitroprusside infusion is required, or when renal failure is present, thiocyanate levels should be measured and maintained below 10 mg percent to avoid toxicity; occasionally, cyanide intoxication has occurred when very high doses of nitroprusside are employed.[11] Adding an infusion of dopamine to nitroprusside particularly when mild hypotension is associated with oliguria (making the renal vasodilator action of this agent useful) may produce favorable effects, and some patients may respond to the use of dopamine[56] or dobutamine[57] alone (see also Ch. 20). Isoproterenol should be avoided because it causes a pronounced increase in heart rate and myocardial oxygen requirements.

Other vasodilator drugs have also been used to treat heart failure after acute myocardial infarction. Phentolamine, started at a dose of 0.1 mg/min and increased to a maximum of 2 mg/min, appears to have effects similar to those of nitroprusside; however, it is expensive, requires high doses, and it may have the disadvantage of provoking relatively more tachycardia (Table 22.1). Nitroglycerin has been used sublingually[42,58] and intravenously.[47] The sublingual effect is transient, and it has been suggested that the intravenous route, using doses of 10 to 75 μg/min, yields greater stability due to better control of drug distribution.[27] Large reductions in pulmonary artery wedge pressure have been encountered with nitroglycerin, but increases in cardiac output have tended to be less and more variable than with nitroprusside, probably because of the more pronounced venodilator action of nitroglycerin[58] (Table 22.1). Occasionally, severe hypotension and bradycardia have complicated the use of nitroglycerin in patients with acute myocardial infarction.[59] As discussed earlier, several experimental and clinical studies have suggested that nitroglycerin has more favorable effects on coronary blood flow and ST segment elevations than nitroprusside, but clinical observations have not been made in those patients with severe heart failure who are most likely to benefit from nitroprusside.

## Cardiogenic Shock

As discussed in Chapter 20, careful hemodynamic monitoring is essential in the management of shock (including measurements of systemic arterial and pulmonary artery wedge pressures and the cardiac output), since hypovolemia as a cause of hypotension must be carefully excluded and vasodilators may have an unfavorable effect in some patients. Cardiogenic shock after myocardial infarction carries a mortality of over 90 percent with conventional treatment. However, some of these patients have responded to vasodilator therapy with nitroprusside and have survived hospitalization; unfortunately, follow-up indicates that late morbidity and mortality are high.[55] While patients with relatively mild degrees of shock can exhibit a favorable response to pharmacologic afterload reduction, if the mean arterial pressure is below 60 mmHg, the systolic pressure below 80 mmHg, or the stroke work index below 10 g-m/m² of body surface area, other therapeutic modalities, such as intraaortic balloon counterpulsation, usually are preferable. In this setting, the initial use of dopamine [56] or dobutamine [57] also may be considered, and the use of dopamine or norepinephrine combined with nitroprusside has been advocated when shock is severe [60] (see Chs. 20 and 21).

### Hypertension After Myocardial Infarction

Significant hypertension sometimes persists in acute myocardial infarction, even after pain and anxiety have been relieved by opiates and diuretic therapy has been administered for signs of pulmonary congestion. In such patients, particularly if hypertension is accompanied by persistent left ventricular failure and/or recurrent pain, it is advisable to consider vasodilator therapy. Thus, a continued systolic pressure overload on the damaged left ventricle contributes to ventricular dysfunction (Fig. 22.4) as well as to augmented oxygen use with its potential for enlarging the ischemic zone. Signs of ischemic damage may lessen when the hypertension is treated.[61] In this setting, vasodilator therapy can improve cardiac function, lower cardiac filling pressure, reduce myocardial oxygen demands, and perhaps prevent the extension of the infarction. Initial administration of nitroprusside intravenously followed by the addition of an oral antihypertensive, if necessary, has usually been successful in reducing the systemic arterial pressure to within the normal range.

### Sudden Severe Mechanical Cardiac Overload Due to Ventricular Septal Rupture or Mitral Regurgitation

When the heart is subjected to an acute, severe pressure or volume overload, the preload reserve becomes exhausted and the left ventricle can be forced onto a descending limb of function.[2] Under such circumstances, the ventricle is confronted with an afterload mismatch (Fig. 22.4) consequent to the increased systolic wall stress associated with acute cardiac dilation and wall thinning. As discussed earlier, the descending limb of function is due to excessive afterload rather than to a true descending

limb of the Frank-Starling relation consequent to sarcomere overstretch (Fig. 22.5).[2]

Although some degree of subendocardial ischemia due to severe cardiac distension may be present in the noninfarcted regions of the heart, myocardial contractility can be relatively well maintained in those regions, and reduced shortening is due to the severe mechanical overload. When acute severe mitral regurgitation follows rupture of one head of a papillary muscle after acute myocardial infarction, or severe ventricular overload is caused by rupture of the interventricular septum, surgical intervention generally will be required. Since the mechanical overload is complicated by myocardial infarction with associated myocardial dysfunction in ischemic and infarcted zones, the degree of pulmonary congestion and reduction of forward cardiac output often are extreme and unresponsive to conventional medical therapy. The clinical response to afterload reduction with nitroprusside in the presence of severe mitral regurgitation can be gratifying.[62,63] By reducing impedance to left ventricular ejection into the aorta, the vasodilator not only increases the forward stroke volume in mitral regurgitation or ventricular septal defect, but also reduces the volume of regurgitation or left to right shunt flow, thereby further reducing pulmonary artery wedge pressure.[63,64] By these mechanisms, the congestive cardiac failure often can be relieved and hemodynamic conditions stabilized until surgical treatment can be performed (Ch. 39).

### Subacute Cardiac Failure

It is advisable to use *intravenous* vasodilator therapy in managing acute left ventricular failure in the early phase of acute myocardial infarction, or in treating the sudden mechanical complications of myocardial infarction. However, when left ventricular failure, unresponsive to digitalis and diuretics, persists later in the hospital course, the addition of an oral vasodilator may be considered. It is advisable to document elevation of pulmonary artery wedge pressure before beginning such therapy. This step may be omitted if clearcut pulmonary congestion is identified on the chest roentgenogram and/or by physical examination, and severely impaired left ventricular function is evident (documented, for example, by a radionuclide ejection fraction), provided the vasodilator is used cautiously with frequent blood pressure monitoring, and care is taken to avoid postural hypotension.

Isosorbide dinitrate, 2.5 to 10 mg in chewable or sublingual form, reduces the pulmonary artery wedge pressure for 90 minutes or more. Oral isosorbide dinitrate in doses of 10 to 60 mg every 4 to 6 hours has also been shown to be effective.[46] Nitroglycerin ointment has similarly prolonged effects. Prazosin, in a dose of 2 to 7 mg every 6 hours, effectively lowers pulmonary artery wedge pressure and systemic vascular resistance;[65] the orthostatic hypotensive response to the initial dose of prazosin (which should not exceed 1 mg) calls for particularly careful use of this drug in the postmyocardial infarction setting. The drug's effects may tend to diminish with time[66] and the increased use of diuretics, such as furosemide, may be required. Hydralazine has not been investigated systematically in postinfarction patients. In a small number of patients with chronic myocardial disease and low-output cardiac failure, hydralazine, in a dose of 50 to 75 mg every 8 hours, was added to digitalis and diuretic therapy;[67] increases averaging 66 percent in cardiac output were accompanied by decreases of 42 percent in systemic vascular resistance, with little change in heart rate and only mild decreases (5 percent) in arterial pressure, although the pulmonary artery wedge pressures remained elevated.[67] Doses of 25 to 100 mg every 8 hours also may be effective,[67,68] and it has been suggested that a twice daily dosage may be sufficient in some patients.[67,68] Since hydralazine has relatively little effect on the venous bed and on pulmonary artery wedge pressure (Table 22.1), the combination of hydralazine with a long-acting nitrate[69] has been advocated in patients who exhibit dyspnea or pulmonary congestion. Long-term use of this agent is known to be accompanied by immunologic and clinical evidence of the lupus syndrome. Other vasodilator drugs[70] and combinations of agents undoubtedly will be forthcoming.

## Reduction of Myocardial Infarct Size

The value of vasodilator therapy for its potential effects on reducing the extent of ischemic injury or infarct size (in the absence of the potential therapeutic indications listed in Table 22.2) has not yet been established. Randomized clinical trials concerned with the use of hyaluronidase or propranolol for this purpose are now underway. Other approaches to limiting ischemic injury, including glucose-potassium-insulin solution, are also under study. Until the results of such investigations are available, the use of vasodilators for this purpose should be considered an experimental form of therapy. Problems in the measurement of infarct size and therapeutic approaches to infarct size reduction are discussed further in the next chapter.

## REFERENCES

1. Braunwald E, Ross J Jr, Sonnenblick EH: Mechanisms of Contraction in the Normal and Failing Heart, 2nd ed. Boston: Little, Brown, 1976.
2. Ross J Jr: Afterload mismatch and preload reserve: A conceptual framework for the analysis of ventricular function. Prog Cardiovasc Dis 18:255–264, 1976.
3. Guyton AC: Determination of cardiac output by equating venous return curves with cardiac response curves. Physiol Rev 35:123–129, 1955.
4. Cohn JN: Vasodilator therapy for heart failure: the influence of impedance on left ventricular performance. Circulation 48:5–7, 1973.
5. Ross J Jr: Effects of afterload or impedance on the heart: Afterload reduction in the treatment of cardiac failure. Cardiovasc Med 2:1115–1132, 1977.
6. Chatterjee K, Massie B, Rubin S, et al: Long-term outpatient vasodilator therapy of congestive heart failure: Consideration of agents at rest and during exercise. Am J Med 65:134–145, 1978.
7. Claus RH, Birtwell WC, Albertal G, et al: Assisted circulation: I. The arterial counterpulsator. J Thorac Cardiovasc Surg 41:447–458, 1961.
8. Spotnitz HN, Covell JW, Ross J Jr, et al: Left ventricular mechanics and oxygen consumption during arterial counterpulsation. Am J Physiol 217:1352–1358, 1969.

9. Austen WG, Buckley MJ, Mundth ED, Sanders CA: Assisted circulation: intra-aortic balloon pumping. Transplant Proc 3:1473–1477, 1971.

10. Ross J Jr: Left ventricular contraction and the therapy of cardiogenic shock (editorial). Circulation 35:611–613, 1967.

11. Chatterjee K, Parmley WW: The role of vasodilator therapy in heart failure. Prog Cardiovasc Dis 19:301–325, 1977.

12. Ross J Jr, Covell JW, Sonnenblick EH, et al: Contractile state of the heart characterized by force-velocity relations in variably afterloaded and isovolumic beats. Circ Res 18:149–163, 1966.

13. Milnor WR: Arterial impedance as ventricular afterload. Circ Res 36:565–570, 1975.

14. Urschel CW, Covell JW, Sonnenblick EH, et al: Effects of decreased aortic compliance on performance of the left ventricle. Am J Physiol 214:298–304, 1968.

15. Pouleur H, Covell JW, Ross J Jr: Effects of alterations in aortic input impedance on the force-velocity-length relationship in the intact canine heart. Circ Res 45:126–136, 1979.

16. Sonnenblick EH: Implications of muscle mechanics in the heart. Fed Proc 21:975–990, 1962.

17. MacGregor DC, Covell JW, Mahler F, et al: Relations between afterload, stroke volume, and descending limb of Starling's curve. Am J Physiol 227:884–890, 1974.

18. Ross J Jr, Braunwald E: The study of left ventricular function in man by increasing resistance to ventricular ejection with angiotensin. Circulation 29:739–749, 1964.

19. Taylor RR, Covell JW, Ross J Jr: Volume-tension diagrams of ejecting and isovolumic contractions in left ventricle. Am J Physiol 216:1097–1102, 1969.

20. Suga H, Sagawa K, Shoukas AA: Load independence of the instantaneous pressure-volume ratio of the canine left ventricle and effects of epinephrine and heart rate on the ratio. Circ Res 32:314–322, 1973.

21. Mahler F, Covell JW, Ross J Jr: Systolic pressure-diameter relations in the normal conscious dog. Cardiovasc Res 9:447–455, 1975.

22. Pouleur H, Covell JW, Ross J Jr: Effects of nitroprusside on venous return and central blood volume in the absence and presence of acute heart failure. Circulation 61:328–337, 1980.

23. Alderman EL, Glantz SA: Acute interventions shift the diastolic pressure-volume curves in man. Circulation 54:662, 1976.

24. Brodie BR, Grossman W, Mann T, McLaurin LP: Effects of sodium nitroprusside on left ventricular diastolic pressure-volume relations. J Clin Invest 59:59, 1977.

25. Shirato K, Shabetai R, Bhargava V, et al: Alteration of the left ventricular diastolic pressure-segment length relation produced by the pericardium: Effects of cardiac distension and afterload reduction in conscious dogs. Circulation 57:1191–1198, 1978.

26. Ross J Jr: Editorial. Acute displacement of the diastolic pressure-volume curve of the left ventricle: Role of the pericardium and the right ventricle. Circulation 59:32–37, 1979.

27. Kjekshus JK: Mechanism for flow distribution in normal and ischemic myocardium during increased ventricular preload in the dog. Circ Res 33:489–499, 1973.

28. Mosher P, Ross J Jr, McFate PA, et al: Control of coronary blood flow by an autoregulatory mechanism. Circ Res 14:250–259, 1964.

29. Tomoike H, Ross J Jr, Franklin D, et al: Improvement by propranolol of regional myocardial dysfunction and abnormal coronary flow pattern in conscious dogs with coronary narrowing. Am J Cardiol 41:689–696, 1978.

30. Bache RJ, McHale PA, Greenfield JC, Jr: Transmural myocardial perfusion during restricted coronary inflow in the awake dog. Am J Physiol 232:H645–H651, 1977.

31. Bache RJ, Cobb FR: Effect of maximal coronary vasodilation on transmural myocardial perfusion during tachycardia in the awake dog. Circ Res 41:648–653, 1977.

32. Boerth RC, Covell JW, Pool PE, et al: Increased myocardial oxygen consumption and contractile state associated with increased heart rate in dogs. Circ Res 24:725–734, 1969.

33. Chiariello M, Gold HK, Leinbach RC, Comparison between the effects of nitroprusside and nitroglycerin on ischemic injury during acute myocardial infarction. Circulation 54:766–773, 1976.

34. Bache RJ: Effect of nitroglycerin and arterial hypertension on myocardial blood flow following acute coronary artery occlusion in the dog. Circulation 57:557–562, 1978.

35. Capurro NL, Kent KM, Smith HM: Acute coronary occlusion: Prolonged increase in collateral flow following brief administration of nitroglycerin and methoxamine. Am J Cardiol 39:679–683, 1977.

36. Most AS, Williams DO, Millard RW: Acute coronary occlusion in the pig: Effect of nitroglycerin

on regional myocardial blood flow. Am J Cardiol 42:947–953, 1978.

37. Cohen MV, Kirk ES: Differential response of large and small coronary arteries to nitroglycerin and angiotensin. Autoregulation and tachyphylaxis. Circ Res 33:445–453, 1973.

38. Armstrong PW, Walker DC, Burton JR, Parker JO: Vasodilator therapy in acute myocardial infarction. A comparison of sodium nitroprusside and nitroglycerin. Circulation 52:1118–1122, 1975.

39. Kirk ES, LeJemtel TH, Nelson GR, et al: Mechanisms of beneficial effects of vasodilators and inotropic stimulation in the experimental failing ischemic heart. Am J Med 65:189–196, 1978.

40. Mann T, Cohn PF, Holman BL, et al: Effect of nitroprusside on regional myocardial blood flow in coronary artery disease. Results in 25 patients and comparison with nitroglycerin. Circulation 57:732–738, 1978.

41. Raabe DS Jr: Combined therapy with digoxin and nitroprusside in heart failure complicating acute myocardial infarction. Am J Cardiol 43:990–994, 1979.

42. Awan NA, Amsterdam EA, Vera Z, et al: Reduction of ischemic injury by sublingual nitroglycerin in patients with acute myocardial infarction. Circulation 54:761–765, 1976.

43. Palmer RF, Lasseter KC: Sodium nitroprusside. N Engl J Med 292:294–297, 1975.

44. Miller RR, Williams DO, Mason DT, et al: Pharmacologic mechanisms for left ventricular unloading in clinical congestive heart failure; differential effects of nitroprusside, phentolamine and nitroglycerin on cardiac function and peripheral circulation. Circ Res 39:127–133, 1976.

45. Mason DT, Braunwald E: The effects of nitroglycerin and amyl nitrite on arteriolar and venous tone in the human forearm. Circulation 32:755–766, 1965.

46. Franciosa JA, Blank RC, Cohn JN, et al: Hemodynamic effects of topical, oral, and sublingual nitroglycerin in left ventricular failure. Curr Ther Res 22:231–245, 1977.

47. Flaherty JT, Reed PR, Kelly DT, et al: Intravenous nitroglycerin in acute myocardial infarction. Circulation 51:132–139, 1975.

48. Majid PA, Sharma B, Taylor SH: Phentolamine for vasodilator treatment of severe heart failure. Lancet 2:719–724, 1971.

49. Khatri I, Uemura N, Notargiacoma A, et al: Direct and reflex cardiostimulating effects of hydralazine. Am J Cardiol 40:38–42, 1977.

50. Franciosa JA, Cohn JN: Hemodynamic responsiveness to short- and long-acting vasodilators in left ventricular failure. Am J Med 65:126–133, 1978.

51. Lowenstein J, Steele J Jr: Prazosin. Am Heart J 95:262–265, 1978.

52. Awan NA, Miller RR, Maxwell K, et al: Effects of prazosin in forearm resistance and capacitance vessels. Clin Pharmacol Ther 22:79–84, 1977.

53. Karliner JS, Ross J Jr.: Left ventricular performance after acute myocardial infarction. Prog Cardiovasc Dis 13:374–391, 1971.

54. Crexells C, Chatterjee K, Forrester JS, et al: Optimal level of filling pressure in the left side of the heart in acute myocardial infarction. N Engl J Med 289:1263–1266, 1973.

55. Chatterjee K, Swan HJC, Kaushik VS, et al: Effects of vasodilator therapy for severe pump failure in acute myocardial infarction on short-term and late prognosis. Circulation 53:797–802, 1976.

56. Holzer J, Karliner JS, O'Rourke R, et al: Effectiveness of dopamine in patients with cardiogenic shock. Am J Cardiol 32:79–84, 1973.

57. Gillespie TA, Ambos HD, Sobel BE, et al: Effects of dobutamine in patients with acute myocardial infarction. Am J Cardiol 39:588–594, 1977.

58. Williams DO, Amsterdam EA, Mason DT: Hemodynamic effects of nitroglycerin in acute myocardial infarction. Circulation 51:421–427, 1975.

59. Come PC, Pitt B: Nitroglycerin-induced severe hypotension and bradycardia in patients with acute myocardial infarction. Circulation 54:624–628, 1976.

60. Mason DT, Amsterdam EA, Miller RR, et al: Medical management of severe left ventricular failure and cardiogenic shock in acute myocardial infarction. In: Clinical Application of Intraaortic Balloon Pump. Balooki H, editor. Futura Publishing Co, Mt Kisco, NY, 1977, p 235.

61. Shell WE, Sobel BE: Protection of jeopardized ischemic myocardium by reduction of ventricular afterload. N Engl J Med 291: 481–486, 1974.

62. Chatterjee K, Parmley WW, Swan HJC, et al: Beneficial effects of vasodilator agents in severe mitral regurgitation due to dysfunction of subvalvar apparatus. Circulation 48:684–690, 1973.

63. Harshaw CW, Grossman W, Munro AB, et al: Reduced systemic vascular resistance as therapy for severe mitral regurgitation of valvular origin. Ann Intern Med 83:312–316, 1975.

64. Goodman DJ, Rossen RM, Holloway EL, et al: Effect of nitroprusside on left ventricular dynam-

ics in mitral regurgitation. Circulation 50:1025–1032, 1974.

65. Awan NA, Miller RR, DeMaria AN, et al: Efficacy of ambulatory systemic vasodilator therapy with oral prazosin in chronic refractory heart failure: concomitant relief of pulmonary congestion and elevation of pump output demonstrated by improvements in symptomatology, exercise tolerance, hemodynamics and echocardiography. Circulation 56:346–354, 1977.

66. Packer M, Meller J, Gorlin R, et al: Hemodynamic and clinical tachyphylaxis to prazosin-mediated afterload reduction in severe chronic congestive heart failure. Circulation 59:531–539, 1979.

67. Chatterjee K, Parmley WW, Massie B, et al: Oral hydralazine therapy for chronic refractory heart failure. Circulation 54:879–883, 1976.

68. O'Malley K, Segal JL, Israili ZH, et al: Duration of hydralazine action in hypertension. Clin Pharmacol Ther 18:581–586, 1975.

69. Massie B, Chatterjee K, Werner J, et al: Hemodynamic advantage of combined administration of hydralazine orally and nitrates nonparenterally in the vasodilator therapy of chronic heart failure. Am J Cardiol 40:794–801, 1977.

70. Dzau VJ, Colucci WS, Williams GH et al: Sustained effectiveness of converting-enzyme inhibition in patients with severe congestive heart failure. N Engl J Med 302:1373–1379, 1980.

## ACKNOWLEDGMENT

This project was supported by NIH Research Grant HL 17682, Ischemic Heart Disease Specialized Center on Research, awarded by the National Heart, Lung and Blood Institute, PHS/DHEW.

# 23 | Approaches to the Protection of Jeopardized Myocardium

P. E. Maroko, M.D.
J. W. Covell, M.D.

## INTRODUCTION

Coronary artery occlusion triggers a sequence of events eventually leading to myocardial cell death. Cell death, which histopathologically constitutes an infarction, is best considered as a dynamic sequence of complex changes. Analysis of this chain of events is complicated by our fragmentary knowledge of the many reactions involved and by certain special characteristics of the process itself. Thus, the necrobiosis should be considered not only from the point of view of the fate of each individual ischemic myocardial cell but also, and perhaps more importantly, from the point of view of the whole population of ischemic cells. The current status of our knowledge concerning the biochemical and histologic events leading to cell death, which is reviewed elsewhere in this text, underlies the assumption that this process can be modified early following coronary occlusion and forms the basis for therapeutic modalities designed to protect the acutely ischemic myocardium. Although the potential reversibility of acute myocardial ischemic injury has been studied extensively, the events that characterize the transition from reversible to irreversible cellular injury remain clouded. The mitochondria demonstrate striking anatomic and metabolic changes as the cells which contain them enter an irreversible phase of injury.[1-3] It is not clear whether such mitochondria are capable of recovery if the ischemia is relieved. Loss of cell volume regulation and increased sarcolemmal permeability have been found to correlate more closely with irreversible injury than has mitochondrial failure,[4] thus suggesting the hypothesis that the primary event leading to irreversibility may be a sarcolemmic defect.

Several studies have been undertaken to examine the problem of how long the ischemic myocardium is still amenable to treatment. The results of this investigation indicate that certain interventions have a significant salutary effect on the ischemic myocardium even when they are administered several hours after coronary artery occlusion.[5-10] Thus, interventions such as the administration of propranolol, changes in arterial pressure, intraaortic balloon counterpulsation, infusion of glucose-insulin-potassium solution plus beta-adrenergic blockade, and glucocorticoids were able to decrease myocardial injury at different time intervals ranging between 3 and 6 hours after coronary artery occlusion.

In a more recent study hyaluronidase was administered at several different intervals following coronary artery occlusion in the dog (20 minutes, 3, 6, and 9 hours).[11] The extent of myocardial necrosis was measured biochemically (myocardial creatine kinase [CK] activity), histologically, and electrocardiographically (changes in QRS configuration 24 hours after coronary artery occlusion).[12] All three methods of measuring necrosis were complementary, and the results of each correlated well with one another. By correlating ST segment elevation shortly after occlusion (15 minutes) with these indices of necrosis at 24 hours, it was demonstrated that the beneficial effects of hyaluronidase declined progressively as the interval between the coronary artery occlusion and the administration of the drug lengthened (Fig. 23.1). However, even when this agent was administered 6 hours after occlusion, a significant beneficial effect was still demonstrable, although it was less than that observed when the drug was given 20 minutes after occlusion. In contrast, hyaluronidase administered 9 hours after occlusion had no discernible beneficial effect. Histochemical studies in the rat are in accordance with these observations.[13] The depletion of oxidative enzymes from the zone destined to necrose was gradual, starting in the center of the ischemic zone and progressing outwards. Following 3 hours of ischemia, 50 per-

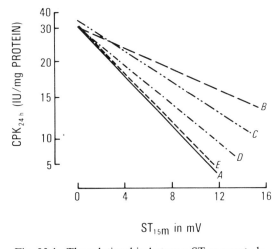

Fig. 23.1 The relationship between ST segment elevation 15 minutes after coronary artery occlusion ($ST_{15M}$) in dogs and log creatine phosphokinase activity values of specimens obtained from subjacent sites 24 hours later ($CPK_{24H}$). Line A, occlusion alone: log CPK = $(-0.064 \pm 0.007)$ $ST_{15m}$ + $(1.49 \pm 0.02)$, n = 14, r = $-0.81 \pm 0.03$. Line B, hyaluronidase treatment 20 minutes after occlusion: log CPK = $(-0.025 \pm 0.003)$ $ST_{15m}$ + $(1.48 \pm 0.02)$, n = 12, r = $-0.72 \pm 0.04$. Line C, hyaluronidase treatment 3 hours after occlusion: log CPK = $(-0.037 \pm 0.005)$ $ST_{15m}$ + $(1.53 \pm 0.01)$, n = 8, r = $-0.85 \pm 0.02$. Line D, hyaluronidase treatment given 6 hours after occlusion: log CPK = $(-0.044 \pm 0.003)$ $ST_{15m}$ + $(1.49 \pm 0.01)$, n = 8, r = $-0.78 \pm 0.03$.

cent of the jeopardized zone still exhibited oxidative enzyme activity. This activity was still 25 percent after 6 hours but was absent 9 and 12 hours after coronary artery occlusion. Thus, histochemically, a zone of salvageable myocardium exists up to 6 hours after occlusion but disappears thereafter under these experimental conditions. It remains possible, however, that a more potent agent or one with a different mechanism of action from that of hyaluronidase might still cause significant myocardial salvage when started at a later time.

Similarly, reperfusion of the coronary artery results in salvage of portions of the ischemic myocardium if it is performed early after occlusion; its effectiveness is reduced as reperfusion is delayed. Thus, in 1972 Maroko et al.[14] and Ginks et al.[15] showed that in anesthetized dogs reperfusion after 3 hours of ischemia resulted in definitive and permanent salvage of jeopardized cells and that concomitantly the contractile function of the initially damaged myocardium improved. The studies of McNamara et al.[16] and Reimer et al.[17] showed in monkeys and dogs, respectively, that the more prolonged the delay in reperfusion, the smaller the salvage.

It is apparent, therefore, that salvage of the myocardium can be induced either pharmacologically or by reperfusion for several hours after coronary artery occlusion, and that the benefit of these interventions decreases over the first 6 hours following occlusion. It should be noted that this progression depends on species differences and on the mechanism of action of the interventions.

## MECHANISMS OF ACTION OF INTERVENTIONS THAT ALTER MYOCARDIAL DAMAGE

In studies begun in 1968, it was shown that the area of ischemic injury, as reflected by epicardial ST segment elevations, can be either increased or decreased by changing the balance between oxygen supply and demand.[6,18] If there are extensive collateral vessels, as in the dog, oxygen supply may be altered by changing systemic arterial pressure and, therefore, coronary collateral flow to the ischemic area. In these experiments, it was found that the extent of acute myocardial injury is inversely proportional to alterations in arterial pressure. Furthermore, changes in myocardial oxygen requirements were shown to be important determinants of the final extent of cell necrosis; interventions that increased oxygen requirements, such as isoproterenol, augmented myocardial injury, whereas interventions that decreased myocardial oxygen requirements, such as propranolol, reduced damage as assessed by both the extent of epicardial ST segment elevation and by myocardial CK activity. It is important to note that, in general, changes in collateral blood flow appeared to override the changes in oxygen requirements. For example, an increase in systemic arterial pressure on the one hand increases the afterload and thereby augments myocardial oxygen consumption, which presumably increases cell damage; on the other hand, this increase in arterial pressure also augments the perfusion pressure in the coronary arteries thereby increasing coronary collateral flow to the ischemic zone and favorably influencing the damaged cells. The net result of these two opposite actions is favorable, at least in the dog, because the effect of an increase in collateral blood flow to the ischemic zone overrides the detrimental effect of the increase in afterload. This indicates the paramount influence of collateral flow in determining the final extent of necrosis.[6] It is important to emphasize that these changes were observed in the dog, an animal that has an extremely rich network of collaterals even in the normal heart. In the pig, an animal that normally has very few collaterals (i.e., without atherosclerosis), the changes in arterial pressure may provoke opposite effects, compared with the dog. Thus, in the pig the increase in arterial pressure will increase cardiac work without an increase in collateral flow, and as a result ischemic injury may increase.[19] The extrapolation of these experimental results to the clinical situation may suggest that each patient, in accordance with the size and number of collateral vessels, has an optimal blood pressure that maximally increases this collateral coronary flow. Further increase in blood pressure, however, will result in an increase in oxygen requirement without

increase in collateral flow, thereby resulting in more ischemia.

Subsequent experimental studies using electrocardiographic, enzymatic, and histologic indices of tissue damage have largely confirmed the initial hypothesis that levels of ischemia may be altered by manipulation of the relationship between $O_2$ supply and demand. Thus, interventions that increased myocardial oxygen requirements increased myocardial damage. These included stimuli that exert positive inotropic or chronotropic actions, such as isoproterenol, glucagon, digitalis in the nonfailing heart (Fig. 23.2), bretylium tosylate, and pacing-induced tachycardia, all of which augment myocardial oxygen needs.[6] Reductions in oxygen delivery to the ischemic myocardium also resulted in extensions of the injury; these reductions could be produced either by hypoxemia[20] or by reducing collateral blood flow to the ischemic zone by lowering the perfusion pressure by means

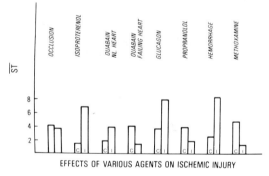

EFFECTS OF VARIOUS AGENTS ON ISCHEMIC INJURY

Fig. 23.2 Average effects on epicardial ST segment elevation of several agents which influence oxygen supply-demand ratio in acutely ischemic dog myocardium. Occlusion represents the effects of repeat 15 minute coronary occlusions one hour apart. ST = average ST segment elevation C = control, I = ST segment following coronary occlusion with the intervention. (Adapted from Maroko PR, Kjekshus JK, Sobel BE, et al: Factors influencing infarct size following coronary artery occlusion. Circulation 43:67–83, 1973; Maroko PR, Libby P Sobel, BE, et al: Effect of glucose-insulin-potassium infusion on myocardial infarction following experimental coronary artery occlusion. Circulation 45:1160–1175, 1972; and Maroko PR, Braunwald E: Effects of metabolic and pharmacologic interventions on myocardial infarct size following coronary occlusion. Circulation 53 (suppl I):162–168, 1976.)

of hemorrhagic hypotension.[6,8] In a canine model in which infarct size was measured anatomically, severe hypotension increased infarct size by 24 percent while moderate hypotension did not change it.[21] Also, myocardial damage can be increased by an unfavorable redistribution of regional myocardial blood flow (i.e., the so called coronary steal) when coronary vasodilators, such as minoxidil[22] and nitroprusside,[23] which act on the resistance vessels, are administered. Thus, it has been suggested that vasodilators that act on the proximal conductance vessels are beneficial,[23,25-31] while those which act on the peripheral resistance vessels are detrimental[22,23,34] because they produce a redistribution of flow away from the ischemic zone.

The recognition that several vasodilators may be detrimental in the setting of experimental acute myocardial infarction may be of considerable clinical importance. The possibility that some vasodilators augment blood flow to the nonischemic zone, where this increase is not necessary, and reduce collateral perfusion of the ischemic zones, where collateral flow is of paramount importance, warrants careful determination of the precise effects of each vasodilator on coronary flow.

In contrast, interventions that increase myocardial oxygen delivery or decrease myocardial oxygen needs reduce the extent of tissue death. Included in this category are: (1) elevation of systemic arterial pressure (which probably acts by increasing coronary perfusion pressure and collateral flow to the ischemic area);[6,8,18,24] (2) administration of coronary vasodilators, such as nitroglycerin, which act on the conductance vessels to increase collateral flow;[23,25-31] (3) administration of coronary vasoconstrictors, such as methoxamine, which probably acts on the coronary resistance vessels, thereby favorably redistributing regional myocardial flow (i.e., the so called reverse coronary steal);[32] and the inhalation of 100 percent nitrogen, which acts by a similar mechanism,[33] i.e., it induces constriction of coronary vessels in the nonischemic zone and increases the collateral coronary blood flow to the ischemic zone.

Other interventions that may decrease injury may act by reducing oxygen needs. These include the beta-adrenergic blockers, such as propranolol[6,8,18,35] practolol, oxprenolol, and timolol,[36,37] halothane, bradycardia, and digitalis in the failing heart.[38,39] As an example, halothane reduced myocardial damage in the canine model of anatomic infarct size. This occurred without an increase in regional myocardial blood flow to the ischemic myocardium and was due to a reduction in contractility and afterload.[40] Some interventions may act both by decreasing myocardial oxygen needs and by increasing coronary perfusion pressure, as in the case of intraaortic balloon counterpulsation.[7,41,42] Of special interest is the action of digitalis, which exhibited opposite effects depending on the inotropic state of the heart.[38,39,43] In the nonfailing heart, digitalis increased damage, while in the same animal, when failure was induced pharmacologically, digitalis reduced injury. It is postulated that in the absence of failure, stimulation of contractility increases oxygen needs, and consequently ischemic injury. In the presence of failure, the reduction in energy requirements resulting from the digitalis-induced decrease in left ventricular size overrides the energy cost of an increase in contractility.

Other studies have shown that many other factors, which do not act by changing myocardial oxygen balance, can also significantly alter infarct size. The infusion of hypertonic glucose, with or without insulin and potassium, reduced the extent of myocardial infarction 24 hours after occlusion.[9] These conclusions were based on the observation that there was less damage in the treated dogs than in the untreated dogs at sites with similar epicardial ST segment elevations. The protection of the ischemic myocardium by the infusion of a glucose-insulin-potassium solution was also evident from the better preservation of cellular ultrastructure in the ischemic zone. The mechanism of action of glucose is debatable, but it may act by increasing substrate availability for glycolysis, by lowering free fatty acid levels that may themselves be deleterious, or both. In contrast, hypoglycemia induced by insulin administration increased myocardial damage.[44] This response to hypoglycemia is probably related to a reduction in available substrate rather than the accompanying adrenergic discharge, since beta-adrenergic blockade with propranolol did not prevent the increase in damage.

Hyaluronidase, an enzyme that depolymerizes mucopolysaccharides, was found to be very effective both in reducing the acute ST segment elevation and the necrosis at 24 hours after occlusion, as analyzed by myocardial CK depletion, histologic appearance, and epicardial ST segment changes [9,11,12] (Fig. 23.3). Moreover, following left coronary artery occlusion in the rat, infarct size in hyaluronidase-treated animals was substantially smaller than in non-treated rats, both when analyzed either by serial histologic sections or by total left ventricular CK activity.[45] This salvage was evident both at 2 and 21 days, thus demonstrating that not only is the necrosis less after 2 days, but also that the final size of the scar, after the process of infarction is complete, is likewise substantially smaller. The mechanism of action of hyaluronidase is still not fully understood. Hyaluronidase has been shown to penetrate the ischemic zone, depolymerizing the mucopolysaccharides even in the center of the infarction.[46] This action may facilitate either the transport of nutrients to the ischemic zone or the washout of harmful metabolites from this area.

An extremely promising group of substances that are strikingly effective in reducing necrosis are drugs that influence the inflammatory process. As the necrotic process evolves, there is usually an increase in capillary permeability, in chemotaxis, and in phagocytosis, each of which plays a role in the transformation of the injured tissue to a scar. We have postulated that contrary to what occurs in other organs or tissues, in the case of the myocardium it may be advantageous to inhibit this process of cellular destruction. Several substances that act on different biologic systems may decrease necrosis by reducing inflammatory reactions. These include glucocorticoids,[5,47] cobra venom factor (CVF),[45,48-50] aprotinin,[51,52] and ibuprofen.[53,54] Glucocorticoids have multiple and complex actions, and the mechanisms by which these agents benefit ischemic myocardium remain to be elucidated. A number of mechanisms of action have been postulated. These include: (1) stabilization of myocardial cell membranes and

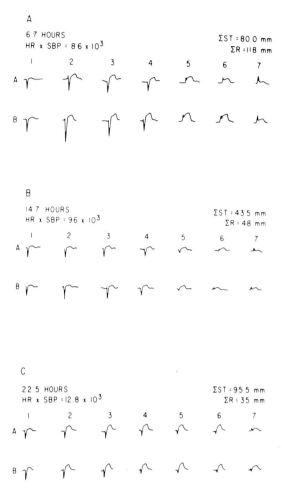

Fig. 23.3 Precordial electrograms from 2 levels (A,B) at 7 sites across the left thorax (V lead designation) from a patient with acute myocardial infarction. (Adapted from Henning H, Hardarson T, Francis G, et al: Approach to the estimation of myocardial infarct size by analysis of precordial ST segment and R wave maps. Am J Cardiol 41:1–8, 1978.)

prevention or delay of the release of lysosomal enzymes;[47,55] (2) stabilization of the phagocytic vacuoles thereby reducing the heterolytic activity of infiltrating inflammatory cells;[5] (3) exertion of other antiinflammatory properties; or (4) increase of collateral blood flow to the ischemic myocardium.[57]

More fascinating, however, are substances that possess only one mechanism of action. Thus, CVF has the specific action of the cleavage, and therefore the depletion of the C3 component of the complement system with the subsequent depletion of other components of this system. It was shown, in the dog,[48,49] rat,[58] and baboon[50] models, that CVF reduced the size of myocardial infarction. It is postulated that this reduction in necrosis is caused by a reduction in capillary permeability and by prevention of both the normal release of chemotactic factor by the C5 component, and of the nonspecific injury to the cells normally induced by the C7 through C9 components. Aprotinin, by inhibiting the kallikrein-kinin system, reduces the effects of the released kinins, which can increase cell permeability. Ibuprofen suppresses prostaglandin-mediated components of inflammation.[53,54] However, indomethacin, which inhibits prostaglandin formation at a different level, increases infarct size.[59] This may be due to the different effect of these two drugs on the synthesis of thromboxanes. The potential advantage of this group of antiinflammatory agents is their relative lack of undesirable side effects.

Other interventions that may have clinical potential for decreasing myocardial necrosis include hyperosmolar substances, such as mannitol,[60,61] which may act by reducing cell swelling and thus facilitate collateral blood flow, and interventions that decrease free fatty acid levels such as betapyridyl-cardinol.[62,63]

A new group of substances, which may be helpful in limiting infarct size, are the calcium blocking agents. Verapamil is the most studied agent, and although the initial reports showed conflicting results,[64,65] it was shown to be an extremely potent intervention, reducing infarct size by over 40 percent when administered to dogs 1 hour after coronary artery occlusion.[54] Nifedipine was also shown to reduce myocardial damage,[66] but its effects seem to be less marked than those of verapamil.

## EFFECTS OF INTERVENTIONS ON SCAR FORMATION

Myocardial tissue death is normally followed by scar formation. Since this healing process is distinct from that of necrosis of the myocardial fibers, it is possible that drugs with a protective effect on the ischemic myocardium may have a detrimental effect on scar formation.[67] In the rat model, the thickness of the scars was examined 3 weeks after coronary occlusion.

Hyaluronidase, reserpine, cobra venom factor, ibuprofen, hydrocortisone, and a single dose of methylprednisolone did not thin the scar. However, when multiple doses of methylprednisolone were administered during the first 24 hours after coronary artery occlusion the scars were excessively thinned.[58] At the time of sacrifice, 21 days after coronary occlusion, these abnormally thin scars had already developed into prominent ventricular aneurysms. In these methylprednisolone-treated rats, the distension of the scar 3 weeks after occlusion may give the false impression that myocardial necrosis has been more extensive than is actually the case. This situation represents expansion (i.e., distension of the scar) rather than extension of infarction due to a true increase in necrosis.[68] This defective healing is also reflected by "mummification" of myocardial cells, which occurs in a great percentage of the necrotic cells that normally should be replaced by fibrotic tissue at this time.[69] Whatever the mechanism of excessive thinning, the hazard of the formation of large ventricular aneurysms is clear. Interestingly, in man, multiple doses of methylprednisolone following acute myocardial infarction have been reported to increase the incidence of ventricular rupture [70] although, so far, this has not been substantiated. Also, in one patient receiving prolonged hydrocortisone therapy following acute myocardial infarction, the development of a ventricular aneurysm was associated with delayed myocardial healing.[71] It is possible that for a more accurate definition of scar formation, biochemical methods of quantification will be used. This approach was attempted by Leon et al.,[72] who measured hydroxyproline and showed that dimethylsulfoxide (DMSO) interferes with the healing process of experimental myocardial infarction.

The present controversy about the role glucocorticoids should play in the treatment of myocardial infarction may be related, at least in part, to their opposite effects on the necrotic and fibrotic processes.[73] One can speculate, therefore, that a dose of glucocorticoids administered minutes after coronary occlusion may act mainly on the necrotic process and be inconsequential to scar formation since the fibrotic process has not begun, while a dose given later may be detrimental by interfering with scar formation. The accurate determination of the temporal sequence of events during the healing process, and the exact phase where the glucocorticoids interfere, will allow a more rational approach to the administration of these agents.

In summary, most experimental and clinical evidence indicates that following coronary occlusion the process of cell death can be considerably attenuated, and that salvage of ischemic myocardium is possible up to 6 hours following coronary occlusion.

## METHODS OF ASSESSING THE RESPONSE TO THERAPY: IMPLICATIONS FOR NEWER THERAPEUTIC APPROACHES

### Enzymatic methods

Serial determinations of creatine kinase (CK) activity in the serum have been used to assess the extent of myocardial tissue necrosis or "infarct size." [74-82] Methods for predicting infarct extent from the early portion of the CK release curve [76,77] also have been applied to study interventions that may alter the magnitude of infarction.[83] Experimental studies have indicated that estimation of myocardial infarction "size" using curves obtained from serial CK samples correlates well with the depletion of this enzyme from the myocardium.[75,82] In man, the integrated area of the CK curve (CK area) also has been employed as an index of the relative size of a myocardial infarction and applied in the evaluation of ECG methods of assessing the extent of myocardial damage.[84] Estimates of infarct "size" using such curves have shown a relation to morbidity, mortality, and alterations in left ventricular performance.[74,77,79,85] Also, in selected patients postmortem measurement of infarct size in man has correlated with estimates of infarct size calculated from serum CK curves.[81] However, Bleifeld et al.[81] concluded that mortality or the development of cardiogenic shock in an individual patient cannot be predicted from enzymatic estimation of infarct "size"; however, such measurements, in conjunction with hemodynamic monitoring

of left ventricular pump function, were considered to be of value in assessing the performance of residual myocardium. Enzymatic estimation of infarct extent has also been correlated with ventricular dysrhythmias, both early and late after myocardial infarction.[86-89] It has been suggested that alterations in predicted CK curves can reflect a beneficial or harmful effect of a particular intervention on the salvage of jeopardized myocardium.[75,76]

The experimental basis for the use of CK curve area determinations as a measure of infarct "size" has been criticized by Roe and his colleagues.[88] They could not distinguish between small and large infarcts produced experimentally, when infarct size was documented by histologic methods and compared to that obtained from enzyme determinations. These investigators also criticized the models that have been proposed to improve CK estimates of the extent of myocardial infarction.[89] These approaches either mathematically fit the serum CK curve for the determination of total release, or assume simple one- or two-compartment models to determine the amount of CK released from the myocardium. They concluded that individualizing disappearance rates or changing the values of other constants in the equations usually employed does not improve the correlation between those estimates and myocardial CK depletion.[90] Others have reached similar conclusions.[91] One possible reason for such discrepancies may reside in the method of calculating CK disappearance. Sobel et al.[92] recently reported that a two-compartment model, using parameters estimated from double exponential fits, provides improved estimates of CK disappearance, accounting for more of the CK released from the heart which appears in the blood after experimental infarction.

Additional factors that may alter CK curves in vivo include infarct extension [80] or expansion,[93] alterations in myocardial blood flow,[88] and administration of drugs such as propranolol [94,95] or digitalis.[43] The independent effects of drugs on serum CK kinetics are of particular importance and must be evaluated in the examination of infarct "size," as determined by CK curve analysis. Other agents, such as morphine, diazepam, or pentobarbital do not seem to alter CK disappearance rates in conscious dogs.[96] Congestive cardiac failure and cardiogenic shock may also alter enzyme curves by influencing CK transport in cardiac lymphatics.[97]

Recently, we assessed the clinical usefulness of serial determinations of serum creatine kinase in the characterization of acute myocardial infarction in man.[98] CK curve areas (112 patients) and peak CK values (154 patients) were determined in subjects with acute myocardial infarction (excluding patients in shock or infarct extension). Two-hour sampling was performed for the first 24 hours or until peak, and a gamma density function was used to calculate curve area from all available samples. The average time from baseline to peak CK was $16.0 \pm 0.5$ hours (SE), and a good correlation (r = 0.93) was found between CK area and peak CK. To establish an approach for detecting peak CK in the clinical setting, a range of sampling intervals (4 to 24 hours) was assessed; 4- and 6-hour sampling intervals for 48 hours produced maximum CK values at or above 85 percent of true peak CK in 92 percent and 89 percent of patients, respectively, and average maximum CK at both sampling intervals exceeded 90 percent of that obtained with 2-hour samplings. Attempts to predict CK curve area, using the portion of the curve prior to peak CK, proved to be inaccurate; not until values 2 hours or more beyond peak CK were utilized did predicted and actual CK areas agree well. Peak CK was higher in patients who died early than in survivors, and both CK area and peak CK were significantly higher in patients with objective evidence of left ventricular failure, indicating the value of these enzyme measures as indices of infarct severity.

The prediction of CK area from the early portions of the curve yielded a wide scatter when compared to the CK area calculated from the total curve. This was true even when predictions were performed up to the peak value. In this approach, each predicted curve was compared with its own "control," i.e., with the true curve obtained from all available data points, rather than with other measures of infarct magnitude such as CK depletion. Our finding casts some doubt on the use of predictive algorithms

for the early estimation of the total CK curve area in man, although it is possible that more frequent sampling might improve the prediction; moreover, use of the MB CK isoenzyme for estimating the extent of myocardial necrosis [99,100] has the advantage in that it is relatively specific for cardiac muscle. However, the potential effects of drug interventions on MB CK disappearance rates have not yet been defined, and the different isoenzymes of CK may exhibit different rates of fractional disappearance.[101]

## Radionuclide Methods

Although radionuclide methods, including $^{99m}$Tc-pyrophosphate scintigrams and positron emission techniques, have been used to assess infarct size in animal studies, these approaches remain largely qualitative and experimental. Nevertheless, radionuclide methods for assessing regional wall motion and regional and global left ventricular performance may be of use in assessing the efficacy of therapeutic interventions designed to limit infarct size.[102] These approaches are discussed in detail in Chapter 28.

## Electrocardiographic Approaches

Although the use of precordial ST segment elevation in patients does not permit the quantitative evaluation of the size of an infarction, the technique is useful for determining whether the myocardial ischemic injury is increasing or decreasing.[102] The precordial ST segment mapping technique has been successfully applied to humans to show that several interventions reduce precordial ST segment elevation more rapidly than expected; this implies that these interventions effectively reduce myocardial injury while it is still in the reversible phase. Such interventions include propranolol,[8,37,91,103] hyaluronidase,[104] nitroglycerin [21,27,28] and the inhalation of a high concentration of oxygen.[68] ST segment elevation can, however, result from other causes, such as pericarditis, epicardial trauma, changes in ionic concentrations (i.e., hyperkalemia), and normal early repolarization. Moreover, ST segments cannot reflect myocardial injury when the QRS complexes are widened.[105] In this instance, the wide QRS complexes cause an opposing displacement of the ST segment, as explained by the gradient theory.[106] This consideration may account for the absence of epicardial ST segment elevation in the center of an ischemic zone where focal block, as defined by a widened QRS complex, is frequently found. The phenomenon of diminished ST segment elevation in the center of an ischemic zone is not observed in dogs without widened QRS complexes [105,107] or in precordial electrocardiograms recorded in patients.

More recently, precordial QRS complex mapping was added to ST segment mapping. By this technique, a fall in R wave amplitude or the appearance of new Q waves are analyzed during the first week following the onset of an infarct in precordial leads that initially (i.e., up to 8 hours after onset of pain) showed ST segment elevations. This approach uses the precordial ST segment recorded as soon as possible after the onset of the clinical event as a predictor of the ultimate fate of the tissue, in a manner analogous to the epicardial ST segment in the experimental animal.[12] The precordial ST segments are compared to subsequent changes in the QRS complexes. These changes are used to assess myocardial necrosis in a manner analogous to the alterations in CK activity or the histologic appearance of the myocardium adjacent to the epicardial electrode in the experimental animal.

While not capable of expressing the mass of infarcted myocardium in quantitative terms, simultaneous analysis of alterations of ST segments and QRS complexes would appear: (1) capable of predicting the surface representation of the expected extent of necrosis while much of the myocardial injury is still in a reversible phase, i.e., at a time of ST segment elevation, prior to the development of changes in the QRS complex; (2) capable of assessing the surface representation of the extent of necrosis that actually develops, as reflected by the change in QRS complexes; and (3) capable of being applied immediately, so as not to delay therapy. Additionally, it is a safe, atraumatic, and relatively inexpensive approach. Nevertheless, it

should be recognized that the "natural history" of alterations in ST segments and R waves must be taken into account when considering the effect of any intervention on these measures [84] (Figs. 23.3 and 23.4).

Using ST segment techniques, the effects of hyaluronidase have been assessed in a multicenter study.[108] Ninety-one patients with anterior infarction were randomized to control (45 patients) or to hyaluronidase-treated (46 patients) groups. A 35-lead precordial electrocardiogram was recorded on admission and 7 days later. Hyaluronidase was administered intravenously after the first electrocardiogram and every 6 hours for 48 hours.

The sum of R wave voltages of vulnerable sites fell more in the control group than in the hyaluronidase group ($70.0 \pm 3.6$ percent) ($\pm$ SE) vs $54.2 \pm 5.0$ percent, $p < 0.01$. Q waves appeared in $59.3 \pm 4.9$ percent of the vulnerable sites in control vs $46.4 \pm 4.9$ percent in hyaluronidase-treated patients ($p < 0.05$). The findings in this study demonstrate that hyaluronidase, when administered within the first 8 hours after the onset of the clinical event, reduces the extent of myocardial necrosis in patients with acute myocardial infarction. Although differences in these electrocardiographic changes between the two groups were approximately 20

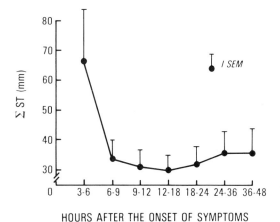

HOURS AFTER THE ONSET OF SYMPTOMS

Fig. 23.4  Natural history of precordial ST segment changes in acute myocardial infarction. (Adapted from Henning H, Hardarson T, Francis G, et al: Approach to the estimation of myocardial infarct size by analysis of precordial ST segment and R wave maps. Am J Cardiol 41:1–8, 1978.)

percent, it should be noted that this type of analysis indicates a directional change in the extent of myocardial infarction, but does not provide quantitative information. The recent observation that changes in precordial ST segments and fall in R wave amplitude correlate qualitatively with the size of infarction in patients with anterior myocardial infarction strengthens the validity of this methodology.[84]

Similarly, after the intravenous administration of propranolol, it was observed that (1) ST segment elevations resolved faster and (2) there was a smaller fall in R wave voltage and less Q wave development 1 week later. Moreover, the administration of propranolol, in many instances, clearly ameliorated morphine-resistant ischemic pain and decreased the accompanying ventricular dysrhythmias.[8,103,108] Thus, propranolol was able to interrupt the ongoing ischemic process, resulting in less necrosis detected electrocardiographically. Nitroglycerin administration was also shown to decrease ST segment elevation and to result in fewer QRS changes.[110] These observations also indicate that, similar to the experimental setting, nitroglycerin is preferable to nitroprusside when afterload and preload must be lowered in the patient with acute myocardial infarction.[23] Also, both intraaortic balloon counterpulsation and oxygen administration were shown to be beneficial.

An extremely important observation was that patients who received propranolol, nitroglycerin, or intraaortic balloon counterpulsation could be divided into groups by degree of response. Patients with a good response have angiographically demonstrable residual blood flow to the infarcting area.[103] Thus, it became clear that propranolol must penetrate the zone in jeopardy and be taken up by the ischemic cells in order to exert its beneficial effects. In the case of nitroglycerin and intraaortic balloon counterpulsation, the existence of collaterals (or subtotal stenoses) permitted the increase in blood flow to the ischemic myocardium; in the absence of these anatomic conduits, an increase in blood flow is impossible. Consequently, benefits to the ischemic myocardium will be limited to the reduction in afterload, and therefore, greatly restricted. There are two corollaries to

this observation: (1) not only may one identify subgroups of patients that will benefit from a specific intervention; but (2) perhaps more importantly, the concept of regional therapy can be advanced.

By selective delivery of drugs to the zone in jeopardy of necrosis, the beneficial effects of a high concentration of the drug can be obtained while adverse reactions in the normal myocardium may be minimal. For example, regional beta-adrenergic blockade of the zone in jeopardy may present advantages over systemic beta blockade, since more drug can be supplied to the ischemic myocardium where it may exert its oxygen-sparing effects while the normal myocardium remains free of the drug and of the undesired negative inotropic side effects. This was attempted in patients with chronic stable angina, who presented with left anterior descending coronary artery stenoses. In these patients the administration of propranolol into the diseased coronary artery effectively delayed the appearance of pacing-induced angina while the administration of the drug into the right coronary artery was ineffective.[111]

It was recently reported that positively charged liposomes can preferentially penetrate the ischemic myocardium.[112] This observation introduced the possibility of delivering higher concentrations of drugs to the ischemic myocardium. It was also shown that the liposomes not only concentrate in the ischemic zone but that they penetrate into the ischemic myocytes.[113] Subsequent studies have demonstrated that ATP can be delivered into the ischemic cells by liposomes,[113] which could potentially reverse the negative energy balance in the ischemic cells.

In summary, it is not possible, at present, to identify the specific intervention likely to be most effective in reducing infarct size in the clinical setting. Indeed, there may not be one single best treatment. Rather, it seems that in the future patients will be carefully, but rapidly, categorized according to the existence of residual flow in the ischemic zone and to their clinical, electrocardiographic, and hemodynamic states, and intervention tailored appropriately. For example, while in hypertensive patients reduction of afterload may be the most effective intervention, and in patients without evidence of myocardial depression, cardiospecific beta-adrenergic blockade may be the treatment of choice, in normotensive or hypotensive patients with pump failure, circulatory support may be desirable. Moreover, all patients with acute infarction, regardless of their hemodynamic state, may benefit from the administration of an anti-inflammatory agent, such as cobra venom factor, ibuprofen, or aprotinin, or from drugs such as hyaluronidase or sulfinpyrazone.[114] The extremely promising experimental results with verapamil raise the possibility of additional potent clinical interventions. Finally, the results of ongoing clinical trials with currently available agents may provide more specific guidelines for use at the bedside in efforts to salvage jeopardized myocardium.

## REFERENCES

1. Jennings RB, Herdson RB, Sommers HM: Structural and functional abnormalities in mitochondria isolated from ischemic dog myocardium. Lab Invest 20:548–557, 1969.
2. Jennings RB, Sommers HM, Herdson PB, et al: Ischemic injury of myocardium. Ann NY Acad Sci 156:61–78, 1969.
3. Jennings RB, Ganote CE: Mitochondrial structure and function in acute myocardial ischemic injury. Circ Res 38 (suppl I):80–89, 1976.
4. Jennings RB: Relationship of acute ischemia to functional defects and irreversibility. Circulation 53 (suppl I): 26–29, 1976.
5. Libby P, Maroko PR, Bloor CM, et al: Reduction of experimental myocardial infarct size by corticosteroid administration. J Clin Invest 52:599–607, 1973.
6. Maroko PR, Kjekshus JK, Sobel BE, et al: Factors influencing infarct size following coronary artery occlusion. Circulation 43:67–83, 1971.
7. Maroko PR, Bernstein EF, Libby P, et al: Effects of intraaortic balloon counterpulsation on the severity of myocardial ischemic injury following acute coronary occlusion. Counterpulsation and myocardial injury. Circulation 45:1150–1159, 1972.
8. Maroko PR, Libby P, Covell JW, et al: Precordial ST segment elevation mapping; an atraumatic method for assessing alterations in the extent of myocardial ischemic injury. The effects of pharmacologic and hemodynamic interventions. Am J Cardiol 29:223–230, 1972.
9. Maroko PR, Libby P, Sobel BE, et al: Effect of glucose-insulin-potassium infusion on myocardial infarction following experimental coronary artery occlusion. Circulation 45:1160–1175, 1972.
10. Maroko PR, Braunwald E: Effects of metabolic and pharmacologic interventions on myocardial infarct size following coronary occlusion. Circulation 53 (suppl I):162–168, 1976.
11. Hillis LD, Fishbein MC, Braunwald E, et al: The influence of the time interval between coronary artery occlusion and the administration of hyaluronidase on salvage of ischemic myocardium in dogs. Circ Res 41:26–31, 1977.
12. Hillis LD, Askenazi J, Braunwald E, et al: Use of changes in the epicardial QRS complex to assess interventions which modify the extent of myocardial necrosis following coronary artery occlusion. Circulation 54:591–598, 1976.
13. Fishbein MC, Hare C, Gissen S, et al: Histochemical identification of quantification of border zones during the evolution of myocardial infarction in the rat. Circulation 55–56 (suppl III):71, 1977.
14. Maroko PR, Libby P, Ginks WR, et al: Coronary artery reperfusion. I. Early effects on local myocardial function and the extent of myocardial necrosis. J Clin Invest 51:2710–2716, 1972.
15. Ginks WR, Sybers HD, Maroko PR, et al: Coronary artery reperfusion. II. Reduction of myocardial infarct size at one week after the coronary occlusion. J Clin Invest 51:2717–2723, 1972.
16. McNamara JJ, Smith GT, Suehiro GT, et al: Myocardial viability after transient ischemia in primates. J Thoracic Cardiovasc Surg 68:248–256, 1974.
17. Reimer KA, Loew JE, Rasmussen MM, et al: The wave front phenomenon of ischemic cell death. I. Myocardial infarct size vs duration of coronary occlusion in dogs. Circulation 56:786–794, 1977.
18. Maroko PR, Braunwald E, Covell JW, et al: Factors influencing the severity of myocardial ischemia following experimental coronary occlusion. Circulation 39–40 (suppl III):111–140, 1969.
19. Carew TE, Johnson A, Covell JW: Effects of blood pressure alterations on ischemic injury in swine with coronary atherosclerosis. Circulation 55–56 (suppl III):526, 1977.
20. Radvany P, Maroko PR, Braunwald E: Effects

of hypoxemia on the extent of myocardial necrosis after experimental coronary occlusion. Am J Cardiol 35:795–800, 1975.

21. Deboer LWV, Davis RF, Rude RE, et al: Effect of arterial hypotension on the size of experimental infarcts. Clin Res 27:162A, 1979.

22. Radvany P, Davis MA, Muller JE, et al: The effect of minoxidil on coronary collateral flow and acute myocardial injury following experimental coronary artery occlusion. Cardiovasc Res 12:120–126, 1978.

23. Chiariello M, Gold HK, Leinbach RC, et al: Comparison between the effects of nitroprusside and nitroglycerin on ischemic injury during acute myocardial infarction. Circulation 54:766–773, 1976.

24. Redwood DR, Smith ER, Epstein SE: Coronary artery occlusion in the conscious dog; effects of alterations in heart rate and arterial pressure on the degree of myocardial ischemia. Circulation 46:323–332, 1972.

25. Bleifeld W, Wende W, Bussman WD, et al: Influence of nitroglycerin on the size of the experimental myocardial infarction. Nauyn Schmiedebergs Arch Pharmacol 277:387–400, 1973.

26. Borer JS, Redwood DR, Levitt B, et al: Reduction in myocardial ischemia with nitroglycerin or nitroglycerin plus phenylephrine administered during acute myocardial infarction. N Engl J Med 293:1008–1012, 1975.

27. Come PC, Flaherty JT, Baird MG, et al: Reversal by phenylephrine of the beneficial effects of intravenous nitroglycerin in patients with acute myocardial infarction. N Engl J Med 293:1003–1007, 1975.

28. Flaherty JT, Rein PR, Kelly DT, et al: Intravenous nitroglycerin in acute myocardial infarction. Circulation 51:132–139, 1975.

29. Gold HK, Leinbach RC, Sanders CA: Use of sublingual nitroglycerin in congestive failure following acute myocardial infarction. Circulation 46:839–845, 1972.

30. Hirshfeld JW Jr, Borer JS, Goldstein RE, et al: Reduction in severity and extent of myocardial infarction when nitroglycerin and methoxamine are administered during coronary occlusion. Circulation 49:291–297, 1974.

31. Smith ER, Redwood DR, McCarron WE, et al: Coronary artery occlusion in the conscious dog. Effects of alterations in arterial pressure produced by nitroglycerin, hemorrhage, and alpha-adrenergic agonists on the degree of myocardial ischemia. Circulation 47:51–57, 1973.

32. Chiariello M, Ribeiro MGT, Davis M, et al: Reverse coronary steal induced by coronary vasoconstriction following coronary artery occlusion in dogs. Circulation 56:809–815, 1977.

33. Ribeiro LGT, Louis EK, Davis MA, et al: Beneficial effect of 100% $O_2$ breathing on redistribution of regional myocardial blood flow. Clin Res 25:248A, 1977.

34. Winbury MM, Howe BB, Hefner MA: Effects of nitrates and other coronary dilators on large and small coronary vessels: An hypothesis for the mechanism of action of nitrates. J Pharmacol Exp Ther 168:70, 1960.

35. Sommers HM, Jennings RB: Ventricular fibrillation and myocardial necrosis after transient ischemia. Arch Intern Med 129:780–789, 1972.

36. Libby P, Maroko PR, Covell JW, et al: Effect of practolol on the extent of myocardial ischemic injury after experimental coronary occlusion and its effects on ventricular function in the normal and ischemic heart. Cardiovasc Res 7:167–173, 1973.

37. Pelides LJ, Reid DW, Thomas M, et al: Inhibition by beta-blockade of the ST segment elevation after acute myocardial infarction in man. Cardiovasc Res 6:295–302, 1972.

38. Maroko PR, Braunwald E, Ross J Jr: The metabolic costs of positive inotropic agents. In: Myocardial Infarction. Corday E, Swan HJC, editors. Williams and Wilkins, Baltimore, 1973, pp. 244–250.

39. Watanabe T, Covell JW, Maroko PR, et al: Effects of increased arterial pressure and positive inotropic agents on the severity of myocardial ischemia in the acutely depressed heart. Am J Cardiol 30:371–377, 1972.

40. Davis RF, Deboer LWV, Rude RE, et al: Effects of halothane anesthesia on the size and geometry of myocardial infarction, hemodynamics and regional myocardial blood flow after experimental coronary artery occlusion. Clin Res 27:161A, 1979.

41. Leinbach RC, Gold HK, Buckley MJ, et al: Reduction of myocardial injury during acute infarction by early application of intraaortic balloon pumping and propranolol. Circulation 47–48 (suppl IV):100, 1973.

42. Levine ID, Maroko PR, Bernstein EF: Comparison of intraaortic balloon pumping and left ventricular decompression on myocardial ischemic injury after experimental coronary artery occlusion. Surg Forum, Clin Congr Am Coll Surg 22:149–150, 1971.

43. Varonkov Y, Shell W, Smirnov V, et al: Aug-

mentation of serum CPK activity by digitalis in patients with acute myocardial infarction. Circulation 55:719–727, 1977.

44. Libby P, Maroko PR, Braunwald E: The effect of hypoglycemia on myocardial ischemic injury during acute experimental coronary artery occlusion. Circulation 51:621–626, 1975.

45. MacLean D, Fishbein MC, Maroko PR, et al: Hyaluronidase induced reductions in myocardial infarct size. Direct quantification of infarction following coronary artery occlusion in the rat. Science 194:199–200, 1976.

46. Maroko PR, Libby P, Bloor CM, et al: Reduction by hyaluronidase of myocardial necrosis following coronary artery occlusion Circulation 46:430–437, 1972.

47. Spath JA Jr, Lane DL, Lefer AM: Protective action of methylprednisolone on the myocardium during experimental myocardial ischemia in the cat. Circ Res 35:44–51, 1974.

48. Maroko PR, Carpenter CB: Reduction in infarct size following acute coronary occlusion by the administration of cobra venom factor. Clin Res 22:298A, 1974.

49. Maroko PR, Carpenter CB, Chiariello M, et al: Reduction by cobra venom factor of myocardial necrosis following coronary artery occlusion. J Clin Invest 61:661–670, 1978.

50. O'Rourke RS, Crawford MH, Ghidoni JJ, et al: Early sarcolemmal complement ($C_3$). Localization in ischemic and infarcted myocardium in the baboon. Clin Res 26:484, 1978.

51. Diaz PE, Fishbein MC, Davis MA, et al: Effect of the kallikrein inhibitor aprotinin on myocardial ischemic injury after coronary occlusion in the dog. Am J Cardiol 40:541–549, 1977.

52. Hartmann JR, Robinson JA, Bunnar RM: Chemotactic activity in the coronary sinus after experimental myocardial infarction: effects of pharmacologic interventions on ischemic injury. Am J Cardiol 40:550–555, 1977.

53. Maclean D, Fishbein MC, Blum RI, et al: Long-term preservation of ischemic myocardium by ibuprofen after experimental coronary artery occlusion. Am J Cardiol 41:394, 1978.

54. Ribeiro LBT, Tasuda T, Lowenstein E, et al: Comparative effects of anatomic infarct size in verapamil, ibuprofen, and morphine-promethazine-chlorpromazine combination. Am J Cardiol 43:396, 1979.

55. Rox AC, Hoffstein S, Weissman G: Lysosomal mechanisms in production of tissue damage during myocardial ischemia and the effects of treatment with steroids. Am Heart J 91:394–397, 1976.

56. Goldstein IM, Malmsten CL, Kaplan HB, et al: Thromboxane generation by stimulated human granulocytes: inhibition by glucocorticoids and superoxide dismutase. Clin Res 25:518A, 1977.

57. Masters TN, Harbold NB, Hall DG, et al: Beneficial metabolic effects of methylprednisolone sodium succinate in acute myocardial ischemia. Am J Cardiol 37:557–563, 1976.

58. Maclean D, Fishbein MC, Braunwald E, et al: Long-term preservation of ischemic myocardium after experimental coronary artery occlusion. J Clin Invest 61:541–551, 1978.

59. Jugdutt BI, Becker LL, Buckley BH, et al: Prostaglandin inhibition increases infarct size after coronary artery occlusion in conscious dogs. Am J Cardiol 41:359, 1979.

60. Powell WJ Jr, Dibona DR, Flores J, et al: Effects of hyperosmotic mannitol in reducing ischemic cell swelling and minimizing myocardial necrosis. Circulation 53 (suppl I):45–49, 1976.

61. Willerson JT, Powell WJ Jr, Cuiney TE, et al: Improvement in myocardial function and coronary blood flow in ischemic myocardium after mannitol. J Clin Invest 51:2989–2998, 1972.

62. Kjekshus JK, Mjos OD: Effect of inhibition of lipolysis on infarct size after experimental coronary artery occlusion. J Clin Invest 52:1770–1778. 1973.

63. Oliver MF: The influence of myocardial metabolism on ischemic damage. Circulation 53 (suppl I):168–170, 1976.

64. Reimer KA, Lowe JE, Jennings RB: Effect of the calcium antagonist verapamil on necrosis following temporary coronary artery occlusion in dogs. Circulation 55:581–587, 1977.

65. Smith HJ, Singh BN, Nisbet HD, et al: Effects of verapamil on infarct size following experimental coronary occlusion. Cardiovasc Res 9:569, 1975.

66. Henry PD, Schuchleib R, Borda LJ, et al: Effects of nifedipine on myocardial perfusion and ischemic injury in dogs. Circ Res 43:372–381, 1978.

67. Green RM, Cohen J, Deweese JA: Short term use of corticosteroids after experimental myocardial infarction: effects of ventricular function and infarct healing. Circulation 50 (suppl III):113, 1974.

68. Hutchins GM, Bulkley BH: Expansion versus extension: two different complications of acute

myocardial infarction. Am J Cardiol 39:323, 1977.

69. Kloner RA, Fishbein MC, Lew H, et al: Mummification of the infarcted myocardium by high dose corticosteroids. Circulation 57:56–63, 1978.

70. Roberts R, Demello V, Sobel BE: Deleterious effects of methylprednisolone in patients with myocardial infarction. Circulation 53 (suppl I):204–206, 1976.

71. Bulkley BH, Roberts WC: Steroid therapy during acute myocardial infarction. A cause of delaying healing and of ventricular aneurysm. Am J Med 56:244–250, 1974.

72. Leon AS, White FC, Bloor CM, et al: Reduced myocardial fibrosis after dimethylsulfoxide (DMSO) treatment of isoproterenol-induced myocardial necrosis in rats. Am J Med Sci 261:41–45, 1971.

73. Sandberg N: Time relationship between administration of cortisone and wound healing in rats. Acta Chirurgica Scand 127:446–455, 1964.

74. Sobel BE, Bresnahan GR, Shell WF, et al: Estimation of infarct size in man and its relation to prognosis. Circulation 46:640–648, 1972.

75. Shell WE, Lavell JF, Covell JW, et al: Early estimation of myocardial damage in conscious dogs and patients with evolving acute myocardial infarction. J Clin Invest 52:2579–2590, 1973.

76. Shell WE, Sobel BE: Protection of jeopardized ischemic myocardium by reduction of ventricular afterload. N Engl J Med 291:481–486, 1974.

77. Mathey P, Bleifeld W, Hanrath P, et al: Attempt to quantitate relation between cardiac function and infarct size in acute myocardial infarction. Br Heart J 35:271–279, 1974.

78. Witteveen SAGJ, Hemker HC, Hollaar L, et al: Quantitation of infarct size in man by means of plasma enzyme levels. Br Heart J 37:795–803, 1975.

79. Mathey D, Bleifeld W, Buss H, et al: Creatine kinase release in acute myocardial infarction: correlation with clinical, electrocardiographic, and pathological findings. Br Heart J 37:1161–1168, 1975.

80. Norris RM, Whitlock RML, Barratt-Boyes C, et al: Clinical measurement of myocardial infarct size. Modification of a method for the estimation of total creatine phosphokinase release after myocardial infarction. Circulation 51:614–620, 1975.

81. Bleifeld W, Mathey D, Hanrath P, et al: Infarct size estimated from serial serum creatine phos-

phokinase in relation to left ventricular hemodynamics. Circulation 55:303–311, 1977.

82. Shell WE, Sobel BE: Deleterious effects of increased heart rate on infarct size in the conscious dog. Am J Cardiol 31:474–479, 1973.

83. Braunwald E, Maroko PR: The reduction in infarct size—an idea whose time (for testing) has come. Circulation 50;206–209, 1974.

84. Henning H, Hardarson T, Francis G, et al: Approach to the estimation of myocardial infarct size by analysis of precordial ST segment and R wave maps. Am J Cardiol 41:1–8, 1978.

85. Kostuk WJ, Ehsani A, Karliner JS, et al: Left ventricular performance after myocardial infarction assessed by radioisotope angiography. Circulation 47:242–249, 1973.

86. Roberts R, Husain A, Ambox D, et al: Relation between infarct size and ventricular arrhythmia. Br Heart J 37:1169–1175, 1975.

87. Ensani AA, Campbell MK, Geltman EM, et al: Correlations between late ventricular dysrhythmias and infarct size. Am J Cardiol 41:424, 1977.

88. Roe CR, Cobb FR, Starmer F: The relationship between enzymatic and histologic estimates of the extent of myocardial infarction in conscious dogs with permanent coronary occlusion. Circulation 55:438–448, 1977.

89. Roe CR, Starmer CF: A sensitivity analysis of enzymatic estimation of infarct size. Circulation 52:1–5, 1975.

90. Roe CR, Starmer CF, Cobb FR: Mathematical modifications fail to improve CPK estimates of extent of infarct. Circulation 55:678–679, 1977.

91. Slutsky AS: Individualized values for the disappearance rate parameter ($K_d$) in the enzymatic estimation of infarct size. Circulation 56:545–547, 1977.

92. Sobel BE, Markham J, Karlsberg RP, et al: The nature of disappearance of creatine kinase from the circulation and its influence on enzymatic estimation of infarct size. Circ Res 41:836–844, 1977.

93. Hutchins GM, Bulkley BH: Infarct expansion versus extension: Two different complications of acute myocardial infarction. Am J Cardiol 41:1127–1132, 1978.

94. Cairns JA, Kalssen GA: The effect of propranolol on canine myocardial CPK distribution space and rate of disappearance. Circulation 56:284–288, 1977.

95. Peter T, Norris RM, Clarke ED, et al: Reduction of enzyme levels by propranolol after acute

myocardial infarction. Circulation 57:1091–1095, 1978.

96. Roberts R, Sobel BE: Effect of selected drugs and myocardial infarction on the disappearance of creatine kinase from the circulation in conscious dogs. Cardiovasc Res 11:103–112, 1977.

97. Clark GL, Roberts R, Sobel BE: The influence of creatine kinase (CK) transport in lymph on plasma CK curves after myocardial infarction. Clin Res 25:213A, 1977.

98. Ryan E, Karliner JS, Gilpin EA, et al: A critical assessment of creatine kinase curve areas in patients with acute myocardial infarction. (Submitted for publication.)

99. Sobel BE, Roberts R, Larson KB: Estimation of infarct size from serum MB creatine phosphokinase activity: applications and limitations. Am J Cardiol 37:474–485, 1976.

100. Rogers WJ, McDaniel HG, Smith LR, et al: Correlation of angiographic estimates of myocardial infarct size and accumulated release of creatine kinase MB isoenzyme in man. Circulation 56:199–204, 1977.

101. Rapaport E: The fractional disappearance rate of the separate isoenzymes of creatine phosphokinase in the dog. Cardiovasc Res 9:473–477, 1975.

102. Beller GA, Smith TW: Radionuclide techniques in the assessment of myocardial ischemia and infarction. Circulation 53 (suppl I):123–125, 1976.

103. Gold HK, Leinbach RC, Maroko PR: Reduction of signs of ischemic injury during acute myocardial infarction by intravenous propranolol. Am J Cardiol 38:689–695, 1976.

104. Maroko PR, Davidson DM, Libby P, et al: Effects of hyaluronidase administration on myocardial ischemic injury in acute infarction. A preliminary study in 24 patients. Ann Intern Med 82:515–520, 1975.

105. Muller JE, Maroko PR, Braunwald E: Evaluation of precordial electrocardiographic mapping as a means of assessing changes in myocardial ischemic injury. Circulation 52:16–27, 1975.

106. Ashman R: The normal human ventricular gradient. IV. The relationship between the magnitudes $A_{QRS}$ and G, the deviations of the RS-T segment. Am Heart J 26:495–510, 1963.

107. Radita L, Borduas JL, Rothman S, et al: Studies on the mechanism of ventricular activity. XII. Early changes in the ST-T segment and QRS complex following acute coronary artery occlusion; experimental study and clinical applications. Am Heart J 48:351–372, 1954.

108. Maroko PR, Hillis LD, Muller JE, et al: Favorable effects of hyaluronidase on electrocardiographic evidence of necrosis in patients with acute myocardial infarction. N Engl J Med 296:898–903, 1977.

109. Gold HK, Leinbach RC, Maroko PR: Reduction of signs of necrosis and preservation of ventricular function by propranolol in acute myocardial infarction. Circulation 57–58 (suppl II):226, 1978.

110. Derrida JP, Sal R, Chiche P: Nitroglycerin infusion in acute myocardial infarction. N Engl J Med 297:336, 1977.

111. Gold HK, Leinbach RC, Maroko PR: Regional beta blockade with intracoronary propranolol. Circulation 54 (suppl II):173, 1976.

112. Caide VJ, Zaret BL: Liposome accumulation in regions of experimental myocardial infarction. Science 198:735–738, 1977.

113. Maroko PR, Ribeiro LGT, Kloner RA, et al: Transport of ATP by liposomes into the ischemic myocardium. Circulation 57–58 (suppl II):218, 1978.

114. Braunwald E: Treatment of the patient after myocardial infarction. The last decade and the next. (Editorial) N Engl J Med 302:290–293, 1980.

# 24 | Incidence, Significance and Approach to the Diagnosis and Therapy of Other Anatomic and Functional Sequelae of Acute Myocardial Infarction

### Ralph Shabetai, M.D.

## PERICARDITIS

Pericarditis occurs in about 10 percent of patients with acute myocardial infarction using clinical criteria [1] but autopsy proves that the true incidence is considerably higher.[2,3] A pericardial friction rub is most common on the second and third days after the onset of myocardial infarction; [1,4,5] less commonly it is audible on the first day and may be heard for up to 1 week after the onset of symptoms. Pericardial friction rubs occurring later than 1 week after the onset of myocardial infarction are rarely caused by simple contiguous pericarditis, but rather they are a sign of generalized pericarditis as a component of Dressler syndrome.[5-8] Pathologic studies show that the pericarditis may be localized over the infarction but may be generalized. It can also occur in nontransmural infarctions and in patients with infarction not affecting the anterior surface of the heart.[4] Autopsy studies have also shown that bleeding may occur from the granulomatous new vessels in acute pericarditis, accounting for tamponade.

A pericardial friction rub is said to be associated with a higher incidence of cardiac failure and dysrhythmias, especially supraventricular dysrhythmias, but the literature does not document the expected outcome of increased complications, i.e., higher mortality in acute myocardial infarction with than without pericarditis.[1,4,5] Nevertheless, pericarditis, when it occurs in the early phase of acute myocardial infarction, poses six important questions to the thoughtful clinician. These relate to chest pain in the days following admission to the Coronary Care Unit; evolution of the ECG pattern; the diagnostic question of extension of the infarction; the question of the systolic murmur of mitral valve dysfunction or ventricular septal defect versus pericardial friction; the safety of anticoagulant therapy when this is otherwise indicated; and predisposition to the Dressler's syndrome. These questions will be examined after the clinical features are considered.

### Clinical Features of Pericarditis in Acute Myocardial Infarction

Because the diagnosis is seldom entertained unless a pericardial friction rub is heard, pericarditis is probably underdiagnosed. One would speculate that pericarditis overlying an anterior myocardial infarction should generate an audible pericardial friction rub, whereas pericarditis over the inferior or posterior aspects of the heart would not. This may not be so, as in some published accounts pericardial friction is as common in inferior as in anterior myocardial infarction.[1,3,4] This serves to underscore our failure to understand the pathophysiology of the friction rub. The simplistic theory that rubs are caused by rubbing of the parietal layer of a serous membrane against the visceral layer will not suffice, because they persist after large pericardial effusions develop.[9] On the other hand, autopsy studies have shown that the region of acute pericarditis may be remote from the site of acute infarction, i.e., it is not always a simple contiguous pericarditis.

The pericardial friction rub is often transient, and, unless the patient's chest is carefully auscultated on several occasions during the first several days after myocardial infarction, it is often missed.[5] It may be present when the patient is supine, only to disappear in the sitting posture. Best results are obtained with firm pressure of the diaphragm chest piece against the chest wall. The typical rub is triphasic, with components in presystole, systole, and diastole.[10] Frequently however, the rub is biphasic, and sometimes it is monophasic, at which time it may be confused with a murmur.

## Chest Pain in the Days Following Myocardial Infarction

Many patients complain of chest pain during the first few days after admission to the coronary care unit. This may not pose a question of diagnosis when the pain and ECG changes are characteristic of myocardial ischemia, or when pulmonary or further myocardial infarction occur in classic fashion. Frequently, the chest pain is atypical in location, radiation, duration, or nature and it may be accompanied by tenderness. Pain of this description is frequently of psychogenic or psychosomatic origin. Except when the pain clearly fits into one of the above categories, the physician should never lose sight of the possibility that it may be, in truth, a manifestation of pericarditis. My own view is that pericarditis is often mistaken for extension of myocardial infarction, thereby adding unnecessarily to the anxiety that any patient feels after learning that he has had a "heart attack."

## ST Segment and T Wave Changes— Ischemia or Pericarditis?

Just as the pain of pericarditis may be mistaken for that of myocardial ischemia, so may ST segment elevation and T wave inversion be ascribed to ischemia or extension of infarction. When these changes occur in the absence of evidence of increased myocardial oxygen demand or serum enzyme elevations compatible with further myocardial necrosis, one should consider the possibility that they are manifestations of pericarditis, and therefore much less ominous. Naturally, suspicion that pericarditis is the cause of repolarization changes is heightened if the patient displays other features of pericarditis: e.g., pain affected by posture or respiration, or referred to the trapezius area; pericardial friction rub; unusually prolonged fever; or evidence of pericardial effusion detected by chest radiographs and echocardiograms.

In severe myocardial ischemia, the QRS-T complex may become virtually monophasic. Nevertheless, it has been found that ST segment elevation tends to be greater in patients with acute myocardial infarction and a pericardial friction rub than in those without evidence of overlying pericarditis.[4] In cases of isolated anterior or inferior myocardial infarction, transient ST segment elevation in leads where one would normally expect "reciprocal" ST segment depression is highly suggestive of complicating generalized pericarditis.[11] Even in the absence of these findings, I believe that patients are quite commonly thought to have suffered new ischemic events based on ST segment and T wave changes that should have been ascribed to pericarditis.

## Friction Rub or Murmur, or Both?

When the patient with acute myocardial infarction is admitted to the CCU, the physician assesses the heart sounds and decides if murmurs and a friction rub are present. He notes the characteristics and intensity of all the sounds and murmurs to use as a baseline for serial auscultation, but recognizes that murmurs and heart sounds may become more distinct and louder as the heart rate slows and recovery from acute infarction commences. The physician is especially alert to the importance of detecting a new systolic murmur, which may signify rupture of the interventricular septum or a portion of the mitral valve apparatus. A pericardial friction rub, loudest at or slightly medial to the apex, can be mistaken for these ominous murmurs, especially when the rub is largely systolic. Systolic murmurs betokening major hemodynamic complications persist and are accompanied by evidence of hemodynamic deterioration. Pericardial friction rubs are transitory and are not associated with hemodynamic deterioration except in the rare event of hemopericardium. Pericardial friction rubs are more "superficial" than murmurs and vary more with posture and with respiration, tending to decrease or disappear when the patient sits up.

Diagnosis is especially difficult when rubs and murmurs coexist. A loud pericardial friction rub is a potent means of obscuring systolic murmurs. The alert physician will not be put off the track of septal rupture or mitral regurgitation when he detects a friction rub, if other evidence points to left-to-right shunt or rapidly advancing cardiac failure.

## Should Anticoagulant Therapy be Discontinued When a Pericardial Friction Rub Develops Early in the Course of Acute Myocardial Infarction?

The place of anticoagulation in the therapeutic regimen of acute myocardial infarction is discussed elsewhere in this volume, and in this chapter I will not add to this controversy. But questions frequently are asked about the safety of continuing (or starting) anticoagulant therapy when a pericardial friction rub is detected.[12-14] The reasons for this concern are as follows. Certain acute pericarditides are associated with hemorrhage and effusion, and when the clotting mechanism is impaired, massive bleeding into the pericardium takes place and may cause cardiac tamponade, which can be fatal. Uremic pericarditis may behave in this fashion.[15] Acute pericarditis overlying a recent myocardial infarction is not a hemorrhagic process and is not thought to be associated with significant pericardial effusion, although serial echocardiograms have not been extensively studied to document this. If anticoagulants are otherwise indicated and there are no other persuasive contraindications, the appearance of a typical pericardial friction rub is not a good reason to discontinue anticoagulation therapy, and it is my practice not to modulate anticoagu-

lation therapy for this reason. On the other hand, unusually persistent pericardial friction, evidence of pericardial effusion, and the late occurrence of pericarditis constitute excellent reasons for promptly discontinuing, or even reversing anticoagulation.

## Cardiac Tamponade Complicating Acute Myocardial Infarction

Cardiac tamponade is difficult to diagnose when it occurs in the setting of acute myocardial infarction, because the cardinal features of cardiac tamponade can be caused by myocardial infarction and cardiac failure. Thus raised venous pressure may be caused by tamponade or cardiac failure; hypotension and tachycardia may equally be manifestations of tamponade or cardiogenic shock, and even pulsus paradoxus may reflect dyspnea and not cardiac tamponade.[16] Thus the key to diagnosis is to remember that cardiac tamponade may occur. Hence, in dealing with complicated myocardial infarction, one must always consider cardiac tamponade. Usually it will be ruled out, but this approach is essential if the physician is not to miss the cases that do occur. For the purpose of this chapter I will divide the syndrome into massive-acute and subacute.

**Massive-Acute Cardiac Tamponade.** This dreaded catastrophe occurs as a consequence of cardiac rupture. Thus the event usually takes place in the first 3 days after the onset of acute infarction, and generally is fatal (Fig. 24.1). Cardiac rupture is said to be more common in patients who resume physical activity too soon after a large myocardial infarction.[17] This is the reason why rupture of the heart has been reported to be more frequent among inmates of mental institutions who frequently fail to report pain when they sustain myocardial infarction.[17]

The patient suddenly collapses and in the most severe cases soon dies. In less severe cases, profound hypotension leads to shock with anuria, obtundation, and greatly increased venous pressure. If the pulse is still palpable, pulsus paradoxus may be appreciated. If the radial pulse is small and thready, it may be impossible to appreciate pulsus paradoxus in this vessel, but

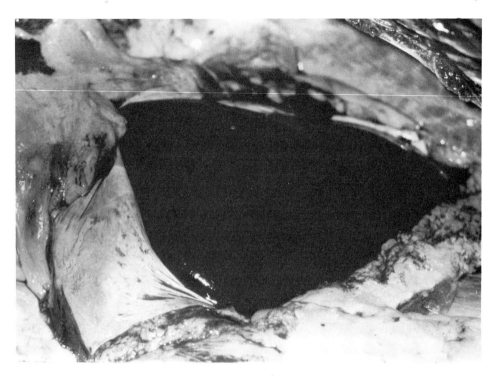

Fig. 24.1 Autopsy photograph of the heart of a patient found dead 2 days after discharge from the coronary care unit where he had spent 3 days with "an uncomplicated inferior wall myocardial infarction." A large tear due to myocardial rupture is shown.

the sign can be elicited from the femoral and carotid pulses.

The skin is cool and often moist, and the patient is either anxious and agitated or drowsy and stuporous. The heart rate is rapid and the heart sounds are impaired, but these findings do not differentiate massive acute tamponade from cardiogenic shock. Palpation of the precordium reveals absent or decreased cardiac activity. This finding favors cardiac tamponade, but in cardiogenic shock the heart's action is very weak, and the cardiac impulse may not be palpable.

Venous pressure is elevated in both conditions, but tends to be higher in cardiac tamponade than in cardiogenic shock. Absence of the Y descent also favors cardiac tamponade.[18,19] It must also be borne in mind that because of the nature of acute massive tamponade complicating acute myocardial infarction, cardiac tamponade and cardiogenic shock may coexist.

Diagnosis depends on maintaining a high index of suspicion. Echocardiography confirms the presence of pericardial effusion and may also show swinging of the heart, a finding that should add strongly to the suspicion of pericardial effusion with tamponade.[20] Electrical alternans of P wave, QRS complex and T wave may be observed and is associated with pendular motion demonstrated by echocardiography.[21] In progressive cardiogenic shock, pulmonary wedge pressure increases more than central venous pressure, widening the difference between these pressures. In cardiac tamponade, this difference narrows and may become zero.

The effusion should be tapped as soon as the diagnosis is made. Anticoagulation, if present, must be promptly reversed. Blood transfusion may be required, but this must be done with careful observation of pulmonary wedge pressure, central venous pressure, and cardiac output because of the severe underlying heart disease. Occasionally, a patient may be saved by prompt pericardiocentesis combined with astute management of the cardiac problem, but, in general, the prognosis is grave and of the few who leave the hospital, only a minority do well.

If one suspects acute massive cardiac tamponade in a moribund patient, it is permissible to perform a bedside needle aspiration of the pericardium. If the suspicion is confirmed, the procedure may be life-saving; if not, little will have been lost. Survival has been reported following emergency infarctectomy carried out immediately after pericardiocentesis and without prior cardiac catheterization and coronary arteriography.[22]

**Subacute Cardiac Tamponade.** Cardiac tamponade may be less rapid and less severe than that described above. Venous pressure is increased and a prominent X, but no Y, descent is observed in the jugular venous pulse contour. In subacute tamponade the normal inspiratory decline in venous pressure is present. The blood pressure may be somewhat decreased but may be normal; pulsus paradoxus, however, is usually easy to appreciate. If pulsus paradoxus is doubtful, the sign can be exaggerated by having the patient breathe slowly, deeply, and quietly, a maneuver the patient with acute massive cardiac tamponade would find impossible to execute.

To measure pulsus paradoxus, the blood pressure is taken with a sphygmomanometer. The cuff is carefully and accurately applied, and most important, the valve on the bulb must be easy to manipulate and must not leak. The pressure is slowly and evenly lowered in the cuff, allowing the examiner to determine the pressure drop between the points at which the first Korotkoff sound is heard only during expiration to that where the sounds are heard throughout the respiratory cycle. This is the measure of pulsus paradoxus,[23] which, under normal circumstances, does not exceed 10 mmHg. In the presence of arterial hypotension (systolic blood pressure < 90 mmHg), pulsus paradoxus may not be evident despite cardiac tamponade. Other causes of pulsus paradoxus include respiratory distress, hypovolemic shock, pulmonary embolism, and positive pressure ventilation.

The clinician may suspect cardiac tamponade for several reasons or in several clinical circumstances: (1) sudden unexpected increase in cardiac size, especially when the lung fields remain relatively clear; (2) the appearance of pulsus paradoxus; (3) clinical deterioration not explicable on other grounds; (4) electrical alternans developing in a patient with acute myocardial infarction, which should always raise the suspicion of complicating cardiac tamponade. Perhaps more important than any of these, the diagnosis is made because the clinician thinks of it. Echocardiography should be performed when cardiac tamponade is suspected. This procedure will determine whether or not pericardial fluid is present, it will provide an estimate of its volume, and it will yield additional information on the pathophysiologic effects of the pericardial effusion that is present. In cardiac tamponade, the heart may swing in the pericardial sac with each cardiac cycle,[20] and the right ventricular dimension often is compressed.[24] In cardiac tamponade, during inspiration the interventricular septum may bulge into the left ventricle, and the EF slope of the mitral valve decreases.[25] "Pseudoprolapse" of the mitral valve has been reported in cardiac tamponade,[26] but it must be recalled that coronary artery disease is a cause of true mitral valve prolapse.

As cardiac tamponade worsens and stroke volume falls, the heart rate may increase. However, "pericardial knock" is a sign of constrictive pericarditis and not of cardiac tamponade [27] and will be sought in vain in such cases.

Hemorrhagic cardiac tamponade has been described in acute myocardial infarction without rupture of the heart or of a coronary artery.[28] Most,[14,29] but certainly not all,[14] reported patients were receiving anticoagulants. Rarely, the atrium may rupture after atrial infarction.[30]

**Treatment of Subacute Cardiac Tamponade in Acute Myocardial Infarction.** Needle exploration of the pericardium to determine whether or not fluid is present has no place in the management of subacute cases. Rather, before the pericardium is explored, the presence, approximate amount, and the location of intrapericardial hemorrhage must be ascertained by echocardiography. As a minimum, a right atrial catheter should be in place and attached to monitoring and recording equipment. Preferably, a double lumen catheter is used to enable the physician to monitor and record pulmonary wedge as well as central venous pressure. In some cases, especially the more critical ones, it is also desirable to place an intraarterial needle or catheter.

The patient is placed in a partly sitting posture, which requires that pressure transducers be carefully positioned to correspond with the middle of the heart. The needle used to tap the pericardium must be long enough to reach the pericardium but should not be of excessive length and flexibility. The length of choice depends on the patient's body build. Electrocardiographic monitoring of the needle position can be performed safely in coronary care units because great care has already been taken with the grounding of monitors, beds, and recording devices.[30] The xiphisternal approach is considered the safest.[31] The needle is placed into the subcutaneous tissue just below and to one side of the xiphoid process. A light cable connects the needle to an electrocardiograph, which is set in the "V" position. A stable electrocardiogram is recorded before the needle is advanced toward the pericardium. If there are sufficient channels, lead II is also monitored. The needle is advanced in a cephalad direction, slightly posteriorly and usually toward one shoulder. When the pericardium is reached, the operator feels a sense of "give," and the needle enters the pericardial space. Blood is now aspirated. Unlike the case of serous pericardial effusion, the blood may clot and its hematocrit may approach that of peripheral blood. These features of pericardial blood make it more difficult to be confident that the needle is in the pericardial space and not in a cardiac chamber—usually the right ventricle.

Correct positioning can best be ascertained by measuring pressure at the needle. The pressure should be close to right atrial pressure and should not have a systolic peak. If a fluoroscope is available, a small volume of radiopaque contrast material, injected through the needle, will outline the pericardial cavity if the needle is properly positioned. If the right ventricle has been entered, the contrast will enter the pulmonary circulation. Entry into the right ventricle should be obviated by observing the needle-monitor lead of the ECG. When the needle contacts the epicardium, the ST segment becomes

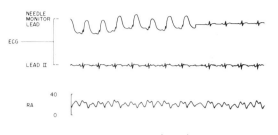

Fig. 24.2 Tracings obtained during pericardiocentesis for the relief of tamponade secondary to a malignant disease. Above, the ECG recorded directly from the pericardiocentesis needle; middle, lead II of the ECG; below, right atrial pressure. When the left side of the figure was being recorded, the needle tip was touching the heart, causing the direct lead to register a monophasic complex, but lead II was not altered. (Shabetai R: Hemodynamics of pericardial disease. In: Cardiac Catheterization and Angiography. Grossman W, editor. Lea and Febiger, Philadelphia, 1980.)

elevated; sometimes the entire ECG complex becomes monophasic. The corresponding ST segment displacement on a standard lead is much less pronounced (Fig. 24.2). Ventricular extrasystoles are also observed. If the diagnosis is correct, the patient's condition will rapidly improve after 50 to 150 ml of blood or bloody fluid have been aspirated. This is because of the steep nature of the pressure-volume curve of the pericardium.[32]

## Unrecognized Intrapericardial Hemorrhage

Undoubtedly, not all bleeding into the pericardial sac after an acute transmural infarction is recognized, and not all of the episodes are fatal. A small hemorrhage may be the precursor of Dressler's syndrome, but in the majority of patients with this syndrome there is no history of pericardial bleeding during the acute stage of the infarct. Myocardial rupture, instead of causing free bleeding into the pericardium, may result in a pseudoaneurysm of the left ventricle; the pericardium, because of previous inflammation, acts as a boundary of the aneurysm and prevents further and generalized bleeding. False aneurysm is usually diagnosed by contrast left ventriculography,[33] or occasionally by two-dimensional echocardiography[34] after the convalescent stage of acute myocardial infarction when the patient is being assessed for cardiac failure or as a candidate for surgical treatment of ischemic heart disease.

False aneurysms of the left ventricle, unlike true aneurysms, tend to have narrow necks and are subject to late enlargement and rupture; they are therefore suitable for surgical resection in symptomatic cases.

## Dressler's Syndrome

Dressler described a syndrome that appears 1 week to several months after acute myocardial infarction.[6,7] The major features are pericarditis, pleurisy, fever, leukocytosis, and pulmonary infiltrates. The pericarditis and pleurisy are usually characterized by significant pleuropericardial pain and by corresponding friction rubs. Pleural effusion and pericardial effusion may occur. Tamponade is rare, but has been described.[35] Constrictive pericarditis is an extremely uncommon sequel.

Dressler's syndrome has many similarities to the postcardiotomy syndrome, post-traumatic pericarditis, and to recurrent idiopathic pericarditis. The precipitating circumstances and associated conditions differ, but all are associated with blood in a pericardial cavity, with some of its living cells injured. All of these syndromes have many of the hallmarks of an autoimmune process. They begin a considerable time after an initiating insult, they are subject to recurrences, they may involve several sites, and they respond to steroid, indomethacin, or aspirin therapy. There is some evidence that antimyocardial antibody may be responsible for Dressler's syndrome.[36]

I believe that there is considerable overlap between pericarditis in the course of acute myocardial infarction and Dressler's syndrome. The former may appear unusually late in some cases, and the latter unusually early. Pericarditis complicating acute myocardial infarction may be localized over the infarction or it may be generalized, and the latter may occur with or without effusion.

The classic presentation is with severe chest pain and general malaise. The patient and the family are apt to attribute the pain to a recurrence of symptoms of ischemic heart disease. However, questioning uncovers the characteristics of pericardial pain: aggravation by breathing or coughing; relief by sitting up; and radiation to the trapezius ridge. The temperature elevation and leukocytosis are too high for myocardial infarction and inconsistent with angina pectoris. A pericardial friction rub is usually appreciated by careful auscultation. Signs of pleurisy and pleural effusion may be detected. Examination of the lungs is usually otherwise negative, but the chest radiograph frequently shows that pulmonary infiltration has occurred. The differential diagnosis then shifts from recurrence of ischemia to pulmonary infarction or pneumonia, but in most instances the diagnosis of Dressler's syndrome is not difficult to make.

Diagnosis in atypical cases may be less straightforward. Failure to detect pericardial friction and occurrence of the syndrome, either in the first days following myocardial infarction or of the first episode several months after myocardial infarction, are features that most commonly serve to make the diagnosis difficult.

If the ECG, especially the ST segments and T waves, has returned to normal, the ECG signs of pericarditis may be helpful, but ST segment elevation with reciprocal depression confined to leads aVR and $V_1$ cannot be counted on to appear when the baseline ECG is grossly abnormal.[37] The amount of pericardial effusion may be too small to detect by chest radiography, but even relatively small effusions can be detected by echocardiography.[38]

Recurrences are common, and the diagnosis then is not difficult because in an individual patient, the pattern tends to be the same or similar on each occasion.

Treatment is nonspecific.[39] First episodes, all highly symptomatic episodes, and pericardial effusion are indications for hospital admission. The patient is observed for evidence of impending cardiac tamponade and for the development and progress of friction rubs, effusions, and pulmonary infiltrates. Aspirin or indomethacin are tried for first episodes; therapeutic failure is an indication for steroid therapy. Prednisone, 60 mg daily, is given until symptoms and signs have abated, usually after several days. The dose is then rapidly tapered to the lowest that will completely suppress the manifestations. After 4 weeks, the dose is tapered to withdrawal.

Some patients respond rapidly, and the treatment regimen is brief. In others, the response is prolonged, raising problems of serious steroid-induced side effects. Recurrences, unless obviously milder than preceeding attacks, are treated with the regimen that was successful earlier.

## SEGMENTAL WALL MOTION DISORDERS

Ischemic heart disease, by its nature, does not affect the heart in a uniform manner. Portions of the ventricular myocardium undergo functional or structural alteration, which is related to diminished capacity of the epicardial coronary arteries to carry blood to regions of the myocardium. The left ventricle is affected more frequently than the right, and the distribution of lesions within the left ventricle corresponds to specific vascular lesions and to areas of myocardium supplied by the narrowed vessels. At one end of the spectrum of ischemic heart disease is the patient whose only manifestation is angina pectoris and who has never sustained a myocardial infarction. In him, left ventricular function studied at rest usually is normal. Thus left ventricular end-diastolic pressure does not exceed 12 mmHg, left ventricular end-diastolic volume is no greater than 90 ml/m$^2$, the ejection fraction is approximately 60 percent, and the isovolumic indices of performance and ventricular diastolic compliance are normal. The left ventriculogram shows that all segments of the left ventricle contract and relax synchronously and to an approximately equal degree. At the other end of the spectrum of ischemic heart disease, is the patient with extensive myocardial fibrosis, who frequently has sustained several myocardial infarctions. In these patients there is global dysfunction of the left ventricle. The ventricle may be of abnormally large volume, but most important its performance is greatly impaired and the ejection fraction may be less than 20 percent. In many of these ventricles, the chamber is so large, the contraction so reduced, and the scarring so widespread that segmental dysfunction can no longer be discerned. There is generalized hypokinesis and the condition has been termed, perhaps not entirely appropriately, ischemic cardiomyopathy. Calcification of the coronary arteries is a most useful means of noninvasively differentiating these patients from those with idiopathic cardiomyopathy.[40] Between these two extreme ends of the spectrum of ischemic heart disease lie the majority of patients with significant coronary artery disease, many of whom have sustained at least one myocardial infarction. In them, contrast left ventriculography shows that some segments of the left ventricular circumference contract normally, whereas in other segments of the left ventricle, contraction is impaired.

Ischemic heart disease is a disorder that usually manifests itself following stress but not when the patient is at rest. Angina and dyspnea are provoked by exercise or emotional stress in individuals in whom physical examination and the electrocardiogram are normal when the patient is at rest. Master [41,42] was among the first to apply the concept that if the ECG is to be used as a tool to diagnose early coronary disease the electrocardiogram at rest must be supplemented by an electrocardiogram obtained during stress. Likewise in the cardiac catheterization laboratory, elevation of the left ventricular end-diastolic pressure during stress is an important hemodynamic marker of ischemia.

The principle that evidence of ischemia may be absent at rest, but present during stress, can be applied to assess the global and segmental function of the left ventricle. In many patients with ischemic heart disease the ejection fraction is normal at rest but fails to increase, or may even decline, during muscular exercise.[43] Likewise, all segments around the left ventricular perimeter may appear to contract and relax normally in a left ventriculogram performed with the patient at rest; but a left ventriculogram made during or immediately following stress, for instance rapid pacing or a spontaneous attack of angina pectoris, may disclose that one or more segments of the left ventricle move in an abnormal fashion.[44] Our ability to detect the development of abnormalities of segmental wall motion disorders in the left ventricle has become one of the most important tools in the assessment of ischemic heart disease. Radiopaque contrast material injected directly into the cavity of the left ventricle is the most specific and sensitive method for the detection of segmental wall motion abnormalities,[45] but often cannot be repeated, and visualization at each examination is limited to a few cardiac cycles. Radionuclide imaging of the heart,[46] at rest and during exercise, and visualization of the left ventricle by two-dimensional ultrasound techniques [47] hold promise that they will allow noninvasive serial studies of segmental wall motion in patients with ischemic heart disease to assess progression and the effects of medical and surgical treatment.

The shape of the left ventricle is somewhat ellipsoidal at end-diastole and the chamber contracts more or less uniformly to about one-third of its end-diastolic volume. Attempts to put this information into quantitative terms are faced with major difficulties. The first requirement is to establish the correct reference frame, but since the heart rotates and shifts during the cardiac cycle, the aortic valve plane is more fixed in some patients than in others, and we do not know the "center of gravity" to which the ventricle is contracting. There is, as yet, no agreement on the correct reference frame. Shortening of an arbitrary long axis from the aortic or mitral valve to the cardiac apex and of a short axis, constructed at right angles to the midpoint of the long axis, can be measured.[48] The long axis may be divided into a series of basal and apical chords and the contraction of the hemichords, anterior and posterior to the long axis, can be measured.[49] Alternatively, the system of Cartesian coordinates may be abandoned altogether, and polar coordinates may be constructed from the center, dividing the left ventricle into a series of pie-shaped segments [50] (Fig. 24.3). The motion of the boundary of each pie is estimated, but there is no agreement on the proper location for the origin of the polar coordinates. In some methods, rotation and translation of the heart are ignored, but in others they are compensated for, different authors using different techniques. The aims are to establish the normal sequence

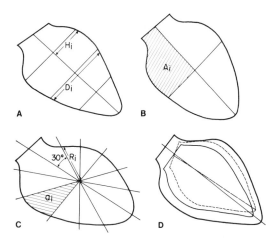

Fig. 24.3 Schematic to outline the principles underlying analysis of regional wall motion of the left ventricle. *(A)* Shortening of the short axis, basal chords and hemichords, and apical chords and hemichords. *(B)* The silhouette is divided into 4 areas so that motion of their boundaries may be related to decrease in the corresponding area; *(C)* The silhouette is divided into pie-shaped segments; shortening is related to changes in area (a) or of the mean radius. *(D)* Apparent wall motion is affected by rotation of the heart.

and range of motion of each segment around the perimeter of the left ventricle. Studies in animals and man using contrast ventriculography, radiopaque markers implanted into the myocardium [52] and ultrasonic dimension gauges sutured into the heart wall are being employed to answer this important question and to establish a universally acceptable reference frame. Radionuclide and two-dimension ultrasound methods require solutions to the same problems and pose more complex problems of their own concerning accurate border detection.

The simplest methods of analysis of segmental wall motion consider only end-diastole and end-systole. More detailed analysis of segmental wall motion involves analysis of the motion of each segment at frequent intervals (for example 10 msec) throughout the cardiac cycle. The large amount of data generated by these techniques requires a computer of considerable capacity for processing.[50]

In spite of the obstacles, considerable progress has been made in the clinical assessment of segmental wall motion disorders in ischemic heart disease because they are usually gross. Herman et al.[53] divided wall motion disorders, which they called asynergy, into hypokinesis, akinesis, and dyskinesis to describe diminished, absent, or paradoxic motion of a segment of the left ventricular wall. Dyskinesis is a systolic bulging and may be seen not only in ventricular aneurysms but in infarctions. These authors introduced the term asynergy to describe disorders of the sequence or timing of shortening of a ventricular segment.

When all segments of the left ventricular myocardium contract normally, a regional wall motion disorder may be unmasked by stress. This may be induced by the physician who may use rapid pacing,[44] exercise, or the administration of pharmacologic agents;[54] or it may occur as a spontaneous attack of angina pectoris.

It would be desirable to know whether impaired segmental wall motion in the individual patient is a manifestation of, on the one hand, irreversible structural myocardial damage by fibrosis or infarction, or on the other hand, is a reversible phenomenon associated with transient myocardial ischemia. Before and during the study of left ventricular segmental wall motion, it is essential to ascertain whether the patient is experiencing angina pectoris, whether the heart rate and left ventricular end-diastolic pressure are changing, and whether the ST segment is displaced from the baseline. There is ample evidence that major global and regional wall motion disorders may be observed when studies are done in the presence of a recent or ongoing episode of myocardial ischemia.[55] It has been hypothesized that segments that contract poorly in normal systoles but improve in postextrasystolic contractions or after the administration of nitroglycerine or other unloading agents, are not permanently damaged; the abnormal contraction is then ascribed to ischemia.[56] A logical extension of this hypothesis is that assessment of regional myocardial performance before and after interventions designed to increase performance or unload the ventricle should separate patients with reversible from irreversible wall motion disorders,[57] and therefore be of importance in predicting the effects of revascularization on regional wall motion.

The limitations in our ability to measure segmental wall motion performance of the left ventricle are more significant when these techniques are used to detect small changes in regional performance following treatment than when they are used in the straightforward diagnosis of gross regional dysfunction. Furthermore, caution is needed in the correct interpretation of the observation that the motion of a segment improves following an intervention; the administration of nitroprusside, for example, may lower tension in the left ventricular myocardium to such an extent that the apparent improvement in segmental motion may be a passive event, and need not imply that the segment itself is capable of improved function.

Recent studies using radioisotope techniques[58] indicate that the long-term oral administration of propranolol improves segmental wall motion performance during muscular exercise. In the light of the foregoing discussion, the thoughtful reader will require confirmation of these and similar results in several large series before modifying therapy.

In summary, segmental wall motion disorders of the left ventricle are so gross in ischemic heart disease that they can be detected and expressed in semiquanititative terms in spite of major unsolved methodologic problems. Segmental abnormalities due to ischemia may be detected only early in systole at rest[58a]; others are uncovered only by stress. The abnormalities associated with previous infarction are apparent at rest, and some abnormalities seen at rest may decrease following interventions that increase inotropy or diminish loading of the ventricle. Biplane contrast left ventriculography affords the most reliable method but has obvious limitations. Radionuclide techniques are less invasive and can be repeated more often, but suffer from problems associated with resolution, background radiation, border detection techniques, smoothing and filtering techniques, selection of "area of interest," and signal averaging. These problems leave the cardiologist overly dependent on computer and statistical techniques; the appropriate response is to view the results critically and to accept them with caution and awareness of the problems and their solutions.

Although most of the above discussion has

been devoted to patients with chronic ischemic heart disease, it is well recognized that acute myocardial infarction is a major cause of abnormal wall motion. However, little information is available concerning the natural history or influence on prognosis of such wall motion abnormalities. It is to be hoped that the application and further development of the techniques discussed above will lead to better understanding and possibly treatment of this aspect of ischemic heart disease.[45]

## RUPTURE OF INTRACARDIAC STRUCTURES

Early in the course of acute myocardial infarction transmural necrosis may result in rupture of the interventricular septum, creating an acute left to right shunt. Similarly, necrosis of an infarcted papillary muscle may result in rupture and massive mitral regurgitation. Both of these catastrophes, which can be difficult to distinguish from each other, are characterized by hemodynamic deterioration and the appearance of a striking systolic murmur, often accompanied by a thrill. The degree and speed of hemodynamic deterioration depend on the magnitude of the accident. Ventricular septal defects in acute myocardial infarction are usually large, but there is a range of orifice sizes; papillary muscle rupture may involve the major belly of the muscle or be limited to a secondary or tertiary division.[59] Hemodynamic deterioration may, therefore, vary from an increase in dyspnea and pulmonary congestion to fulminating uncontrollable cardiac failure, which may be rapidly fatal. These myocardial catastrophes are associated with extensive infarctions and thus often take place in the already unfavorable setting of left ventricular failure and pulmonary congestion, contributing significantly to the grim prognosis. Very extensive myocardial necrosis may cause rupture of both the interventricular septum and the mitral valve apparatus in the same patient. In some patients, myocardial rupture extends from the ventricular septum to one of the free walls of the left or right ventricle, superimposing evidence for pericarditis, ventricular aneurysm (which may be true

or false), or cardiac tamponade on an already complex clinical picture. The location of this acquired variety of ventricular septal defect does not correspond with the usual congenital defects but is dictated by the distribution of muscular necrosis. The membranous septum consequently is not involved, but rupture of the muscular septum (Fig. 24.4) may be high or

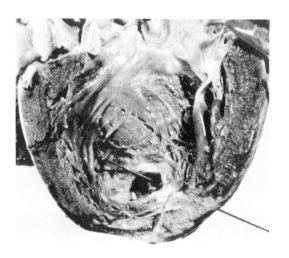

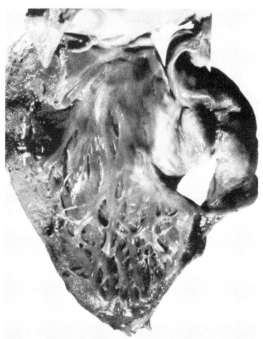

Fig. 24.4  Postmortem photographs of two hearts with rupture of the muscular ventricular septum after acute myocardial infarction. (Bloor CM: Cardiac Pathology. JB Lippincott Company, Philadelphia, 1978.)

low, anterior or posterior, simple or complex. This variable anatomy explains the variable location and radiation of the murmur among patients, and why these characteristics are often unlike those of the usual congenital defect of the membranous septum.[60] Striking differences between patients with congenital and acquired defects of the ventricular septum also exist in the pulmonary circulation. Sudden rupture of the ventricular septum allows a hyperacute left to right shunt into a pulmonary vasculature characterized by "adult" pulmonary arterioles. This difference confers the disadvantage that the lungs are not protected by arterioles with a high wall-to-lumen ratio from flooding by torrential shunts, and the advantage that the Eisenmenger reaction does not occur in arterioles that have fully evolved from the fetal to the adult configuration. Another factor that imparts an important difference between congenital ventricular septal defects and those acquired in the course of acute myocardial infarction is that in the former pulmonary venous pressure is normal and congestion therefore absent; in the latter, pulmonary venous hypertension and pulmonary congestion are present and modify the clinical and radiographic examination.

## Rupture of the Ventricular Septum

The blood supply to the ventricular septum is delivered by the septal perforating branches of both the anterior and posterior descending branches of the coronary arterial tree. Rupture of the ventricular septum may, therefore, complicate both anterior and inferior wall myocardial infarctions, an observation that greatly diminishes the importance to the clinician of the reported distribution of coronary arterial lesions and the locations of myocardial infarction in published accounts of ruptured interventricular septum.[61] In any case, an overwhelming predeliction to one or other site has not been shown and there is considerable variation between series. Thus the clinician faced with a patient whose hemodynamic condition is deteriorating and who has developed a new murmur during the course of an acute myocardial infarction should not be influenced by the anatomic loca-

tion of the infarction when considering the diagnosis of rupture of the ventricular septum.

The incidence of this complication, 2 to 3 percent, is higher than clinical experience and the numbers of cases constituting published series would suggest, because a good many of the patients die and not all cases are recognized clinically. Necropsy may not be performed and the literature has concentrated on that subset of patients for whom surgical closure of the defect must be considered.

Rupture of the ventricular septum is swiftly followed by an increase in the symptoms and signs of pulmonary congestion and tissue hypoperfusion.[60,61] Dyspnea increases and the general appearance of the patient deteriorates with the appearance of tachypnea, pallor or cyanosis, increased tachycardia and hypotension, anxiety, and oliguria. These changes are not specific, and in this setting they may be related to the size of the infarction, acute ischemia, progression of the infarction, cardiac tamponade, and pulmonary embolism, to name some of the leading causes. The diagnostic probabilities are sharply reduced to rupture of the ventricular septum or the mitral valve apparatus when these changes are accompanied by the advent of a new, loud pansystolic murmur and thrill.[61] If the murmur is loudest along the lower left sternal border, rupture of the ventricular septum is the most likely diagnosis. If the murmur is louder at the apex than at the lower left sternal border, it is impossible, on this account alone, to distinguish from rupture of a papillary muscle. This is an important distinction between the differential diagnosis of these two complications of myocardial infarction on the one hand, and the differential diagnosis of congenital ventricular septal defect versus mitral regurgitation on the other. The variable location and radiation of the murmur of these acquired defects of the ventricular septum, and the frequent location of its maximal intensity at the cardiac apex result from the variable locations of ruptures in the substance of the muscular septum (Fig. 24.4) with sparing of the relatively avascular membranous septum. The murmur is often accompanied by a third heart sound, but because of preexisting tachycardia and a fourth heart sound, this is usually appreciated as a summation gallop, but when the shunt is large, a distinct mitral diastolic rumble can be heard.

The electrocardiogram is not helpful, dominated as it is by the signs of infarction, ischemia, and dysrhythmia. Conduction defects are uncommon, but persistent ST segment elevation due to associated ventricular aneurysm is quite common.[61] The appearance of the chest radiograph confirms deterioration, the lung field opacity being increased. Careful scrutiny allows detection of evidence for pulmonary arterial overcirculation (left-to-right shunt) superimposed on the evidence of pulmonary congestion: redistribution of flow towards the upper lung fields, enlargement of the pulmonary veins, edema of the interstitium or alveoli, and Kerley B lines. Frequently the patient is too ill to hold an inspiration, and indeed ventilation may be with the help of a respirator; also, electrodes or an endotracheal tube may obscure the lung fields, and at best portable techniques will have been employed in taking the chest radiographs. These factors combine to decrease the likelihood that the chest radiograph will be important in establishing the correct diagnosis. The reader will appreciate that in clinical practice, suspicion that the ventricular septum has ruptured is an urgent indication for catheterization of the right side of the heart. This holds true even when the patient is apparently in a stable and apparently satisfactory state because deterioration may be rapid and profound. Discussion of the subtleties of congestion versus overcirculation of the lungs and of timing of the gallop can properly be postponed until after the diagnosis has been established by right-heart catheterization.

Catheterization is usually performed in the coronary care unit, using a balloon-tipped "floating" catheter. The position of the catheter tip in the right atrium or superior vena cava, right ventricle, and pulmonary artery can be ascertained by inspection of the pressure monitor. However, since diagnosis depends on localizing the site of a step-up of oxygen saturation, fluoroscopy is preferred. The catheter is advanced to the superior vena cava where a pressure reading and duplicate blood samples are obtained. If possible, the catheter tip is then manipulated into the inferior vena cava and duplicate blood samples are again obtained. The tip is next withdrawn into the right atrium. Pressures and blood samples are obtained from high, mid, and low right atrial positions.

Analysis of blood oxygen content or tension shows an increase in oxygen when right ventricular and pulmonary arterial samples are compared with caval and right atrial samples. Usually the step-up is found in the ventricle, but right heart failure with tricuspid regurgitation may cause the shunt to be detected at the atrial level. In some cases sampling errors may occur because of inadequate mixing of the systemic venous return with the left-to-right shunt flow, so that the step-up is not detected until the catheter is in the pulmonary artery. These difficulties can be reduced by analyzing multiple samples in duplicate from the several sites. It should also be recalled that there are normal differences in oxygen content because of streamlined flow. Superior vena caval blood has a lower oxygen content than inferior vena caval blood, which carries a large volume of relatively saturated blood from the renal veins. Coronary sinus blood, which also drains into the right atrium, is highly unsaturated. These three streams do not mix well until they join in the pulmonary artery. For this reason, slightly higher oxygen contents can be found in normal subjects and patients without left-to-right shunts when samples are successively obtained from the superior vena cava, right atrium, right ventricle, and pulmonary artery. Samples from the inferior vena cava may normally be more highly saturated than samples of right atrial blood. Mixed venous blood in patients without left-to-right shunts is sampled from the pulmonary artery. In patients with left-to-right shunting at the ventricular level, the oxygen content of mixed venous blood must be estimated from the average of samples from the right atrium, or by taking three times the average oxygen concentration in the superior vena cava, adding the average inferior vena caval oxygen content and dividing the answer by four.

In practice, there should be no difficulty in establishing the diagnosis of rupture of the ventricular septum by blood oxygen analysis because the oxygen saturation of the venous return blood is low, an expression of diminished cardiac output, whereas oxygen saturation in the right ventricle and pulmonary artery is very high. Because these defects are large, the pulmonary vascular resistance is only modestly elevated and the shunt is, in consequence, large. Mixed venous blood is about 75 percent saturated with oxygen in normal subjects (pO$_2$ 40 Torr) but values of 50 to 65 percent are common in acute myocardial infarction with "pump failure." These values differ sharply from those found in samples from the right ventricle and pulmonary artery when the ventricular septum has ruptured. Here values in the 80 to 93 percent range are common.

The diagnosis may also be established rapidly by the hydrogen curve technique (Fig. 24.5). A platinum-tipped catheter is advanced to the pulmonary artery and is connected to an electrocardiograph. The patient inhales a single breath of hydrogen, which immediately diffuses into the pulmonary capillaries and rapidly appears in the left ventricle. If hydrogen-bearing blood enters the right ventricle through a septal defect, a large polarizing voltage is recorded from the platinum electrode a few seconds after the patient has inhaled the hydrogen (Fig. 24.5). When the ventricular septum is intact, a greatly attenuated signal occurs after the transit time from left to right ventricle through the systemic circulation is completed.

**Pressure Measurement in the Right Side of the Heart.** Central venous pressure is commonly elevated, reflecting failure of the right side of the heart; pulmonary wedge and arterial pressures are elevated, reflecting left ventricular failure and the consequent pulmonary hypertension (Fig. 24.6). The waveform of the pulmonary arterial and wedge pressure tracings is unremarkable in the absence of associated mitral regurgitation.

**Management.** With the diagnosis established, the physician's attention is next directed first to the short-term survival and then to the long-term prognosis of the patient. When the infarction is massive and destruction of the septum

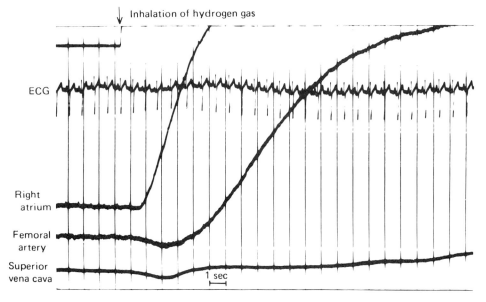

Fig. 24.5 Use of inhaled hydrogen gas to demonstrate a left to right shunt, on this occasion at the atrial level. Following inhalation hydrogen appeared earlier in the right atrium than in the femoral artery (1 second and 3.5 seconds, respectively). The femoral artery sensor serves as a standard. Appearance of hydrogen in the superior vena cava, which was proximal to the shunt, occurred more than 12 seconds after its inhalation and represented the systemic circulation time. In rupture of the ventricular septum early appearance is detected in the right ventricle and appearance in the right atrium is greatly prolonged because "circulation time" is lengthened. (Fowler N: Cardiac Diagnosis and Treatment, third ed., Harper & Row, Publishers, Inc., New York, 1980.)

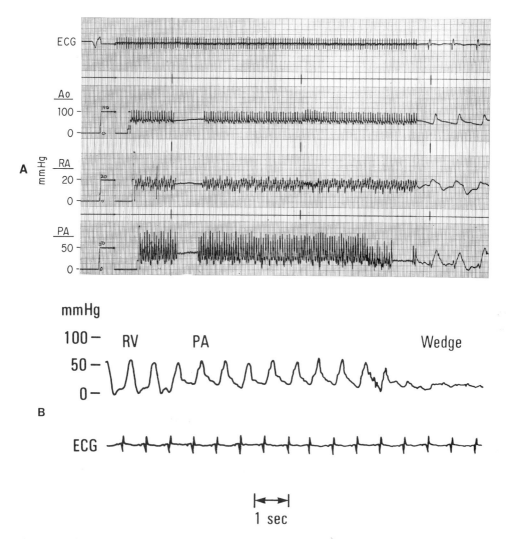

Fig. 24.6  *(A)* Pressures recorded in the coronary care unit from a patient with ruptured ventricular septum. The systolic arterial pressure is 80 mmHg, the right atrial mean pressure 17 mmHg, the pulmonary arterial pressure mean pressure 30 mmHg *(left side of figure)* and the pulmonary wedge pressure *(right side of figure)* is 20 mmHg. *(B)* From the same patient as illustrated in *(A)*: Data obtained during cardiac catheterization performed 3 weeks later and 1 day preceeding successful closure of the defect and coronary arterial bypass grafting. The record is recorded as the catheter is advanced from the right ventricle, through the pulmonary artery to the pulmonary wedge position.

extensive, the outcome usually will be fatal, often rapidly so, in spite of the physician's best supportive efforts. Three basic principles underly the therapeutic plan. The first is to treat tissue hypoperfusion, pulmonary congestion, dysrhythmia, and conduction disturbance vigorously and effectively using guidelines applicable to patients with acute myocardial infarction without rupture of the interventricular septum. The second principle is to intervene to reduce

the shunt and increase cardiac output. The final principle is that the ventricular septum must be repaired at the optimal time in the patient's course. The objectives of the first two principles are accomplished by afterload reduction therapy.[62] Arteriolar vasodilatation not only helps to preserve ischemic myocardium and reduce ventricular volume, it also enhances the ability of the left ventricle to pump into the aorta, thereby at once increasing cardiac output and proportionately reducing the magnitude of the left-to-right shunt.

The intravenous administration of nitroprusside should be started as soon as the diagnosis is established, provided this therapy is not contraindicated by prohibitive shock. Afterload is even more effectively lowered by intraaortic balloon counterpulsation,[63] which possesses the additional advantage of increasing aortic diastolic pressure and thereby coronary arterial blood flow. In my opinion, this therapy should be instituted early and should be maintained until the ventricular septum can be closed surgically. In selecting the time when the septum should be repaired, one is forced to compromise between factors necessitating early closure of the defect and those that predict a more favorable outcome if operative treatment can be postponed.[64] With each day that passes after infarction and septal rupture, hemodynamic stress and volume overload continue. In spite of the best and most intensive care that can be offered, the tendency is toward hemodynamic deterioration, often slowly progressive but accelerated by acute episodes. During this period, tolerance and side effects of drug therapy may develop; the balloon-tip cathether, vital to adequate monitoring, must be replaced through different veins; difficulties may arise with the intraaortic balloon counterpulsation system or at the site of its insertion through the skin; and pulmonary complications may appear. On the other hand, with each passing day the infarct heals, enabling the myocardium to hold sutures better and decreasing the risk that inevitably accompanies the performance of a major surgical operation shortly after extensive acute myocardial infarction. The ideal time to operate is about 3 weeks following the acute event, but there can be no absolute rule. If hemodynamic deterioration is rapid in spite of maximal therapy, and in the medical team's judgment the patient is likely to die or develop irreversible heart failure and this risk exceeds that of early operation, surgical treatment cannot be postponed for 3 weeks but may be performed 2 weeks, 1 week, or days after the septal rupture.[65] Some patients are stable after 3 weeks and no longer require supportive therapy. In this small minority, operation should be postponed beyond 3 weeks. As soon as the diagnosis is established the patient must be jointly managed by cardiologic and surgical teams. The latter must be in a position to perform the operation at short notice, and, in practice, the decision whether to prolong medical treatment or to operate is reconsidered once or twice a day.

**Preparation For Surgical Treatment.** When the decision has been reached that operation should be undertaken within the next 24 to 72 hours, definitive studies should be carried out in the cardiac catheterization laboratory. These studies are often carried out while intraaortic balloon counterpulsation is continued. The first priority is to obtain coronary arteriograms to enable the surgeon to decide which, if any, vessels to bypass with a saphenous vein graft at the time of the operation. If the patient has tolerated coronary arteriography well, the next step is to obtain a left ventriculogram to demonstrate true or false ventricular aneurysms requiring resection, to evaluate the competency of the mitral valve, and to outline the anatomy of the septal tear.

**Surgical Treatment.** The ventricular septal defects are closed either with a patch, or by direct sutures reinforced with pledgets to help prevent them tearing through necrotic myocardium. Ventricular aneurysms are excised or imbricated and all significant coronary stenoses are bypassed unless the vessel supplies an area of scar or aneurysm. If a major degree of mitral regurgitation was identified by left ventriculography, the mitral valve is replaced.

When the team is driven to early surgical treatment, the risk is increased, often to 30 percent and certainly more if the patient is critically ill, but dramatic saves have been recorded. The risk may be 15 percent when it is possible to treat the patient medically for 3 weeks before embarking on operative treatment. In patients who can wait a full 2 to 3 months without intensive drug support, the risk should not exceed 5 to 10 percent.

## Rupture of the Papillary Muscle

This complication of acute myocardial infarction bears many similarities to rupture of the interventricular septum; the prognosis however is even less favorable.

In the first few days after acute myocardial infarction, an acute, dramatic deterioration appears accompanied by a new pansystolic murmur. The murmur is usually at the cardiac apex, but occasionally may be louder medial to the apex. The murmur of acute mitral regurgitation is less likely than the murmur of a rupture of the ventricular septum to be accompanied by a thrill.[61] A loud third heart sound is commonly audible. This filling sound is sometimes long enough to justify its designation as a diastolic murmur. Frequently there is a preexisting fourth heart sound, and when tachycardia is also present, the third and fourth heart sounds merge into a summation gallop.

**Pathophysiology.** Rupture of the mitral valve apparatus creates instantaneous mitral regurgitation, a lesion that is exceptionally poorly tolerated.[66]

The left atrium cannot appreciably dilate in response to a hyperacute hemodynamic strain, and this chamber therefore retains the dimensions present immediately before the acute insult. In this group of patients, the left atrium is usually normal in size or slightly enlarged. In a few of the patients, it is considerably larger owing to the existence of prior chronic mitral regurgitation, usually associated with ischemic scarring of papillary muscles or extreme cardiac dilatation.[67] Free regurgitation into a left atrium that has not dilated and therefore is operating at the top end of a steep pressure-volume relation differs from chronic mitral regurgitation in which the left atrium progressively enlarges and may become quite compliant. In papillary muscle rupture, the left atrium is stiff and fails to act as a damping chamber between the left ventricle and the pulmonary veins during systole. A systolic pressure wave, frequently only a few millimeters of mercury below peak left ventricular pressure in amplitude, therefore occurs in the left atrium and pulmonary veins. The sudden appearance of massive pulmonary venous hypertension leads to acute pulmonary congestion, which is often overwhelming, accompanied as it is by a precipitous drop in cardiac output. If a primary belly ruptures, both leaflets of the mitral valve become flail because

chordae tendineae arising from both of the papillary muscles insert into both leaflets (Fig. 24.7). This degree of mitral regurgitation is seldom compatible with life beyond a few hours or days. Rupture of secondary and tertiary papillary muscle bellies causes proportionately less severe mitral regurgitation.

The sudden appearance of a volume overload on the left side of the heart does not allow the left atrium and ventricle to dilate, as they would when chronically volume loaded. It has been speculated that acute dilatation is prevented by

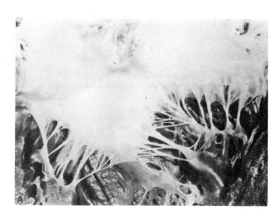

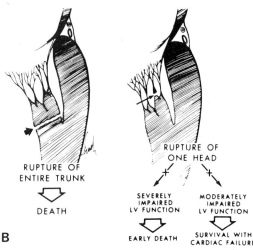

Fig. 24.7 *(A)* Arrangement of the papillary muscles, chordae tendiniae, and leaflets of the mitral valve showing that rupture of a main belly causes both leaflets to become incompetent. *(B)* The spectrum of papillary muscle rupture in acute myocardial infarction. (Roberts WC, Perloff JK: A clinicopathologic survey of the conditions causing the mitral valve to function abnormally. Ann Intern Med 77:939, 1978.)

the pericardium that strongly resists sudden stretching. Indeed, protection of the heart from acute overdistension is one of the postulated functions of the pericardium. The restraining action of the pericardium has been demonstrated in patients with ruptured chordae tendiniae studied soon after the acute event.[68] Not only the large left atrial systolic wave was shown, but so were equal diastolic pressures in the two atria and ventricles, with diastolic pressure waveforms showing early an diastolic dip and a late diastolic plateau reminiscent of constrictive pericarditis (Fig. 24.8). The pathology is illustrated in Figure 24.9.

**Diagnosis.** The clinical problem and the differential diagnosis are essentially the same as in rupture of the ventricular septum. In both situations, while it is interesting to weigh the fine points of clinical and radiologic examina-

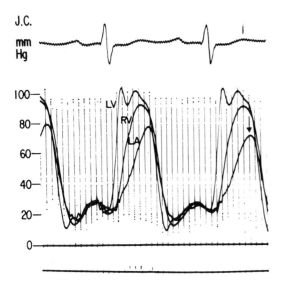

Fig. 24.8  Pressure recording from a patient with acute mitral regurgitation secondary to rupture of the mitral valve apparatus. Note the tall pointed V waves characteristic of this condition. Note also that the left and right ventricular filling pressures are equal, and the wave forms are similar to those of constrictive pericarditis. This suggests that the pericardium restrains cardiac volume in the face of a massive acute volume overload. Arrow points to tall V wave in the left atrial pressure pulse. (Bartle SH, Hermann HJ: Acute mitral regurgitation in man. Hemodynamic evidence and observations indicating an early role for the pericardium. Circulation 36:839, 1967.)

tion, early recourse to catheterization of the right side of the heart is prudent.[69] When the papillary muscle has ruptured, a shunt will not be found, but the pulmonary wedge pressure tracing is characterized by a tall, narrow systolic peak (Fig. 24.8). In many of the cases, this systolic peak is also seen in the pulmonary arterial tracing as a second peak following peak systolic pressure (Fig. 24.8). Cardiac output is depressed, often to values below 2 l/min/m². Severe pulmonary arterial hypertension is the rule, and frequently its sudden onset leads to failure of the right side of the heart manifest by an elevated right heart filling pressure.

The chest radiograph is not helpful because the abnormalities are nonspecific; there is little if any increase in the size of cardiac silhouette as a whole, and the left atrium does not enlarge. Pulmonary congestion is severe and may amount to florid pulmonary alveolar and interstitial edema. There are no ECG changes that particularly point to papillary muscle rupture. The echocardiogram does not show acute changes in the left atrial and left ventricular dimensions, but the flail leaflet or leaflets can be demonstrated, sometimes in dramatic fashion (Fig. 24.10).

**Management.** Almost always there is nothing the physician can do to alter the relentless path to a fatal outcome in the most severe cases.[70] The principles of therapy are straightforward in their aims but less so in execution, and are similar to those underlying the treatment of ruptured ventricular septum. The principles are (1) to optimize the treatment of the infarction itself, combatting cardiogenic shock, pulmonary congestion, dysrhythmia, and hypoperfusion of the critical vascular beds; (2) mitral regurgitation must be reduced and cardiac output increased; and (3) when these measures succeed, late surgical correction of mitral regurgitation will be required.

As with septal rupture, afterload reduction therapy conveys the double advantage of increasing forward ejection by the left ventricle at the expense of the regurgitant fraction, which is proportionately reduced.[63] As in ventricular rupture, hypotension may prevent the successful administration of nitroprusside. Counterpulation by means of an intraaortic balloon then

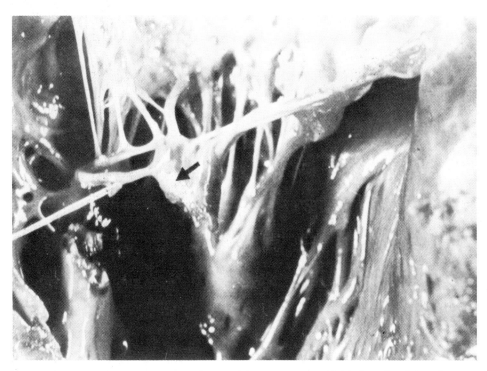

Fig. 24.9  Papillary muscle rupture in a heart with acute myocardial infarct involving the posterior left ventricular wall and the posterior papillary muscle. The *black arrow* points to the ruptured posterior papillary muscle belly. The patient died within 24 hours.

becomes the appropriate mode of afterload reduction.[63] This method confers the additional advantage of raising the aortic diastolic pressure, which, together with the lowered left ventricular diastolic pressure, increases coronary blood flow.

The rare patient who responds favorably should be studied in the cardiac catheterization laboratory, 24 to 48 hours before mitral valve replacement.[71] Left ventriculography defines the distribution and location of segmental wall abnormalities and quantifies overall left ventricular function. This study also confirms the diagnosis and rules out associated lesions, such as ventricular septal rupture and ventricular aneurysms, which may be true or false. Coronary arteriography must be accomplished, because it is important that at the time of valve replacement the surgeon bypass all severe lesions technically amenable to this procedure, that occur in vessels supplying viable myocardium. When possible, operative treatment should be delayed for 3 weeks, but hemody-

namic deterioration in the face of maximal medical treatment may be the signal to attempt earlier operative intervention at high risk and as a last resort.[70]

## Combined Rupture of the Interventricular Septum and a Papillary Muscle

This diagnosis is virtually impossible using ordinary bedside clinical tools. In practice, the physician must recall that a massive infarction may cause necrosis of both structures and that both may rupture—not necessarily at the same time. At times, the site of septal rupture and a flail mitral valve may both be visualized by real time echocardiography. The diagnosis is usually made by the physician who is cognizant that these two dreaded complications of myocardial infarction can coexist and therefore diligently searches out a shunt and also obtains optimal quality pulmonary wedge pressure tracings in every patient in whom one of these diagnoses is suspected. The occurrence of tall nar-

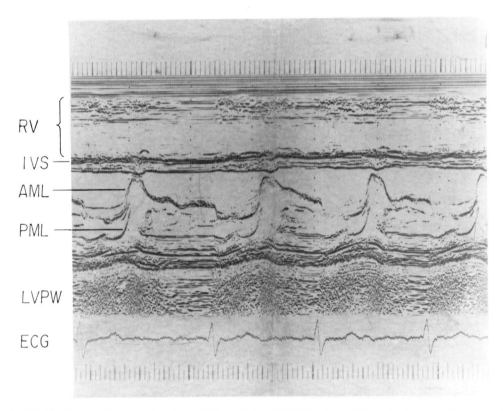

Fig. 24.10 Echocardiogram showing a flail posterior (PML) leaflet of the mitral valve. The posterior leaflet moves sharply anteriorly during diastole, in parallel with the D-E slope of the anterior leaflet (AML). In systole, the posterior leaflet is nowhere close to apposition with the anterior leaflet, but sags in a posterior direction.

row systolic peaks of pulmonary wedge pressure and a step-up of oxygen saturation in the right ventricle constitute acceptable hemodynamic evidence of the combined lesion.

Mitral regurgitation may accompany rupture of the interventricular septum even when the papillary muscle is not itself ruptured. The basis for mitral regurgitation in such cases may be cardiac dilatation, or necrosis and fibrosis of the papillary muscles. The systolic wave in the pulmonary wedge pressure tracing is of lower amplitude and greater duration than that of papillary muscle rupture.

Severe mitral regurgitation of any mechanism in the setting of rupture of the ventricular septum is an indication to replace the mitral valve at the time of septal repair because the chances of survival are even less when a major hemodynamic lesion remains uncorrected.

In patients with overt tricuspid regurgitation, one must consider the possible presence of rup-

ture of a portion of the tricuspid valve apparatus.[72]

## THROMBOEMBOLIC COMPLICATIONS OF ACUTE MYOCARDIAL INFARCTION

Major illnesses associated with a hypercoagulable state and which mandate bed rest for treatment are associated with a high risk of thromboembolic complications. Acute myocardial infarction furnishes a common and important example of this problem.

More than 30 years after Wright's publication [73] on the effectiveness of anticoagulant therapy for "coronary thrombosis with myocardial infarction," the controversy that was sparked remains unsettled, although radical changes have ensued in our thinking about the role of thrombosis in myocardial infarction. Indeed, the term coronary thrombosis now strikes a quaint note. At present there is no authoritative opinion on whether to administer anticoagulants to patients with acute myocardial infarction; certainly the duration of and means for administration differ from those promulgated three decades ago. Few, if any, authors now claim that anticoagulant therapy influences the course of the infarction itself and particularly that it can prevent extension of the infarction. The notion that anticoagulant therapy should be routinely administered for months or years after uncomplicated myocardial infarction has long since been abandoned.

## Deep Vein Thrombosis and Pulmonary Embolism

Authorities who advise anticoagulation as a standard component of therapy for acute myocardial infarction base their recommendation on the prevention of thromboembolism, especially pulmonary embolism, and not on the hypothesis that anticoagulants can modify the progress of the infarction itself. Thrombosis of the calf veins can be demonstrated within the first few days [74] when sensitive techniques, such as [125]I-labeled fibrinogen [75,76] or electric impedance plethysmography [77] are used for their detection, but clinical examination is notoriously inadequate. Thrombosis of calf vessels can be prevented by low-dose heparin, but in any case, it is not a direct cause of pulmonary embolism.[78] Unfortunately, in 20 percent of cases with calf vein thrombosis, which usually begins in the soleal vein, propagation into the politeal, femoral, and iliac veins occurs, and this is the source of pulmonary embolism. It has been estimated that pulmonary embolism may complicate 50 percent of cases with deep vein thrombosis,[79] and that perhaps half of these prove fatal. Frishman [74] has estimated that national use of anticoagulant therapy in the setting of acute myocardial infarction may save more than 8,000 lives a year in the United States.

Several factors increase the predisposition to

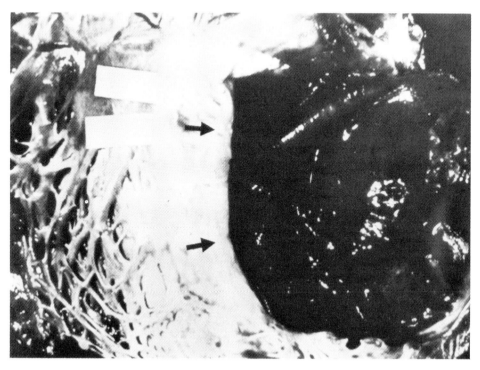

Fig. 24.11 Ventricular aneurysm in a heart 6 months after acute myocardial infarction. A massive aneurysm has developed in the posterior portion of the interventricular septum and the posterior ventricular wall *(dark arrows)*. A large mural thrombus is adherent to the wall of the aneurysm *(white arrow, top)*.

deep vein thrombosis and pulmonary embolism in the early stage of acute myocardial infarction; these include, shock, left ventricular failure, old age, obesity, varicose veins, and any other circumstance that prevents early ambulation.[80] Low-dose heparin depresses the coagulation process by decreasing the rate at which circulating antithrombin III inactivates activated factor X. This explains why low-dose heparin therapy, to be effective in preventing calf vein thrombosis, must be started immediately after the patient is admitted to the hospital, and why this form of anticoagulant therapy is powerless to halt an ongoing thrombotic process. Although low-dose heparin does not lack for advocates and substantially reduces the incidence of deep vein thrombosis,[81,82] it has not been shown to reduce the incidence of pulmonary embolism after acute myocardial infarction. Anticoagulant therapy for acute myocardial infarction therefore ordinarily means therapeutic doses of heparin given intravenously together with, and followed by, warfarin sodium or a similar oral anticoagulant. Clinical practice varies widely from the routine administration of warfarin sodium for 1 month to all patients without a specific contraindication, to witholding anticoagulants unless there is a specific individual indication. Anticoagulant therapy is used less commonly in academic centers, where, because of imperfections in the published trials,[82,83] skepticism is high, than in community hospitals where the majority of patients are treated. Most authorities treat patients who are at increased risk of thromboembolic complications with conventional intravenous doses of heparin given as boluses every 4 to 6 hours or by drip. Usually 20,000 to 60,000 units per 24 hours is needed.

The dose is regulated by maintaining the activated partial thromboplastin time 1.5 to 2 times normal. Heparin therapy is discontinued after 72 hours and warfarin is given to maintain the prothrombin time twice as high as control. Opinion remains divided on whether or not to treat patients who are not at increased risk of thromboembolism in the same manner. My own practice, at best, is to individualize the decision for each patient, at worst it is capricious. I am unlikely to prescribe anticoagulant therapy for young patients with a straightforward inferior wall myocardial infarction; I would prescribe anticoagulants for an 80-year-old, debilitated, obese patient who has varicose veins with a large anterior myocardial infarction. I am easily deterred from prescribing anticoagulants by reasonable evidence of a bleeding diathesis, or by a late or prolonged pericardial friction rub, and I am easily swayed by a house officer with strong convictions in either direction.

**Alternative Modes of Therapy.** The most effective means of preventing deep vein thrombosis is early ambulation,[84] but the very patients for whom this is most desirable are the ones in whom early mobilization is not possible. Intermittent pneumatic compression of the calf has been advocated,[85] but there is little clinical experience with this method. Elastic stockings [86] are used extensively, but there is

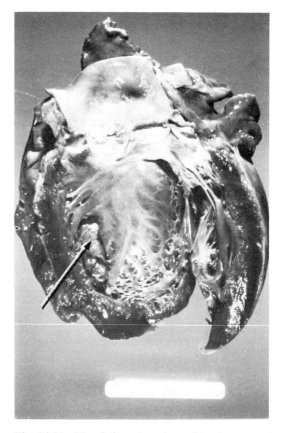

Fig. 24.12 Mural thrombus *(arrow)* in the apex of a greatly dilated left ventricle. The patient died from a massive cerebral embolus, which occurred 3 weeks before he died.

little proof that they are effective, and usually they are improperly applied.

## Mural Thrombi

Mural thrombi develop over the site of infarction in perhaps the majority of patients,[80,82] more commonly in the left than in the right ventricle (Figs. 24.11, 24.12). These give rise to systemic emboli and are responsible for a small proportion of pulmonary emboli. Fortunately, massive systemic embolism is not a common complication of acute myocardial infarction. Cerebral embolus occurs in 5 percent [74] and less commonly emboli lodge in the renal or mesenteric arteries or at the aortic bifurcation and in peripheral arteries. The risk to an individual is low, but the large number of potential cases is used as an additional argument by those who favor routine anticoagulation for myocardial infarction. Patients with a documented ventricular aneurysm should always be anticoagulated, unless there is a specific contraindication.

## SUGGESTED READINGS

Bloor CM: Cardiac pathology. JB Lippincott, Philadelphia, 1978.

Gelberg HJ, Brundage BH, Glanz S, et al: Quantitative left ventricular wall motion analysis. A comparison of area, chord and radial methods. *Circulation* 59:991, 1977.

Spodick DH: Acute pericarditis. Grune and Stratton, New York, 1959.

Spodick DH: Pericardial diseases. FA Davis, Philadelphia, 1976.

## REFERENCES

1. Thadani U, Chopra MP, Aber CP: Pericarditis after acute myocardial infarction. Br Med J 2:135, 1971.
2. Parkinson J, Bedford DR: Cardiac infarction and coronary thrombosis. Lancet 1:4, 1928.
3. Stewart CF, Turner KB: A note on pericardial involvement in coronary thrombosis. Am Heart J 15:232, 1938.
4. Lichstein E, Liu HM, Gupta P: Pericarditis complicating acute myocardial infarction. Incidence of complications and significance of electrocardiogram on admission. Am Heart J 87:246, 1973.
5. Khan AH: Pericarditis of acute myocardial infarction: review of the literature with case presentation. Am Heart J 90:288, 1975.
6. Dressler W: Management of pericarditis secondary to myocardial infarction. Prog Cardiovasc Dis 3:13, 1960.
7. Dressler W: The post-myocardial infarction syndrome: A report on 44 cases. Arch Intern Med 103:28, 1956.
8. Miarchos AP, McKendrich CS: Prognosis of pericarditis after acute myocardial infarction. Br Heart J 35:49, 1973.
9. Shabetai R: Diseases of the pericardium. In: Quick Reference to Cardiovascular Disease. Chung K, editor. Lippincott, Philadelphia, 1977.
10. Spodick DH: Acoustic phenomena in pericardial disease. Am Heart J 81:114, 1971.
11. Langendorf R: The effect of diffuse pericarditis on the electrocardiographic pattern of recent myocardial infarction. Am Heart J 22:86, 1941.
12. Aarseth S, Lange HF: The influence of anticoagulant therapy on the occurrence of cardiac rupture and hemopericardium following heart infarction. Am Heart J 56:250, 1958.
13. Lange HF, Aarseth S: The influence of anticoagulant therapy on the occurrence of cardiac rupture and hemopericardium following heart infarction. A controlled study of a selected treated group based on 1044 autopsies. Am Heart J 56:257, 1958.
14. Miller R: Hemopericardium with use of anticoagulant therapy. JAMA 209:1362, 1969.
15. Luft FC, Kleit SA, Smith RN, et al: Uremic pericarditis with tamponade. Arch Intern Med 134:488, 1974.
16. Shabetai R, Fowler NO, Gueron M: The effects of respiration on aortic pressure and flow. Am Heart J 65:412, 1963.
17. Jetter WW, White PO: Rupture of the heart in patients in mental institutions. Ann Intern Med 21:783, 1944.
18. Degiristofaro D, Liu CK: The hemodynamics of tamponade and blood volume overload in dogs. Cardiovasc Res 23:349, 1969.
19. Shabetai R, Fowler NO, Guntheroth WG: The hemodynamics of cardiac tamponade and constrictive pericarditis. Am J Cardiol 26:480, 1970.
20. Feigenbaum H, Zaky A, Grabhorn LL: Cardiac motion in patients with pericardial effusion. A study using reflected ultrasound. Circulation 34:611, 1966.

21. Spodick DH: Electrical alternation of the heart. Its relation to the kinetics and physiology of the heart during cardiac tamponade. Am J Cardiol 10:155, 1962.
22. Eisman B, Bareiss P, Pacifico AD, et al: Anatomic, clinical and therapeutic features of acute cardiac rupture. Successful surgical management fourteen hours after myocardial infarction. J Thorac Cardiovasc Surg 76:78, 1978.
23. Shabetai R: The pathophysiology of cardiac tamponade and constriction. Cardiovasc Clin 7:67, 1976.
24. Schiller NB, Botvinick EH: Right ventricular compression as a sign of cardiac tamponade. An analysis of electrocardiographic ventricular dimensions and their clinical implications. Circulation 66:774, 1977.
25. D'Cruz IA, Cohen HC, Prabhu R, et al: Diagnosis of cardiac tamponade by echocardiography. Changes in mitral valve motion and ventricular dimensions with special reference to paradoxical pulse. Circulation 52:460, 1975.
26. Settle HP, Adolph RJ, Fowler NO, et al: Echocardiographic study of cardiac tamponade. Circulation 56:951, 1977.
27. Shabetai R: Cardiac tamponade and constrictive pericarditis Med Ann DC 41:635, 1972.
28. Anderson MW, Christensen NA: Hemopericardium complicating myocardial infarction in the absence of cardiac rupture. Arch Intern Med 90:634, 1952.
29. Goldstein R, Wolff L: Hemorrhagic pericarditis in acute myocardial infarction treated with bishydroxycourmarin. JAMA 146:616, 1951.
30. Bishop LH, Estes EH, McIntosh H: The electrocardiogram as a safeguard in pericardiocentesis. JAMA 162:264, 1956.
31. Shabetai R: Cardiac tamponade. In: Cardiac Emergencies. Mason D, ed. Williams and Wilkins, Baltimore, 1978.
32. Shabetai R: Hemodynamics of pericardial disease. In: Cardiac Catheterization and Angiography. Grossman W, editor. Lea and Febiger, Philadelphia, 1980.
33. Yakierevitch V, Vione B, Melamed R, et al: False aneurysm of the left ventricle: Surgical treatment. J Thorac Cardiovasc Surg 78:556, 1978.
34. Cristal IP, Inbar-Yana, I: Atrial infarction leading to rupture. Br Heart J 41:350, 1979.
35. Tew FT, Mantle JA, Russell RO, et al: Cardiac tamponade with nonhemorrhagic pericardial fluid complicating Dresslers syndrome. Chest 72:93, 1974.
36. Fowler NO: Autoimmune heart disease. Circulation 44:159, 1971.
37. Goldberger AL: Myocardial Infarction: Electrocardiographic Differential Diagnosis. CV Mosby, St Louis, 1979.
38. Prakash R, Moorthy K, Del Vicario M, et al: Reliability of echocardiography in quantitating pericardial effusion: A prospective study. J Clin Ultrasound 6:398, 1977.
39. Khan AH: Post myocardial infarction syndrome. Cardiology 63:188, 1978.
40. Johnson AD, Laiken SL, Shabetai R: Non-invasive diagnosis of ischemic cardiomyopathy by fluoroscopic detection of coronary calcification. Am Heart J 96:521, 1978.
41. Master AM, Friedman R, Dack S: The electrocardiogram after standard exercise as a fundamental test of the heart. Am Heart J 24:777, 1942.
42. Master AM, Rosenfeldt I: Master two-step exercise test. JAMA 172:265, 1969.
43. Borer JS, Bucharach SL, Green MV, et al: Effect of nitroglycerine on exercise induced abnormalities of regional left ventricular function and ejection fraction in coronary artery disease. Circulation 57:314, 1978.
44. Pasternac A, Gorlin R, Sonnenblick EH, et al: Abnormalities of left ventricular motion induced by atrial pacing in coronary artery disease. Circulation 45:1195, 1972.
45. Rigaud M, Rocha P, Boschat J, et al: Regional left ventricular function assessed by contrast angiography in acute myocardial infarction. Circulation 60:130, 1979.
46. Zaret BL, Strauss WH, Martin MD, et al: Noninvasive regional myocardial perfusion with radioactive potassium. N Engl Med 288:809, 1973.
47. Carr KW, Engler RL, Forsythe JR, et al: Measurement of left ventricular ejection fraction by mechanical cross sectional echocardiography. Circulation 59:1196, 1979.
48. Chatman BR, Bristow DJ, Rahimtoola SH: Left ventricular wall motion assessed by using fixed external reference systems. Circulation 48:1043, 1973.
49. Sniderman AD, Marpole D, Fallen EL: Regional contraction patterns in the normal and ischemic left ventricle in man. Am J Cardiol 31:484, 1973.
50. Smalling RW, Skolnick MH, Myers D, et al: Digital boundary detection: Volumetric wall motion analysis of left ventricular cine angiograms. Comput Biol Med 6:73, 1976.
51. Leighton RF, Wilt SM, Lewis RP: Detection of hypokinesis by a quantitative analysis of left

ventricular cineangiograms. Circulation 50:121, 1974.

52. McDonald IG: The shape and movements of the human left ventricle during systole. Am J Cardiol 26:221, 1970.

53. Herman MV, Heinle RA, Klein MD, et al: Localized disorders in myocardial contraction. Asynergy and its role in congestive heart failure. N Engl J Med 277:222, 1967.

54. Klausner SC, Ratshin RA, Tyberg JV, et al: The similarity of changes in segmental contraction patterns induced by postextrasystolic potentiation and nitroglycerine. Circulation 54:615, 1976.

55. Maseri A, Severi S, De Ness M, Variant angina: One aspect of a continuous spectrum of vasospastic myocardial ischemia. Am J Cardiol 42:1019, 1978.

56. Banka VS, Bodenheimer MM, Shah R, et al: Intervention ventriculography. Comparative value of nitroglycerine, post-extrasystolic potentiation and nitroglycerine plus post-extrasystolic potentiation. Circulation 53:632, 1976.

57. Helfant RH, Pine R, Meister SG, et al: Nitroglycerine to unmask reversible asynergy. Correlation with post coronary bypass ventriculography. Circulation 50:108, 1974.

58. Mehta J, Pepine CJ: Assessment of cardiac performance with quantitative radionuclide angiography. Effects of oral propranolol on global and regional left ventricular function in coronary artery disease. Circulation 58:808, 1978.

58a. Slutsky R, Karliner JS, Battler A et al: Comparison of early systolic and holosystolic ejection phase indexes by contrast ventriculography in patients with coronary artery disease. Circulation 61:1083, 1980.

59. Roberts WC, Perloff JK: A clinicopathologic survey of the conditions causing the mitral valve to function abnormally. Ann Intern Med 77:939, 1978.

60. Champion BC, Harrison CE, Guiliani ER, et al: Ventricular septal defect after myocardial infarction. Ann Intern Med 70:251, 1969.

61. Selzer A, Berbode F, Kerth WJ: Clinical hemodynamic and surgical considerations of rupture of the ventricular septum after myocardial infarction. Am Heart J 78:598, 1969.

62. Tecklenberg PL, Fitzgerald J, Alderman EL, et al: Afterload reduction in the management of post infarction ventricular septal defect. Am J Cardiol 38:956, 1976.

63. Gold HK, Leinbach RC, Sanders CA, et al: Intra-aortic balloon pumping for ventricular septal defect or mitral regurgitation complicating acute myocardial infarction. Circulation 47:1191, 1973.

64. Schumacher HB: Suggestions concerning the operative management of post infarction septal defects. J Thorac Cardiovasc Surg 64:452, 1972.

65. Kahn JC, Rigaud M, Gandjbakheh I, et al: Posterior rupture of the interventricular septum after acute myocardial infarction: successful early surgical repair. Ann Thorac Surg 23:483, 1977.

66. DeBusk RF, Harrison DC: The clinical spectrum of papillary muscle disease. N Engl J Med 281:1458, 1969.

67. Bashour RA: Mitral regurgitation following myocardial infarction: the syndrome of papillary mitral regurgitation. Dis Chest 48:113, 1965.

68. Bartle SH, Hermann HJ: Acute mitral regurgitation in man. Hemodynamic evidence and observations indicating an early role for the pericardium. Circulation 36:839, 1967.

69. Meister SG, Helfant RH: Rapid bedside differentiation of ruptured interventricular septum from acute mitral insufficiency. N Engl J Med 287:1024, 1972.

70. Wei JY, Hutchins GC, Bulkley B: Papillary rupture in fatal acute myocardial infarction. A potentially treatable form of cardiogenic shock. Ann Intern Med 90:149, 1979.

71. Cheng TO, Bashour T, Adkins PC: Acute severe mitral regurgitation from papillary muscle dysfunction in acute myocardial infarction. Circulation 46:491, 1972.

72. Eisenberg S, Suyemeto J: Rupture of a papillary muscle of the tricuspid valve. Report of a case. Circulation 30:588, 1964.

73. Wright IS, Marple CD, Beck CF: Report of the committee for evaluation of anticoagulants in the treatment of coronary thrombosis with myocardial infarction. Am Heart J 36:801, 1948.

74. Frishman WH, Ribner HS: Anticoagulation in myocardial infarction: modern approach to an old problem. Am J Cardiol 43:1207, 1979.

75. Gallus AS, Hirsh J, Tuttle RJ, et al: Small subcutaneous doses of heparin in prevention of venous thrombosis. N Engl J Med 288:545, 1973.

76. Wray R, Maurer B, Shillingford J: Prophylactic anticoagulant therapy in the prevention of calf vein thrombosis after myocardial infarction. N Engl J Med 288:815, 1973.

77. Sasahara AA, Sharma GVRK, Parisi AF: New developments in the detection and prevention of venous thromboembolism. Am J Cardiol 43:1214, 1979.

78. Rogers PH, Sherry S: Current status of antithrombotic therapy in cardiovascular disease. Prog Cardiovasc Dis 19:235, 1976.

79. Kakkar VV, Flanc C, Howe CT, et al: Natural history of post operative deep vein thrombosis. Lancet 2:230, 1969.

80. Ebert RV: Anticoagulants in acute myocardial infarction. Results of a cooperative clinical trail. JAMA 225:724, 1973.

81. Warlow C, Terry G, Kenmure ACF, et al: A double blind trial of low doses of subcutaneous heparin in the prevention of deep vein thrombosis after myocardial infarction. Lancet 2:934, 1973.

82. Gifford RH, Feinstein AR: A critique of methodology in the studies of anticoagulant therapy for acute myocardial infarction. N Engl J Med 280:351, 1969.

83. Goldman L, Feinstein AR: Anticoagulants and myocardial infarction. Ann Intern Med 90:92, 1979.

84. Miller RR, Lies JE, Carretta RF, et al: Prevention of lower extremeity venous thrombosis by early mobilization. Ann Intern Med 84:700, 1976.

85. Hill NJ, Pflug JJ, Jeyasingh K, et al: Prevention of deep vein thrombosis by intermittent pneumatic compression of the calf. Br Med J 1:131, 1972.

86. Holford GP: Graded compression for preventing deep vein thrombosis. Br Med J 2:969, 1976.

# 25 | *Unstable and Variant Angina: Approach to Diagnosis and Treatment*

*John Watkins, M.B.*
*Allen D. Johnson, M.D.*

## UNSTABLE ANGINA

### INTRODUCTION

Of the estimated one and a half million Americans per annum who sustain a myocardial infarction, between 30 and 60 percent have some premonitory symptoms.[1-3] The most common prodrome is one of increasingly frequent and severe attacks of angina pectoris, known as unstable angina. This syndrome has been recognized since the turn of the century[4] and has stimulated immense interest ever since, because it identifies a population at risk for myocardial infarction. Since more than half of those who die as a result of acute myocardial infarction do so before they reach a hospital,[5] the manifestation of unstable angina offers a unique opportunity for early therapeutic interventions aimed at reducing the incidence, morbidity, and mortality of myocardial infarction.

By no means, however, do all patients with unstable angina go on to develop myocardial infarction—nor is it possible to predict its occurrence in an individual case. Thus, some of the alternative names for this condition, such as "preinfarction angina" and "impending myocardial infarction," which prejudge the outcome, are misleading and best avoided. Other terms, such as "crescendo angina," "acute coronary insufficiency," and "status anginosus" are still occasionally used in contemporary accounts of this syndrome; but most authors have now adopted the term "unstable angina," in accordance with the precepts of the National Cooperative Study comparing medical and surgical therapy in this condition.[6]

### DEFINITION

Unstable angina represents the broad spectrum of symptomatic manifestations of myocardial ischemia intermediate in severity between stable, effort-induced angina and angina leading to inevitable myocardial infarction.

The following clinical presentations of unstable angina are recognized:

1. Angina of recent onset, usually within the preceding month. This includes patients who develop angina within a month of a documented myocardial infarction.
2. Angina of effort with a changing pattern. This may be an increase in the frequency, severity, or duration of previously stable effort angina or a reduction in the stress required to precipitate pain. The pain may radiate to a new location or be accompanied for the first time by diaphoresis or nausea. Nitroglycerin may be less effective in relieving chest pain than had previously been the case.
3. Angina occurring at rest. Some of these patients develop reversible ST segment elevation on the electrocardiogram taken during pain—a syndrome known as variant angina. This syndrome appears to result from a pri-

mary abnormality of coronary vasomotion in a major coronary artery, usually superimposed on an atheromatous narrowing. (The role of "coronary vasospasm" in unstable angina is complex and does not seem to be entirely confined to patients with ST segment elevation on the electrocardiogram.[7,8] The possible mechanisms underlying this phenomenon and their implications in diagnosis and therapy are considered in detail under the heading "Variant Angina" later in this chapter.) The remaining patients have either no ST segment shift or ST segment depression on the ECG taken during pain.

Neither the clinical nor the pathologic interface between unstable angina and acute myocardial infarction is clearly defined, however. Most, if not all, of these clinical features can also accompany acute myocardial infarction. Also, differentiation from unstable angina is not always possible, even when sophisticated laboratory techniques are used. Indeed, it is now recognized that subclinical myocardial necrosis ("microinfarction") can occur in patients with unstable angina,[9,10] so that its differentiation from acute myocardial infarction is, to some extent, semantic and dependent upon the sensitivity of the tests employed.

## PATHOGENESIS

There appears to be no specific pathoanatomical substrate for unstable angina. An autopsy study performed on patients who died after coronary artery bypass surgery showed no difference in the severity or distribution of coronary atherosclerosis between patients with stable angina and patients with unstable angina. Histologic evidence of localized myocardial necrosis, however, was more commonly found in the group with unstable angina.[11] Angiographic studies have also shown a comparable spectrum of coronary disease in both syndromes. Approximately 30 percent of patients each have single-, double-, or triple-vessel disease, and the remaining 10 percent have apparently normal coronary arteries.[12] Left main coronary disease is found in 15 percent of cases, and the left anterior descending coronary artery is involved in more

than 70 percent of cases.[13,14] The same distribution and severity of coronary disease are also found in patients with either ST segment elevation or depression on the ECG taken during pain.[15]

Thus, the distribution of atherosclerotic disease in the coronary tree, per se, explains neither the pathogenesis of unstable angina nor the predisposition to myocardial infarction. One possible explanation is that collateral channels are less well developed around coronary lesions causing unstable angina, implying that the atherosclerotic process is of more recent onset or progresses more rapidly than in comparable lesions causing stable angina. Some angiographic observations lend support to this suggestion,[16] as does the finding that the velocity of retrograde coronary blood flow measured at operation appears to be slower in patients with unstable angina than in those with stable angina.[17]

In physiologic terms, angina results from an imbalance between myocardial oxygen supply (coronary blood flow) and demand. Most cases of exercise-induced angina result from an increase in myocardial oxygen consumption, which cannot be balanced by a further increase in coronary blood flow because of the high coronary vascular resistance imposed by atherosclerotic disease.[18,19] In many cases of angina at rest, however, no changes in the determinants of myocardial oxygen demand are seen prior to the onset of pain, suggesting that a reduction in coronary blood flow is the initiating event.[7,20] This is undoubtedly due to localized coronary vasospasm in some patients with unstable angina;[8] in other patients, however, more generalized reflex coronary vasoconstriction of an inappropriate degree, in response to stimuli such as cold, may be important.[21] The hemodynamic response to rest pain tends to differ between those who show concomitant ST segment depression on the ECG and those who show ST segment elevation (variant angina). In the group of patients showing ST segment depression, left ventricular stroke work index and other measures of ventricular performance tend to fall initially, but then steadily rise until the pain remits.[7] In those showing ST segment elevation during pain, however, left ventricular performance tends to remain depressed throughout the ischemic episode,[7] as is seen after acute coronary occlusion in the dog.[22] This may be because myocardial ischemia is more severe in patients with ST segment elevation (transmural rather than subendocardial ischemia),[23] so that reflex autonomic influences cannot augment left ventricular performance as effectively.

Platelets synthesize a prostaglandin-like compound called thromboxane $A_2$, which causes profound vasoconstriction and is also the most potent platelet aggregating substance known. Thromboxane $A_2$ appears to be involved in some cases of unstable angina where coronary spasm is implicated.[24] The cause-and-effect relationship between changes in coronary vascular resistance and changes in thromboxane $A_2$ activity are not yet established, however. (See Pathogenesis of Variant Angina.)

## INCIDENCE AND NATURAL HISTORY

The incidence of unstable angina is unknown, but it is clearly of great clinical and socioeconomic importance, accounting for some 20 percent of all patients admitted to the coronary care unit[25] and nearly 15 percent of all patients requiring coronary artery bypass surgery.[26] Approximately half of all patients with unstable angina have recent onset of angina on minimal effort or at rest.[12] Unstable angina occurs most frequently in males between 40 and 60 years of age, as is the case with stable, effort-induced angina. In the subgroup with variant angina and normal coronary arteries, however, premenopausal women tend to predominate.[27] Of those patients with rest pain, 25 percent have concomitant ST segment elevation on the ECG (variant angina).[16]

The two major therapeutic measures currently used in the treatment of unstable angina—$\beta$-adrenergic blockade and coronary artery bypass surgery—were not widely available in the United States until about ten years ago. Consequently, an analysis of series reported prior to that time offers some insight into the natural history of this condition (see Table 25.1.) The mean incidence of myocardial infarction three months after the onset of unstable angina was 40 percent but ranged from 22 to 80 percent in these series. Mortality over the same period ranged from 1 to 60 percent, with a mean value of 17 percent. Long-term follow-up indicated an annual attrition rate of about 8 percent, the mortality being highest in patients who presented with pain at rest for more than 48 hours.[32] (These morbidity and mortality figures are not strictly comparable to contemporary reports, since earlier series did not tend to include patients with recent onset angina unless other criteria for unstable angina were present. Theoretically, these patients present at an earlier stage in the natural history of their coronary disease and might therefore be expected to have a more favorable prognosis.)

## DIAGNOSIS

It is not usually difficult to distinguish between unstable and stable angina on historical grounds alone. However, any definition of unstable angina that attempts to embrace all its clinical forms will necessarily result in some overlap

**Table 25.1  The Natural History of Unstable Angina, Based on Series Reported Prior to 1964 ***

| Author | No. of Patients | Mean Follow-up (Months) | Non Fatal MIs % | Deaths % |
|---|---|---|---|---|
| Levy [28] | 158 | 2 | 39 | 32 |
| Beamish [29] | 15 | 1.5 | 80 | 60 |
| Wood [30] | 50 | 2 | 22 | 16 |
| Vakil [31] | 251 | 3 | 37 | 1 |
| Vakil [1] | 156 | 3 | 49 | 24 |
| Total | 630 | 2.6 † | 40% | 17% |

* i.e., no propranolol therapy or coronary artery bypass surgery.
† = mean individual follow-up
MI = myocardial infarction
(Adapted from Cairns JA et al: Unstable angina pectoris. Am Heart J 92:373, 1976.)

with the definition of stable angina. The inclusion of patients with angina of recent onset within the definition of unstable angina, even if such individuals are symptomatically stable, is a case in point.

The diagnostic priority, however, is to exclude acute myocardial infarction. This is done by repeated clinical examinations, ECGs, cardiac enzyme determinations, and possibly radionuclide studies, during the first 48 hours of hospital admission. Other nonischemic chest pain syndromes must also be excluded.

## Clinical Features

Chest pain is the single, unifying feature of unstable angina. The patient's description of the pain is usually that of typical myocardial ischemia. One or more characteristics of the pain (frequency, intensity, duration, etc.—see definition) has usually worsened, which should alert one to the diagnosis. Symptomatic deterioration may occur over a few hours or several months. With variant angina particularly, attacks of rest pain may have a regular diurnal rhythm, often occurring in the early morning and waking the patient from sleep.[27]

Physical examination during an attack of pain may be helpful in differentiating unstable angina from other nonexertional chest pain syndromes. The finding of a transient third or fourth heart sound, the emergence of a palpable abnormality of left ventricular wall motion, the presence of a mitral systolic murmur, reversed splitting of the second heart sound, or an arrhythmia would each suggest that the pain is due to myocardial ischemia. Prolonged hypotension or frank cardiogenic shock almost always imply that acute myocardial infarction has occurred. Persistent pyrexia is also indicative of myocardial necrosis. As mentioned earlier, arterial pressure and heart rate may not change prior to the onset of pain, signifying that a reduction in coronary blood flow is the initiating event. Sometimes, however, a small increase in arterial pressure and/or heart rate is seen just before the pain commences, with further increases once the pain is established.[33]

Other conditions which might precipitate or exacerbate angina, such as thyrotoxicosis, ane-

mia, and hypertension, must also be considered and ruled out at the initial evaluation.

## Electrocardiographic Changes

Focal or diffuse changes are almost invariably seen in the electrocardiogram of patients with unstable angina. In fact, a completely normal ECG makes the diagnosis of unstable angina unlikely.[15] T wave changes, such as flattening, peaking, or inversion, are seen in the ECGs of most patients during pain. Symmetrical and steeply inverted T waves are characteristic. ST segment depression is found in 60 to 90 percent of cases during pain,[6,16] and ST segment elevation is present in approximately 25 percent.[14] However, both ST segment elevation and depression may occur in serial ECGs taken from the same patient and may vary from one episode of pain to the next or even change polarity during a single episode of pain.[8] The evolution of persistent Q waves implies myocardial necrosis and excludes the diagnosis of unstable angina, although the transient appearance of Q waves during pain without other evidence of myocardial infarction has been reported with variant angina.[34] Serious arrhythmias during pain are more commonly associated with variant angina than with other forms of unstable angina.

The electrocardiogram between attacks of pain is commonly abnormal, showing nonspecific repolarization abnormalities and sometimes evidence of previous myocardial infarction. The ST segment shifts seen during unstable angina are usually transient but occasionally persist for several hours in the absence of myocardial infarction. Thus, with the exception of unequivocal, persistent new Q waves, electrocardiographic changes are frequently unhelpful in differentiating unstable angina from acute myocardial infarction. Moreover, the electrocardiographic changes during pain are poor predictors of coronary angiographic findings,[9] except in the setting of variant angina.

## Cardiac Enzymes

Serial determinations of cardiac enzymes currently provide the most sensitive means of excluding myocardial necrosis. At least three separate determinations of creatine kinase (CK) and one determination of lactate dehydrogenase (LDH) should be performed within the first 24 hours after admission. Elevation of one or both of these enzymes to levels diagnostic of myocardial infarction (see Ch. 11), coupled with an increase of the appropriate isoenzyme activity, by definition excludes the diagnosis of unstable angina. However, an increase of up to 50 percent over initial enzyme levels, if still within the normal range, is considered compatible with the diagnosis of unstable angina. It has been speculated that these nondiagnostic elevations of cardiac enzyme levels might represent subclinical myocardial necrosis [9,35] or "microinfarction." The recent development of specific and highly sensitive assays for measuring cardiac isoenzymes, especially MB-CK,[36] has produced further evidence to support this contention. The phenomenon of "microinfarction" may also occur after repeated episodes of stable, effort-induced angina.[37] Clinical and angiographic features do not appear to differ between those patients with a slight elevation of cardiac enzymes and those without,[16] but a recent study has shown that a nondiagnostic elevation of cardiac enzymes in this condition is associated with a higher incidence of subsequent overt myocardial infarction and death.[38]

These observations underscore the problem of defining the point at which unstable angina stops and acute myocardial infarction begins in the continuum of myocardial ischemia.

## Radionuclide Studies

Pyrophosphate labeled with [99m]Tc is avidly taken up by acutely infarcted myocardium, and this is seen as a "hot spot" on a left ventricular scintigram. The ability of this method to differentiate unstable angina from acute myocardial infarction, however, has been questioned. "False positive" pyrophosphate scans have been reported in up to 40 percent of patients with unstable angina without other evidence of myocardial infarction.[39-41] This has been attributed to tracer uptake in noninfarcted but critically ischemic myocardium, such as is found in the periinfarction zone.[42] However, Jaffe et al. compared the results of pyrophosphate infarct scanning with serial estimates of MB-CK, a highly sensitive indicator of myocardial necrosis, in 116 patients with unstable angina.[10] In this study, only 8 percent of the scans were false positives (i.e., not accompanied by a diagnostic elevation of MB-CK levels). In the absence of other causes for false positive studies [43] (Table 25.2) this suggests that pyrophosphate scanning might in fact be more specific for myocardial necrosis than has previously been thought. Moreover, it may be the only means of detecting myocardial necrosis if the patient does not present until after the MB-CK levels have returned to normal. Thus, as with MB-CK determinations, a negative scan is very helpful in confirming the absence of myocardial infarction, but a positive scan can result from a degree of myocardial cell death that may not be clinically relevant and that would not be diagnosed as acute myocardial infarction by other criteria. Further, it is not clear whether any therapeutic advantage is gained from the knowledge that subclinical myocardial necrosis has occurred. At the time of this writing, this dilemma has not been resolved.

In contrast to infarct-avid radiotracers such

Table 25.2   Other Causes of "False Positive" [99m]Tc Pyrophosphate Scans

| Cardiac | Noncardiac |
| --- | --- |
| Cardiomyopathy | Skeletal muscle damage after electrical |
| Valve calcification | cardioversion or cardiopulmonary |
| Left ventricular aneurysm or large | resuscitation |
| dyskinetic segment | Rib fractures |
| Myocardial contusion | Calcified costal cartilages |
|  | Breast tumors |

(Adapted from Wynne J et al: Myocardial scintigraphy by infarct-avid radiotracers. In: Principles of Cardiovascular Nuclear Medicine. Holman et al., editors, Grune and Stratton, New York, 1978.)

as $^{99m}$Tc-labeled pyrophosphate, $^{201}$Tl is taken up preferentially by nonischemic myocardial cells in direct proportion to the level of myocardial perfusion. Thus, acutely ischemic, acutely infarcted, and previously infarcted myocardium all appear as "cold spots" on $^{201}$Tl scintigraphy of the left ventricle.

Within the first 6 hours after the onset of pain, $^{201}$Tl scanning is a highly sensitive indicator of myocardial ischemia and may become positive in unstable angina or myocardial infarction before any ECG or cardiac enzyme changes occur.[44] A positive scan may also be useful in excluding other nonischemic causes for chest pain at rest. However, acute $^{201}$Tl imaging will not differentiate between unstable angina and acute myocardial infarction. Serial $^{201}$Tl scanning may show reperfusion of a reversibly ischemic zone of myocardium between attacks of unstable angina; however, some degree of reperfusion occurs as a function of time even in acute myocardial infarction,[45] so that interpretation can be difficult (see Fig. 25.1). Recent studies suggest that $^{201}$Tl cellular release rather than accumulation may be a better indicator

of irreversible myocardial ischemia.[46] Development of a method for quantifying this phenomenon would clearly have important diagnostic potential in the setting of unstable angina. Perhaps its most valuable application is in variant angina, when $^{201}$Tl given during an episode of pain is not taken up in the region supplied by the vasopastic artery, but repeat scintigraphy *immediately* after the pain resolves shows reperfusion of the previously ischemic zone.[8,47]

Finally, gated cardiac blood pool imaging permits a noninvasive assessment of ventricular function by calculation of the ejection fraction and ventricular volumes and also by the evaluation of wall motion abnormalities. Either the patient's own red cells or human serum albumin are labeled with $^{99m}$Tc to delineate the blood pool. While the demonstration of impaired ventricular performance during pain supports the diagnosis of myocardial ischemia, as with perfusion imaging, only serial studies showing resolution of these abnormalities, in conjunction with serial ECGs and enzyme determinations, are helpful in distinguishing between unstable angina and acute myocardial infarction.

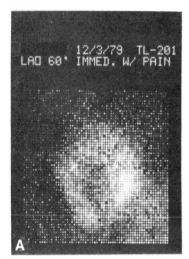 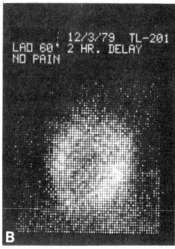 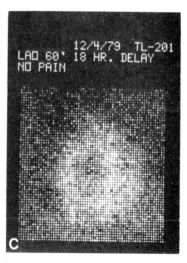

Fig. 25.1   $^{201}$Tl scintigraphy in a patient with unstable angina (all views in 60° LAO projection). $^{201}$Tl was given immediately after an episode of chest pain at rest associated with only minor T-wave inversion on the ECG. The initial study *(A)* showed an anteroapical perfusion defect. The pain resolved within 15 minutes and a repeat study at 2 hours *(B)* showed partial reperfusion of this region. A final study 18 hours later *(C)* showed normal perfusion of the previously ischemic area. Cardiac enzyme determinations were within normal limits during and following this episode. Subsequent angiography revealed a 90 percent stenosis in the proximal left anterior descending coronary artery, with normal LV wall motion.

## Stress Testing

Exercise and other forms of stress testing are contraindicated in unstable angina because of the risk of precipitating myocardial infarction. There are, however, two possible exceptions to this rule. The first exception is that group of patients who have persistently normal ECGs during pain with no clinical or enzymatic evidence of myocardial ischemia and in whom the diagnosis of angina, let alone unstable angina, is based purely on the clinical history. Even in these patients, stress testing should be considered only after other measures (e.g., $^{201}$Tl scintigraphy) have failed to demonstrate myocardial ischemia at rest.

The second is that group of patients with variant angina. In these patients, exercise testing, pharmacologic provocation tests, and cold pressor stimulation have all been used as aids to diagnosis, with variable degrees of safety and success. (See section on Diagnosis of Variant Angina.)

In both groups, however, stress testing should not even be considered until the acute episode has been vigorously treated and the patient's symptoms have been stabilized.

## INITIAL MANAGEMENT

Unstable angina is a medical emergency. The primary objective of therapy is to prevent myocardial infarction or minimize its sequelae. Of equal importance, however, is control of the clinical manifestations of severe ischemia—i.e., angina, heart failure, and arrhythmias.

Patients with unstable angina should be admitted urgently to a hospital—preferably to a well-equipped and fully staffed coronary care unit. It is not usually possible to confidently exclude myocardial infarction on admission, so initial therapy must be applicable to both situations until the diagnosis is established. Rapid differentiation of these two conditions is particularly important from the standpoint of emergency coronary artery bypass surgery. At the present time, this technique is widely used in certain patients with unstable angina, but it is still considered experimental and potentially very hazardous in patients with established

acute myocardial infarction. (Recent studies, however, suggest that emergency surgical revascularization within 5 hours of acute transmural myocardial infarction can be undertaken relatively safely in selected patients.[48])

Patients with unstable angina should have the highest priority for admission to a coronary care unit because, with intensive management, myocardial infarction can be prevented rather than merely limited or palliated. Facilities should be available for continuous clinical and electrocardiographic monitoring and, when indicated, for monitoring of hemodynamic parameters such as arterial, right heart, and left ventricular filling pressures. Ideally, it should also be possible to undertake both coronary arteriography and cardiac surgery at the admitting hospital.

While the diagnosis of unstable angina is being confirmed as previously outlined, initial therapeutic measures are commenced (Table 25.3). Even if emergency coronary artery bypass surgery is indicated, it is usually advisable to initiate intensive medical therapy as an interim measure (see $\beta$-Adrenergic Blockade).

## General Considerations

Marked anxiety and a fear of imminent death are common accompaniments of unstable angina. The resulting sympathetic hyperfunction may actually contribute to a realization of the patient's fears. Continual reassurance from the medical and nursing staff is therefore essential. The purpose of monitoring and resuscitation equipment in the coronary care unit should be explained to the patient at the earliest opportunity. Agents that reduce anxiety, such as diazepam, should be given as regularly as necessary, provided there are no hemodynamic contraindications to their use. The sedative and euphoric properties of nitrous oxide and opiate analgesics are also valuable in this context.

Smoking must obviously be discontinued, as should all sympathomimetic drugs such as nasal decongestants. The patient must be confined to bed initially. A decision about the relative stresses of using a bedpan or a bedside commode must be made for each patient individually. Ideally, the diet should comprise about 1500 calo-

**Table 25.3  Initial Management of the Patient with Unstable Angina**

| Therapeutic Measures | Diagnostic Aims |
|---|---|
| Bed rest | 1) Exclude myocardial infarction |
| Reassurance |    a) clinically |
| Prohibit smoking |    b) by serial electrocardiograms, cardiac enzyme |
| Oxygen |       determinations and radionuclide studies. |
| Analgesia | 2) Exclude: |
| Sedation |    a) non ischemic chest pain syndromes (e.g., peptic ulceration) |
| β-adrenergic blockade |    b) other cardiac diseases (e.g., hypertrophic cardiomyopathy, anemia, thyrotoxicosis) |
| Nitrates | |
| Calcium transport inhibitors | 3) Definition of hemodynamic status by appropriate (e.g., invasive) techniques. |
| Anticoagulants | |
| Antiarrhythmic therapy | |
| Treatment of heart failure including intraaortic balloon counterpulsation | |
| Antihypertensive therapy if indicated. | |

ries per day, with no added salt. Constipation can be avoided by the inclusion of high-residue food in the diet and by the use of stool-softening agents. Prompt recognition and treatment of coexistent medical conditions is essential. Some conditions may restrict the choice of therapy while others, especially uncontrolled systemic hypertension, may seriously affect the overall prognosis.[49]

## Analgesics

A 50 percent mixture of nitrous oxide and oxygen delivered by nasal prongs is often effective in relieving myocardial ischemic pain and also has useful sedative and euphoric properties.[50] Morphine or analogs such as meperidine are commonly administered for severe or prolonged attacks of pain. These drugs should be given intravenously in small doses every 20 to 30 minutes until the pain is abolished, unless respiratory depression occurs. An antiemetic agent (e.g., prochlorperazine) may sometimes be necessary after repeated doses of opiate analgesics.

## Oxygen

Supplemental oxygen therapy may also be given by nasal prongs. In acute myocardial ischemia, coronary vasoconstriction occurs in vessels supplying adequately oxygenated re-

gions of myocardium. If coronary blood flow is already maximal and remains constant, this results in improved perfusion of ischemic zones. A small increase in arterial oxygen extraction may also occur in the ischemic regions.[51] Thus, systemic arterial oxygen desaturation is an undisputed indication for supplemental oxygen therapy. However, the rationale for its use in patients without hypoxia is less clear.

Certain electrocardiographic manifestations of acute myocardial ischemia can be abolished by administration of 100 percent oxygen,[52] but a controlled trial of supplemental oxygen therapy showed no benefit in terms of mortality and morbidity in patients with acute myocardial infarction.[53] Thus, supplemental oxygen therapy is not of proven value in all patients with unstable angina, but it appears to be safe and has some theoretical benefits.

## β-Adrenergic Blocking Agents

β-adrenergic blocking agents are the mainstay of initial therapy in unstable angina. However, the usual absolute or relative contraindications to their use (obstructive airways disease, bradycardia, heart failure, etc.) still apply. The widest experience has been with propranolol, which has had such a beneficial impact on both morbidity and mortality in unstable angina that a placebo-controlled trial of its efficacy has never been undertaken. The antianginal effects of β-adrenergic blockade result from a reduction in myocardial oxygen consumption, principally due to a decrease in heart rate.[54] Therefore, the dose should be increased until the patient is pain-free or until the resting heart rate is less than 60 beats per minute. Further increases in dose are unlikely to be beneficial and may precipitate heart failure or bradyarrhythmias. Using these guidelines, Fischl et al. have reported successful initial control of pain with propranolol in more than 80 percent of patients with unstable angina.[16]

This group used an initial starting dose of 80 mg of propranolol daily by mouth, increasing to 360 to 480 mg/day, depending on the heart rate and blood pressure response. In a few patients, intravenous propranolol (initial dose 0.5 mg) may be considered necessary to achieve rapid $\beta$-adrenergic blockade. The total dose probably should not exceed 0.1 mg/kg by the intravenous route, although little information is available regarding this mode of administration in patients with unstable angina. It appears safe and theoretically advantageous to continue $\beta$-adrenergic blocking drugs through coronary arteriography and even through anesthetic induction and intubation prior to coronary artery bypass surgery, provided left ventricular failure has not occurred.[55] These are two occasions when catecholamine-mediated increases in myocardial oxygen consumption are particularly likely to occur, with disastrous consequences. Theoretically, cardioselective $\beta_1$ antagonists such as metoprolol may be preferable to propranolol, since coronary sympathetic vasodilator tone is probably mediated largely by $\beta_2$ receptors. This may be especially relevant if coronary spasm is suspected.

## Nitrates

These drugs exert their major antianginal effect by reducing preload and, to a lesser extent, afterload on the left ventricle, which leads to a reduction in myocardial oxygen consumption. In addition, nitrates may also redistribute coronary blood flow from normally perfused to underperfused areas of myocardium and thus limit the extent of ischemic injury.[56] The reflex tachycardia that accompanies systemic vasodi-

lation is blocked by concomitant $\beta$-adrenergic blockade, so that large doses of nitrates may be used. Nitrates assume a unique importance in variant angina and are probably the most effective spasmolytic agents currently available. (The role of nitrates in the management of coronary spasm is discussed in detail under "variant angina.") Sublingual nitroglycerin (0.3 to 0.6 mg) is usually given for acute relief of pain, and either 2 percent nitroglycerin paste (0.5 to 1.5 inches) or a long-acting nitrate such as isosorbide dinitrate (10 to 30 mg) is administered every 3 to 6 hours as prophylaxis. The dose should be increased until limited by a supine blood pressure of approximately 100 mm Hg systolic or 60 mm Hg diastolic, or until a headache develops that the patient is unable to tolerate. Further increases in dose may reduce coronary artery perfusion pressure and even precipitate myocardial infarction, so careful clinical monitoring is essential. The dose may need to be reduced at night to enable the patient to sleep. Nitroglycerin can be administered intravenously if rapid unloading of the left ventricle is indicated (initial infusion rate of 5 $\mu$g/minute, with 5 to 10 $\mu$g/minute increments every 2 to 3 minutes to a rate of 30 to 100 $\mu$g/minute). A recent report of the effects of intravenous nitroglycerin in 45 patients with unstable angina indicated that 40 were symptomatically improved within a few hours, even though in 20 patients angina had been refractory to sublingual nitroglycerin.[56a]

However, the caveats attendant upon the use of nitroglycerin paste are even more applicable to intravenous administration. Further, intravenous nitroglycerin is not yet commercially available in the United States, and each hospital pharmacy must prepare its own.

## Calcium Transport Inhibitors

Calcium transport inhibitors antagonize calcium ion flux in both myocardial and smooth muscle cells. This results in a decrease in myocardial contractility and also causes coronary vasodilation by inhibiting smooth muscle contraction.[57]

Both nifedipine[58] and verapamil[59] have been

successfully used in the management of patients
with coronary vasospasm (see variant angina).
In addition, there is evidence to suggest that,
like the nitrates, they may have myocardial protective effects in acute ischemia and might
therefore limit infarct size should myocardial
infarction occur.[60] Thus, calcium transport inhibitors appear to be a rational adjunct to therapy in all patients with unstable angina, but
whether they offer any major therapeutic advantages over the nitrates has not yet been established.

## Anticoagulants

The use of full anticoagulant doses of heparin
to prevent coronary thrombosis in patients with
unstable angina is highly controversial. Present
evidence indicates that coronary thrombosis
may be a consequence rather than a cause of
myocardial infarction,[61] so that the pathologic
basis for anticoagulant therapy is not sound.
However, there is some evidence in the animal
model to suggest that the extent of myocardial
necrosis after acute coronary occlusion can be
limited by pretreatment with heparin.[62] In addition, four clinical studies performed in the early
1960s all concluded that anticoagulation did
prevent myocardial infarction in patients with
unstable angina.[1,29,30,63] The controversy lies in
the fact that none of these trials was adequately
controlled, leaving serious doubt about the validity of the conclusions. The only controlled
study from that era showed no benefit from
antiocoagulants.[64]

Indeed, there is now evidence to suggest that
heparin therapy in patients with angina may
even predispose them to myocardial infarction
by releasing thromboxane $A_2$ (a potent platelet
aggregator and coronary vasoconstrictor) into
the peripheral circulation.[65] The introduction
of early and effective therapy in unstable angina,
in the form of $\beta$-adrenergic blockade and coronary artery bypass surgery, makes it unlikely
that a definitive study of the value of heparin
will ever be undertaken. Our policy has been
to use low-dose, subcutaneous heparin as prophylaxis against deep venous thrombosis while
the patient is confined to bed, but not to fully
anticoagulate with heparin.

## Therapy of Cardiac Failure

The development of left ventricular failure
in a patient with unstable angina often, but not
invariably, signifies that acute myocardial infarction has occurred. Recurrent ventricular
tachyarrhythmias and high-dose $\beta$-blockade
may both predispose to heart failure in the absence of infarction, a situation with important
therapeutic implications. Inotropic support
with drugs such as isoproterenol, epinephrine,
aminophylline, and dopamine can only be effected at the expense of further increases in
myocardial oxygen consumption. The safety of
digoxin in this context is also questionable.[66]
Left ventricular filling pressures can be more
safely reduced with intravenous furosemide
and/or morphine, but careful hemodynamic
monitoring is essential. Nitrates will further reduce preload but, unless adequate $\beta$-adrenergic
blockade has been achieved, these agents may
in some instances cause a reflex tachycardia.
It is recognized that the use of $\beta$-adrenergic
blockade in this situation is potentially hazardous; however, where heart failure is presumed
to be present purely on the basis of acute myocardial ischemia, $\beta$-blocking drugs may actually
improve ventricular performance by alleviating
the ischemia. If heart failure is unresponsive
to these initial measures, then nitroprusside infusion or intraaortic balloon counterpulsation
is indicated (see Refractory Unstable Angina).

## Antiarrhythmic Therapy

Tachyarrhythmias, even sinus tachycardia,
must be vigorously treated because of the unattainable increase in oxygen demand they place
upon the critically ischemic myocardium. Prolonged arrhythmic episodes in these patients
may lead to syncope, heart failure, myocardial
infarction, or death. Relief of the underlying
myocardial ischemia is often necessary before
specific antiarrhythmic therapy is effective. The
indications for both pharmacologic and electrical antiarrhythmic therapy are identical to
those in patients with acute myocardial infarction (see Ch. 15 and 16). Ventricular tachycardia refractory to conventional therapy may
sometimes be terminated by intraaortic balloon

counterpulsation, so that emergency coronary arteriography can be performed.

## FURTHER MANAGEMENT

Rational selection of further treatment for this condition requires a detailed knowledge of both the extent and location of the underlying coronary disease. We therefore advise that coronary arteriography and left ventriculography be performed in all patients with unstable angina, except in those who are considered from the outset to be unsuitable for coronary artery surgery.

### Controlled Unstable Angina

In those patients whose angina and/or hemodynamic disturbances come under control within 24 to 48 hours of intensive medical therapy, we continue this treatment regime and perform coronary arteriography semielectively, usually no later than 7 days after admission to hospital. Patients remain on restricted activity in hospital while awaiting this procedure. This semielective approach has been adopted whenever possible, because of the additional morbidity and mortality associated with coronary arteriography performed in the acute phase of unstable angina.[13,67]

### Refractory Unstable Angina

In 20 to 50 percent of patients, however, unstable angina is refractory to initial medical therapy, and chest pain is continuous or recurs frequently in the first 12 to 24 hours after admission.[26] Recurrent arrhythmias and left ventricular failure may further complicate management in this group. Despite the increased risks, urgent coronary arteriography is required in such patients, with a view to performing emergency coronary bypass surgery if anatomically feasible.

Intraaortic balloon counterpulsation has greatly reduced the risks attending coronary angiography in refractory unstable angina,[68] especially in those patients with postinfarction angina.[69] Its judicious use may even allow coronary arteriography (and coronary artery sur-

gery, if indicated) to be performed semielectively. The two major beneficial effects are an improvement in coronary artery diastolic perfusion pressure and a reduction of left ventricular afterload. In one large study of balloon counterpulsation, however, the device could not be passed from the femoral or iliac vessels in 13 percent of patients, and a further 10 percent of patients developed serious peripheral arterial ischemic complications once the balloon was in place.[70] Not surprisingly, the risks of irreversible ischemia in the lower limbs are even greater in patients with coexistent peripheral vascular disease. These potential hazards have precluded the more widespread use of balloon counterpulsation in patients with unstable angina.

Nitroprusside infusion (10 to 150 $\mu$g/minute) provides an effective alternative to balloon counterpulsation in patients with refractory unstable angina. In addition to afterload reduction, nitroprusside also reduces left ventricular preload and causes direct coronary vasodilation.[71] Unlike balloon counterpulsation though, nitroprusside infusion does not augment diastolic coronary artery perfusion pressure. However, nitroprusside infusion has the advantage of being almost immediately effective, and the short half-life of this agent permits minute-to-minute titration of the hemodynamic response. As with all vasodilators, constant clinical monitoring is necessary to ensure that diastolic arterial pressure does not fall precipitously and further prejudice myocardial perfusion. Coronary steal is a further theoretical hazard of nitroprusside therapy in this situation.

### The Relative Merits of Medical and Surgical Therapy

Following coronary arteriography in any patient with unstable angina, a choice must be made as to the more appropriate form of therapy—medical or surgical. The available evidence on which this decision must be based is confusing and often contradictory. We have therefore attempted an analysis of the nonanecdotal studies of medical and surgical therapy in unstable angina.

When coronary artery bypass grafting was

introduced in the early 1970s, it was widely acclaimed as the treatment of choice in unstable angina. This initial enthusiasm for surgical therapy was not surprising when one considers that prior to that time the only treatments available were nitroglycerin, bed rest, and anticoagulation. Surgery offered a potential for rapid and often complete reversal of the underlying myocardial ischemia in a condition with an otherwise dismal prognosis. Initial reports of operative mortality were high,[72] possibly because some patients were evolving an acute myocardial infarct prior to surgery. Further experience with the technique, however, showed that emergency coronary bypass surgery could be performed with a mortality rate of less than 5 percent in many centers.[73-75]

The advancing wave of enthusiasm for coronary surgery was paralleled by a recognition of the beneficial effects of propranolol in patients with unstable angina.[16,76] Medical therapy also had the major advantages of being more widely available and far less expensive than surgery. Both medical and surgical therapy were clearly effective, but comparative studies of their efficacy were needed. Several studies were subsequently performed in which the results of coronary artery bypass surgery were compared to those of medical therapy in the same institution (see Table 25.4).[13,16,67,77-79] By summating the data from these studies, it may be seen that the mean mortality during an average follow-up of 20 months was 10 percent in surgically treated patients and 20 percent in the medically treated group. Nonfatal myocardial infarctions were diagnosed in 14 percent of those treated surgically but in 21 percent of those treated medically. Most strikingly, however, these studies indicated that only 11 percent of medically treated patients became pain free, whereas surgery rendered 60 percent of patients pain-free on no medical therapy. Moreover, four times as many medically treated patients either were unimproved or still had severe angina on follow-up at 20 months.

However, treatment was not randomized in any of these studies. The larger number of surgically treated patients in all but one of the studies cited attests to the preference for this form of therapy. Consequently, the medically treated

groups invariably contained patients who were inoperable by virtue of either poor left ventricular function or diffuse coronary artery disease. Also, there was no standardization of therapy in the medically treated patients.

Thus, serious doubts remained as to whether the apparent superiority of surgical therapy, both in terms of survival and relief of symptoms, was merely an artifact of patient selection. In a prospective study comparing the results of medical therapy in patients considered operable with those of patients considered technically inoperable, myocardial infarction and death were found to be twice as frequent in the inoperable group.[80] Furthermore, the results in the potentially operable group (14 percent suffered nonfatal myocardial infarctions and 9.5 percent died after 12 months of treatment) were similar to the contemporary results of coronary artery bypass surgery in unstable angina (Table 25.4).

From the earliest days of coronary artery surgery, the need for a controlled trial of medical and surgical therapy in unstable angina was recognized. Thus a multicenter prospective study was initiated in 1972 by the National Heart, Lung and Blood Institute.[6,14] In this study, and in two smaller independent studies,[81,82] therapy was randomized after coronary arteriography had been performed, so that patients requiring obligatory medical or surgical therapy by virtue of their angiographic findings could be excluded from the trials.

Table 25.5 shows a summary of the results from these studies. In contrast to the nonrandomized studies, after a mean follow-up of 26 months the overall incidence of nonfatal myocardial infarction was 27 percent in the surgically treated group, but only 17 percent in the medically treated group. Mortality was comparable in both groups (8 to 9 percent), but symptomatic improvement was still undoubtedly superior in the surgically treated patients.

## NHLBI Study

The large patient population (288) in the NHLBI study permitted further comparison of medical and surgical therapy according to the extent of the underlying coronary disease (Figs. 25.2 and 3). Hospital mortality was lower in

Table 25.4 Nonrandomized Studies Comparing Medical and Surgical Therapy for Unstable Angina in the Same Institution

| Author | Medical Therapy | | | | | | Surgical Therapy | | | | | |
|---|---|---|---|---|---|---|---|---|---|---|---|---|
| | # of pts. | Mean follow-up (mths.) | Non fatal MIs | Deaths | # of pain free pts. | # of pts. with severe angina | # of pts. | Mean follow-up (mths.) | Non fatal MIs | Deaths | # of pain free pts. | # of pts. with severe angina |
| Goodin et al.[77] | 7 | 10 | 2 | 3 | 0 | 2 | 12 | 10 | 1 | 1 | 5 | 0 |
| Fischl et al.[16] | 9 | 32 | 0 | 3 | 1 | 5 | 14 | 22 | 1 | 1 | 10 | 0 |
| Scanlon et al.[67] | 22 | ? | 13 | 6 | 3 | 3 | 39 | ? | 10 | 4 | 25 | 12 |
| Conti et al.[13] | 15 | 10 | 1 | 1 | 0 | 8 | 40 | 17 | 1 | 9 | 21 | 1 |
| Bender et al.[78] | 35 | 20 | 6 | 4 | 0 | 21 | 53 | 20 | 6 | 3 | 35 | 1 |
| Hultgren et al.[79] | 66 | 23 | 11 | 14 | 13 | 23 | 52 | 24 | 10 | 3 | 31 | 6 |
| Totals | 154 | 21* | 33 (21%) | 31 (20%) | 17 (11%) | 62 (40%) | 210 | 20* | 29 (14%) | 21 (10%) | 127 (60%) | 20 (10%) |

MI = myocardial infarction
* = mean individual follow-up
pts = patients

Table 25.5 Randomized Studies Comparing Medical and Surgical Therapy for Unstable Angina in the Same Institution

| Author | Medical Therapy | | | | | | Surgical Therapy | | | | | |
|---|---|---|---|---|---|---|---|---|---|---|---|---|
| | # of pts. | Mean follow-up (mths.) | Non-fatal MIs | Deaths | # of pain free pts. | # of pts. with severe angina | # of pts. | Mean follow-up (mths.) | Non fatal MIs | Deaths | # of pain free pts. | # of pts. with severe angina |
| Pugh et al.[81] | 14 | 19 | 0 | 1 | 1 | 5 | 13 | 18 | 2 | 1 | 7 | 0 |
| Selden et al.[82] | 19 | 4 | 2 | 0 | 2 | 12 | 21 | 4 | 3 | 1 | 9 | 1 |
| NHLBI Study [6,14] | 147 | 30 | 28 | 14 | 65+ | 21 | 141 | 30 | 42 | 14 | 67† | 11 |
| Totals | 180 | 26* | 30 (17%) | 15 (8%) | 68 (38%) | 38 (21%) | 175 | 26* | 47 (27%) | 16 (9%) | 83 (47%) | 12 (7%) |

MI = myocardial infarction
* = mean individual follow-up
† = patients able to work at least part time but ? pain free
pts = patients

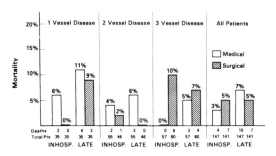

Fig. 25.2 Mortality rates in hospital (INHOSP) and after an average follow-up of 30 months (LATE) for medically and surgically treated patients in the NHLBI comparative study. (Unstable angina pectoris: National cooperative study group to compare medical and surgical therapy. Am J Cardiol 42:839, 1978.)

surgically treated patients with single-vessel disease and in medically treated patients with triple-vessel disease; however, these differences were not significant, and overall hospital mortality was comparable with both forms of therapy (3 to 5 percent). In the last four years of the study, however, hospital mortality fell to only 2 percent in medically treated patients and to 3 percent in those treated surgically. After a mean follow-up of 30 months, no significant differences in mortality were observed between medically and surgically treated patients with single-, double-, or triple-vessel disease.

The overall incidence of in-hospital myocardial infarction was significantly higher in pa-

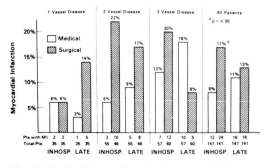

Fig. 25.3 Incidence of nonfatal myocardial infarction in hospital (INHOSP) and after an average follow-up of 30 months (LATE) for medically and surgically treated patients in the NHLBI comparative study. (Unstable angina pectoris: National cooperative study group to compare medical and surgical therapy. Am J Cardiol 42:839, 1978.)

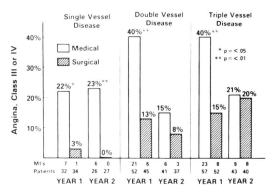

Fig. 25.4 Worst degree of angina (Class III or IV) at any follow-up during the first and second years after randomization in the NHLBI comparative study. (Unstable angina pectoris: National cooperative study group to compare medical and surgical therapy. Am J Cardiol 42:839, 1978.)

tients treated surgically (17 percent as compared to 8 percent in medically treated patients), but there was no apparent difference in those patients with single-vessel disease (6 percent for both forms of treatment). Late myocardial infarction occurred more commonly in surgically treated patients with single- and double-vessel disease but was more common in medically treated patients with triple-vessel disease. Overall, the incidence of late myocardial infarction was comparable with both forms of therapy (11 to 13 percent).

Symptomatic improvement was assessed by comparing the number of patients with New York Heart Association functional Class III or IV angina in each group, one and two years after randomization (Fig 25.4). Severe angina was found to be significantly more common in all medically treated patients after one year (36 percent, as compared to 11 percent in those who underwent surgery) but only in medically treated patients with single-vessel disease after two years (23 percent as compared to none of those treated surgically). The overall incidence of severe angina at two years was 19 percent in patients managed medically and 11 percent in those who had surgery. However, 31 percent of patients initially randomized to medical therapy had crossed over within two years and underwent surgery because of intolerable symptoms, so that the true incidence of severe angina

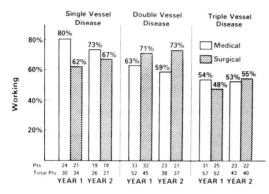

Fig. 25.5 Percentage of patients working at least part-time after one and two years of follow-up in the NHLBI comparative study. (Unstable angina pectoris: National cooperative study group to compare medical and surgical therapy. Am J Cardiol 42:839, 1978.)

in patients treated medically was much higher than 19 percent.

The ability of patients to work, at least part-time, was used as a further index of therapeutic success (Fig 25.5). There was no significant difference between the work status of the two groups one and two years after randomization, but patients with triple-vessel disease were less commonly able to work than those with single- and double-vessel disease, regardless of the mode of treatment.

In the subgroup of patients with refractory unstable angina, one randomized study showed that medical therapy was attended by a significantly higher mortality than surgical therapy after 8 months of follow-up.[83] In this study, however, therapy was randomized *before* coronary arteriography had been performed, and left main coronary disease was not considered an indication for obligatory surgical therapy. Consequently, the survival figures in this series are not directly comparable to those of the NHLBI sponsored study.

In summary, the NHLBI study showed no difference in mortality between medically and surgically treated patients with unstable angina. However, an unspecified number of patients were excluded from the study because their angiographic findings were felt to warrant obligatory medical or surgical therapy (see An Approach to Selection of Therapy). The incidence of in-hospital myocardial infarction was higher

in surgically treated patients, but surgery afforded a better prospect for significant and lasting symptomatic improvement. Other studies have shown that surgical therapy appears more effective in reversing ischemic impairment of left ventricular function,[84,85] which may explain the better long-term symptomatic results after surgery. In view of the comparable survival figures associated with medical and surgical therapy, considerable attention has been devoted to their relative cost effectiveness.

A recent survey of patients employed before the onset of unstable angina has shown that 68 percent of those treated medically and 53 percent of those treated surgically were gainfully employed after a mean follow-up period of 38 months.[86] Patients who underwent initial surgery also had the largest reduction in personal income over that period. The in-patient costs of coronary artery bypass surgery were approximately $10,000—more than double those of medical treatment—but the final cost to patients requiring later surgery after an initial trial of medical therapy was over $20,000.[87]

## An Approach to Selection of Therapy

In approximately 10 percent of patients presenting with unstable angina, no significant coronary artery lesions are demonstrable at angiography.[12] These patients are therefore obliged to continue intensive medical therapy as already outlined (see also Variant Angina). Others may require chronic medical therapy because they are found to have inoperable coronary artery disease (small-caliber distal vessels, posterior location, or diffuse lesions). Patients with a left ventricular ejection fraction of less than 30 percent and an end-diastolic volume greater than 125 ml/m² body surface area are also considered inoperable in most centers and are obliged to continue medical therapy.[14]

Conversely, 15 percent of patients are found to have a 50 percent or greater luminal narrowing of the left main coronary artery,[12] an absolute indication for surgical treatment. This is because of the now well-established superiority of surgical therapy in improving the prognosis of this condition.[88] In addition, unremitting pain with widespread ischemic ECG changes,

**Table 25.6   An Approach to Selection of Medical or Surgical Treatment in Unstable Angina**

| Medical Treatment | Surgical Treatment |
|---|---|
| *Absolute indications* | *Absolute indications* |
| Inoperable coronary disease. | Left main coronary disease. |
| Very poor left ventricular function. | Angina at rest, arrhythmias or heart failure refractory to intensive medical therapy. |
| No coronary disease. | |
| Hemodynamically insignificant coronary disease. | Recurrence of intolerable symptoms whilst on optimal medical therapy. |
| Coexistent medical conditions that preclude surgery. | |
| *Relative indications* | *Relative indications* |
| Coronary vasospasm. | Multiple-vessel disease. |
| Single-vessel disease. | Moderate impairment of left ventricular function. |
| Rapid and persistent improvement following initial medical therapy. | Postinfarction angina. |
| | Previous myocardial infarction. |
| Recent onset of effort induced angina. | Young patients. |
| Elderly patients. | Contraindication to $\beta$-adrenergic blockade. |
| Reluctance to have surgery. | Home or work remote from a major medical center. |
| | Heavy manual occupation. |

refractory arrhythmias, or intractable heart failure are all considered absolute indications for urgent surgical revascularization if anatomically feasible.[14]

In the remaining patients, we generally advise a trial of continuing medical therapy on an outpatient basis and resort to later surgery only if symptoms recur or persist. For socioeconomic as well as clinical reasons, however, our threshold for advising elective surgery is low, especially in younger patients. Several other factors may also influence the decision to offer surgery without a preliminary trial of medical therapy (see Table 25.6).

## Results of Therapy

The results of surgery in patients controlled by initial medical therapy are broadly comparable to those of surgery for chronic stable angina (90 percent survival at seven years, with 80 percent of patients able to return to work in one series.[26]) Preliminary experience suggests that delaying coronary bypass surgery for up to two years does not adversely affect outcome in this group.[14] Operative mortality is higher in patients whose symptoms are refractory to initial medical therapy (5.5 percent compared to 1.8 percent), but 80 percent are still alive seven years after surgery.[26]

The results of medical therapy in those patients who have no coronary atheromatous disease are not well established. Some will have variant angina, but in others no pathogenetic mechanism can be identified. The overall prognosis in such patients with chronic stable angina is good,[89] but it may be unwise to assume that this is also the case in patients with unstable angina.[90] Those with operable coronary disease whose symptoms remain controlled by medical therapy are apparently at no greater risk from death or late myocardial infarction than those treated by initial surgery.[14] By contrast, those with inoperable coronary disease and/or poor left ventricular function are twice as likely to die or suffer a myocardial infarct within 12 months of presentation.[80] Reports on the in-hospital mortality of medically treated patients with fixed coronary stenoses have varied from 0 to 27 percent,[13,16,67] but there were considerable variations in both the type and dose of drugs used, the total duration of therapy, and the severity of underlying coronary disease. In the last few years, however, an upward trend has been noted in the survival associated with medical therapy, which may reflect an improvement in the treatment regimes employed.[14]

## CONCLUSIONS

Unstable angina is not a discrete clinical entity, but rather a diverse collection of clinical syndromes resulting from severe myocardial ischemia. The severity of the myocardial ischemia is variable, and the overlap with stable angina on the one hand and acute myocardial infarction on the other is ill defined. Even the presumed mechanisms of myocardial ischemia vary from case to case. It is therefore not surprising that the results of therapy in this condition have been wide-ranging and have often been frankly contradictory.

Further improvements in the management of patients with unstable angina will depend to a large extent on the identification of homogeneous clinical and pathological subgroups. This has been clearly demonstrated in the case of patients with coronary spasm and also in those with left main coronary disease. At the present time, however, there are no totally reliable clinical markers of these pathologic entities, and coronary arteriography remains necessary in all patients with unstable angina.

Coronary artery surgery has emerged as a relatively safe and effective, albeit costly, alternative to medical therapy, with apparent superior long-term symptomatic improvement. It remains to be seen whether this holds true for all the clinicopathologic subgroups of unstable angina, however. It is also possible that recent improvements in medical therapy will redress the balance with respect to long-term relief from angina.

Since prognosis appears comparable with both medical and surgical therapy in the majority of patients with controlled unstable angina, the attending physician must make a reasoned decision about whether or not to advise surgery and, if so, when. Until more is known about the various subgroups of unstable angina, it seems reasonable to reserve elective surgical therapy for those patients whose lifestyle or personality would be unsuited to continued supervised medical treatment.

## VARIANT ANGINA AND OTHER MANIFESTATIONS OF CORONARY SPASM

### INTRODUCTION

Coronary spasm was first alluded to as a possible cause of myocardial ischemia in 1768 by Heberden.[91] In 1910, Osler stated that "spasm or narrowing of a coronary artery or even of one branch, may so modify the action of a section of the heart that it works with disturbed tension . . . sufficient to arouse painful sensations."[4] Despite these observations, the prevailing view for the next 50 years was that angina invariably resulted from a primary increase in myocardial oxygen demand rather than from a decrease in oxygen supply.

Then, in 1959, Prinzmetal et al. described a group of patients with a variant form of angina[92] in whom there was no apparent increase in myocardial oxygen demand prior to the onset of pain. The clinical syndrome was one of increasingly frequent attacks of severe angina at rest, associated with ST segment elevation on the electrocardiogram taken during pain. Nearly 40 percent of Prinzmetal's patients went on to suffer myocardial infarction, and 10 percent died, the autopsy specimens all showing significant proximal coronary atherosclerosis. Prinzmetal concluded that coronary spasm at the site of athermatous lesions was the probable cause of this syndrome, leading to transient coronary artery occlusion. Numerous angiographic studies during episodes of Prinzmetal's angina have subsequently confirmed beyond doubt that coronary vasospasm does occur in the vicinity of proximal atherosclerotic lesions leading to reversible, but often complete, coronary occlusion (Fig 25.6).[27,93-95]

Coronary vasospasm, however, has now been implicated in a wide range of clinical syndromes other than that which Prinzmetal et al. originally described. It has been shown to occur spontaneously in large, proximal coronary arteries that are totally free from coronary atheroma and also in those arteries with only mild, nonobstructive atherosclerotic lesions.[96-100] In each instance, spasm may lead to transient coronary occlusion. Coronary spasm has been documented in patients in the absence of anginal pain,[94,101] in the absence of ST segment or T wave changes on the ECG (Fig 25.7),[102] and in both nonexertional and exercise-induced angina associated with ST segment *depression* on the ECG. Further, it has been observed that, in certain patients with documented coronary spasm, the direction and magnitude of ST segment changes on the ECG may vary from one episode of pain to the next or change pro-

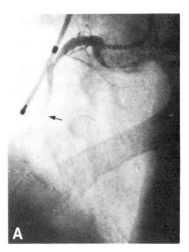 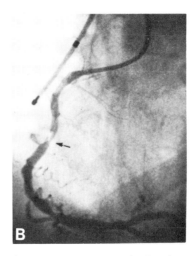

Fig. 25.6 *(A)* Selective right coronary anteriogram during a spontaneous attack of variant angina associated with ST segment elevation of the inferior ECG limb leads and total occlusion of the artery in its mid third *(arrow)*. Following sublingual nitroglycerin, the ST segments became isoelectric and pain resolved. A repeat injection *(B)* showed antegrade flow past a significant anterosclerotic obstruction at the site of the previous spasm (arrow). (Johnson AD et al: Variant angina pectoris: Clinical presentations, coronary angiographic patterns and the results of medical and surgical management in 42 consecutive patients. Chest 73:786, 1978.) MacAlpin (Am J Cardiol 46:143, 1980) has suggested that in most patients coronary spasm is intimately associated with organic coronary stenosis.

gressively during a single episode. Mitral valve prolapse has also been seen in association with both spontaneous and pharmacologically induced coronary spasm.[105,106] In addition, coronary spasm superimposed on a high-grade atherosclerotic lesion has been reported in 6 of 15 patients within 6 hours of acute myocardial infarction,[107] but whether this was cause or effect was not established. Finally, coronary spasm has been proposed as a possible etiologic factor in the sudden death syndrome. Recurrent ventricular tachyarrhythmias may sometimes be precipitated by coronary spasm;[108] and it is by no means unusual for the coronary arteries to be only minimally diseased or even free from atherosclerosis in cases of sudden death. Thus, variant angina is by no means the only consequence of coronary spasm. Indeed, it appears to be implicated across the entire clinical spectrum of acute myocardial ischemia.

## DEFINITION

Variant angina may be defined as chest pain associated with ST segment elevation on the electrocardiogram which occurs at rest and which is usually reversed by the administration of nitroglycerin. The term variant angina has been used synonymously with Prinzmetal's angina; this is not strictly correct, however, since Prinzmetal described a group of patients who were all presumed to have severe coronary atherosclerosis. Although this distinction may appear semantic, much confusion in the literature on coronary spasm has stemmed from imprecise definition. Variant angina, as defined above, is a broader, entirely clinical definition and makes no assumptions regarding underlying pathology. It includes patients both with and without coexistent fixed obstructive coronary disease. Note that, although coronary vasospasm is not mentioned in the definition either, to date no other pathogenetic basis for variant angina has been demonstrated. In an attempt to describe a clinically homogeneous group of patients, this definition excludes those who have nonexertional angina that is associated exclusively with ST segment depression but that is nonetheless reversed by nitroglycerin.[7,94] In some of these patients at least, coronary spasm is undoubtedly implicated; thus, for diagnostic and therapeutic purposes, they may be considered comparable

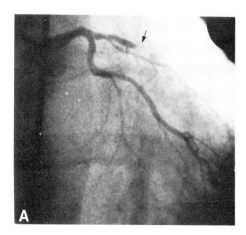 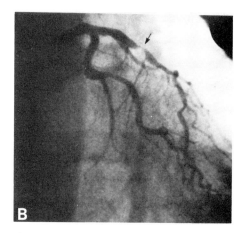

Fig. 25.7 *(A)* Selective left coronary arteriogram during a spontaneous attack of angina at rest, with no associated ST segment shift on the ECG, and a total proximal occlusion of the left anterior descending artery. After initial sublingual nitroglycerin, the pain resolved and the ECG remained normal. However, a repeat injection *(B)* showed antegrade distal filling of the anterior descending artery past a high-grade atherosclerotic lesion at the site of the previous spasm. (Johnson AD et al: Variant angina pectoris: Clinical presentations, coronary angiographic patterns and the results of medical and surgical management in 42 consecutive patients. Chest 73:786, 1978.)

Further support for the concept of intermittent coronary artery obstruction due to vasospasm and/or reversible platelet aggregation as a cause of unstable angina has been provided by Neill et al., who obtained sequential coronary angiograms in patients at the time of acute coronary insufficiency and then several months later. Patients with stable angina served as a control group. New occlusions in the patients with unstable angina occurred in severely narrowed arteries previously correlated with regional ST-T changes; these obstructed vessels had normal baseline collaterals, thus providing indirect evidence that the acute coronary-insufficiency syndrome commonly represents intermittent transient coronary artery occlusion and a threat of new permanent occlusion of the same artery. (Neill WA, Wharton TP Jr, Fluri-Lundeen J, Cohen IS: Acute coronary insufficiency—coronary occlusion after intermittent ischemic attacks. N Engl J Med 302:1157, 1980.)

to those with variant angina. Whether or not this holds true for prognostic considerations, however, is less clear. The myriad of clinical and electrocardiographic manifestations that can be produced by coronary spasm precludes a more precise definition.

## POSSIBLE CAUSES OF CORONARY SPASM

Current evidence points overwhelmingly to an abnormality of autonomic nervous system regulation as the principal mechanism of coronary spasm. In particular, $\alpha$-adrenergic receptors on large epicardial coronary arteries seem to be involved. Stimulation of these receptors in vitro causes marked vasoconstriction.[109] Several studies have further shown that a significant basal level of $\alpha$-adrenergic vasoconstrictor tone, capable of independently altering coronary vascular resistance, exists in the coronary tree.[110,111] Yasue et al. were able to consistently initiate coronary spasm similar to spontaneous attacks in four patients with variant angina by infusion of $\alpha$-receptor agonists.[112] Ricci et al. showed that $\alpha$-adrenergic antagonists could be used to abruptly terminate spontaneous coronary spasm in some cases and to prevent recurrent spasm in others.[115] Recent data suggest that both exercise-induced[113] and cold-induced[21] coronary spasm may also be $\alpha$-receptor mediated. Indeed, ergonovine maleate, an ergot alkaloid with $\alpha$-adrenergic agonist properties, has been widely used as a provocative test for coronary spasm. (See Pharmacological Provocation of Coronary Spasm).

Human coronary arteries are also rich in $\beta_2$ receptors, whose stimulation causes vasodilatation. Pharmacologic blockade of these receptors might be expected to worsen coronary spasm because of the unopposed $\alpha$-receptor mediated coronary vasoconstriction.[114] While there have been reports of coronary spasm precipitated by propranolol administration,[101] this finding has not been universal. Although there is good indirect evidence for an abnormality of sympathetic nervous regulation in the pathogenesis of coronary spasm,[115] Robertson et al. were unable to show an increase in plasma or urinary catecholamines during or after spontaneous coronary spasm.[101] An increase in $\alpha$-adrenoceptor sensitivity in that portion of the vessel affected by coronary spasm would be consistent with all these observations, but there are currently no data to support this hypothesis.

Some evidence implicates the parasympathetic nervous system in the genesis of coronary spasm. Cholinergic drugs such as methacholaline can precipitate coronary spasm, and atropine is an effective spasmolytic agent.[116] Under normal circumstances, vagal stimulation appears to augment sympathetic coronary vasoconstrictor tone, possibly through presynaptic cholinergic receptors, the activation of which facilitate local norepinephrine release.[116] Moreover, parasympathetic tone is subject to marked circadian variation, being greatest at night,[117] when spontaneous coronary spasm is most frequent.

Three other possible mechanisms for the induction of coronary spasm deserve mention. First, it has been suggested that the myotatic reflex in the tunica media of coronary vessels subject to spasm is abnormally sensitive. Catheter-induced spasm, particularly in the proximal portion of the right coronary artery, may be triggered by this myotatic reflex.

The second possibility concerns the recent discovery of $\alpha_2$ receptors on human platelets.[118] It is possible that, under the influence of circulating catecholamines, platelets are sensitized to thrombin and other local tissue factors, facilitating the release of thromboxane $A_2$, which has marked platelet aggregating and vasoconstrictor properties. In support of this hypothesis, abnormally high levels of thromboxane $A_2$ metabolites have been found in peripheral blood samples after coronary spasm.[24]

The third possibility is that one of the many locally vasoactive substances found in the heart—e.g., adenosine, lactate, and histamine—may be involved in either the initiation or the termination of coronary spasm.[118a] These effects may be mediated via an inhibition of inward current in coronary smooth muscle associated with calcium ion flux.[118b] Additional evidence implicating histamine comes from the recent identification of $H_1$ receptors on human coronary arteries, whose stimulation in vitro leads to profound vasoconstriction.[119] In conclusion, it seems probable that, once a coronary vessel becomes predisposed to vasospasm, a variety of physical, pharmacological and neurohumoral influences can precipitate its recurrence. Thus, some if not all of the causes of coronary spasm that have been identified to date (Table 25.7) above may merely be secondary phenomena.

## PATHOGENESIS OF VARIANT ANGINA

As with other forms of unstable angina, the spectrum of underlying coronary disease in variant angina ranges from no atherosclerosis to diffuse triple-vessel disease. In the NHLBI study of unstable angina, the severity and distribution of coronary atherosclerosis were not significantly different in the subgroup of 79 pa-

Table 25.7  **Factors Which Have Been Shown to Precipitate Coronary Vasospasm in Man**

| Pharmacologic Factors | Physical Factors |
|---|---|
| $\alpha$-adrenergic agonists | Exercise |
| $\beta$-adrenergic antagonists | Cold |
| Ergot alkaloids | Catheter manipulation in coronary |
| Norepinephrine | ostium |
| Epinephrine | Hyperventilation |
| Alcohol | |
| Smoking | |

tients with variant angina.[120] Johnson et al.[102] compared the coronary angiographic findings in 42 patients who had variant angina with those of age- and sex-matched controls who had chest pain at rest without ST segment elevation on the ECG. In this study, normal coronary arteries, trivial disease, and single-vessel disease were more common in patients with variant angina, while left main and triple-vessel disease were more frequent in those with decubitus angina (see Fig. 25.8). Significant coronary atherosclerosis has been reported in 40 to 100 percent of patients with variant angina, being apparently more common in the United States and Western Europe than in Japan.[94,121-124] To date, no epidemiologic explanation for this disparity has been found. Proximal single-vessel disease is frequently found in the ischemic territory suggested by the ECG, but is often not sufficiently severe to explain the patient's symptoms.[121] Atherosclerotic lesions presumably serve as a focus for superimposed coronary spasm in such cases, although the cause-and-effect relationship between these two entities is by no means clear-cut. Indeed, Marzilli et al. have suggested that recurrent coronary vasospasm may be important in the pathogenesis of fixed atherosclerotic coronary disease.[124a]

The angiographic demonstration of spontaneous coronary vasospasm has been reported in about 20 percent of patients with variant angina; however, in series where pharmacologic provocation tests have been employed to induce spasm, the overall yield is nearer 90 percent. Coronary spasm is usually seen in the epicardial portion of a single coronary vessel, but occasionally multiple vasopastic areas are found.[108] It has been suggested that the right coronary artery is especially vulnerable to spasm,[120] but review of a large number of case reports suggests that it is at least as common in the left anterior descending artery. It is not known whether the distal vessel beyond the demonstrated site of occlusion is also vasospastic, but direct observation of coronary vasospasm during surgery suggests that it may occur over a segment of up to 4 cm in length.[121] As previously mentioned, the hemodynamic changes occurring with rest pain induced by coronary spasm tend to differ from those found in other cases of nonexertional angina. Systemic arterial pressure, heart rate, and left ventricular filling pressure do not appear to rise prior to the onset of variant angina,[7] suggesting that a reduction of coronary blood flow, rather than an increase in myocardial oxygen consumption, is the initiating event. Moreover, left ventricular function remains depressed throughout the ischemic episode, and autonomic reflex augmentation of left ventricular contractility, commonly seen in other cases of unstable angina, does not usually occur.[7] Transient localized dyskinesis in the region of the left ventricle supplied by the vasospastic vessel may sometimes be demonstrated angiographically during such an attack (Fig. 25.9).[125]

Spontaneous resolution of the pain is often accompanied by an overshoot of blood pressure and heart rate, which return to normal within a few minutes after the electrocardiographic ST segments become isoelectric. These hemodynamic findings are all very similar to those following experimental acute coronary occlusion in the conscious dog.[22]

Thus, coronary spasm, either alone or superimposed on an atheromatous lesion, appears to be the pathophysiologic basis for variant angina, with the ST segment elevation implying transmural myocardial ischemia. The occurrence of ST segment depression with similar hemodynamic changes can also result from coronary

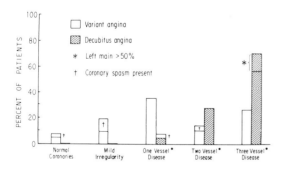

Fig. 25.8  A comparison of the distribution of coronary atheroma in patients with variant and decubitus angina. (Johnson AD et al: Variant angina pectoris: Clinical presentations, coronary angiographic patterns and the results of medical and surgical management in 42 consecutive patients. Chest 73:786, 1978.)

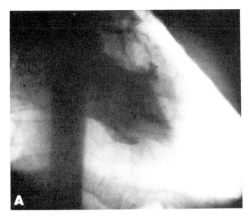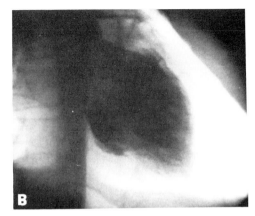

Fig. 25.9   Left ventriculogram (30° RAO projection) revealing a transient inferior wall motion abnormality during an episode of variant angina. (*A* in systole, *B* in diastole.)

spasm, but the resulting myocardial ischemia is presumably restricted to the subendocardial zone in such cases.

## INCIDENCE AND NATURAL HISTORY

The incidence of variant angina is unknown, but it accounts for approximately 25 percent of all cases of unstable angina.[14] The natural history seems to largely depend on the severity and location of any coexistent coronary atheroma. In the past, different interpretations of the definition of variant angina obscured this fact. As previously noted, Prinzmetal's patients had a poor prognosis, with a 10 percent mortality, and a 40 percent incidence of myocardial infarction over an unspecified period.[92] Coronary pathology was not defined in the survivors, but the autopsy findings in those who died revealed severe proximal atherosclerotic coronary disease. Silverman and Flamm's review[122] indicated an even worse prognosis, with almost 60 percent of patients suffering myocardial infarction or death within one year of presentation. Once more, however, the extent of underlying coronary atheroma in these patients was not always known. Selzer et al. attempted to clarify this issue by comparing the outcome of patients without significant coronary atheroma to that of patients having severe coronary disease.[126] They concluded that variant angina without severe coronary disease generally ran a benign course, since there were no deaths on follow-up in this group. The small but definite risk

for such patients was myocardial infarction associated with serious arrhythmias. The prognosis of the group with high-grade coronary disease, however, was not good despite medical therapy, with a 15 percent mortality and a 20 percent incidence of myocardial infarction over the same period.

Sudden death not due to myocardial infarction in patients with variant angina has been found to occur most frequently in those with left anterior descending coronary disease, and ventricular arrhythmias are often diagnosed prior to death.[121]

The long-term outlook for patients with variant angina is unpredictable, but several cases have been reported where symptoms regressed or even disappeared with time, despite the coexistence of coronary atherosclerosis.[126-128]

## DIAGNOSIS

The diagnosis of variant angina should be considered in any patient who presents with angina at rest. This diagnosis is confirmed by the finding of reversible ST segment elevation in the standard leads of an ECG taken during pain. Long periods of bed rest or ambulatory monitoring may be necessary to document this finding. In order to ascertain the diagnosis, it is also often necessary to withdraw any medications, especially nitrates, which might inhibit coronary vasospasm.

As with other forms of unstable angina, the

diagnostic priority is to exclude acute myocardial infarction, which it may closely resemble. (The methods by which this is accomplished are detailed earlier in the section dealing with unstable angina. Only those features specific to the diagnosis of variant angina are further discussed here.)

## Clinical and Electrocardiographic Features

The clinical and electrocardiographic features of variant angina tend to differ slightly, depending on whether or not severe atheromatous coronary disease is present. Table 25.8 shows some of the differences that have been reported [27,126] although it should be emphasized that none of these are absolute and that other studies have failed to show any differences between the two groups.[129] The character and radiation of the pain are identical to those found in classical, effort-induced angina. While no obvious precipitant is found in most cases, smoking,[130] alcohol,[131] or prolonged emotional stress [90] may all initiate an attack in predisposed individuals.

Classically, exercise is said not to induce chest pain or ST segment elevation on the ECG in patients with variant angina.[121] However, it is now clear that some patients can suffer both resting and exercise-induced coronary vasospasm.[132,133] Until recently, it was not clear whether such patients constituted yet another "coronary spasm syndrome" distinct from variant angina. However, Yasue et al.[134] have now shown a circadian variation in the exercise capacity of patients with variant angina, both with and without coronary atherosclerosis. When exercised early in the morning, his patients consistently suffered chest pain with ST segment elevation on the ECG. Identical exercise stress in the afternoon, however, failed to induce angina or ECG changes in every case. Thus, it may be that exercise-induced coronary spasm with diurnal variation is an integral feature of variant angina that explains the so-called "warm-up effect" of exercise in this condition.[135]

The rest pain, too, has a diurnal rhythm, often occurring in the early morning, waking the patient from sleep.[27] Other manifestations of abnormal arterial vasomotion should also be inquired into (e.g., migraine, Raynaud's phenomenon) since these are particularly common in patients with variant angina.[136]

As with other forms of unstable angina, the diagnosis of variant angina is more often confused with acute myocardial infarction than with stable angina. Indeed, if the attack is not terminated, myocardial infarction, ventricular tachycardia, or death may ensue.

**Table 25.8   Some Features of Variant Angina Which May Differ Between Patients with and without Severe Coronary Atherosclerosis**

| Little or No Coronary Atherosclerosis | Severe Coronary Atherosclerosis (Prinzmetal's angina) |
| --- | --- |
| More common in premenopausal women. | More common in men aged 40–60 years, similar to stable angina. |
| Previous myocardial infarct uncommon. | Previous effort related angina and/or myocardial infarct common. |
| ECG may be normal between attacks. | ST segment depression and T wave inversion common between attacks. |
| Long history, with stable frequency and severity of pain. | Short history, with crescendo in frequency and severity of pain. |
| Attacks often of short duration (less than 1 minute). | Attacks of pain often last 10 minutes or more. |
| ST segment elevation commonly is seen in inferior ECG leads. | ST segment elevation more common in anterior and lateral ECG leads. |
| Right coronary artery frequently involved. | Left anterior descending or circumflex coronary arteries frequently involved. |
| Bradycardia or heart block more common during pain. | Ventricular tachyarrhythmias more common during pain. |
| Good prognosis if serious arrhythmias not present. | Poor prognosis without treatment. |

There are no clinical features that will reliably differentiate between variant angina and acute myocardial infarction, but variant angina is more frequently improved by the administration of nitroglycerin.[101] Physical examination between attacks may be unremarkable, but the absence of an increase in blood pressure or heart rate prior to or during an attack of pain is highly suggestive of variant angina.[136] (See Pathogenesis of Variant Angina.)

Patients with variant angina share the unifying electrocardiographic abnormality of ST segment elevation during chest pain at rest in the territory of a single, major coronary vessel. Reciprocal ST segment depression is also seen in the appropriate leads, mimicking acute myocardial infarction. The ST segment elevation is often very marked, implying transmural ischemia,[23] and the resultant complexes sometimes resemble a monophasic intracellular action potential. ST segment depression may occur in the same ECG leads during a single episode of pain (Fig. 25.10). ST segment alternans, another marker of severe transmural ischemia, has also been described in this condition.[137] Abnormalities of the QRS complex are often seen in the same distribution. These include: an increase in amplitude and duration of the R wave;[127] less commonly, a reduction of R wave voltage;[138] and the transient appearance of Q waves[34] during pain, without confirmatory evidence of myocardial necrosis. The ECG between attacks may be normal, but frequently it shows ST-segment depression and T-wave inversion in the same distribution as the changes seen during pain. While an abnormal ECG between attacks is a poor guide to the presence of underlying coronary atherosclerosis, an entirely normal record often signifies no atheromatous coronary disease.[126] Approximately 50 percent of patients experience arrhythmias during an attack, usually when the pain is at its

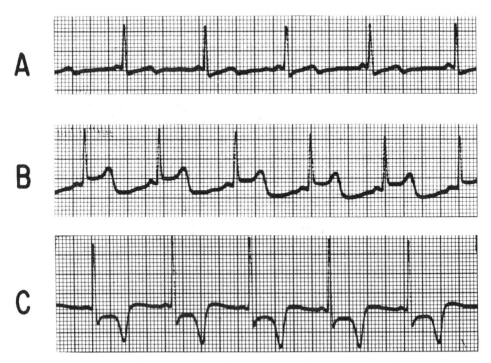

Fig. 25.10 Serial electrocardiograms (monitoring lead) taken from a patient with variant angina. *(A)* Prior to the onset of pain, there was 1 mm ST segment depression. *(B)* Thirty seconds before the onset of pain, ST segment elevation developed and persisted throughout the attack. *(C)* Sixty seconds after 0.5 mg. sublingual nitroglycerin, 2 mm ST segment depression was seen with deep T-wave inversion. R-wave amplitude was also increased compared to strips A and B. Within 3 minutes, the electrocardiogram resumed the configuration seen in strip A.

most severe (Fig. 25.11).[139] Ventricular tachyarrhythmias occur most commonly in patients with underlying atherosclerotic coronary disease,[140] while sinus bradycardia and occasionally heart block tend to predominate in those with normal coronary vessels.[126] This is probably because of the relatively higher frequency with which the right coronary artery, which usually supplies the sinus and atrioventricular

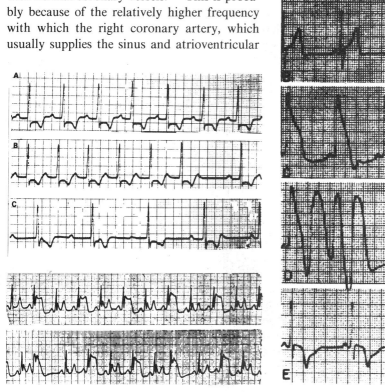

Fig. 25.11   Arrhythmias and depolarization abnormalities.
*(Upper left)* Noncontinuous rhythm strips (monitor lead) taken during an attack of variant angina, showing first-degree A-V block *(A)*, Mobitz type I second-degree A-V block *(B)*, and third-degree A-V block *(C)*. (Bharati S et al: Conduction system in a patient with Prinzmetal's angina and transient atrioventricular block. Am J Cardiol 39:120, 1977.)
*(Lower left)* Monitor lead recording of 2:1 ST segment elevation alternans during an episode of variant angina. (Williams RR et al: ST segment alternans in Prinzmetal's angina: A report of two cases. Ann Intern Med 81:51, 1974.) *(Right)* Noncontinuous monitor lead recordings: *(A)* Before attack. *(B)* At onset of pain showing ST segment elevation. *(C)* The ST segment elevation becomes progressively more marked. *(D)* Episodes of tachycardia follow, which are probably ventricular in origin. *(E)* Steep T-wave inversion is seen after the tachycardia has resolved. (Smithen C et al:Variant angina pectoris. Am Heart J 89:87, 1975.)

nodal branches, is the vessel affected by spasm in patients with otherwise normal arteries.[126]

## Coronary Angiography

All patients fulfilling the ECG and clinical prerequisites for the diagnosis of variant angina should undergo selective coronary arteriography. This is necessary to determine the severity and extent of the underlying coronary atherosclerosis (if any) which has a major bearing on both prognosis and treatment. It is also undertaken with the objective of demonstrating coronary vasospasm in the vessel supplying the ischemic territory suggested from the ST segment elevation on the ECG. The angiographic demonstration of spontaneous coronary spasm is to some extent fortuitous, and pharmacologic spasm provocation may therefore be indicated to confirm the diagnosis in selected cases.

However, many features of the routine technique of coronary arteriography can potentially obscure the demonstration of coronary spasm, so some modifications of technique and some simple precautions are usually necessary. Firstly, the angiographic study should be scheduled at the time of day when spontaneous attacks of pain are most common. Next, premedications of any sort, especially those containing diazepam or atropine, should be avoided wherever possible. This is because both drugs have a spasmolytic effect on the coronary arteries.[141,142] The practice of giving nitroglycerin just prior to injecting contrast medium into the coronary tree should clearly also be avoided for the same reason. The total dose of angiographic contrast medium should be kept to a minimum since it, too, has direct coronary vasodilator properties. Therefore coronary arteriography should ideally be performed prior to left ventriculography, and the vessel suspected from the ST segment elevation on the ECG should be delineated first if possible. Catheter manipulation should be kept to a minimum to avoid the possibility of catheter-induced spasm, to which the patient's symptoms might be wrongly ascribed.

The use of a Sones coronary catheter introduced through a right brachial arteriotomy is preferable, since it facilitates rapid sequential study of right and left coronary vessels without the need for a change of catheters.

Finally, if an episode of pain or ST segment elevation on the ECG occurs during the procedure, prompt but cautious selective angiographic definition of the appropriate vessel should be attempted. Vasospasm often occludes the vessel totally, whether or not there is coexistent atherosclerotic disease. After the demonstration of spasm, nitroglycerin should be given either sublingually or intravenously, and the angiogram should be repeated to confirm that the spasm has been reversed. If nitroglycerin does not relieve the spasm, an intravenous infusion of sodium nitroprusside should be commenced immediately. Special attention must be paid to accurately documenting the site and severity of any atheroma in the vessel involved. In the absence of pain or ST segment changes in the ECG during baseline angiography, it is still necessary to repeat the study after the injection of nitroglycerin if any coronary narrowing has been seen, to rule out spasm as the cause. Arrhythmias must be anticipated and treated appropriately, equipment for DC cardioversion should be available, and a temporary pacing wire should be inserted prophylactically at the start of the procedure in any patient who has previously demonstrated bradyarrhythmias during pain.

## Pharmacological Provocation of Coronary Spasm

Even when all the precautions cited above are observed, spontaneous coronary spasm is found in fewer than 3 percent of unselected patients being investigated for angina pectoris[143] and only in about 20 percent of patients with variant angina.[144] Angiographic confirmation of coronary spasm can be an extremely important factor in selecting therapy in patients with variant angina, especially in those with moderate or severe coronary atherosclerosis. It is for this reason that coronary spasm provocation tests have been developed.

Ergonovine maleate, an ergot alkaloid, is currently the most widely used agent for inducing coronary vasospasm in patients with variant angina. It has a direct vasoconstrictor effect on smooth muscle,[145] but is also an α-adrenergic agonist both centrally and peripherally.[146] The relative importance of these two actions in producing coronary spasm is not established. Ergotamine tartrate and methacholine have also had their advocates, but neither has been used on such a large scale. Ergonovine given in sufficiently large doses will produce coronary vasoconstriction and angina pectoris in most patients with coronary atherosclerosis.[147] However, ergonovine in doses of 0.05 to 0.15 mg given by peripheral intravenous bolus injection appears to be a highly sensitive and specific provocation test for coronary spasm in patients with variant angina.[103,148] Moreover, at this dose level, ergonovine has no consistent hemodynamic effects.[147]

A commonly employed protocol is to give 0.05 mg ergonovine after baseline coronary arteriography while continously monitoring the ECG. After 5 minutes or immediately following the onset of either chest pain or ST segment elevation on the ECG, selective coronary injections are made to document the spasm. Nitroglycerin is then administered, and the arteriogram repeated to confirm that the spasm has been reversed. If no effect is seen five minutes after 0.05 mg ergonovine, the injection is repeated at a dose of 0.1 mg. A further 0.15 mg may be given if necessary (Fig. 25.12). As with the angiographic demonstration of spontaneous coronary spasm, a defibrillator, pacing equipment, nitroprusside infusion, a full range of antiarrhythmic drugs, and resuscitation equipment must all be readily available before ergonovine is administered. A parenteral preparation of nitroglycerin also should be available for intravenous or direct intracoronary infusion.[56a]

Most centers report a 90 percent or greater sensitivity for ergonovine-induced spasm in patients with variant angina,[148,149] with virtually 100 percent specificity.[103,148] Moreover, the subjective experience, ECG changes, and angiographic appearance of ergonovine-induced spasm appear almost identical to those resulting from spontaneous episodes.[149] The degree of inhibition of coronary blood flow following ergonovine also appears comparable to that which accompanies spontaneous coronary spasm.[150] However, there have been reports of serious complications, including hypertension, ventricular arrhythmias, myocardial infarction, and death following the use of this agent, although usually with individual doses larger than 0.25 mg.[151-153]

No studies have yet evaluated the additional risk of performing an ergonovine provocation test at the time of coronary arteriography, but reports from groups who have used *cumulative* doses of erogonovine no greater than 0.3 mg, suggest that this test is safe.[103,148,149] An initial dose or increments larger than 0.05 mg appear to be associated with an increased risk.[153a]

Because of the inherent risks, opinion is divided as to the indications for ergonovine provocation testing. Some clinicians feel that, in those patients with classical ECG and clinical features of variant angina, the finding of an entirely normal coronary arteriogram is sufficient to make a presumptive diagnosis of coronary spasm and commence appropriate therapy.

Similarly, in those patients who have coronary atherosclerosis of a severity that would not be expected to cause ischemic symptoms per se (50 percent or less reduction in luminal diameter), some clinicians feel that a fairly confident diagnosis of coronary spasm at the site of the stenosis can be made without the need for ergonovine testing, especially if one of the vessels involved supplies the territory suspected from the ECG. An alternative approach has been to perform the ergonovine provocation test in such patients well after angiography, in the coronary care unit.[154] (In general, however, we do not recommend the use of ergonovine outside the catheterization laboratory.) Other clinicians routinely employ ergonovine provocation at the time of catheterization in such patients, on the grounds that the information obtained is essential for long-term management.

It is more generally agreed, however, that ergonovine provocation testing is contraindicated in patients with severe triple-vessel atheromatous disease and in those with disease of the left main coronary artery. Many people also regard any hemodynamically significant atheromatous lesion (occluding more than 70 percent of the vessel lumen) as a contraindication to this test. The approach we have adopted in selecting patients for ergonovine spasm provocation testing is summarized in Table 25.9.

### ²⁰¹Tl Scintigraphy

This technique is complementary to coronary angiography, which remains the definitive investigation in patients with variant angina. Serial ²⁰¹Tl scintigrams, however, have been used to successfully document *reversible* reductions of transmural blood flow during both spontaneous and ergonovine-induced coronary vasospasm.[47,94,155] In these studies, the area of reduced blood flow on the scintigram corresponded closely to that suspected from the

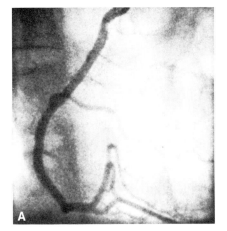

RIGHT CORONARY INJECTION
3-26-75

Fig. 25.12A Coronary angiographic findings in a young man with variant angina. At the time of his first study (3–26–75) he was 23 years old and had sustained a high lateral myocardial infarct three months earlier. This examination revealed no coronary atherosclerosis or spontaneous vasospasm, but spasm provocation was not attempted. (A shows the right coronary artery at that time.) Five months later, the patient sustained a second myocardial infarct (subendocardial inferior). Over the next year he experienced numerous episodes of rest pain, which were always relieved by nitroglycerin.

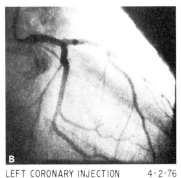

LEFT CORONARY INJECTION    4-2-76
BASAL STATE

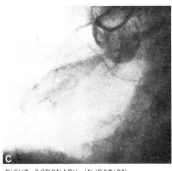

RIGHT CORONARY INJECTION
4-2-76

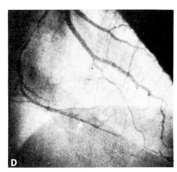

LEFT CORONARY INJECTION
4-2-76

B–D At the time of the second study (4–2–76), the patient had been admitted following a prolonged attack of rest pain during which anterior ST segment elevation was noted on his ECG. This examination revealed a normal left coronary artery in the basal state (B) but a proximal occlusion of the previously normal right coronary artery (C), the distal portion filling retrogradely via collaterals from the left coronary system (D).

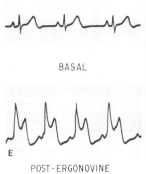

BASAL

POST-ERGONOVINE
LEAD I,  4-2-76

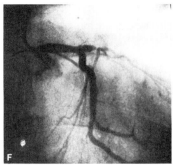

LEFT CORONARY INJECTION    4-2-76
POST-ERGONOVINE

E–F After administration of 0.05 mg i.v. ergonovine, ST segment elevation was immediately observed on his ECG (E). He then developed chest pain, and severe localized spasm was documented in the proximal left anterior descending artery (F) which was subsequently reversed by sublingual nitroglycerin. (Johnson AD and Detweiler JH: Coronary spasm, variant angina and recurrent myocardial infarctions. Circulation 55:947, 1977.)

Table 25.9   An Approach to the Investigation of Patients with Suspected Coronary Vasopasm

1. Stabilize patient.
2. Document ST segment elevation, preferably with a 12 lead ECG taken during a spontaneous episode of pain.
3. Undertake coronary arteriography using the modifications of standard technique detailed in the text.
4. Use ergonovine and nitroglycerin as follows:

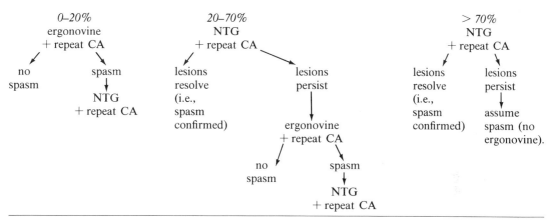

*Worst lesion demonstrated at baseline CA (% reduction in luminal diameter)*

CA = coronary angiography
NTG = nitroglycerin

ECG. Although the coronary anatomy is not directly visualized, this method appears useful in detecting coronary spasm and eliminates the potential hazards of injecting contrast material into the coronary tree during an ischemic episode. False negative studies due to contrast or premedication-induced vasodilation of the coronary bed can also be avoided.

Finally, [201]Tl scintigraphy has the advantage that it can be initiated *after* the onset of pain. Theoretically, this should enable more studies to be performed during spontaneous coronary spasm than can be achieved with coronary arteriography, so that the need for ergonovine provocation testing is reduced. In practice, however, there are major limitations as to the specificity of this method for demonstrating reversible myocardial ischemia (see Unstable Angina).

Exercise and Other Physical Stress Tests

It is now established that exercise can precipitate coronary vasospasm associated with electrocardiographic ST segment elevation and chest pain in certain individuals,[133,134] but whether or not this too should be called variant angina is debatable. Coronary spasm has also been reported following cessation of exercise in such patients.[156] The traditional view, however, has been that exercise does not usually precipitate variant angina.[121] The recently described circadian variation of exercise capacity in this condition may explain these conflicting reports.[134]

Dynamic exercise has been used as a provocative test in patients prone to variant angina[157,158] but it has not proved nearly as specific or sensitive as ergonovine provocation. In an analysis of the effects of exercise in this condition, Waters et al.[159] found that ST segment elevation occurred in approximately one third of patients on exercise, always accompanied by pain and always in the same distribution as that occurring in spontaneous episodes. ST segment depression was seen in a further 25 percent of patients during exercise but was not invariably accompanied by pain. In 5 out of 9 cases, ST segment depression occurred in different leads from those showing ST segment elevation during spontaneous pain. ST segment shifts of either polarity on exercise occurred with equal frequency in patients with and without significant fixed coronary stenoses, so that they were not in themselves predictive of coronary atherosclerosis. The combination of effort-induced pain and ST segment depression, however, especially in a lead not showing ST segment elevation during spontaneous pain, was highly suggestive of fixed coronary disease.

There are obvious potential dangers inherent in exercise testing of such patients and, as with ergonovine provocation, resuscitation equipment and parenteral spasmolytic therapy must be on hand before exercise is commenced. We do not routinely employ exercise testing in this situation, however, since it does not appear sufficiently reliable to obviate the need for coronary arteriography. Nevertheless, we do not regard variant angina as an absolute contraindication to exercise testing; with proper precautions, it can be a valuable means of assessing the response to therapy in patients who have both spontaneous and exercise-induced angina.[160]

The value of atrial pacing as a stress test in patients with variant angina is unknown, but it has been suggested that it is safer than exercise testing.[161] Finally, it has been proposed that cold pressor testing might precipitate coronary spasm in some patients, especially those with fixed coronary disease,[162] but there are no reports of its diagnostic specificity or safety in patients with variant angina.

## TREATMENT OF VARIANT ANGINA

The general management principles of unstable angina are equally applicable to patients with variant angina. As with the diagnostic considerations, only those aspects of therapy that pertain specifically to variant angina will be further discussed. Although the objectives of therapy in variant angina are those of unstable angina generally, the therapeutic approach differs in several important respects.

Pharmacologic interventions in most cases of unstable angina are directed toward a reduction in myocardial oxygen consumption. In variant angina, however, these measures are often ineffective and therapy must be directed toward reversal of the spasm-induced reduction in coronary blood flow. To date, no uniformly

effective treatment has been found, and the clinical responses to the drug regimes described below are extremely variable. Thus, it is usually necessary to modify the therapeutic regime in an individual patient on the basis of the response to therapy.

Ergonovine provocation testing has been advocated as a means of predicting the response to certain drugs, but reports of its reliability have been conflicting.[163,164]

### Nitrates

The coronary vasodilator action of nitroglycerin and other nitrates appears to be a relatively unimportant factor in the relief of chronic stable angina; the major benefit is derived from a reduction in cardiac preload, which in turn reduces myocardial oxygen requirements.[165] In variant angina, however, nitrates appear to exert their major therapeutic effect by reversing the underlying coronary vasospasm.

There is abundant clinical and angiographic evidence to confirm that nitroglycerin can acutely reverse both spontaneous and ergonovine-induced coronary vasospasm.[27,94,99-102] Evidence that nitrates can prevent rather than reverse coronary spasm is less conclusive, however, since spontaneous fluctuations in the frequency of variant angina are common and controlled studies have not been performed. Nevertheless, sublingual nitroglycerin, isosorbide dinitrate, and erithrityl pentanitrate have all been used with apparent success in the prevention of variant angina.[121] Several studies have shown, however, that as many as 50 percent of patients are not significantly improved by chronic nitrate therapy.[27,102] The optimal dose of nitroglycerin is highly variable, but in general the use of larger doses is limited by the baroreflex-mediated tachycardia that attends its peripheral vasodilator effects and thereby increases myocardial oxygen requirements. Increases of coronary vessel caliber of approximately 20 percent have been reported after 150 $\mu$g of sublingual nitroglycerin with no associated peripheral hemodynamic effects.[166] Concomitant $\beta$-adrenergic blockade can limit the reflex tachycardia associated with larger doses of nitrates, but this renders the patient particularly vulnerable to orthostatic hypotension and its sequelae. $\beta$-adrenergic blockade may also precipitate coronary vasospasm in some individuals.

In cases of variant angina considered suitable for coronary artery bypass surgery, parenteral nitroglycerin may be given throughout the operation to prevent coronary vasospasm. Even if chronic nitrate therapy proves to be an effective prophylaxis against variant angina, lifelong treatment with these drugs at high doses must be approached with a certain degree of caution. There is some evidence that tolerance develops to the effects of chronic nitrate therapy, so that progressively higher doses are necessary to achieve the same pharmacologic response. Most of these reports are anecdotal, however,[167] and the phenomenon has not been described in patients with variant angina. By contrast, nitrate dependence has been substantiated in a large number of munitions workers chronically exposed to nitrates.[167] Withdrawal from the nitrate-rich environment has led to severe headache, angina, myocardial infarction, and even sudden death in some of these workers.[168] Moreover, several of these victims had no coronary atheromatous lesions at autopsy.[169] The presumed mechanism for this effect is a rebound vasoconstriction which involves the coronary arteries. Withdrawal effects have never been reported in patients receiving therapeutic doses of nitrates, but, as Reichek has pointed out, high-dose, long-acting nitrates are now used on a wide scale in cardiologic practice and nitrate withdrawal effects would be extremely easily overlooked in individuals with symptomatic ischemic heart disease.[170]

One final caveat regarding chronic oral nitrate therapy concerns the suggestion that it might predispose to gastric carcinoma by facilitating nitrosamine formation within the stomach.[171] This is a purely theoretical risk, however, and there are no clinical findings to support this contention.

## $\alpha$-Adrenergic Blockade

This form of therapy is based upon a consideration of the likely role of the coronary artery $\alpha$-receptor in the pathogenesis of coronary spasm. Intravenous phentolamine (5 mg) has been successfully used to reverse acute coronary spasm, and it has been claimed that oral phenoxybenzamine reduces the frequency of attacks.[115] As with the nitrates, however, an almost equal number of case reports attest to the ineffectiveness of chronic $\alpha$-adrenergic blockade in this situation.[57] Myocardial oxygen consumption can be markedly increased by the reflex tachycardia that accompanies $\alpha$-adrenergic blockade, especially on standing. This effect may be less marked with the specific $\alpha_1$ receptor antagonist prazosin,[172] and studies are under way to evaluate this drug in patients with variant angina. There are currently no controlled studies of the effects of $\alpha$-adrenergic antagonists in variant angina, however, and the total number of anecdotal case reports is small. Moreover, we have found the postural hypotension associated with chronic $\alpha$-adrenergic blockade to seriously limit its usefulness in this context.

## Calcium Transport Inhibitors

This relatively new group of compounds has been extensively evaluated in Europe and Asia and has been found to be reasonably effective at controlling both the pain and the associated arrhythmias of variant angina. Preliminary studies in this country have also been encouraging, and it is likely that one or more of these drugs will become commercially available in the United States. Their probable mode of action is to reverse coronary vasospasm by inhibiting smooth muscle contraction in the arterial wall.[57] Nifedipine 30 to 180 mg daily has been reported to reduce or abolish attacks of variant angina in 66 to 78 percent of patients in uncontrolled studies.[58,99,173] In a review of the collective clinical experience of nifedipine therapy in the United States, Antman et al. reported the following observations among 127 symptomatic patients: 110 had at least a 50 percent reduction in the frequency of anginal attacks; in 80 the attacks were totally abolished; and in only 5 was the frequency of attacks not reduced by at least 10 percent.[173]

Patients with coronary spasm and no atherosclerotic disease seem to respond at least as well as those with coexistent fixed coronary lesions.[99] Several patients have been described with variant angina unresponsive to medical and surgical treatment, who were ultimately improved by nifedipine therapy.[57,99] Verapamil has also been used in patients with variant angina, in doses ranging from 120 to 480 mg/day, with symptomatic improvement reported in 75 to 88 percent of cases.[59,174] The results with perhexilene maleate have been less encouraging. In one series, 75 percent of patients were asymptomatic after 5 days of therapy; however, the drug had to be withdrawn in 24 percent because of serious adverse reactions and a further 34 percent developed less severe but dose-limiting side effects.[175] Furthermore, in a comparative study of calcium antagonists in patients with variant angina, perhexilene was found to be less effective than nifedipine, verapamil, or diltiazem at preventing ergonovine-induced coronary spasm.[164] Diltiazem is the most recently introduced of the calcium antagonists; 360 mg daily appears to be roughly equipotent with 480 mg of verapamil in preventing ergonovine-induced coronary spasm.[164]

Chronic perhexilene therapy has been associated with hepatocellular damage, peripheral neuropathy, ataxia, and weight loss,[176] but these effects have not been seen following chronic therapy with nifedipine or verapamil. Both drugs are negatively inotropic to a mild degree, however, and this effect may be seriously potentiated by coadministration of $\beta$-adrenergic blocking drugs. Worsening of angina has also been reported in association with nifedipine therapy, but the circumstances were not sufficiently clear-cut to indict nifedipine as the cause.[177]

In conclusion, the available evidence suggests that calcium transport inhibitors may complement nitrate therapy in the management of variant angina, the latter being used primarily for reversing acute attacks and the former being used as prophylaxis. However, further studies of their long-term safety and efficacy are needed.

## $\beta$-Adrenergic Blockade

The therapeutic role of $\beta$-adrenergic blockade in patients with variant angina is controversial. Theoretically, it should precipitate or worsen coronary vasospasm, since sympathetic coronary vasodilation appears to be mediated via $\beta_2$ receptors. Several studies have reported this effect,[101,116,178] but the majority of studies have shown no benefit[27,93,97,99,108,129] and some have even reported symptomatic improvement after propranolol.[124,179,180] "Cardioselective" $\beta$-blocking agents such as metoprolol, which have predominantly $\beta_1$ antagonist effects at low doses, might potentially be of benefit by reducing myocardial oxygen consumption without blocking coronary vasodilator sympathetic tone. No studies comparing selective and nonselective $\beta$-blocking drugs have been performed in patients with variant angina, however.

In the light of current evidence, we believe that $\beta$-adrenergic blockade should be avoided or used with extreme caution in patients with variant angina and then only in conjunction with a coronary vasodilator such as nitroglycerin.

## Other Drugs

A variety of other drugs—including atropine, clonidine, propantheline, nylidrin, dipyridamole, hydralazine, and various ergot derivatives—have been used in an attempt to reverse or prevent coronary vasospasm.[57] With the possible exception of atropine, none of these appears to be clinically useful.[99]

## Surgery

Attempts at coronary artery bypass surgery in patients with variant angina have been generally unsuccessful, especially in those without fixed coronary stenoses. A recent analysis of 18 series of surgically treated patients revealed a 13 percent incidence of hospital deaths and a further 15 percent incidence of nonfatal myocardial infarctions.[181] These results compare very unfavorably with the results of surgery for all other forms of ischemic heart disease. The likely reason for these poor results is that the vessel at or distal to the insertion of the vein graft continues to be vasospastic, since myocardial ischemia or infarction almost invariably appears in the territory of the operated vessel. Surgery has been reported by some authors to be beneficial, however, in patients with

Table 25.10 Comparison of Medical and Surgical Therapy in Patients with Variant Angina (From NHLBI Study)

| Treatment | # of Patients | In-Hospital | | Late | | Late Angina—NYHA Class | | | |
|---|---|---|---|---|---|---|---|---|---|
| | | MI | Death | MI | Death | 1 | 2 | 3 | 4 |
| Medical | 42 | 4 (10%) | 2 (5%) | 7 (17%) | 1 (2%) | 10 (24%) | 15 (36%) | 8 (19%) | 0 |
| Surgical | 37 | 5 (14%) | 2 (5%) | 3 (8%) | 3 (8%) | 26 * (70%) | 2 (5%) | 0 | 1 (3%) |

MI = myocardial infarction; * p < 0.05

(No significant differences between patients with variant angina and those with unstable angina as a whole, in this study.)

(Schroeder et al: Unstable angina pectoris—National randomized study of surgical vs. medical therapy. Results in Prinzmetal type angina. Am J Cardiol 41:397, 1978.)

triple-vessel atherosclerotic disease and in those with less severe or even no fixed coronary stenoses but with symptoms or arrhythmias refractory to maximum medical therapy.[102] Indeed, the surgical results in patients with fixed coronary stenoses in the NHLBI study were comparable to those of patients with unstable angina generally.[120] Another approach has been to try to ablate the presumed vasospastic mechanism by cardiac denervation, usually in combination with coronary bypass grafting. Indeed, one comparative study has shown better symptomatic and functional improvement following combined coronary denervation and bypass surgery than following bypass alone.[181a] Cardiac sympathectomy[182] and autotransplantation[183] have both been used with apparent success in a few patients, but the overall experience is too small to permit a critical evaluation of these methods. Thus, coronary artery bypass surgery seems to be more appropriate in patients with fixed coronary stenoses, both in terms of symptom relief and prognosis; however, this operation seems indicated only as a last resort in patients without significant coronary atherosclerosis.

## RESULTS OF THERAPY

In the NHBLI-sponsored study of unstable angina, 79 of the 288 patients had variant angina, but only those with one or more operable fixed coronary lesions were included. In these patients, there was no difference in early or late deaths or nonfatal myocardial infarctions between medically and surgically treated pa-

tients[120] (Table 25.10). Moreover, although the published data do not allow a comparison between those with and those without variant angina, there were no differences at early or late follow-up between the subset with variant angina and the study population as a whole. As with other forms of unstable angina, however, symptomatic improvement was significantly better at 30 months of follow-up in those who were treated surgically.

Longer-term results of either form of therapy are less clear and, especially in patients with fixed coronary stenoses, the risks of myocardial infarction or sudden death are not abolished.[184] The influence of cardiac denervation on the late results of surgery and of calcium transport inhibitors on the effects of long-term medical therapy have yet to be determined.

## CONCLUSIONS

Variant angina has been elevated from the realm of curiosity to the forefront of cardiologic interest since it has been shown to be a manifestation of coronary vasospasm. Several other clinical syndromes involving coronary vasospasm have subsequently been identified and yet more have been postulated. Maseri et al. have put the pathogenetic role of coronary spasm in perspective by calling variant angina "one aspect of a continuous spectrum of vasospastic myocardial ischemia."[8]

The identification of coronary spasm as a pathophysiological entity has finally offered a plausible explanation for the occurrence of angina pectoris, malignant arrhythmias, myocardial infarction, and sudden death in patients with apparently normal coronary arteries. However, coronary spasm may not be the only cause of myocardial ischemia in the absence of fixed coronary stenoses. In some patients with normal coronary arteries but a history of chest pain suggestive of myocardial ischemia, previous myocardial infarction or angina without electrocardiographic changes during pain, ergonovine testing has failed to provoke coronary spasm.[144]

Abnormalities of the microvasculature, myocardial metabolism, the hemoglobin-oxygen dissociation curve, and platelet survival have all been proposed as alternative explanations for myocardial ischemia in these patients.[130,185-189] The better prognosis of patients with angina and normal coronary arteries, but without the electrocardiographic features of variant angina, supports the contention that coronary vasospasm may not be the underlying cause in this group.[190]

While the occurrence of coronary spasm is now beyond dispute, its pathogenesis remains unclear. This is reflected in the diversity of the therapeutic approaches that have been tried. Coronary artery $\alpha$-receptors appear to be involved, but pharmacological antagonism of these receptors has not been consistently successful in preventing coronary spasm. Thromboxane $A_2$ also appears to be involved in some patients, but clinical studies with its physiologic antagonist, prostacyclin, have not yet been undertaken in this condition.

The diversity of physiologic and pharmacologic precipitants all point toward a common intracellular mechanism for coronary spasm, capable of activation by a variety of cell surface membrane receptors.

Nevertheless, significant advances in the treatment of coronary spasm have been made in the last few years, but none can yet be considered universally effective. Further progress will be partly dependent upon the elucidation of the pathogenetic basis of coronary spasm but also upon the development of a safe and effective means of confirming or excluding coronary spasm in all patients with suspected myocardial ischemia.

## REFERENCES

1. Vakil RJ: Preinfarction syndrome—management and follow-up. Am J Cardiol 14:55, 1964.
2. Mounsey P: Prodromal symptoms in myocardial infarction. Br Heart J. 13:215, 1951.
3. Fulton M, Lutz W, Donald KW, Kirby BJ, Duncan B, Morrison SL, Kerr F, Julian DG: Natural history of unstable angina. Lancet 1:860, 1972.
4. Osler W: The Lumleian lectures on angina pectoris. Lancet 1:839, 1910.
5. Armstrong A, Duncan B, Oliver MF, Julian DG, Donald KW, Fulton M, Lutz W, Morrison SL: Natural History of acute coronary heart attacks. A community study. Br Heart J 34:67, 1972.
6. Unstable Angina Pectoris. National cooperative study group to compare medical and surgical therapy. 1. Report of protocol and patient population. Am J Cardiol 37:896, 1976.
7. Guazzi M, Polese A, Fiorentini C, Magrini F, Olivari MT, Bartorelli C: Left and right heart haemodynamics during spontaneous angina pectoris. Comparison between angina with ST segment depression and angina with ST segment elevation. Br Heart J 37:401, 1975.
8. Maseri A, Severi S, De Nes M, L'Abbatte A, Chierchia S, Marzilli M, Ballestra AM, Parodi O, Biagini A, Distante A: "Variant" angina: one aspect of a continuous spectrum of vasospastic myocardial ischemia. Am J Cardiol 42:1019, 1978.
9. Plotnick GD, Conti CR: Transient ST segment elevation in unstable angina. Clinical and hemodynamic significance. Circulation 51:1015, 1975.
10. Jaffe AS, Klein MS, Patel BR, Siegel BA, Roberts R: Abnormal technetium–99m pyrophosphate images in unstable angina: ischemia vs. infarction? Am J Cardiol 44:1035, 1979.
11. Guthrie RB, Vlodaver Z, Nicoloff DM, Edwards JE: Pathology of stable and unstable angina pectoris. Circulation 51:1059, 1975.
12. Cairns JA, Fantus IG, Klassen GA: Unstable angina pectoris. Am Heart J 92:373, 1976.
13. Conti RC, Brawley RK, Griffith LS, Pitt B, Humphries JO, Gott VL, Ross RS: Unstable angina: morbidity and mortality in 57 consecutive patients evaluated angiographically. Am. J. Cardiol. 32:745, 1973.
14. Unstable Angina Pectoris. National cooperative study group to compare medical and surgical

therapy. II. In-hospital experience and initial follow-up results in patients with one, two and three vessel disease. Am J Cardiol 42:839, 1978.

15. Cohn LH, Medical/surgical treatment of unstable angina. In: The Treatment of Acute Myocardial Ischemia, an Integrated Medical/Surgical Approach. Eds: Cohn PF, Cohn LH: Futura Press, New York, 1979.

16. Fischl S, Herman MV, Gorlin R: The intermediate coronary syndrome: clinical, angiographic and therapeutic aspects. New Engl J Med 288:1193, 1973.

17. Parker FB Jr, Neville JF Jr, Hanson EL, Webb WR: Retrograde and antegrade pressures and flows in preinfarction syndrome. Circulation 49 and 50 (suppl 2):122, 1974.

18. Braunwald E: Control of myocardial oxygen consumption. Am J Cardiol 27:416, 1971.

19. Gorlin R: Pathophysiology of cardiac pain. Circulation 32:138, 1965.

20. Berndt TB, Fitzgerald J, Harrison DC, Schroeder JS: Hemodynamic changes at the onset of spontaneous versus pacing-induced angina. Am J Cardiol 39:784, 1977.

21. Mudge GH Jr, Grossman W, Mills RM Jr, Lesch M, Braunwald E: Reflex increase in coronary vascular resistance in patients with ischemic heart disease. N Engl J Med 295:1333, 1976.

22. Bishop VS, Kaspar RL, Barnes GE, Kardon MB: Left ventricular function during acute regional myocardial ischemia in the conscious dog. J Appl Physiol 37:785, 1974.

23. Braunwald E: Coronary spasm and acute myocardial infarction—new possibility for treatment and prevention. N Engl J Med 299:1301, 1978.

24. Levy RI, Wiener L, Smith JB, Walinsky P, Silver MJ: Measurement of plasma thromboxane in peripheral blood of Prinzmetal's angina patients. Circulation 59 and 60 (suppl 2):248, 1979.

25. Helfant RH, Banka VS: Unstable angina. In: A Clinical and Angiographic Approach to Coronary Heart Disease. Helfant RH and Banka VS, editors. F.A. Davis Co., Philadelphia, 1978.

26. Cohn LH, Alpert J, Koster JK Jr, Mee RB, Collins JJ Jr: Changing indications for the surgical treatment of unstable angina. Arch Surg 113:1312, 1978.

27. Higgins CB, Wexler L, Silverman JF, Schroeder JS: Clinical and arteriographic features of Prinzmetal's variant angina: documentation of etiologic factors. Am J Cardiol 37:831, 1976.

28. Levy H: The natural history of changing patterns of angina pectoris, Ann Intern Med 44:1123, 1956.

29. Beamish RE, Storrie VM: Impending myocardial infarction, Recognition and management. Circulation 21:1107, 1960.

30. Wood P: Acute and subacute coronary insufficiency. Br Med J 1:1779, 1961.

31. Vakil RJ: Intermediate coronary syndrome. Circulation 24:557, 1961.

32. Gazes PC, Mobley EM, Jr, Faris HM Jr, Duncan RC, Humphries GB: Preinfarctional (unstable) angina—a prospective study—ten year follow-up. Prognostic significance of electrocardiographic changes. Circulation 48:331, 1973.

33. Roughgarden JW: Circulatory changes associated with spontaneous angina pectoris. Am J Med 41:947, 1966.

34. Widlansky S, McHenry PL, Corya BC, Phillips JF: Coronary angiographic, echocardiographic and electrocardiographic studies on a patient with variant angina due to coronary artery spasm. Am Heart J 90:631, 1975.

35. Resnik WH: Preinfarction angina Part 1: The transaminase test—a diagnostic aid. Mod Con Cardiovasc Dis 31:751, 1962.

36. Roberts R, Sobel BE, Parker CW: Radioimmunoassay for creatine kinase isoenzymes. Science 194:855, 1976.

37. Allison RB, Rodriguez FL, Higgins EA Jr, Leddy JP, Abelmann WH, Ellis LB, Robbins SL: Clinicopathological correlations in coronary atherosclerosis. Four hundred thirty patients studied with postmortem coronary angiography. Circulation 27:170, 1963.

38. Armstrong PW, Chiong MA, Parker JO: The spectrum of unstable angina. Circulation 59 and 60 (suppl 2):248, 1979.

39. Abdulla AM, Canedo MI, Cortez BC, McGinnis KD, Wilhelm SK: Detection of unstable angina by $^{99m}$technetium pyrophosphate myocardial scintigraphy. Chest 69:168, 1976.

40. Knutsen KM, Otterstad JE, Strøm O: Myocardial scintigraphy with $^{99m}$technetium stannous pyrophosphate in patients with possible acute myocardial infarction. Acta Med Scand 202:107, 1977.

41. Walsh WF, Karunaratne HB, Resnekov L, Fill HR, Harper PV: Assessment of diagnostic value of technetium-99m pyrophosphate myocardial scintigraphy in 80 patients with possible acute myocardial infarction. Br Heart J. 39:974, 1977.

42. Zweiman FG, Holman BL, O'Keefe A, Idoine J: Selective uptake of $^{99m}$Tc complexes and $^{67}$Ga in acutely infarcted myocardium. J Nuc Med 16:975, 1975.

43. Wynne J, Holman BL, Lesch M: Myocardial scintigraphy by infarct-avid radiotracers. In: Principles of Cardiovascular Nuclear Medicine. Holman BL, Sonnenblick EH and Lesch M, editors. Grune and Stratton, New York, 1978.

44. Wackers FJ, Sokole EB, Samson G, Schoot JB, Lie KI, Liem KL, Wellens HJ: Value and limitations of thallium 201 scintigraphy in the acute phase of myocardial infarction. N Engl J Med 295:1, 1976.

45. Lange RC, Umbach RE, Lee JC, Zaret BL: Temporal changes in sequential quantitative thallium 201 ($^{201}$Tl) imaging following myocardial infarction in dogs. Comparison of four hour and twenty four hour infarct images. Circulation 56 (suppl 3):108, 1977.

46. Ingwall J, Kramer M, Kloner RA, Alpert NM, Newell JB, Pohost GM: Tl$^+$ accumulation. Differentiation between reversible and irreversible myocardial injury. Circulation 59 and 60 (suppl 2):173, 1979.

47. Maseri A, Parodi O, Severi S, Pesola A: Transient transmural reduction of myocardial blood flow demonstrated by thallium-201 scintigraphy, as a cause of variant angina. Circulation 54:280, 1976.

48. DeWood MA, Spores J, Notske RN, Lang HT, Shields JP, Simpson CS, Rudy LW, Grunwald R: Medical and surgical management of myocardial infarction. Am J Cardiol 44:1356, 1979.

49. Wiles JC, Peduzzi PN, Hammond GL, Cohen LS, Langou RA: Preoperative predictors of operative mortality for coronary bypass grafting in patients with unstable angina pectoris. Am J Cardiol 39:939, 1977.

50. Thompson PL, Lown B: Nitrous oxide as an analgesic in acute myocardial infarction. JAMA 235:924, 1976.

51. Weber KT, Janicki JS: The metabolic demand and oxygen supply of the heart: Physiologic and clinical considerations. Am J Cardiol 44:722, 1979.

52. Madias JE, Madias NE, Hood WB, Jr: Precordial ST-segment mapping. 2. Effects of oxygen inhalation on ischemic injury in patients with acute myocardial infarction. Circulation 53:411, 1976.

53. Rawles JM, Kenmure AC: Controlled trial of oxygen in uncomplicated myocardial infarction. Br Med J 1:1121, 1976.

54. Wolfson S, Gorlin R: Cardiovascular pharmacology of propranolol in man. Circulation 40:501, 1969.

55. Manners JM, Walters FJ: Beta adrenoceptor blockade and anaesthesia Anaesth 1:3, 1979.

56. Cohn PF, Gorlin R: Physiologic and clinical actions of nitroglycerin. Med Clin N Amer 58:407, 1974.

56a. Mikolich JR, Nicoloff NB, Robinson PH, Logue RB: Relief of refractory angina with continuous intravenous infusion of nitroglycerin. Chest 77:375, 1980.

57. Heupler FA Jr, Proudfit WL: Nifedipine therapy for refractory coronary arterial spasm. Am J Cardiol 44:798, 1979.

58. Goldberg S, Reichek N, Wilson J, Hirschfeld JW Jr, Muller J, Kastor JA: Nifedipine in the treatment of Prinzmental's (variant) angina. Am J Cardiol 44:804, 1979.

59. Parodi O, Maseri A, Simonetti I: Management of unstable angina at rest by verapamil. Br Heart J 41:167, 1979.

60. Clark RE, Christlieb IY, Henry PD, Fischer AE, Nora JD, Williamson JR, Sobel BE: Nifedipine: A myocardial protective agent. Am J Cardiol 44:825, 1979.

61. Roberts WC: Coronary thrombosis and fatal myocardial ischemia. Circulation 49:1, 1974.

62. Saliba MJ Jr, Covell JW, Bloor CM: Effects of heparin in large doses on the extent of myocardial ischemia after acute coronary occlusion in the dog. Am J Cardiol 37:599, 1976.

63. Nichol ES, Phillips WC, Casten GG: Virtue of prompt anticoagulant therapy in impending myocardial infarction: Experiences with 318 patients during a 10-year period. Ann Intern Med 50:1158, 1959.

64. Master AM: The treatment of impending infarction (premonitory phase of coronary occlusion). Chest 43:302, 1963.

65. Lewy RI, Wiener L, Smith JB, Walinsky P, Silver MJ: Intravenous heparin initiates in vivo synthesis and release of thromboxane in angina pectoris. Lancet 2:97, 1979.

66. Forrester JS, Chatterjee K: Preservation of ischemic myocardium. In: Advances in Cardiology Vol 2. A perspective on new techniques in congenital and acquired heart disease. Vogel JH, editor. Karger, Basel, 1974.

67. Scanlon PJ, Nemickas R, Moran JF, Talano JV, Amirparviz F, Pifarre R: Accelerated angina pectoris. Clinical, hemodynamic, arteriographic and therapeutic experience in 85 patients. Circulation 47:19, 1973.

68. Weintraub RM, Voukydis PC, Aroesty JM, Cohen SI, Ford P, Kurland GS, LaRaia PJ, Morkin E, Paulin S: Treatment of preinfarction angina with intra-aortic balloon counterpulsation and surgery. Am J. Cardiol 34:809, 1974.

69. Gold HK, Leinbach RC, Sanders CA, Buckley MJ, Mundth ED, Austen WG: Intra-aortic balloon pumping for control of recurrent myocardial ischemia. Circulation 47:1197, 1973.

70. LeFemine AA, Kosowsky B, Madoff I, Black H, Lewis M: Results and complications of intra-aortic balloon pumping in surgical and medical patients. Am J Cardiol 40:416, 1977.

71. Yeh BK, Gosselin AJ, Swaye PS, Larsen PB, Gentsch TD, Traad EA, Faraldo AR: Sodium nitroprusside as a coronary vasodilator in man. Am Heart J 93:610, 1977.

72. Favoloro RG, Effler DB, Cheanvechai C, Quint RA, Sones FM Jr: Acute coronary insufficiency (impending myocardial infarction and myocardial infarction). Surgical treatment by the saphenous vein graft technique. Am J Cardiol 28:598, 1971.

73. Langou RA, Wiles JC, Cohen LS: Coronary surgery for unstable angina. Incidence and mortality of perioperative myocardial infarction. Br Heart J 40:767, 1978.

74. Golding LA, Loop FD, Sheldon WC, Taylor PC, Groves LK, Cosgrove DM: Emergency revasularization for unstable angina. Circulation 58:1163, 1978.

75. Bonchek LI, Rahimtoola SH, Anderson RP, McAnulty JA, Rosch J, Bristow JD, Starr A: Late results following emergency saphenous vein bypass grafting for unstable angina. Circulation 50:972, 1974.

76. Master AM, Jaffe HL: Propranolol vs. saphenous vein graft bypass for impending infarction (pre-infarction syndrome). Am Heart J 87:321, 1974.

77. Goodin PR, Ingelsby TV, Lansing, AM, Wheat MW Jr: Preinfarction angina pectoris—a surgical emergency. J Thorac Cardiovasc Surg 66:934, 1973.

78. Bender HW Jr, Fisher RD, Faulkner SL, Friesinger, GC: Unstable coronary artery disease: Comparison of medical and surgical treatment. Ann Thorac Surg 19:521, 1975.

79. Hultgren HN, Pfeifer JF, Angell WW, Lipton, MJ, Bilisoly J: Unstable angina: comparison of medical and surgical management. Am J Cardiol 39:734, 1977.

80. Plotnick GD, Conti CR: Unstable angina: Angiography, short and long term morbidity, mortality and symptomatic status of medically treated patients. Am J Med 63:870, 1977.

81. Pugh B, Platt MR, Mills LJ, Crumbo D, Poliner LR, Curry GC, Blomqvist GC, Parkey RW, Buja LM, Willerson JT: Unstable angina pectoris: a randomized study of patients treated medically and surgically. Am J Cardiol 41:1291, 1978.

82. Selden R, Neill WA, Ritzmann LW, Okies JE, Anderson RP: Medical versus surgical therapy for acute coronary insufficiency. A randomized study. N Engl J Med 293:1329, 1975.

83. Bertolasi CA, Trongé JE, Carreño CA, Jalon J, Vega MR, Unstable angina—Prospective and randomized study of its evolution, with and without surgery. Preliminary report. Am J Cardiol 33:201, 1974.

84. Priest MF, Curry GC, Smith LR, Rogers WJ, Mantle JA, Rackley CE, Kouchoukos NT, Russell RO Jr: Changes in left ventricular segmental wall motion following randomization to medicine or surgery in patients with unstable angina. Circulation 58 (suppl 1):62, 1977.

85. Chatterjee K, Swan HJ, Parmley WW, Sustaita H, Marcus H, Matloff J: Depression of left ventricular function due to acute myocardial ischemia and its reversal after aortocoronary saphenous-vein bypass. N Engl J Med 286:1117, 1972.

86. Russell RO Jr, Wayne JB, Kronenfeld J, Charles ED, Oberman A, Kouchoukos NT, White C, Rogers W, Mantle JA, Rackley CE: Surgical versus medical therapy for treatment of unstable angina: Changes in work status and family income. Am J Cardiol 45:134, 1980.

87. Charles ED Jr, Kronenfeld JJ, Wayne JB, Kouchoukos NT, Oberman A, Rogers WJ, Mantle JA, Rackley CE, Russell RO Jr: Unstable angina pectoris: a comparison of the cost of medical and surgical treatment. Am J Cardiol 44:112, 1979.

88. Taroko T, Hultgren HN, Lipton MJ, Detre KM: The VA cooperative randomized study of surgery for coronary arterial occlusive disease. II. Subgroup with significant left main lesions. Circulation 54 (suppl 3):107, 1976.

89. Kemp HG Jr, Vokonas PS, Cohn PF, Gorlin R: The anginal syndrome associated with normal coronary arteriograms. Report of a six year experience. Am J Med 54:735, 1973.

90. Carey RJ: Self predicted fatal myocardial infarction in absence of coronary artery disease. Lancet 1:159, 1980.

91. Heberden W: Some account of a disorder of

the breast. Trans. Roy Coll Physicians 2:59, 1768.

92. Prinzmetal M, Kennamer R, Merliss R, Wada T, Bor N: Angina pectoris: A variant form of angina pectoris: Preliminary report. Am J Med 27:375, 1959.

93. Dhurandhar RW, Watt DL, Silver MD, Trimble AS, Adelman AG: Prinzmetal's variant form of angina with arteriographic evidence of coronary arterial spasm. Am J Cardiol 30:902, 1972.

94. Maseri A, Mimmo R, Chierchia S, Marchesi C, Pesola A, L'Abbatte A: Coronary artery spasm as a cause of acute myocardial ischemia in man. Chest 68:625, 1975.

95. Maseri A, Pesola A, Marzilli M, Severi S, Parodi O, L'Abbate A, Ballestra AM, Maltini G, De Nes DM, Biagini A: Coronary vasospasm in angina pectoris. Lancet 1:714, 1977.

96. Oliva PB, Potts DE, Pluss RG: Coronary arterial spasm in Prinzmetal's angina: documentation by coronary arteriography. N Engl J Med 288:745, 1973.

97. Whiting RB, Klein MD, Veer JV, Lown B: Variant angina pectoris. N Engl J Med 282:709, 1970.

98. Cheng TO, Bashour T, Kelser GA, Weiss L, Bacos J: Variant angina of Prinzmetal with normal coronary arteriograms. A variant of the variant. Circulation 47:476, 1973.

99. Endo M, Kanda I, Hosoda S, Hayashi H, Hirosawa K, Konno S: Prinzmetal's variant form of angina pectoris: re-evaluation of mechanisms. Circulation 52:33, 1975.

100. Gianelly R, Mugler F, Harrison DC: Prinzmetal's variant of angina pectoris with only slight coronary atherosclerosis. Calif Med 108:129, 1968.

101. Robertson D, Robertson RM, Nies AS, Oates JA, Freisinger GC: Variant angina pectoris: Investigation of indexes of sympathetic nervous system function. Am J Cardiol 43:1080, 1979.

102. Johnson AD, Stroud HA, Vieweg WV, Ross J Jr: Variant angina pectoris. Clinical presentations, coronary angiographic patterns and the results of medical and surgical management in 42 consecutive patients. Chest 73:786, 1978.

103. Schroeder JS, Bolen JL, Quint RA, Clark DA, Hayden WG, Higgins CB, Wexler L: Provocation of coronary spasm with ergonovine maleate. New test with results in 57 patients undergoing coronary arteriography. Am J Cardiol 40:487, 1977.

104. Clark DA, Quint RA, Bolen J, Schroeder JS: The angiographic demonstration of coronary artery spasm in patients with suspected variant angina: method and therapeutic implications. Am J Cardiol 35:127, 1975.

105. Buda AJ, Levene DL, Myers MG, Chisholm AW, Shane SJ: Coronary artery spasm and mitral valve prolapse. Am Heart J 95:457, 1978.

106. Sabom MB, Curry RC Jr, Pepine, CJ, Christie LG, Conti CR: Ergonovine testing for coronary artery spasm in patients with angiographic mitral valve prolapse. Cathet Cardiovasc Diag 4:265, 1978.

107. Oliva PB, Breckinridge JC, Arteriographic evidence of coronary artery spasm in acute myocardial infarction. Circulation 56:366, 1977.

108. Wiener L, Kasparian H, Duca PR, Walinsky P, Gottlieb RS, Hanckel F, Brest AN: Spectrum of coronary arterial spasm. Clinical, angiographic and myocardial metabolic experience in 29 cases. Am J Cardiol 38:945, 1976.

109. Ross G, Stinson EB, Schroeder J, Ginsburg R: Vasoactivity of human large coronary arteries in vitro. Circulation 59 and 60 (suppl 2):260, 1979.

110. Vatner SF, Franklin D, Higgins CB, Patrick T, White S, Van Citters RL: Coronary dynamics in unrestrained conscious baboons. Am J Physiol 221:1396, 1971.

111. Orlick AE, Ricci DR, Alderman EL, Stinson EB, Harrison DC: Effects of alpha adrenergic blockade upon coronary hemodynamics. J Clin Invest 62:459, 1978.

112. Yasue H, Touyama M, Kato H, Tanaka S, Akiyama F: Prinzmetal's variant form of angina as a manifestation of alpha adrenergic receptor-mediated coronary artery spasm: Documentation by coronary arteriography. Am Heart J 91:148, 1976.

113. Freedman B, Dunn RF, Kelly DT: Exercise induced coronary spasm: $\alpha$–adrenergic mechanism? Circulation 59 and 60 (Suppl 2):265, 1979.

114. Hillis LD, Braunwald E: Coronary artery spasm. N Engl J Med 299:695, 1978.

115. Ricci DR, Orlick AE, Cipriano PR, Guthaner DF, Harrison DC: Altered adrenergic activity in coronary arterial spasm: Insight into mechanism based on study of coronary hemodynamics and the electrocardiogram. Am J Cardiol 43:1073, 1979.

116. Yasue H, Touyama M, Shimamoto M, Kato M, Tanaka S, Akiyama F: Role of autonomic nervous system in the pathogenesis of Prinzmetal's variant form of angina. Circulation 50:534, 1974.

117. Glick G, Braunwald E: Relative roles of the sympathetic and parasympathetic nervous systems in the reflex control of heart rate. Circ Res 16:363, 1965.

118. Alexander RW, Cooper B, Handin RI: Characterization of the human platelet $\alpha$–adrenergic receptor: correlation of [$^3$H] dihydroergocryptine binding with aggregation and adenylate cyclase inhibition. J Clin Invest 61:1136, 1978.

118a. Conti RC, Pepine CJ, Curry RC Jr: Coronary artery spasm: An important mechanism in the pathophysiology of ischemic heart disease. Current Problems in Cardiology 4:18, 1979.

118b. Fleckenstein A, Nakayama K, Fleckenstein–Grun G, Byon Y: Interaction of vasoactive ions and drugs and Ca-dependent excitation contraction coupling in vascular smooth muscle. In: Calcium Transport in Contraction and Secretion. Carafol E, ed. North Holland Publishing Co., Amsterdam, 1975.

119. Ginsburg R, Bristow MR, Harrison DC, Stinson EB: Are histamine receptors present in human coronary arteries? Circulation 59 and 60 (Suppl 2):101, 1979.

120. Schroeder JS, Russell RO, Jr, Resnekov L, Wolk M, Hutter AM, Rosati RA, Conti CR, Becker LC, Biddle T, Kaplan EM, Gilbert JP, Mock MB: Unstable angina pectoris—National randomized study of surgical vs. medical therapy. Results in Prinzmetal type angina. Am J Cardiol 41:397, 1978.

121. MacAlpin RN, Kattus AA, Alvaro AB: Angina pectoris at rest with preservation of exercise capacity. Prinzmetal's variant angina. Circulation 47:946, 1973.

122. Silverman ME, Flamm MD Jr: Variant angina pectoris. Ann Intern Med 75:339, 1971.

123. Murao M: Research of variant forms of angina pectoris in Japan (in Japanese). Heart 5:1029, 1973.

124. Allaire BI, Schroeder JS: Prinzmetal's angina: clinical and anatomic aspects. West J Med 122:187, 1975.

124a. Marzilli M, Goldstein S, Trivella MG, Palumbo C, Maseri A: Some clinical considerations regarding the relation of coronary vasospasm to coronary atherosclerosis. A hypothetical pathogenesis. Am J Cardiol 45:882, 1980.

125. Johnson AD, Detwiler JH: Coronary spasm, variant angina and recurrent myocardial infarctions. Circulation 55:947, 1977.

126. Selzer A, Langston M, Ruggeroli C, Cohn K: Clinical syndrome of variant angina with normal coronary arteriogram. N Engl J Med 295:1343, 1976.

127. Bouvrain Y, Fortin P, Coumel P: Modifications inhabituelles de l'électrocardiogramme au cours de crises d'angines de poitrine spontanées de decubitus. Arch Mal Coeur 56:961, 1963.

128. Calzavara G, Lusiani GB, Saraceni G: Contributo clinico alla conoscenza della "variant form" di angina pectoris. Folia Cardiol (Milano) 25:283, 1966.

129. Shubrooks SJ, Bete JM, Hutter AM Jr, Block PC, Buckley MJ, Daggett WM, Mundth ED: Variant angina pectoris: clinical and anatomic spectrum and results of coronary bypass surgery. Am J Cardiol 36:142, 1975.

130. Eliott RS, Bratt A: The paradox of myocardial ischemia and necrosis in young women with normal coronary arteriograms. Relation to abnormal hemoglobin oxygen dissociation. Am J Cardiol 23:633, 1969.

131. Fernandez D, Rosenthal JE, Cohen LS, Hammond G, Wolfson S: Alcohol induced Prinzmetal variant angina. Am J Cardiol 32:238, 1973.

132. Kemp GL: Value of treadmill stress testing in variant angina pectoris. Am J Cardiol 30:781, 1972.

133. Specchia A, deServi S, Falcone C, Bramucci E, Angoli L, Mussini A, Martinoni GP, Montemartini C, Bobba P: Coronary arterial spasm as a cause of exercise induced ST-segment elevation in patients with variant angina. Circulation 59:948, 1979.

134. Yasue M, Omote S, Takazawa A, Nagao M, Miwa K, Tasaka S: Circadian variation of exercise capacity in patients with Prinzmetal's variant angina: role of exercise-induced coronary arterial spasm. Circulation 59:938, 1979.

135. MacAlpin RN, Kattus AA: Adaptation to exercise in angina pectoris: The electrocardiogram during treadmill walking and coronary angiographic findings. Circulation 33:183, 1966.

136. Proudfit W: Types of spasm and their diagnosis. Am J Cardiol 44:841, 1979.

137. Kleinfeld MJ, Rozanski JJ, Alternans of the ST segment in Prinzmetal's angina. Circulation 55:574, 1977.

138. Roesler H, Dressler W: Transient electrocardiographic changes identical with those in acute myocardial infarction accompanying attacks of angina pectoris. Am Heart J 47:520, 1954.

139. Raynaud R, Brochier M, Morand P, Fauchier J-P, Raynaud P, Chatelain B: Une forme clinique de l'angine de poitrine: l'angor de Prinzmetal. Semaine des Hôpitaux de Paris 45:2662, 1969.

139a. Smithen C, Wilner G, Baltaxe H, Gay W Jr,

Killip T: Variant angina pectoris. Am Heart J 89:87, 1975.

139b. Williams RR, Wagner GS, Peter RH: ST segment alternans in Prinzmetal's angina. A report of two cases. Ann Intern Med 81:51, 1974.

139c. Bharati S, Dhingra RC, Lev M, Towne WD, Rahimtoola SH, Rosen KM: Conduction system in a patient with Prinzmetal's angina and transient atrioventricular block. Am J Cardiol 39:120, 1977.

140. Levi GF, Proto C: Ventricular fibrillation in the course of Prinzmetal's angina pectoris. Br Heart J 35:601, 1975.

141. Bennett KR, Coronary artery spasm: the effects of cardiovascular laboratory premedication practice. Cath Cardiovasc Diag 2:321, 1976.

142. Côté P, Gueret P, Bourassa MG: Systemic and coronary hemodynamic effects of diazepam in patients with normal and diseased coronary arteries. Circulation 50:1210, 1974.

143. Chahine RA, Raizner AE, Ishimori T, Luchi RJ, McIntosh MD: The incidence and clinical implications of coronary artery spasm. Circulation 52:972, 1975.

144. Heupler FA, Proudfit WL, Razavi M, Shirey EK, Greenstreet R, Sheldon WC: Ergonovine maleate provocation test for coronary arterial spasm. Am J Cardiol 41:631, 1978.

145. Brown GL, Dale H, The pharmacology of ergometrine. Proc Roy Soc Lond (Biol) 118:446, 1935.

146. Innes IR: Identification of the smooth muscle excitatory receptors for ergot alkaloids. Br J Pharmacol 19:120, 1962.

147. Stein I, Weistein J: Further studies of effect of ergonovine on coronary circulation. J Lab Clin Med 36:66, 1950.

148. Heupler F, Proudfit W, Siegel W, Shirey E, Razavi M, Sones FM: The ergonovine maleate test for the provocation of coronary artery spasm. Circulation 52 (suppl 2):11, 1975.

149. Curry RC, Pepine CJ, Sabom MB, Feldman RL, Christie LG, Conti CR: Effects of ergonovine in patients with and without coronary artery disease. Circulation 56:803, 1977.

150. Ricci DR, Orlick AE, Doherty PW, Cipriano PR, Harrison DC: Reduction of coronary blood flow during coronary artery spasm occurring spontaneously and after provocation by ergonovine maleate. Circulation 57:392, 1978.

151. Wright EN, Graiewski SJ: Ergonovine sensitivity and/or toxicity: Report of a case. Obstet and Gynecol 6:347, 1955.

152. Forman JB, Sullivan RL: The effects of intravenous injection of ergonovine and methergine on the post partum patient. Am J Obstet Gyn 63:640, 1952.

153. Scherf D, Perlman A, Schlachman M: Effect of dihydroergocornine on the heart. Proc Soc Exp Biol Med 71:420, 1949.

153a. Buxton A, Goldberg S, Hirschfeld JW, Wilson J, Mann T, Williams DO, Oliva P, Kastor JA: Refractory ergonovine induced coronary vasospasm: importance of intracoronary nitroglycerin. Am J Cardiol 45:390, 1980.

154. Nelson C, Nowak B, Childs H, Weinrauch L, Forwand S: Provocative testing for coronary arterial spasm: Rationale, risk and clinical illustrations. Am J Cardiol 40:624, 1977.

155. McLaughlin PR, Docherty PW, Martin RP, Goris ML, Harrison DC, Myocardial imaging in a patient with reproducible variant angina Am J Cardiol 39:126, 1977.

156. Broustet JP, Griffo R, Seriès P, Guern P, Laylavoix F: Angor de Prinzmetal déclenché par l'arrêt de l'effort. Arch Mal Coeur 72:391, 1979.

157. Fortuin NJ, Freisinger GC: Exercise induced ST segment elevation. Clinical, electrocardiographic and arteriographic studies in 12 patients. Am J Med 49:459, 1970.

158. Detry JM, Mengeot P, Rousseau MF, Cosyns J, Ponlot R, Brasseur LA: Maximal exercise testing in patients with spontaneous angina pectoris associated with transient ST segment elevation: Risks and electrocardiographic findings. Br Heart J 37:897, 1975.

159. Waters DD, Chaitman BR, Théroux P, Dauve F, Mizgala HF: Exercise testing in variant angina. Circulation 59 and 60 (suppl 2):265, 1979.

160. Ellestad MH: Contraindications to testing and safety precautions. In: Stress Testing, Principles and Practice. Ellestad MH, ed; FA Davis Co., Philadelphia, 1976.

161. Linhart JW: Atrial pacing in coronary artery disease, including preinfarction angina and postoperative studies. Am J Cardiol 30:603, 1972.

162. Mudge GH Jr, Grossman W, Mills RM Jr, Lesch M, Braunwald E: Evidence for reflex coronary artery spasm in patients with ischemic heart disease. Trans Assoc Am Phys 89:225, 1976.

163. Previtali M, Salerno JA, Medici A, Chimenti M, Ray M, Tavazzi L, Bobba P: Poor predictability of ergonovine maleate test in predicting response to treatment in angina at rest. Circulation 59 and 60 (suppl 2):249, 1979.

164. Waters DD, Théroux P, Dauwe F, Crittin J,

Affaki G, Mizgala HF: Ergonovine testing to assess the effects of calcium antagonist drugs in variant angina. Circulation 59 and 60 (suppl 2):248, 1979.

165. Goldstein RE, Epstein SE: Medical management of patients with angina pectoris. Prog Cardiovasc. Dis 14:360, 1972.

166. Feldman RL, Pepine CJ, Curry RC Jr, Conti RC: Coronary arterial responses to graded doses of nitroglycerin. Am J Cardiol 43:91, 1979.

167. Abrams J: Nitrate tolerance and dependence. Am Heart J 99:113, 1980.

168. Symanski M: Schwere gesundheits-schädigungen durch berufliche nitroglykoleinwirkung. Arch Hyg Bakt 136:139, 1952.

169. Lange RL, Reid MS, Tresch DD, Keelan MH, Bernhard VM, Coolidge G: Non-atheromatous ischemic heart disease following withdrawal from chronic industrial nitroglycerin exposure. Circulation 46:666, 1972.

170. Reichek N: Long-acting nitrates in the treatment of angina pectoris. JAMA 236:1399, 1976.

171. Editorial comment. Anon. Brit Med J 1:163, 1980.

172. Cambridge D, Davey MJ, Massingham R: Prazosin, a selective antagonist of post-synaptic α-adrenoceptors. Br J Pharmacol 59:514P, 1977.

173. Antman E, Muller J, Goldberg S, MacAlpin R, Rubenfire M, Tabaznik B, Liang C, Heupler F, Achuff S, Reichek N et al: Nifedipine therapy for coronary-artery spasm. Experience in 127 patients. N Engl J Med 302:1269, 1980.)

174. Freedman B, Dunn RF, Richmond DR, Kelly DT: Coronary artery spasm—treatment with verapamil: Circulation 59, 60 (Suppl 2):249, 1979.

175. Mizgala HF, Crittin J, Waters DD, Théroux P: Results of immediate and long term treatment of variant angina (VA) with perhexilene maleate. Circulation 59 and 60, (suppl 2):181, 1979.

176. Adverse Reactions Series. No. 15 (Perhexilene) Committee on the Safety of Medicines, London, 1977.

177. Jariwalla AG, Anderson EG: Production of ischemic cardiac pain by nifedipine. Br Med J 1:1181, 1978.

178. Black MM, Black A, Huntington P: Prinzmetal's variant angina with syncope: treatment with permanent demand pacemaker. NY State J Med 76:255, 1976.

179. Donsky MS, Harris MD, Curry GC, Blomqvist CG, Willerson JT, Mullins CB: Variant angina pectoris: a clinical and coronary arteriographic spectrum. Am Heart J 89:571, 1975.

180. Guazzi M, Fiorentini C, Polese A, Magrini F, Olivari MT: Treatment of spontaneous angina pectoris with beta blocking agents: a clinical, electrocardiographic and haemodynamic appraisal. Br Heart J 37:1235, 1975.

181. Conti CR, Curry RC Jr: Therapy of unstable angina. In: Diagnosis and Therapy of Coronary Artery Disease. Cohn PF, editor. Little Brown and Co., Boston, 1979.

181a. Bertrand ME, LaBlanche JM, Rousseau MF, Warembourg HH Jr, Stankowtak C, Soots G: Surgical treatment of variant angina: use of plexectomy with aortocoronary bypass. Circulation 61:877, 1980.

182. Grondin CM, Limet R: Sympathetic denervation in association with coronary artery grafting in patients with Prinzmetal's angina. Ann Thorac Surg 23:111, 1977.

183. Clark DA, Quint RA, Mitchell RL, Angell WW: Coronary artery spasm. Medical management, surgical denervation and autotransplantation. J Thorac Cardiovasc Surg 73:332, 1977.

184. Curry RC Jr., Pepine CJ, Feldman RC, Whittle JL, Conti CR: Frequency of myocardial infarction and sudden death in 44 variant angina patients: a high risk ischemic heart disease subset. Am J Cardiol 45:454, 1980.

185. James TN: Angina without coronary disease. Circulation 42:189, 1970.

186. Steele P, Rainwater J, Vogel R: Abnormal platelet survival time in men with myocardial infarction and normal coronary arteriogram. Am. J. Cardiol. 41:60, 1978.

187. Boudoulas H, Cobb TC, Leighton RF, Wilt SM: Myocardial lactate production in patients with angina like chest pain and angiographically normal coronary arteries and left ventricle. Am J Cardiol 34:501, 1974.

188. Neill WA, Kassebaum DA, Judkins MP: Myocardial hypoxia as the basis for angina pectoris in a patient with normal coronary arteriograms. N Engl J Med 279:789, 1968.

189. Likoff W, Segal BL, Kasparian H: Paradox of normal selective coronary arteriograms in patients considered to have unmistakable coronary heart disease. N Engl J Med 276:1063, 1967.

190. Bemiller CR, Pepine CJ, Rogers AK: Long term observations in patients with angina and normal coronary arteriograms. Circulation 47:36, 1973.

# Section 6
# ADDITIONAL MONITORING AND DIAGNOSTIC METHODS

# 26 | The Chest Radiograph in Acute Myocardial Infarction

*Charles B. Higgins, M.D.*
*Alexander Battler, M.D.*

The chest radiograph is one of the most frequently performed diagnostic studies in patients in the coronary care unit. It has been, and remains, a basic modality for assessing the severity of left ventricular dysfunction, detecting complications of acute myocardial infarction (AMI), and monitoring responses to therapy. Recent studies suggest that certain findings on the chest radiograph in patients with AMI have important prognostic implications. However, a limitation to the value of the radiograph in patients with AMI is that it is usually technically less than ideal due to the exigencies of the clinical status of the critically ill patient. Portable anteroposterior radiographs of the chest obtained with the patient in the supine or in a semiupright position for only a short time preclude accurate interpretation of some valuable radiographic signs.

This chapter will deal with the utility of the chest radiograph in evaluating the severity of acute myocardial infarction, for monitoring therapy, for estimating immediate and long-term prognosis, and for detecting complications of this disorder. As the status of patients in the coronary care unit is usually critical, portable chest x-rays are required. This type of radiographic study imposes diagnostic limitations that will be considered at the outset.

## SUPINE ANTEROPOSTERIOR CHEST RADIOGRAPHS

These radiographs are usually obtained with a portable radiographic unit in which the tube (focus) to x-ray film distance is 36 to 40 inches, rather than the 72-inch focus-to-film distance used with the standard upright posteroanterior radiograph. Because of this shorter focus-film distance and the anteroposterior direction of the x-ray beam, magnification of the heart and anterior mediastinum is 15 to 20 percent compared to 5 to 8 percent in the standard posteroanterior radiograph. Since the heart lies anterior in the thorax, it is magnified to a relatively greater extent on the anteroposterior than on the posteroanterior radiograph; the upper limits of 0.50 for a normal cardiothoracic ratio on the standard radiograph cannot be applied for the portable radiograph with the same degree of reliability. However, it was of interest that in a recent study separation of patients with acute myocardial infarction into groups, based on a cardiothoracic ratio of less than or greater than 0.50 on portable radiographs, showed a 2.5-fold greater early and late mortality in those with a ratio greater than 0.50.[1] In order to provide a uniform method for estimating the size of the left ventricle in supine anteroposterior

603

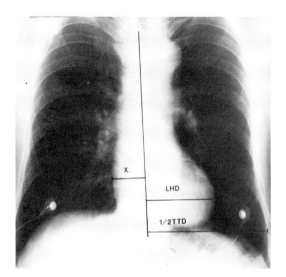

Fig. 26.1 Method for measuring the left heart dimension (LHD). The measurement is obtained on an anteroposterior supine radiograph exposed at end-diastole and at a tidal volume of 1 l. Left heart dimension is the horizontal distance from the anterior midline (line joining lead markers) to the widest point on left side of cardiac silhouette. (Battler A et al.: The initial chest x-ray in acute myocardial infarction. Prediction of early and late mortality and survival. Circulation 61:1004, 1980.)

radiographs, the left heart dimension (LHD) was devised.[2] The LHD is a measure of the distance from the mid-spinal line to the most lateral point on the left side of the cardiac silhouette, which is standardized for body surface area (Fig. 26.1). The supine radiographs are obtained after a measured 1 liter inspiration and are exposed at end-diastole.

The supine radiograph also results in some accentuation in the size of the azygos vein and the pulmonary veins, which are used as indicators of systemic and pulmonary venous hypertension, respectively. The average diameter of the azygos vein in normal patients is 7 mm (upper normal, 10 mm) on upright radiographs[3] but may be twice this diameter on supine radiographs. Likewise, pulmonary veins are larger overall in the supine position as a consequence of an approximately 30-percent greater pulmonary blood flow in the supine position. The differences in the size of the pulmonary vessels are particularly noticeable in the upper lobes due to the reduced gravitational

effect in this position. Consequently, redistribution of pulmonary blood flow cannot be relied upon as a sign of early or mild congestive heart failure in the supine chest radiograph.

## POSITION OF CARDIOPULMONARY MONITORING AND ASSIST DEVICES

The treatment of many patients in the coronary care unit entails the placement of a variety of wires, tubes, and catheters for monitoring important hemodynamic parameters and for cardiopulmonary support. The accuracy of hemodynamic measurements is critically dependent on the proper position of monitoring catheters. Moreover, support devices must be properly positioned to be effective. Indeed, improper insertion and/or position of these devices has been a frequent cause of major complications in these patients. With these considerations in mind, it is important to document the position of these various devices by obtaining at least a frontal chest radiograph immediately after their insertion. If monitoring catheters are apparently in proper position on the frontal chest radiograph but pressure recordings seem anomalous, an intraluminal position should be confirmed by the injection of iodinated contrast material into the catheter during exposure of the radiograph (Fig. 26.2).

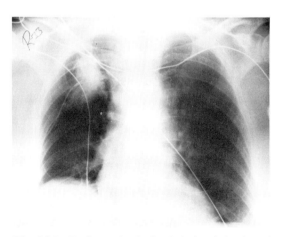

Fig. 26.2 Radiograph obtained during injection of contrast material into the central venous pressure catheter shows extravasation of contrast material indicating extravascular position of catheter tip.

Although contrast materials can have important electrophysiologic and hemodynamic actions, a small volume ($<$10 ml) injected on the venous side of the circulation is unlikely to have any important cardiac effects, even in the patient with ischemic heart disease. The position of these devices must be carefully assessed on subsequent chest radiographs as well, since they may change position as a result of change in the patient's position, inadvertent traction, or manipulation by physicians.

There is an ideal position on the frontal radiograph for each of the cardiopulmonary monitoring and assist devices. This position is shown in Table 26.1. The tip of the central venous pressure (CVP) line should lie in the superior vena cava. When the catheter has been intro-duced into a peripheral vein of the upper extremity, the catheter tip must be medial to the location of the proximal valve in the subclavian vein, which approximates the medial border of the anterior first rib on the frontal radiograph, in order to record true CVP.[4] Through this route of insertion, the most frequent improper positions are in the jugular vein (Fig. 26.3), hepatic vein, or within the right sided cardiac chambers. The latter position may induce dysrhythmias. A study that recorded the initial position of CVP catheters revealed aberrant position in more than one-third of the patients.[5] Aberrantly positioned catheters have resulted in thromboplebitis of smaller veins, pneumothorax, chylothorax, glucothorax, pericardial tamponade, dysrhythmia, and infusion of poten-

**Table 26.1   The Chest Radiograph in Identifying Coronary Complications**

| Tube or Catheter | Optimal Position | Complication Identified on Chest Radiograph |
|---|---|---|
| CVP catheter | Superior vena cava | Cardiac perforation<br>Hemothorax, hydrothorax<br>Hydromediastinum<br>Venous thrombosis–subclavian or superior vena cava obstruction, embolism<br>Infection (abscess)<br>Pneumomediastinum<br>Pneumothorax (percutaneous subclavian catheterization)<br>Phrenic or brachial plexus neural injury (subclavian catheterization) |
| Swan-Ganz catheter | Right or left pulmonary artery | As above<br>Pulmonary infarction<br>Knotting of catheter |
| Intraaortic counter-pulsation balloon | Aortic knob | Aortic dissection<br>Cerebral embolization<br>Occlusion of left subclavian artery<br>Hemolysis |
| Transvenous pacing catheter | Apex of right ventricle (anterior position on lateral view) | Aberrant position (coronary sinus)<br>Myocardial perforation<br>Wire fracture |
| Endotracheal tube | Mid-trachea (5–7 cm above carina) | Right upper lobe atelectasis or left lung atelectasis (malposition in right bronchus)<br>Interstitial emphysema<br>Pneumomediastinum<br>Pneumothorax<br>Gastric dilatation<br>Aspiration<br>Pharyngeal or esophageal perforation<br>Atelectasis |

CVP = central venous pressure

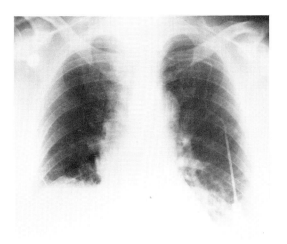

Fig. 26.3 The most frequent aberrant position of a central venous pressure catheter is the jugular vein.

tially damaging solutions into pulmonary and hepatic vessels.

When the CVP catheter is inserted by direct percutaneous puncture of the subclavian vein, a chest radiograph should be immediately obtained to again define the position of the catheter tip and also to exclude any complications from this procedure. Since the most frequent complication of this approach is pneumothorax, an upright radiograph, preferably in expiration, should be obtained. This should be done before catheterization of the contralateral subclavian vein is attempted after an initial unsuccessful attempt on one side. Less frequently, a pneumomediastinum is observed; pneumomediastinum may be associated with chest pain and be mistaken for persistent angina in the patient with ischemic heart disease.

The appearance of extrapleural, intrapleural, or mediastinal fluid collection after subclavian vein catheterization is usually indicative of either vascular injury with hemorrhage or an extravascular location of the catheter tip with extravascular infusion of intravenous fluids (Fig. 26.4).

The tip of the Swan-Ganz catheter ideally should be positioned in the central right or left pulmonary artery. The catheter should not be coiled in the superior vena cava or within the heart in order to minimize the risk of inadvertent movement into the distal pulmonary artery. A distal position in a segmental pulmonary ar-

tery (Fig. 26.5) should be avoided. A distal position of this catheter for a protracted period has been associated with pulmonary infarction [6-8] either from failure to deflate the balloon with the tip in a segmental pulmonary artery or wedging of the tip into a subsegmental artery (Fig. 26.5). In one retrospective study, pulmonary infarction as a complication of the use of this catheter was documented in 7.2 percent of 125 patients.[6] Excessive coiling of the catheter in cardiac chambers may also cause dysrhythmias or knotting of the catheter. A rare cause of dense opacification of the lung on a chest radiograph, in a patient with a Swan-Ganz catheter in place, is rupture of a pulmonary artery

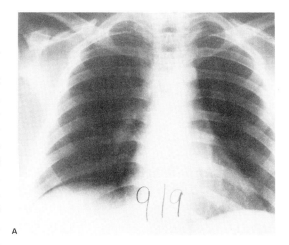

A

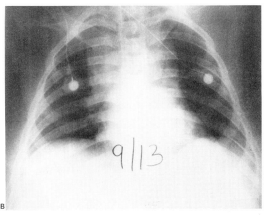

B

Fig. 26.4 Chest radiograph (A) obtained several days prior to unsuccessful efforts were made to catheterize the subclavian vein. Chest radiograph (B) 6 hours after the unsuccessful catheterization reveals enlargement of superior mediastinum. Vascular injury caused a large mediastinal hematoma.

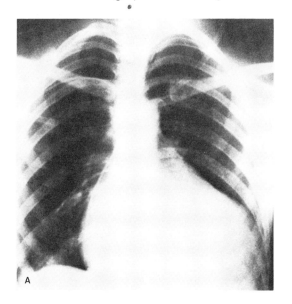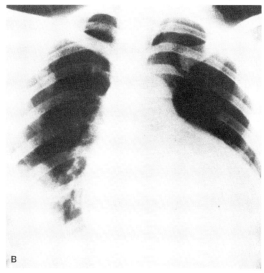

Fig. 26.5   Radiograph *(A)* shows distal position of Swan-Ganz catheter. A later radiograph *(B)* in the same patient shows a pulmonary density characteristic of a pulmonary infarction. Infarction is in the region of the lung corresponding to the distribution of the segmental artery occluded by the catheter.

during inflation of the balloon. This is a potentially fatal complication.

The tip of the intraaortic circulatory assist balloon catheter should be ideally positioned just distal to the origin of the left subclavian artery;[4,9] on the frontal radiograph this position corresponds to the aortic knob. A position in the aorta proximal to this point entails the danger of cerebral embolization, while an inadvertent position in one of the arch vessels may obstruct or damage the artery with subsequent thrombosis. The radiograph may give evidence of aortic dissection after transfemoral arterial insertion of this catheter. This complication is disclosed by loss of definition of the descending aortic shadow; lateral displacement of the paraspinal line; and/or appearance of an extrapleural collection above the apex of the left lung.

Transvenous pacing catheters may not function after implantation due to malposition of the electrode tip. On the frontal radiograph, the tip of the catheter should be at the apex of the right ventricle and should be directed anteriorly on the lateral view. A common aberrant position is when the tip enters the coronary sinus. This position is suggested, on the frontal radiograph, by a superior orientation of the tip of the catheter rather than the inferior orienta-

tion observed when it lies in the right ventricular apex. The lateral view demonstrates that the tip is directed posteriorly rather than anteriorly.

Myocardial perforation by the catheter can be suspected on the radiograph.[10] The catheter tip lies clearly outside or at the margin of the cardiac silhouette. Although an abrupt increase in the cardiac silhouette would suggest myocardial perforation causing hemopericardium, acute pericardial fluid collections seldom cause any substantial increase in the cardiac silhouette.

The endotracheal tube is visible on most frontal radiographs. The tip of this tube should lie approximately midway between the thoracic outlet and the carina, a location approximately 5 to 7 cm above the carina.[11,12] Flexion and lateral rotation of the neck causes the tip of the endotracheal tube to descend approximately 2 cm, while extension of the neck causes the tip to retract approximately 2 cm. Therefore, the tip of the tube should be no less than 2.5 cm above the carina when the head is in a neutral position to insure that the tube does not enter the bronchus during flexion.

Occasionally, the carina cannot be visualized with certainty on a frontal radiograph; in these instances, the position of the tip of the endotra-

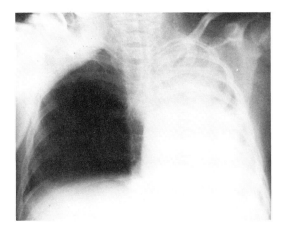

Fig. 26.6 Chest radiograph shows inadvertent intubation of right bronchus causing collapse of the left lung and overexpansion of the right lung.

cheal tube can be related to the thoracic vertebral bodies (T). In over 90 percent of adult patients, the carina is situated at or within one vertebral body of $T_6$.[12] Therefore, when the carina cannot be visualized, one should ascertain that the tip of the endotracheal tube is at the level of $T_2$ to $T_4$.[12]

Intubation of the right mainstem bronchus, which is reported to occur in 10 to 15 percent of intubations, most frequently results in partial or complete collapse of the left lung and/or right upper lobe (Fig. 26.6). Ventilation of only

one lung may result in ipsilateral interstitial emphysema or pneumothorax. Intubation of the esophagus may be suspected if gastric dilatation occurs.

Tracheal stenosis and malacia from tracheal intubation have been related to the use of high intracuff pressure (>24 mmHg).[13] High intracuff pressure can be suspected by the observation of a circular configuration of the balloon cuff, particularly when its margin projects beyond the edges of tracheal air space above and below the level of the cuff.

Mechanical ventilation is occasionally required in patients in the coronary care unit. In this clinical situation, the thoracic radiograph may provide the initial indication of an extra-alveolar air leak. Interstitial emphysema and subpleural blebs are frequently followed by tension pneumothorax in adults on assisted ventilation.[11,14] Extension of pneumomediastinum into the peritoneum or extraperitoneal space is not uncommon in adult patients.[14]

## PULMONARY VENOUS HYPERTENSION

Chest radiographs have commonly been used to gauge the severity of pulmonary venous hypertension, which, in AMI, occurs as a result of

Table 26.2 Classification of Pulmonary Venous Hypertension (PVH)

| PVH | Radiographic Findings | Pulmonary Wedge Pressure (mean) |
| --- | --- | --- |
| Grade I | Redistribution of pulmonary vascularity<br>Loss of right hilar angle | 12 to 20 mmHg |
| Grade II | Kerley's B lines (interstitial pulmonary edema)<br>Prominent interstitial markings<br>Hilar haze<br>Peribronchial and perivascular thickening | 20 to 25 mm Hg |
| Grade III | Perihilar alveolar infiltrate (perihilar pulmonary edema)<br>Generalized alveolar infiltrate (generalized pulmonary edema) | 25 mmHg |

left ventricular failure or diminished left ventricular compliance. The radiographic manifestations of pulmonary venous hypertension (PVH) have been empirically divided into three grades of severity (Table 26.2). Defining the radiographic grade of PVH (Fig. 26.7) permits a rough estimate of the pulmonary venous pressure or left ventricular end-diastolic pressure.

However, reservations must be stated regarding any estimate of hemodynamics from the radiographic signs of PVH because of temporal differences in the rate of hemodynamic and radiographic changes.

Simultaneously measured pulmonary artery wedge (PAW) pressure and radiographic estimates of the severity of PVH have shown a rough correlation,[15-17] but examples of both overestimation and underestimation of the level of PAW pressure from the radiographic grade of PVH are not infrequent. Several studies have attempted to relate the radiographic severity of PVH to the hemodynamic severity (PAW pressure)[16,17] and to the extravascular water content.[18] PAW pressure greater than 18 mmHg was almost invariably associated with distinct radiographic signs of PVH (Fig. 26.8). On the other hand, when PAW pressure was greater than 12 mmHg but less than 18 mmHg, normal lung fields were observed nearly as often as any sign of PVH. This is not unexpected, since radiographs in patients with AMI are usually less than ideal for detecting early or minor changes indicative of grade I PVH. The detection of redistribution of pulmonary blood flow

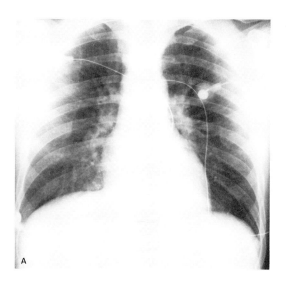

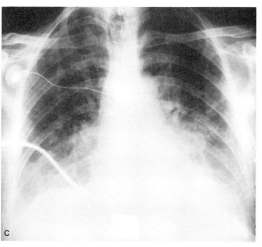

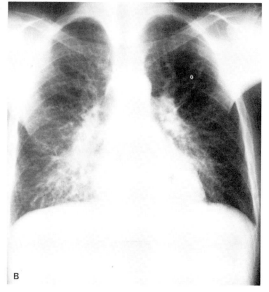

Fig. 26.7 Radiograph displays the grades of severity of pulmonary venous hypertension. Grade I *(A)* is characterized by redistribution of pulmonary vascularity and loss of distinct right hilar angle. Grade II *(B)* is characterized by Kerley's B lines (interstitial pulmonary edema), hilar haze, peribronchial and perivascular cuffing. Grade IV *(C)* is characterized by confluent alveolar edema. Grade III (localized pulmonary edema—not shown) is characterized by confluent alveolar infiltrates in the perihilar areas and lower lung fields. (Battler A et al.: The initial chest x-ray in acute myocardial infarction. Prediction of early and late mortality and survival. Circulation 61:1004, 1980.)

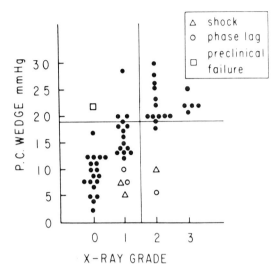

Fig. 26.8 Graph shows the pulmonary capillary (PC) wedge pressure plotted against the x-ray grade of pulmonary venous hypertension for individual patients with acute myocardial infarction. (McHugh TF, Forrester JS, Adler L, Zion D, Swan HJG: Pulmonary vascular congestion in acute myocardial infarction: Hemodynamic and radiologic correlations. Ann Intern Med 76:29, 1972.)

is frequently precluded by the supine or semiupright position of the patient or suboptimal degree of inspiration during exposure of the radiograph.

However, the major reason for the lack of a more precise correlation between the chest radiograph and hemodynamic measurements in AMI is the nearly immediate change in pulmonary venous pressure resulting both from the ischemic myocardial damage and the response to therapy, while a newly attained level of PVH must be present for some time before it is reflected on the radiograph. Many of the radiographic signs of PVH depend on the flux of fluid from the vascular to the extravascular space; therefore, the radiographic signs of PVH correlate better with increased pulmonary extravascular water.[18] The period of time required for sufficient fluid to accumulate in the interstitial or alveolar spaces of the lungs after the pulmonary venous pressure is elevated in order to permit radiographic detection has been referred to as a "diagnostic phase lag."[16,17] Kostuk et al.[17] documented a 12-hour lag between a measured elevation in PAW pressure and the

radiographic reflection of this abnormal level of pressure in a number of patients with AMI. These and other investigators[16,17] have also demonstrated a "post-therapeutic phase lag," which is the time required for the reappearance of a normal radiograph after elevated PAW pressures fall to normal levels in response to therapy. This phenomenon was observed in nearly 25 percent of patients, and, in some instances, up to 4 days elapsed between normalization of the PAW pressure and the radiograph.

Pulmonary venous hypertension is observed within the initial 24 hours after AMI in one-third to nearly one-half of patients.[1,16,17] Frequently, pulmonary edema occurs in the absence of obvious cardiomegaly (Fig. 26.7). However, heart size may be difficult to gauge on initial chest radiographs after AMI, as these are usually anteroposterior portable radiographs with the patient in a supine or semiupright position. The occurrence of PVH in the absence of left ventricular or overall cardiac enlargement may be a reflection of the diminished compliance of the left ventricle, which characterizes ischemic LV dysfunction.[19,20]

The presence and severity of PVH on chest radiographs within the initial 24 hours after AMI has been found to have prognostic implications;[1] early and late mortality were significantly higher in patients with any degree of PVH (Fig. 26.9). Without PVH, mortality was less than 10 percent, while with any degree of PVH it was greater than 30 percent. In those with generalized alveolar edema, mortality rates within the first month and the first year were unusually high. Generally, the presence and severity of PVH have shown an inverse relation to systolic blood pressure, stroke volume, and cardiac index and a direct relation to arteriovenous oxygen difference and infarct "size," as assessed by serial enzyme studies.[21]

The radiographic signs of PVH or pulmonary edema in elderly patients occasionally are atypical. Several factors influence the accumulation of pulmonary extravascular fluid, including gravity (patient lying continuously on one side); underlying pulmonary parenchymal disease (chronic obstructive pulmonary disease); and status of the pulmonary vascular bed (chronic obstructive pulmonary disease, pulmonary em-

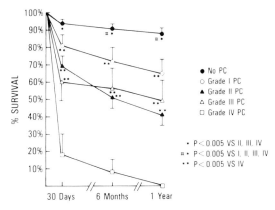

Fig. 26.9 Graph displays the relationship between early and late survival and the severity of pulmonary venous hypertension on the initial chest radiograph after acute myocardial infarction. (Battler A et al.: The initial chest x-ray in acute myocardial infarction. Prediction of early and late mortality and survival. Circulation: 1004, 1980.)

bolism). A frequent concurrent disease with AMI is emphysema, which may alter the appearance of the lung fields to an extent that pulmonary edema may be difficult to detect. Hublitz and Shapiro [22] recognized two atypical patterns of pulmonary edema in patients with emphysema. One pattern was alveolar edema in a nonuniform distribution because of regional obliteration of the vascular bed. In the other pattern, fluid collects almost exclusively in the interstitial space and produces a cloudy reticular or nodular pattern. Heart size may be small and remain so as a consequence of the chronic obstructive pulmonary disease.

## Heart Size

Most patients with a single myocardial infarction have a normal heart size. Nevertheless, it is not infrequent to find pulmonary edema in the presence of a normal heart size (Fig. 26.7).

Cardiomegaly has been observed in approximately 40 percent,[23-25] and an abnormally large left ventricle (as gauged by the left heart dimension (LHD)) in 54 percent,[26] of patients incurring an AMI. Cardiomegaly or the presence of an enlarged left ventricle have some prognostic value. Several studies have revealed a combined early and late mortality of over 50 percent in patients with persistent cardiomegaly after AMI compared to a rate of half this in patients with normal heart size on chest radiographs.[23-25] An enlarged left heart dimension has likewise been associated with a several-fold higher early and late mortality compared to that observed with a normal LHD.[1,21]

Cardiomegaly generally indicates severe coronary obstructive disease with ischemic dysfunction of at least the anterior or anterolateral wall of the left ventricle, as a consequence of occlusion of the left anterior descending coronary artery.[27] The presence of cardiomegaly, along with either radiographic or clinical evidence of congestive heart failure, has been indicative of a low ejection fraction, usually less than 0.30.[27,28]

### Complications

#### Cardiogenic Shock.

This complication may be predicted based on the volume of infarcted myocardium. Infarction of greater than 40 percent of the left ventricular myocardium is usually found in patients succumbing from cardiogenic shock.[29,30] Most patients with this syndrome have occlusion of at least the left anterior descending coronary artery.[30]

While in some patients with cardiogenic shock there is an increased left ventricular end-diastolic volume,[30] it is not uncommon to find shock in the absence of cardiomegaly.[26] Serial radiographs are utilized in the evaluation of patients during the treatment of cardiogenic shock by intraaortic balloon pumping. Improvement in the roentgenographic degree of heart failure within 24 hours or less of balloon pumping suggests the likelihood of immediate survival.[31] On the other hand, in those patients who show deteriorating or unchanging chest X-ray findings, the volume of nonischemic myocardium is insufficient to allow survival.

#### Ventricular Dysrhythmias

Radiography has little role in this regard, except to demonstrate the presence of a ventricular aneurysm. Ventricular aneurysm may be the focus of origin of recurrent and intractable ventricular tachycardia.

## Cardiac Rupture

Rupture of an infarct freely into the pericardial sac is usually associated with precipitous demise from exanguination and/or tamponade. If rupture is contained by fused pericardial layers, a localized sacculation (false aneurysm) extending from the cardiac margin may be observed.[32-34]

## Ventricular Septal Rupture

Ventricular septal rupture has been found at postmortem examination in 1 to 2 percent of fatal MIs. It usually occurs between 4 to 21 days after the onset of the acute MI but may occur within the first 24 hours after AMI.[35-37] This complication has been associated with a 90 percent mortality.[35] Ventricular septal rupture occurs with both anteroseptal and posteroseptal MIs.[36] The septal defect is always in the muscular portion of the septum. Rupture in the posterior portion of the septum usually results from occlusion of the right coronary artery and has been associated with akinesis of the diaphragmatic or posterobasal segment. Anterior septal rupture has been associated with anterior or apical akinesis. Infarction of the right ventricle, mitral regurgitation and aneurysms of the left ventricle have been frequently encountered in association with this complication.[36] These associated complications and the fact that a large volume of muscle has usually been irreversibly damaged are contributing factors to the high mortality reported with postinfarction ventricular septal defect. Pathologic studies suggest that septal rupture is the result of a large transmural infarction with a paucity of collateral vessels or collateral vessels arising from arteries with significant proximal obstructive disease.[37]

The chest radiograph generally reveals a dramatic change with the occurrence of septal rupture. The superimposition of a large left to right shunt on even a moderate size MI produces the rapid onset of signs of severe pulmonary venous congestion or generalized alveolar pulmonary edema (Fig. 26.10). In 33 patients with postinfarction ventricular septal defect, the chest radiograph showed interstitial or alveolar pulmonary edema in 78 percent and left ventricular enlargement in 82 percent. Less severe hemodynamic compromise allows time for the

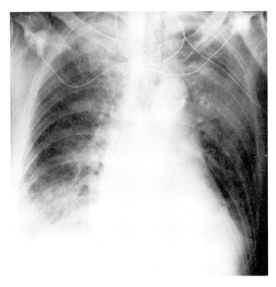

Fig. 26.10 Chest radiograph of a patient with a large myocardial infarction complicated by rupture of the interventricular septum shows severe pulmonary edema. Bilateral alveolar infiltrate obscures the pulmonary vascularity which complicates detection of shunt vascularity.

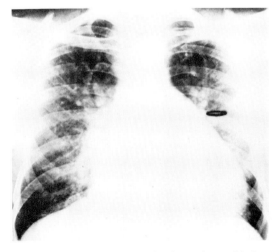

Fig. 26.11 Chest radiograph of a patient with less severe hemodynamic compromise from postinfarction interventricular septal rupture. In this instance pulmonary arterial overcirculation (shunt vascularity) is apparent.

appearance of pulmonary plethora and an increase in cardiac size during the early recovery phase (Fig. 26.11).

## Papillary Muscle Rupture

The frequency with and time at which this complication occurs is similar to that of rupture of the ventricular septum.[38-40] This complication is most frequent with posterior or diaphragmatic MI where dysfunction involves the posteromedial papillary muscle but rupture of the anterior papillary muscle after AMI does occur. Eighty percent of patients with acute rupture of papillary muscles die within 2 weeks of the event.

Acute papillary muscle rupture is manifested radiographically by the abrupt appearance of pulmonary edema. Most frequently, pulmonary edema exists with a heart size that is normal or only slightly increased. Likewise, left atrial enlargement is usually not evident.

## Ventricular Aneurysms

The aneurysm is usually a true one but rarely may be false. An attempt to differentiate between the two is important because of the possibility of a late rupture of false aneurysms.[33]

## True Aneurysm

These usually involve the anterolateral or apical portions of the left ventricle and result from occlusion of the left anterior descending coronary artery or one of its branches.[41,42] Many true aneurysms produce no perceptible abnormality of the cardiac silhouette. An abnormal evagination along the cardiac shadow, when present, is usually located along the lower left cardiac border on the frontal view and anteriorly on the lateral view (anterior double density, Fig. 26.12). Occasionally, calcification in the wall of the aneurysm is observed along the anterior or apical portion of the ventricular contour.

## False Aneurysm

This aneurysmal sac results from the localized containment of a ventricular rupture by the fused layers of the visceral and parietal pericardium.[32,33] The site of origin of the aneurysm is most frequently from the posterolateral or diaphragmatic segments of the left ventricle

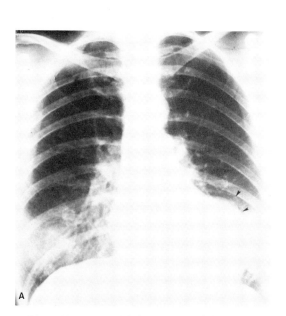 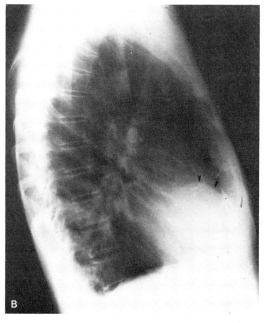

Fig. 26.12 Frontal *(A)* and lateral *(B)* chest radiographs demonstrate a true aneurysm of the anterolateral segment of the left ventricle. The lateral view shows the double density located anteriorly which is characteristic of an aneurysm.

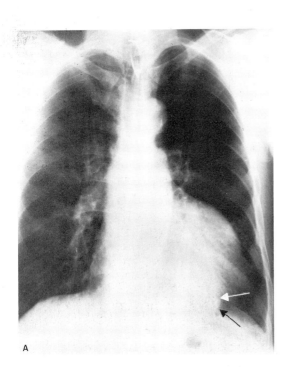

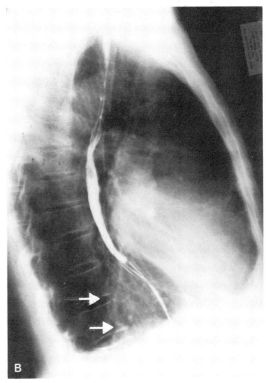

Fig. 26.13   Frontal *(A)* and lateral *(B)* chest radiographs reveal a large false aneurysm arising from the posterior region of the left ventricle. The frontal veiw demonstrates the left retrocardiac double density *(arrows)*. The lateral view reveals the enormous size and posterior location of the aneurysm *(arrows)* which are features suggestive of a false aneurysm.

as a result of occlusion of the circumflex or right coronary arteries.[34] Consequently, the abnormal evagination on the lateral radiograph is frequently from the posterior border of the heart (Fig. 26.13). This location may cause a left retrocardiac double density on the frontal view (Fig. 26.13). False aneurysms tend to be large or even enormous in size compared to true aneurysms. Sequential radiographs frequently reveal a perceptible increase in size. Angiography defines the posterior or diaphragmatic location of the aneurysm, enormous size, and, in some instances, one or more small ostia between the left ventricle and the aneurysm.[34]

## RADIOGRAPHIC CLUES IN THE DIFFERENTIAL DIAGNOSIS OF ACUTE CHEST PAIN

A multitude of other diseases may cause the acute onset of chest pain and thereby mimic

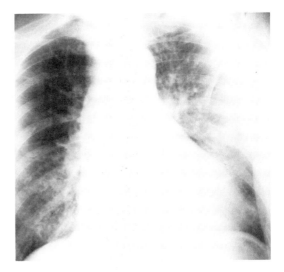

Fig. 26.14   Frontal chest radiograph in a patient with acute dissection of the aorta reveals substantial enlargement of the ascending aorta and pulmonary venous hypertension. Dissecting aneurysm should be a diagnostic consideration in a patient with chest pain and a markedly enlarged ascending aorta.

ischemic heart disease. The chest radiograph may reveal signs suggestive of or diagnostic for these conditions.

Dissecting aneurysm causes abnormal findings on the posteroanterior chest radiograph in nearly 90 percent of patients, of which the most frequent are enlargement of the ascending aorta and widening of the superior mediastinum (Fig. 26.14).[43] The significance of the latter finding on the anteroposterior (portable) radiograph is difficult to determine because of the greater magnification of the anterior mediastinum in this projection. The intramural and perivascular hematoma causes displacement of nearby structures. The chest radiograph may show rightward displacement of the trachea; downward displacement of the left bronchus; and lateral displacement of the paraspinal line. Additional radiographic clues are obscuration of the margin of the aortic knob and/or descending aorta (Fig. 26.14) and left pleural effusion.

Acute pericarditis commonly causes no radiographic abnormalities. Infrequently, the associated pericardial effusion is sufficiently large to cause a positive fat-pad sign, i.e., separation of the lucent strip of substernal fat from the lucent strip of subepicardial fat by water density on the lateral chest radiograph. Usually, the small volume of effusion in this affliction is detectable only by M-mode or real-time echocardiography.

Pulmonary embolism produces abnormalities on the chest radiograph in a majority of patients; however, usually the findings are minor and nonspecific.[44] The classic pleural-based density in a wedge-shaped configuration is infrequently observed. Likewise, the Westermark sign of abrupt termination of a pulmonary vascular shadow along with lucency of the lung field beyond it is relatively specific but infrequently observed. However, consideration of pulmonary embolism should be aroused by the less specific findings of persistent elevation of a hemidiaphragm, pleural effusion, and persistent discoid atelectasis (Fleischner lines).

Other abnormalities that produce chest pain and can be easily detected on the chest radiograph are spontaneous pneumothorax,[45] pneumomediastinum (post-tussive or with acute

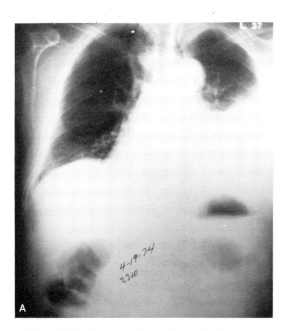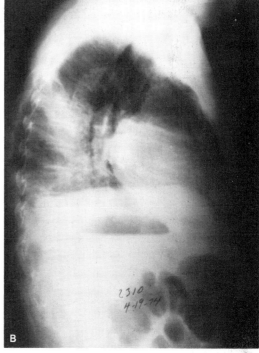

Fig. 26.15 Frontal *(A)* and lateral *(B)* radiographs in a patient with Boerhaave syndrome, showing mediastinal emphysema and left pleural effusion. These findings are almost diagnostic of this entity.

asthma),[46] and rupture of the esophagus (Boerhaave syndrome).[47,48] The most frequent site of esophageal rupture is the left posterolateral aspect of the esophagus. Consequently, it generally results in a left pleural effusion and pneumomediastinum (Fig. 26.15). This catastrophe usually results from retching or vomiting, or from the ingestion of a foreign body.

## REFERENCES

1. Battler A, Karliner JS, Higgins CB, et al: The initial chest X-ray in acute myocardial infarction: Prediction of early and late mortality and survival. Circulation, 61:1004, 1980.
2. Kazamias TM, Gander MP, Gault JH, et al: Roentgenographic assessment of left ventricular size in man: A standardized method. J Appl Physiol 32:881, 1972.
3. Keats TE, Lipscomb GE, Betts CS III: Mensuration of the azygos vein and its application to the study of cardiopulmonary disease. Radiology 90:990, 1968.
4. Ravin CE, Putman CE, McCloud TC: Hazards of the intensive care unit. Am J Roentgenol 126:423, 1976.
5. Langson CS: The aberrant central venous catheter and its complications. Radiology 100:55, 1971.
6. Foote GA, Schabel SI, Hodges M: Pulmonary complications of the flow-directed balloon tipped catheter. N Engl J Med 290:927, 1974.
7. McCloud TC, Putman CE: Radiology of the Swan-Ganz catheter and associated pulmonary complications. Radiology 116:19, 1975.
8. Reinke RT, Higgins CB, Atkin TW: Pulmonary infarction complicating the use of Swan-Ganz catheters. Br J Radiol 48:885, 1975.
9. Hyson EA, Ravin CE, Kelley MJ, et al: The intraaortic counterpulsation balloon: Radiographic considerations. Am J Roentgenol 128:915, 1977.
10. Ormond RS, Rubenfire M, Anbe DT, et al: Radiographic demonstration of myocardial penetration by permanent endocardial pacemakers. Radiology 98:35, 1971.
11. Goodman LR: Pulmonary support and monitoring apparatus. In: Intensive Care Radiology. Goodman LR, Putman CE, Mosby CV, editors. St Louis, 1978.
12. Goodman LR, Conrardy PA, Laing F, et al: Radiographic evaluation of endotracheal tube position. Am J Roentgenol 127:433, 1976.
13. Ching NP, Ayres SM, Spina RC, et al: Endotracheal damage during continuous ventilatory support. Ann Surg 179:123, 1974.
14. Rohlfing BM, Webb WR, Schlobohm RM: Ventilator-related extra-alveolar air in adults. Radiology 121:25, 1976.
15. Harrison MO, Conte PJ, Heitzman ER: Radiological detection of clinically occult cardiac failure following myocardial infarction. Br J Radiol 44:265, 1971.
16. McHugh TF, Forrester JS, Adler L, et al: Pulmonary vascular congestion in acute myocardial infarction: Hemodynamic and radiologic correlations. Ann Intern Med 76:29, 1972.
17. Kostuk W, Barr JW, Simon AL, et al: Correlations between the chest film and hemodynamics in acute myocardial infarction. Circulation 48:624, 1973.
18. Luepker RV, Caralis DG, Voigt GC, et al: Detection of pulmonary edema in acute myocardial infarction. Am J Cardiol 39:146, 1977.
19. Dwyer EM: Left ventricular pressure-volume alterations and regional disorders of contraction during myocardial ischemia induced by atrial pacing. Circulation 42:1111, 1970.
20. Diamond G, Forrester JS: Effect of coronary artery disease and acute myocardial infarction on left ventricular compliance in man. Circulation 45:11, 1972.
21. Battler A, Higgins CB, Karliner JS, et al: The initial chest X-ray in acute myocardial infarction: Relation of pulmonary congestion to heart size and to hemodynamic data. Submitted for publication.
22. Hublitz UF, Shapiro JH: Atypical pulmonary patterns of congestive failure in chronic lung disease. Radiology 93:995, 1969.
23. Norris RM, Caughey DE, Mercer CJ, et al: Coronary prognostic index for predicting survival after recovery from acute myocardial infarction. Lancet 2:485, 1970.
24. Amundsen P: The diagnostic value of conventional radiological examination of the heart in adults. Acta Radiol 181 (suppl): 1, 1959.
25. Waris EK, Siitonen L, Himanka E: Heart size and prognosis in myocardial infarction. Am Heart J 71:187, 1966.
26. Kostuk WF, Kazamias TM, Gander MP, et al: Left ventricular size after acute myocardial infarction. Serial changes and their prognostic significance. Circulation 47:1174, 1973.
27. Aintablian A, Hanby RI, Garsman J: Correlation of heart size with clinical and hemodynamic

findings in patients with coronary artery disease. Am Heart J 91:21, 1976.

28. Field BJ, Russell RO, Moraski RE, et al: Left ventricular size and function and heart size in the year following myocardial infarction. Circulation 50:331, 1971.

29. Page DL, Caulfield JB, Kastor JA, et al: Myocardial changes associated with cardiogenic shock. N Engl J Med 285:133, 1971.

30. Leinbach RC, Dinsmore RE, Mundth, Buckley MJ, et al: Selective coronary and left ventricular cineangiography during intraaortic balloon pumping for cardiogenic shock. Circulation 45:845, 1972.

31. Cascade PN, Kantrowitz A, Wajszczuk SW, et al: The chest X-ray in acute left ventricular power failure: An aid to determining prognosis of patients supported by intraaortic balloon pumping. Am J Roentgenol 126:1147, 1976.

32. Van Tassel RA, Edwards JE: Rupture of heart complicating myocardial infarction. Analysis of 40 cases including nine examples of left ventricular false aneurysm. Chest 61:104, 1972.

33. Vlodaver Z, Coe JI, Edwards JE: True and false left ventricular aneurysms. Propensity for the latter to rupture. Circulation 51:567, 1975.

34. Higgins CB, Lipton MJ, Johnson AD, et al: False aneurysms of the left ventricle: Identification of distinctive clinical, radiographic, and angiographic features. Radiology 127:21, 1978.

35. Heikkila J, Karesoja M, Luomanmaki K: Ruptured interventricular septum complicating acute myocardial infarction. Chest 66:675, 1974.

36. Miller SW, Dinsmore RE, Greene RE, et al: Coronary, ventricular and pulmonary abnormalities associated with rupture of the interventricular septum complicating myocardial infarction. Am J Roentgenol 131:571, 1978.

37. Hutchins GM: Rupture of the interventricular septum complicating myocardial infarction: Pathological analysis of 10 patients with clinically diagnosed perforations. Am Heart J 97:165, 1979.

38. Sanders RJ, Neubuerger KT, Ravin A: Rupture of papillary muscles. Occurrence of rupture of the posterior muscle in posterior myocardial infarction. Dis Chest 31:316, 1957.

39. Heikkilu J: Mitral incompetence as a complication of acute myocardial infarction. Acta Med Scand (Suppl) 475:7, 1967.

40. DeBusk RF, Harrison DC: The clinical spectrum of papillary muscle disease. N Engl J Med 281:1458, 1969.

41. Baron MG: Postinfarctional aneurysm of the left ventricle. Circulation 43:762, 1971.

42. Kittredge RD, Gamboa B, Kemp HG: Radiographic visualization of left ventricular aneurysms on lateral chest film. Am J Roentgenol 126:1140, 1976.

43. Beachley MC, Ranniger K, Roght FJ: Roentgenographic evaluation of dissecting aneurysms of the aorta. Am J Roentgenol 121:617, 1974.

44. Kelley MJ, Elliott LP: The radiologic evaluation of the patient with suspected pulmonary thromboembolic disease. Med Clin NA 59:3, 1975.

45. Mills M, Baisch BG: Spontaneous pneumothorax. A series of 400 cases. Ann Thoracic Surg 1:286, 1965.

46. Munsell WP: Pneumomediastinum: A report of 28 cases and review of literature. JAMA 202:689, 1967.

47. Abbott OA, Mansour KA, Logan WD, et al: A traumatic so-called "spontaneous" rupture of the esophagus: A review of 47 personal cases with a new method of surgical therapy. J Thorac Cardiovasc Surg 49:67, 1970.

48. Rogers LF, Puig AW, Dooley BN, et al: Diagnostic considerations in mediastinal emphysema: A pathophysiologic-roentgenologic approach to Boerhaave's syndrome and spontaneous pneumomediastinum. Am J Roentgenol 115:495, 1972.

# 27 | Hemodynamic Monitoring in the Coronary Care Unit

## Gabriel Gregoratos, M.D.

During the first 10 years of the coronary care unit era, emphasis was placed on early detection, prevention, and treatment of cardiac arrhythmias that developed after an acute myocardial infarction. The use of drugs to prevent and terminate potentially lethal arrhythmias and electric defibrillation applied in the setting of continuous electrocardiographic monitoring resulted in a marked reduction in the incidence of primary dysrhythmic deaths after acute myocardial infarction. As a result, myocardial "pump failure" has become the major cause of death in patients hospitalized with acute myocardial infarction.[1] The 1970s were characterized by the widespread application of hemodynamic monitoring techniques in the coronary care unit in response to the need to understand the hemodynamic alterations produced by myocardial infarction and to assess the results of therapeutic interventions.

The technique of bedside cardiac catheterization came into its own in 1970 with the introduction of balloon flotation catheters by Swan, Ganz, and their associates.[2] Based on an original idea of Lategola and Rahn,[3] the impetus for the development of balloon flotation catheters stemmed initially from the realization that measurement of the central venous pressure, although a good index of right ventricular filling pressure, was, at best, an imprecise and often a highly misleading index of left ventricular filling pressure in acute myocardial infarction.[4] In early attempts to perform right heart catheterization at the bedside, fine, small-lumen, highly flexible catheters composed of various materials (nylon, silastic, tygon, and so on) were used.[5,6] These catheters were introduced into an antecubital vein and advanced gently through the venous system into the right heart chambers. They were light and flexible enough to be carried into the pulmonary artery by blood flow. The use of these "microcatheters" had several disadvantages, including the induction of ventricular ectopy as the catheter traversed the right ventricle and, mainly, their relative unreliability. In 15 to 20 percent of cases there was failure to catheterize the right ventricle and pulmonary artery. Furthermore, long periods of manipulation were required before successful flotation into the pulmonary artery could be accomplished. It was the combination of the poor reliability of pulmonary artery catheterization by means of the small catheters described above and the unreliability of the central venous pressure as an index of left ventricular filling pressure that spurred development of the balloon flotation catheter in 1970.[4]

Since its inception, the balloon-flotation catheter has undergone many changes. Catheters are now available with multiple lumens for the simultaneous recording of pressures from two different cardiac chambers; many catheters incorporate a thermistor bead to measure cardiac output by the thermodilution principle, and others include electrodes to record intracardiac electrograms as well as to pace the atria and/

or the ventricles. The major utility of the balloon-flotation catheter, however, remains the ability of the user to catheterize the pulmonary artery safely and quickly (without the aid of fluoroscopy) and to obtain pressure recordings from the pulmonary artery and pulmonary artery wedge position, as will be described later in this chapter. The techniques of bedside right-heart catheterization, arterial catheter introduction, and measurement of important variables, utilizing these methods as well as a discussion of the potential complications of these techniques, form the basis for the remainder of this chapter.

## INDICATIONS FOR HEMODYNAMIC MONITORING IN ACUTE MYOCARDIAL INFARCTION

Our current indications for hemodynamic monitoring in patients with an acute myocardial infarction are listed in Table 27.1. Invasive hemodynamic monitoring is not recommended for the patient with an uncomplicated myocardial infarction unless the patient is participating in a formal investigation designed to evaluate new forms of treatment or prognosis after the infarct.

Patients who manifest even minor degrees of hypotension and other signs of early circula-

Table 27.1   Indications for Invasive Hemodynamic Monitoring

Uncomplicated Infarction
  1. Prognostic evaluation *
  2. Evaluation of new/investigational treatment methods *

Complicated Infarction
  1. Diagnostic uncertainty as to hemodynamic status
  2. Hypotension (pump failure vs hypovolemia) †
  3. Congestive heart failure
  4. Unstable angina, post infarction
  5. Hypoxemia (pulmonary vs cardiac in origin) †
  6. Suspected cardiac tamponade
  7. Suspected structural defects (ventricular septal defect, acute mitral regurgitation) †
  8. Monitoring of vasodilator and/or inotropic drug administration

* Patients on approved investigational protocols only
† See text for discussion

tory collapse should undergo prompt right-heart catheterization to measure left ventricular filling pressure and cardiac output. The purpose of this early intervention is to define precisely the presence of early "pump failure" and to exclude the possibility of hypovolemia, a readily treatable and rapidly reversible cause of circulatory collapse.[7] This is particularly important in older patients on chronic diuretic therapy. Such patients will often have a chronically reduced plasma volume and may show significant hypotension, even in the presence of a minor myocardial insult. Plasma volume expansion may rapidly reverse the circulatory collapse in this setting. Similarly, in the presence of signs of right or left ventricular failure, the early insertion of a right-heart catheter to measure right and left ventricular filling pressures is recommended. In the setting of pulmonary edema, continuous monitoring of left ventricular filling pressure provides the physician with invaluable help in adjusting diuretic and/or vasodilator therapy. The availability of left ventricular filling pressure measurements becomes even more important during the recovery phase from acute pulmonary edema. In this setting it is well recognized that a time of lag of as much as 48 hours may exist between hemodynamic stabilization and resolution of the physical and radiographic signs of pulmonary edema.[8,9] If this time lag is not recognized and vigorous diuretic therapy is continued, it is possible to reduce left ventricular filling pressures to such an extent that effective cardiac output may decline. Similarly, in the setting of elevated jugular venous pressure with clear lungs, the introduction of a balloon flotation catheter through the cardiac chambers of the right side will help resolve the question of right ventricular infarction versus cardiac tamponade.

A major indication for invasive hemodynamic evaluation and monitoring of the myocardial infarction patient is the existence of diagnostic uncertainty as to the patient's hemodynamic status. Although thorough and repeated examinations by alert clinicians often provide valuable clues regarding the development or progression of postmyocardial infarction pump failure, the dynamic and complex nature of this process requires the more objective quantitative assessment of hemodynamic measurements. Discrepancies between clinical and hemodynamic assessment have been amply documented.[9,10] Another common diagnostic dilemma arises when a patient with chronic obstructive lung disease develops an acute myocardial infarction. In this setting, it is often exceedingly difficult to decide whether the physical, radiographic, and laboratory signs (including arterial hypoxemia) are due to chronic lung disease or to left ventricular failure. Measurement of left ventricular filling pressures will almost certainly dispel the uncertainty.

The presence of a new systolic murmur in the postmyocardial infarction period is usually due to the development of mitral regurgitation or rupture of the interventricular septum. Although the diagnosis of interventricular septal rupture can usually be made clinically, its confirmation requires right-heart catheterization. Management of the subsequent worsening hemodynamic state requires the ability to monitor pulmonary artery and pulmonary artery wedge pressures and systemic and pulmonary arterial oxygen content. The murmur of acute mitral regurgitation due to rupture of chordae tendineae or a head of a papillary muscle is often not typically holosystolic but may simulate an ejection aortic murmur because of a late systolic decrease in intensity and radiation towards the base of the heart.[11] Furthermore, in low cardiac output states, the intensity of the systolic murmur correlates poorly with the severity of mitral regurgitation.[7] The introduction of a balloon-flotation catheter in the pulmonary artery and the recording of a pulmonary artery wedge pressure with a dominant systolic wave can therefore be of great value in confirming the diagnosis of acute mitral regurgitation.

From the above discussion, one may easily draw the conclusion that hemodynamic monitoring in the setting of acute myocardial infarction is applicable in a variety of clinical situations and that the indications are fairly liberal. One must remember, however, that hemodynamic monitoring is an invasive procedure. Not only is the skin penetrated, but catheters are placed in the central circulation and the right-sided cardiac chambers. Although the risk of invasive hemodynamic monitoring is, in practi-

cal terms, negligible, complications do occur. Therefore, the rational application of invasive hemodynamic studies requires that this procedure be undertaken to acquire specific predetermined information necessary to establish a full diagnosis, decide on the most rational form of therapy, or allow rapid appraisal of the results of therapy being employed. In addition, this specific information may not be obtainable with sufficient precision by available noninvasive techniques.

## AVAILABLE HEMODYNAMIC DATA AND THEIR SIGNIFICANCE

Using current monitoring techniques, the following information can be obtained at the bedside: (1) pressure data, (2) blood flow data (cardiac output), and (3) metabolic and respiratory data.

Pressure data commonly obtained include systemic arterial, right atrial, right ventricular, pulmonary arterial, and pulmonary artery wedge pressures. [Pulmonary capillary wedge pressure is a term that has been used synonymously with pulmonary artery wedge pressure to indicate the pressure recorded from a proximally occluded secondary or tertiary pulmonary artery branch. Since the mean pulmonary artery wedge pressure has been found to be essentially identical to pressure in the next active vascular compartment (the pulmonary veins)[7] and since it does not represent a direct measurement of pressure in the pulmonary capillary bed, we prefer the term pulmonary artery wedge pressure, omitting the word capillary.]

Direct left ventricular pressure data are usually not obtainable at the bedside because retrograde crossing of the aortic valve frequently requires fluoroscopic guidance of the catheter. Left ventricular catheterization, therefore, remains in the province of the cardiac catheterization laboratory. However, it is rarely necessary to obtain direct left ventricular pressures for monitoring purposes, as will become evident from the subsequent discussion.

Cardiac output in liters per minute is usually obtained at the bedside by the indicator dilution technique and most commonly by the thermodilution technique (see below). It is customary to normalize cardiac output data by dividing them by the patient's body surface area so that blood flow data among patients of varying size can be compared. Heart rate is obtained by continuous electrocardiographic monitoring.

Metabolic and respiratory data obtainable include arterial blood gases ($PaO_2$, $PaCO_2$, pH), arterial oxygen content, mixed venous blood gases and oxygen content (in the absence of a left to right shunt mixed venous blood samples are optimally obtained from the pulmonary artery), serum lactate levels, arterial base excess, and central core temperature.

From the measured pressure and flow data, a number of derived hemodynamic parameters can be calculated. These are the cardiac index (CI), stroke volume (SV), stroke index (SI), stroke work index (SWI), systemic vascular resistence (SVR), and pulmonary arteriolar resistance (PAR). The most commonly measured and derived hemodynamic parameters are listed along with methods of calculation in Table 27.2. A detailed treatment of the derivation and calculation of these hemodynamic parameters can be found in standard cardiac catheterization reference texts.[12]

A major objective of invasive hemodynamic monitoring, of the type discussed above, is the evaluation of the heart as a pump. Such an evaluation relates parameters of ventricular work performed, such as cardiac output, stroke volume, or stroke work, to the degree of myocardial fiber stretch, a clinical extension of the Frank-Starling principle.[1] Although left ventricular end-diastolic volume is the measurement that relates most closely to end-diastolic myocardial fiber stretch[13] in the intact heart, determination of this parameter requires angiographic techniques rarely available outside the cardiac catheterization laboratory. Consequently, most clinical hemodynamic studies continue to utilize the left ventricular end-diastolic pressure as an index of end-diastolic volume and tension. The limitations of ventricular end-diastolic pressure in the assessment of ventricular function were clearly described many years ago.[13] These limitations relate to the shape of ventricular function curves and ventricular pressure-volume curves, which indicate that when the end-diastolic pressure is in the normal or near normal range it is a relatively insensitive index of end-diastolic volume. In this setting, large changes in ventricular stroke work or ventricular end-diastolic volume may be associated with relatively small changes in ventricular end-diastolic pressure. Conversely, in patients with increased ventricular stiffness (whether due to concentric myocardial hypertrophy, pericardial constriction, or a restrictive myocardial defect) the ventricular end-diastolic pressure may be markedly elevated in the presence of normal end-diastolic and end-systolic ventricular volumes.[14] Despite these limitations, judicious interpretation of left ventricular end-diastolic pressure remains a useful clinical tool, especially during cardiac catheterization. Since direct left ventricular end-diastolic pressure is not commonly measured at the bedside in the intensive care unit, we must address the question of whether pulmonary artery wedge or pulmonary artery diastolic pressures accurately reflect this measurement.

Frahm and Braunwald[15] established that in normals the difference between mean left atrial pressure and left ventricular end-diastolic pressure was of small magnitude, ranging from +4 to −5 mmHg and averaging 0.2 mmHg. In patients with left ventricular hypertrophy or left ventricular failure, however, left ventricular end-diastolic pressure exceeded mean left atrial pressure by 1 to 18 mmHg, and the difference averaged 9 mmHg. This relationship has been confirmed repeatedly and can be seen regularly in the catheterization laboratory. On the other hand, the mean left atrial pressure is rather closely related to the *mean* left ventricular diastolic pressure, exceeding it by 2 to 6 mmHg, depending on the functional state of the left ventricle and its pressure-volume relationships (provided mitral valve function is normal).[7] The mean left ventricular diastolic pressure is also a significant determinant of left ventricular function as it reflects the state of compliance of the left ventricular wall and the left ventricular diastolic volume. It remains, therefore, to examine the relationship between left atrial and pulmonary artery wedge pressures.

The pulmonary artery wedge pressure is used widely, both in the catheterization laboratory

**Table 27.2  Hemodynamic Data Calculations**

**1. Cardiac Output**

Fick: $CO(l/min) = \dfrac{\dot{V}O_2(ml/min)}{a\text{-}vDO_2(vol\ \%) \times 10}$

$\dot{V}O_2$ = Oxygen consumption
a-vDO$_2$ = Arteriovenous oxygen content difference

Indicator-Dilution: $CO(l/min) = \dfrac{I \times 60}{\overline{C} \times t}$

I = Indicator amount injected (mg)
60 = Conversion factor seconds to minutes
$\overline{C}$ = Mean concentration of indicator (mg/l)
t = Time of curve duration (sec)

Thermodilution: $CO(l/min) = \dfrac{(1.08)Ct(60)V_i(T_b - T_i)}{\displaystyle\int_0^\infty \Delta T_b(t)dt}$

1.08 = Factor derived from specific heat and density of 5% glucose and blood
Ct = Correction factor for injectate temperature rise during injection
60 = Conversion factor seconds to minutes
$V_i$ = Volume of injectate
$T_b$ = Initial temperature of blood (°C)
$T_i$ = Initial temperature of injectate (°C)
$\displaystyle\int_0^\infty \Delta T_b(t)dt$ = Integral of blood temperature change (°C-sec)

**2. Derived Data**

$CI = \dfrac{CO}{BSA}$

CI = cardiac index (l/min/m²)
CO = cardiac output (l/min)
BSA = body surface area (m²)

$SV = \dfrac{CO}{HR}$

SV = stroke volume (ml/beat)
HR = heart rate (beats/min)

$SI = \dfrac{SV}{BSA}$

SI = stroke index (ml/beat/m²)

$SVR = \dfrac{\overline{SAP} - \overline{RAP}}{CO}$

SVR = systemic vascular resistance (hybrid units)
$\overline{SAP}$ = mean systemic arterial pressure (mm Hg)
$\overline{RAP}$ = mean right atrial pressure (mm Hg)
CO = cardiac output (l/min)

$TPR = \dfrac{\overline{MPA}}{CO}$

$\overline{MPA}$ = mean pulmonary artery pressure (mm Hg)
TPR = total pulmonary resistance (hybrid units)

$PAR = \dfrac{\overline{MPA} - \overline{PAW}}{CO}$

PAR = Pulmonary arteriolar or vascular resistance (hybrid units)
$\overline{PAW}$ = Mean pulmonary artery wedge pressure (mm Hg)

NOTE: 1 hybrid resistance unit = 80 dynes·sec·cm$^{-5}$

and at the bedside as an index of left atrial pressure. It is generally considered to accurately reflect mean left atrial pressure and, therefore, in the absence of mitral valve disease, to be a useful and reliable indicator of left ventricular diastolic dynamics.[16] However, it is recognized that there are intrinsic limitations in the interpretation of the pulmonary artery wedge pressure. Walston and Kendall,[17] in a retrospective analysis of 700 patients with various forms of cardiac disease, compared the pulmonary artery wedge pressure with the left atrial pressure measured directly by transseptal left atrial puncture. An overall correlation coefficient of 0.93 was found. However, it was also found that scatter increased as the wedge and left atrial pressures rose. At mean wedge pressures above 25 mmHg, statistically significant differences ($p < 0.05$) were found between pulmonary artery wedge and left atrial pressures. This progressive loss of correlation at higher levels may in part be explainable by the findings of Caro et al.[18] These investigators demonstrated, in the experimental animal, that high transcapillary pressures produced an alteration in the ratio of pulmonary arterial and pulmonary venous compliance, thereby promoting asymmetric transmission of pressure waves across the pulmonary vascular bed. Other investigators have recorded similar discrepancies between mean wedge and mean left atrial pressures and have recommended the employment of a correction factor,[19] which, however, is rarely used in clinical practice.

In the presence of severe pulmonary arterial hypertension, a number of investigators have noted technical difficulties in obtaining a satisfactory pulmonary artery wedge waveform.[20-22] The use of flow-directed balloon-tipped catheters has obviated some of these difficulties, although we and others have noted that the phasic characteristics of wedge pressures obtained in patients with pulmonary hypertension are often suboptimal.

Patients with obstructive pulmonary disease commonly demonstrate substantial alterations in pleural pressure during respiration, which can influence the recorded absolute wedge pressure. Rice and coworkers[23] have recommended the use of an "effective pulmonary wedge pres-

sure" to obviate this problem, i.e., the difference between pulmonary wedge pressure and intrathoracic pressure, which is simultaneously recorded via an esophageal balloon. However, in critically ill patients even this approach presents technical and interpretive problems. An analogous situation arises when the patient is ventilated mechanically, and it is therefore customary to briefly disconnect the patient from the mechanical ventilator, if at all possible, while pulmonary artery wedge pressure is recorded.

The author of this chapter agrees with the position of Kaplan,[24] namely, that the pulmonary artery wedge pressure is usually a satisfactory approximation of the left atrial pressure, although it is frequently affected by artifacts and respiratory variation. The concordance of pulmonary artery wedge and left atrial pressures improves when mean pressures are compared, even though considerable variation in the phasic characteristics of these pressures may exist. It has been found that the mean pulmonary artery wedge pressure is usually closely related to the mean left atrial pressure and does not ordinarily exceed that value by more than 1 to 2 mmHg.[7] In my opinion, the clinical utility of the pulmonary artery wedge pressure is enormous, especially when it is used to ascertain directional changes. However, careful analysis of wedge pressures obtained in patients with pulmonary vascular disease is essential, as is constant recognition of the pitfalls and problems of this measurement.[25]

The pulmonary artery end-diastolic pressure is also thought to reflect mean left atrial pressure closely, except in patients with preexisting pulmonary hypertension.[16] Investigations have indicated that a pressure gradient of 5 mmHg or less between pulmonary artery diastolic and mean pulmonary artery wedge pressure indicates normal pulmonary arteriolar resistance.[26] Whether, in fact, pulmonary artery end-diastolic pressure faithfully reflects left ventricular end-diastolic pressure is disputed by several investigators.[27,28] In acute myocardial infarction, atrial contraction makes a large contribution to left ventricular end-diastolic pressure. Therefore, left ventricular end-diastolic and mean left atrial pressures are usually not equal, and there is no equalization of pressures between the pulmonary artery and the left ventricle at end-diastole. In addition, increases in pulmonary vascular resistance will also cause differences between pulmonary artery end-diastolic and mean pulmonary artery wedge pressures. It is therefore necessary to ascertain the relationship between pulmonary arterial end-diastolic and mean pulmonary artery wedge pressures in the individual patient before relying on pulmonary artery end-diastolic pressure as a precise indicator of either left atrial mean pressure or left ventricular end-diastolic pressure.

Monitoring systemic arterial blood pressure is an integral part of hemodynamic monitoring in the cardiac care unit. It is as important as monitoring left ventricular filling pressures but considerably less complex. In most situations, arterial blood pressure can be determined accurately by the sphygmomanometer. However, in a setting of low cardiac output, peripheral pulses are poorly palpable and Korotkoff sounds hard to hear when, in fact, the intraarterial pressure may be only modestly reduced.[29] Therefore, monitoring of direct intraarterial pressure by the percutaneous insertion of a plastic cannula into a radial, brachial, or femoral artery is often necessary. In the setting of circulatory collapse and peripheral vasoconstriction, there is diminution or even disappearance of peripheral pulses, probably the result of reduced stroke volume and increased arterial wall stiffness.[30] In this setting, therefore, intraarterial radial or brachial artery pressures may not accurately reflect central aortic pressure.[1] In this situation, we have customarily employed a 24-inch plastic cannula inserted percutaneously into the femoral artery and advanced to the aortic bifurcation. Other approaches include the insertion of a similar cannula by brachial arterial cutdown and advancement to the subclavian artery. Our personal preference is to stay clear of the braciocephalic vessels because of the ever-present risk of embolization. In the absence of shock, however, a short 18- or 20-gauge plastic cannula, inserted percutaneously in the radial artery, will provide satisfactory pressure monitoring. It is important to recognize that even in the presence of normal physiology, differences exist between peripheral and

**Table 27.3   Central Aortic and Brachial Artery Pressures in the Normal ***

1. Mean aortic pressure exceeds mean brachial artery pressure by 2 to 4 mmHg
2. Systolic brachial artery pressure exceeds systolic aortic pressure by 5 to 10 mmHg
3. Diastolic aortic pressure exceeds diastolic brachial artery pressure by 2 to 4 mmHg
4. Brachial artery pulse pressure exceeds aortic pulse pressure by a few mmHg

* Adapted from Grossman [16]

central aortic systemic pressures, which must be taken into account whenever critical decisions depend on the level of arterial blood pressure. The usually accepted relationships between central aortic and brachial artery pressures are listed in Table 27.3.

The presence of an intraarterial line provides the monitoring physician with additional benefits. The most important is probably the ability to obtain blood samples and measure arterial blood gases as often as necessary, obviating serial arterial punctures, which may be both uncomfortable and distressing to the critically ill patient.[31] Furthermore, it has been shown that the area enclosed by the aortic pressure pulse tends to vary directly with left ventricular stroke volume. Computer analysis was applied to this concept by Warner and methods have been developed for continuous stroke volume monitoring.[32] However, this type of monitoring technique has not become widely accepted, both because of the sophisticated and expensive instrumentation required and because it has been shown that this beat-to-beat analysis presupposes a stable vascular impedance, which is seldom present in patients requiring such monitoring.[33]

## BEDSIDE CATHETERIZATION OF THE RIGHT CARDIAC CHAMBERS

### Technique of Catheter Insertion

The introduction of a balloon-tipped flow-directed catheter can be accomplished by cutdown on a superficial or deep antecubital vein, or percutaneously utilizing the internal jugular, subclavian, or femoral vein by the Seldinger technique. Certainly a cutdown on a superficial antecubital vein is simple and carries practically no risk. On the other hand, superficial veins of critically ill patients are often collapsed or thrombosed from repeated use, and often some difficulty is encountered in advancing the catheter past the shoulder.

Recently, the percutaneous cannulation of the internal jugular vein has been advocated as easier and accompanied by fewer complications than percutaneous puncture of the subclavian vein.[34-36] It is stated that internal jugular venous cannulation is easier technically because of the more definite landmarks (the sternal and clavicular portions of the sternocleidomastoid muscle and the clavicle) and because of its more superficial location. Additionally, it has been our experience that once internal jugular vein cannulation has been accomplished, a balloon-flotation catheter can be advanced into the right atrium and across the tricuspid valve with great ease. Complications of this approach are said to be fewer than with percutaneous cannulation of the subclavian vein, but they still occur. They include the development of hematomas and a 1 to 2 percent incidence of carotid artery puncture. Pneumothorax, the most common complication of subclavian vein cannulation, has not been reported in several series of internal jugular vein cannulation; however, the author is aware of two cases of massive hemopneumothorax, which occurred as a result of improper internal jugular vein puncture. Lethal air embolization has been reported,[34] and it has been therefore emphasized that if the neck veins are not distended, placement of the patient in a head-down position is essential to avoid this complication.

The author prefers to use the femoral vein to insert balloon-flotation catheters into the right side of the heart. The advantages of this approach are that the femoral vein lies outside and not in proximity to major body cavities, can be easily compressed to prevent hematoma formation and, most importantly, allows the patient free use of his arms and neck, which are otherwise encumbered with catheters, stopcocks, and manifolds. The major disadvantages of using the femoral vein approach are two: (1) difficulty puncturing the femoral vein in ex-

tremely obese patients, and (2) difficulty manipulating the balloon-flotation catheter across the tricuspid valve and right ventricle into the pulmonary artery in patients with dilated right heart chambers and low cardiac output. It is clear therefore that selection of the site of entry into the venous system for catheterization of the right-sided cardiac chambers must be individualized and will depend on the experience of the operator as well as the anatomic and hemodynamic features of the patient. In the discussion that follows, the femoral venous approach is utilized as an example.

After the procedure has been explained to the patient in some detail, and consent has been obtained, the right inguinal area is shaved and surgically scrubbed with an iodine preparation, such as Providone-Iodine Complex (Betadine). The operator is scrubbed, gloved, and gowned as if for a minor surgical procedure. We insist on meticulous observance of sterile technique in order to minimize sepsis, one of the major problems with indwelling venous and arterial lines. The patient's right inguinal area is then draped with sterile towels, leaving exposed an area of approximately $10 \times 10$ cm starting 2 cm above the inguinal ligament and extending inferiorly over the anterior surface of the thigh. The inguinal ligament is identified by palpation of the anterior superior iliac spine and the symphysis pubis. The inguinal crease is subsequently identified, usually 1 to 2 cm below and parallel to the inguinal ligament. The operator then palpates and locates the femoral artery at a point immediately below the inguinal crease. The femoral artery is gently retracted with the palpating fingers of the left hand laterally, since it often partially overlies the femoral vein. Another helpful maneuver to allow better exposure of the femoral vein is to have the patient externally rotate the right foot. The skin and subcutaneous tissues are then infiltrated with 2 percent lidocaine (Xylocaine) starting at a point approximately 2 cm below the inguinal crease. The area is explored with the infiltrating needle (usually a 20- or 22-gauge, 1½- or 2-inch needle) and an attempt is made to puncture the femoral vein and aspirate blood at a level of 1 to 2 cm below the inguinal crease and just medial to the femoral artery pulse, which the physician continuously monitors with the fingers of his left hand. Once the femoral vein is located with the infiltrating needle, the needle is withdrawn from the vein and further lidocaine infiltration is accomplished as the needle is withdrawn to the skin. Pressure is exerted for 1 or 2 minutes over the femoral vein to prevent the development of a hematoma. With a number 11 surgical blade, a 2 to 3 mm incision is made in the skin directly over the course of the femoral vein. A small straight hemostat is then inserted in the incision and gently opened to separate the subcutaneous fat and establish a small tract down to the level of the fascia. In extremely thin patients, care must be exercised not to injure the underlying vessels. Once the subcutaneous tract has been established, a standard 18-gauge arterial puncture needle, with an obturator, is inserted and directed towards the femoral vein just medial to the palpable pulse of the femoral artery. The needle is directed slightly cephalad and allowed to form a 60° angle with the horizontal plane. If the landmarks have been correctly identified, a single quick advance of the needle will puncture both the anterior and posterior walls of the femoral vein and the tip may reach the periostium. If the patient experiences discomfort, additional lidocaine is infiltrated at this point once the obturator has been removed. It is, of course, always necessary to aspirate first before injecting lidocaine to prevent intravascular injection. A 5- or 10-ml syringe, partially filled with heparinized saline solution, is then attached to the needle, and the entire needle-syringe assembly is tilted gently caudad until it forms only a 20° to 30° angle with the horizontal plane. Gentle suction is then generated with the barrel of the syringe, and the entire needle-syringe assembly is gradually withdrawn. As the tip of the needle is withdrawn through the posterior wall of the femoral vein and into its lumen, venous blood will be aspirated into the syringe, confirming the position of the tip in the lumen of the vein. At this point, the needle is held steady with the left hand, the syringe is detached from the needle, and a standard 40-cm, 0.035-in spring guidewire (USCI, Cook and other manufacturers) is introduced through the needle, flexible end first. If the tip of the

needle is squarely in the lumen of the vessel, the spring guidewire should advance easily for 15 to 20 cm in the vein. If any obstruction is encountered, gentle changes in the lateral orientation of the needle may allow advancement of the guidewire. Under no circumstances should force be used to advance the guidewire since the need for force indicates that the tip of the needle is not squarely in the lumen of the vessel and that most likely it is abutting the intima of the posterior or side walls of the femoral vein. Similarly the guidewire should never be forcibly withdrawn through the needle as it is possible to amputate its flexible tip against the sharp edges of the puncture needle. If the operator decides to withdraw, both the spring guidewire and needle should be removed simultaneously. Once the spring guidewire is in place, the needle is withdrawn with the right hand, while the operator is exerting pressure over the puncture site with the third, fourth, and fifth digits of his left hand and, at the same time, grasping the wire with the thumb and forefinger of the left hand to prevent its inadvertant removal from the vein. The wire is wiped clean of blood with a sponge wetted in heparinized saline solution, and a standard introducer-sheath assembly (USCI, Cook, Cordis and others) is then advanced over the wire and, with gentle rotational pressure, introduced into the vein. The wire and introducer are then removed and a 10-ml syringe filled with heparinized flush solution attached to the sheath, which is flushed clear of blood. The size of the introducer-sheath set will vary from 5 to 8 French, depending on the size of the particular balloon-flotation catheter it must accommodate. It must be kept in mind that even though the most common triple-lumen balloon-flotation catheters used in adults are of the 7 French size, most will not pass through a 7 French sheath because the balloon diameter, even in the deflated state, will exceed the diameter of the body of the catheter. We commonly employ a 7.5 French introducer-sheath assembly with 7 French triple lumen thermodilution balloon-flotation catheters.

It is now time to insert the balloon-flotation catheter into the venous system. The catheter has been previously checked and the balloon has been inflated with the required amount of air, under sterile water, to check for leaks. Both lumens have been flushed with heparinized saline and the lumen leading to the distal tip is connected to the pressure transducer via a fluid-filled connector. The lumen leading to the proximal part is filled with heparinized saline and a three-way stopcock is placed proximally to prevent the backflow of blood. The catheter is wiped gently with a sponge wetted in heparinized saline to remove any foreign particles from its surface. If one is using a thermodilution catheter, the integrity of the thermistor system is best checked before the catheter is introduced into the vascular system by connecting the thermistor wires to the thermodilution cardiac output device being employed and checking for integrity of the circuit. Once the catheter is prepared and is ready for insertion, the syringe is disconnected from the venous sheath and the catheter tip is introduced and advanced gently into the femoral and thence into the iliac vein. Advancement should be easy and require no force. It is often aided by imparting to the cath-

eter a slight rotational movement with thumb and forefinger. Once the catheter has been introduced approximately 20 cm and is presumably at or near the bifurcation of the inferior vena cava, the balloon is partially inflated (½ to ¾ of its capacity) to aid its further advancement through the inferior vena cava. At this point, pressure should be monitored on the oscilloscope and should be seen as a damped atrial pressure of 2 to 6 mmHg under normal conditions.

Further advance of the catheter will bring the balloon into the right atrium. The position of the catheter tip in the right atrium is recognized by observing not only improved pressure waveforms on the oscilloscope, with recognizable A and V waves (Fig. 27.1A) if the patient is in sinus rhythm, but also by the development of fairly prominent respiratory oscillations once the catheter tip is above the diaphragm. At this point, a preliminary recording of the right atrial pressure is obtained. It is assumed that the amplifier-transducer system has been appropriately

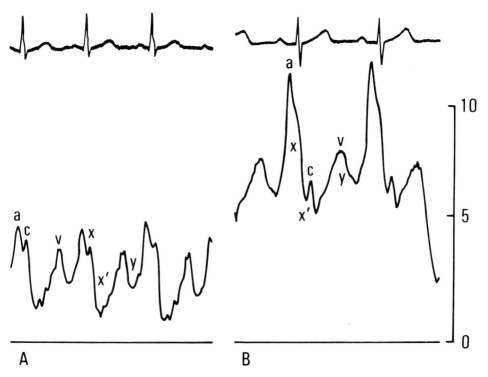

Fig. 27.1  Right atrial pressure tracings. *(A)* Normal tracing demonstrating a slightly dominant A wave, as well as C and V waves and X and Y descents. *(B)* From a case of valvular pulmonic stenosis with severe right ventricular hypertrophy. Tracing demonstrates "giant" A waves.

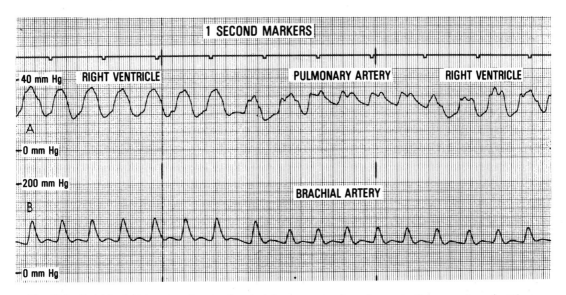

Fig. 27.2 Bedside right heart and systemic arterial pressure tracings demonstrating a number of artifacts. *(A)* Tip of balloon flotation catheter is at the pulmonic valve level and is intermittently recording right ventricular and pulmonary artery pressures. Improper calibration has resulted in spuriously elevated systolic and diastolic pressures. Despite the artifact note the change in level and configuration of diastolic pressure as catheter passes from right ventricle to pulmonary artery. *(B)* Systemic arterial pressure tracing is damped by partial occlusion of the cannula tip against the vessel intima.

balanced and calibrated (as discussed later) before the procedure is initiated. At this point the balloon is inflated to the maximum recommended volume for the particular catheter being used. Under continuous electrocardiographic and pressure monitoring, the catheter is advanced slowly. Imparting a slight clockwise torque to the catheter will help to bring the balloon towards the tricuspid valve and allow it to enter the right ventricle. With the catheter tip in the right ventricle, a distinct change in pressure will be recognized on the monitoring oscilloscope (Fig. 27.2). If no ectopy is produced by the catheter, at this point a recording is obtained of the right ventricular pressure and the catheter is then further advanced while imparting additional clockwise torque to allow it to traverse the right ventricular outflow tract, cross the pulmonary valve, and enter the pulmonary artery. A change in the pressure waveform, and specifically a change in diastolic pressure, will signal the passing of the catheter tip from the right ventricle into the pulmonary artery (Fig. 27.2). Further advance of the catheter will bring it into the pulmonary artery wedge position, which will be recognized because of

its usually damped nature and wide respiratory oscillations (Fig. 27.3). A recording is made of the pulmonary artery wedge pressure and while the pressure recording is continued, the balloon is deflated. After deflation, the catheter tip will usually recoil into the main pulmonary artery and, perhaps, as far back as the right ventricular outflow tract (Fig. 27.2). It is therefore necessary to advance the catheter an additional 1 to 2 cm while deflating the balloon.

It is important to recognize clearly the difference between pulmonary artery wedge and pulmonary arterial pressure and not to allow the catheter to remain in a permanently wedged position as this may result in complications, which will be discussed later. The tip of the catheter is properly placed in a branch of the pulmonary artery if, with the balloon deflated, clear undamped pulmonary artery pressure tracings are obtained and if good quality wedge pressure tracings are obtained by inflating the balloon to three-fourths of the full specified volume. It is important, always, to inflate the balloon very slowly and immediately stop inflation as the pressure tracing changes from that of the pulmonary artery to one of the pulmonary

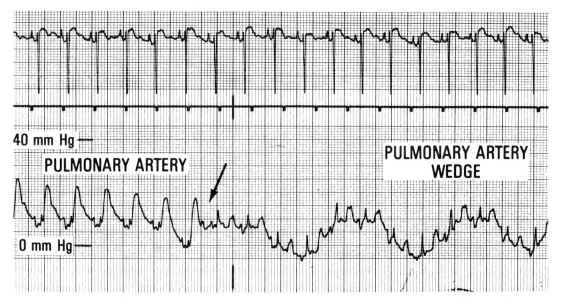

Fig. 27.3 Pulmonary artery and wedge pressure tracings. Arrow denotes inflation of the balloon. Note the wedge pressure characteristics: Lower pressure level than in the pulmonary artery, development of A and V waves, respiratory variation.

artery wedge position. A properly located catheter will record wedge pressure tracings of good phasic quality with recognizable A and V waves (Fig. 27.4). If the catheter tip is located peripherally, inflation of the balloon may completely damp the obtainable pressure and result in an unrecognizable tracing (Fig. 27.5). It is particularly important to avoid overdistension of a peripheral pulmonary artery branch, as this may lead to rupture of the vessel, particularly in patients with pulmonary hypertension. Rupture of a pulmonary arterial branch in anticoagulated patients may be a lethal complication and is discussed later in this chapter. Continuous monitoring of the catheter-tip pressure is essential because as the catheter becomes softer in response to body temperature, the loop of the catheter through the right atrium and right ventricle may become attenuated; the catheter tip then may migrate into a permanently wedged position, which may cause pulmonary infarction in a short period of time. The catheter is never withdrawn while the balloon is inflated, as this may cause vascular intimal damage; if it is withdrawn across a valve it may cause valvular rupture.

Once the operator is satisfied with the proper location of the catheter tip, the venous sheath

is removed from the vein, pressure is exerted over the point of catheter entry, and the catheter is secured to the inguinal area either by a single suture through the skin or with the application of sterile adhesive tape. A firm pressure dressing is applied over the point of venous puncture, and for this purpose, we employ several strips of elastic adhesive (Elastoplast) to hold in place a firm dressing of 4 × 4 inch gauze pads. If simultaneous monitoring of right atrial pressure is required, the proximal lumen orifice is attached to a second pressure transducer. Otherwise, the proximal lumen is connected to a slow infusion of heparinized solution to maintain patency and insure its availability for blood sample withdrawal, performance of thermodilution studies, and so on. A small amount of an antibacterial ointment (for example Betadine Ointment, Mycitracin, and so on) is applied to the skin puncture before the dressing is applied. It is helpful to keep the first 4 or 5 inches of catheter outside the body in a sterile condition in case the catheter must be subsequently manipulated. Since maintenance of sterility is difficult under these circumstances, however, it is preferable not to advance the catheter after the original insertion. Luminal patency is maintained through the use of a heparinized flush

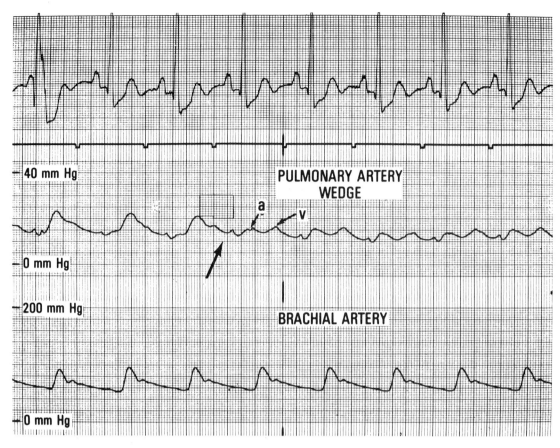

Fig. 27.4   Pulmonary artery wedge pressure tracing of good quality with recognizable phasic characteristics (A and V waves). Arrow indicates balloon inflation.

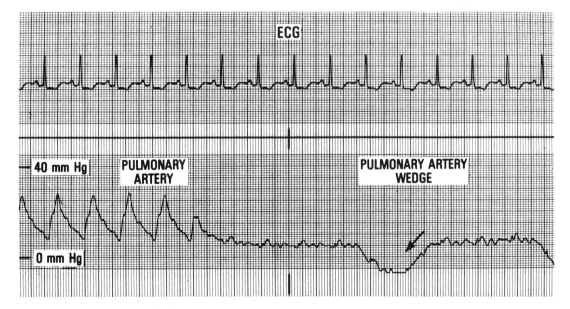

Fig. 27.5   Overdamped pulmonary artery wedge pressure tracing with poor phasic characteristics. Arrow indicates wedge pressure decline as a result of an exaggerated inspiratory effort.

solution administered via a continuous flush device (Sorenson Intraflow, and others).

## Interpretation of Pressure Data

Interpretation of the pressure data obtained during bedside catheterization depends on recognition of alterations in the magnitude and morphology of the pressure waves recorded. Thus, knowledge of the normal range of pressures in the right side of the heart is essential and therefore these are listed in some detail in Table 27.4. Equally important are the qualitative alterations reflected in changes of the

**Table 27.4   Common Values Used in Cardiac Catheterization ***

| | Normal Oxygen Values—Adults | |
| --- | --- | --- |
| | *Oxygen Content (vol %)* | *Oxygen Saturation (%)* |
| Superior vena cava | 14.0 ± 1 | 70 ± 5 |
| Inferior vena cava | 16.0 ± 1 | 80 ± 5 |
| Right atrium | 15.0 ± 1 | 75 ± 5 |
| Right ventricle | 15.2 ± 1 | 75 ± 5 |
| Pulmonary artery | 15.2 ± 1 | 75 ± 5 |
| Pulmonary vein | 19.7 to 20.1 | 98 to 100 |
| Brachial artery | 19.1 to 19.5 | 95 to 97 |
| A-V oxygen content difference | 3.5 to 5.5 | |
| Oxygen capacity | Hgb × 1.39 | |

| | Resting Normal Pressure Values (mmHg)—Right Heart—Adults | |
| --- | --- | --- |
| | *Range* | *Average* |
| Right atrium | 'a' wave | 3–7 | 6 |
| | 'c' wave | 2–6 | 4 |
| | 'v' wave | 2–8 | 5 |
| | Mean | 0–5 | 3 |
| Right ventricle | Systolic | 17–30 | 25 |
| | End diastolic | 0–6 | 4 |
| Pulmonary artery | Systolic | 15–29 | 23 |
| | Diastolic | 5–13 | 9 |
| | Mean | 10–18 | 14 |
| Pulmonary artery "wedge" | Mean | 2–12 | 8 |

| | Resting Normal Pressure Values (mmHg)—Left Heart—Adults | |
| --- | --- | --- |
| | *Range* | *Average* |
| Left atrium | Mean | 1–12 | 8 |
| | 'a' wave | 4–16 | 10 |
| | 'v' wave | 6–20 | 13 |
| Left ventricle | Systolic | 90–140 | 110 |
| | End diastolic | 5–12 | 9 |
| Brachial artery | Systolic | 100–150 | 125 |
| | Diastolic | 60–90 | 80 |
| Aorta | Systolic | 100–140 | 120 |
| | Diastolic | 60–80 | 70 |
| | Mean | 70–90 | 80 |

* Adapted from Zimermann [24] and Grossman [16]

morphology of pressure pulses in diverse conditions. A brief discussion of these alterations follows, but the interested reader is referred to standard cardiac catheterization textbooks for a more complete analysis.[12,16,24] As the CCU changes from a Coronary Care to a Cardiac Intensive Care Unit, it is necessary for persons undertaking hemodynamic monitoring to be familiar not only with basic cardiac catheterization techniques but also with pressure waveform analysis.

**Right Atrial Pressure.** The right atrial pressure corresponds to both right ventricular diastolic pressure and central venous pressure. Subnormal right atrial pressures are usually recorded in hypovolemia and shock. Elevation of right atrial pressure is usually the result of one of four major abnormalities: (1) right ventricular failure of any origin (in patients with coronary artery disease left ventricular failure and right ventricular infarction are the common causes); (2) tricuspid valve disease, both stenosis and regurgitation; (3) cardiac tamponade; and (4) constrictive pericarditis.

The normal right atrial pressure consists of three positive waves and two descents (Fig. 27.1*A*). The A wave is the result of atrial systole and, by definition, must therefore follow the P wave of the electrocardiogram. Depending on the length of the recording catheter, the peak of the A wave may be delayed, because of the time required to transmit the pressure pulse to the transducer, and may therefore correspond to the PR segment or even the QRS complex of the electrocardiogram. The descent to baseline of the pressure pulse following the A wave represents the decline in pressure following atrial systole and has been labeled the X descent. The X descent is usually interrupted by a second smaller positive deflection called the C wave, which is thought to represent transmission of the rising right ventricular systolic pressure through the closed tricuspid valve; its peak indicates the opening of the pulmonic valve. Following the C wave, the pressure pulse continues its decline towards the baseline, and this portion of the pressure curve has been labeled the X' descent. From the nadir of the X' descent, the pressure pulse rises again to its third peak, the V wave, which represents

filling of the right atrium by systemic venous return. At the peak of the V wave, the tricuspid valve opens, allowing the right atrium to empty into the right ventricle, and the atrial pressure pulse again descends towards baseline; this portion is labeled the Y descent. Normally, the right atrial A wave exceeds the V wave by 1 to 3 mmHg.

Numerous clues can be obtained by inspecting the changes in right atrial pressure pulse morphology. For example, giant A waves (Fig. 27.1*B*) are recorded in conditions of increased right ventricular stiffness (valvular pulmonic stenosis, severe pulmonary hypertension, and so on), in cases of severe tricuspid stenosis, or whenever the right atrium is contracting against a closed tricuspid valve because of a dysrhythmia (ventricular ectopic beats, ventricular tachycardia with atrioventricular dissociation, complete heart block, and so on). In the presence of severe tricuspid regurgitation, the V wave becomes more prominent and occurs earlier in systole, merging with the C wave. In this setting the V wave has been called CV or S (for systolic) wave. In severe tricuspid regurgitation, complete ventricularization of the right atrial pressure pulse may be seen (Fig. 27.6).

In both cardiac tamponade and constrictive pericarditis, the right atrial pressure is elevated and there is near equalization of right atrial mean, right ventricular end-diastolic, pulmonary arterial end-diastolic, mean pulmonary artery wedge, and left ventricular end-diastolic pressures (Fig. 27.7). However, in cardiac tamponade a prominent Y descent, commonly found in constrictive pericarditis, is not seen [37] (Figs. 27.8 and 27.9).

Right ventricular infarction has been recently reported to produce hemodynamics which may be misinterpreted as those of cardiac tamponade.[38] However, the authors point out that in the setting of right ventricular infarction, the elevated right atrial pressure pulse more closely simulated the pressure pulse of constrictive pericarditis with a dominant Y descent and an inspiratory increase in right atrial pressure (Kussmaul sign), findings not commonly seen in cardiac tamponade.

**Right Ventricular Pressure.** The normal right ventricular systolic pressure in the adult

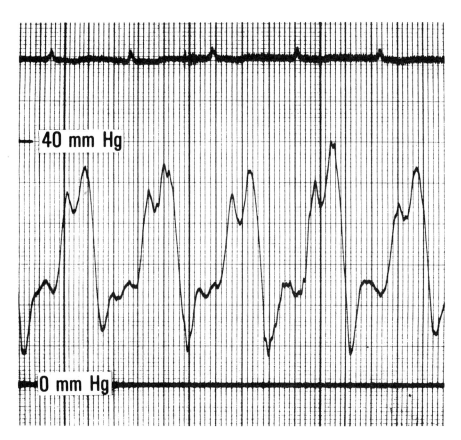

Fig. 27.6   Right atrial pressure tracing from a patient with severe tricuspid regurgitation. The right atrial pressure has become almost entirely "ventricularized" and consists of a dominant CV wave.

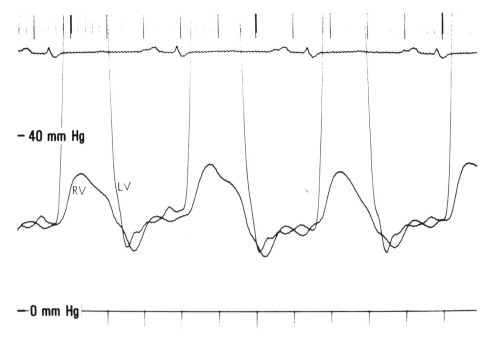

Fig. 27.7   Simultaneous right (RV) and left (LV) ventricular pressure tracings from a case of constrictive pericarditis. The pressures were recorded by fluid filled catheters connected to transducer-amplifier systems whose gains were matched. Note the equilibration of RV and LV pressures in diastole.

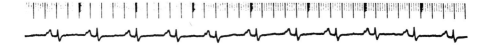

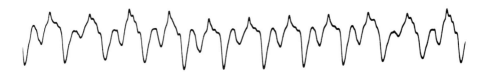

**– 40 mm Hg**

**–0 mm Hg**

Fig. 27.8   Right atrial pressure recording in constrictive pericarditis. The pressure is elevated and exhibits prominent X and Y descents.

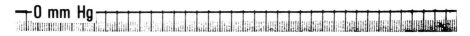

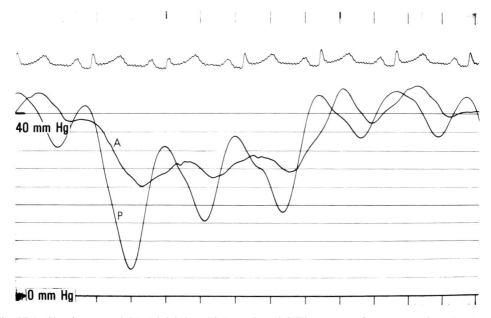

**40 mm Hg**

A

P

**0 mm Hg**

Fig. 27.9   Simultaneous right atrial (A) and intrapericardial (P) pressures from a case of cardiac tamponade. Note the blunted right atrial pressure wave form, the exaggerated respiratory oscillations, and the marked decline in intrapericardial pressure with each ventricular ejection.

ranges from 17 to 30 mmHg. Right ventricular end-diastolic pressure is usually less than 6 mmHg. The onset of the steep rise of the right ventricular systolic pressure denotes isovolumetric systole and coincides with S1 and the latter portion of the QRS complex. However, due to delays in the transmission of pressure pulse through variable length catheters, the onset of right ventricular systolic pressure rise may be delayed 40 to 80 msec and may therefore coincide with the ST segment of the electrocardiogram.

A higher than normal right ventricular systolic pressure is seen in patients with pulmonary hypertension of any cause, right ventricular outflow obstruction (valvular, subvalvular or supravalvular pulmonic stenosis), left ventricular failure, constrictive pericarditis, and ventricular septal defect with a large left-to-right shunt. In isolated right ventricular failure, the systolic pressure in the right ventricle may be normal.[38]

The right ventricular end-diastolic pressure will be elevated in instances of right ventricular or biventricular failure, right ventricular infarction, constrictive pericarditis, and cardiac tamponade. In constrictive pericarditis and right

ventricular infarction, a sharp early diastolic dip of the right ventricular diastolic pressure is usually recorded and this is followed by a plateau phase (Fig. 27.10). On the other hand, in cardiac tamponade, the "dip and plateau" diastolic right ventricular pressure pulse configuration is rarely seen [37,38] (Fig. 27.11).

**Pulmonary Artery Pressure.** Pulmonary artery pressure equals right ventricular pressure during systole when the pulmonic valve is open. In the adult, the normal systolic pulmonary artery pressure ranges from 15 to 29 mmHg. It is elevated in the presence of increased pulmonary vascular resistance (pulmonary arterial hypertension, mitral stenosis, pulmonary embolism, and so on), left ventricular failure of any cause, and in the presence of a large left-to-right shunt.

The pulmonary artery end-diastolic pressure ranges from 5 to 13 mmHg and when pulmonary arteriolar resistance is normal, it very nearly equals the mean pulmonary artery wedge pressure. Therefore, the pulmonary artery diastolic pressure will also nearly equal left ventricular diastolic pressure, if left ventricular compliance is normal. In the face of severe left

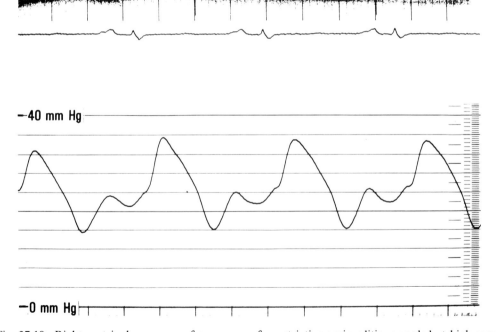

Fig. 27.10   Right ventricular pressure, from a case of constrictive pericarditis, recorded at high speed. Note the early diastolic "dip" followed by a "plateau" in late diastole.

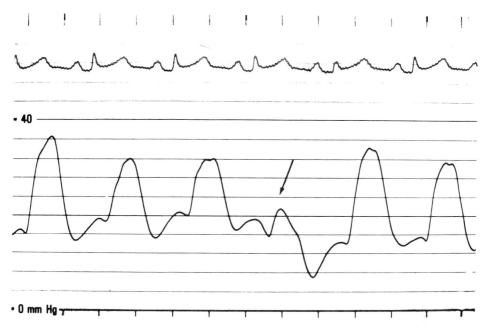

Fig. 27.11 Right ventricular pressure from a case of cardiac tamponade. Diastolic pressure is elevated but does not exhibit typical dip and plateau configuration of constriction. During inspiration (arrow) there is a marked decline in RV systolic pressure.

ventricular hypertrophy and decreased left ventricular compliance, the left ventricular end-diastolic pressure will almost always exceed the pulmonary artery end-diastolic pressure and the mean pulmonary artery wedge pressure (Fig. 27.12). When the pulmonary vascular resistance is increased, pulmonary arterial end-diastolic pressure will exceed mean pulmonary wedge pressure by more than 5 mmHg, and this distinction can be of diagnostic value in differentiating cardiogenic shock from pulmonary embolism, since in the latter case pulmonary arterial diastolic pressure may be elevated in the face of normal pulmonary artery wedge pressure. In cardiogenic shock both pressures are usually elevated and nearly equal.[8]

Examination of the morphology of the pulmonary arterial pressure pulse may be of value in the diagnosis of acute mitral regurgitation. In this setting the pulmonary arterial pressure waveform may be distorted by a giant regurgitant CV wave transmitted through the low resistance pulmonary vascular bed.[8] However, critical evaluation of the pulmonary arterial pressure waveform is often hindered by a variety of artifacts, which are discussed later.

**Pulmonary Artery Wedge Pressure.** The pulmonary artery wedge pressure waveform closely parallels that of the directly recorded left atrial pressure, although it is commonly saddled with artifacts (Fig. 27.13). It is also very similar to the right atrial pressure waveform in that it is composed of A and V waves. However, in contrast to the right atrial pressure waveform, the V wave is dominant in the left atrial and pulmonary artery wedge pressure pulses. The C wave is not commonly seen in either direct left atrial or indirect pulmonary artery wedge pressure tracings. The left atrial V wave, and therefore the pulmonary artery wedge pressure V wave, may occasionally be unusually prominent, reaching a magnitude of 20 mmHg in the absence of other abnormalities. Mean pulmonary artery wedge and left atrial pressures are almost always equal and normally should not exceed 12 mmHg. Because of the further delay in pressure pulse transmission through the pulmonary venous and capillary vascular beds, there is commonly a delay of 20 to 80 msec in the pulmonary artery wedge pressure tracing when compared with a direct left atrial pressure tracing. Elevation of the pulmonary arterial wedge

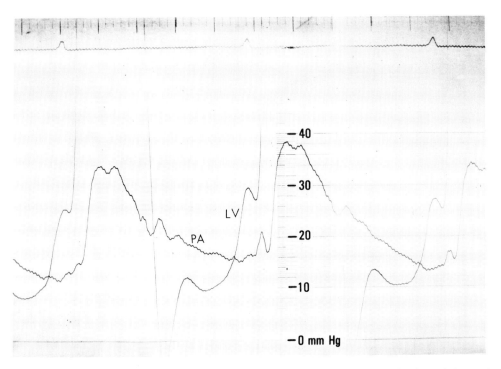

Fig. 27.12 Simultaneous recording on equisensitive amplifiers of pulmonary artery (PA) and left ventricular (LV) pressures in a patient with severe left ventricular hypertrophy. Note that LV end-diastolic pressure (EDP) exceeds PAEDP by more than 10 mmHg.

pressure is seen in the presence of left ventricular failure, mitral stenosis and mitral insufficiency, and either thrombus or tumor obstruction of the pulmonary veins.

In the setting of acute myocardial infarction, the pulmonary artery wedge pressure is probably the most critical hemodynamic measurement in assessing the patient's clinical status.[8] This is so because the pulmonary artery wedge pressure is, in fact, the hydrostatic pressure that distends the pulmonary capillary bed and forces fluid into the interstitial and alveolar spaces. It can therefore be considered to be the hemodynamic determinant of pulmonary congestion and pulmonary edema. Secondly, within the limitations discussed previously, the pulmonary artery wedge pressure closely parallels left ventricular diastolic pressure and can serve as an index of myocardial fiber stretch and therefore of left ventricular function. As an easily obtainable measurement of left ventricular filling pressure, the pulmonary artery wedge pressure is often used to construct ventricular function curves. An increase in pulmonary artery wedge

pressure usually reflects diminished left ventricular systolic function and an increased left ventricular volume.[39] However, acute myocardial infarction is also commonly followed by an increase in left ventricular stiffness,[40,41] which, in turn, will cause an increase in left ventricular diastolic pressure and probably pulmonary artery wedge pressure.[8]

It is now generally accepted that pulmonary artery wedge pressure is the best measure for assessing the risk of pulmonary congestion during fluid administration to a patient. The previous practice of using the central venous pressure for this purpose can be misleading, since right atrial pressure reflects predominantly *right* ventricular filling pressure and therefore *right* ventricular function. When right and left ventricular function are comparable, as in a normal heart or in a patient with chronic biventricular failure, then right atrial pressure will reflect the level of left ventricular filling pressure and an approximation of this measure can be obtained by adding 7 mmHg to the mean right atrial pressure.[8] However, when right ventricular

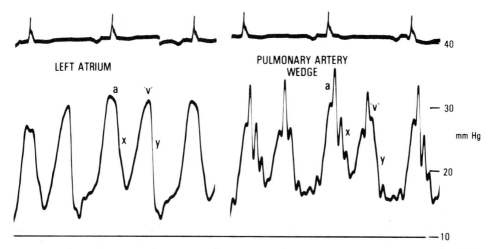

Fig. 27.13 Left atrial and pulmonary wedge pressure tracings from a patient with left ventricular failure. Pressures were recorded with the same transducer-amplifier system in rapid sequence. Note the similarity in pressure wave-form and magnitude. Also note the artifactual sharp peaks of the wedge pressure tracing, presumably due to catheter "fling" (see text).

function differs substantially from left ventricular function, as in most cases of acute myocardial infarction, this relation becomes invalid. Thus, the right atrial pressure may be elevated in the presence of normal pulmonary artery wedge pressure when right ventricular performance is impaired, as in pulmonary embolism, right ventricular infarction, or chronic obstructive pulmonary disease. Conversely, pulmonary artery wedge pressure will be significantly higher than right atrial pressure when left ventricular dysfunction predominates, as in most cases of acute myocardial infarction.[42] Therefore, although the right atrial pressure measurement remains a useful index of the magnitude of right heart failure, we and others have often observed a normal right atrial pressure in the presence of florid pulmonary edema.[43]

Recognition that the catheter tip is recording a reliable pulmonary artery wedge pressure, and not a hybrid of pulmonary artery wedge and pulmonary arterial pressures, rests on the following criteria: (1) mean pulmonary artery wedge pressure is less than mean pulmonary artery pressure; (2) the pulmonary artery wedge pressure demonstrates a clearly bifid waveform due to transmitted A and V waves of the left atrial pressure pulse (in the presence of sinus rhythm); and (3) an abrupt rise in pressure level and change in waveform will be appreciated on sudden deflation of the balloon. When one is confident that the recording is that of a pulmonary arterial wedge pressure, an analysis of the waveform may be most useful in the setting of acute myocardial infarction. Acute mitral regurgitation will alter the waveform of the pulmonary arterial wedge tracing from a bifid form to one with a single monophasic systolic wave—the transmitted giant CV wave of acute mitral regurgitation. Differentiation can be made between the CV wave of mitral regurgitation and the usual pulmonary arterial pressure waveform, using the following criteria: (1) the CV wave of the pulmonary artery wedge pressure is narrower and more sharply peaked than the usual pulmonary arterial systolic pressure wave; (2) it peaks later in systole than the pulmonary artery pressure waveform, usually after the end of the T wave; and (3) there is no discernible dicrotic notch, as is commonly seen in the pulmonary arterial pressure tracing (Fig. 27.14). By allowing systolic flow into a small noncompliant left atrium, acute mitral regurgitation may raise pressure in the left atrium and, consequently, the pulmonary artery wedge pressure to remarkable levels. Gratifying responses can be obtained in these life-threatening situations with the prompt use of vasodilator agents (Fig. 27.15A and B).

In summary, the measurement and analysis

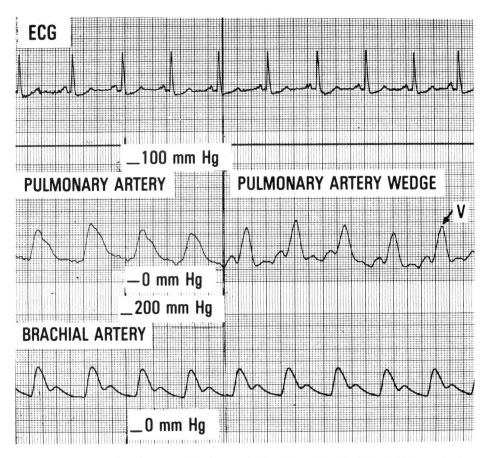

Fig. 27.14 Pressure tracings in acute mitral regurgitation. Note that the V (or CV) wave in the wedge position equals the pulmonary artery pressure wave in systole. The morphology however is entirely different (see text for discussion).

of the contour of the pulmonary artery wedge pressure are of great value in the hemodynamic assessment of patients with acute myocardial infarction. However, the constraints on the interpretation of pulmonary artery wedge pressure, as discussed above, should always be kept in mind. In addition, one should be constantly aware of the potential technical pitfalls of this particular measurement, as discussed later in this chapter.

## SYSTEMIC ARTERIAL PRESSURE MONITORING

### Technique for Arterial Catheter Insertion

The technique for inserting a cannula or catheter for intraarterial pressure monitoring will vary, depending on whether the radial, brachial, or femoral artery is used and the particular type of needle-cannula assembly available.

If direct intraarterial pressure monitoring is being performed for reasons other than circulatory collapse or shock, we prefer to insert a short (2 or 2½-inch) plastic cannula into the radial artery. For this purpose, we employ one of the several commercially available cannula-over-needle systems (Angiocath, Cathlon IV, and others). The radial artery is used in preference to the brachial artery, as it allows the patient greater arm mobility.

Before a radial artery cannula is inserted, the patency of both the radial and ulnar arteries must be assessed by the Allen test,[44] a Doppler ultrasonic flowmeter, or both.[45] The wrist is then hyperextended, the radial artery localized by palpation, and a small area over the radial

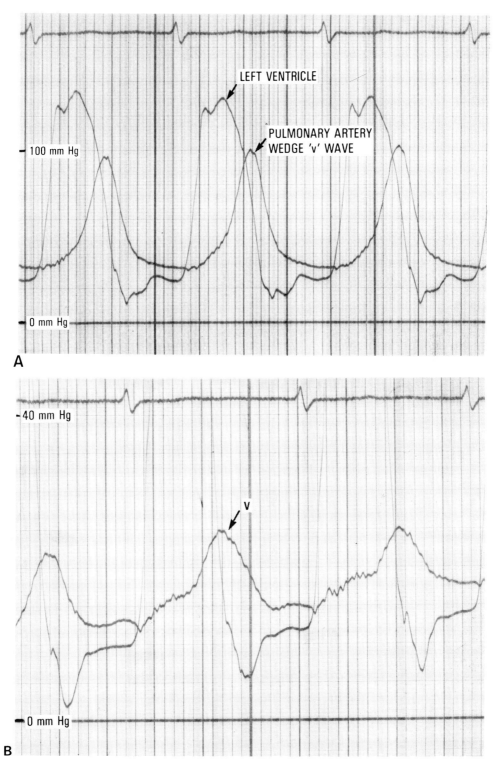

Fig. 27.15  Simultaneous left ventricular and pulmonary artery wedge pressures from a case of acute mitral regurgitation, recorded on equisensitive amplifiers. *(A)* Baseline recording with V wave amplitude almost 100 mmHg. The left ventricular end-diastolic pressure (LVEDP) is also elevated at 28 mmHg. *(B)* Following institution of nitroprusside infusion both the V wave and the LVEDP have returned to near normal levels.

artery cleansed with an iodine containing tincture. Lidocaine hydrochloride, 1.0 percent, is infiltrated intradermally over the proposed puncture site and on either side of the radial artery, taking care to avoid puncturing the radial artery or introducing so much anesthetic agent that palpation of the pulse becomes difficult. The operator is gloved but is not necessarily wearing a mask or gown. A small nick, 1.0 mm in depth, is made in the skin with a No. 11 Bard-Parker blade directly over the radial artery and the cannula-needle assembly is then inserted together, without a stylette. The orientation of the needle is cephalad, parallel to the course of the radial artery and in a plane approximately 30° from the plane of the forearm. When the anterior wall of the radial artery is cleanly punctured, pulsatile retrograde blood flow will occur. Both needle and cannula are advanced slightly and the cannula is then advanced further while the needle is held steadily in place with the other hand. With this maneuver, the cannula should enter the radial artery securely for a distance of 1½ to 2 inches. The needle is then removed from the cannula, and the position of the cannula in the radial artery is confirmed, either by observing pulsatile retrograde blood flow again or by connecting the cannula to a pressure transducer and observing a clean, undamped, arterial pressure waveform on the oscilloscope. It often helps to interpose a stopcock between the pressure monitoring line and the cannula so that arterial blood samples can be withdrawn. The hub of the cannula and the stopcock are then secured to the patient either with a single silk suture through the skin or preferably by applying sterile adhesive strips. A small amount of an antibacterial ointment (Betadine, Neosporin, and others) is applied over the puncture site of the skin and a gauze pad with an elastic pressure dressing is then applied to control bleeding and prevent the formation of a hematoma.

In patients who are in shock or who are potential shock candidates, it is preferable to monitor arterial pressure from a central location, as discussed previously. In this setting, we prefer to use the femoral artery and avoid placing long catheters in the subclavian artery near the origins of the craniocerebral vessels. The technique for inserting a femoral artery catheter varies with the equipment on hand. Standard catheterization techniques can be used with a Cournand needle and a spring guidewire, with subsequent insertion of a previously prepared clear Teflon or polyethylene tubing, long enough to reach the aortic bifurcation, over the guidewire. More commonly, however, an 18- to 24-inch disposable catheter (Deseret Intracath and others) is inserted through a needle. Several sizes are available, but for the average adult, an 18-gauge catheter inserted through a 16-gauge needle is usually adequate. The technique used to insert the catheter through the needle is not appreciably different from that described above for radial artery catheterization. The femoral arterial puncture must be clean and the tip of the needle must be squarely in the lumen of the femoral artery; otherwise the catheter will not advance. If the catheter does not advance easily, force should not be exerted, as intimal damage to the vessel may occur.

Whether arterial catheterization is performed via the radial or femoral arteries, the integrity of the arterial circulation distal to the point of insertion must be ascertained immediately after the procedure and periodically thereafter. In case of radial artery cannulation, the integrity of the distal arterial circulation must be confirmed either by palpating the ulnar pulse or by periodically checking the capillary filling time of the nail beds. In case of femoral arterial catheterization, periodic checks of the dorsalis pedis and posterior tibial pulses will provide a good index of arterial blood flow distal to the point of catheterization.

Maintenance of catheter patency is usually a greater problem with arterial than with venous catheters. We routinely connect all arterial and venous catheters to a Sorenson Intraflow device to deliver 3 to 6 ml/hr of heparinized solution through the catheter. When connected to a flush system, this device is designed to provide a small amount of fluid flow through the catheter to maintain patency while pressure is being recorded. For arterial lines, it must be used in conjunction with a pressurized bag system. The concentration of heparin commonly employed in our unit is 1,000 units/500 ml of infusate. Others have recommended higher concentrations.[45-47] Despite the continuous infusion of heparinized solution, damping of pressure is often seen secondary to sludging of formed blood elements at the tip of the catheter. We therefore recommend the use of the rapid flush valve of the Sorenson Intraflow device every 2 hours to deliver a few milliliters of heparinized solution rapidly into the arterial cannula. However, care must be exercised as cerebral embolization can result from excessively vigorous flushing of radial artery cannulas.[48] Since thrombus formation at the cannula tip almost invariably occurs, at least to a small degree, it is preferable to aspirate 2 to 3 ml of blood firmly with a syringe before flushing the catheter either manually or via the rapid flush valve of the Intraflow device.

## Interpretation of Arterial Pressure Data

The normal systemic arterial pressure waveform is sharp, has a rapid upstroke, a definite dicrotic notch, and a clear end-diastolic point

(Fig. 27.14). In the presence of a normal aortic valve, peak systolic pressure in the radial artery is usually 5 to 10 mmHg higher than peak left ventricular systolic pressure. The upstroke of the arterial pressure pulse is delayed in cases of low cardiac output and especially in instances of fixed left ventricular outflow obstruction (e.g., valvular aortic stenosis). Conversely, the upstroke of the arterial pressure pulse becomes rapid in patients with hyperdynamic circulation, high cardiac output, and hypertrophic obstructive cardiomyopathy.

In addition to measurement of the absolute value of the systemic arterial pressure, identification of other alterations of the pressure pulse may be helpful in monitoring the critically ill patient. For example, in patients with severe left ventricular dysfunction, pulsus alternans may be recorded. Under these circumstances, peak systolic arterial pressure may alternate by as much as 10 to 20 mmHg (Fig. 27.16). Similarly, in cardiac tamponade monitoring of systemic arterial pressure will demonstrate pulsus paradoxus with an inspiratory decline in peak

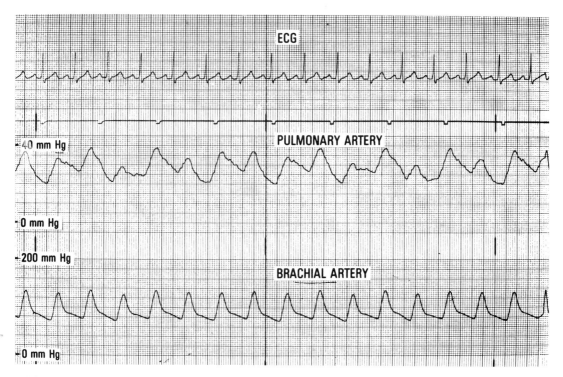

Fig. 27.16 Brachial and pulmonary artery pressure recording in a case of biventricular failure. Alternation of systolic pressure is evident in both tracings.

systolic arterial pressure in excess of 10 mmHg (Fig. 27.17). In the presence of severe aortic stenosis, the upstroke of the arterial pulse may be deformed by an anacrotic notch and a high frequency artifact may be recorded at peak systole (Fig. 27.18).

The most common cause of deformation of the systemic arterial pressure contour during

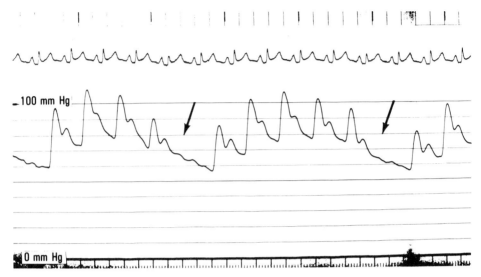

Fig. 27.17  Brachial artery pressure recording from a case of cardiac tamponade. There is marked pulsus paradoxus with almost total obliteration of the systemic arterial pulse during inspiration *(arrows)*.

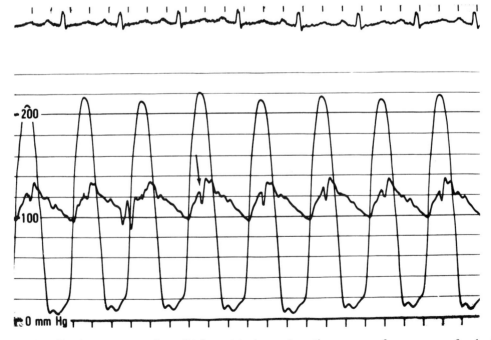

Fig. 27.18  Simultaneous recording of left ventricular and aortic pressures from a case of valvular aortic stenosis. Recordings made on equisensitive amplifiers. In addition to the obvious pressure gradient between the left ventricle and the aorta *(arrow)*, note the slow upstroke and the "anacrotic notch" *(arrow)* of the aortic pressure wave form.

bedside hemodynamic monitoring is undoubtedly damping due to the formation of thrombus at the tip of the cannula or due to partial occlusion of the cannula tip by adjacent intimal tissue. These considerations are discussed in more detail later in this chapter.

Reductions in systemic arterial pressure are commonly seen during the early phase of an acute myocardial infarction. Systolic blood pressure may decline to 90 mmHg or less and yet the patient may be well perfused peripherally, maintain adequate urinary output, and, by definition, is not in cardiogenic shock.[49] It is therefore clear that although measurement of systemic arterial pressure is an important hemodynamic parameter in the setting of acute myocardial infarction, this measurement must be related to cardiac output and systemic vascular resistance before conclusions regarding the presence or absence of cardiogenic shock are reached. On the other hand, the prognostic value of the intraarterial diastolic pressure in left ventricular pump failure due to acute myocardial infarction has been recently investigated.[50] If the diastolic pressure was 55 mmHg or greater at the time of the initial hemodynamic study, survival was predicted with a 68 percent reliability. Addition of arterial blood lactate concentration to the equation increased the reliability of prognostic prediction to 80 percent.

## DETERMINATION AND MONITORING OF CARDIAC OUTPUT

Cardiac output is defined as the volume of blood ejected by the ventricles per unit time and is commonly reported in liters per minute. Under normal circumstances, right and left ventricular outputs are nearly equal. Significant differences, however, occur in the presence of an intracardiac shunt. The importance of including blood flow measurements (cardiac output determination) in evaluating left ventricular performance is well recognized. Even more important is the determination of serial cardiac outputs in assessing a patient's response to therapy. It is customary to normalize cardiac output data by dividing by the patient's body surface area to allow comparisons between patients of

different sizes. The patient's body surface area, according to standard tables, is calculated from the formula developed by Dubois in 1926 for use in metabolic studies:[51]

$$\text{Body surface area (m}^2) = \text{weight}^{0.425}\text{ (kg)}$$
$$\times \text{ height}^{0.725}\text{(cm)} \times 0.007184$$

Until recently, cardiac output determinations were confined to the cardiac catheterization laboratory, because of their complexity. Newer technical developments, however, have made this procedure easily available at the bedside. The three common methods used to determine cardiac output are: (1) the Fick principle method, (2) the indicator-dilution method, and (3) the thermodilution method. Other less commonly used techniques include angiographic measurements, radioisotope techniques, and the pulse contour method.

### The Fick Method

To calculate cardiac output by the Fick method, it is necessary to measure oxygen consumption and arteriovenous oxygen difference (Table 27.2). Arteriovenous oxygen difference can be calculated easily by measuring oxygen content in systemic arterial and mixed venous (usually pulmonary arterial) blood samples. The measurement of oxygen consumption, however, is more cumbersome and requires collection of expired air for a period of 3 to 5 minutes. This is done by having the patient exhale through a tightly fitting mouthpiece and a one-way valve into a Tissot spirometer or a Douglas bag. The total volume of expired air over a period of time is measured and its oxygen concentration analyzed by one of several techniques (mass spectrography, Scholander analysis, and so on). If the patient has been inspiring ambient air, the difference between the oxygen concentration of ambient air (21 percent) and expired air allows one to calculate oxygen consumption.

The Fick method of cardiac output measurement has long been considered the "gold standard" of all cardiac output techniques because of its accuracy. It is particularly useful because it gives accurate results, even in the presence of low cardiac output, valvular regurgitation, and intracardiac shunts. On the other hand, the Fick method has several disadvantages. It requires that the patient be in a steady state and cooperate in collecting expired air. This may be particularly difficult in a critically ill patient, who may be either agitated or obtunded. Furthermore, since most patients in the coronary care unit are on some form of oxygen therapy and since it is practically impossible to calculate oxygen concentration of inspired air accurately in the presence of mask or nasal prong oxygen administration, accurate oxygen consumption measurement is difficult. Even in a cooperative patient who is breathing ambient air, oxygen consumption may be spuriously elevated by anxiety and hyperventilation. In view of the above disadvantages, collection of expired air and direct measurement of oxygen consumption are rarely practiced in clinical coronary care units. However, oxygen consumption can be estimated by multiplying the patient's body surface area by 130 ml, an average value of oxygen consumption per square meter for normometabolic adults whose body weight is estimated to consist of 15 percent or more fat. If fat content is estimated at 5 percent or less, 140 ml/m$^2$ is used.[52]

The arteriovenous oxygen content difference is best calculated by direct measurement of oxygen content of arterial and mixed venous blood samples either by the Van Slyke manometric technique or its more modern modifications (LEX-02-CON Instrument, and so on). Since this type of direct measurement requires both time and expertise in manometric analysis, a simplified—but less accurate—method can be used. This method involves estimating the oxygen carrying capacity of blood by multiplying the patient's hemoglobin value by 1.39.[53] Systemic arterial and mixed venous hemoglobin oxygen saturations are then measured, either directly by the use of an oximeter or indirectly by calculating saturation from oxygen tension. Oxygen carrying capacity is then multiplied by the saturation to obtain the oxygen content of arterial and mixed venous blood samples; the difference between these two figures constitutes the arteriovenous oxygen difference. It must be clearly recognized that this method involves

several assumptions and introduces potential errors at several points along the way.

Although the assumptions and short cuts outlined above inevitably produce errors in the measurement of cardiac output, these techniques are useful for estimating serial changes in the cardiac output of a given patient. Since the arteriovenous oxygen difference is inversely related to cardiac output, serial determinations of this parameter may be used to approximate serial changes in the cardiac output of individual patients.

### Indicator-Dilution Techniques

The indicator-dilution technique is based on the well-recognized principle that if a known amount of an indicator is added to an unknown volume of fluid and adequate time is allowed for complete mixing, the volume of fluid may be determined by analyzing a sample of the fluid for indicator concentration. Stewart, in 1897, was the first to demonstrate that this principle is also applicable to fluids in motion, and Henriques and Hamilton subsequently further refined and validated this concept.[51] The clinical determination of cardiac output is accomplished by injecting into the venous system, preferably the pulmonary artery, a known amount of an indicator whose concentration is subsequently monitored continuously on the arterial side of the circulation by an appropriate instrument. The most common indicator used in clinical practice today is indocyanine green dye (Cardiogreen) and its concentration in the arterial system is usually monitored by withdrawing arterial blood through a densitometer that records a time-concentration curve as the indicator passes through the circulation. As the first molecules of the dye reach the sampling site, the densitometer detects their presence and begins to record the time-concentration curve (Fig. 27.19). The concentration of dye rises rapidly to its peak height and then declines exponentially. Because of recirculation, the time-concentration curve does not return to the baseline, and depending on the sensitivity of the recording system, a discrete second curve may be recorded. The densitometer used with indocyanine green dye is an optical instrument that

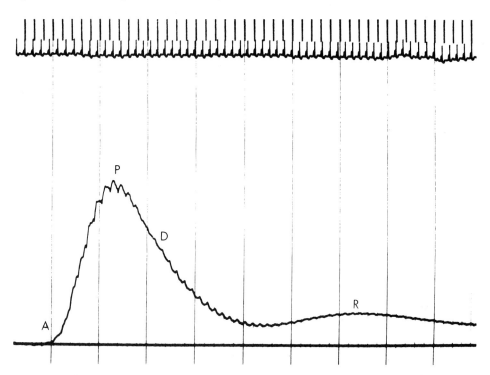

Fig. 27.19 Typical indocyanine green dilution curve. The indicator was injected in the pulmonary artery and sampled from the brachial artery. A = appearance, P = peak concentration, D = exponential decay, R = recirculation curve.

records light transmission through flowing blood. When indocyamine green dye is mixed with blood being sampled, reduced transmission of light occurs and this is recorded by the densitometer as a time-concentration curve.

A variety of other indicators may be used, including thermal (cold or hot), electrical (saline), chemical (hydrogen or ascorbic acid), radioactive, and other optical agents. By far the most common techniqe is to use an optical indicator, usually indocyanine green, in conjunction with an optical densitometer.

As indicated in the formula for calculating cardiac output by the indicator-dilution principle (Table 27.2), it is necessary to calculate the mean concentration of the indicator during the time of the total curve inscription. Since recirculation of the indocyanine green precludes the return of the time-concentration curve to the baseline, it is necessary to replot the descending limb of the curve on semilogarithmic paper and then exclude the recirculation curve. This particularly tedious technique may be avoided by using a small computer. If the com-

puter has been appropriately calibrated, it will immediately calculate cardiac output and eliminate the need for manual measurement of the dye curve. A variety of shortcuts have been developed for the hand calculation of indicator-dilution curves, and the interested reader is referred to standard textbooks for further details.[51,54]

The measurement of cardiac output by the indicator-dilution technique is advantageous because it can be performed more rapidly than by the Fick method, serial measurements are easily performed, and use of a small computer can give results immediately. Furthermore, this method is not affected by oxygen administration to the patient. Its relative disadvantages include the requirement for venous and arterial catheters and the need for an appropriate recording device. If computer analysis is not available, rather tedious hand measurement and calculation of the time-concentration curves is necessary. The technique is less accurate than the Fick method in patients with low cardiac output, and the presence of severe valvular insufficiency or large intracardiac shunts introduces significant errors. Similarly, the presence of rapid recirculation may affect the calculations. The need to withdraw 15 to 25 ml of blood for each determination is certainly a limiting factor in the number of cardiac outputs that may be serially measured.

## Thermodilution Technique

The thermodilution technique is actually an extension of the indicator-dilution principle discussed earlier. The measurement of cardiac output by thermodilution was first described in 1954 by Fegler.[55] The indicator used is commonly 5 percent dextrose solution of a known temperature, usually cooler than body temperature. A small amount (usually 10 ml for adults) is injected into the right atrium and the blood temperature change is recorded downstream, commonly in the pulmonary artery. The thermodilution method came into its own with the development by Ganz and Swan [56] of flow-directed multilumen catheters that incorporated a thermistor distally and allowed the simple, safe, and accurate measurement of cardiac output in the clinical setting. The equation for calculating cardiac output by the thermodilution method is listed in Table 27.2. The interested reader is referred to the papers by Ganz and Swan,[56] and Maruschak et al.[57] for a more detailed mathematical description of the principle.

The cool solution must be injected quickly and smoothly through the proximal port of the balloon-flotation catheter in the right atrium to allow for uniform mixing of the injectate with the venous return. Although the time-temperature curve generated by the thermistor can be recorded (Fig. 27.20) and cardiac output may be calculated manually, such a calculation involves considerable mathematic tedium. One of several commercially available small computers may be used to calculate and display the cardiac output immediately. Because of the rapidity of this determination and the virtual absence of recirculation (heat is dissipated entirely after one circulation through the body), serial measurements may be made as often as once every 60 seconds. Reproducibility is usually good, especially when duplicate determinations are performed to detect variations.[58] It is obvious that the thermodilution technique, as clinically employed with injection of the cool solution in the right atrium and recording of temperature changes in the pulmonary artery, measures, in fact, right ventricular output. In the absence of a central shunt, right ventricular output will nearly equal left ventricular output and therefore the technique is applicable in all instances of left or right ventricular failure. The advantages of the thermodilution method are several, and for this reason it has become the method of choice for the bedside estimation of cardiac output. Only one catheter is required and the catheter can usually be inserted at the bedside without the use of fluoroscopy. Blood withdrawal is not required and the measurement can be performed rapidly with good reproducibility. The method is not affected by recirculation or by oxygen administration. It can be performed simply and easily by one person. If one of the newer, calibrated thermistor beads is used, an additional advantage of the technique is the ability to record central core body temperature. The disadvantages of the technique include the potential electric hazards that may result from damaged thermistor wires in the catheter and the potential hazard of an indwelling pulmonary artery catheter. The technique is not accurate with extremely low cardiac output, or in the presence of intracardiac shunts and pulmonary or tricuspid regurgitation. A number of potential sources of error are discussed below.

## Interpretation of Cardiac Output Data

A reduction in cardiac output is usually the result of several mechanisms operating concurrently. In the setting of acute myocardial infarction, the most common factors are a decrease in contracting muscle mass (either infarcted or ischemic and noncontractile) and cardiac dysrhythmias.[59,60] Less frequently, cardiac output may be diminished because of specific structural cardiac defects, such as rupture of the interventricular septum or the development of acute mitral regurgitation. Noncardiac factors that may contribute to the reduction in cardiac output in acute myocardial infarction include hy-

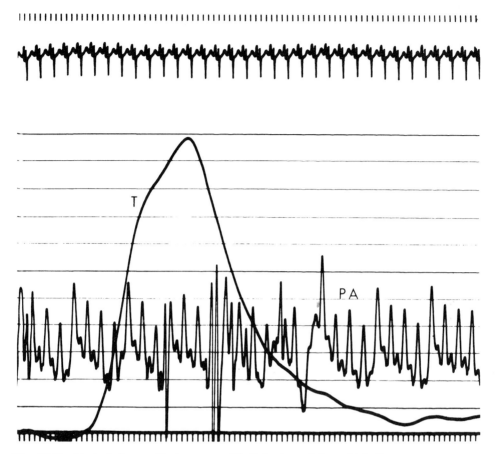

Fig. 27.20   Typical thermodilution curve (T). Injection of the cold indicator was made in the right atrium and the thermistor recorded blood temperature changes in the pulmonary artery. Note the absence of recirculation with this technique. Pulmonary artery pressure (PA) was recorded simultaneously.

povolemia and increased systemic vascular resistance.

Organ hypoperfusion has been related to cardiac output as follows: cardiac index of 2.7 to 4.3 l/min/m² is the usual normal range; a cardiac index of 2.2 to 2.7 indicates subclinical depression of cardiac output; values of 1.8 to 2.2 indicate the onset of clinical hypoperfusion; and values below 1.8 l/min/m² are usually associated with cardiogenic shock.[9] In a setting of acute myocardial infarction, determination of cardiac output may be of prognostic value. In the study of Ratshin et al.[61] a cardiac index of less than 2.3 l/min/m² in the presence of a left ventricular filling pressure of greater than 15 mmHg was associated with 100 percent mortality.

In the presence of a ventricular septal defect due to rupture of the interventricular septum with associated left-to-right shunting, the normally smooth exponential downslope of an indicator-dilution or thermodilution curve will be altered. Specifically, the thermodilution curve downslope will be deformed by the appearance of a second peak resulting from the reappearance, in the pulmonary circuit, of cooled blood that has traversed the pulmonary vascular bed and reentered the right side of the heart through the ventricular septal defect.[9] This early recirculation curve is diagnostic of a left-to-right shunt. However, it will cause most currently available thermodilution cardiac output computers to miscalculate cardiac output by including shunt flow in the computation. Under these circumstances, the curve must be calculated manually. The presence of a left-to-right shunt at the ven-

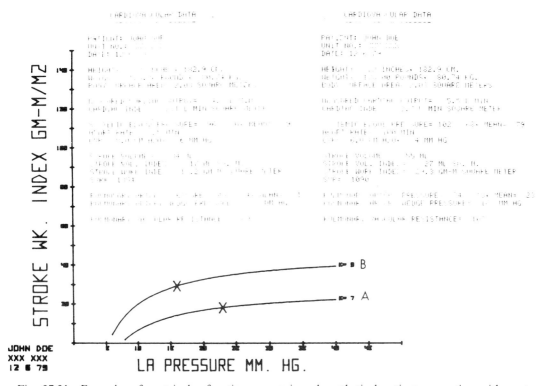

Fig. 27.21 Examples of ventricular function curves in a hypothetical patient presenting with post myocardial infarction pump failure and following treatment with nitroprusside infusion. Data and curves were computed and recorded on a Hewlett-Packard 9830 programmable calculator and plotter. (Program developed by Dr. T. P. Clemmer, Director Critical Care Medicine, Latter Day Saints Hospital, Salt Lake City, Utah.)

tricular level may be confirmed by withdrawing blood samples from the right ventricle, or pulmonary artery and right atrium, and demonstrating an increase in oxygen content of at least 0.9 volumes percent from the right atrium to the right ventricle.[12]

The availability of cardiac output measurements, along with right atrial and pulmonary artery wedge pressure measurements, makes the construction of ventricular function curves feasible. For teaching purposes, we have used the equations for hyperbolas proposed by Guyton [51] to construct serial ventricular function curves as the patient's hemodynamic status changes with therapy (Fig. 27.21). Although the construction of a ventricular function curve from a single cardiac output and filling pressure measurement is open to many theoretical objections, we have found this visual display of great value in teaching hemodynamics to medical students and nursing staff.

## PITFALLS IN HEMODYNAMIC MONITORING

A large number of potential pitfalls exist in the acquisition and interpretation of pressure and flow data during bedside hemodynamic monitoring. The problem is compounded by the fact that many physicians and nurses who engage in bedside hemodynamic monitoring have had no formal training in this technique.[62] It is likely that most bedside hemodynamic monitoring in coronary care units is performed under the supervision, at least, of persons experienced in cardiac catheterization techniques. Even so, great differences exist between the acquisition of data in the catheterization laboratory and at the bedside. The potential pitfalls of hemodynamic monitoring fall into two categories: technical and interpretive. Table 27.5 lists the usual sources of technical errors and artifacts. It must be obvious from perusing these factors that

Table 27.5  Sources of Error and Artifact in Pressure
Monitoring

**Table 27.5  Sources of Error and Artifact in Pressure
Monitoring**

1. Inadequate system frequency response
2. Improper calibration
3. Improper balancing of transducer-amplifier
   system
4. Improper zero reference
5. Underdamping
6. Overdamping
7. Catheter movement (whip)
8. Catheter tip occlusion (partial)
9. Extraneous influences (respiratory variations)
10. Improper catheter tip location in the heart.

most of them apply to the commonly used fluid-filled catheter systems attached to external pressure transducers (damping problems, improper zero reference point selection, inadequate system frequency response). Although a detailed discussion of these technical factors is beyond the scope of this chapter, a few points deserve emphasis.

It has been shown that in order to faithfully reproduce intravascular pressures in the human, a catheter transducer system with a flat frequency response to 20 Hz is necessary.[16] Most of the flow-directed balloon-tipped catheters used for bedside catheterization of the right side of the heart have a frequency response of 10 to 15 Hz.[63] Consequently, certain high frequency events of the pressure waveform (such as the dicrotic notch of the pulmonary artery pressure) may be attenuated or completely lost. Fortunately this is of no great import if bedside hemodynamic monitoring is being undertaken mainly to ascertain mean left ventricular filling pressures, since, for this purpose, the frequency response of available systems is more than adequate.

Of more practical importance are damping problems, particularly overdamping. The introduction of even a small amount of blood or a small air bubble in the tubing connecting the intravascular catheter to the external pressure transducer may drastically alter the damping characteristics of the system and result in overdamping. In our experience this is not an uncommon problem, particularly when blood samples are being withdrawn from the distal or proximal ports of the balloon-flotation catheter with subsequent inadequate flushing, or the

inadvertent introduction of air into the system.

Improper location of the zero reference point is also a common source of error during bedside hemodynamic monitoring, because patients frequently move about and the head of the bed is often elevated or depressed. We commonly take the zero reference point to be at the midchest position and use a carpenter's level to be certain that the transducer diaphragm is at the proper reference height. Optimally, recordings should be made with the patient in the horizontal position, although the patient's clinical condition frequently requires that the head of the bed be elevated 30° to 45°. In this situation there may be a vertical distance of 5 to 8 cm between the tip of a flow-directed catheter in the pulmonary artery and the zero reference point taken at the approximate right atrial level (the midaxillary line at the fourth interspace). Remembering that the pressure of 1.0 cm of water equals 0.74 mmHg, an error of 4 to 6 mmHg is possible. This error is of sufficient magnitude to make a difference between normal and elevated pulmonary artery diastolic pressures. Problems related to damping, frequency response, and catheter location within the heart may be largely obviated by the use of a catheter-tip micromanometer (Fig. 27.22). Unfortunately, to date, such catheter-tip micromanometers must be inserted with the aid of fluoroscopy and are not available in the usual clinical bedside setting.

Improper location of a balloon-flotation catheter tip in a distal pulmonary artery branch may result in a spuriously high wedge pressure.[64] In this situation, inflation of the balloon may cause occlusion of the catheter tip and result in a spuriously high (up to 15 mmHg) and damped tracing devoid of typical phasic contours.

Another common problem is the improper calibration of the transducer-amplifier system. Although most modern pressure amplifiers incorporate an electric calibration signal, the accuracy of this signal should always be checked against a mercury manometer. Similarly, even though a transducer-amplifier system may be properly calibrated, if a different transducer is attached to the amplifier, recalibration must be carried out. Our practice includes the initial

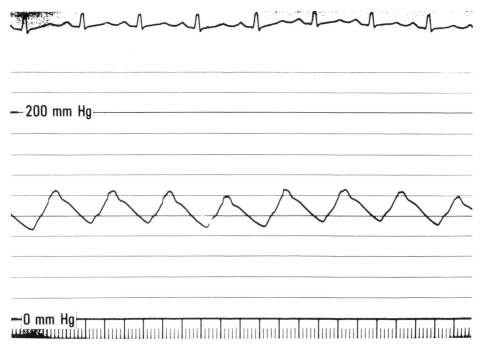

Fig. 27.22   High fidelity catheter tip micromanometer recording of aortic pressure in a case of severe aortic stenosis. This is from the same patient in Figure 27.18. Note the marked diminution of the anacrotic notch and the absence of other high frequency artifacts.

mercury calibration of a pressure amplifier system at the onset of a monitoring procedure. Mercury calibration is repeated at the change of every nursing shift (every 8 hours). In addition, before any pressure recording is made, the transducer is opened to air (stopcocks to the catheter and the flush solution must be turned off) and the electric calibration is rechecked.

Additional problems exist because of the introduction of extraneous influences on the catheter and the transducer-amplifier system. One of the most common problems with catheters in the right side of the heart is the presence of catheter movement (catheter whip or fling, Fig. 27.23). This is a particular problem in persons with hyperdynamic circulation and whenever underdamped catheter systems are used. Excessive motion of the catheter tip within the pulmonary artery may cause cyclic acceleration and deceleration of the fluid contained within the catheter and transmission of this artifactual pressure to the transducer. Errors of up to 50 mmHg are possible. Catheter fling artifacts are particularly difficult to eliminate in catheterization of the right side of the heart and one may

have to be satisfied with mean pressure measurements. Another common extraneous influence on pressures in the right side of the heart is the superimposition of a high negative or positive intrapleural pressure. This is a particular problem in patients who are dyspneic and in respiratory distress, in patients with severe obstructive pulmonary disease, and in patients on mechanical ventilatory assistance (Fig. 27.23).

Partial occlusion of the catheter or cannula tip by a small thrombus or by close apposition of the cannula tip to the vessel intima may grossly distort the pressure waveform but may be entirely missed unless the transition has been observed (Fig. 27.2). In our experience, this is a particular problem with the use of small-lumen, flexible polyethylene or Teflon catheters in the brachial or femoral artery.

Of equal importance are interpretive errors. These can present a particular problem to the physician, nurse, or technician who is not accustomed to dealing with pressure waveform analysis. One of the most common interpretive problems consists of failure to recognize the large systolic (V or CV) wave of mitral regurgitation in the pulmonary artery wedge position (Fig. 27.14). A balloon-flotation catheter may be improperly placed just at the level of the pulmonic valve, and a pressure recording may be a hybrid of right ventricular and pulmonary arterial pressures (Fig. 27.2). In addition to the potential complications that such a catheter position may produce, for example ventricular dysrhythmias, such a hybrid recording, if unrecognized, may lead to erroneous conclusions regarding the level of pulmonary artery diastolic pressure. Constant vigilance, and a good deal of experience in analyzing pressure waveforms are necessary if one is to avoid serious interpretive errors during cardiac catheterization at the bedside. Even so, examples of erroneously interpreted pressure waveforms have been published.[65,66]

The technique of cardiac output determination by thermodilution is relatively simple. Despite this simplicity there are several pitfalls that may introduce a significant error in the output determination. It has been stated that the position of the catheter tip bearing the thermistor bead in the pulmonary arterial tree has no effect on the accuracy of cardiac output measurement unless the catheter tip becomes wedged.[29] On the other hand, in the cardiac catheterization laboratory we have observed variations in cardiac output measurements by this technique of as much as 20 percent, depending on whether the catheter tip is stable in the pulmonary arterial tree or whether it has an excessive motion and is alternating between the main pulmonary artery and one of its branches.

In a recent study, Sobol et al.[67] demonstrated that significant errors may be introduced by a number of variables. These investigators determined the accuracy and reproducibility of the thermodilution technique by measuring constant blood flow via a heart-lung machine pump. They found that a variation of $\pm0.5$ ml in the recommended quantity of the injectate (10 ml) resulted in a $\pm8$ percent error in cardiac output. Similarly, they found that if the injection time was 6 seconds, instead of the recommended 3 to 4 seconds, an error of minus 16 percent in cardiac output could be identified. If the injectate syringe was taken out of the ice bath and held for 30 seconds encircled by the operator's hand prior to the injection, allowing a brief period of rewarming, a +9 percent error in cardiac output could be measured. Although these variations are small, when they are added to the known limitations of the thermodilution technique in low output states, they may become clinically significant. Therefore, strict adherence to the technique recommended

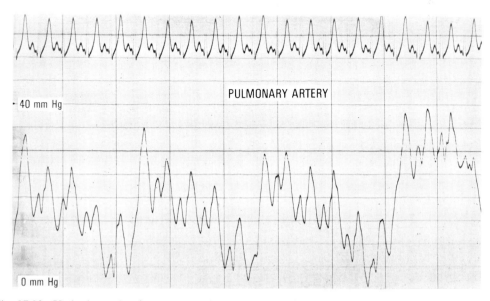

Fig. 27.23 Underdamped pulmonary artery pressure recording demonstrating catheter "whip" artifact as well as excessive oscillations due to labored respirations.

by the manufacturer of the system being used is absolutely essential.

## COMPLICATIONS OF HEMODYNAMIC MONITORING

As indicated earlier in this chapter, hemodynamic monitoring at the bedside constitutes an invasive procedure. Consequently, complications can be expected and do occur. The incidence of such complications is probably very low considering the estimate that between 1 and 2 million bedside catheterizations, using a balloon-flotation catheter, have been performed since its introduction in 1970.[62] On the other hand, it is likely that many such complications are not reported. Awareness, therefore, of the potential complications of invasive hemodynamic monitoring is essential as is strict ad-

herence to established guidelines for these procedures.[68]

The reported and potential complications of hemodynamic monitoring are listed in Table 27.6. It is evident that some of these complications are related to the technique of insertion of the catheter or cannula, whereas others result from limitations of catheter design, inappropriate monitoring and maintenance of the indwelling catheter, and erroneous interpretation of the data being obtained.

With reference to the technique for inserting balloon-flotation catheters into the right side of the heart, the safest avenue is via a small cutdown on a median basilic vein in the right or left antecubital fossa. Such a cutdown may be performed safely and expeditiously under local anesthesia by almost any physician who has adequate training in the technique. Although isolation of a median basilic vein is easy,

**Table 27.6  Complications of Hemodynamic Monitoring**

| Right Heart Balloon Flotation Catheters | Systemic Arterial Pressure Monitoring |
|---|---|
| 1. Thrombophlebitis, localized | 1. Hematoma formation |
| 2. Sepsis | 2. Arterial dissection |
| 3. Endocarditis<br>Septic<br>Aseptic | 3. Arterial thrombosis |
| 4. Vein perforation<br>Hematoma<br>Hemothorax<br>Pneumothorax | 4. Arterial embolization |
| 5. Cardiac Perforation<br>Tamponade | 5. Distal ischemia |
| 6. Heart Block/RBBB | 6. Cerebral embolization |
| 7. Dysrhythmias<br>Atrial<br>Ventricular | 7. Arterial aneurysm formation |
| 8. Intracardiac catheter knotting | 8. Nerve injury |
| 9. Pulmonary embolism | 9. Sepsis |
| 10. Pulmonary infarction | |
| 11. Pulmonary artery tear | |
| 12. Balloon fragment embolism | |
| 13. Air embolism | |
| 14. Valvular damage<br>Pulmonic valve<br>Tricuspid valve | |
| 15. In situ thrombosis<br>Superior vena cava<br>Right sided cardiac chambers | |
| 16. Electrical hazards | |
| 17. Information: Inadequate<br>Erroneous | |

insertion of the catheter into the right side of the heart from this approach may be unsuccessful in 10 percent of cases, due either to retrograde entry of the catheter into the internal jugular vein or to obstruction to the catheter's passage in the axillary vein.[69] Venospasm may occur and further delay the passage of the catheter. For these reasons, percutaneous insertion of catheters into the right side of the heart, via the femoral, subclavian, or internal jugular vein, has become commonplace. Only personnel who have had appropriate training in these procedures should attempt the percutaneous puncture of a large vein, since the potential for serious complications exists, especially when either the subclavian or internal jugular vein is cannulated. Complications secondary to puncture of the subclavian vein have included pneumothorax, hemothorax, air embolization, massive subcutaneous emphysema as well as injuries to the subclavian artery and brachial plexus.[70] Complications of internal jugular vein puncture are less common. Jernigan et al.[71] have reported only three serious complications in approximately 1,000 internal jugular vein punctures. These complications included air embolism, thrombophlebitis of the internal jugular vein, and perforation of the vein with resultant infusion of fluid into the mediastinal space. Air embolism secondary to internal jugular vein puncture should be almost entirely eliminated if patients are placed in the Trendelenburg position and puncture is carried out during the straining phase of a Valsalva maneuver. The femoral vein approach is, in our opinion, safer, since this vessel is located away from vital structures and can be easily compressed to prevent hematoma formation. However, thrombophlebitis of the femoral vein has been reported following the introduction of venous catheters, with subsequent thromboembolic complications. For this reason, systemic anticoagulation is probably necessary if long-term monitoring is undertaken utilizing the femoral vein approach in patients with reduced cardiac output.

Insertion of a radial artery cannula for pressure monitoring can generally be accomplished with few complications.[45,72] Arterial dissection, trauma to the nerves of the hand or wrist, hematoma formation and/or excessive bleeding re-

quiring transfusion and surgical intervention have been reported in association with radial artery cannulation.[45] Reduction of radial artery blood flow following serial unsuccessful insertion attempts has been reported,[45] and for this reason it has been recommended that if cannulation attempts are not immediately successful, recurrent probing for the artery should be abandoned. If a patient is receiving anticoagulant therapy, it may be necessary to "sandbag" the insertion site and, in addition, apply the usual elastic pressure dressing to prevent clinically important hematoma formation.

Once the balloon-flotation catheter has gained access into the venous system, and while it is being advanced to the pulmonary artery, the potential for a number of additional complications exists. These include perforation of a vein, cardiac perforation with tamponade, development of transient right bundle branch block [73] or heart block,[74] development of dysrhythmias, and intracardiac knotting of the catheter.[4] Although cardiac dysrhythmias are rare, one study reported the development of occasional premature ventricular contractions during 17 percent of balloon-flotation catheter placements.[75] These commonly occurred when the distal tip of the catheter was in the right ventricle or pulmonary outflow tract. Premature ventricular contractions are usually self-limited and resolve with the forward progress of the catheter into the pulmonary artery. In addition, several instances of more serious dysrhythmias have been reported: ventricular fibrillation and paroxysmal ventricular tachycardia may occur,[4] particularly in a setting of acute myocardial infarction and pronounced myocardial ischemia.

Intracardiac knotting of the catheter associated with continued manipulation was reported early after the introduction of balloon-flotation catheters.[4] The incidence of catheter knotting is said to be inversely proportional to the size of the catheter, since the smallest catheters are the most flexible and therefore more prone to coil and knot in the right atrium. The risk for intracardiac knotting of a balloon-flotation catheter can be minimized if manipulation is kept to a minimum. The operator must estimate the length of the catheter that would allow its tip to pass across the tricuspid valve. Persistence in advancing the catheter beyond this estimated length, associated with vigorous manipulation and induction of torque, are probably responsible for most instances of intracardiac knotting. Fortunately, although knotting is certainly a source of concern and embarassment, it has not been reported to result in serious complications. The knotted catheter can usually be withdrawn gently to the site of insertion and, if necessary, a small venotomy may be carried out so that the tightened knot can be removed. Preferably, if fluoroscopy is available, the introduction of a flexible guidewire in the lumen of the catheter and manipulation of the knot in the right atrium by an experienced operator may result in its resolution.[76]

Probably the most common and potentially most serious complications associated with long-term pulmonary artery catheterization by balloon-flotation catheters are related to damage of lung parenchyma. Several reports have appeared in the literature of fatal pulmonary hemorrhage related to tear of a pulmonary arterial radicle by a balloon-flotation catheter.[77-80] It appears likely that this complication is the result of overdistension and tearing of a pulmonary artery branch by inappropriate inflation of the catheter balloon. Systemic anticoagulation, and especially the presence of pulmonary hypertension, contribute to the development of this dreaded complication.[62,68] Slow inflation of the balloon with the minimal amount of air required to change the tracing of pulmonary artery pressure to that of pulmonary wedge pressure and limiting wedging time to a minimum should provide a measure of protection against this complication. In general, the guidelines established by Swan and Ganz[68] and reproduced in Table 27.7 should be followed carefully.

Pulmonary embolization and infarction may also complicate long-term pulmonary arterial catheterization. In one reported series, pulmonary embolization, possibly related to the presence of a pulmonary artery catheter, was suspected in 16 of 392 critically ill patients.[75] Most often, pulmonary infarction is the result of undetected long-term "wedging" of a pulmonary artery catheter (Fig. 27.24). It is therefore important to monitor catheter-tip pressure continuously or at frequent intervals (15 to 30 minutes).[4] It is unwise to attempt to monitor pulmonary artery wedge pressure continuously. It is our practice not to allow the catheter to remain in the wedge position for more than 15 to 30 seconds at any one time, even in the absence of pulmonary hypertension. The user should recognize that balloon-flotation catheters have the intrinsic propensity to become softer in vivo. This results in a reduction of the diameter of the catheter loop in the cham-

**Table 27.7   Guidelines for the Safe Use of Balloon-Tipped Catheters ***

1. Keep "wedge" time to a minimum, especially in patients with pulmonary hypertension (preferably 10 to 15 sec).
2. When the balloon is reinflated for recording wedge pressure, the inflation medium (carbon dioxide or air) must be added slowly under continuous monitoring of the pulmonary artery pressure waveform. Inflation *must* be stopped immediately when the pulmonary artery pressure tracing is seen to change to pulmonary wedge pressure.
3. If fluoroscopy is available (as in the cardiac catheterization laboratory), refloat the catheter tip from the central pulmonary artery for each wedge pressure measurement.
4. Careful note of the balloon inflation volume must be made. If "wedge" is recorded with a balloon volume significantly below that indicated on the catheter shaft, pull the catheter gradually into a position in which full or near full inflation volume produces a wedge tracing.
5. Anticipate spontaneous catheter tip migration toward the periphery of the pulmonary bed. To avoid possible damage to the pulmonary artery, monitor the pressure tracing during every balloon inflation.
6. Spontaneous catheter tip migration into wedge position may also induce pulmonary infarction. Continuous or frequent monitoring of the catheter tip pressure is therefore necessary.
7. Do not use liquids for balloon inflation; they may be irretrievable and may prevent balloon deflation.
8. Keep a syringe on the balloon lumen of the catheter to prevent accidental injection of liquids into the balloon.

* Adapted from Swan and Ganz [68]

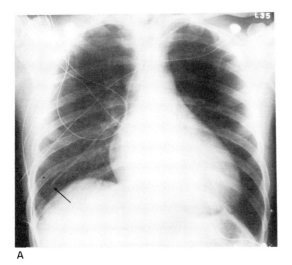

A

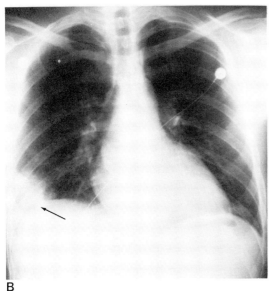

B

Fig. 27.24 Chest radiographs illustrating a pulmonary complication of flow-directed catheters. *(A)* The catheter tip has migrated spontaneously to a peripheral pulmonary artery *(arrow)*. Note the tight catheter loop in the right atrium and right ventricle. *(B)* Forty-eight hours later a pulmonary infarct *(arrow)* has developed distal to the artery presumably occluded by the flow-directed catheter.

bers of the right side of the heart and allows its tip to migrate distally, even when the balloon is not inflated. For this reason, if damping of the pressure tracing is observed, the catheter should be gently withdrawn 1 to 2 cm and a small quantity of fluid injected to insure patency of the catheter lumen. Even if a good

phasic pulmonary arterial pressure tracing is being obtained, it is important to ascertain the location of the catheter tip periodically by a chest roentgenogram. During long-term pulmonary artery catheterization, it is our practice to attempt to maintain the tip of the balloon-flotation catheter in the right pulmonary artery just beyond the mediastinal border (Fig. 27.25). From this point, inflation of the balloon will allow the catheter tip to migrate distally into the wedge position. When the balloon is deflated, the catheter tip will usually return to its original position.

Thromboembolic complications following the long-term use of indwelling balloon-flotation catheters have been reported.[4] Many instances of thrombus formation on the balloon or the body of the catheter have been recognized, and instances of pulmonary infarction secondary to distal embolization of such thrombus have been suspected. Thrombus formation on the catheter is particularly likely to occur in the seriously ill cardiac patient in whom a hypercoagulable state develops during the course of illness.[4] Similarly, the possibility of

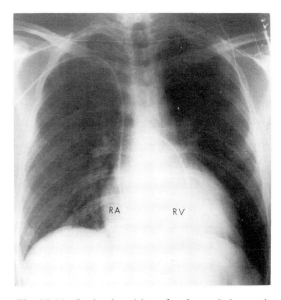

Fig. 27.25 Optimal position of catheter tip in proximal right pulmonary artery for long-term pressure monitoring. Note the relaxed loop of the catheter in the right atrium (RA) and right ventricle (RV) in comparison to the catheter illustrated in Figure 27.24*A*.

thromboembolic complications increases with the length of catheterization. It is therefore important to limit the duration of catheterization to the minimum period of time required by the patient's condition. It is our practice to place all patients undergoing prophylactic hemodynamic monitoring on low-dose subcutaneous heparin therapy (5,000 units every 12 hours). In patients who are critically ill, who appear to be candidates for the development of a hypercoagulable state, or who will require prolonged hemodynamic monitoring, full-dose systemic heparinization is usually undertaken. Localized thrombophlebitis is occasionally seen, especially when the balloon-flotation catheter has been inserted through a peripheral vein. This complication is usually related to inadequate skin preparation prior to the insertion of the catheter. Local thrombophlebitis necessitates removal of the catheter and usually responds to local measures of heat and elevation. It is rarely of serious import.

Rupture of the balloon occurs occasionally, and this may result in minor air embolization or embolization of balloon fragments. This complication seems to be fairly common (5 percent) with catheters that have been subjected to multiple uses.[4] Exposure of the balloon to the atmosphere, improper handling during insertion, as well as the absorption of lipoproteins by the latex membrane of the balloon are all factors that increase the likelihood of rupture.[4,63] Single use of balloon-flotation catheters is recommended along with limitation of the cannulation time to 48 hours, if possible. In the absence of an intracardiac shunt, the introduction of 1 to 1.5 ml of air in the venous system does not appear to be a hazardous complication, nor has it been reported to produce symptoms or adverse consequences. However, even a minimal amount of air entering the left side of the heart poses the risk of coronary or cerebral air embolization with catastrophic consequences. For this reason, in a setting of intracardiac shunts, the use of carbon dioxide is recommended for inflation of the catheter balloon.

A less common but potentially serious complication is damage to the pulmonic or tricuspid valve by the indwelling catheter. Both septic and aseptic endocardial vegetations have been reported following prolonged pulmonary artery catheterization.[81-83] Disruption of the pulmonic valve with resulting pulmonic insufficiency in the absence of sepsis has been reported recently in association with pulmonary artery pressure monitoring via a balloon-tipped catheter.[84] Although mechanical trauma to valvular structures by the indwelling catheter has been invoked, it is possible that an underlying defect of the endocardium may be necessary before valve cusps can be seriously damaged by the catheter.[84]

Septicemia related to indwelling venous and arterial lines was well recognized before the advent of balloon-flotation catheters. In one study, indwelling venous catheters were thought to be responsible for 43 percent of hospital-acquired septicemias.[85] With the explosion of hemodynamic monitoring during the past 10 years, nosocomial infections related to hemodynamic monitoring have become a health hazard of major proportions. It is estimated that hospital-acquired infections occur in 5 to 15 percent of the 40 million patients admitted annually to hospitals in this country.[86] Most of these infections appear to be related causally to surgery or invasive procedures, such as urethral catheterization, endotracheal intubation, or vascular cannulation. The incidence of nosocomial infection has been highest among patients in intensive care units.[87] Although most of these patients are hospitalized for multiorgan failure and consequently are not directly comparable to patients hospitalized in coronary care units, the potential for the development of sepsis exists in any patient undergoing invasive monitoring.

Several avenues of bacterial contamination exist during hemodynamic monitoring. The most obvious is the patient's skin, especially if it has not been properly cleansed prior to invasion. Fortunately most health practitioners are well aware of the requirement for proper skin cleansing and strict aseptic technique during the insertion of arterial or venous cannulae. Contamination at the time of catheter insertion does not appear to be a major source of sepsis.[86] To the contrary, most episodes of sepsis appear to be related to infusion or are secondary to contamination of the monitoring equipment.

The development of disposable tubing connecting the catheter to the pressure transducer, and more recently the development of disposable transducer "domes," have not eliminated the risk of contamination and infection.[88] In two separate studies outbreaks of sepsis in patients being monitored hemodynamically were ascribed to contaminated pressure transducers connected to intravascular catheters.[89,90] Sepsis occurred despite the use of disposable domes. Two mechanisms have been postulated: (1) possible contamination at the time of initial equipment assembly and (2) contamination of the monitoring lines across the membrane of the disposable dome, which was rendered defective as the equipment was being assembled. Pressure transducers should therefore be considered potential sources of infection, even if they are used with disposable pressure domes. Routine disinfection of the nondisposable transducer heads with gluteraldehyde has been recommended. Similarly the substitution of a few drops of 70 percent isopropyl alcohol for dextrose-containing solutions to establish fluid coupling between the diaphragm of the transducer and the membrane of the disposable dome has been suggested.[89] The long-term effects of isopropyl alcohol on the diaphragm of the transducer are unknown. Furthermore, the risk of bacteremia may be decreased by using fluids for flushing that do not contain glucose [89] and by changing the tubing and fluids in the monitoring system at regular intervals, possibly every 24 hours.[91,92] Another major source of infection appears to be the stopcock, which is usually inserted between the intravascular catheter and the connecting fluid-filled tubing. It is customary to occlude the extra stopcock port, when it is not in use, with a sterile cap or syringe. The extra port is used to aspirate blood samples and to inject flushing solution, medications, and so forth. Despite careful attention to technique, stopcocks are frequently contaminated. In one study, 48 percent of stopcocks cultured were found to be contaminated. Stopcocks on venous lines had a 59 percent contamination rate, while arterial stopcocks had a 38 percent rate of contamination.[92] Of interest is the finding that stopcocks on antecubital lines had a higher incidence of contamination than stopcocks on femoral lines. Several hypotheses have been advanced to explain this discrepancy, but it appears likely that increased handling of the antecubital-line stopcocks was responsible for their higher contamination rate.

Constant vigilance, observance of sterile technique, use of disposable equipment as much as possible, and limitation of the length of hemodynamic monitoring will almost certainly decrease the incidence of nosocomial sepsis related to invasive monitoring. In the study of Prachar et al.,[93] the incidence of bacterial contamination of pulmonary artery catheters decreased from 45 percent in 1974 to 18 percent in 1976.

Other less common complications of hemodynamic monitoring include cardiac perforation, catheter fragment embolism, and in situ thrombosis of large veins or of the right side of the heart. Cardiac perforation was more commonly seen with straight polyethylene central venous pressure catheters than with contemporary balloon-tipped catheters. If the flow-directed catheter is properly manipulated across the right atrium and right ventricle with the balloon inflated, the risk of cardiac perforation is practically nil, since the balloon projects beyond the catheter tip and pressure exerted on the endocardium is distributed over a larger surface area. Similarly, catheter embolism, which was rather common with straight polyethylene catheters, is extremely uncommon with the use of flow-directed balloon catheters, except for the possible embolization of balloon fragments. Massive in situ thrombosis associated with the use of a flow-directed catheter has been reported [94] and is probably related to the existence of a hypercoagulable state.

The most serious complication of long-term arterial catheterization is thrombosis, with or without distal embolization, and clinical signs of ischemia. Thrombus formation has been previously reported to occur in 40 to 60 percent of cases.[46] As experience has been gained, however, the incidence of complications from arterial cannulation has decreased markedly. In a study of 531 patients in whom the radial artery was cannulated for central arterial monitoring, Gardner et al.[46] reported hematoma formation in 9.3 percent of patients and thrombosis requiring thrombectomy in only 0.56 percent of patients. It appears that total occlusion of the radial artery by thrombus was related to the following three factors: (1) the indwelling catheter was left in situ for 6 or more days; (2) hypotension was present; and (3) patients were receiving vasoactive drugs, resulting in severe peripheral vasoconstriction. Follow-up study of 280 patients with a Doppler ultrasonic flowmeter demonstrated detectable flow reductions in the radial artery in 19 percent of cases. Downs et al.[95] studied the incidence of thrombotic embolization after a short cannula was inserted in the radial artery of 32 patients. The study was carried out by performing portable arteriograms via the indwelling radial artery cannula, shortly after insertion and daily thereafter, until the cannula was removed. A 23 percent incidence of thromboembolism was found. Thromboemboli were seen in the brachial, interosseous, ulnar, and digital arteries and were frequently multiple. Of interest is that only one instance of clinical symptoms could be related to the occurrence of thromboembolism. Of even geater interest is that an arteriogram performed on a 15-year-old patient by the injection of 3 ml of contrast solution demonstrated that the contrast material reached the subclavian-axillary artery junction. Furthermore, the authors pointed out that the lowest incidence of thromboembolic complications occurred when a 20-gauge Longdwell (Becton Dickinson and Company) nontapered cannula was used. In a study of brachial artery cannulation, using a similar Teflon cannula, Barnes et al,[96] using the Doppler technique, found evidence of localized arterial obstruction in the forearm below the site of cannulation in 3 of 54 patients. None of these patients had low cardiac output, none had received vasopressor therapy, and none were symptomatic. It appears, therefore, that the incidence of thromboembolic complications of arterial cannulation varies widely and depends on technique, type of cannula, site of cannulation, as well as the physiologic state of the patient.

The risk of cerebral or coronary embolism from the vigorous retrograde flushing of arterial cannulae has been raised by Lowenstein et al.[48] A more recent study by Gardner et al.[97] suggested that the problem is minimal. In a simulated system, these investigators demonstrated that vigorous manual injection of dye resulted in retrograde migration of the injectate to a maximum of 4.8 cm when the injection was made against a forward flow of 1.7 l/min. The discrepancy is probably related to the experimental design of the study, wherein the injection was made through an arterial catheter 1m long, with an internal diameter of 0.5 mm. The length and diameter of such a catheter impart sufficient resistance to the injection as to successfully preclude distal flow of a manually injected flush. On the other hand, the vigorous injection of a volume of flush solution into a short radial or brachial cannula may well cause the material to reach the brachiocephalic vessels, as the angiographic study of Downs et al.[95] demonstrated. Despite this controversy, the risk of air embolism of the arterial side of the circulation is such that careful monitoring of pressurized constant flush systems is necessary to avoid this potentially lethal complication.

Finally, it is important to recognize that all intravascular catheters provide a low impedance pathway to the central circulation by means of an electrolytic fluid column. The risk of electrically induced cardiac dysrhythmias is ever present, and proper isolation of all electric devices connected to these catheters is essential. The subject is discussed in detail in Chapter 6.

## MONITORING EQUIPMENT

A multitude of monitoring equipment components are available from numerous manufacturers in the United States and abroad. This section will serve as a brief review of available equipment, attempting at the same time to point out desirable and undesirable features. No attempt will be made to compare equipment of different manufacturers or to rate similar components. The user must establish his needs and then "shop around" for those items of equipment that best meet his requirements. Probably the single most important element in deciding on one manufacturer versus another is the reputation of the local representative regarding promptness and service. Even institutions with large biomedical engineering sections must often avail themselves of the services of the manufacturer's local representative. Hence, in my opinion, service is probably the most important element in deciding on a particular manufacturer.

## Right Heart Catheters

As mentioned earlier in this chapter, the era of hemodynamic monitoring actually began with the introduction by Swan and Ganz of balloon-flotation catheters for bedside pulmonary artery catheterization.[2] Balloon-tipped flow-directed (Swan-Ganz and others) catheters are available in a variety of sizes and specifications. They are generally constructed of soft, flexible polyvinyl chloride and, in the basic version, consist of a double-lumen catheter with an outside diameter of approximately 1.5 mm (5 French). The monitoring lumen has a cross-sectional area of 0.8 mm² and a frequency response of 10 Hz. The smaller lumen is approximately 0.4 mm in diameter and is used to inflate a small latex balloon positioned at the catheter tip (Fig. 27.26). The inflation capacity of the balloon is 0.8 ml and the length of the adult 5 French, double-lumen catheter is usually 110 cm. Six French and 7 French catheters are available with larger monitoring lumens and higher frequency responses up to 25 Hz. The

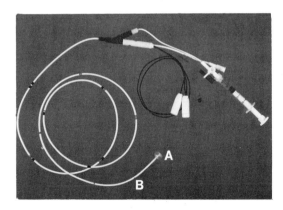

Fig. 27.26 Example of a triple-lumen, thermodilution, balloon flotation catheter. The balloon is inflated with 1 ml of air *(A)*. The thermistor bead is located 4 cm proximal to the catheter tip *(B)*. The proximal termination of the three lumens and the thermistor leads are seen in the upper right hand corner of the figure.

basic flow-directed balloon-tipped catheter is used to monitor solely pulmonary artery and pulmonary artery wedge pressures.

Triple-lumen balloon-flotation catheters are commonly available in a 7 French size. These catheters have a third lumen (in addition to the tip lumen and to the lumen leading to the latex balloon) that terminates at a side port located 20 or 30 cm from the tip, for monitoring right atrial or central venous pressure. The cross-sectional areas of the monitoring lumens vary from 0.5 to 0.75 mm² and the frequency response from 10.5 to 30 Hz, depending on the manufacturer. The user must remember that the diameter of the deflated balloon at the tip is usually one or one-half French size larger than the diameter of the catheter shaft; therefore one must use an introducer-sheath assembly of a size larger than the nominal size of the catheter to avoid damaging the latex balloon as it passes through the sheath.

An additional modification of the basic balloon-tipped flow-directed catheter is the positioning of a thermistor temperature detector on the catheter surface 4 cm proximal to the catheter tip. A fourth small lumen in the catheter carries the electric leads for the thermistor and terminates proximally in an electric "plug" (Fig. 27.26) that must be connected via an appropriate cable to the cardiac output "computer" used to measure thermodilution cardiac output. The luminal cross-sectional areas of quadruple-lumen thermistor balloon-tipped catheters vary from 0.5 to 0.8 mm² and the nominal frequency responses from 10.5 to 22 Hz.

Although all manufacturers provide precalibrated thermistors with resistance data included on a catheter tag, some manufacturers provide thermistor beads of a similar resistance and temperature coefficient of resistance. These catheters are then interchangeable, with no need to recalibrate the thermodilution measurement system. Other manufacturers provide thermistors that are calibrated but vary considerably in resistance and coefficient of resistance; therefore the thermodilution measurement system must be recalibrated as catheters are changed. In general, catheters recommended by the manufacturer of the thermodilution measurement system should be used. Double, triple, and thermodilution balloon-flotation catheters are manufactured by Edwards Laboratories, Electrocatheter Corporation, American Catheter Corporation, Extracorporeal Medical Specialties, and others.

## Arterial Cannulae

A large number of devices for monitoring intraarterial pressure are available. For radial artery cannulation, our preference is a 2- to $2\frac{1}{2}$-inch, 18- or 20-gauge nontapered polyethylene cannula fitted to the outside of a smaller needle. For femoral artery cannulation, we employ a 12- to 24-inch, 18- or 20-gauge polyethylene catheter within a larger needle. A longer catheter is desirable to insure its stability within the femoral artery, and, more importantly, to allow it to reach the bifurcation of the aorta and thus monitor true central aortic pressure.

## Pressure Transducers

A pressure transducer is an electromechanical device designed to recognize changes in pressure and convert this biologic event to a usable electrical signal. In general, most pressure transducers operate on the principle of the strain gauge. This principle involves the deformation of a series of resistance wires interconnected to form a Wheatstone bridge. As the length of the resistance wires increases or decreases, these changes unbalance the Wheatstone bridge, causing a voltage change proportional to the pressure signal that caused the deformation. These changes in voltage signal are then amplified, measured, and recorded as the electrical manifestation of the biologic pressure event.

Most commonly used pressure transducers (Fig. 27.27) are devices mounted externally and connected to an intravascular catheter through a fluid-filled tubing system. A fluid-filled chamber or "dome" is connected to the catheter fluid column so that pressure changes transmitted via the fluid-filled system can be directly reflected on the diaphragm of the strain gauge. Newer strain gauges employ disposable domes attached to the transducer and coupled to the

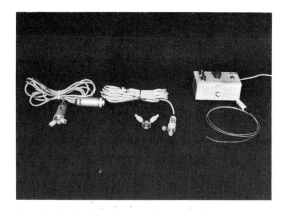

Fig. 27.27 Some commonly available pressure transducers. *(A)* External strain gauge manufactured by Hewlett-Packard. *(B)* External strain gauge with an extra disposable dome manufactured by Statham-Gould. *(C)* High fidelity micromanometer mounted on the tip of a 5 French catheter by Millar instruments.

diaphragm of the transducer with one or two drops of saline. The advantage of disposable domes is that they are prepackaged sterile and, theoretically at least, minimize the risk of infection, obviating the need for sterilizing the entire transducer. However, serious questions have been raised as to the efficacy of disposable domes in preventing infection, as discussed earlier in this chapter. An additional benefit of disposable domes is that they provide electrical isolation between strain gauge and patient.

Other available pressure devices are miniaturized external transducers that can be attached directly to the arterial cannula or the proximal end of a catheter, obviating the need for long fluid-filled tubing. The highest fidelity pressure recordings are obtainable by means of miniature catheter-tip mounted transducers that can be inserted directly into the cardiovascular system (Fig. 27.27). At this writing, these catheter tip transducers have not been mounted on flow-directed catheters. They therefore require manipulation with the aid of fluoroscopy and are rarely used at the bedside.

External pressure transducers are commonly mounted on an appropriate holder, the height of which can be changed to bring the transducer diaphragm level with the midchest position of the patient being monitored (Fig. 27.28). A continuous flush device (Sorensen Intraflow and

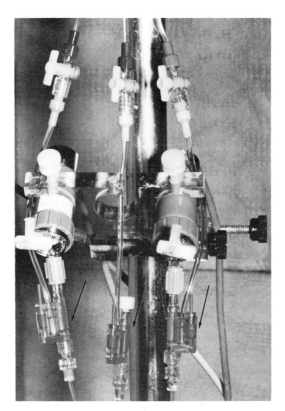

Fig. 27.28  Two pressure transducers mounted on a bedside IV pole via an adjustable holder so that their level may be adjusted to correspond to the patient's right atrial level. Intraflow devices are interposed between the transducer and the intravascular catheters *(arrows)*. The center Intraflow is connected to the proximal lumen of the Swan-Ganz catheter to maintain patency.

others) is frequently interposed between transducer and catheter tubing to provide a constant slow (3 to 6 ml/hr) flow of heparinized saline to maintain catheter lumen patency.

Desirable pressure transducer characteristics include a small volume dome and a linear response exceeding the usual physiologic range of intravascular pressures, e.g., from −30 to +300 mmHg.

## Amplifying and Recording Systems

More than any other component of the monitoring system, the amplifier, with its display oscilloscope and recorder, requires careful choice by the user because of the high initial cost and critical nature of the task it performs.

As with all other components, a large number of amplifier recording systems in diverse configurations are available from a variety of manufacturers.

Our preference is for portable self-contained systems that can be moved from bedside to bedside as the need for hemodynamic monitoring arises. This configuration is advantageous because of a much lower initial cost than if each bedside were equipped with a stationary amplifier-recorder system. Although hemodynamic monitoring has become commonplace in coronary care units, in our experience two pressure monitoring systems will suffice in the average 6- or 8-bed unit. Of course, the requirements will vary depending on the nature of the coronary care unit. A medical center CCU designed to accept in transfer critically ill patients for hemodynamic monitoring [98] will require a greater monitoring capability than a community hospital CCU.

The amplifier-recording system should include at least two pressure amplifiers with variable gain ranges, in order to display optimally both low and high pressures. A minimum of three different gain ranges are necessary, for example, 0–40, 0–100, and 0–200 mmHg. In addition, it is desirable to include an electrocardiographic amplifier in the system so that the electrocardiogram can be displayed simultaneously with the pressures. This is necessary in order to time accurately certain pressure events, such as A and V waves in the right atrial and pulmonary artery wedge pressure tracings. Most modern pressure amplifiers will incorporate some type of a digital or analog readout that will display readings of systolic, diastolic, and mean pressures, recorded either sequentially or simultaneously. The pressure amplifiers should incorporate easy to use zero and gain controls, and most amplifiers today have an integrated electric calibration circuit. It is important to remember that calibration cannot be carried out unless the strain gauge is attached to the amplifier. Because strain gauge electric characteristics vary, recalibration must be carried out if a different pressure transducer is connected to a particular amplifier.

A multichannel oscilloscope should be an integral part of the pressure recording system so that the electrocardiogram and the pressure waveforms are continuously displayed. This is essential if artifacts in the pressure tracings are to be recognized early and corrected promptly. Our preference is for oscilloscopes that allow the electron beams to cross and therefore display pressure waveforms in an expanded mode for better recognition and analysis.

Even though the pressure amplifiers may provide electronic readouts of pressure values, it is important for the monitoring system to include a hard copy recorder so that pressure waveforms may be recorded and carefully measured and analyzed. For bedside hemodynamic monitoring, a direct-writer multichannel recorder appears to be the simplest and most convenient to use. The recorder should incorporate subsidiary amplifier controls so that pressure tracings being recorded may be accurately calibrated on paper. In addition, it should be capable of a variety of recording speeds from 1 to 100 mm/sec. Slow paper speeds are useful for continuously recording pressures that are being monitored and committing to paper long-term trends following management interventions. Rapid paper speeds, on the other hand, are often useful in analyzing complex waveforms. An example of mobile bedside pressure monitoring equipment is illustrated in Figure 27.29.

## Cardiac Output Measuring Devices

In the majority of intensive care units today, cardiac output is determined by the thermodilution principle. A large number of devices are available, which, operating on the computer principle, will immediately calculate the thermodilution curve parameters and display the cardiac output results in liters per minute.

Simplicity of use is extremely important in the performance of bedside cardiac output determinations. Many of the newer cardiac output computers offer practically a one- or two-button operating procedure. They automatically measure the core temperature of the patient, via the thermistor in the pulmonary artery, as well as the temperature of the injectate by means of a separate temperature probe. The circuits are balanced automatically and the user often has only to depress the balance button and then

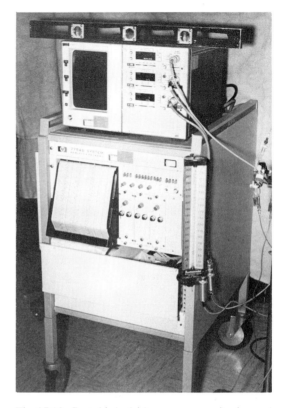

Fig. 27.29 Portable bedside pressure monitoring and recording cart. It incorporates a 4-channel oscilloscope, two pressure amplifiers and one electrocardiograph amplifier and a 4-channel direct writer. The pressure amplifiers display digitally the systolic, diastolic or mean pressures being monitored. Note the ancillary equipment: mercury manometer and level (see text for discussion).

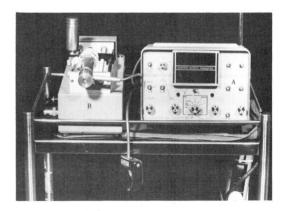

Fig. 27.30 An Electronics for Medicine-Lyons dual thermodilution and indicator dilution cardiac output computer (A). A constant rate withdrawal pump (B) and the photoelectric cuvette (C) complete the system.

inject the cold saline when the computer gives the signal. Some manufacturers provide devices that combine a thermodilution and an indicator-dilution cardiac output computer (Fig. 27.30). These instruments provide flexibility in that cardiac output may be measured by two different techniques. They are usually somewhat more complex and require greater technical expertise to operate. If cardiac output is being measured by the indicator-dilution technique, the system must incorporate a photoelectric cuvette and a constant rate withdrawal pump to draw blood through the cuvette.

Some intensive care units are equipped with general purpose digital computers designed to perform such "housekeeping chores" as storage and retrieval of patient related data, arterial blood gases, and so on. Such computers may easily be adapted to the calculation of the thermodilution cardiac output. All that is necessary

is the appropriate software and an electronic interface to connect the thermodilution catheter to the computer. Additional software may be written so that derived parameters of cardiovascular function may be instantly calculated by entering "off line" pressure data after the cardiac output determination (Fig. 27.31). The role of computers in intensive care monitoring is expanding rapidly; a detailed discussion of this topic, however, falls beyond the scope of this chapter.

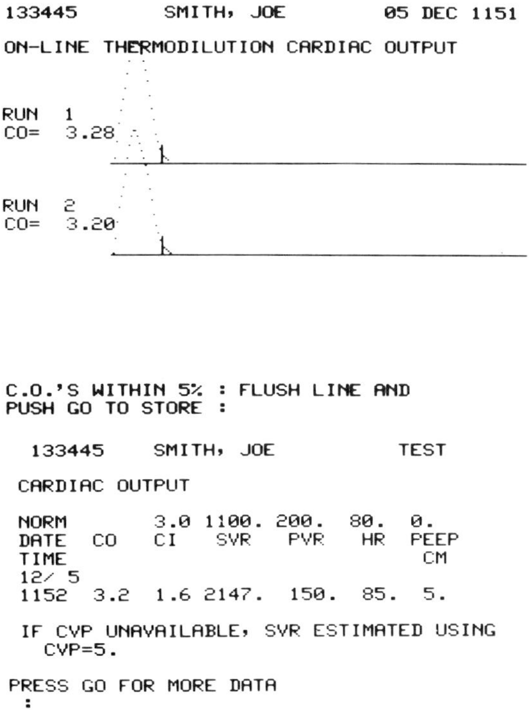

## Ancillary Equipment

A variety of additional equipment is necessary to institute hemodynamic monitoring at the bedside. Equipment such as syringes, tubing, stopcocks, ice bath, and so on, will vary from unit to unit and must be collected and organized efficiently by the unit personnel for their purposes. A few comments only will be made in this connection.

Tubing used to connect fluid-filled catheters to pressure transducers must be of relatively small internal diameter and low compliance to transmit pressures faithfully. Large volume, high compliance tubing will cause overdamping and distortion of transmitted pressures. The length of such connecting tubing should be kept to a minimum, consistent with the patient's requirements to be able to move about in bed.

A mercury manometer is an essential part of the monitoring equipment (Fig 27.29). Despite the availability of electric calibration signals on most modern amplifiers, mercury calibration should be carried out regularly as a check of the electric calibration, since the latter may fluctuate from time to time. A system of short rubber tubing and stopcocks is necessary to connect the mercury manometer to the transducer for proper calibration. Similarly, a level 2 to 3 feet long is an invaluable aid in checking and adjusting the height of the transducers, which should be kept at the approximate level of the mid-right atrium (Fig. 27.29).

Introducer-sheath assemblies come prepackaged and include a short guidewire, vessel dilator, and the venous sheath. A sheath with a side port may prove valuable in certain circumstances, by allowing blood withdrawal and/or

```
133445        SMITH, JOE          05 DEC 1151
ON-LINE THERMODILUTION CARDIAC OUTPUT


RUN  1
CO=  3.28


RUN  2
CO=  3.20


C.O.'S WITHIN 5% : FLUSH LINE AND
PUSH GO TO STORE :

  133445       SMITH, JOE            TEST

CARDIAC OUTPUT

NORM         3.0 1100. 200.  80.   0.
DATE   CO   CI   SVR   PVR    HR  PEEP
TIME                               CM
12/ 5
1152   3.2  1.6 2147.  150.  85.   5.

IF CVP UNAVAILABLE, SVR ESTIMATED USING
  CVP=5.

PRESS GO FOR MORE DATA
  :
```

Fig. 27.31  Example of hard copy printout of computer generated cardiovascular data. Two simulated thermodilution curves were entered "on line" and pressure data had been previously entered "off-line." (Patient monitoring project, UCSD; supported by USPHS grant GM 17284).

infusion directly into a large vein without interrupting the pressure monitoring functions of the catheter.

## REFERENCES

1. Walinsky P: Hemodynamic monitoring in acute myocardial infarction. Cardiovasc Clin 7:61, 1975.
2. Swan HJC, Ganz W, Forrester J, et al: Catheterization of the heart in man with the use of a flow-directed balloon-tipped catheter. N Eng J Med 283:447, 1970.
3. Lategola M, Rahn H: A self-guiding catheter for cardiac and pulmonary arterial catheterization and occlusion. Proc Soc Exp Bio Med 84:667, 1953.
4. Swan HJC, Ganz W: Use of balloon flotation catheters in critically ill patients. Surg Clin NA 55:501, 1975.
5. Fife WP, Lee BS: Construction and use of a self-guiding, right heart and pulmonary artery catheter. J Appl Physiol 120:148, 1965.
6. Scheinman MM, Abbot JA, Rapaport E: Clinical uses of a flow-directed right heart catheter. Arch Intern Med 114:19, 1969.
7. Swan HJC: What is the role of invasive monitoring procedures in the management of the critically ill? Cardiovasc Clin 8:103, 1977.
8. Simon M: The pulmonary vasculature in congenital heart disease. Radiol Clin NA: 6:303, 1968.
9. Forrester JS, Diamond G, Chatterjee K, et al: Medical therapy of acute myocardial infarction by the application of hemodynamic subsets. N Eng J Med 295:1356 and 1404, 1976.
10. Chatterjee K, Swan HJC: Hemodynamic profile of acute myocardial infarction. In: Myocardial Infarction. Corday E, Swan HJC, editors. Williams and Wilkins, Baltimore, 1973.
11. Ronan JA, Steelman RB, DeLeon AC, et al: The clinical diagnosis of acute severe mitral insufficiency. Am J Cardiol 27:284, 1971.
12. Yang SS, Bentivoglio LG, Marañhao V, et al: From cardiac catheterization data to hemodynamic parameters. 2nd Ed. FA Davis, Philadelphia, 1978.
13. Braunwald E, Ross J Jr: The ventricular end-diastolic pressure: Appraisal of its value in the recognition of ventricular failure in man. Am J Med 34:147, 1963.
14. Folse R, Braunwald E: A method for the determination of the fraction of left ventricular volume ejected per beat and of the ventricular end-diastolic and residual volumes. Circulation 25:674, 1962.
15. Braunwald E, Frahm CJ: Studies on Starling's law of the heart. IV. Observations on the hemodynamic functions of the left atrium in man. Circulation 24:633, 1961.
16. Grossman W (Ed): Cardiac Catheterization and Angiography. Lea and Febiger, Philadelphia, 1974.
17. Walston A, Kendall ME: Comparison of pulmonary wedge and left atrial pressure in man. Am Heart J 86:159, 1973.
18. Caro CG, Bergel DH, Seed WA: Forward and backward transmission of pressure waves in the pulmonary vascular bed of the dog. Circ Res 20:185, 1967.
19. Luchsinger PC, Seipp HW Jr, Patel DJ: Relationship of pulmonary artery-wedge pressure to left atrial pressure in man. Circ Res 21:315, 1962.
20. Fowler NO, Black-Schaffer B, Scott RC, et al: Idiopathic and thromboembolic pulmonary hypertension. Am J Med 40:331, 1966.
21. Yu PN: Primary pulmonary hypertension: Report of six cases and review of the literature. Ann Intern Med 49:1138, 1958.
22. Trell E: Pulmonary hypertension in disorders of the left heart. Scand J Clin Lab Invest 31:409, 1973.
23. Rice DL, Awe RJ, Gaash WH, et al: Wedge pressure measurement in obstructive pulmonary disease. Chest 66:628, 1974.
24. Kaplan S: Pressure curve analysis. In: Intravascular Catheterization. Zimermann HA, editor. 2nd Ed. Charles C Thomas, Springfield, Ill, 1966.
25. Bernstein WH, Fierer EM, Laszlo MH, et al: The interpretation of pulmonary artery wedge pressures. Br Heart J 22:37, 1960.
26. Manjuran RS, Agarwal JB, Roy SB: Relationship of pulmonary artery diastolic and pulmonary artery wedge pressures in mitral stenosis. Am Heart J 89:207, 1975.
27. Bouchard RJ, Gault JH, Ross J Jr: Evaluation of pulmonary arterial end-diastolic pressure as an estimate of left ventricular end-diastolic pressure in patients with normal and abnormal left ventricular performance. Circulation 44:1072, 1971.
28. Rahimtoola SH, Loeb HS, Ehsani A, et al: Relationship of pulmonary artery to left ventricular diastolic pressures in acute myocardial infarction. Circulation 46:283, 1972.
29. Buchbinder N, Ganz W: Hemodynamic moni-

toring: Invasive techniques. Anesthesiology 45:146, 1976.

30. Cohn JN: Blood pressure monitoring in shock: Mechanism of inaccuracy in auscultatory and palpatory methods. JAMA 199:972, 1967.

31. DelGuercio LRM, Cohn JD: Monitoring: Methods and significance. Surg Clin NA 56:977, 1976.

32. Warner H: The role of computers in medical research. JAMA 196:944, 1966.

33. McDonald DA, Kouchoukos NT, Shepard LC, et al: Estimation of stroke volume and cardiac output from the central arterial pulse contour in postoperative patients. Circulation 38(suppl 6):118, 1968.

34. Daily PO, Griepp RB, Shumway NE: Percutaneous internal jugular vein cannulation. Arch Surg 101:534, 1970.

35. Kaplan JA, Miller ED: Internal jugular vein catheterization. Anesthesiol Rev 3:21, 1976.

36. Baker JD, Wallace CT: Internal jugular central venous pressure monitoring—a panacea? Anesthesiol Rev 3:15, 1976.

37. Fowler NO: Diseases of the pericardium. Curr Probl Cardiol 2:13, 1978.

38. Lorell B, Leinbach RC, Pohost GM, et al: Right ventricular infarction. Clinical diagnosis and differentiation from cardiac tamponade and pericardial constriction. Am J Cardiol 43:465, 1979.

39. Swan HJC, Forrester JS, Diamond G, et al: Hemodynamic spectrum of myocardial infarction and cardiogenic shock. A conceptual model. Circulation 45:1097, 1972.

40. Diamond G, Forrester JS: Effect of coronary artery disease and acute myocardial infarction on left ventricular compliance in man. Circulation 45:11, 1972.

41. Smith M, Ratshin RA, Russell RO Jr, et al: Early consecutive left ventricular compliance changes after acute myocardial infarction. Am J Cardiol 31:158, 1973.

42. Forrester JS, Diamond G, McHugh TJ, et al: Filling pressures in the right and left sides of the heart in acute myocardial infarction: A reappraisal of central venous pressure monitoring. N Eng J Med 285:190, 1971.

43. Forrester JS, Diamond G, Swan HJC: Bedside diagnosis of latent cardiac complications in acutely ill patients. JAMA 30:338, 1972.

44. Allen EV: Thromboangitis obliterans: Methods of diagnosis of chronic occlusive arterial lesions distal to the wrist with illustrative cases. Am J Med Sci 178:237, 1929.

45. Gardner RM, Schwartz RN, Wong HC, et al: Percutaneous indwelling radial-artery catheters for monitoring cardiovascular function. N Engl J Med 290:1227, 1974.

46. Smith RN: Invasive pressure monitoring. Am J Nurs 78:1514, 1978.

47. Bedford RF: Percutaneous radial-artery cannulation: Increased safety using teflon catheters. Anesthesiology 42:219, 1975.

48. Lowenstein E, Little JW III, Lo HH: Prevention of cerebral embolization from flushing radial-artery cannulas. N Engl J Med 285:1414, 1971.

49. Gazes PC, Gaddy JE: Bedside management of acute myocardial infarction. Am Heart J 97:782, 1979.

50. Afifi A, Chang PC, Liu VY, et al: Prognostic indexes in acute myocardial infarction complicated by shock. Am J Cardiol 33:826, 1974.

51. Guyton AC: Circulatory Physiology: Cardiac Output and Its Regulation. WB Saunders, Philadelphia, 1963.

52. Altman PL, Dittmer D (Eds): Respiration and Circulation. Biological Handbooks. Federation of American Societies for Experimental Biology, Bethesda, 1971.

53. Brobeck JR (Ed): Best and Taylor's Physiological Basis of Medical Practice. 10th Ed. Williams and Wilkins, Baltimore, 1979.

54. Schroeder JS, Daily EK: Techniques in Bedside Hemodynamic Monitoring. CV Mosby Company, St Louis, 1976.

55. Fegler G: Measurement of cardiac output in anesthetized animals by a thermodilution method. QJ Exp Physiol 39:153, 1954.

56. Ganz W, Swan HJC: Measurement of blood flow by thermodilution. Am J Cardiol 29:241, 1972.

57. Maruschak GF, Meathe EA, Schauble JF, et al: A simplified equation for thermal dilution cardiac output. J Appl Physiol 37:414, 1974.

58. Vandermoten P, Bernard R, de Hemptinne J, et al: Cardiac output monitoring during the acute phase of myocardial infarction: Accuracy and precision of the thermodilution method. Cardiology 62:291, 1977.

59. Hood WB Jr: Pathophysiology of ischemic heart disease. Prog Cardiovasc Dis 14:297, 1971.

60. Lassers BW, George M, Anderton JL, et al: Left ventricular failure in acute myocardial infarction. Am J Cardiol 25:511, 1970.

61. Ratshin RA, Rackley CE, Russell RO Jr: Hemodynamic evaluation of left ventricular function in shock complicating myocardial infarction. Circulation 45:127, 1972.

62. Swan HJC, Ganz W: Complications with flow-

directed balloon-tipped catheters. Ann Intern Med 91:494, 1979.

63. Swan-Ganz ® flow directed monitoring catheters specifications. Published by Edwards Laboratories, Santa Ana, California, 1977.

64. Meister SG, Engel TR, Fischer HA, et al: Potential artifact in measurement of left ventricular pressure with flow-directed catheters. Catheter CV Diagn 2:175, 1976.

65. Schaerf RHM, de Campo T, Civetta JM: Hemodynamic alterations and rapid diagnosis in a case of amniotic fluid embolus. Anesthesiology 46:155, 1977.

66. Chambers DA, Kaplan JA: Tracings of left heart failure—not mitral regurgitation. Anesthesiology 47:395, 1977.

67. Sobol S: Potential errors in bedside cardiac output determinations by the thermodilution technique. Personal communication, 1976.

68. Swan HJC, Ganz W: Guidelines for use of balloon-tipped catheters. Am J Cardiol 34:119, 1974.

69. Dane TEB, King EG: Fatal cardiac tamponade and other mechanical complications of central venous catheters. Br J Surg 62:6, 1975.

70. Borja AR, Hinshaw JR: A safe way to perform infraclavicular vein catheterization. Surg Gynecol Obstet 130:673, 1970.

71. Jernigan WR, Gardner WC, Mahr MM, et al: Use of the internal jugular vein for placement of central venous catheter. Surg Gynecol Obstet 130:520, 1970.

72. Mathieu A, Dalton B, Fischer JE, et al: Expanding aneurysm of the radial artery after frequent puncture. Anesthesiology 38:401, 1973.

73. Luck JC, Engel TF: Transient right bundle branch block with "Swan-Ganz" catheterization. Am Heart J 92:263, 1976.

74. Abernathy WS: Complete heart block caused by the Swan-Ganz catheter. Chest 65:349, 1974.

75. Katz JD, Cronan LH, Barash PG, et al: Pulmonary artery flow-guided catheters in the perioperative period. Indications and complications. JAMA 237:2832, 1977.

76. Mond HG, Clark DW, Nesbitt SJ, et al: A technique for unknotting an intracardiac flow-directed balloon catheter. Chest 67:731, 1975.

77. Golden MS, Pinder T Jr, Anderson WT, et al: Fatal pulmonary hemorrhage complicating use of a flow directed catheter in a patient receiving anticoagulant therapy. Am J Cardiol 32:865, 1973.

78. Lapin ES, Murray JA: Hemoptysis with flow-directed cardiac catheterization. JAMA 220:1246, 1972.

79. Lemen R, Jones JG: A mechanism of pulmonary artery perforation by Swan-Ganz catheters. N Engl J Med 291:260, 1974.

80. Pape LA, Haffajee CI, Markis JE, et al: Fatal pulmonary hemorrhage after use of the flow-directed balloon-tipped catheter. Ann Intern Med 90:344, 1979.

81. Greene JR Jr, Fitzwater JE, Clemmer TP: Septic endocarditis and indwelling pulmonary artery catheters. JAMA 233:891, 1975.

82. Greene JF Jr, Cummings KC: Aseptic thrombotic endocardial vegetations: A complication of indwelling pulmonary artery catheters. JAMA 225:1525, 1973.

83. Pace NL, Horton W: Indwelling pulmonary artery catheters: Their relationship to aseptic thrombotic endocardial vegetations. JAMA 233:893, 1975.

84. O'Toole JD, Wurtzbacher JJ, Wearner NE, et al: Pulmonary valve injury and insufficiency during pulmonary-artery catheterization. N Engl J Med 301:116, 1979.

85. Bentley DW, Lepper MH: Septicemia related to indwelling venous catheter. JAMA 206:1749, 1968.

86. Maki DG, Band JD: Septicemia from disposable pressure-monitoring chamber domes. Chest 74:486, 1978.

87. Schimpff SC, Miller RM, Polakavetz S, et al: Infection in the severely traumatized patient. Ann Surg 179:352, 1974.

88. Retailliau HF, Dixon RE: Letter to the editor. Heart and Lung 8:154, 1979.

89. Buxton AE, Anderson RL, Klimek J, et al: Failure of disposable domes to prevent septicemia acquired from contaminated pressure transducers. Chest 74:508, 1978.

90. Donowitz LG, Marsik FJ, Hoyt JW, et al: Serratia marcescens bacteremia from contaminated pressure transducers. JAMA 242:1749, 1979.

91. Weinstein RA, Stamm WE, Kramer L, et al: Pressure monitoring devices. Overlooked source of nosocomial infection. JAMA 236:936, 1976.

92. Walrath JM, Abbott NK, Caplan E, et al: Stopcock bacterial contamination in invasive monitoring systems. Heart and Lung 8:100, 1979.

93. Prachar H, Dittel M, Jobst C, et al: Bacterial contamination of pulmonary artery catheters. Intens Care Med 4:79, 1978.

94. Yorra FH, Oblath R, Jaffe H, et al: Massive thrombosis associated with use of the Swan-Ganz catheter. Chest 65:682, 1974.

95. Downs JB, Rackstein AD, Klein EF, et al: Hazards of radial artery catheterization. Anesthesiology 38:283, 1973.

96. Barnes RW, Foster EJ, Janssen GA, et al: Safety of brachial arterial catheters as monitors in the intensive care unit. Prospective evaluation with the Doppler ultrasonic velocity detector. Anesthesiology 44:260, 1976.

97. Gardner RM, Bond EL, Clark JS: Safety and efficacy of continuous flush systems for arterial and pulmonary artery catheters. Ann Thorac Surg 23:534, 1977.

98. Carabello B, Cohn P, Alpert JS: Hemodynamic monitoring in patients with hypotension after myocardial infarction. The role of the medical center in relation to the community hospital. Chest 74:5, 1978.

# 28 | Additional Nuclear Cardiology Techniques: Computer Applications and Evaluation of Cardiac Function in Ischemic Heart Disease

### Kathryn F. Witztum, M.D.
### William L. Ashburn, M.D.

". . . the blood in the animal body moves around in a circle continuously, and . . . the action or function of the heart is to accomplish this by pumping. *THIS IS THE ONLY REASON FOR THE MOTION AND BEAT OF THE HEART*"

> William Harvey, M.D., 1628 *

## INTRODUCTION: HISTORICAL SURVEY AND BASIC PRINCIPLES

Nuclear cardiology, in the span of a single short decade, has become one of the most dynamic and exciting areas of medicine. This recent explosion of technology and information tends to obscure the fact that, just as in any other scientific endeavor, progress in this field would not be possible without the elegant and lucid groundwork of our predecessors. This is nowhere more applicable than in the radioisotopic study of cardiac function. Accordingly, it seems both appropriate and interesting to recall a few historical events relating ischemic heart disease and nuclear medicine.

The "modern" experimental and clinical concepts of ischemic heart disease may be traced to the work of Chirac, who in 1698 first ligated a coronary artery in a dog and observed that the heart soon after ceased to beat.[1] In 1743, Morgagni and others [2-4] described ". . . a disorder of the breast marked with strong and peculiar symptoms, considerable for the kind of danger belonging to it, and not extremely rare. . . . The seat of, and sense of strangling and anxiety with which it is attended, may make it not improperly be called *angina pectoris.*"

By the early 1800s, this "new" disease entity was well recognized and established, and the possible relationship of the pain to relative myocardial ischemia had been formally proposed by Burns in 1809.[5] But even earlier, in 1793, Edward Jenner had also noted a clinical syndrome, which he termed "syncope anginosa," in his friend John Hunter, whose symptoms he documented through their progression to Hunter's death. During this period, Jenner conceived the notion that this symptom complex might be due to "ossification" or some similar occlusive disease of the coronary arteries. He was proven correct, at least anatomically, at the time of Hunter's autopsy. However, because of his reluctance to report on the case history of a close friend, his ideas were not published until after the turn of that century.[6] Subsequently, in 1842, Erichsen [7] performed the first careful experimental study on a dog heart in vivo, in which he recorded specific details of

---

* From Harvey W: DeMotu Cordis, 5th edition, 14:204, translated by Chauncey D. Leake, Charles C. Thomas, Publisher, Springfield, Illinois, 1970. (Emphasis on the last sentence by Chapter authors).

the effect of coronary ligation on heart rate, at precise time intervals from ligation to cardiac standstill. It should also be noted that the lipid infiltration and thrombogenic theories of the etiology of atherosclerosis were first propounded in this remarkable era—in 1862 by R. Virchow[8] and in 1852 by Rokitansky.[9]

Following Erickson's dog work in 1842, many similar studies[10-12] were performed; added variables such as changing intraventricular pressure, coronary venous occlusion, and ligation of differing combinations and levels of the coronary arteries were introduced. The reported results in these papers were frequently at odds. Therefore, in 1894, W. Townsend Porter, in an effort to clarify and resolve these disputes, succeeded in ligating the left anterior descending coronary artery without the accompanying veins, and made exact manometric recordings of the decreasing left ventricular systolic pressure curves.[13] Thereafter, in 1932, Orias[14] reported reduced duration of ventricular systole with ischemia; and in 1935, the classic work of Tennant and Wiggers,[15] employing myographic measurements of segment length in the dog heart, demonstrated significant abbreviation of systole in the ischemic ventricle within 14 beats after coronary artery ligation, followed by frank systolic bulging of the affected area within 60 beats.

With the ensuing increased sophistication of instrumentation and technique, the findings of those early investigators have been confirmed and expanded.[16-26] Certain important aspects of this more recent work bear mentioning:

1. In human subjects with coronary heart disease, kinetocardiograms frequently demonstrated a "disorganized pattern of contraction," for which Harrison coined the term "asynergy."[16]
2. Herman et al.[17] further characterized abnormal myocardial contractile patterns using the terms hypokinesis, asyneresis, dyskinesis, and asynchrony. They also suggested that, if sufficient focal asynergy occurred, global ventricular contractile effort would suffer, such that congestive heart failure might result.

3. Klien et al.,[18] on the basis of a theoretical model, proposed further that, if noncontracting myocardium approached 20 to 25 percent of left ventricular surface area, the extent of shortening required of the remaining functioning left ventricular muscle would begin to exceed physiologic limits, and consequently either stroke volume would fall or ventricular dilation would ensue. These events would constitute the first steps leading to congestive failure.
4. Detailed studies,[19-26] in vitro and in vivo of the mechanics of cardiac contraction under acutely ischemic (hypoxic) conditions have demonstrated the following major effects:
   a. Decreased rate of isometric force development.[19]
   b. Decreased duration of contraction.[19]
   c. Decreased magnitude of peak force.[19]
   d. Reduced regional systolic wall thickening[20] and decreased active segment shortening within 5 seconds[21-22] of coronary artery occlusion.
   e. (d) above progresses to an ejection systolic bulge by 30 seconds, and finally to a holosystolic bulge at 3 minutes after occlusion.
   f. Graded reductions in regional coronary perfusion pressure and blood flow result in precise, stepwise decrements in systolic myocardial shortening measured by the pressure-length loop method; thus, four clearly identifiable loop patterns can be related to four specific, abnormal myocardial contraction patterns: dyssynchrony, hypokinesis, akinesis, and paradoxic holosystolic expansion. These changes begin within seconds of induction of ischemia, and progress consistently to a stable state over 1 to 3 minutes; following immediate reperfusion, normal function returns in essentially the reverse order.[24]
5. The abnormal myocardial mechanics described above during acute ischemia have also been shown to be accompanied by a prompt and significant fall in left ventricular ejection fraction.[25]

6. If graded ischemia is applied sufficient to produce only minimal segmental dysfunction at rest, further degradation of segmental function will occur with exercise stress.[26]

These and other investigations provide extensive evidence that regional and global ventricular dysfunction are extremely sensitive indices of myocardial ischemia, which may be exacerbated or unmasked by exercise or other stress.

With currently available invasive and noninvasive techniques, a number of parameters reflecting the status of cardiac pump function may be measured. Among these parameters, the left ventricular ejection fraction has proved to be a very sensitive and clinically useful indicator of global ventricular performance in patients with ischemic heart disease.[27-31] Ventricular ejection fraction (EF) is defined as stroke volume (SV) divided by end-diastolic volume (EDV) where SV equals EDV minus end systolic volume (ESV). Thus, the formula is simply:

$$EF = \frac{SV}{EDV} = \frac{EDV - ESV}{EDV}$$

The combined assessment of segmental wall motion, an index of regional ventricular function (as discussed above), and EF, an index of global function, represents an important approach in the evaluation of ischemic heart disease.

Left ventricular EF (LVEF) and LV wall motion were initially evaluated by means of contrast ventriculography, using planimetry according to the method of Sandler and Dodge.[32-33] Prior to the development of the radioisotope techniques discussed in this chapter, there had been no noninvasive method to assess EF *and* wall motion in the intact human subject. The use of radioactive materials for evaluating the cardiovascular system, however, predates contrast ventriculography (which was first used clinically in the late 1950s).[34] The pioneering work of Blumgart and Weiss on the measurement of blood flow in man was published in 1927–1931 [35,36] at a time when the only radioactive substances available were the radium products. Employing the radionuclide generator

principle 35 years in advance of its current implementation,[†] they studied pulmonary transit time as a measure of pulmonary vascular volume in congestive heart failure, utilizing a cloud chamber detector and the short-lived daughter products of the radium kept for treatment of various cancers.

Thereafter, further significant advances in nuclear cardiology did not occur until "radiocardiography" was introduced by Prinzmetal, et al., in 1948. In this new approach, scintillation probes (with sodium iodide crystals) were positioned over the precordium and used to study blood flow through the cardiac chambers in human beings.[38] More quantitative approaches and the basic concept of the radionuclide ejection fraction by probe techniques were advanced in 1962 by Donato [39] and Folse et al.[40] However, it was not until the development and refinement of the Anger scintillation camera [41,42] and the appropriate short-lived radioisotopes [43,44] that nuclear cardiology began to reach toward its full potential. Thus, radioisotope scintiphotography of a dynamic series of events made it possible to view the passage of a radiotracer bolus through the central venous and arterial circulations.[45-46] By interfacing a videorecording system to an Anger camera, Ashburn, Mason and Mullins [47-49] determined ventricular volume by this "first-pass" radioisotope-angiography method. Subsequently, Zaret and Strauss et al.[50-52] combined first-pass and gated equilibrium techniques to determine ventricular volumes, ejection fraction, and ventricular wall motion by planimetry, and reported good correlation with contrast ventriculography.

In 1972–73, Secker-Walker and associates [53-54] extended the gated equilibrium technique to the minidigital computer. Based on the assumption that, with complete mixing, the number of counts obtained in the end-diastolic and end-systolic images were proportional to blood volumes (given constant acquisition time

---

† The first modern generator-produced nuclide, $^{132}$I, obtained from $^{132}$Te, was used in 1962 for functional studies of the thyroid [37]. See Chapter 12 for discussion of the generator principle.

for each image), it was possible to calculate the LVEF from count information alone, thus avoiding planimetry; again correlation with contrast ventriculography was good. This conceptional advance was also extended with good results to computer analysis of first-pass time activity curves, as reported by Schelbert, et al.[55] With the introduction of computer technology into nuclear cardiology, recent advances in this area, paralleling rapid instrumentation development, have come with exponential frequency. The new concepts and clinical potential of radionuclide angiography are exciting and far-reaching; it is a field whose time has come.

We have suggested, at the beginning of Chapter 12 of this text, that one must have an understanding of the technology of nuclear cardiology in order to appreciate the application of these tests and the implications of their results. This is perhaps most important in the approach to nuclear medicine methods for functional evaluation of the heart. The fundamentals of nuclear physics, scintillation imaging and general instrumentation, counting statistics, and radiopharmaceuticals have been discussed in Chapter 12. In this chapter we will present:

1. an overview of computer methodology and terminology, as applicable to rest and stress nuclear cardiac function studies; 2. an explanation of how computers interact with cameras and physiologic synchronizers; 3. a description of radiopharmaceutical options; 4. an outline of general quality control for nuclear cardiology procedures; 5. a short résumé of general applications of radionuclide angiography in various clinical settings; and 6. a survey of the literature regarding the current use of radionuclide techniques in the assessment and care of acute myocardial infarction patients.

## DIGITAL COMPUTER METHODS AND VOCABULARY

### Historical Background

A glance at the etymology of the word "compute" (from which "computer" derives), is almost like tracing the history of the origin of the computer. Note the following, as taken from a standard Webster's Collegiate Dictionary:

1. *compute:* to determine by calculation; to reckon (from the Latin word *computare,* meaning "to reckon or think").
2. *reckon:* to count; or to name one by one, or by groups, so as to ascertain the whole number of units in a collection; to number (from the Anglo-Saxon word *gerecenian,* meaning "to explain").
3. *calculate:* to determine by mathematical processes (from the Latin word *calculus,* which was a "stone" used in reckoning; Latin *calcis,* or "limestone").
4. *mathematics:* the science of the exact relations existing between quantities and operations; and the methods by which (according to these rules or relations) an unknown quantity may be learned from other known or assumed quantities (from the Latin word *mathemata,* meaning "things learned").

We may imagine, then, that when prehistoric man began to "think," to communicate with his fellows, and to try "to explain" his thoughts to others, the need to "count or reckon" things arose. This probably occurred when he began keeping flocks or growing his own crops, and it is likely that the first things he used in order to "keep tally" of his counting were small stones. Probably much later, it occurred to him that his fingers and toes could stand in place of stones, at least to a total count of 20 "domestic" animals! (Hence, the origin of the word *digital,* from the Latin word *digitus,* meaning a finger or toe; *digit* still means a finger or toe, but also a *number.*) Or perhaps fingers and toes came *before* stones in this ancient counting system; but the stone idea was eventually translated into what might be considered the first "computer"—the ancient Chinese abacus, which is still used today. The abacus, consisting of beads (or fancy "stones") strung on a series of parallel vertical rods, may be used to perform very complicated calculations by moving the beads along the rods into specified groups and positions.

The invention of the first mechanical adding machine is attributed to Pascal, who in the early seventeenth century developed a "modern" version of the abacus, consisting of wheels labeled with the numbers 0 through 9, and a handcrank for turning the wheels in proper sequence.[56] Subsequently, in the nineteenth century, an English mathematician, Charles Babbage, conceived the notion of "programming" weaving machines using holes punched in cardboard cards, so that no human operator would be needed. Because his plan required many elaborate moving parts, the new technology of the time could not meet the demands of his design, and his "computerized weaver" was not yet feasible. However, his concepts were essentially sound, and he is therefore credited with establishing the basic principles from which modern computers evolved.[56]

The development of current computer technology began in the 1950s after the invention of the vacuum tube. Vacuum tubes permitted much faster operations than mechanical devices but were unreliable and more often "down" than working. However, transistors, which became available in the early 1960s, proved reliable, conserved power, and were smaller and cheaper. With this innovation, computer capacity increased while costs decreased; and with the advent of integrated circuit technology, dedicated minicomputers became cost-effective and more generally available. Further recent refinements have produced microprocessors, in which the circuitry of a minicomputer has been reduced to the size of a small silicon wafer, or "chip," which may cost as little as a few dollars. Thus, computer applications have become extensive in many fields, among them nuclear medicine.

While most of us are impressed, and often overwhelmed, by the pervasiveness of computers in almost every aspect of our lives, it is well to remember that a computer is virtually useless without being programmed to perform a task; *human* ingenuity is necessary to *define* the "problem," conceptualize an approach to the solution, and then write the programs that instruct the computer as to what operations need to be performed in order to produce an "answer." Furthermore, even after a computer has been programmed appropriately, it is still not invulnerable to "operator error." In prosaic terms, *the computer is only as smart as the opera-*

*tor using it!* Since a very important part of nuclear cardiology—i.e., radionuclide angiography—is in large part dependent on the "answers" generated by a variety of computer systems and programs now in broad use, it is important to have a basic understanding of what these systems are and how they work. This is becoming true not only for physicians who perform and interpret these procedures, but also for those who request such studies for their patients. To this end, we have directed this part of the chapter.

## General Configuration of Computers

A computer or *central processing unit (CPU)* may be thought of as being organized in five major divisions, as shown schematically in Figure 28.1: (1) the control unit; (2) the memory unit; (3) the arithmetic and logic unit (ALU); (4) the input unit; and (5) the output unit. The latter two units are sometimes the same device, or separate devices, and are generally lumped under the heading of input/output *(I/O)* devices. All information passing to or from the CPU is transmitted by these devices, which include a wide variety of mechanisms such as those listed in Table 28.1.

The *ALU* is the powerful part of the computer that is capable of performing all mathematical functions as well as many other specialized manipulations, each in a matter of $\mu$sec (millionths of a second). The internal speed with

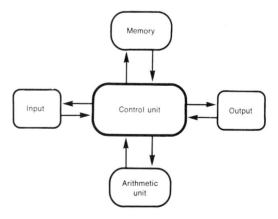

Fig. 28.1 General organization of the five divisions of a small computer. (Lieberman, DE: Computer Methods. C.V. Mosby Co., St. Louis, Mo., 1977.)

**Table 28.1  Typical I/O Devices for Computer Systems**

| Input Devices | Output Devices |
| --- | --- |
| 1. Terminal keyboards | 1. Terminal printer |
| 2. Punch card reader | 2. Punch card punch |
| 3. Paper tape reader | 3. Paper tape punch |
| 4. Toggle switches | 4. Digital plotter |
| 5. Lightpen | 5. Line printer |
| 6. Joystick | 6. Display screen |

which mathematical operations are performed is due to the use of *registers* or *accumulators,* which are separate from and much faster than direct use of *memory* for such functions. The *memory* contains thousands of programmable cells or *bits,* in which are stored data and/or instructions to direct the computer activity. The memory is divided into discrete locations or *words,* which are composed of a specific number of bits, depending on the particular computer. Many *nuclear medicine* computers are based on a *16-bit word;* other computers may have 8, 12, 18, 32 or even more bits per word. This is determined by the demands placed on the system from the specific discipline(s) for which it is designed. Another commonly used term in describing the divisions of computer memory is the *byte,* consisting of *8 bits,* or one-half word in a 16-bit-word computer. The modern prototype of memory is *core memory,* so called because each memory bit consists of a magnetizable "core" or ring, through the center of which pass wires potentially capable of carrying current (see Fig. 28.2). When electrical current passes through these wires, an electromagnetic field is induced, which magnetizes the core ring; with *no* current, the core is demagnetized. This

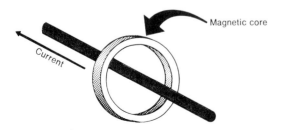

Fig. 28.2  Representation of core memory structure. (Lieberman DE: Computer Methods. C.V. Mosby Co., St. Louis, Mo., 1977.)

situation is analogous to an "on/off" switch (which is an "either/or," all-or-none phenomenon), and is of primary importance in understanding the *binary language* of digital computers (to be discussed below). (An alternative to core memory is semiconductor memory, which is generally cheaper and faster than core.) The *controller (control unit)* directs the flow of data to and from other parts of the CPU, by means of following specific instructions (programs) supplied by the manufacturer (or the operator), which may be called from memory to allow the performance of any of the available operations.

In addition to the CPU and I/O devices described above, nuclear medicine computer systems also usually include the following: 1. some sort of bulk storage device for saving image data (such as rigid or floppy disks, multiplatter disk systems, magnetic tape, and occasionally videorecorders); 2. one or more display devices (such as CRTs or TV monitors); 3. a device for interfacing the imaging system (usually a gamma camera) to the CPU. (Such a system is shown in Fig. 28.3.) The signals originating from the gamma camera are *analog* in nature. Thus, voltage changes as a function of time and may assume any shape, ranging from a typical sine wave pattern to a waveform which may have no characteristic shape (more often the latter). By contrast, *digital* signals must behave such that the voltage at any given instant may assume *only* one of two values, with the transition time between values being extremely small (nanoseconds)—i.e., a digital signal appears as a "square wave." It is apparent that the interface between the camera and the computer would be termed an *analog to digital converter (ADC)*.

In general, ADCs are of two types: *ramp ADCs* and *successive approximation ADCs.* The latter has more complex circuitry but is also much faster, and is therefore required to avoid computer dead-time limitations which would impose count-rate limitations *exceeding* the camera count-rate limitations (and which would, therefore, be undesirable). To further protect against computer dead-time losses, especially in first-pass studies, some ADCs are analog buffered by means of a *derandomizing sam-*

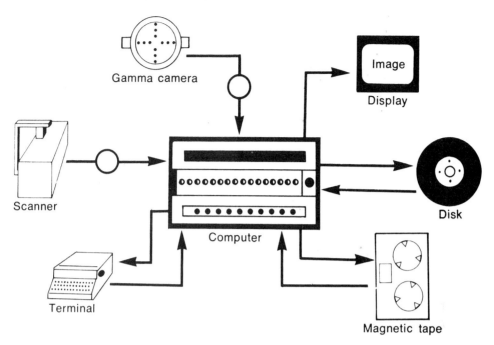

Fig. 28.3  Schematic diagram of the configuration of a typical nuclear medicine computer system. (Lieberman DE: Computer Methods. C.V. Mosby Co., St. Louis, Mo., 1977.)

*ple and hold circuit* interposed between the camera and the ADC, which allows for recording of bursts of data occurring at a rate that would be too fast for the typical ADC. (For further discussion of ADCs, the reader is referred to the text on digital nuclear medicine by Lieberman,[56] and the monograph on data processing in nuclear cardiology by Bachrach et al.,[57] listed in the Reference section.) In addition to *speed*, ADCs are also characterized by *accuracy*, which is related to the number of bits per word that the ADCs use to digitize the camera signals (x and y). The number of bits per word utilized by the ADCs to encode the x and y signals from the camera directly determine the maximum possible matrix size of the *computer* image. The accuracy of the ADCs and, therefore, the potential matrix size for images, should be at least twice the resolution capability of the camera. However, accuracy and speed in ADCs are usually inversely related. Thus, the particular combination of resolution and speed required by the camera determines the type and cost of the ADCs required for the computer; the overall performance of the system is obviously highly interrelated.

All the above-discussed components of a computer system are termed, in the jargon of the trade, *hardware,* which are the physical pieces of equipment which "can be seen, touched or broken!"[56] *Software* refers to the programs which may be entered into the memory to control the computer. The earliest data-analysis systems in nuclear medicine used pre-programmed circuits (known as "hard-wired" computers) instead of true computers; these systems are usually limited and inflexible, but simple to operate by push button, with minimal operator interaction. In our opinion, a flexible, programmable computer system (such as described in some detail above) is preferable, not only because it is vastly more versatile for general use, but also because we believe that human judgment must be allowed to interact with sophisticated technology in order to achieve the best clinical results.

## The Binary Number System

In order to comprehend the nature of digital computer image matrices and the limitations of these systems, a passing knowledge of "machine language," or binary numbers, is necessary. As was implied earlier, the electrical encoding of information into computer memory resembles an "either-or"/"on-off" switch and, therefore, the choice of conditions is *binary.* The binary number system is based on two basic premises:

1. Numbers may be formed using *only the two* digits *1* or *0* (i.e., "on" or "off").
2. These two digits may only be raised to powers of 2 (i.e., $n \times 2^0$, $n \times 2^1$, $n \times 2^2$, etc., where n may only assume values of 0 or 1).

These principles are illustrated in Table 28.2. It may be seen from this table that the power of *two* to which a particular binary digit is raised is related to the position of that digit with respect to an imaginary decimal (which would be located at the far right-hand side of the string of binary digits). Thus, a digit *adjacent* to the "decimal" is considered *zero distance* from the decimal and is, therefore, multiplied by $2^0$, whereas a digit in the *third* position from the decimal is considered *two places* removed from the zero position and so is raised to $2^2$. It is also apparent that, if the binary digit is zero, the decimal equivalent of that number position is always zero, no matter the location, since zero times anything (including any $2^n$) is always zero. Therefore, one need really only calculate the decimal values of all the binary positions containing the digit *one,* add up the total decimal value, and that is the decimal equivalent of the binary string of digits. Therefore, if we add up the decimal value of a string of *16* binary digits, all containing ones, which would be $(1 \times 2^0) + (1 \times 2^1) + (1 \times 2^2) + \ldots (1 \times 2^{15})$, the total is 65,279—while a similar operation on a string of *8* binary digits (all ones) yields 255. The importance of these two numbers will become apparent in the following discussion of computer acquisition matrices for nuclear images.

## Computer Matrices: Static and Dynamic Digital Nuclear Imaging

In our survey of static myocardial imaging in Chapter 12, we did not attempt to discuss the various computer processing methods which have been advocated. These range from various background subtraction, contrast enhancement, and cinematic or tomographic methods for thallium imaging;[58-60, 65-68] to myocardial count-rate analysis by histogram, threshold, or circumferential profile routines;[61-64] to suppression of unwanted anatomical structures or infarct sizing in pyrophosphate imaging.[69,70] While these or other data processing methods for static imaging may have real merit (see future directions to be discussed later), at the present time, these techniques appear to require broader application and validation before definitive statements may be made as to their clinical utility. However, the general concepts of static digital nuclear imaging bear examining, because they relate also to methods of dynamic data acquisition.

The most common mode of static digital image recording is the *frame* or *histogram* mode, as illustrated in Figure 28.4. In this method, the digital picture is "built-up" in the computer memory as follows: A part of the computer memory is organized as an x, y grid or "matrix" of digital numbers called "pixels" (contraction of "picture elements"). For illustration purposes, we may imagine that this grid (whatever its x, y dimensions in pixels) is superimposed on the face of the camera crystal, such that x max = y max = the diameter of the crystal face. A photon interacting with the crystal produces, by way of the camera electronics (see Ch. 12), analog signals representing the x and y coordinates of that event on the crystal surface. It is an easy concept, then, to see that these analog x, y signals may be converted by the ADCs to digital x, y signals corresponding to the same x, y coordinates (or "address") in the computer matrix. Therefore, each time the z-signal from one of these scintillation events passes the pulse-height analysis test, the appropriate pixel in the computer matrix is incremented by exactly one count. Subsequent events may increment the same address, or any other matrix address, such that, by totaling the number of events in each pixel, a digital map of the image is generated. This "map" may be visually represented in a print-out of the *decimal values* of each pixel (even though the

**Table 28.2  Principles Governing the Binary vs. the Decimal Number System**

| Standard Decimal Number | 0 | 1 | 2 | 3 | 4 | 5 | 6 | 7 | 8 | 9 | 10 |
|---|---|---|---|---|---|---|---|---|---|---|---|
| Binary Equivalent | 0 | 1 | 10 | 11 | 100 | 101 | 110 | 111 | 1000 | 1001 | 1010 |
| Binary to Decimal Conversion | $0 \times 2^0 = 0$ | $1 \times 2^0$ | $0 \times 2^0 = 0$<br>$1 \times 2^1 = 2$ | $1 \times 2^0 = 1$<br>$1 \times 2^1 = 2$ | $0 \times 2^0 = 0$<br>$0 \times 2^1 = 0$<br>$1 \times 2^2 = 4$ | $1 \times 2^0 = 1$<br>$0 \times 2^1 = 0$<br>$1 \times 2^2 = 4$ | $0 \times 2^0 = 0$<br>$1 \times 2^1 = 2$<br>$1 \times 2^2 = 4$ | $1 \times 2^0 = 1$<br>$1 \times 2^1 = 2$<br>$1 \times 2^2 = 4$ | $0 \times 2^0 = 0$<br>$0 \times 2^1 = 0$<br>$0 \times 2^2 = 0$<br>$1 \times 2^3 = 8$ | $1 \times 2^0 = 1$<br>$0 \times 2^1 = 0$<br>$0 \times 2^2 = 0$<br>$1 \times 2^3 = 8$ | $0 \times 2^0 = 0$<br>$1 \times 2^1 = 2$<br>$0 \times 2^2 = 0$<br>$1 \times 2^3 = 8$ |
| | $=0$ | $=1$ | $=2$ | $=3$ | $=4$ | $=5$ | $=6$ | $=7$ | $=8$ | $=9$ | $=10$ |

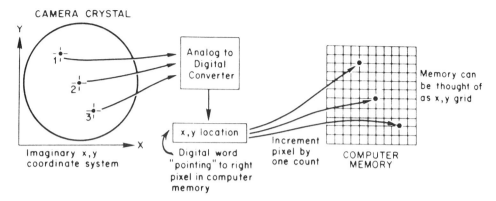

Fig. 28.4 Schematic representation of digital data acquisition in the histogram or frame mode. Each acceptable event is routed from the camera electronics to the computer storage location corresponding to the x, y location of that event within the camera crystal. A specified area in computer memory is thus created which is a 1:1 matrix map of the crystal face. (Lewis et al: Physics and instrumentation. In Clinical Nuclear Cardiology, Parkey et al, eds., Appleton-Century-Crofts, 1979. Used by permission.)

actual count information in each pixel is coded in *binary* numbers); or, the map may be displayed as a digital image on a video device, in which the count information is displayed as shades of a gray or color scale. Each binary digit in a pixel requires one bit; in a 16-bit-word computer, possible matrix sizes would be as shown in Table 28.3, depending on the amount of memory available. Byte mode versus word mode acquisition may be conceptualized as shown in Figure 28.5. Note that in byte mode acquisition, twice as many *images* may be stored for the same number of memory words, as compared to word mode. However, in byte mode, since only eight bits per pixel are available for encoding count information, byte mode images may have a maximum count per pixel of 255 counts (see binary numbers discussed earlier), before pixel overflow would occur; while in word mode images, with 16 bits per pixel, over 65,000 counts per pixel may be registered before pixel overflow occurs. Thus, byte mode acquisition is ideal for dynamic frame mode studies in which rapid sequence images with relatively low count rate statistics will suffice (such as brain dynamic studies) and, therefore, will require half the space on the bulk storage unit (e.g., disk) as compared to word mode. For high count rate statistics, whether for static or dynamic images, word mode acquisition is usually required, and the size of the matrix and number of frames are then limited by the

amount of memory and bulk storage available. These two types of *frame* mode dynamic acquisition are frequently encountered in nuclear angiography studies. For static acquisition, 128 × 128 matrices are generally the minimal requirement for current camera resolution capability.[71]

The second type of digital data storage is *list* or *serial mode* acquisition. In its simplest form, this method may be thought of as simply a *direct transfer* of x, y coordinates from the camera crystal face into computer memory (or

**Table 28.3  Common Matrix Sizes for Digital Nuclear Imaging**

| Matrix Mode | Number of Pixels in Matrix | Number of Memory Words Required |
|---|---|---|
| 32 × 32 byte | 1,024 | 512 |
| 32 × 32 word | 1,024 | 1,024 |
| 64 × 64 word | 4,096 | 4,096 |
| 64 × 64 byte | 4,096 | 2,048 |
| 128 × 128 word | 16,384 | 16,384 |
| 128 × 128 byte | 16,384 | 8,192 |
| 256 × 256 word | 65,536 | 65,536 |
| 256 × 256 byte | 65,536 | 32,768 |

(From Lieberman DE: Computer Methods, The Fundamentals of Digital Nuclear Medicine, C. V. Mosby Company, St. Louis, 1977, p. 55. Courtesy of C. V. Mosby Company.)

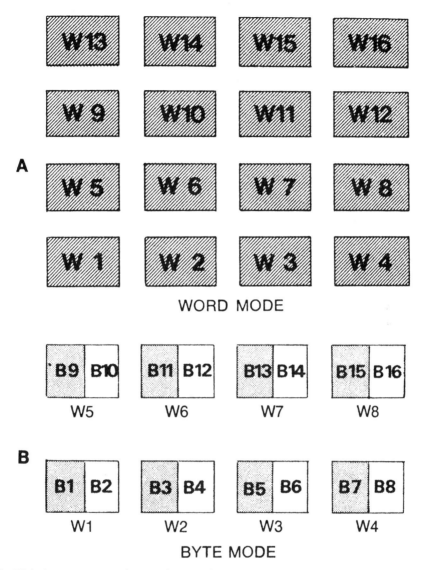

WORD MODE

BYTE MODE

Fig. 28.5   Digital computer matrix organization. *(A)* Matrix elements stored as full words. *(B)* Matrix elements stored as half-words or bytes. (Note that byte mode storage holds twice as many images for the same number of memory words.) (Lieberman DE: Computer Methods. C.V. Mosby Co., St. Louis, Mo., 1977.)

onto disk or tape), in the *sequential order* in which the events occurred, without any effort at constructing image matrices at the time of acquisition. In a somewhat more complex form of list mode data, other types of data may be inserted into the list of x, y addresses, such as clock time markers (or physiologic trigger markers). This method is illustrated in Figure 28.6. This type of data can be formatted a posteriori into digital image matrices, as described above. The advantages and disadvantages of these two acquisition modes for nuclear cardiology studies will be discussed in the context of clinical applications.

### Further Hardware and Software Considerations

A few additional points regarding the "mechanics" of the nuclear medicine computer sys-

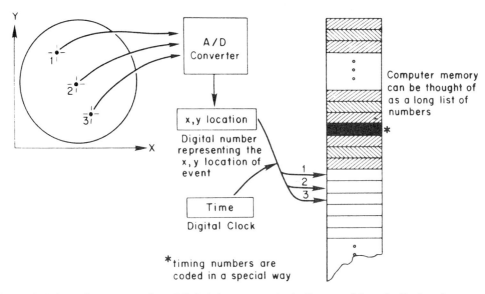

Fig. 28.6 Schematic representation of digital data storage in the list or serial mode. Rather than accumulating the count data in the form of a picture in computer memory, the x, y location of each acceptable event is stored *as it occurs* in the next available spot on either disk or magnetic tape, along with coded timing markers. Images are produced after the fact: A desired time interval is selected, then, a matrix map for histogram data is created by using the list of events from disk or tape as the input data (instead of using events directly from the camera). (Lewis et al: Physics and Instrumentation. In Clinical Nuclear Cardiology, Parkey et al, Appleton-Century-Crofts, 1979. Used by permission.)

tem should be briefly mentioned as desirable features:

**Basic software supplied by the manufacturer.** In short, with the multiplicity of minicomputer systems currently being marketed, there should be available with almost any system virtually all the necessary programs for acquiring and processing the various dynamic and static studies now commonly employed in nuclear medicine, including: smoothing, contrast enhancement, and other image manipulations; profile selection; and dynamic curve generation, display, and manipulation. Each system should come with adequate documentation and system-user prompts for ease of use. (Acceptable exceptions might be those systems which are designed solely for nuclear cardiology studies, and which are frequently incorporated as part of a mobile camera unit.)

**Hardware zoom.** This is a feature of the ADCs which allows for higher digital resolution without decreasing the framing rate, by means of amplification of the x, y analog signals. (For further technical explanation, see discussion presented in reference 57.) The essence of this feature is in effect to "magnify" a *portion* of the camera's field of view, so that a smaller matrix array size will have equivalent pixel resolution to that of the original full field resolution, while at the same time requiring *less memory* for digitization than the full field. This principle is demonstrated in Figure 28.7. A further useful feature is analog offset controls, which allow the zoomed area to become any portion of the camera's field of view, rather than only a central portion.

**Display requirements.**
1. Capability of displaying relatively low-resolution images (e.g., 32 × 32 or 64 × 64 dynamic acquisition) as visually acceptable images.
2. Flicker-free movie format and multiple static image display.
3. Between 32 and 256 shades of gray.
4. Interpolation, if needed, must be "on-the-fly" hardware interpolation.
5. "Gray-scale look-up table," for easy adjustment of gray-scale translation table.

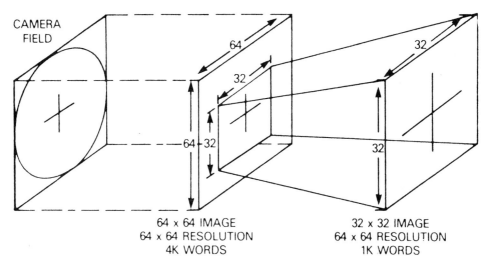

CAMERA
FIELD

64 x 64 IMAGE
64 x 64 RESOLUTION
4K WORDS

32 x 32 IMAGE
64 x 64 RESOLUTION
1K WORDS

Fig. 28.7   Schematic illustration of the principle of hardware "zoom." The field of view of the camera shown on the left has been digitized in a 64 × 64 array of pixels (also called a "4K" array, since 64 × 64 = 4096). The zoom feature allows a portion of this array (in this case, a 32 × 32 or 1K portion), to be magnified up to the same physical size as the original 64 × 64 array. The spatial resolution in the 32 × 32 array is the same as in the 64 × 64 array; however, storage of a 1K array rather than the 4K array takes only ¼ as much memory space, with no loss in resolution. (Bachrach et al: Seminars In Nuclear Medicine IX:257, Oct. 1979. Used by permission.)

(For more detail on display requirements, see References 56 and 57.)

**Region-of-interest (ROI) selection options.** Lightpen, joystick, automatic.

**Additional options.** Useful when *programming* capability is desired are higher-level language compilers (such as for Fortran and Basic); hardware multiply and divide and hardware floating point for greater speed of repetitive processing. These are also important in expediting filtering routines for data processing.

## CLINICAL TECHNIQUES IN RADIONUCLIDE ANGIOGRAPHY

There are two general categories of radionuclide techniques commonly employed for assessment of ventricular performance: "first-pass" and "equilibrium" methods. This terminology refers to the status of the radiopharmaceutical during the study, which is inherent to each technique. Both methods are currently implemented with some kind of computer-assisted analysis to measure various indices of cardiac performance.

### First-Pass Technique

First-pass studies typically consist of rapid-sequence recording of the passage of a bolus of radioactivity through the right and left sides of the heart. Suppose the heart were simply a two-sided, nonpulsatile viscus, with the two sides in series and the lungs interposed between. Recording of this transit of a tight, small bolus of radioactivity through the two sides would be expected to produce a two-phase, but otherwise rather ordinary, time-activity curve (time on the abscissa, activity, or count rate on the ordinate), much like a "two-humped" version of the dynamic curves ordinarily obtained with rapid imaging of any vascular structure, such as kidney or brain (Figure 28.8*A*). Considering activity as the count rate perceived by the detector at a given point in time, then the curve peaks when maximum activity (or count rate) is present within the organ "viewed" by the detector—that is, when most of the bolus is present within the organ. Because the transit time through the pulmonary circulation is normally short, the two humps of the curve (representing right and left heart, in temporal sequence) actually would superimpose somewhat

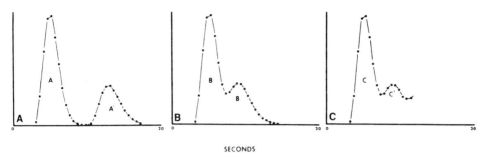

SECONDS

Fig. 28.8  First-pass time-activity curves, low framing rate. *(A)* Time-activity curve produced by passage of a bolus of activity through the two chambers of a hypothetical hollow, nonpulsating viscus; the two chambers are in series with regard to passage of the bolus, but both are in the field of view of the detector, while the connecting line between the chambers may be thought of as being primarily out of the detector field of view. With a connection line of capacity larger than the bolus volume, the two chambers will appear as two discrete activity "humps" on the curve, as shown by A and A'. (We assume the activity drains away from the system after A', so no subsequent transits occur.) *(B)* If the connecting volume between the two chambers is made smaller than the volume of the bolus (the remainder of the system being unchanged), the second chamber's activity hump becomes partially superimposed on the first (as in B and B'). *(C)* If the activity is no longer drained out, but is allowed to recirculate (as in the real case), the curves in B take on the appearance of C and C'. (Adapted from Parker and Treves: Radionuclide Studies of Cardiac Shunts. In Holman et al: Principles of Cardiovascular Nuclear Medicine, Grune & Stratton, New York, 1978. Used by permission.)

on each other, as shown in Figure 28.8*B*. Let us assume that our radioactive tracer will remain in the blood pool; since we are dealing with a closed-return system (the peripheral circulation) in this theoretical model, recirculation of the initial bolus would ultimately occur, producing curves such as those shown in Figure 28.8*C*. In point of fact, with a sufficiently slow image-framing rate, such as two frames per second, a normal pulmonary dilution curve very much like that shown in Figure 28.8*C* is actually obtained; and when these curves are fit with a least-squares gamma variate function, this method may be very successfully used in detection and quantification of left-to-right intra- or extracardiac shunts.[72]

Now let us impose on the above "theoretical" model the following conditions and assumptions:

1. The two-sided hollow viscus is actually pulsatile at a rate of about 60 cycles per minute.
2. We will record our time-activity data at a much more rapid rate, such as 25 data points per second (which would be 25 data points per cycle with the above heart rate).
3. The radioactive bolus is still small and tight, but is also homogeneously mixed with blood

as it enters the right side of our "pulsating hollow viscus."

Under the above-described conditions, the resulting time-activity curves for the first transit of tracer through the right and left ventricles would be expected to appear as shown in Figure 28.9. In this case, the general form of the two-phase curve is maintained as before, but superimposed on this are the multiple oscillations in count rate resulting from the chamber pulsations. With adequate mixing of tracer and blood, it may be assumed that count rate at any given point in time is proportional to chamber volume and, therefore, that changes in count rate (as reflected in the "peaks" and "valleys" of the multiple oscillations) are proportional to change in volume (or stroke volume) for the chamber in question. It is apparent, then, that from such data one may calculate ejection fraction (EF) values for multiple beats from the right and left ventricle(s) (RV and LV), which may be averaged to obtain the global RVEF and LVEF for the sample time interval.

Certain aspects of the first-pass method, which we have described in very general terms above, should be further considered:

1. A data sampling rate of at least 25 times

per second has been found optimum for first-pass determination of ventricular ejection fraction.[73]

2. When these rapid sequence count data are acquired with a scintillation imaging device, there are two schools of thought regarding the best position of the camera in relation to the patient (although, in theory, first-pass studies may be performed in any view.):

    a. The 20 to 30° right anterior oblique projection (RAO) is preferred by some, as it appears to provide the best separation of ventricles both from the atria and from the aortic and pulmonic outflow tracts[74] (see Fig. 28.10).

    b. Others feel the straight anterior view provides adequate anatomical separation of structures in conjunction with the *temporal* separation of right and left sides of the heart which is inherent in the method, while at the same time placing the heart closer to the detector (camera) face for greater counting efficiency.[75]

    c. Regardless of which view is chosen, serial studies should be performed in the same position for best reproducibility of results.[75]

3. Good bolus injection technique is of critical importance, as discussed elsewhere.[74,75] We prefer using a 19- to 20-gauge, 1 ½-inch indwelling polyethylene catheter inserted into a large right medial antecubital vein. The catheter is attached to an extension tubing of less than 3 ml volume, into which the bolus (of less than 1 ml volume) is loaded, for rapid-flush injection with 10 to 20 ml of saline.

4. A number of imaging and nonimaging devices may be used for acquiring first-pass data, including current single crystal gamma cameras, multicrystal scintillation cameras, or nonimaging probes.[74-76,82] The primary requirements of the device chosen are that the system provide adequate temporal and spatial resolution with acceptable counting statistics. The best combination of these factors for first-pass studies appears to be provided by the multicrystal cameras. There is an inherent statistical uncertainty produced by the more limited peak-count rates (in the range of 30,000 to 60,000 counts per second) achieved with the standard gamma camera (beyond which camera dead-time losses intervene); however, this may be reduced by means of curve processing with one of several mathematical techniques, as discussed by Ashburn et al.[74]

5. Computer storage of these data is usually accomplished either in list mode (for single- *or* multicrystal cameras) or rapid-frame byte mode (for single-crystal cameras), since the

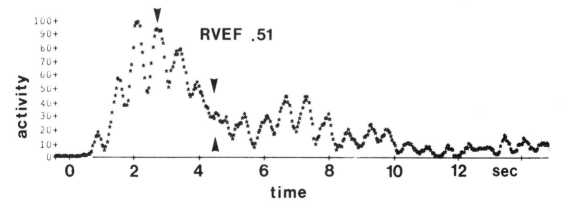

Fig. 28.9 First-pass time activity curves, rapid framing rate. The general shape of a "two-humped" curve is retained, as in Figure 28.8C; however, in a pulsating system (i.e., the heart), the changing count rate in the chambers due to contraction and relaxation are shown as fluctuations in activity level, superimposed on the general curve form (as shown). The left hump is produced as the bolus of activity passes through the right ventricle; the right hump represents transit through the left ventricle. Ejection fraction may be calculated from the fluctuations on each half of the curve (see text). RVEF, calculated by averaging the three beats shown between the upper arrows, is 0.51.

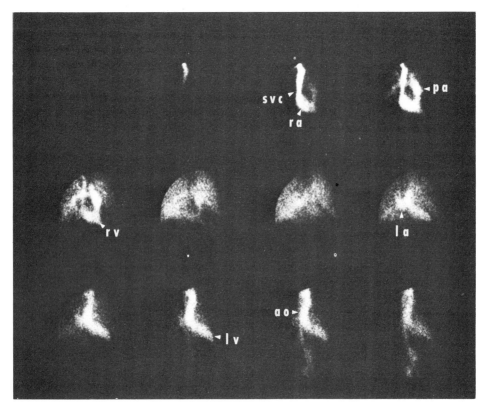

Fig. 28.10 First-pass radionuclide angiogram performed in the 20 to 30° right anterior oblique view with good intravenous bolus injection technique of 20 mCi of Tc-99m-pertechnetate. Sequential 2-sec images, shown from upper left to right, allow clear identification of the superior vena cava (svc), right atrium (ra), right ventricle (rv), pulmonary artery (pa), left atrium (la), left ventricle (lv), and ascending aorta (ao).

number of counts per pixel per image at 25 frames per second is relatively low. A series of summed frames sufficient to demonstrate discrete right and left heart anatomy are used to allow for computer-lightpen or joystick assignment of regions of interest for right and left ventricles and an appropriate background area (see discussion of choices of background assignment in Berger et al.[75]). These regions of interest (ROIs) are used like a template or window to be passed through the raw data to generate the time-activity curves, so that only those parts of the raw data "seen" by the ROI are allowed to contribute to the data points; and the raw data for each chamber is analyzed only for that part of the acquisition time when activity is in that chamber. Typical ROIs generated on digitized, summed LV and RV images from a single crystal camera are shown in Figure 28.11.

6. Calculation of ejection fraction is performed by averaging several beats at the peak of the background-corrected ventricular time-activity curves for the right and left ventricles (as shown in Fig. 28.12 for LVEF). Comparison of results from this technique to LVEF by biplane contrast ventriculography shows good agreement (r = from 0.87 to 0.95), and excellent intra- and interobserver reproducibilities in the hands of numerous investigators (see further references as given by Ashburn et al. and Berger et al.).[74,75]

7. Virtually any [99m]Tc-labeled radiopharmaceutical may be used as a first-pass agent. However, if sequential studies are desired, an agent which is cleared rapidly from the blood, such as [99m]Tc-sulfur colloid (cleared by liver) or

⁹⁹ᵐTc-DTPA (cleared by kidneys) is preferred. If the first-pass study is to be performed in conjunction with an equilibrium study, any of the standard blood pool imaging agents may be used initially as the first-pass agent, provided good bolus technique is used.

## Gated Equilibrium Techniques

In the above description of current first-pass techniques, it is apparent that, although a number of beats may be averaged for EF determination, the essence of the method is that it permits beat-to-beat analysis of high-frequency information by means of very short-duration, high-frequency recording (with certain statistical limitations imposed by the use of a standard, single-crystal gamma camera). Gated equilibrium studies, on the other hand, differ fundamentally from first-pass methods, in that gated studies actively combine many cardiac cycles during the acquisition period (which may extend over several minutes), so that *all* measurements resulting from such studies are by definition *average* parameters from the time period included during the study. Thus, some of the high-frequency information may be sacrificed, but much greater statistical certainty results.

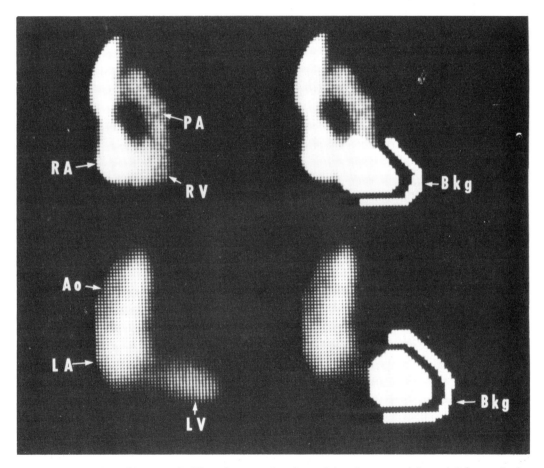

Fig. 28.11 Region-of-interest (ROI) assignment for determining first-pass right and left ventricular ejection fractions. Summed images in 64 × 64 digital matrices show right heart *(top left)* and left heart *(bottom left)* anatomical features. In the images shown on the right, a computer light pen has been used to flag right ventricular and background (bkg) ROIs *(top right),* and left ventricular and bkg ROIs *(bottom right).* The ROIs are subsequently used to generate time-activity curves (see text) for beat-to-beat analysis. (PA = pulmonary artery; RA = right atrium; RV = right ventricle; Ao = ascending aorta; LA = left atrium; LV = left ventricle.)

LEFT VENTRICULAR TIME-ACTIVITY CURVE

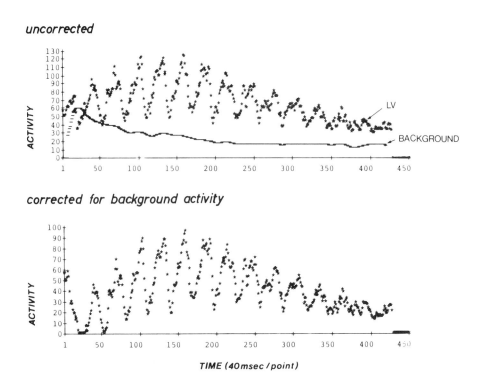

Fig. 28.12  Time-activity curves produced from ROIs for the left ventricle (LV) and background with first-pass data. The upper panel shows the unsmoothed LV curve, and the background curve which has been 5-point smoothed. The lower panel shows the background-corrected LV curve, which may be used for calculation of LVEF.

The simplest form of a gated blood-pool study is to record only two views of the heart—one at end-diastole and one at end-systole, as determined by interfacing the electrocardiogram to the imaging device for use as a "triggering" mechanism. In this manner, the ECG "gates" the camera, so that it is allowed to accumulate counts only during a short "time-window" at the end of diastole (corresponding to the early part of ventricular depolarization, or the peak of the R wave on the ECG), and for a short time interval at the end of systole (corresponding to the downslope of the T wave). Thus, by recording counts in these time-windows over a series of many consecutive cardiac cycles, sufficient counts in each of the two images can be accumulated to produce highly discriminant views of the heart at maximum and minimum ventricular volume. These images may be obtained in any position desired, and may be recorded in a number of ways—e.g., by using Polaroid or X-ray film images taken from the camera persistence scope; by means of videotape; or by digitizing the images in computer matrices. Left ventricular ejection fraction (LVEF) may be calculated from any of these methods, either by the area-length method of Sandler and Dodge,[32,33] or by the count-based method from the computer images, in the LAO view. Also, these two frames may be superimposed or played as a two-frame movie, for a rough assessment of wall motion. The computer method for lightpen region-of-interest (ROI) assignment to determine LVEF is illustrated in Figure 28.13. Left ventricular end-diastolic (LVED) ROIs, left ventricular end-systolic (LVES) ROIs, and background ROIs are required, so that background corrected LVED and LVES counts may be used to calculate LVEF, based on assumptions of complete mixing of tracer, count/volume proportionality, and stability of tracer in the blood pool over the acquisition time interval. The formula for calculation of LVEF becomes:

$$LVEF = \frac{(LVED\ cts - BKg\ cts) - (LVES\ cts - BKg\ cts)}{(LVED\ cts - BKg\ cts)}$$

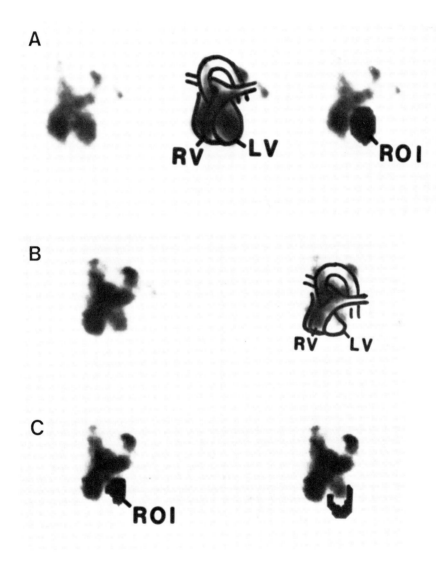

Fig. 28.13   End-diastolic and end-systolic gated LAO equilibrium images for calculation of LVEF. *(A)* shows the digitized end-diastolic image, with superimposed schematic illustrating the anatomy; a computer lightpen has been used to assign the LV end-diastolic ROI. *(B)* and *(C)* show end-systolic anatomy, and ROIs for the LV and background at end-systole. LVEF is calculated from background-corrected, end-diastolic and end-systolic counts. (Courtesy James W. Fletcher, M.D., St. Louis University School of Medicine, St. Louis, Mo.)

In the numerator, the "BKg cts" (background counts) cancel, so that we are left with:

$$LVEF = \frac{LVED\ cts - LVES\ cts}{LVED\ cts - BKg\ cts}$$

In such computer acquisitions, the ECG gates both the camera and the computer, so that the ECG becomes the "physiologic synchronizer."

It is conceptually easy, although technically sophisticated, to step from the simple gating approach described above to the *multiple* gating technique in common usage at the present time. This type of study can only be performed with the aid of computer acquisition and analysis. Consider the following: Assume that we wish to record, rather than only two images, a series of from 14 to even 80 or 100 frames throughout the cardiac cycle—i.e., from R wave to R wave—and that these images will be acquired in frame mode, such that each picture represents a portion of the cardiac cycle, unique in its temporal relation to the preceding R wave, but equal in *time length* to all other images in the series. This may be accomplished by first allowing the computer to average a series of R-R intervals (as triggered by the ECG synchronizer), so as to arrive at a "standard" R-R interval for the particular study to be performed. Then, if, for example, the R-R interval is found to be one sec, and the number of images we wish to acquire per cardiac cycle (or in this case frames per sec) is to be 25, then the computer calculates the time per frame (TPF) as:

$$TPF = \frac{R\text{-}R\ interval\ in\ sec}{\substack{number\ of\ frames\ to\\be\ acquired}}$$

$$TPF = \frac{1.0}{25} = 0.04\ sec\ per\ frame$$

This means that, at the onset of the first cycle, the operator and computer have designated a series of 25 consecutive image buffers, in which the images of the heart will be stored, starting with the first 0.04 sec of the cycle in the first image buffer, the second 0.04 sec of the cycle in the second image buffer, etc., until the entire cardiac cycle is stored in image form in 25 sequential data buffers in the computer. All subse-

quent cycles (i.e., each time a new R wave triggers the system) are acquired in the same manner, into the *same* 25 image buffers; thus, over a period of several hundred cardiac cycles, the total number of counts in *each image* becomes several hundred thousand. Thus, we would have a "composite" cardiac cycle, in the form of 25 images from R wave to R wave, each image of the series representing 0.04 sec of the cardiac cycle and containing highly statistically significant count information. It is therefore apparent that these studies often require word mode or zoomed byte mode acquisition to avoid pixel count overflow. The multiple gating concept is illustrated in Figure 28.14. This series of images may also be displayed in an endless-loop movie mode (as shown schematically in Fig. 28.15), to enable excellent assessment of wall motion from any number of studies acquired in several different views.

The calculation of left ventricular ejection fraction (LVEF) from such a series of images is in principle the same as for the simple, two-view gated study—except that, in the multi-image study, we must first define in which image of the series end-systole occurs. This is most often accomplished by using a first-frame ROI over the left ventricle, which is then "passed through" the entire series of images as a "fixed-first-frame" ROI, or template, to construct a time-activity curve from the changing counts in the left ventricle as "seen" by the ROI. From this curve, the end-systolic frame can be determined. At this point, we could take the same simplistic approach as described above and manually (with lightpen or joystick) define the LVED, LVES, and background ROIs from which LVEF may be calculated as before. In most current systems, however, one or more semiautomated computer algorithms are available for determining the "edge" of the LV in each of the 25 frames. From these circumferential edges, 25 ROIs would be produced and an automatically defined and positioned background ROI would be assigned, both for subsequent calculation of LVEF and for construction of a composite ventricular volume curve, as illustrated by the graphic output of a typical computer system shown in Figure 28.16.

There are a number of theoretical methods

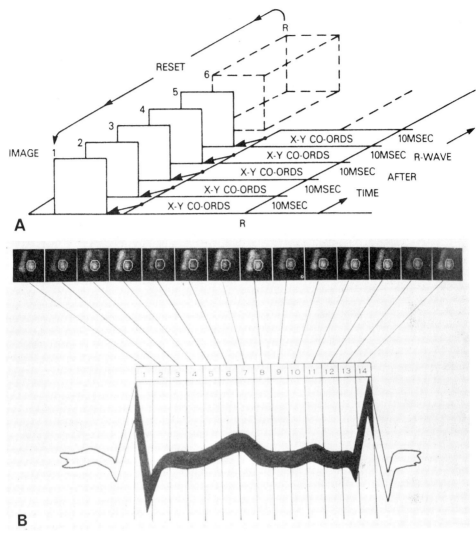

Fig. 28.14 Creation of an R-wave gated sequence of images spanning the R-R interval. Scintillation data (x, y coordinates) occurring during consecutive, equal-time intervals, are additively sorted into the image whose location in the sequence is determined by the elapsed time from the R-wave. For example, in *(A)*, all x, y coordinates occurring between 30 and 40 msec after the R-wave are sorted into the proper locations in Image 4 of the series. When the next R-wave is detected, the sorting process is reset to Image 1, and so on for each subsequent beat. The time per image for the sequence (shown as 10 msec in *(A)* is determined by the length of the average R-R interval, and by the number of images desired in the sequence. Thus, in *(B)*, the R-R interval has been divided into 14 equal temporal divisions, each with a corresponding image of the heart during that part of the cardiac cycle, arranged sequentially in the computer's memory. *(A,* used by permission, from Bachrach et al, Seminars in Nuclear Medicine IX:257, Oct., 1979; *B,* courtesy of James W. Fletcher, M.D., St. Louis University School of Medicine, St. Louis, Mo.)

for automatic edge detection, some of which are discussed in a recent publication by Chang et al.[77] Two points should be made regarding the algorithms most commonly utilized in current systems:

1. In general, the less operator interaction in the edge-detection/ROI assignment process, the better will be the interstudy and intra- and interobserver reproducibility of results, as generated on a given computer system.

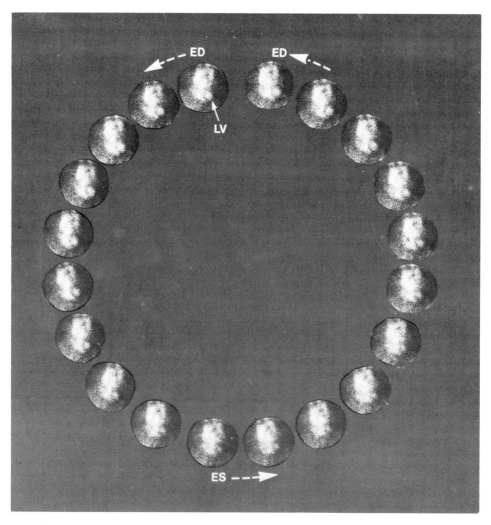

Fig. 28.15 Illustration of the principle of an "endless loop" cine display of a sequence of 21 images from R wave to R wave (or from end-diastole (ED) to end-diastole). In this case, left ventricular (LV) end-systole (ES) occurs about half-way through the cycle.

2. On the other hand, many of these current algorithms have limitations based on theoretical/mathematical considerations, not the least of which is poor signal-to-noise ratio (or poor ventricular versus background count ratio), usually resulting from inadequate counting statistics (too few counts per image due to short acquisition time and/or low tracer concentration in the blood pool). The obvious solution to these problems is to optimize the potential for good counting statistics *before* the study acquisition begins. This can be accomplished by the following means: maximum *safe* tracer concentration; maximum sensitivity collimation that still preserves minimum resolution requirements; and maximum possible acquisition time (which depends on the particular application for which the study is being performed— e.g., rest/exercise or drug or other intervention). Studies performed in our institution have demonstrated that, with approximately 10,000 counts in the background-corrected LVED blood pool and 5,000 LVES background-corrected counts, the LVEF = 0.50 ± 0.012 (±one standard deviation).[78] This means that, 95.4 percent of the time, the "true" LVEF will fall between 0.476 and 0.524 (see discussion of statistics in Ch. 12). With fewer counts in the LVED and LVES

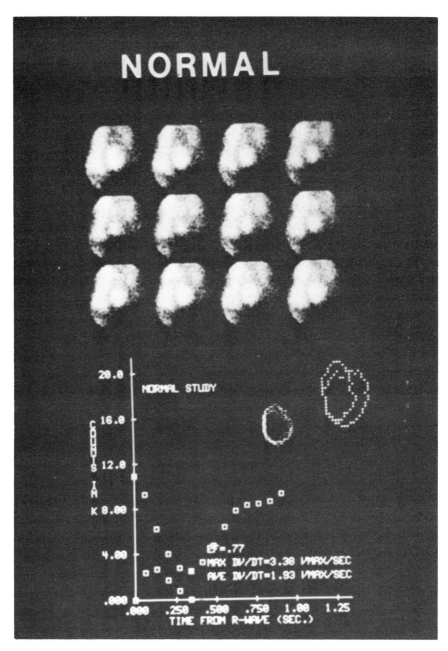

Fig. 28.16 A typical computer graphic display of the time-activity curve generated from multiple ROIs for the left ventricle with 14 frames from R wave to R-wave. (12 of the 14 images are shown above.) The time-activity curve represents a composite cardiac cycle resulting from the integration of several hundred actual cycles; each data point on the curve represents background-corrected LV counts from each of the 14 images of the study sequence. LVEF is calculated from the end-diastolic and end-systolic data points. The smaller curve at the bottom is the first derivative of the time-activity curve, from which are derived the maximum and average ejection rates (Max dV/dt and ave dV/dt). LVEF here is 0.77. The composite edges shown in the upper right corner of the graph are generated from the LV "activity pool" by the computer edge-detection algorithm (see text); the smaller composite shows all 14 edges superimposed while the larger is composed of only the end-diastolic and end-systolic edges. These may be used for a rough "static" evaluation of wall motion. (Algorithms courtesy of Medical Data Systems).

regions, for any of the above-listed reasons, the standard deviation and, therefore, the "true value" range, increases (i.e., poorer statistical reliability of the LVEF value). This diminished statistical reliability also relates directly to less accurate edge detection because images with poor ventricular blood-pool statistics also generally have reduced signal-to-noise ratios. The point is that, *after* a study has been acquired, it may be found that the edge detection algorithm has been inaccurate due to poor count rate statistics, resulting in edge assignment which includes nonventricular vascular structures in the ROI (e.g., left atrial appendage or aortic outflow tract). If this is the case, it seems only reasonable to allow greater operator interaction (i.e., judgment) in ROI assignment— even to the point of *manual* ROI assignment—in those cases where the algorithm may fail completely (e.g., with a very small LVES volume). The upshot of this argument is that appropriately educated humans generally know anatomy better than computer edge-detection algorithms! Therefore, an "educated subjectivity" is not inappropriate when attempting to assess cardiac function on the basis of such studies. This entire process, whether automated or manual, is greatly facilitated by *viewing the movie display of wall motion before attempting to analyze the study for a numerical value.* Furthermore, as has been pointed out by Pierson et al.[79] and Borer et al.,[80] subtle abnormalities of wall motion may be the earliest clues to the presence of coronary artery disease (especially as elicited by stress-intervention studies). Such abnormalities may only be appreciated by the human eye and may not be detected by the *numerical* output of the digital computer, because no significant abnormality in global ejection fraction is present. With further sophistication and refinement in computer hardware and software, it may eventually be possible to default entirely to a computer-derived decision on the question of normality versus abnormality in these studies of cardiac function. However, in the current state of this art, it perhaps should be said that all that is reproducible may not

necessarily be good, especially when it involves deriving reasonable and clinically relevant information upon which may be based important judgments concerning the care of the individual patient. But, finally, *subjective criteria* for defining abnormality with a given test should also be compared with some standard of "goodness" for sensitivity, specificity, and reproducibility of results (perhaps even more stringently than *objective* criteria). All of these considerations bear importantly on the subject of limitations and quality control of these testing procedures.

In general, the experience of many investigators with gated blood-pool studies of good quality has been that the results of ejection fraction and wall motion analysis using this technique are reproducible and correlate well with both contrast angiography and first-pass studies in a variety of clinical conditions.[79,80,83-125a] Gated equilibrium studies have also been performed both on a "beat-to-beat" basis, and by the "cumulative composite cycle" approach, utilizing a nonimaging probe device, with apparent good results.[76,82]

## ADVANTAGES, LIMITATIONS AND GENERAL CLINICAL APPLICATIONS OF FIRST-PASS AND GATED EQUILIBRIUM RADIONUCLIDE ANGIOGRAPHY

As shown in Table 28.4, each of these two techniques has advantages and disadvantages. Perhaps the most important advantage of the first-pass method is that it is theoretically the most accurate available method for determining RVEF, because there is little or no interference either from the right atrium or from background, and because it is virtually independent of geometric assumptions. Further, the first-pass method requires minimal patient cooperation because of short acquisition time. However, the greatest advantage of gated blood-pool studies is the ability to evaluate the effects of a variety of interventions (see below) over prolonged time periods with a single isotope injection. A brief survey of the current applications of these techniques follows:

## Characteristics of Wall Motion Abnormalities

Among the earliest and most straightforward uses for gated blood-pool imaging was to determine in patients with congestive heart failure (CHF) whether the etiology of the CHF was diffuse asynergy versus discrete aneurysm which could be surgically treated.[85,86] Excellent agreement in determining focal versus diffuse abnormality and extent and location of focal disease (especially on the anterolateral and apical surfaces) has been found when comparing contrast angiography to either gated studies [87,88] or first-pass techniques.[89-91] Figure 28.17 shows stop-motion images at end-diastole and end-systole of a large anteroapical aneurysm in two views of a gated equilibrium study. In general, it may be said that *focal* wall motion abnormalities suggest coronary artery disease, whereas *diffuse* asynergy more likely represents cardiomyopathy, or possibly severe multivessel coronary artery disease. Additional conditions which have been diagnosed on the basis of wall motion analysis and/or filling patterns with either first-pass or gated studies include left ventricular false aneurysm [92,93] and idiopathic hypertrophic subaortic stenosis (IHSS).[81] In IHSS, a typical pattern is described consisting of septal

**Table 28.4   Comparison of First-Pass and Gated Equilibrium Radionuclide Angiography**

|  | First Pass | Gated Equilibrium |
|---|---|---|
| 1. *Acquisition Time* | *Rapid*—usually less than 30 seconds per study. | *More prolonged*—usually requires at least 2 (or more) minutes. |
| 2. *Anatomical Features* | a.) Temporal separation allows optimum viewing of all 4 chambers. | a.) Four chambers best separated only in modified LAO view, and then not completely. |
|  | b.) Limited to single view per study. | b.) Unlimited additional views possible for wall motion assessment. |
|  | c.) Pulmonary transit and shunt evaluation. | c.) Not possible with equilibrium studies. |
| 3. *Counting Statistics* | Count-rate limited, unless using multicrystal camera. | Good statistics possible with more prolonged acquisition time. |
| 4. *Intervention Studies* | Limited due to limited number of injections (usually no more than 3). | Unlimited number of acquisitions possible over several hours. |
| 5. *Effect of arrhythmias*<br>a.) *Occasional* | a.) *May* limit study if occurs at peak of bolus, but usually have sufficient "good" beats. | a.) May be "filtered" out or "absorbed" into many cycles, without detriment. |
| b.) *Frequent* | b.) *May* average selected beats of similar R-R length, but reliability reduced with fewer beats analyzed. | b.) Gated studies unreliable with frequent arrhythmia. |
| 6. *Isotope Techniques* | Requires good bolus injection which may be difficult with severe pulmonary hypertension or tricuspid regurgitation; any $^{99m}$Tc compound may be used. | No bolus injection needed; but must use radiopharmaceuticals which remain stable in the blood pool over prolonged periods. (See discussion of pharmaceuticals and quality control in this chapter; see also Ch. 12.) |

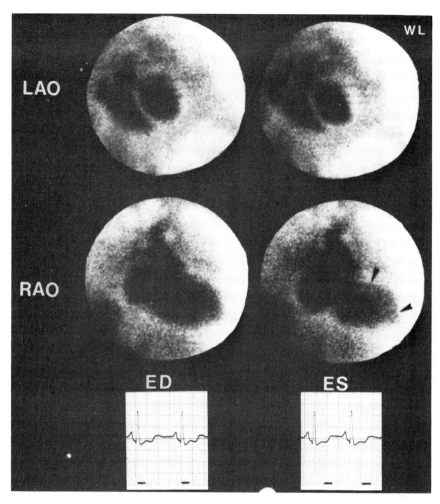

Fig. 28.17  Stop-motion images of a large antero-apical aneurysm of the left ventricle. The LAO (top) and RAO (bottom) views are the end-diastolic (left) and end-systolic (right) frames from a standard gated equilibrium blood pool image sequence of 28 frames from R-wave to R-wave. The gating markers for end-diastole and end-systole are shown on the ECG strips below the images. The arrows indicate the dyskinetic area (seen best here on the RAO view, but also apparent inferolaterally on the LAO end-systolic image).

straightening with upper septal thickening and LV cavity obliteration during systole.

## Intervention Radionuclide Angiography: Rest/Exercise Studies, Nitroglycerin Studies, Propranolol Studies

A number of investigators have compared the response of ejection fraction and wall motion during maximal exercise with resting results, as an approach to improve the sensitivity and specificity of these techniques for the detection and classification of coronary artery disease (CAD). Characteristic responses of normals versus abnormals to various types of stress (including supine and upright bicycle and handgrip exercise) have been defined.[94-98] In normal subjects, there is ordinarily at least a 10 percent rise in peak exercise LVEF over the resting value (generally in the range of 0.67 $\pm$ 0.07),[143] with no evidence of abnormal wall motion.[98] In CAD patients whose exercise is limited by fatigue, the LVEF will show little or no change from rest to maximum exercise; and in CAD patients limited by angina, LVEF actually tends to decrease with exercise.[98] Coronary patients also frequently develop new or worsened regional dysfunction (wall motion) with exercise stress.[94] Preliminary results also suggest that there is a direct relationship between the *number* of diseased vessels and the magnitude of fall in EF and the incidence of induced wall motion abnormalities.[107] It should be noted that, according to Baysian theory, the ability of any test to detect a specific abnormality in a given patient population depends in part on the prior probability of that abnormality existing in the population to be tested.[171] When currently available data are evaluated, it appears that the sensitivity of these techniques for diagnosing coronary artery disease approaches 90 percent using ejection fraction alone, and 95 percent when wall motion analysis is added.[95]

Several more complex computer approaches using gated studies have also been employed with some success to improve diagnostic accuracy. Among these newer methods are determination of *regional* ejection fraction [99,100] at rest and exercise; stroke volume [100,101] and ejection fraction imaging; [102] paradox imaging; [103] assessment of radionuclide-determined changes in pulmonary blood volume with exercise; [104] non-invasive measurement of ventricular pressure during systole, by means of integrated ventricular volume curve analysis; [105] and evaluation of the first one-third of systole for the partial ejection fraction from resting first-pass studies.[106] Many of these techniques appear quite promising, but most will require further validation to confirm their clinical utility.

Additional diagnostic approaches have incorporated these radioisotope techniques with one of several pharmacologic interventions. The earliest of these studies involved attempts at determining the extent of retrievable ventricular function (either global and/or regional) by assessing the effect of nitroglycerin, first in the context of contrast ventriculography. (The concept originated with reports concerning the epinephrine ventriculogram and the analysis of postextrasystolic potentiation during angiographic studies.) [108-111] The theory behind these interventions is that, if wall motion and/or ejection fraction improve under the influence of

nitroglycerin (NTG), there will likely be similar improvement as a result of revascularization of the compromised coronary circulation. (Preliminary studies utilizing two-view intervention radionuclide angiography [172] pre- and postoperatively suggest that this may indeed be a useful approach.) On an even more fundamental level, this kind of response may be taken as an indication, at least, of the need for *medical* prophylaxis or therapeutic trial. This type of intervention study has been combined with rest and/or exercise gated blood-pool studies in CAD patients, with the following results: [112-117]

1. Regional dyssynergy at rest that improves with NTG is usually in an area *without* prior infarction.
2. An abnormal resting EF that improves with NTG does so by a decrease of ventricular volumes both at end-systole and end-diastole but often more so at end-systole.
3. Abnormalities in regional wall motion and EF which are induced by exercise will be improved when exercise is performed after NTG.
4. Normal subjects, who show a *normal* increase in EF with exercise, show *no* further increase in EF when exercising without NTG.
5. In studies of patients who experience spontaneous resting angina, ejection fraction and stroke volume may decrease before actual subjective pain is reported; after administration of sublingual NTG, both ejection fraction and stroke volume increase, peaking at about 6 to 8 minutes, with the total effect lasting about one hour; improvement in these functional parameters also tends to be evident *prior* to the time the patients report relief of pain.
6. In patients with LV aneurysms, if the resting LVEF is less than 40 percent, sublingual isosorbide dinitrate does not improve exercise functional reserve; but, if resting EF exceeds 40 percent, about 50 percent of patients will show improved exercise reserve with the drug.

A second kind of pharmacologic intervention which has been studied in conjunction with radionuclide angiography is the effect of propranolol, both in normals and patients with CAD. The results have been controversial, perhaps in part due to methodological differences—i.e., oral vs. intravenous administration of drug. For example, some investigators have found that the *normal* heart responds to oral propranolol by showing a "blunting" or decrease in LVEF and cardiac output, both at rest and with exercise.[117,118] A similar blunted response of LVEF to supine bicycle exercise has been reported in normal men after i.v. propranolol.[119] It has been suggested that these changes are primarily due to decreased heart rate resulting from this drug intervention. Conversely, others have found that i.v. infusion of the drug resulted in *increased* LVEF and ejection rate in normal resting subjects.[120] In coronary artery disease patients, however, it has been variously shown either that there is no change in these functional parameters at rest while on therapeutic antianginal doses of *oral* propranolol,[121,122] or that there is a fall in ejection fraction under these conditions.[123] General agreement does seem to hold that exercise function improves in CAD patients with propranolol.[124,125] It is advisable to be aware of the discrepancies as noted above, and perhaps a cautious approach to interpretation of these data is warranted until further investigation clarifies these issues.

## Additional Pharmacologic and Clinical Studies; RVEF; Ventricular Volumes

Other preliminary reports utilizing these radioisotope techniques include studies of various digitalis preparations[126-128] and terbutaline.[129] In addition, other specific groups of patients have been evaluated, with promising results. For example, among patients undergoing coronary artery bypass grafting, it has been shown that, while postoperative resting function may not differ significantly from preoperative resting function, exercise LVEF and exercise wall motion generally show improvement in patients who experience symptomatic improvement post-operatively.[130] The severity of valvular regurgitation has also been assessed by the left-to-right ventricular stroke index ratio determined from gated blood-pool studies; this method has shown good agreement in human subjects in whom regurgitation was estimated qualitatively by angiography,[131] and in a dog model in which regurgitant fraction was estimated by electromagnetic flowmeter.[132] Further, in patients receiving doxorubicin hydrochloride therapy for various cancers, serial assessment of LVEF appears to be a sensitive method for detecting cardiotoxicity prior to clinical manifestations of heart failure.[133,134]

Another area of recent interest and some disagreement is the assessment of *right* ventricular ejection fraction in patients with CAD. Earlier studies employed only first-pass techniques. However, methods for determining RVEF from gated blood-pool imaging have been recently described.[135,136] The normal RVEF by these techniques is in close agreement (0.49 ± 0.10 by one group, and 0.48 ± 0.05 by the other).[135,136] Both of these values are generally lower than the normal LVEF by the gated blood-pool technique (in the range of 0.63 ± 0.08 to 0.67 ± 0.07).[135,143] (All values are mean ± one SD.) There appears to be general agreement, with either first-pass or gated blood-pool techniques, that *resting* RVEF is not substantially different from normal in CAD patients.[135-140] However, the response of RVEF to exercise in coronary artery disease patients has been reported by some investigators to be primarily dependent on the concomitant LV response, rather than on the presence or absence of proximal right coronary stenosis; [136,140] while other studies suggest that a dissociation of the exercise response of the right and left ventricles may occur when the right coronary artery is not involved.[138,139] Again, these discrepancies may be due in part to differences in methodology or patient selection which will require further evaluation to resolve. Slutsky and associates [136] have proposed that RV dysfunction during exercise in CAD may in fact be caused *in part* by local ischemia *as well as* by altered loading conditions due to LV dysfunction. One study of RVEF in chronic obstructive pulmonary disease showed that 19 of 36 patients had an abnormal RVEF, whereas only 10 of the 19 abnormal RVEF values occurred in patients with cor pulmonale.[141] The authors suggested that the RVEF may therefore be more sensitive to early RV dysfunction than other clinical criteria for detecting incipient cor pulmonale. This is most interesting in view of the hypothesis that RV dysfunction may result from increased afterload due to LV dysfunction with exercise. The most important point to be made, however, is that many of these parameters for assessing cardiac function are probably very sensitive to a *number* of cardiopulmonary disorders and therefore become *less specific* for any single occult cause of dysfunction. Further refinements in methodology may therefore be required to overcome this problem.

Finally, it has been shown recently that absolute ventricular volumes may be calculated from gated blood pool studies, by comparing ventricular activity (as "seen" by the computer) to activity counted from a blood sample obtained from the patient during image acquisition. After normalizing to time per frame and number of cardiac cycles acquired, and after making any necessary decay corrections with regard to blood count rate, the resulting volume index may be compared to contrast angiographic results by means of linear regression analysis, yielding an LV volume value in ml.[142-144] By this method, it has been shown that the normal response of LVEF to exercise is due to increased stroke volume by virtue of a decrease in end-systolic volume (ESV); in CAD patients *without* angina, LVEF showed no change, due to no change in ESV.[143] In CAD patients *with* angina, both ESV *and* EDV increased with exercise, but ESV increased more, which accounted for the resulting decrease in LV stroke volume and LVEF. The ESV response of the left ventricle to exercise was found to be almost as sensitive as LVEF for revealing the presence of CAD.[143] This latter diagnostic potential assumes increasing importance in view of recent reports that certain *normal* subjects (usually presenting with complaints of atypical chest pain) may *fail* to demonstrate the "normal" increase in LVEF with exercise.[107,173] Further, Slutsky and associates have shown that, although LV volumes in CAD patients still *increase* abnormally during exercise after sublingual nitroglycerin, the abnormal response is diminished by nitroglycerin (thus accounting for the improved LVEF as discussed earlier).[174]

These innovative methods, along with others described above, offer great potential in the noninvasive study of cardiopulmonary physiology and pathophysiology under a wide variety of conditions, and should in future be applicable to patients with myocardial infarction during both the acute and the convalescent phase.

## EVALUATION OF THE ACUTE MYOCARDIAL INFARCTION PATIENT WITH RADIONUCLIDE ANGIOGRAPHY

It has been well established by means of contrast angiography that left ventricular performance is an extremely powerful predictor of survival in CAD patients, both in medically and surgically treated groups.[145-151] However, use of this modality for serial evaluation of the seriously ill patient has been impractical, due to the invasive nature of cardiac catheterization, and because the hypertonic contrast media utilized have been shown to produce transient impairment of myocardial function.[152] On the other hand, the noninvasive, atraumatic, and safely repeated assessment which is possible with radioisotope techniques, has made these procedures ideally suited for use in such patients as the acute myocardial infarction (AMI) group.

One of the earliest studies of left ventricular function in acute infarction was by Kostuk et al.,[153] who employed "real time" video tape recording of first-pass data, with simultaneous ECG recording on the audio track. The image data thus acquired were subsequently "reconstructed" with reference to the R and T waves, so as to obtain arrhythmia-filtered, end-diastolic and end-systolic composite images with high count information. These images were photographed on 35-mm film and then projected in enlarged format with a size calibration image for planimetry and volume determination by the standard Sandler-Dodge method. Sixty-four acute infarction patients and 15 patients without acute illness were studied; the latter group also underwent contrast angiography within 24 hours after the isotope study, in order to compare results obtained by the two techniques.

(Good agreement for end-diastolic volume (r = 0.87) and LVEF (r = 0.94) was obtained, as well as for identification of wall motion abnormalities). Infarction patients were studied from 6 hours to 1 month after the acute episode. Results in the AMI group showed the following:

1. 47 of 64 patients had an elevated LV end-diastolic volume.
2. 58 of 64 patients had a reduced initial LV ejection fraction (0.38 ± 0.03, mean ± one standard deviation).
3. 53 survivors had an EF averaging 0.40 ± 0.02, compared to 0.26 ± 0.07 in 11 patients who died within one month (p < 0.05).
4. EF correlated inversely with infarct size as estimated by serial serum CK analysis in 42 patients (r = −0.71).
5. 47 of 64 patients showed wall motion abnormalities on both radionuclide ventriculography and radarkymography.
6. Serial isotope studies from 6 hours to 1 month showed improvement of function in 30 of 55 patients, with no change in 12, and deterioration in 13.

Subsequently, Rigo and associates [154] performed first-pass and gated equilibrium studies, also using the simple gated technique. They recorded biplane images directly on 35-mm film for subsequent planimetry. Thirty-eight AMI patients were studied within 48 hours of onset of symptoms. Again, results showed elevated end-diastolic *and* end-systolic LV volumes in all 38 patients; mean LVEF was 0.38 ± 0.08. Thirty-six of 38 had akinetic areas ranging from 15 to 59 percent of the LV wall by perimeter measurement. Followup in 20 patients at 1 week to 3 months after the acute event showed significant improvement in LVEF (0.38 to 0.45, p < 0.001) in those 14 patients who improved clinically, while those 6 who failed to improve or worsened showed persistently low LVEF (0.30). The percent akinesis was also smaller in those who subsequently improved clinically; however, no attempt was made to compare percent akinesis to infarct size by other (enzymatic) parameters.

Rigo et al.[155] also studied *right* ventricular

dysfunction in acute infarction, including 14 patients with inferior MI and 13 with anterior MI. Simple gated cardiac blood-pool images were obtained in the manner described above. From the LAO end-diastolic view, an index of RV volume was obtained by calculating the area of the RV and comparing it to the area of the *LV* in the same view. LV volumes and ejection fraction were planimetered from biplane images as in the earlier study. These values, as well as RV/LV area ratio from the MI patients, were compared to similar data obtained from 10 normal volunteers. The RV/LV area ratio in normals was found to be 1.11 ± .66; in *anterior* infarction patients, the ratio dropped to 0.75 ± 0.12 (p < .05). This reduction was presumed to be due to LV enlargement. In inferior infarctions, the ratio was 1.12 ± 0.23, which was greater than in patients with anterior MI (p < .05), but *not* significantly different from normal. This latter finding was felt to be due to enlargement of *both* ventricles in inferior MI. Similarly, in 6 additional patients with cardiogenic shock, 3 each with inferior and anterior MI, the area ratio dropped even further in anterior MI with shock (to 0.62), but rose to an impressive 2.05 in inferior MI with shock, suggesting a greater degree of RV dilatation and dysfunction. The authors pointed out that the relatively high incidence of RV dysfunction in their patients with inferior MI was consistent with autopsy findings of up to 40 percent incidence of RV scarring in cases of inferior MI. They further suggested that the ability to diagnose RV dysfunction (and RV infarction) in patients with inferior MI complicated by cardiogenic shock would be of particular importance, since shock associated with RV infarction is potentially reversible with volume loading therapy.

It is of interest to note that Steele and his coinvestigators observed apparently different results in the series of patients in whom they studied RV function.[137] In 29 men with an inferior infarction, the *mean* RVEF was not different from the 14 normals in their study. In fact, only 7 of 29 (or 24 percent) with inferior MI had a depressed RVEF; of these, 4 had triple vessel CAD. They concluded, therefore, that RVEF was relatively preserved except in multiple vessel disease associated with MI. There are two critical points to be noted, however, in comparing these two papers: First, the patients of Steele et al. were all *stable* and *without a history of of recent MI* at the time of study. And second, in none of their patients was RV infarction recognized clinically at the time of the acute event. Therefore, these two studies are not necessarily at odds; in fact, taken together, they seem to reinforce the conclusion that RV dysfunction in acute inferior MI probably indicates RV infarction.

Subsequent investigations published by three different groups have supported and expanded these conclusions: Sharpe et al.,[156] employing the RV/LV area ratio method, showed in 15 patients with acute inferior transmural MI that RV dysfunction (by the radioisotope method as well as by echocardiography and mean RV filling pressure) was most evident in those 6 patients who had RV infarction; the diagnosis was confirmed by RV free wall segmental asynergy and/or by RV free wall uptake of pyrophosphate (see chapter 12 for discussion of "hot spot" acute infarction imaging.) Tobinick and associates,[157] utilizing the first-pass technique for determining RVEF, showed that a single injection of Tc-99m-pyrophosphate could be used to:

1. demonstrate RV dysfunction (RVEF = $0.39 \pm 0.05$ in 7 of 19 inferior MIs vs. RVEF = $0.52 \pm 0.04$ in normals, $p < 0.001$); and 2. image the infarcted RV free wall in those patients with inferior MI involving the RV. LVEF was also depressed significantly below normal in the 19 inferior MI patients; but RVEF was abnormal only in those with scintigraphic evidence for RV infarction. Carrying the assessment of ventricular performance further into the immediate post-MI period was the logical next step pursued by Reduto and coworkers.[158] They performed sequential first-pass studies in 31 patients with uncomplicated (Killip Class I and II) acute transmural MI (13 anterior and 18 inferior). Studies were performed on all patients on days 1, 3, 5, and approximately day 13 after the acute event (the latter study being within 3 days of discharge). They also found that inferior MI resulted in a significantly greater reduction in RVEF than

anterior MI, while anterior MI produced greater depression in LVEF. Furthermore, throughout hospitalization there was no significant change in global EF or regional wall motion in either group.

Serial measurements of LVEF by first-pass radioisotope angiography were also obtained by Schelbert et al in 43 acute MI patients, with followup extended up to 39 months after the acute event.[159] Early after infarction (during the first 5 days) the extent of LVEF depression correlated directly with the extent of LV failure (LVEF tending toward normal in uncomplicated infarction). LVEF also reflected regional function in this study; normal wall motion was accompanied by a significantly higher EF ($0.53 \pm 0.08$) than was regional asynergy (LVEF = $0.41 \pm 0.10$, $p < 0.0001$). Improvement in LVEF in the first 5 days was noted in 54 percent of these patients, while 20 percent showed no change and 26 percent deteriorated; improvement was seen only in those patients who were treated with diuretics, digitalis, and/or antihypertensive drugs. In contrast, improvement in LVEF in the *late* followup period was observed only in patients who required *no* drug therapy. Thus, the early improvement in LV performance appeared to be due to drug-related alterations in ventricular loading conditions, or enhanced contractile state of the remaining intact myocardium. Further, LVEF improved over time in patients whose wall motion abnormalities or left heart dimension decreased or normalized; whereas in those who manifested new segmental dysfunction or persistent cardiomegaly, LVEF tended to remain adnormal. Serial changes in ejection fraction were also closely related to subsequent morbidity and mortality. Patients with an initially low or decreasing LVEF had a significantly greater incidence of early mortality (secondary to recurrent MI within the first 60 days) and LV dysfunction ($p < 0.02$), than those whose EF was normal, or improved to normal early after infarction. Again, we should point out that differences in patient selection criteria (inclusion of patients with LV failure, up to and including overt pulmonary edema in the Schelbert study, versus only Class I and II patients in the Reduto study), may explain the inconsistencies noted when comparing the results reported in the above papers.

In the patients evaluated by Shah and colleagues [160] with gated equilibrium cardiac blood pool scintigraphy, 27 of 56 with acute infarction (anterior and inferior), developed one or more complications during the hospital course. The mean LVEF in this group was lower ($0.34 \pm 0.10$) than in the 29 patients with an uncomplicated course ($0.52 \pm 0.13$, p $<$ 0.001). Seven patients died (of either pump failure or arrhythmia) within the first 14 days post-MI; the initial LVEF was lower in these nonsurvivors than in survivors. Death due to pump failure occurred in 55 percent of patients with an EF of 0.30 or less. Further, in a study by Schulze et al.,[161] patients were classified according to gated blood-pool LVEF, percent LV akinesis, infarct size (by peak CK), and incidence of VPCs during 24-hour ambulatory ECG monitoring within 2 to 4 weeks after acute MI. With regard to the incidence of VPCs, patients in Classes II, III, and IV—i.e., patients with more than 30 unifocal VPCs per hour, or multifocal VPCs, or coupled VPCs including ventricular tachycardia—had significantly lower mean EF ($30.5 \pm 2.3$ vs. $49.6 \pm 4.0$), higher mean percent akinesis ($28.1 \pm 2.2$ vs. $16.9 \pm 3.7$), and higher mean peak CK ($1350 \pm 187$ vs. $721 \pm 155$ I.U.), than did Class 0 and I patients (0 to $<$ 30 unifocal VPCs per hour). A similar trend toward lower LVEF was noted by Ritchie et al.[162] in survivors of sudden cardiac death due to ventricular fibrillation; these investigators also utilized the gated equilibrium method. Using first-pass data, Slutsky and associates [163] found that not only total global LVEF, but also early systolic (first third of systole) LVEF had important predictive value regarding morbidity and mortality early after acute infarction: a total LVEF of $< 0.52$ predicted significantly increased morbidity from congestive heart failure and mortality during the first year post-MI, and a first third EF of $< 0.17$ also predicted increased mortality in the first year. The authors point out that, while in one third of patients studied early after admission for acute MI the total LVEF may fail to indicate LV dysfunction, the first third EF appeared to be highly sensitive for detecting early ventricular dysfunction.

And, finally, by assessing regional ejection fraction from gated blood-pool studies in patients within 4 days after first acute transmural MI, Wynne et al.[164] found, as might be expected, that prognosis and functional class were related to depressed regional function in *infarcted* zones. However, they also observed that apparently *noninfarcted* zones (defined by ECG) showed depressed function, particularly in patients with anterior MI and/or severe pump failure. Thus, depressed mechanical performance in regions beyond the peri-infarction ischemic zone occurs for unknown reasons and may contribute to global LV dysfunction after acute MI.

From the above, it is apparent that a number of important parameters of cardiac function can be measured in the acute myocardial infarction patient. Also, nitroglycerin (NTG) intervention radionuclide studies using first-pass techniques have been recently reported within 6 to 24 hours after acute infarction;[165] other patients with a remote MI (more than 1 year old) were also studied. All infarcted zones showed asynergy under ordinary resting conditions. However, after administration of sublingual NTG, acutely infarcted areas showed improved contraction in 20 of 23 patients, but no significant improvement was seen in areas of old infarction in a separate group of 6 patients. Furthermore, when the acutely infarcted areas were serially examined in this manner—within 24 hours, after 5 to 7 days, and again after 4 to 6 weeks—*without* NTG, there was no apparent difference in the serial studies. But *with* NTG, within 24 hours after infarction, as noted above, there was significant improvement in segmental contraction; at 5 to 7 days, somewhat *less* improvement was demonstrated; and after 4 to 6 weeks, *no* significant improvement in contraction could be detected in the infarcted zones with NTG.[166] These and other studies suggest that a variety of intervention radionuclide methods might also be used, singly or in combination (as tolerated by the patient), in order to assess (1) response of the acutely infarcted heart to drug therapies, such as digoxin; [166a]    (2) the incidence of infarct extension;    (3) development and extent of ventricular aneurysm; and (4) for prognostication.

For example, *submaximal* exercise testing has previously been combined with radionuclide angiography in patients 2 to 3 weeks after acute infarction, demonstrating differences in functional ventricular response when comparing anterior infarction to inferior or nontransmural infarction.[167] However, several more recent studies utilizing *symptom limited* exercise testing (but without incorporating isotope techniques) have produced the following very important information:

1. Cardiovascular responses to symptom-limited exercise testing (e.g., frequency of exercise-induced ischemic ST-segment depression, angina pectoris, premature ventricular complexes; peak systolic pressure; rate-pressure product) are highly reproducible from 3 weeks to 3 months after uncomplicated MI; therefore, changes in the response to treadmill exercise tests performed several weeks apart reflect real alterations in cardiovascular performance.[168]

2. Symptom-limited, exercise-induced ST-segment depression $\geq 0.2$ mV 3 weeks after uncomplicated acute MI (patients without clinical heart failure or unstable angina) is significantly more prevalent in, and predictive of, subsequent cardiac arrest, recurrent MI, sudden death, or coronary artery bypass surgery, within 2 years of infarction.[169,170]

3. Exercise-induced ventricular ectopy on a *single* test at 3 weeks post-MI was *not* a powerful predictor of subsequent cardiac events.[169,170]

4. However, exercise-induced ventricular arrhythmia on *multiple* tests 5 to 52 weeks after MI was more prevalent in patients with recurrent MI.[169]

5. Maximal work load < 4 METS at 3 weeks (in conjunction with ST-segment depression as above) was predictive of *medical* events.[170]

6. However, *angina pectoris* at 3 weeks (in conjunction with ST-segment depression) was predictive of *surgical* events.[170]

It is most intriguing to speculate as to how the addition of certain parameters—such as LVEF, RVEF, regional wall motion, regional EF, ventricular volumes, and first-third EF—and changes in these factors with time, exercise, NTG, or other drug interventions—would affect the predictive values resulting from multivariate analysis as outlined above. The potential of this type of approach remains to be defined by future clinical studies similar to those of Borer et al.[170a]

## QUALITY CONTROL IN BRIEF: RADIOPHARMACEUTICALS, EQUIPMENT, EXERCISE TESTING, STUDY INTERPRETATION

### Radiopharmaceuticals

We have outlined in Chapter 12 the basic requirements for quality control of any radiopharmaceutical that is to be used in human studies. As we have already indicated, almost any available Tc-99m-labeled pharmaceutical may be utilized to perform first-pass studies, depending on the kind of additional information desired from the study. However, specific mention should be made here of the three primary agents currently available for obtaining gated equilibrium cardiac blood-pool studies, along with some of the advantages and limitations of each.

**Tc-99m Human Serum Albumin.** As with virtually all methods for labeling a given pharmaceutical with technetium, the pertechnetate ion as it is eluted from a generator in the $+7$ oxidation state must be reduced to a $+3$, $+4$, or $+5$ state before it can effectively be bound to the desired ligand—in this instance, human serum albumin (HSA). This reduction reaction for HSA labeling may be accomplished by an electrolytic process or, in the typical lyophylized kit system, with stannous ion as the reducing agent.[175] The degree and nature of technetium binding with the albumin varies with the method of preparation, and the agent usually carries with it a certain unavoidable quantity of free, unbound Tc-99m-pertechnetate and reduced hydrolyzed technetium. These latter characteristics alter the blood clearance properties of the preparation, which may seriously affect the in vivo distribution of the technetium label.[175] These three forms of the label may be separated and quantitated fairly easily by instant thin-layer chromatography. In most commercially available kits, there is, after appropriate preparation, greater than 90 percent bound technetium. Nevertheless, standard in vitro quality control methods (as described above) may not accurately reflect the actual blood clearance characteristics in vivo. Thus, two preparations that have similar in vitro characteristics may differ considerably in vivo.[175] The precise reason for this spectrum of clearances is not readily apparent. In view of these considerations, it is evident that studies that require repeated determinations of ejection fraction or ventricular volumes over prolonged periods of time, or studies that require computation of blood volume by the dilution principle, will be less than ideal if the properties of the radiopharmaceutical change unpredictably with time. In addition to radioactive decay, leakage into the intravascular space may account in part for alterations in activity. Obviously, if one of these agents is to be used, the product with the slowest clearance is desirable. In man, on the average, about 80 percent of the activity administered with these agents remains intravascular at 15 min, and 75 percent at 30 min. Subsequently, biologic clearance occurs with a T½ of about 15 hours, with urinary clearance averaging about 40 to 50 percent at 24 hours.[175]

**In Vivo Red Cell Labeling with TC-99m.** This is perhaps the most commonly used and easily accomplished of the blood-pool labeling techniques. In essence, the patient's blood pool becomes the "kit" by virtue of "pretinning" of the red cells with microgram quantities of stannous ion. This is accomplished by injecting i.v. a vial of stannous pyrophosphate which has been reconstituted from the lyophylized form with normal saline (rather than in the usual manner in which Tc-99m-pyrophosphate is prepared for bone imaging purposes). After an incubation period of 20 to 30 min (during which time the stannous ion may cause the induction of oxidative enzymes in the red cells),[175] the Tc-99m pertechnetate is injected i.v. It is then reduced, and it associates with the red cells almost immediately, to the extent of 80 to 90 percent labeling efficiency. In rats, the biologic

T½ of red cells labeled in this manner is 19.5 hours, and the T½ is even longer in humans. Thus, this is an easy and efficient method for achieving a stable blood-pool label that is excellent for equilibrium studies over a prolonged period of time. During injection of the pertechnetate, one may also accomplish a first-pass study, provided good bolus injection technique is observed. The primary difficulty with this method is that in certain clinical circumstances—such as the presence of liver disease and in anticoagulant therapy with heparin—there is major interference with labeling efficiency.

**In Vitro Red Cell Labeling with Tc-99m.** The principle here is essentially the same as in the in vivo method, except that a sample of the patient's blood is "pretinned," then labeled with Tc-99m-pertechnetate entirely in vitro, and subsequently reinjected to become the blood-pool label. Labeling efficiency of 95 percent has been reported with this technique, and the label is also stable in the blood pool over prolonged periods of time. However, the lesser convenience of this method has made it of secondary importance. A lyophylized kit for more convenient and sterile performance of in vitro red cell labeling has been produced by Richards et al; however, if excess carrier Tc-99 is present in the generator eluate, this will be detrimental to the labelling efficiency.[175]

It is apparent from the above discussion that the method of choice currently seems to be the in vivo red cell labeling, except where patients are anticoagulated, in which instance Tc-HSA is preferred.

## Equipment

Throughout this chapter we have attempted to emphasize that the quality of nuclear cardiology procedures depends heavily on appropriate choices of systems for performing such studies. Cameras and collimators must have the optimum combination of resolution and sensitivity, and must be interfaced appropriately to the optimum computer system—which has in turn been programmed to acquire, process (if necessary), and display the images in the optimum mode. It should by now be obvious that no single set of choices in the above option list will be ideal, or even adequate, for all types of nuclear cardiology procedures. Choices must be based on informed understanding of the technical aspects of this field, which have been presented briefly in this chapter and in Chapter 12. Similarly, the adequacy of exercise testing as an integral part of these methods depends in part on the quality of the equipment used.

In general, any current state-of-the-art Anger-type gamma scintillation camera may be used satisfactorily for gated equilibrium or first-pass radionuclide angiograms. If the choice is between a camera with 37-photomultiplier (37-pm) tubes with a *standard* size (10-inch diameter) field of view vs. a camera with 37-pm tubes and a *large* field of view (15 inch diameter), the standard field of view is probably a better choice, because the heart occupies a greater portion of the field of view. This choice would maximize both resolution and counting efficiency for *cardiac* activity. First-pass studies are usually performed with a *high sensitivity,* parallel-hole collimator, to maximize counts during the bolus passage. Gated equilibrium studies *may* be performed with *any* parallel-hole collimator. However, some investigators feel that a high-sensitivity collimator is preferable, in order to maximize counting efficiency, especially for shorter studies (e.g., during exercise). Others feel that resolution and sensitivity are of equal importance in producing technically optimal gated images. Therefore, some prefer a *general purpose* collimator. Standard quality control and maintenance measures for gamma cameras are of course mandatory. (Further discussion in this regard is beyond the scope of this chapter.) (Also see under Study Interpretation below for further brief discussion of technical adequacy of studies.) It is also helpful to determine by bar phantom and field flood studies how resolution and sensitivity differ, at the *face* of the collimator, and at a depth approximately equal to the "average" depth of a heart in situ, comparing high-sensitivity and general purpose collimators, so that a reasonable choice of collimator can be made.

The choice of nuclear cardiology equipment is clearly an area where the expertise and inter-action of both nuclear medicine physicians and cardiologists can be an invaluable cooperative effort.

## Exercise Testing

Any discussion of quality control in this area is of necessity a direct extension of the above comments. Exercise nuclear cardiology procedures, no matter how expertly the imaging may be performed, are only as good as the exercise test. As pointed out by Pierson et al.,[176] the reputation of nuclear cardiology is at stake when we attempt to draw conclusions based on studies performed with suboptimal exercise testing. This is supported by a recent study from Brady and associates [177] which showed that some patients with CAD may have a normal ventricular response at inadequate, submaximal exercise levels; and to attain a high degree of sensitivity in these tests, adequate symptom-limited maximum or submaximum exercise must be performed. The primary reason for inadequate exercise in this series was leg fatigue. This latter fact bears directly on the choice of exercise equipment. For example, if supine bicycle equipment is to be used, the pedal mechanism and shoulder supports should be movable into a variety of heights and positions, so as to comfortably accommodate any body habitus, thereby minimizing leg fatigue. (One such system is shown in Fig. 28.18.) Also, a number of recent studies have been published regarding the adequacy of gating, and its effects on data collection during rest and exercise cardiac blood-pool studies.[178-180]

Brash et al.[178] showed by computer modeling that a linear relationship exists between the percent of ectopic beats and the underestimation of ejection fraction, when data are collected in an R-wave-triggered, forward-frame mode. One ectopic beat in 10 led to a 5% underestimation of EF, which could be rectified when R-wave filtering was applied. The authors suggest that in chronic ischemic heart disease there is a 7 percent incidence of extrasystoles, which is even greater in the acute infarction population. This point is of obvious import in any discussion of the efficacy of these techniques in evaluating the acute infarction patient. How-

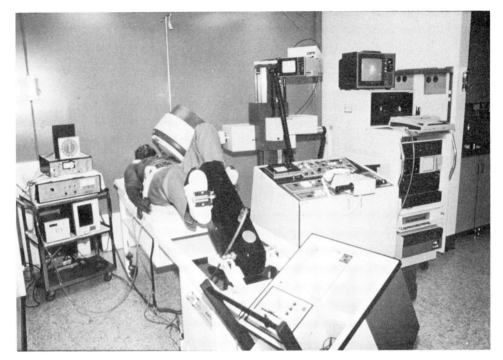

Fig. 28.18  A typical equipment configuration for performing exercise gated equilibrium cardiac blood pool studies. The computer is seen on the far right (with TV monitor), and the mobile gamma camera console next to the computer. The camera detector head is shown placed over the subject's left chest, in the LAO position. The supine bicycle table (with the ergometer to the left), and a standard 12-lead electrocardiograph (at end of table) complete the set-up seen here. (Not shown is the emergency resuscitation equipment, which is always at hand for any exercise procedures.)

ever, most current nuclear cardiology computer systems are not capable of performing efficient R-wave filtering.[180] Again, the need for collaboration between Nuclear Medicine and Cardiology is apparent, if we are to find solutions to these and other problems in this field.

## STUDY INTERPRETATION: A SYSTEMATIC APPROACH TO THE GATED EQUILIBRIUM BLOOD-POOL SCAN

The first step in interpreting a gated equilibrium study is to assess the technical adequacy of the study. Good-quality images show well-demarcated edges of cardiac structures. Factors that can degrade image quality are as follows:

1. *Patient motion.* Shoulder supports and a thoracic harness may be used to minimize this; however, caution must be used so that,

during exercise when the patient is breathing more rapidly and deeply, uncomfortable constriction is not produced.

2. *Inadequate tracer complex formation.* This may be "diagnosed" by observing the equilibrium count rate over the precordium with time, looking for deterioration of count rate that occurs more rapidly than can be accounted for on the basis of radioactive decay. Also, increased activity in thyroid, stomach, kidneys, or urinary bladder indicates excessive free Tc-99m-pertechnetate.

3. *Marked obesity.* Not much can be done about this on a short-term basis!

4. *Inadequate collimator resolution at depth.* (See discussion above).

5. *Improper pulse-height analyzer setting.* Generally, the best compromise between sensitivity and resolution for pulse-height analysis of $^{99m}$Tc is obtained with a 20 percent window setting about the 140 keV photopeak.

Gating problems in a study may be assessed by looking at the spread of the R-R interval histogram (if available from the computer) and by checking the total counts in each image of the study. If there is more than a 10 percent variation in total counts per frame, when comparing each frame to all other frames in the study, it is likely due to suboptimal gating.[81] (See further discussion under exercise testing above.)

After determining the technical adequacy of the study, interpretation is carried out in two general phases: (1) inspection of the study in cine mode; and (2) calculation of parameters to quantify ventricular function (usually primarily global ventricular ejection fraction). This discussion will be confined to the kinds of observations that may be made in the first of these two phases. (For further detailed discussion, see Reference 81.)

1. *Low-contrast cine display.* May be useful in judging the thickness of the myocardial silhouette.
2. *High-contrast cine display.* Useful for defining valve planes and chamber borders.
3. *Synchrony of contraction.* The two ventricles should be in phase; the two atria in phase; and the ventricles in opposite phase to the atria. Although the degree of ventricular contraction is not the same at all points, all surfaces of the ventricles should move *inward* at the onset of systole. The *apex* of the LV normally contributes importantly to stroke volume, and therefore "apical lag," which is sometimes said to be within normal limits on contrast ventriculography, is *not* a normal finding on a gated equilibrium radionuclide study.
4. *Right atrium and tricuspid valve.* The right atrium is usually easily seen in the standard LAO view, at the end of ventricular systole; the tricuspid valve plane is seen best tangentially on a 30° RAO view. Enlargement of the right atrium often produces bulging in the lateral and superoinferior directions, which may be appreciated on LAO and RAO views.
5. *Left atrium and mitral valve.* The left atrium may be seen on the LAO (left atrial append-

age seen primarily at the end of ventricular systole), left lateral, and LPO views. The mitral valve plane is best seen on the latter two views. In the 45 to 50° LAO view, the atrial appendage appears superior to the LV, and inferior to the left pulmonary vascular structures. If this space remains "active" throughout the entire cardiac cycle, and the patient is not in atrial fibrillation, then one may postulate left atrial enlargement; the possibility of mitral regurgitation should also be considered.

6. *Right ventricle.* Although the normal RV is pyramid-shaped, it may appear almost semilunar in the LAO view. In the RAO view, the tricuspid valve plane may be seen to move *toward* the RV during ventricular systole. The RV apex moves slightly toward its base during systole, but the majority of RV stroke volume is produced by motion of the free wall. Because of the limited muscle mass of this chamber, an acute increase in volume or pressure usually produces acute dilation.
7. *Left ventricle.* The normal LV myocardium is sufficiently thick to be well defined at end-diastole. The walls should normally thicken from diastole to systole; this may be used, along with wall motion, to assess the presence of ischemia and/or scarring. Papillary muscles may occasionally be seen as indentations in the posterior and septal walls in the LAO view. The antero- and posterolateral walls usually move somewhat more vigorously than the inferior (or septal) surfaces. During contraction the normal septum thickens, shortens, and moves slightly toward the left ventricular posterior wall. Significant LV dilation or hypertrophy can usually be detected on inspection.

## FUTURE DEVELOPMENTS

The future objectives in the field of nuclear cardiology are centered around efforts to obtain more and better anatomical and functional information with shorter acquisition times and less patient radiation exposure. While some of these points may seem mutually exclusive, tremendous strides are already being taken toward these goals. A few of the methods being developed are as follows:

1. *Tomography.* This approach—which uses multiplanar longitudinal gated tomography of the cardiac blood pools in the LAO and RAO views with 7-pinhole reconstruction from a wide-field camera, and 1-cm cuts— has been presented by Vogel et al.[181] Tomography appears to permit segmental wall motion analysis in three dimensions for both ventricles, as well as comparison of diastolic and systolic myocardial wall dimensions.

2. *Image filtration and background subtraction techniques.* These appear to offer great potential for improving signal-to-noise ratio on low-count images. Some of the techniques are: interpolative background subtraction;[182] nonstationary, adaptive two-dimensional image filtration for edge enhancement;[183-184] and Fourier filtering routines for phase analysis.[185,186] Verba and associates,[186] by means of Fourier filtering in both the space and time domains and using very low-count data, have been able to achieve fully automated, global and regional time-activity curve generation from all four cardiac chambers. Further, by analyzing time-activity curves on a pixel-by-pixel basis, they have been able to map the onset and progression of ventricular mechanical systole, to the extent of even detecting the site of an abnormal focus of ectopic depolarization.

3. *Coded-aperture imaging.*[187] This technique appears to combine the advantages of tomography with good sensitivity, high resolution, and accurate size scaling, and is adaptable to small, portable cameras for bedside use.

It is apparent from the above that most of these newer developments depend increasingly on computer interactions and applications. It therefore becomes even more important for the medical community at large to be at least familiar with computer "jargon," and to have some concept of the operational nature of these machines.

Nuclear cardiology is a dynamic and rapidly growing speciality, with important advances appearing almost with every new publication in the area. But more significant is its potential for contributing to patient care through the noninvasive assessment of cardiac disease and response to therapy.

## REFERENCES

1. Chirac P: De motu cordis, adversaria analytica, 1698, p. 121. Cited by Porter WT: On the results of ligation of the coronary arteries. J Physiol 15:5, 1894.
2. Morgagni JB: De sedibus et causis morborum, per anatomen indagatis, Venetiis 1761, Lib II.XXIV. 16, p. 252. Cited by Porter WT: On the results of ligation of the coronary arteries. J Physiol 15:5, 1894.
3. Heberden W: Pectoris dolor. In Commentaries on the History and Cure of Diseases. Hafner Publishing Company, New York (Facsimile edition 1962 of original 1802 edition, (p. 362).
4. Rougnon NF. Pathologisch-semiotische Betrachtungen aller Verrichtungen des menschlichen Körpers. Translated from the Latin by KG Kühn. Halle & Leipzig, 1801, Bd. I. S. 202. Cited by Porter WT: On the results of ligation of the coronary arteries. J Physiol 15:5, 1894.
5. Burns A: Observations on some of the most frequent and important diseases of the heart. Edinburgh, TT Brice, 1809. Cited in Leibowitz JO: The History of Coronary Heart Disease. University of California Press, Los Angeles, 1970.
6. Jenner E: In Parry CH: An inquiry into the symptoms and causes of the syncope anginosa, commonly called angina pectoris. R Crutwell, Bath and London, 1799.
7. Erichsen JE: On the influence of the coronary circulation on the action of the heart. The London Medical Gazette, II:561–564, 1842. Cited by Porter WT: On the results of ligation of the coronary arteries. J Physiol 15:5, 1894.
8. Virchow R: Gesammelte Abhandlungen zur wissenschaftlichen Medicin G Grote, Hamm, 1862, pp. 458,500,521.
9. Rokitansky. Cited by Duguid JB: The thrombogenic hypothesis and its implications. Postgrad Med J 36:226, 1960.
10. Bezold AV, Breymann E: Von den Veränderungen des Herzschlages nach Verschliessung der Coronarterien. Hall M: On the mutual relations between Anatomy, Physiology, Pathology, and Therapeutics. Gulstonian Lectures read at the

British Association for the Advancement of Science, June 24, 1842. Untersuchungen aus dem physiologischen Laboratorium in Wurzburg, 1867, II. S. 288–313. Cited by Porter WT: On the results of ligation of the coronary arteries. J Physiol 15:122, 1894.

11. Samuelson B: Ueber den Einfluss der Coronar-Arterien-Verschliessung auf die Herzaction. Zeitschrift fur klinische Medicin, 1881,Bd. II. S. 12–33. Cited by Porter WT: On the results of ligation of the coronary arteries. J Physiol 15:124, 1894.

12. Cohnheim J und A V Schulthess-Rechberg: Ueber die Folgen der Kranz-Arterien-Verschliessung für das Herz. Virchow's Archive, 1881, Bd. 85,S. 503–537. Cited by Porter WT: On the results of ligation of the coronary arteries. J Physiol 15:124, 1894.

13. Porter WT: On the results of ligation of the coronary arteries. J Physiol 15:121, 1894.

14. Orias O: Dynamic changes in ventricles following ligation of the ramus descendens anterior. Am J Physiol 100:629, 1932.

15. Tennant R, Wiggers CJ: The effect of coronary occlusion on myocardial contraction. Am J Physiol 112:351, 1935.

16. Harrison TR: Some unanswered questions concerning enlargement and failure of the heart. Am Heart J 69:100, 1965.

17. Klien MD, Heiman MV, Gorlin R: Hemodynamic study of left ventricular aneurysm. Circulation 35:614, 1967.

18. Herman MV, Heinle RA, Klein MD, Gorlin R: Localized disorders in myocardial contraction. N Engl J Med 277:222, 1967.

19. Tyberg JV, Yeatman LA, Parmley WW, et al: Effects of hypoxia on mechanics of cardiac contraction. Am J Physiol 218:1780, 1970.

20. Goldstein S, de Jong JW: Changes in left ventricular wall dimensions during regional myocardial ischemia. Am J Cardiol 34:56, 1974.

21. Theroux P, Franklin D, Ross J, et al: Regional myocardial function during acute coronary occlusion and its modification by pharmacologic agents in the dog. Circ Res 35:896, 1974.

22. Theroux P, Ross J, Franklin D, et al: Regional myocardial function in the conscious dog during acute coronary occlusion and responses to morphine, propranolol, nitroglycerin and lidocaine. Circulation 53:302, 1976.

23. Wyatt HL, Forrester JS, Tyberg JV, et al: Effect of graded reductions in regional coronary perfusion on regional and total cardiac function. Am J Cardiol 36:185, 1975.

24. Forrester JS, Wyatt HL, da Luz PL, et al: Functional significance of regional ischemic contraction abnormalities. Circulation 54:64, 1976.

25. Banka VS, Bodenheimer MM, Helfant RH: Relation between progressive decreases in regional coronary perfusion and contractile abnormalities. Am J Cardiol 40:200, 1977.

26. Tomoike H, Franklin D, McKown D et al: Regional myocardial dysfunction and hemodynamic abnormalities during strenuous exercise in dogs with limited coronary flow. Circ Res 42:487, 1978.

27. Rigo P, Murray M, Strauss HW, et al: Left ventricular function in acute myocardial infarction evaluated by gated scintiphotography. Circulation 50:540, 1974.

28. Cohn PF, Gorlin R, Cohn LH, et al: Left ventricular ejection fraction as a prognostic guide in the surgical treatment of coronary and valvular heart disease. Am J Cardiol 34:136, 1974.

29. Cohn PF, Gorlin R, Herman MV, et al: Relation between contractile reserve and prognosis in patients with coronary artery disease and a depressed ejection fraction. Circulation 51:414, 1975.

30. Nelson GR, Cohn PF, Gorlin R: Prognosis in medically-treated coronary artery disease. Circulation 52:408, 1975.

31. Schelbert HR, Henning H, Ashburn WL, et al: Serial measurements of left ventricular ejection fraction by radionuclide angiography early and late after myocardial infarction. Am J Cardiol 38:407, 1976.

32. Dodge HT, Sandler H, Ballew DW, et al: The use of biplane angiocardiography for the measurement of left ventricular volume in man. Am Heart J 60:762, 1960.

33. Sandler H, Dodge HG: Use of single plane angiocardiograms for the calculation of left ventricular volume in man. Am Heart J 75:325, 1968.

34. Sones FM Jr, Shirey FK: Cine coronary arteriography. Modern Concepts Cardiovasc Dis 31:735, 1962.

35. Blumgart HL, Weiss S: Studies on the velocity of blood flow: VI. The method of collecting the active deposits of radium and its preparation for intravenous injection. J Clin Invest 4:389, 1927.

36. Blumgart HL: The velocity of blood flow in health and disease. Medicine 10:1, 1931.

37. McAfee JG, Subranmanian G: Radioactive agents for imaging. In Clinical Scintillation Im-

aging. Freeman LM, Johnson PM, editors. Grune & Stratton, 1975.

38. Prinzmetal M, Corday E, Bergman HC, et al: Radiocardiography: A new method for studying the blood flow through the chambers of the heart in human beings. Science 108:340, 1948.

39. Donato L: Selective quantitative radiocardiography. Prog Cardiovasc Dis 5:1, 1962.

40. Folse R, Braunwald E: Determination of fraction of left ventricular volume ejected per beat of ventricular end-diastolic and residual volumes. Circulation 25:674, 1962.

41. Anger HO: Scintillation camera. Rev. Scint Instruments 29:27, 1958.

42. Anger HO: Gamma ray and position scintillation camera. Nucleonics 21:56, 1963.

43. Harper PV, Lathrop KA, Jiminez F et al: Technetium-99m as a scanning agent. Radiology 85:101, 1965.

44. Richards P: The technetium-99m generator. In Radioactive Pharmaceuticals. Andrews GA, Kinseley RM, Wagner HN Jr, editors. Washington, D.C., U.S. Atomic Energy Commission, 1966, pp 323–334.

45. Gottschalk A: Radioisotope scintigraphy with technetium-99m and gamma scintillation camera. Am J Roentgenol 97:860, 1966.

46. Kriss JP, Yeh SH, Farrer PA, McKean JA: Radioisotope angiography. J Nucl Med 7:367, 1966.

47. Ashburn WL, Harbert JC, Whitehouse WC et al: A video system for recording dynamic radioisotope studies with the Anger scintillation camera. J Nucl Med 9:554, 1968.

48. Mason DT, Ashburn WL, Harbert JC et al: Rapid sequential visualization of the heart and great vessels in man using the wide-field Anger scintillation camera: radioisotope-angiography following the injection of technetium-99m. Circulation 39:19, 1969.

49. Mullins CB, Mason DT, Ashburn WL, Ross J Jr: Determination of ventricular volume by radioisotope-angiography. Am J Cardiol 24:72, 1969.

50. Zaret BL, Strauss HW, Hurley PJ et al: Left ventricular ejection fraction and regional myocardial performance in man without cardiac catheterization. Circulation 42 (suppl III):120, 1970.

51. Zaret BL, Strauss HW, Hurley PJ et al: A noninvasive scintiphotographic method for detecting regional ventricular dysfunction in man. N Engl J Med 284:1165, 1971.

52. Strauss HW, Zaret BL, Hurley PJ et al: A scintiphotographic method for measuring left ventricular ejection fraction in man without cardiac catheterization. Am J Cardiol 28:575, 1971.

53. Parker JA, Secker-Walker R, Hill R et al: A new technique for the calculation of left ventricular ejection fraction. Nucl Med 13:649, 1972.

54. Secker-Walker RH, Resnick L, Kunz H et al: Measurement of left ventricular ejection fraction. J Nucl Med 14 (II):789, 1972.

55. Schelbert HR, Verba JW, Johnson AD et al: Nontraumatic determination of left ventricular ejection fraction by radionuclide angiocardiography. Circulation 51:902, 1975.

56. Lieberman DE: The fundamentals of digital nuclear medicine in Computer Methods. The C.V. Mosby Company, Saint Louis, 1977, p. 3.

57. Bachrach SL, Green MV, Borer JS: Instrumentation and data processing in cardiovascular nuclear medicine: Evaluation of ventricular function. Semin in Nucl Med 9:257, 1979.

58. Goris ML, Daspit SG, McLaughlin P, Kriss JP: Interpolative background subtraction. J Nucl Med 17:744, 1976.

59. Narahara KA, Hamilton GW, Williams DL et al: Myocardial imaging with thallium-201: An experimental model for analysis of true myocardial and background image components. J Nucl Med 18:781, 1977.

60. Pohost GM, Alpert NM, Ingwall JS et al: Thallium redistribution: mechanisms and clinical utility. Semin Nucl Med 10:70, 1980.

61. Faris JV, Burt RW, Graham MC, Knoebel SB: Improved sensitivity in detecting coronary artery disease using computer statistical analysis of thallium-201 scans. World Federation of Nuclear Medicine and Biology: Second International Congress Washington DC, Sept. 17–21, 1978, p. 93.

62. Fletcher JW, Walter KE, Witztum KF et al: Diagnosis of coronary artery disease with 201Tl: Computer analysis of myocardial perfusion images. Radiology 128:423, 1978.

63. Buell U, Kleinhans E, Seiderer M, Strauer BE: Quantitative assessment of thallium-201 images. Cardiovasc Rad 2:183,1979.

64. Folland ED, Hamilton GW, Larson SM, Kennedy JW, Williams DL, Ritchie JL: The radionuclide ejection fraction: a comparison of three radionuclide techniques with contrast angiography. J Nucl Med 18:1159, 1977.

65. Alderson PO, Wagner HN, Gomez-Moeiras JJ

et al: Simultaneous detection of myocardial perfusion and wall motion abnormalities by cinematic 201 Tl imaging. Radiology 127:531, 1978.

66. Vogel RA, Kirch D, LeFree M et al: A new method of multiplanar emission tomography using a seven pinhole collimator and an anger scintillation camera. J Nucl Med 19:648, 1978.

67. Jengo JA, Mena I, Blaufuss A et al: Evaluation of left ventricular function (ejection fraction and segmental wall motion) by single pass radioisotope angiography. Circulation 57:326, 1978.

68. Dymond DS, Jarritt PH, Britton KE et al: Detection of post infarction left ventricular aneurysm by first pass radionuclide ventriculography using a multicrystal gamma camera. Br Heart J 41:68, 1979.

69. Stokley EM, Parkey RW, Lewis SE et al: Computer processing of $^{99m}$Tc-Phosphate myocardial scintigram. Proceedings IV, International Conference on Information Processing in Scintigraphy, Paris, 1975, p. 164.

70. Kronenberg MW, Wooten NE, Friesinger GC: Scintigraphic characteristics of experimental myocardial infarct extension. Circulation 60:1130, 1979.

70a. Lewis SE, Willerson JT, Parkey RW et al: Scintigraphic methods for sizing myocardial infarction. In Clinical Nuclear Cardiology. Parkey RW, Bonte FJ, Buja LM, Willerson JT, editors. Appleton-Century-Crofts, 1979.

71. Lewis SE, Stokely EM, Bonte FJ: Physics and instrumentation. In Clinical Nuclear Cardiology. Parkey RW, Bonte FJ, Buja LM, Willerson JT, editors. Appleton-Century-Crofts, 1979.

72. Parker JA, Treves S: Radionuclide detection, localization and quantitation of intracardiac shunts and shunts between the great arteries. In Principles of Cardiovascular Nuclear Medicine. Grune & Stratton, New York, 1978, p 189.

73. Hamilton GW, Williams DL, Caldwell JH: Frame rate requirements for recording time-activity curves by radionuclide angiography. In Nuclear Cardiology: Selected Computer Aspects. Society of Nuclear Medicine, New York, 1978, p 75.

74. Ashburn WL, Schelbert HR, Verba JW: Left ventricular ejection fraction: a review of several radionuclide angiographic approaches using the scintillation camera. In Principles of Cardiovascular Nuclear Medicine. Grune & Stratton, New York, 1978, p 171.

75. Berger HJ, Matthay RA, Pylik LM et al: First-pass radionuclide assessment of right and left ventricular performance in patients with cardiac and pulmonary disease. Semin Nucl Med 9:275, 1979.

76. Wagner HN, Rigo P, Baxter RH et al: Monitoring ventricular function at rest and during exercise with a non-imaging nuclear detector. Am J Cardiol 43:975, 1979.

77. Chang W, Henkin RE, Hale DJ, Hall D: Methods for detection of left ventricular edges. Semin Nucl Med 10:39, 1980.

78. Pfisterer ME, Ricci DR, Schuler G et al: Validity of left-ventricular ejection fractions measured at rest and peak exercise by equilibrium radionuclide angiography using short acquisition times. J Nucl Med 20:484, 1979.

79. Pierson RN, Friedman MI, Tansey WA et al: Cardiovascular nuclear medicine: an overview. Semin Nucl Med 9:224, 1979.

80. Borer JS, Bachrach SL, Green MV et al: Real time radionuclide cine-angiography in the non-invasive evaluation of global and regional left ventricular function at rest and during exercise in patients with coronary artery disease. N Engl J Med 296:839, 1977.

81. Strauss HW, McKusick KA, Boucher CA: Of linens and lace—the eighth anniversary of the gated blood pool scan. Semin Nucl Med 9:296, 1979.

82. Wexler JP, Blaufox MD: Radionuclide evaluation of left ventricular function with nonimaging probes. Semin Nucl Med 9:296, 1979.

83. Burow RD, Strauss HW, Singleton R et al: Analysis of left ventricular function from multiple gated acquisition cardiac blood pool imaging. Comparison to contrast angiography. Circulation 56:1024, 1977.

84. Wackers FJTh, Berger HJ, Johnstone DE et al: Multiple gated cardiac blood pool imaging for left ventricular ejection fraction: Validation of the technique and assessment of variability. Am J Cardiol 43:1159, 1979.

85. Strauss HW, Zaret BL, Hurley PJ et al: A scintiphotographic method for measuring left ventricular ejection fraction in man without cardiac catheterization. Am J Cardiol 28:575, 1971.

86. Zaret BL, Strauss HW, Hurley PJ et al: A non-invasive scintiphotographic method for detecting regional ventricular dysfunction in man. N Engl J Med 284:1165, 1971.

87. Rigo P, Murray M, Strauss HW et al: Scintiphotographic evaluation of patients with sus-

pected left ventricular aneurysm. Circulation 50:985, 1974.

88. Berman DS, Salel AF, DeNardo GL et al: Clinical assessment of left ventricular regional contraction patterns and ejection fraction by high resolution gated scintigraphy. J Nucl Med 16:865, 1976.

89. Jengo JA, Mena I, Blaufuss A et al: Evaluation of left ventricular function (ejection fraction and segmental wall motion) by single pass radioisotope angiography. Circulation 57:326, 1978.

90. Marshall RC, Berger HJ, Reduto LA et al: Variability in sequential measures of left ventricular performance assessed with radionuclide angiocardiography. Am J Cardiol 41:531, 1978.

91. Dymond DS, Jarritt PH, Britton KE et al: Detection of post infarction left ventricular aneurysm by first pass radionuclide ventriculography using a multicrystal gamma camera. Br Heart J 41:68, 1979.

92. Botvinick EH, Shames D, Hutchinson JC et al: Noninvasive diagnosis of a false left ventricular aneurysm with radioisotope gated cardiac blood pool imaging. Differentiation from true aneurysm. Am J Cardiol 37:1089, 1976.

93. Sweet SE, Sterling R, McCormick JR et al: Left ventricular false aneurysm after coronary bypass surgery: Radionuclide diagnosis and surgical resection. Am J Cardiol 43:154, 1979.

94. Borer JS, Bacharach SL, Green MV et al: Real-time radionuclide cineangiography in the noninvasive evaluation of global and regional left ventricular function at rest and during exercise in patients with coronary-artery disease. N Engl J Med 296:839, 1977.

95. Borer J, Kent K, Bacharach S et al: Sensitivity, specificity and predictive accuracy of radionuclide cineangiography during exercise in patients with coronary artery disease. Comparison with exercise electrocardiography. Circulation 60:572, 1979.

96. Jengo J, Oren V, Conant R et al: Effects of maximal exercise stress on left ventricular function in patients with coronary artery disease using first pass radionuclide angiocardiography. A rapid, noninvasive technique for determining ejection fraction and segmental wall motion. Circulation 59:60, 1979.

97. Berger H, Reduto L, Johnstone D, et al: Global and regional left ventricular response to bicycle exercise in coronary artery disease. Assessment by quantitative radionuclide angiography. Am J Med 66:13, 1979.

98. Pfisterer ME, Battler A, Swanson SM, et al: Reproducibility of ejection-fraction determinations by equilibrium radionuclide angiography in response to supine bicycle exercise: concise communication. J Nucl Med 20:491, 1979.

99. Bodenheimer M, Banka V, Fooshee C et al: Comparison of wall motion and regional ejection fraction at rest and during isometric exercise: concise communication. J Nucl Med 20:724, 1979.

100. Maddox DE, Wynne J, Uren R et al: Regional ejection fraction: A quantitative radionuclide index of regional left ventricular performance. Circulation 59:1001, 1979.

101. Schad N: Nontraumatic assessment of left ventricular wall motion and regional stroke volume after myocardial infarction. J Nucl Med 18:333, 1977.

102. Maddox DE, Holman BL, Wynne J et al: Ejection fraction image: A noninvasive index of regional left ventricular wall motion. Am J Cardiol 41:1230, 1978.

103. Holman BL, Wynne J, Idoine J, et al: The paradox image: A noninvasive index of regional left-ventricular dyskinesis. J Nucl Med 20:1237, 1979.

104. Okada RD, Pohost GM, Kirshenbaum HD, et al: Radionuclide-determined change in pulmonary blood volume with exercise. Improved sensitivity of multigated blood-pool scanning in detecting coronary-artery disease. N Engl J Med 301:569, 1979.

105. Bourguignon MH, Wagner HN Jr: Noninvasive measurement of ventricular pressure throughout systole. Am J Cardiol 44:466, 1979.

106. Slutsky R, Gordon D, Karliner J et al: Assessment of early ventricular systole by first pass radionuclide angiography: Useful method for detection of left ventricular dysfunction at rest in patients with coronary artery disease. Am J Cardiol 44:459, 1979.

107. McEwan P, Newman G, Portwood J et al: Correlation of rest and exercise radionuclide angiocardiographic ventricular function with the number of significantly stenosed vessels in 230 patients with coronary artery disease. J Nucl Med 20:687, 1979 (Abstr.).

108. Bryson AL, Aycock AC, Flamm MD et al: Changes in regional ventricular contraction of the arteriosclerotic heart following nitroglycerin administration—surgical correlation. Circulation 50 (suppl III):44, 1974 (Abstr).

109. Pine R, Meister RG, Helfant RH et al: Nitroglycerine to unmask reversible asynergy: Coro-

lation with post coronary bypass ventriculography. Circulation 50:108, 1974.

110. McAnulty JH, Hattenhauer MT, Rosch J et al: Improvement in left ventricular wall motion following nitroglycerin. Circulation 51:140, 1975.

111. Salel AF, Berman DS, DeNardo GL et al: Radionuclide assessment of nitroglycerin influence on abnormal left ventricular segmental contraction in patients with coronary heart disease. Circulation 53:975, 1976.

112. Berman D, Maddahi J, Charuzi Y, et al: Evaluation of left ventricular function during sitting bicycle exercise by multiple gated scintigraphy: Validation and clinical application in coronary disease. J Nucl Med 19:771, 1978 (Abstr).

113. Borer JS, Bacharach SL, Green MV et al: Effect of nitroglycerin on exercise-induced abnormalities of left ventricular regional function and ejection fraction in coronary artery disease. Assessment by radionuclide cineangiography in symptomatic and asymptomatic patients. Circulation 57:314, 1978.

114. Ritchie JL, Sorensen SG, Kennedy JW et al: Radionuclide angiography: Noninvasive assessment of hemodynamic changes after administration of nitroglycerin. Am J Cardiol 43:278, 1979.

115. Slutsky R, Curtis G, Battler, A et al: Effect of sublingual nitroglycerin on left ventricular function at rest and during spontaneous angina pectoris: Assessment with a radionuclide approach. Am J Cardiol 44:1365, 1979.

116. Stephens JD, Dymond DS, Spurrell RAJ: Radionuclide and hemodynamic assessment of left ventricular functional reserve in patients with left ventricular aneurysm and congestive cardiac failure. Response to exercise stress and isosorbide dinitrate. Circulation 61:536, 1980.

117. Port S, Cobb FR, Jones RH: Effects of propranolol on left ventricular function in normal men. Circulation 61:358, 1980.

118. Port S, Cobb FR, Jones RH: Effects of propranolol on left ventricular function in normal men. (Abstr) Circulation 59,60 (suppl II):351, 1979.

119. Sorensen SG, Ritchie JL, Caldwell JH: Serial exercise radionuclide angiography. Validation of count-derived changes in cardiac output and quantitation of maximal exercise ventricular volume change after nitroglycerin and propranolol in normal men. Circulation 61:600, 1980.

120. Marshall RC, Berger HJ, Costin JC et al: As-

sessment of cardiac performance with quantitative radionuclide angiocardiography. Sequential left ventricular ejection fraction, normalized left ventricular ejection rate, and regional wall motion. Circulation 56:820, 1977.

121. Marshall, RC, Berger HJ, Reduto, LA et al: Assessment of cardiac performance with quantitative radionuclide angiocardiography. Effects of oral propranolol on global and regional left ventricular function in coronary artery disease. Circulation 58:808, 1978.

122. Reduto LA, Berger HJ, Geha A, et al: Radionuclide assessment of ventricular performance during propranolol withdrawal prior to aortocoronary bypass surgery. Am Heart J 96:714, 1978.

123. Steele PP, Maddoux G, Kirsch DL et al: Effects of propranolol and nitroglycerin on left ventricular performance in patients with coronary artery disease. Chest 73:19, 1978.

124. Marshall RC, Wisenberg G, Schelbert H et al: Radionuclide evaluation of the effect of oral propranolol on left ventricular function during exercise in patients with coronary artery disease. Am J Cardiol 43:398, 1979 (Abstr).

125. Battler A, Ross Jr, J, Slutsky R et al: Improvement of exercise-induced left ventricular dysfunction with oral propranolol in patients with coronary heart disease. Am J Cardiol 44:318, 1979.

125a. Slutsky R, Karliner J, Battler A et al: Reproducibility of ejection fraction in ventricular volume by gated radionuclide angiography after myocardial infarction. Radiology 132:155, 1979.

126. Podrid P, Zielonka J, Wynne J et al: The effects of rapid digitalization on left ventricular function. (Abstr) Circulation 59,60 (suppl II):348, 1979.

127. Morton M, McNulty J, Rahimtoola S: Acute digitalization shifts the ventricular function curve in man. (Abstr) Circulation 59,60 (suppl II):349, 1979.

128. Nixon JV, Harper J, Jones J, Mullins CB: Effects of acute digitalization on left and right ventricular function in chronic pulmonary hypertension. (Abstr) Circulation 59,60 (suppl II):499, 1979.

129. Slutsky, R, Gerber, K, Hooper, W, et al.: The effect of subcutaneous terbutaline on the left ventricle; evidence for an inotropic effect. Chest, in press.

130. Kent KM, Borer JS, Green MV, et al: Effects of coronary-artery bypass on global and re-

gional left ventricular function during exercise. N Engl J Med 298:1434, 1978.

131. Rigo P, Alderson PO, Robertson RM et al: Measurement of aortic and mitral regurgitation by gated cardiac blood pool scans. Circulation 60:306, 1979.

132. Baxter RH, Becker LC, Alderson PO et al: Quantification of aortic valvular regurgitation in dogs by nuclear imaging. Circulation 61:404, 1980.

133. Alexander J, Dainiak N, Berger HJ, et al: Serial assessment of doxorubicin cardiotoxicity with quantitative radionuclide angiocardiography. N Engl J Med 300:278, 1979.

134. Henderson IC, Frei E III: Adriamycin and the heart. N Engl J Med 300:310, 1979.

135. Maddahi J, Berman DS, Matsuoka DT et al: A new technique for assessing right ventricular ejection fraction using rapid multiple-gated equilibrium cardiac blood pool scintigraphy. Circulation 60:581, 1979.

136. Slutsky R, Hooper K, Gerber K et al: Assessment of right ventricular function at rest and during exercise in patients with coronary heart disease: a new approach using equilibrium radionuclide angiography. Am J Cardiol 45:63, 1980.

137. Steele P, Kirch D, LeFree M et al: Measurement of right and left ventricular ejection fractions by radionuclide angiocardiography in coronary artery disease. Chest 70:51, 1976.

138. Maddahi J, Berman D, Matsuoka D et al: Right ventricular ejection fraction at rest and during exercise in normals and in coronary artery disease patients: Assessment by multiple gated equilibrium scintigraphy. J Nucl Med 20:625, 1979.

139. Johnson LL, McCarthy DM, Sciacca RR et al: Right ventricular ejection fraction during exercise in patients with coronary artery disease. Circulation 60:1284, 1979.

140. Berger HJ, Johnstone DE, Sands JM et al: Response of right ventricular ejection fraction to upright bicycle exercise in coronary artery disease. Circulation 60:1292, 1979.

141. Berger HJ, Matthay RA, Loke J et al: Assessment of cardiac performance with quantitative radionuclide angiocardiography: Right ventricular ejection fraction with reference to findings in chronic obstructive pulmonary disease. Am J Cardiol 41:897, 1978.

142. Slutsky R, Karliner J, Ricci D et al: Left ventricular volumes by gated equilibrium radionu-

clide angiography: A new Method. Circulation 60:556, 1979.

143. Slutsky R, Karliner J, Ricci D et al: Response of left ventricular volume to exercise in man assessed by radionuclide equilibrium angiography. Circulation 60:565, 1979.

144. Dehmer GJ, Lewis SE, Hillis LD et al: Nongeometric determination of left ventricular volumes from equilibrium blood pool scans. Am J Cardiol 45:293, 1980.

145. Bruschke AVG, Proudfit WL, Sones FM Jr: Progress study of 590 consecutive nonsurgical cases of coronary disease followed 5-9 years. II. Ventriculographic and other correlations. Circulation 47:1154, 1973.

146. Murray JA, Chinn N, Peterson DR: Influence of left ventricular function on early prognosis in atherosclerotic heart disease. Am J Cardiol 33:159, 1974.

147. Nelson GR, Cohn PF, Gorlin R: Prognosis in medically-treated coronary artery disease. Circulation 52:408, 1975.

148. Lea RE, Tector AJ, Flemma RJ et al: Prognostic significance of a reduced ejection fraction in coronary artery surgery. Circulation 46 (suppl II):49, 1972.

149. Hammermeister KE, Kennedy JW: Predictors of surgical mortality in patients undergoing direct myocardial revascularization. Circulation 50 (suppl II):112, 1974.

150. Cohn PF, Gorlin R, Cohn LH et al: Left ventricular ejection fraction as a prognostic guide in the surgical treatment of coronary and valvular heart disease. Am J Cardiol 34:136, 1974.

151. Cohn PF, Gorlin R, Herman MV et al: Relation between contractile reserve and prognosis in patients with coronary artery disease and a depressed ejection fraction. Circulation 51:414, 1975.

152. Karliner JS, Bouchard RJ, Gault JH: Hemodynamic effects of radiographic contrast media in man: A beat by beat analysis. Br Heart J 34:347, 1972.

153. Kostuk WJ, Ehsani AA, Karliner JS et al. Left ventricular performance after myocardial infarction assessed by radioisotope angiocardiography. Circulation 47:242, 1973.

154. Rigo P, Murray M, Strauss HW et al: Left ventricular function in acute myocardial infarction evaluated by gated scintiphotography. Circulation 50:678, 1974.

155. Rigo P, Murray M, Taylor DR et al: Right ventricular dysfunction detected by gated scin-

tiphotography in patients with acute inferior myocardial infarction. Circulation 52:268, 1975.

156. Sharpe DN, Botvinick Eh, Shames DM, et al: The noninvasive diagnosis of right ventricular infarction. Circulation 57:483, 1978.

157. Tobinick E, Schelbert HR, Henning H, et al: Right ventricular ejection fraction in patients with acute anterior and inferior myocardial infarction assessed by radionuclide angiography. Circulation 57:1078, 1978.

158. Reduto LA, Berger HJ, Cohen LS, et al: Sequential radionuclide assessment of left and right ventricular performance after acute transmural myocardial infarction. Ann of Intern Med 89:441, 1978.

159. Schelbert HR, Henning H, Ashburn WL et al: Serial measurements of left ventricular ejection fraction by radionuclide angiography early and late after myocardial infarction. Am J Cardiol 38:407, 1976.

160. Shah PK, Pichler M, Berman DS et al: Left ventricular ejection fraction determined by radionuclide ventriculography in early stages of first transmural myocardial infarction. Relation to short-term prognosis. Am J Cardiol 45:542, 1980.

161. Schulze RA Jr, Rouleau J, Rigo P et al: Ventricular arrhythmias in the late hospital phase of acute myocardial infarction. Relation to left ventricular function detected by gated cardiac blood pool scanning. Circulation 52:1006, 1975.

162. Ritchie JL, Hamilton GW, Trobaugh GB et al: Myocardial imaging and radionuclide angiography in survivors of sudden cardiac death due to ventricular fibrillation: preliminary report. Am J Cardiol 39:852, 1977.

163. Battler A, Slutsky R, Karliner J et al: Left ventricular ejection fraction early after acute myocardial infarction: Value for predicting mortality and morbidity. Am J Cardiol 45:197, 1980.

164. Wynne J, Sayres M, Maddox DE et al: Regional left ventricular function in acute myocardial infarction: evaluation with quantitative radionuclide ventriculography. Am J Cardiol 45:203, 1980.

165. Ramanathan KB, Bodenheimer MM, Banka VS et al. Severity of contraction abnormalities after acute myocardial infarction in man: response to nitroglycerin. Circulation 60:1230, 1979.

166. Bodenheimer M, Banka V, Helfant R: Nuclear Cardiology. I. Radionuclide angiographic assessment of left ventricular contraction: uses,

limitations and future directions. Am J Cardiol 45:661, 1980.

166a. Morrison J, Coromilas J, Robbins M et al: Digitalis and myocardial infarction in man. Circulation 62:8, 1980.

167. Pulido JI, Doss J, Tweig D et al: Submaximal exercise testing after acute myocardial infarction: myocardial scintigraphic and electrocardiographic observations. Am J Cardiol 42:19, 1978.

168. Haskell WL, DeBusk R: Cardiovascular responses to repeated treadmill exercise testing soon after myocardial infarction. Circulation 60:1247, 1979.

169. Sami M, Kraemer H, DeBusk RF: The prognostic significance of serial exercise testing after myocardial infarction. Circulation 60:1238, 1979.

170. Davidson DM, DeBusk RF: Prognostic value of a single exercise test 3 weeks after uncomplicated myocardial infarction. Circulation 61:236, 1980.

170a. Borer JS, Rosing DR, Miller RH, et al: Natural history of left ventricular function during one year after acute myocardial infarction: Comparison with clinical, electrocardiographic and bio-chemical determinations. Am J Cardiol 46:1, 1980.

171. Hamilton GW: Myocardial imaging with thallium-201: the controversy over its clinical usefulness in ischemic heart disease. J Nucl Med 20:1201, 1979.

172. Hellman C, Carpenter J, Garner T et al: Reversible left ventricular dysfunction: unmasking by 2-view radionuclide angiography. (Abstr) J Nucl Med 20:662, 1979.

173. Caldwell J, Ritchie J, Hamilton G et al: Comparative sensitivity and specificity of exercise radionuclide ventriculography and rest-exercise thallium imaging in the detection of coronary artery disease. (Abstr) J Nucl Med 20:687, 1979.

174. Slutsky R, Battler A, Gerber K et al: Effect of nitrates on left ventricular size and function during exercise: comparison of sublingual nitroglycerin and nitroglycerin paste. Am J Cardiol 45:831, 1980.

175. Chervu LR: Radiopharmaceuticals in cardiovascular nuclear medicine. Semin Nucl Med 9:241, 1979.

176. Pierson RN Jr, Friedman MI, Tansey WA et al: Cardiovascular nuclear medicine: an overview. Semin Nucl Med 9:224, 1979.

177. Brady TJ, Thrall JH, Lo K et al: Sensitivity

of exercise radionuclide ventriculography in coronary artery disease detection: importance of adequate exercise. (Abstr) J Nucl Med 20:687, 1979.

178. Brash HM, Wraith PK, Hannan WJ, Dewhurst NG, Muir AL. The influence of ectopic heart beats in gated ventricular blood pool studies. J Nucl Med 21:391, 1980.

179. Bacharach SL, Green MV, Borer JS, Ostrow HG, Bonow RO, Farkas SP, Johnston GS. Beat-by-beat validation of ECG gating. J Nucl Med 21:307, 1980.

180. Murphy PH, ECG gating: Does it adequately monitor ventricular contraction? (Editorial) J Nucl Med 21:399, 1980.

181. Vogel RA, Krich DL LeFree MT, Rainwater JO, Jensen DO, Steele PP: Tomographic gated blood pool scintigraphy using a wide-field scintillation camera. J Nucl Med 20:643, 1979.

182. Goris ML, Daspit SG, McLaughlin P, et al: Interpolative background subtraction. Proc. Sixth Symp on Sharing of Comp Progs and Tech in Nucl Med, Atlanta, 1976, pp. 350–360.

183. Chesler DA: Resolution enhancement by variable filtering. Massachusetts General Hospital Physics Laboratory Report, January 1969 (unpublished).

184. Chesler DA: An algorithm for non-stationary filtering of scintigrams. Massachusetts General Hospital Laboratory Communication, 1975 (unpublished).

185. Adam WE, Tarkowska A, Bitter F et al: Equilibrium (gated) radionuclide ventriculography. Cardiovascular Radiology 2:161, 1979.

186. Verba JW, Bornstein I, Bhargava V et al: Complete cycle global and regional volume analysis of gated radionuclide cardiac studies. Proc Soc Nucl Med 3rd Ann West Reg Mtg, Vancouver, B. C., 1978, H2 (abstract).

187. Rogers, WL, Koral KF, Mayans R et al: Coded-aperture imaging of the heart. J Nucl Med 21:371, 1980.

# 29 | *M-Mode Echocardiography*

*Michael H. Crawford, M.D.*

Repeated evaluations of cardiac anatomy and performance in patients suffering from acute myocardial infarction would be of considerable value for planning treatment and assessing prognosis. In the setting of an acute myocardial infarction, this would be best accomplished by a noninvasive technique. There are certain obvious advantages of M-mode echocardiography for this purpose: (1) in comparison to plain radiographic or radionuclide angiographic studies, more specific anatomic detail can be learned from an echocardiographic examination; (2) there is no radiation hazard with echocardiography; and (3) the equipment used for M-mode echocardiography is much more portable and considerably less costly than radiographic or radionuclide equipment. Therefore, echocardiography would seem to be an ideal technique for evaluating cardiac anatomy and performance during acute myocardial infarction.

To fulfill this potential, M-mode echocardiography ideally should provide certain types of information: (1) an estimate of the extent of tissue damage due to the acute myocardial infarction; (2) an evaluation of overall left ventricular performance; (3) an assessment of the various complications of myocardial infarction, such as heart failure, papillary muscle dysfunction, myocardial rupture, thrombus formation, and pericarditis; and (4) the echocardiogram should provide prognostic information that would be of value in planning the overall approach to the patient. The purpose of this chapter is to discuss how well M-mode echocardiography meets the above goals of a noninvasive technique for evaluating cardiac anatomy and performance following acute myocardial infarction

## TECHNIQUE

The basic technique of M-mode echocardiography is to (1) apply a high frequency sound-emitting transducer to the chest wall; (2) send pulses of sound through the tissue; and (3) subsequently receive echoes back from the tissue, which can then be translated into anatomic information. The type of transducer is very important for the evaluation of a patient with myocardial infarction. Many such patients are heavy smokers, since this is a risk factor for coronary artery disease, and they have varying degrees of chronic obstructive pulmonary disease. This disease is often associated with increased expansion of the lungs, which tends to push the heart more centrally in the chest behind the relatively echo-dense sternum. Also, the amount of lung tissue between the anterior chest wall and the heart is increased. Since sound waves do not travel well through air, the lungs serve as a barrier to the penetration of high frequency ultrasound. For this reason, it is often useful to use lower frequency transducers that tend to penetrate air better than the higher frequency

717

transducers. For example, we find that a 1.9 mHz transducer is much more useful in these patients than is the standard 2.25 mHz transducer. Occasionally, in an extremely difficult patient, a 1.6 mHz transducer will be necessary. Transducers of a lower frequency than 1.6 mHz usually do not provide sufficient image clarity to be used for cardiac work. Also, the diameter of the crystal face on the transducer is important for penetration. With a larger diameter (within certain limits), there is less dispersion of the sound waves, allowing the sound beam to penetrate deeper. Therefore, a ¾-inch diameter transducer is often better than a ¼-inch transducer for this type of work. Also, a transducer focused at 10 cm is better than one focused at the standard 7 cm because of the deeper penetration necessary. Thus, careful transducer selection can be an important aspect of achieving high quality M-mode echocardiograms in patients with acute myocardial infarction.

In the usual M-mode echocardiographic evaluation, the transducer is placed along the left sternal border in the second, third, fourth, or fifth interspaces until the mitral valve can be visualized without extreme angulation of the transducer. This has been called the standard interspace technique and serves as a reference for identifying other structures and for measuring left ventricular dimensions at the minor axis of the presumed elliptical left ventricle.[1] Often, it is necessary, with this transducer placement, to roll the patient in the left lateral decubitus position so that the heart is further to the left side. This is especially important for visualizing the right ventricle and the interventricular septum as part of the evaluation of the left ventricle. In patients with obstructive lung disease and medial position of the heart, it is often easier to visualize the left ventricle from the subxyphoid transducer position.[2] This is best accomplished by positioning the patient's upper torso at a 30° angle, flexing the knees somewhat to relax the abdomen, and placing the transducer where the cardiac impulse is felt in the subxyphoid area. Again, the mitral valve should be located as the reference point for this examination. The right and left ventricles are easily seen by angulating the transducer inferior to the mi-

tral valve. The great vessels and left atrium are less well appreciated from this position because they are parallel to the sound beam.[3]

Once the appropriate transducer is selected and the proper position is found for the patient and the transducer, it is then necessary to select different views to provide the anatomic and functional information sought. One of the more useful procedures is the slow sector-scan sweep, where the transducer is first placed perpendicular to the chest wall such that the mitral valve can be seen, and then is slowly angulated superomedially until the aortic valve and left atrium are visualized. Subsequently, the transducer is angulated inferolaterally until the left ventricle at the level of the chordae tendineae is seen. Usually at the three different levels, that is the aorta/left atrium, the mitral valve, and the left ventricle at the chordal level, several recordings are made without moving the transducer. Another useful technique is the linear scan, wherein the transducer is slowly moved over the chest wall along the long axis of the heart in order to visualize more of the left ventricular apex or the great vessels, depending on the area of interest. This can be useful in searching for aortic dissection or left ventricular abnormalities near the apex.

In order to do a high quality M-mode echocardiographic study, it is necessary to have a strip chart recorder attached to the ultrasonograph. This enables one to continuously run paper and record during transducer movement. Most recorders are now supplied with a choice of different types of paper to suit various needs. There are also a variety of methods for developing the paper. Another important feature of the recording equipment should be the ability to record other cardiac events such as the electrocardiogram, phonocardiogram, and various external pulse waves. This is very important for a complete echocardiographic evaluation since the heart sounds and pulse waves are very useful for timing purposes, and both can add important additional information. In our laboratory we routinely record electrocardiographic lead II, the phonocardiogram at the base, and the carotid pulse tracing with each echocardiogram.

## MEASUREMENTS

From the echocardiographic recordings described above, certain measurements have been made, which appear to have clinical utility. The normal left ventricle is best described by a prolate ellipse formula in which the major axis (L) equals two times the minor axis (D). If one assumes that the left ventricular echo at the level of the chordae tendineae approximates the minor axis of the left ventricular ellipse, then the volume (V) of the ventricle can be calculated in both systole and diastole utilizing the formulae described below:

$$V = \frac{\pi}{6} D^2 L$$

$$V = \frac{\pi}{6} D^2 2D$$

$$V = 1.047 \, D^3$$

$$V \simeq D^3$$

Thus, left ventricular volumes can be approximated from a very simple expression. From volume calculations in systole (s) and diastole (d), one can calculate the ejection fraction (EF) and the stroke volume (SV):

$$EF = \frac{D^3 d - D^3 s}{D^3 d} \times 100\%$$

$$SV = D^3 \text{diastole} - D^3 \text{systole}$$

Recently, there has been some controversy over how exactly to measure the end-diastolic and end-systolic dimensions of the left ventricle, and there is no clear consensus.[4,5] Since there is no evidence showing the clear superiority of one technique over another, our current technique, which has been validated versus both biplane and single plane cineangiography,[4,6] is described below. The end-diastolic dimension is measured at the peak of the R wave of the QRS complex on the simultaneously recorded electrocardiogram, using the inner or apposing edges of the endocardium of the interventricular septum and posterior left ventricular wall. End-systole is measured in the same fashion as the smallest dimension in systole, whether or not the two walls are exactly apposed. These measurements are illustrated in Figure 29.1

The estimation of left ventricular volumes by echocardiography has been relatively accurate in most laboratories where it has been compared with the results of cineangiography.[7-9] However, some laboratories have noted that in large spherical ventricles the relationship between the minor and major axis is different from that of an ellipse. Therefore, the ellipse formula tends to overestimate volume. Similarly, in very small ventricles, as in patients with mitral stenosis, the ventricle is more cigar-shaped than elliptical and the formula tends to underestimate left ventricular volumes. For this reason, some laboratories have developed regression equations to account for these discrepancies.[10,11] However, each of these equations is different and no uniformly acceptable regression equation has been established.[12] Therefore, we recommend using the ellipse formula described above, realizing its limitations in ventricles that are very large or very small.

Another problem with the elliptical model for the left ventricle occurs in patients with

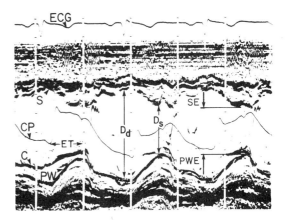

Fig. 29.1 Left ventricular echogram at the level of the chordae illustrates various measurements (see text). C = chordae tendineae; CP = indirect carotid pulse tracing; Dd = left ventricular end-diastolic dimension; Ds = left ventricular end-systolic dimension; ECG = electrocardiogram; ET = ejection time; S = interventricular septum; SE = septal excursion. PW = posterior wall; PWE = posterior wall excursion.

ischemic heart disease. Often, such patients have segmental contraction abnormalities that produce gross distortions in chamber shape. These distortions are most marked in systole, where areas may move very sluggishly (hypokinetic), not move at all (akinetic), or paradoxically bulge during systole (dyskinetic). These aberrations in shape not only make volume estimates based on an elliptical formula inaccurate, but one minor dimension measured by M-mode echocardiography may be grossly inaccurate as a reflection of overall left ventricular performance due to wall motion abnormalities in this or other areas not in the echo beam.[13] Therefore, the estimate of end-systolic size in patients with coronary artery disease, especially those who have sustained a myocardial infarction, is unreliable. The estimation of end-diastolic size, however, should be more accurate since wall motion abnormalities are not evident in diastole unless there is aneurysm formation. Therefore, in the setting of acute myocardial infarction, we are limited to estimating left ventricular end-diastolic volume alone, realizing the limitations of this estimate in extremely large or very small ventricles, and in those with aneurysm formation.

Measuring the dimensions of other chambers also provides useful information in the assessment of patients with acute myocardial infarction. The left atrium is measured at the point where the aortic leaflets are visualized. This measurement is usually taken at end-systole, when the atrium is largest, from the inner edge of the posterior aortic wall to the inner edge of the posterior left atrial wall. This value is less than 4 cm in normal adults.[14] The aorta at the same location is customarily measured at end-diastole, from the outer edge of its anterior wall to the inner edge of its posterior wall. The upper limit for this measurement in an adult is also 4 cm.[15] The right ventricle is usually measured at the same location as the left ventricle, where the chordae tendineae of the left ventricle are visualized from the standard interspace. For this measurement, the apposing endocardial surfaces of the right ventricle are measured at end-diastole. Because of the irregular shape of the right ventricle, no suitable formulae have been derived for use with M-mode

echocardiography to estimate volume. Consequently, systolic size is rarely measured. The upper limit of normal for the diastolic right ventricular dimension in the left lateral decubitis position in an adult is 2.6 cm.[15]

In addition to measurements of overall chamber size, M-mode echocardiography has been used to assess the functional status of small regions of the left ventricle. One early measurement of regional performance was wall excursion, which is the amplitude of wall motion from end-diastole to end-systole (Fig. 29.1). Because of the anterior motion of the entire heart during systole, posterior wall endocardial excursion is greater than that of the interventricular septum. Normal posterior wall excursion at the level of the chordae tendineae is 1.0 to 1.4 cm and normal septal excursion at the same location is 0.5 to 1.0 cm (unpublished data). If the left ventricular ejection time (ET) has been measured via an indirect carotid pulse tracing, one can calculate velocity (Vel) of motion of the posterior wall or the septum by the following formula:

$$\text{Vel} = \frac{\text{wall excursion}}{\text{ET}}$$

These velocities can also be normalized for the size of the left ventricle by dividing the result by the end-diastolic dimension. Posterior wall velocity ranges from 2.7 to 5.2 cm/sec and normalized posterior wall velocity is between 0.52 and 1.04 $\text{sec}^{-1}$ in normal individuals.[16] These amplitude and velocity measurements are quite useful in defining the function of individual segments of the myocardium, but do not reflect overall left ventricular performance, especially in patients with segmental myocardial disease.[17]

Studies in animals have shown that one of the earliest changes after acute myocardial infarction is a lack of contractile function of the involved myocardium. This results in the thinning of this segment of the myocardium and a lack of systolic thickening. These changes, which have been detected by M-mode echo in dogs and man,[18] can be quantitated by measuring wall thickness at end-diastole and end-systole and calculating the percent change in thickness. Posterior wall thickness is usually measured from the cavity side of the endocar-

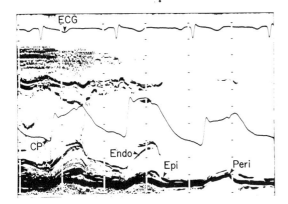

Fig. 29.2 Left ventricular echogram during progressive gain decrease to identify the various layers of the heart. Endo = endocardium; Epi = epicardium; Peri = pericardium.

dial echo to the myocardial side of the left ventricular epicardium. Accurate assessment of wall thickness is enhanced by decreasing the ultrasound gain to clearly identify various structures adjacent to the walls (Fig. 29.2). The thickness of the posterior wall and septum are usually less than 1.2 cm.[15] Percent thickening is usually higher for the posterior wall, averaging about 84 percent versus 49 percent for the septum.[19]

Several problems inherent in measuring the thickness of ventricular walls should be taken into consideration when evaluating the measurements. First, reproducibility has not been high.[19] Part of the reason for this is that the resolution of M-mode echocardiography is about 1 mm and the structure being measured is about 10 mm. Thus, there is an inherent 10 percent baseline error in the technique. Also, there are problems with echo dropout due to poor angle of incidence of the sound beam, which is a very vexing problem, particularly with weak echo-producing structures such as the endocardium of the posterior wall.[20]

Because of the problems of using the dimensional measurements of the left ventricle during systole as a measure of overall left ventricular performance in patients with coronary artery disease, there has been considerable interest in evaluating the motion pattern of other structures that may reflect the performance of the left ventricle. The major structure evaluated in this regard is the motion of the mitral valve.

Studies have examined the amplitude of anterior leaflet opening, the timing of the diastolic motion and systolic motion of the leaflets, and the position of the mitral valve in the ventricle.[21] The AC segment of the normal mitral valve anterior leaflet echogram, which represents the time period between atrial contraction and closure of the mitral leaflets during early systole, has been found to be a useful tool for estimating left ventricular end-diastolic pressure.[22] Often in patients with increased left ventricular end-diastolic pressure, there is a bump produced in the otherwise smooth descent of the leaflet from the A point to the C point, which has been labeled the B-hump (Fig. 29.3). This abnormality is usually accompanied by a prolongation of the AC interval in relationship to the electrocardiographic PR interval. The normal PR-AC interval is usually more than 60 msec. Although a short PR-AC interval usually indicates impairment of left ventricular performance, the exact left ventricular end-diastolic pressure cannot be predicted from this measure.[23]

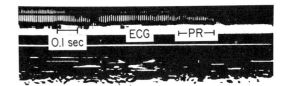

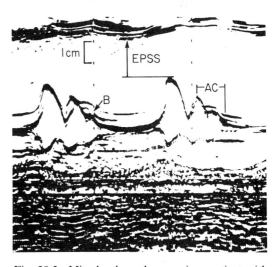

Fig. 29.3 Mitral valve echogram in a patient with reduced left ventricular performance following an anteroseptal myocardial infarction (see text). EPSS = E point septal separation.

Another feature of left ventricular failure is spherical dilatation of the ventricle, which places the mitral valve leaflets toward the center of the left ventricular cavity. This increases the distance between the E point (maximum early diastolic opening) and the interventricular septum (Fig. 29.3). This E point septal separation is usually less than 5 mm in normal individuals; larger values have been found to correlate fairly well with left ventricular ejection fraction in patients with chronic ischemic heart disease.[24]

Finally, M-mode echocardiography can be extremely useful for detecting pericardial effusion. For this examination, the damping or gain of the echocardiograph is progressively decreased until only the strongest echo-producing structures can be visualized. One of these structures is the pericardium. When it is identified, the gain is then returned and the relationship of the pericardium to the myocardium is evaluated. A space between these two structures, especially if the pericardium does not move along with the rest of the myocardium, is highly suggestive of pericardial effusion and is very sensitive for detecting a small amount of pericardial fluid[25] (Fig. 29.4). This examination should be done at the level of the left ventricle, where the heart is surrounded by lung, which serves as an excellent backdrop for visualizing the pericardium clearly. If the more basal segments of the heart are utilized, echoes from mediastinal structures, such as the esophagus, can cause confusion. Another potential source of error

is the presence of a pleural effusion. It is best if one has a chest X-ray film to examine in advance to be sure that a pleural effusion on the left side is not falsely producing the diagnosis of pericardial fluid.

## GENERAL APPLICATIONS IN PATIENTS WITH ACUTE MYOCARDIAL INFARCTION

One of the first questions to be discussed is whether the M-mode echocardiographic techniques described above can be useful for the diagnosis of acute myocardial infarction. As discussed, patients with acute myocardial infarction would be expected to have an area of decreased thickness and reduced thickening during systole. Corya and associates[26] have commented that systolic thinning is seen almost exclusively in patients with acute myocardial infarction. This finding was most common in the septum of patients with anterior infarction

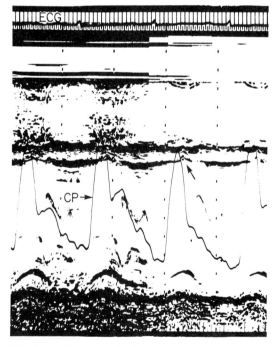

Fig. 29.5 Left ventricular echogram in a patient with stable angina pectoris that demonstrates systolic thinning and paradoxical motion of the septum. (Note arrow during the third systole from the left on the left side of the septum.)

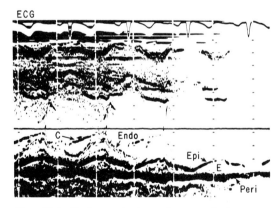

Fig. 29.4 Left ventricular echogram during progressive gain decrease to identify the pericardium in a patient with a small pericardial effusion (E). (Compare to Fig. 29.2.)

and was seen less frequently in the posterior wall. Similar findings were reported by Fujii et al.[27] However, systolic thinning is not completely specific for acute infarction and has been observed in some patients with chronic coronary artery disease (Fig. 29.5). Furthermore, not all patients with acute myocardial infarction exhibit systolic thinning.

A more common finding in patients with acute myocardial infarction has been some area of abnormal wall excursion. Heikkila and Nieminen,[28] using multiple transducer positions, found some evidence of abnormal wall motion in all 30 of their patients with acute myocardial infarction. Corya and associates [29] found that 84 percent of 64 patients with acute myocardial infarction had detectable wall motion abnormalities, using linear scanning. Para-

doxical septal motion was frequently seen in patients with anterior infarction (Fig. 29.5), whereas posteroinferior infarctions usually showed hypokinesis or akinesis. Another interesting finding was the frequent detection of increased wall excursion in the noninvolved areas of the myocardium (Fig. 29.6).

Follow-up studies of patients with acute myocardial infarction have shown that these wall motion abnormalities decrease with time, but abnormal excursion and thickening of the involved walls persists in many cases.[27,29] Some patients develop thin walls with increased echo density, which has been shown to be scar tissue in selected patients [30] (Fig. 29.7). These features have been used to detect chronic ischemic heart disease and identify areas of previous myocardial infarction in patients suspected of having

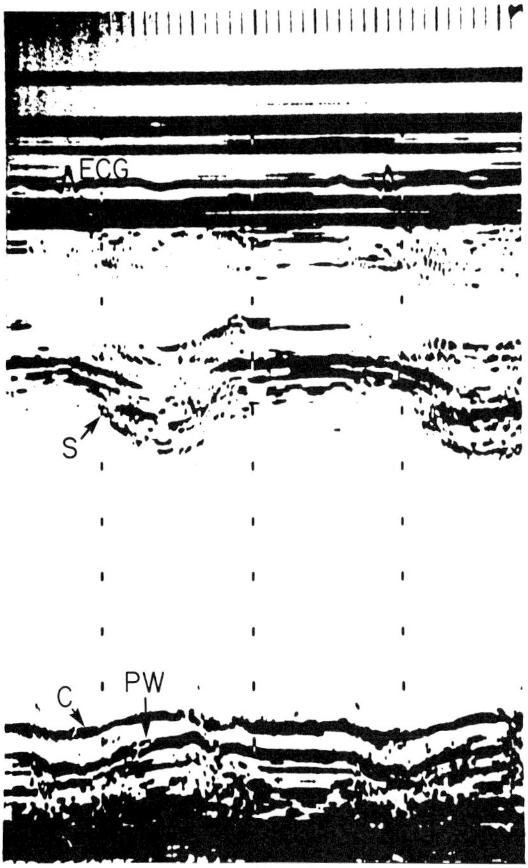

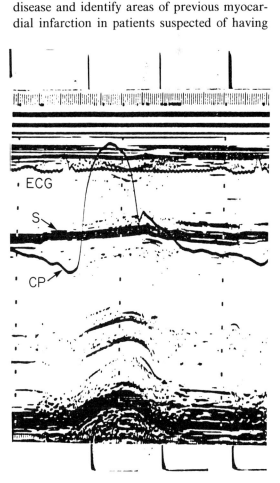

Fig. 29.6 Left ventricular echogram showing hypercontractile function of the interventricular septum with reduced motion of the posterior wall in a patient with an inferior myocardial infarction.

Fig. 29.7 Left ventricular echogram showing a thin dense septal echo in a patient with a previous anteroseptal infarction, which probably represents scar tissue.

coronary artery disease.[31-34] Except for the almost exclusive finding of wall thinning in the patient with acute myocardial infarction, the echocardiogram alone cannot distinguish chronic from acute coronary artery disease nor can it reliably distinguish patients with primary cardiomyopathy and other types of diseases of the myocardium from those with coronary artery disease.[35] Therefore, M-mode echocardiography is unlikely to be useful for supporting the diagnosis of myocardial infarction unless thinning of a ventricular segment is seen during systole.

Another potential application of M-mode echocardiography is to determine the extent or size of the myocardial damage caused by an acute infarction. Two approaches to this question have been used. One is multiple transducer positions with analysis of the subsequent recordings of individual areas of the left ventricle; the other technique has been the utilization of linear scans recorded at very slow paper speeds

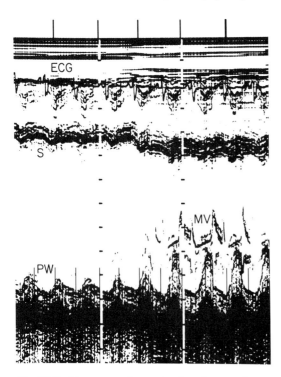

Fig. 29.8 Linear scan demonstrating abrupt enlargement of the left ventricular dimension and reduction in posterior wall excursion below the mitral valve apparatus in a patient with acute myocardial infarction.

(Fig. 29.8). Although such analyses can often be accomplished in patients with acute myocardial infarction, these techniques have never been compared to other methods for determining the size or extent of myocardial infarction, such as radionuclide myocardial imaging or the analysis of creatine kinase release by the myocardium. Another drawback to echocardiography is that unless wall thinning is noted, one cannot tell the difference between acute and chronic changes. Thus, the only reliable assessment that can be made is the overall extent of damage due to coronary artery disease.

This raises the question of whether overall left ventricular performance can be assessed by M-mode echocardiography in a patient with acute myocardial infarction. Heikkila and Nieminen [28] examined multiple areas of the myocardium using different transducer positions and found that some areas had reduced excursion and others had increased excursion of the ventricular walls. They utilized a summation of all these excursions and found that this sum compared favorably with the clinical assessment of left ventricular performance.[36] However, there was considerable overlap in the data. For example, the highest sum in patients with pulmonary edema and shock was equal to the lowest sum in patients with uncomplicated infarctions. Also, the study was not controlled for other therapy, and some of the patients in failure were on inotropic agents such as dopamine. Therefore, it would appear that the evaluation of multiple individual areas of wall motion in the ventricle is going to result in a crude appraisal of overall left ventricular performance.

Measuring left ventricular minor axis dimensions and calculating ejection phase indices as an estimate of overall left ventricular performance has been done despite problems with this limited view of the ventricle. Nieminen and Heikkila [37] noted a relationship between ejection phase indices and the clinical assessment of the patient, but there was no statistical correlation between these indices and clinical class. In one patient we studied, cardiogenic shock developed after an extension of a 2-day-old apical infarction. However, the M-mode echocardiographic ejection phase indices were unchanged, despite a fall in his radionuclide ejection fraction from 50 to 37 percent. Therefore, calculation of the standard ejection phase indices will not be very helpful for estimating left ventricular performance in patients with acute myocardial infarction.

Measurement of the left ventricular end-diastolic dimension, which should not be influenced by systolic wall motion abnormalities, seems to be a simple approach to separating patients with abnormal left ventricular performance from those with normal performance, since heart size usually increases as ventricular performance decreases. However, in the setting of acute myocardial infarction, changes in heart size do not always reflect ventricular performance. Left ventricular dimensions have been found to be generally increased in Class III and IV patients, but there is considerable scatter in these data.[29,36-38] Also, it has been noted that left ventricular end-diastolic dimension is larger in patients with uncomplicated anterior myocardial infarction, compared to other uncomplicated infarctions.[37] One explanation for these problems with predicting left ventricular performance based on the end-diastolic dimension is that extensive infarction of the apical part of the ventricle will not be seen in the usual minor dimension measurement, and such patients may be in Class III or IV with a normal left ventricular end-diastolic dimension. Therefore, it appears that the left ventricular end-diastolic dimension is a crude index of overall left ventricular performance in patients with acute myocardial infarction and cannot be reliably used to predict their functional class.

The electrocardiographic PR interval minus the AC interval on the mitral valve recording has potential use in evaluating left ventricular performance in patients with acute myocardial infarction by estimating left ventricular filling pressure. Unfortunately, this index has not correlated well with the clinical assessment of left ventricular performance.[29] Also, two studies reported difficulty in measuring the PR-AC interval in approximately 25 percent of patients with acute myocardial infarction.[29,39] Furthermore, if the data on patients with chronic heart disease are any indication of some of the problems that may be encountered with estimating

left ventricular pressures from the PR-AC interval, it is unlikely that the accuracy will be better in the patient with acute myocardial infarction. Thus, it remains to be shown that the PR-AC interval is of value in evaluating patients with acute myocardial infarction.

The E point-septal separation measurement is obtainable in almost all patients with acute myocardial infarction and is simple to interpret. Lew and associates[40] examined this measure in 38 patients with acute myocardial infarction and found that if it was greater than 5.5 mm, a low ejection fraction determined by radionuclide angiography was correctly predicted 95 percent of the time (specificity). However, the number of patients with low ejection fractions detected (sensitivity) was only 65 percent. Since this measure was less accurate in patients with severe wall motion abnormalities, it was postulated that the high number of falsely negative results may have occurred because wall motion abnormalities affected the position of the mitral valve in the ventricle. Other investigators have noted a relationship between the size of the left ventricle and the amount of E point-septal separation and suggested that left ventricular outflow tract dilatation is relatively more important than reduced mitral valve excursion in producing this abnormality.[41] These considerations may explain the high number of falsely negative results, especially if the left ventricular apex is extensively damaged in the infarction. The basal portion of the ventricle may compensatorily increase its performance, which could lead to normal positioning of the mitral valve despite a reduced overall ejection fraction. Therefore, an increase in the mitral echogram E point-septal separation is of some value for predicting reduced left ventricular performance in the setting of acute myocardial infarction, but a normal value does not exclude abnormal ventricular function.

## ASSESSMENT OF COMPLICATIONS

Another issue is whether the complications of myocardial infarction can be assessed by M-mode echocardiography. The most common complication of myocardial infarction is arrhythmia. Since an ECG should be included on the echocardiogram, the operator should always be alert for arrhythmias when studying patients with acute myocardial infarction. Thus, if there is a sudden change in the quality of the echocardiogram on the viewing scope, the operator should check the ECG to exclude a ventricular tachyarrhythmia as the cause of the deterioration in ventricular wall motion. Arrhythmias tend to be more common in patients with enlarged left ventricles with poor performance after myocardial infarction so that the echocardiogram may be useful for identifying patients who are at increased risk for arrhythmias.

The second most common complication of myocardial infarction is left ventricular failure. We have discussed above the utility of M-mode echocardiography for evaluating regional and overall left ventricular performance and have concluded that it could be used as a crude index of left ventricular function, which may aid in identifying patients at risk for developing overt pump failure.

Another common complication of myocardial infarction is involvement of the papillary muscles with resultant papillary muscle dysfunction. Little data exist analyzing this complication of myocardial infarction by M-mode echocardiography, but it has been reported that the usual mitral valve prolapse pattern is not seen on the mitral valve echogram in patients with papillary muscle dysfunction.[29] A sudden dramatic change in anterior mitral valve leaflet early diastolic amplitude, or slope, may be found in some cases of papillary muscle dysfunction,[42] but this has not been a consistent finding.[43] One potential use of M-mode echocardiography is to distinguish whether mitral regurgitation is due to isolated ischemic damage of the muscle or to gross enlargement of the left ventricle and malalignment of the papillary muscles, or both. Thus, evaluation of papillary muscle dysfunction can be aided by the echocardiogram because it can exclude other causes of mitral valve disease and may give some clue as to the etiology of the problem.

Rupture of the myocardium is an infrequent, often fatal, complication of myocardial infarc-

tion. There have been a few reported cases of survival after rupture of the free wall of the myocardium when immediate cardiac surgery has been performed. Also, an occasional patient seals off the rupture with the pericardium and survives. A potential use of M-mode echocardiography is to detect the false aneurysm formation that follows myocardial rupture sealed by the pericardium.[44] Early detection of these pseudoaneurysms may improve patient survival because they need to be repaired surgically before they rupture.

Rupture of the ventricular septum will result in acute right and left heart failure, usually associated with an increase in the size of the right ventricle, which may be detected by M-mode echocardiography.[45] The usual septal rupture is low in the muscular septum and is not ordinarily visualized by the M-mode beam. The acute change in right ventricular size is not specific for ventricular septal defect and can be produced by left ventricular failure or right ventricular infarction alone.[46] Thus, clinical evaluation is probably more important than echocardiography in the diagnosis of ruptured septum, although management may be aided by following ventricular size on M-mode echo.

Rupture of part of the papillary muscle apparatus results in flail mitral valve leaflets. There is a distinctive pattern on the mitral valve echogram, which suggests flail leaflet: pansystolic prolapse followed by coarse fluttering and abnormal movements of the involved leaflets in diastole.[47] Therefore, M-mode echocardiography can be extremely useful in confirming the diagnosis of flail mitral valve leaflet due to supporting apparatus disruption.

Emboli, both systemic and pulmonary, can be complications of myocardial infarction. Pulmonary embolus is perhaps the most common and may give rise to pulmonary hypertension, which can be detected on echocardiography by the lack of an "a" wave in the pulmonary valve tracing and may be suggested by the development of an increase in right ventricular size.[48] The source of systemic emboli is presumably mural thrombi overlying the infarcted segment. It has been commented that one often sees an increase in background echoes adjacent to akinetic left ventricular walls.[49] Whether or not this "fuzz" represents mural thrombi has not been definitely established. Also, it is well known that patients with large left ventricles and large left atria due to myocardial disease of any kind have a higher incidence of systemic emboli. Thus, M-mode echocardiography can help confirm the diagnosis of pulmonary hypertension due to pulmonary emboli and may identify patients at increased risk for systemic emboli following myocardial infarction.

Pericarditis is a frequent accompaniment of the acute myocardial infarction process, especially if the infarction is transmural. This form of acute transmural injury pericarditis usually does not result in cardiac tamponade, but may give rise to pain and discomfort. This condition can usually be diagnosed by the typical pleuritic chest pain and rub on auscultation, and can be confirmed on echocardiography by the finding of pericardial fluid. Perhaps more important is the unusual late development of pericarditis, weeks to months after myocardial infarction, which has been called Dressler's syndrome. This probably represents an autoimmune phenomenon that can lead to chronic pericarditis, tamponade, constriction and other complica-

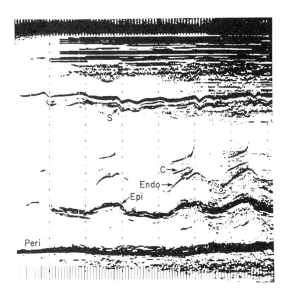

Fig. 29.9 Left ventricular echogram showing a large posterior pericardial effusion in a patient with cardiomegaly on a chest radiograph 6 weeks following an anteroseptal myocardial infarction.

tions, and is readily diagnosed with echocardiography by the presence of pericardial fluid (Fig. 29.9). Also, the echocardiogram can be very useful in following such patients to detect changes in the amount of fluid and confirm potential compression of ventricular chambers.

## PROGNOSIS

One important aspect of acute myocardial infarction care is estimating the prognosis of the patient in order to make reasonable plans for hospital management and rehabilitation. It is well known that an increase in left ventricular size following a myocardial infarction is a poor prognostic sign.[50] Hence, enlargement of the left ventricular end-diastolic dimension on the echocardiogram indicates a poorer prognosis as compared to patients who have a normal left ventricular minor axis dimension. As one would anticipate from the discussion above, a normal end-diastolic dimension does not always indicate a good prognosis because this dimension may not evaluate areas of the myocardium that are diseased. The PR-AC interval has also been found to be of some prognostic value. Again, this is a reflection of the performance of the ventricle, and the lower the performance, the worse the prognosis. However, combination of both these measures has been shown to predict mortality and future ischemic events with a reasonable degree of accuracy.[29,38] Therefore, it is likely that signs of left ventricular dysfunction, detected by M-mode echocardiography, will augur a poor prognosis in patients following acute myocardial infarction. Of course, the absence of such findings does not insure a benign course.

## SUMMARY

M-mode echocardiography is useful for measuring the dimensions of cardiac chambers and the thickness of the interventricular septum and posterior wall. Since myocardial infarction impairs wall thickening and movement, echocardiography can be used to confirm the diagnosis and assess the extent of damage. Myocardial infarction often leads to a deterioration in left ventricular performance, which can be detected by measuring ventricular dimensions and assessing the timing and motion of the mitral valve in diastole.

Echocardiography is especially useful for distinguishing pericardial fluid from left ventricular enlargement in the patient with cardiomegaly on chest X-ray examination after myocardial infarction. Also, it can aid in the diagnosis of right ventricular dysfunction due to infarction or ventricular septal rupture. Finally, signs of left ventricular dysfunction and enlargement will augur a poor prognosis in patients with acute myocardial infarction, but it must be pointed out that a normal M-mode echocardiographic evaluation does not exclude left ventricular dysfunction, since not all segments of the left ventricular myocardium can be visualized by the single sound beam. Furthermore, all of the M-mode echocardiographic findings discussed above are not specific for acute myocardial infarction and can be found in other conditions. Therefore, M-mode echocardiography is best utilized as an adjunct to the total clinical evaluation of the patient and should not be considered diagnostic by itself.

## REFERENCES

1. Popp RL, Filly K, Brown, OR, et al: Effect of transducer placement on echocardiographic measurement of left ventricular dimensions. Am J Cardiol 35:537, 1975.
2. Kline LE, Crawford MH, McDonald WJ Jr., et al: Non-invasive assessment of left ventricular performance in patients with chronic obstructive pulmonary disease. Chest 72:558, 1977.
3. Feigenbaum H: Echocardiography. 2nd ed. Lea and Febiger, Philadelphia, 1976, p 79.
4. Crawford MH, Grant D, O'Rourke RA, et al: Accuracy and reproducibility of new M-mode echocardiographic recommendations for measuring left venticular dimensions. Circulation 61:137, 1980.
5. Sahn DJ, DeMaria A, Kisslo J, et al: Recommendations regarding quantitation in M-mode echocardiography: Results of a survey of echocardio-

graphic measurements. Circulation 58:1072, 1978.
6. Cooper RH, O'Rourke RA, Karliner JS, et al: Comparison of ultrasound and cineangiographic measurements of mean rate of circumferential fiber shortening in man. Circulation 46:914, 1972.
7. Belenkie I, Nutter DO, Clark DW, et al: Assessment of left ventricular dimensions and function by echocardiography. Am. J Cardiol 31:755, 1973.
8. Murray JA, Johnston W, Reid JM: Echocardiographic determination of left ventricular dimensions, volumes and performance. *Am J Cardiol* 30:252, 1972.
9. Pombo JF, Troy BL, Russell, RO Jr, et al: Left ventricular volumes and ejection fraction by echocardiography. Circulation 43:480, 1971.
10. Fortúin NH, Hood WP, Sherman ME, et al: Determination of left ventricular volumes by ultrasound. Circulation 44:575, 1971.
11. Teichholz LE, Kreulen T, Herman, MV, et al: Problems in echocardiographic volume determinations: Echocardiographic-angiographic correlations in the presence or absence of asynergy. Am J Cardiol 37:7, 1976.
12. Linhart JW, Mintz, GS, Segal BL, et al: Left ventricular volume measurement by echocardiography: Fact or fiction? Am J Cardiol 36:114, 1975.
13. Henning H, Schelbert H, Crawford MH, et al: Left ventricular performance assessed by radionuclide angiocardiography and echocardiography in patients with previous myocardial infarction. Circulation 52:1069, 1975.
14. Brown OR, Harrison DC, Popp RL: An improved method for echographic detection of left atrial enlargement. Circulation 50:58, 1974.
15. Feigenbaum H: Echocardiography. 2nd ed. Lea and Febiger, Philadelphia, 1976, p 463.
16. Hirshleifer J, Crawford M, O'Rourke RA, et al: Influence of acute alterations in heart rate and systemic arterial pressure on echocardiographic measures of left ventricular performance in normal human subjects. Circulation 52:835, 1975.
17. Ludbrook P, Karliner JS, London A, et al: Posterior wall velocity: An unreliable index of total left ventricular performance in patients with coronary artery disease. Am J Cardiol 33:475, 1974.
18. Kerber RE, Marcus ML: Evaluation of regional myocardial function in ischemic heart disease by echocardiography. Progress in Cardiovascular Diseases, 20:441, 1978.

19. Monoson PA, O'Rourke RA, Crawford MH, et al: Measurements of left ventricular wall thickness and systolic thickening by M-mode echocardiography: Interobserver and intrapatient variability. J Clin Ultrasound 6:252, 1978.
20. Roelandt J, vanDorp WG, Bom N, et al: Resolution problems in echocardiology: A source of interpretation errors. Am J Cardiol 37:256, 1976.
21. Feigenbaum H: Echocardiography. 2nd ed. Lea and Febiger, Philadelphia, 1976, p. 93.
22. Konecke LL, Feigenbaum H, Chang S, et al: Abnormal mitral valve motion in patients with elevated left ventricular diastolic pressures. Circulation 47:989, 1973.
23. Lewis JR, Parker JO, Burggraf GW: Mitral valve motion and changes in left ventricular end-diastolic pressure: A correlative study of the PR-AC interval. Am J Cardiol 42:383, 1978.
24. Massie BM, Schiller NB, Ratshin RA, et al: Mitral-septal separation: New echocardiographic index of left ventricular function. Am J Cardiol 39:1008, 1977.
25. Horowitz MS, Schultz CS, Stinson EB, et al: Sensitivity and specificity of echocardiographic diagnosis of pericardial effusion. Circulation 50:239, 1974.
26. Corya BC, Rasmussen S, Feigenbaum H, et al: Systolic thickening and thinning of the septum and posterior wall in patients with coronary artery disease, congestive cardiomyopathy, and atrial septal defect. Circulation 55:109, 1977.
27. Fujii J, Watanabe H, Kato K: Detection of the site and extent of the left ventricular asynergy in myocardial infarction by echocardiography and B-scan imaging. Jap Heart J 17:630, 1976.
28. Heikkila J, Nieminen M: Echoventriculographic detection, localization, and quantification of left ventricular asynergy in acute myocardial infarction. Br Heart J 37:46, 1975.
29. Corya BC, Rasmussen S, Knoebel SB, et al: Echocardiography in acute myocardial infarction. Am J Cardiol 36:1, 1975.
30. Rasmussen S, Corya BC, Feigenbaum H, et al: Detection of myocardial scar tissue by M-mode echocardiography. Circulation 57:230, 1978.
31. Dortimer AC, DeJoseph RL, Shiroff RA, et al: Distribution of coronary artery disease: Prediction by echocardiography. Circulation 54:724, 1976.
32. Gordon MH, Kerber RE: Interventricular septal motion in patients with proximal and distal left anterior descending coronary artery lesions. Circulation 55:338, 1977.
33. Joffe CD, Brik H, Teichholz LE, et al: Echocardiographic diagnosis of left anterior descending coronary artery disease. Am J Cardiol 40:11, 1977.
34. Kolibash AJ, Beaver BM, Fulkerson PK, et al: The relationship between abnormal echocardiographic septal motion and myocardial perfusion in patients with significant obstruction of the left anterior descending artery. Circulation 56:780, 1977.
35. Corya B, Feigenbaum H, Rasmussen S, et al: Echocardiographic features of congestive cardiomyopathy compared with normal subjects and patients with coronary artery disease. Circulation 49:1153, 1974.
36. Nieminen M, Hiekkila J: Echoventriculography in acute myocardial infarction III. Clinical correlations and implication of the noninfarcted myocardium. Am J Cardiol 38:1, 1976.
37. Nieminen M, Heikkila J: Echoventriculography in acute myocardial infarction II: Monitoring of left ventricular performance. Br Heart J 38:271, 1976.
38. Nixon JV, Blomqvist CG, Willerson JT, et al: Serial echocardiography in patients with acute myocardial infarction: Its value and prognostic significance. Eur J Cardiol 9:161, 1979.
39. Wiener I, Meller J, Packer M, et al: Prognostic value of echocardiographic evaluation of septal function in acute anteroseptal myocardial infarction. Am Heart J 97:726, 1979.
40. Lew W, Henning H, Schelbert H, et al: Assessment of mitral valve E point-septal separation as an index of left ventricular performance in patients with acute and previous myocardial infarction. Am J Cardiol 41:836, 1978.
41. D'Cruz IA, Lalmalani GG, Sambasivan B, et al: The superiority of mitral E point-ventricular septum separation to other echocardiographic indicators of left ventricular performance. Clin Cardiol 2:140, 1979.
42. Talhury VK, DePasquale NP, Burch GE: The echocardiogram in papillary muscle dysfunction. Am Heart J 83:12, 1972.
43. Bergeron GA, Cohen MV, Teichholz LE, et al: Echocardiographic analysis of mitral valve motion after acute myocardial infarction. Circulation 51:82, 1975.
44. Roelandt J, van den Brand M, Vletter WB, et al: Echocardiographic diagnosis of pseudoaneurysm of the left ventricle. Circulation 52:466, 1975.
45. Chandraratna PAN, Balachandran PK, Shah PM, et al: Echocardiographic observations on

ventricular septal rupture complicating acute myocardial infarction. Circulation 51:506, 1975.

46. Sharpe DN, Botvinick EH, Shames DM, et al: The noninvasive diagnosis of right ventricular infarction. Circulation 57:483, 1978.

47. Sweatman T, Selzer A, Kamagaki M, Cohn K: Echocardiographic diagnosis of mitral regurgitation due to ruptured chordae tendineae. Circulation 46:580, 1972.

48. Weyman AE, Dillon JC, Feigenbaum H, et al: Echocardiographic patterns of pulmonic valve motion with pulmonary hypertension. Circulation 50:905, 1974.

49. Feigenbaum H: Echocardiography. 2nd ed. Lea and Febiger, Philadelphia, 1976, p 350.

50. Kostuk WJ, Kazamias TM, Gander MP, et al: Left ventricular size after acute myocardial infarction. Circulation 47:1174, 1973.

# 30 | Cross-Sectional Echocardiography in Patients with Acute Myocardial Infarction

## Joseph S. Alpert, M.D.

Prognosis after myocardial infarction is determined by residual left ventricular function.[1,2] There is a reciprocal relationship between the extent of myocardial necrosis and the amount of residual functioning myocardium. Thus, patients with large infarctions (or multiple smaller infarcts) will have less functioning myocardium than individuals with a single small area of myocardial necrosis. Also of importance in determining postinfarction left ventricular function and, hence, prognosis is the state of the coronary arterial circulation, which supplies functioning zones of myocardium.[3] Functioning but ischemic or potentially ischemic myocardium is less advantageous to the patient than functional myocardium with a normal coronary blood supply.

Myocardial cells must have vigorous aerobic production of high energy phosphate compounds in order to contract normally. Ischemia results in abnormally reduced or even absent myocardial contractility.[4,5] Thus, examination of the contractile pattern of the left ventricle in patients with acute myocardial infarction might yield information about prognosis and the state of the underlying coronary circulation.

Cross-sectional echocardiography is one technique capable of defining left ventricular wall motion in patients with acute myocardial infarction.[6-8] It can be done at the patient's bedside in the coronary care unit and is safe and reproducible. This technique has the advantage, compared with M-mode echocardiography, of sampling all wall regions of the left ventricle.

Two different systems of cross-sectional echocardiography have been employed in patients with myocardial infarction: mechanical sector scanning and phased-array scanning. Both methods produce real-time images at 30 frames/sec with a field of view of 80° to 90°. Images are recorded on videotapes and/or stopframe photographs. As yet, it is unclear which of these two techniques will become preeminent in clinical studies.

Patients are examined primarily with left parasternal and apical views of the left ventricle. Subxiphoid or four chamber views are frequently attempted, but visualization is sometimes less successful than with the two earlier mentioned windows. The usual study consists of a longitudinal cut and several transverse cuts of the left ventricle at different levels (Fig. 30.1). Five left ventricular wall regions can be identified with these cross-sectional views: anterolateral, posterolateral, apical, anteroseptal, and inferior. Technically, adequate studies can be obtained in approximately 90 percent of patients with acute myocardial infarction.[6] The average study requires 10 minutes.

Exact quantitative analysis of left ventricular volume and ejection phase indices is more difficult with cross-sectional than with M-mode echocardiography. Nevertheless, recent reports have indicated that in most patients, including those with abnormal wall motion due to coro-

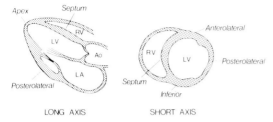

Fig. 30.1 Longitudal and transverse views of the left ventricle as seen by cross-sectional echocardiography. Five anatomic regions can be identified: anteroseptal, anterolateral, posterolateral, apical, and inferior. The long axis view is shown schematically; the aortic root and apex are not in the same plane and hence are not usually visualized simultaneously. Ao = aorta, LA = left atrium, LV = left ventricle and RV = right ventricle.

nary artery disease, careful analysis of two-dimensional echocardiograms can yield useful information relative to left ventricular end-systolic volume and ejection fraction when compared to left ventricular angiography in the same patients.[9,10] It should be appreciated, however, that cross-sectional echocardiography, regardless of the views employed, tends to underestimate left ventricular end-diastolic volume.[9,10]

In patients with acute myocardial infarction, most investigators have employed a more sub-

Table 30.1   Scoring System for Left Ventricular Wall
Motion by Cross-sectional Echocardiography *

1. Each of the 5 left ventricular regions is assigned a score based on the following scale:

     0 = hyperkinetic wall motion
     1 = normokinetic wall motion
     2 = hypokinetic wall motion
     3 = akinetic wall motion
     4 = paradoxical wall motion

2. Regions are scored by comparison with each other and with studies from known normal individuals.
3. Some zones demonstrate mixtures of different types of wall motion (e.g., hypokinesis and akinesis). An average of all such scores is taken as the overall score for that zone.
4. Scores from the 5 left ventricular regions are summed to produce a semiquantitative estimate of global left ventricular wall motion.

* Adapted from Wynne J, Birnholz J, Finberg H, et al: Assessment of regional left ventricular wall motion in acute myocardial infarction by two-dimensional echocardiography.

jective system, consisting of visual assessment and grading of the adequacy of left ventricular wall motion in the five regions noted above. A typical, but not the only system, is recorded in Table 30.1. The reproducibility of such a scoring system has been evaluated. Approximately 85 percent of regional wall motion scores are reproduced identically or with only a minor change at delayed repeat analysis.[6] Global left ventricular wall motion scores are also very reproducible. Regional and global estimates of left ventricular function by cross-sectional echocardiography correlate well with radionuclide ventriculographic measurements of regional and global left ventricular function (Fig. 30.2). Evaluation of left ventricular function by radionuclide ventriculography has repeatedly correlated with similar determinations made at the time of cardiac catherization. Hence, radionuclide ventriculography serves as an adequate substitute (gold standard) for comparison with cross-sectional echocardiography.

Regional left ventricular wall motion abnormalities are noted in over 90 percent of patients with acute myocardial infarction, who were studied within 72 hours of infarction.[6,7] Smaller infarctions, transmural and nontransmural,

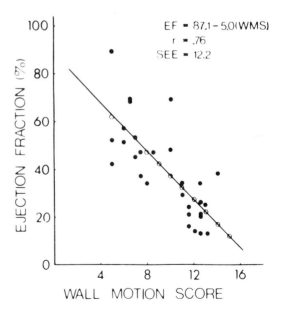

$$EF = 87.1 - 5.0(WMS)$$
$$r = .76$$
$$SEE = 12.2$$

Fig. 30.2 Global left ventricular wall motion score by echocardiography plotted against ejection fraction by gated blood-pool radionuclide ventriculography.

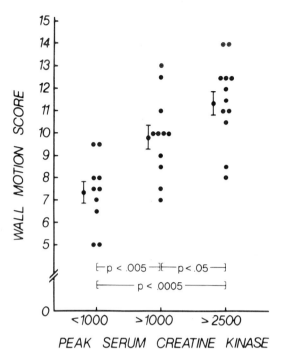

Fig. 30.3  Global left ventricular wall motion score by cross-sectional echocardiography in 18 patients with acute transmural myocardial infarction plotted against infarct size as gauged from peak serum creatine kinase values.

may be associated with normal regional wall motion by this technique. In patients with transmural infarction, 91 percent of zones with significant Q waves on the EKG demonstrate wall motion abnormalities (hypokinesis and/or akinesis) by cross-sectional echocardiography.[6] Only 9 percent of zones with transmural infarction by EKG have normal wall motion. Half of these occur in patients with inferior infarction. Of great interest is the finding that 49 percent of electrocardiographically normal left ventricular regions also demonstrate hypoki-

nesis and/or akinesis on the cross-sectional echocardiogram.[6]

A consistent relationship exists between the size of a particular infarction (judged roughly by peak serum creatine kinase levels) and the severity of abnormal left ventricular wall motion (Fig. 30.3). Moreover, patients whose infarcts are not complicated by left ventricular failure (Killip Class I) have less abnormal wall motion than individuals with heart failure (Killip Classes II, III and IV). This relationship can be seen in Table 30.2.[6] The number of patients studied is as yet too small to determine if individuals who subsequently succumb as a result of their infarction can be prospectively identified by cross-sectional echocardiography.

Modest, gradual improvement in global left ventricular function can be demonstrated in patients with acute infarction studied over 2 to 3 weeks.[6] Improvement in wall motion occurs in both infarcted and noninfarcted zones. A small number of patients demonstrate deterioration in wall motion without obvious clinical evidence of extension of infarction. Almost 90 percent of patients with transmural myocardial infarction demonstrate improved regional wall motion in at least one noninfarcted zone.[6]

Compensatory hyperkinetic wall motion occurs in only 13 percent of patients with acute myocardial infarction. Paradoxical wall motion is seen in 19 percent of infarcted regions, all of which demonstrated Q waves on the EKG. Abnormal diastolic left ventricular wall motion, corresponding to easily audible third and fourth heart sounds, can be noted in an occasional patient. Abnormal left ventricular cavity echoes, suggestive of mural thrombus, can also be seen, on occasion, in regions of transmural infarction.[6]

**Table 30.2  Clinical Classification of Infarct Patients Compared with Echocardiographic Wall Motion Score \***

| Killip Class | Wall Motion Score (mean ± SD) | Number of Patients | p (Student's t test) |
|---|---|---|---|
| I | 8.4 ± 2.4 | 24 | I vs II, $p < .005$ |
| II | 10.8 ± 2.0 | 13 | I vs II, III and IV, $p < .005$ |
| III | 10.2 ± 1.4 | 6 | |
| IV | 10.8 ± 3.3 | 3 | |

\* Adapted from Wynne J, Birnholz J, Finberg H, et al: Assessment of regional left ventricular wall motion in acute myocardial infarction by two-dimensional echocardiography.

In a recent study, Hutchins and Bulkley [11] distinguished between infarct *expansion* and infarct *extension* in patients studied at necropsy. They defined infarct expansion as "acute dilatation and thinning of the area of infarction not explained by additional myocardial necrosis" and extension as "more recent foci of contraction band necrosis around an infarct" as seen histologically. In their study, 72 percent of patients dying within 30 days of acute myocardial infarction exhibited some thinning and dilatation of infarcted myocardium; in one-third of the hearts with transmural infarcts, marked expansion of the infarcted zone resulted in obvious cardiac dilatation.[11] Subsequently, Eaton et al reported a prospective two-dimensional echocardiographic study, using a computer-aided semiautomated system for analysis.[12] Of the 28 patients studied, 8 showed infarct expansion, with disproportionate dilatation and transmural thinning in the infarcted zone days to weeks following the infarct. Four of these 8 patients died of progressive heart failure over a period of 1 to 7 weeks and the other 4 were in functional Class II or III at follow-up examination. None of the other 20 patients died, and none exhibited progressive congestive cardiac failure. The authors speculated that if patients in whom regional infarct dilatation develops could be identified early by sequential two-dimensional echocardiography, conventional management could be altered in favor of closer and more prolonged monitoring, with later rather than earlier ambulation. Whether there are any pharmacologic interventions that could prevent or arrest regional infarct dilatation remains an issue to be investigated. In addition, the pathogenesis of infarct expansion, as opposed to infarct extension, is open to speculation.[13] This issue may at least, in part, be resolved by careful correlation of two-dimensional echocardiographic studies with serial estimations of the MB isoenzyme of creatine kinase.[14]

In summary, left ventricular function can be accurately and reproducibly estimated at the bedside in patients with acute myocardial infarction using cross-sectional echocardiography. Abnormal wall motion occurs in electrocardiographically infarcted, as well as noninfarcted, zones. Patients with large infarctions

and individuals with left ventricular failure demonstrate reduced left ventricular function, compared with individuals with smaller infarcts or patients without heart failure. Sequential studies of left ventricular function after infarction reveal gradual improvement in wall motion with time. Cross-sectional echocardiography is a promising technique for identifying, quantifying, and evaluating global and regional left ventricular wall motion abnormalities in patients with acute myocardial infarction (Fig. 30.4 and 30.5).

Recent studies have identified additional potential uses of two-dimensional echocardiography in patients with acute myocardial infarction. Using this technique it is possible to delineate alterations in right ventricular chamber size and wall motion in cases of right ventricular infarction.[15] Of considerable potential therapeutic importance is the ability to identify mural thrombi in all four cardiac chambers by two-dimensional echocardiography reported by Dobrac et al.[16] These investigators also carried out an in vitro study using clots prepared from fibrin, whole blood, and platelets as well as an organized thrombus obtained at surgery. Using two-dimensional echocardiography, they were able to detect all clots regardless of composition and could visualize clots as small as 2 mm in diameter.[16] In the left ventricle, mural thrombi appear to be associated with dyskinesis, both in patients with acute as well as chronic ischemic heart disease.[17,18] Further, in patients with acute myocardial infarction, Asinger et al. reported that mural thrombi tend to develop at the apex of the left ventricle in dyskinetic areas produced by anterior infarction.[18] Thus, in the future it should be possible to use two-dimensional echocardiography: (1) to determine whether present conventional anticoagulation regimes (e.g., low-dose subcutaneous heparin) are efficacious in preventing the development of mural thrombi; (2) to characterize the natural history of mural thrombi; and, possibly, (3) to identify a subset of patients in whom long-term anticoagulation may be of benefit in preventing systemic embolization.

Two-dimensional echocardiography may also be useful in the detection and management of some of the serious and often catastrophic com-

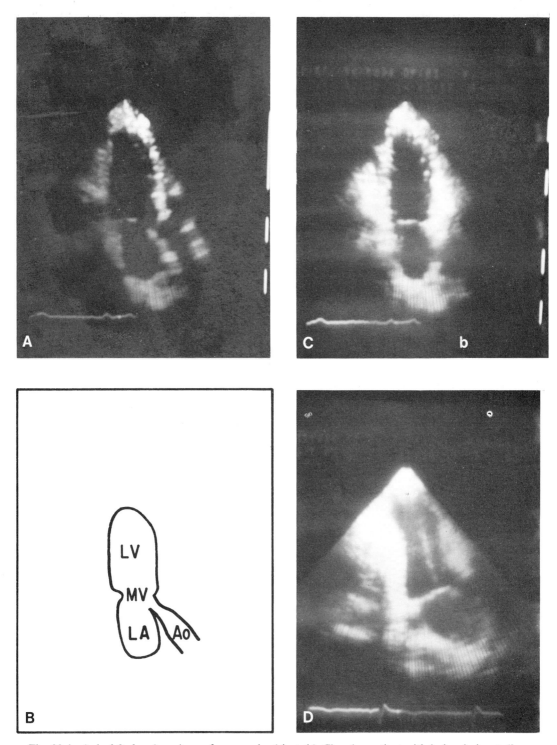

Fig. 30.4  Apical 2-chamber views of a normal subject *(A–C)* and a patient with ischemic heart disease
*(D)*. *(A)* End-diastolic frame from a normal subject. *(B)* Schematic outline of the major structures
seen in *A*. LV = left ventricle; MV = mitral valve; LA = left atrium; Ao = aorta. *(C)* End-systolic
frame obtained in the same normal subject. Note the symmetrical wall motion and the much smaller
size of the left ventricular cavity. The mitral valve is closed. *(D)* End-systolic frame from a patient
with ischemic heart disease. There is asynergy—particularly at the apex of the left ventricle—and reduced
wall motion is present throughout. (Courtesy of Dr. Arthur Hagan.)

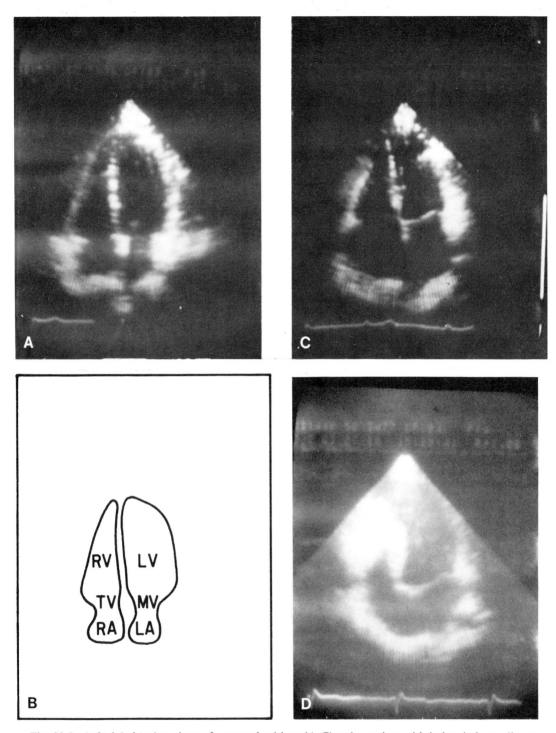

Fig. 30.5 Apical 4-chamber views of a normal subject *(A–C)* and a patient with ischemic heart disease *(D). (A)* End-diastolic frame from a normal subject. *(B)* Schematic outline of the major structures seen in *A*. LV = left ventricle; MV = mitral valve; LA = left atrium; RV = right ventricle; TV = tricuspid valve; RA = right atrium. *(C)* End-systolic frame obtained in the same normal subject. As in Fig. 30.4, note the symmetrical wall motion and the reduced size of both the left and right ventricular cavities. The mitral valve is closed. The tricuspid valve is not seen, and the interatrial septum is only partially visualized. *(D)* End-systolic frame from a patient with ischemic heart disease. There is marked asynergy—especially at the left ventricular apex—and reduced wall motion is present throughout. (Courtesy of Dr. Arthur Hagan.)

plications of acute myocardial infarction. Thus, Farcot et al. reported that this technique could be used to successfully visualize the defect after septal rupture in three patients with acute anterior myocardial infarction.[19] In addition, they used negative contrast echoventriculography to identify a left-to-right shunt at the ventricular level. Two-dimensional echocardiography appears to be superior to M-mode echocardiography in the detection of flail mitral leaflets,[20] and thus the two-dimensional approach should be helpful in assessing patients who develop acute mitral regurgitation due to papillary muscle rupture or dysfunction after acute myocardial infarction.

Finally, improved two-dimensional ultrasound techniques may permit easier visualization of the left main coronary artery.[21] Noninvasive identification of obstruction to this vessel would aid greatly in the management of unstable and variant angina as well as in the selection of patients for coronary arteriography early after recovery from acute myocardial infarction.

## REFERENCES

1. Sobel BE, Bresnahan GF, Shell WE, et al: Estimation of infarct size in man and its relation to prognosis. Circulation 46:640, 1972.
2. Luria MH, Knoke JD, Margolis RM, et al: Acute myocardial infarction: Prognosis after recovery. Ann Intern Med 85:561, 1976.
3. Bruschke AVG, Proudfit WL, Sones FM Jr: Progress Study of 590 consecutive nonsurgical cases of coronary disease followed 5–9 years. II. Ventriculographic and other correlations. Circulation 47:1154, 1973.
4. Waters, DD, Forrester, JS: Myocardial ischemia: detection and quantitation. Ann Intern Med 88:239, 1978.
5. Wyatt, HL, Forrester, JS, Tyberg, JV, et al: Effect of graded reductions in regional coronary perfusion on regional and total cardiac function. Am J Cardiol 36:185, 1975.
6. Wynne J, Birnholz J, Finberg H, et al: Assessment of regional left ventricular wall motion in acute myocardial infarction by two-dimensional echocardiography. Submitted.
7. Heger JJ, Weyman AE, Warn LS, et al: Cross-sectional echocardiography in acute myocardial infarction: Detection and localization of regional left ventricular asynergy. Circulation 60:531, 1979.
8. Weiss JL, Bulkley BH, Hutchins GM, Mason SJ: Correlation of real time 2-dimensional echocardiography with post-mortem studies (abstract). Am J Cardiol 41:369, 1978.
9. Carr KW, Engler RL, Forsythe JR, Johnson AD, Gosink B: Measurement of left ventricular enjection fraction by mechanical cross-sectional echocardiography. Circulation 59:1188, 1979.
10. Schiller NB, Acquatella H, Ports TA, Drew D, Goerke J, Rinquetz H, Silverman NH, Brundage B, Botvinick EH, Boswell R, Carlsson E, Parmley WW: Left ventricular volume from paired biplane two-dimensional echocardiography. Circulation 60:547, 1979.
11. Hutchins GM, Bulkely BH: Infarct expansion versus extension: two different complications of acute myocardial infarction. Am J Cardiol 41:1127, 1978.
12. Eaton LW, Weiss JL, Bulkley BH, Garrison JB, Weisfeldt ML: Regional cardiac dilation after acute myocardial infarction. N Engl J Med 300:57, 1979.
13. Willerson JT: Echocardiography after acute myocardial infarction (editorial). N Engl J Med 300:87, 1979.
14. Rothkopf M, Boerner J, Stone MJ, Smitherman TG, Buja LM, Parkey RW, Willerson JT: Detection of myocardial infarction extension by CK-B radioimmunoassay. Circulation 59:268, 1979.
15. D'Arey BJ, Bapineedu G, Nanda NC, Gatewood RP, Biddle T: Real time two-dimensional echocardiography in right ventricular infarction. Am J Cardiol (abstract) 45:436, 1980.
16. Drobuc M, Rakowski W, Gilbert BW, Glynn MX, Silver MD: Two-dimensional echocardiographic recognition of mural thrombi: in-vivo and in-vitro studies. Am J Cardiol (abstract) 45:435, 1980.
17. Quinones MA, Nelson JG, Winters Jr. WL, Waggoner AD, Rosenfeld SP, Young JB, Miller RR: Clinical spectrum of left ventricular mural thrombi in a large cardiac population: assessment by two-dimensional echocardiography. Am J Cardiol (abstract) 45:435, 1980.
18. Asinger RW, Mikell FL, Francis G, Elsperger J, Hodges M, Sharmu B: Serial evaluation for left ventricular thrombus during acute transmural myocardial infarction using two-dimensional echocardiography (2 DE). Am J Cardiol (abstract) 45:483, 1980.

19. Farcot JC, Boisante L, Rigaud M, Bardet J, Bourdarias JP: Two-dimensional echocardiographic visualization of ventricular septal rupture after acute anterior myocardial infarction. Am J Cardiol 45:370, 1980.

20. Mintz G Kotler MN, Parry WR, Segal BL: Statistical comparison of M mode and two dimensional echocardiographic diagnosis of flail mitral leaflets. Am J Cardiol 45:253, 1980.

21. Rink LD, Feigenbaum H, Marshall JE, Godley RW, Doty D, Dillon JC, Weyman AE: Improved echocardiographic technique for examining the left main coronary artery. Am J Cardiol (abstract) 45:435, 1980.

# Section 7
# FURTHER ASPECTS
# OF THERAPY

# 31 | Cardiopulmonary Resuscitation

## Martin M. LeWinter, M.D.
## Robert L. Engler, M.D.

As has been discussed in other chapters, the major contribution of the coronary care unit toward the reduction of in-hospital mortality of ischemic heart disease is the result of the prompt treatment of potentially lethal cardiac dysrhythmias. Modern techniques of cardiopulmonary resuscitation (CPR), including the use of direct current countershock, have been, in large measure, directly responsible for this major benefit of intensive coronary care. Thus, the effective management of cardiac arrest may be regarded as one of the most important functions of a coronary care unit. Entire books, national conferences, one journal (Resuscitation), and a very large body of literature that includes both original reports and review articles have been concerned solely with CPR. It is therefore beyond the scope of this chapter to deal comprehensively with all aspects of CPR. Rather, an attempt will be made to synthesize available information in a comprehensible fashion and provide an introduction that may be used as the framework for more in-depth study. A basic operating assumption for most of this chapter is that the description of CPR techniques that follows is applicable to a modern, well-equipped coronary care unit. Thus, it is assumed that a variety of laboratory and diagnostic tests as well as therapeutic modalities are readily available and that therapy can be instituted within seconds of the time of cardiac arrest.

## THE ETIOLOGY AND CLINICAL CORRELATES OF CARDIAC ARREST IN THE CORONARY CARE UNIT

By far, the most common cause of cardiac arrest in the coronary care unit is dysrhythmia. Most such potentially lethal dysrhythmias occur in patients admitted with acute myocardial infarction. Their incidence appears to be highest early after myocardial infarction and then decreases after the first 48 to 72 hours.[1-4] Thus, the earlier after the onset of symptoms a patient with myocardial infarction is admitted, the higher is the risk for sudden, lethal dysrhythmias. Although it is possible, in patients with acute myocardial infarction, to use certain criteria, particularly the presence of heart failure and prior myocardial infarction, to designate relatively high and low risk groups for cardiac arrest, it is at present not possible to predict with confidence which patients will develop this complication.[5-7] The experience of Cobb and coworkers [8-10] indicates that a significant proportion of patients with "sudden death" who are resuscitated outside of the hospital and subsequently admitted to a coronary care unit do not go on to evolve a myocardial infarction. These patients have been found to subsequently be at considerably higher risk for sudden death than similar patients who do evolve a myocardial infarction, presumably because they remain vulnerable to electrical instability of the heart. If rapidly available mobile coronary care units staffed with trained personnel become widely used, a significant number of patients admitted to coronary care units in the future are likely to be from this group with "sudden death" in the absence of myocardial infarction. This group would then constitute a different type of patient in the coronary care unit, one at major risk from lethal dysrhythmias. The risk in patients admitted to the coronary care unit with unstable angina patterns has not been carefully studied, but it is certainly considerably less than that of patients with myocardial infarction. Finally, a heterogenous group of patients admitted to a coronary care unit for monitoring of known or suspected dysrhythmias of any etiology will also, of course, be at significant but variable risk.

The most commonly encountered dysrhythmia in patients with acute myocardial infarction and cardiac arrest, and, in fact, in all patients suffering cardiac arrest in the coronary care unit setting, is ventricular fibrillation.[2,3,5-7,11-15] As discussed elsewhere, this rhythm is generally initiated either by a single premature ventricular contraction or a run of ventricular tachycardia, which rapidly degenerates into ventricular fibrillation. Ventricular fibrillation may also be considered a primary or secondary rhythm disturbance, the latter implying it occurs as a terminal event in patients with severe pump failure.[11]

Ventricular fibrillation is occasionally associated with bradydysrhythmias, it may be preceded by less malignant ventricular dysrhythmias, or it may occur without any prior evidence of electrical instability. Thus, many patients do not develop warning signs of approaching ventricular fibrillation. Less frequently, sustained ventricular tachycardia at a rate sufficient to result in cardiovascular collapse does not degenerate rapidly into ventricular fibrillation and is the rhythm encountered when therapy for cardiac arrest is begun.

Much less commonly, sudden bradydysrhythmias are responsible for circulatory collapse, requiring CPR in the coronary care unit. The most important example of the latter is complete heart block.[16-22] As discussed in other chapters, this conduction disturbance is a frequent complication of acute inferior wall myocardial infarction, but is usually well-tolerated and is associated with escape rhythms adequate to sustain an effective circulation. Complete heart block is encountered much less frequently after anterior myocardial infarction, but often results in cardiovascular collapse, if untreated, because the site of the block is in the distal conduction system and escape pacemakers may therefore not become activated or may have exceedingly slow rates. After anterior myocardial infarction, complete heart block may be heralded by various combinations of fascicular blocks or it may occur without premonitory electrocardiographic signs. Sudden complete heart block may of course also occur in patients admitted to the coronary care unit for monitoring in whom complete heart block of any etiology is suspected. Occasional patients in the coronary care unit may suffer circulatory collapse resulting from primary asystole or marked sinus bradycardia with very slow escape pacemakers, and require CPR. These dysrhythmias, when they occur as a primary event, are often the result of a profound vagal discharge, which may occur in several settings. For instance, patients with inferior wall myocardial infarction (who as a group appear to have increased vagal tone) may suffer bouts of severe sinus slowing or asystole, resulting in circulatory collapse. However, it must be stressed that sinus slowing to this extent is rare. In fact, sinus bradycardia, in general, does not appear to be associated with a worse prognosis.[22-27] Additionally, occasional patients who receive nitrates may have paradoxical sinus slowing, which may also result in circulatory collapse.[27]

A number of other dysrhythmias, to be discussed subsequently, are encountered during the course of cardiopulmonary resuscitation but are rarely the primary cause of circulatory collapse or the first rhythm encountered when treatment is initiated within seconds, as should be routine in any coronary care unit.

There are a variety of other settings in which sudden dysrhythmias may result in circulatory collapse in the coronary care unit, for instance, digitalis toxicity, quinidine toxicity, and various electrolyte disorders. Since these are usually complications of therapy rather than of the basic cardiac disorder, they will not be considered further in this section, but of course must be kept in mind in all patients.

Dysrhythmias are not the only cause of circulatory collapse requiring resuscitative efforts in the coronary care unit. Obviously, patients with severe pump failure can and do have circulatory collapse without a dysrhythmic basis, although secondary lethal dysrhythmias are often terminal events in such cases. A subset of such patients develop severe pump failure and electromechanical dissociation abruptly, presumably as a result of an acute worsening of myocardial ischemia leading to global dysfunction.[29] Two other less common, but well-defined complications of myocardial infarction present as abrupt circulatory collapse with electromechanical dissociation: (1) rupture of the free wall of the left ventricle [30,31] and (2) rupture of the belly of a papillary muscle.[32] These may be suspected when there is sudden development of electromechanical dissociation. Both of these events are similar from a pathologic standpoint, usually occurring 3 to 4 days after the onset of symptoms when the area of necrosis is thought to be most vulnerable to rupture. Except in rare circumstances, these complications are incompatible with life and resuscitative efforts are unrewarding. Another complication, now relatively rare in the coronary care unit but which may result in abrupt circulatory collapse without dysrhythmia, is massive pulmonary embolism. The incidence of thromboembolic phenomena appears to have been markedly reduced due to early ambulation of patients with myocardial infarction and the judicious use of heparin therapy.

## Pathophysiologic Considerations Relating to Abrupt Circulatory Collapse

The metabolic, functional and anatomic derangements of various organ systems that follow circulatory collapse have been studied extensively.[33] Except in unusual circumstances (for instance, rupture of the left ventricular free wall), it should be possible, in the coronary care unit, to rapidly restore an effective circulation, using cardiopulmonary resuscitation techniques. Therefore, a number of the organ system derangements that follow the abrupt loss of effective circulation become relatively less important.

The most important general pathophysiologic considerations in formulating an effective plan for cardiopulmonary resuscitation in the coronary care unit are the effects of loss of circulation on (1) central and autonomic nervous system function, (2) cardiovascular function, and (3) metabolic status. As will be seen, these three areas are intimately related. With sudden cardiac arrest, a predictable sequence of events is initiated. Initially, there is a profound stress reaction, with an outpouring of catecholamines and corticosteroids.[33] The former may have important consequences with regard to the possibility of restoring spontaneous effective cardiac activity. Thus, for instance, high levels of sympathetic stimulation may favorably influence the ability to subsequently defibrillate the heart in a patient with ventricular fibrillation by increasing the amplitude of fibrillatory waves.[34,35] On the other hand, if defibrillation is successful, the tendency for ventricular fibrillation to recur may be increased in the presence of increased sympathetic stimulation.[36-39] In patients in whom the primary mechanism of cardiac arrest is a bradydysrhythmia or asystole, an increase in sympathetic stimulation may obviously help to restore spontaneous cardiac electrical activity. With respect to cardiac function, the increase in sympathetic stimulation may be a mixed blessing in patients with ischemic heart disease. If effective electrical activity is restored, intense sympathetic stimulation may help to restore mechanical function to the initially depressed myocardium but may subsequently result in increased myocardial oxygen demands.[40] Although the distribution of blood flow following the restoration of cardiac activity after sudden cardiac arrest has not been specifically studied, it is likely that the stress reaction and its associated autonomic nervous system alterations, along with local metabolic effects related to tissue ischemia, result in shunting of blood to critical organs, such as the brain, and away from tissue such as skeletal muscle.[41]

In addition to the phenomenon of generalized tissue ischemia, an invariable accompaniment of cardiac arrest is the development of metabolic acidosis, which is, of course, additive to the obligatory respiratory acidosis that occurs in this setting. As a result, one of the most important tenets of cardiopulmonary resuscitation is the administration of appropriate amounts of base in the form of sodium bicarbonate, which will be discussed in more detail subsequently. However, if CPR is instituted rapidly in the coronary care unit, acidosis, both metabolic and respiratory, should be minimal.[42] Additionally, the well-documented depressant effects of acidosis on myocardial function [43-46] should also be minimal.

Respiration ceases promptly after abrupt circulatory collapse. Therefore, arterial hypoxemia is another invariable accompaniment of cardiac arrest, which undoubtedly plays a major role in the generalized stress reaction. Acute hypoxemia alone, independently of ischemia, results in reflex sympathetic stimulation and an outpouring of catecholamines with a resulting increase in systemic vascular resistance and shunting of blood to critical organs.[47-50] Pulmonary vascular resistance also markedly increases with acute hypoxemia.[51] Although it is difficult to sort out the effects of hypoxemia independent of tissue ischemia and other elements of a generalized stress reaction in this setting, correction of hypoxemia is a prime goal in all resuscitative efforts.

In summary, then, the effects of the sudden cessation of cardiac activity are rapid suspension of respiration, resulting in marked hypoxemia and respiratory acidosis; generalized tissue ischemia, resulting in metabolic acidosis; and a profound stress reaction, resulting in intense sympathetic stimulation. Accompanying these effects are alterations in systemic vascular resistence that produce maximal vasodilatation in critical organs, such as the brain, and vasoconstriction in tissue such as skeletal muscle. The latter adaptations are obviously teleologically useful and help to shunt blood to critical organs when circulation is restored either by artificial means or by the resumption of spontaneous cardiac activity. Total systemic vascular resistance and myocardial sympathetic stimulation are increased as a result of the latter adaptation. As a consequence, patients in whom cardiac arrest results from dysrhythmias and who have no major problems with myocardial pump function, often develop a surprisingly high systemic arterial pressure when effective cardiac activity is promptly restored.

The brain, particularly the higher cortical centers, is particularly susceptible to the cessation of blood flow. It is generally accepted that the critical time period for the restoration of blood flow to the brain is about 4 minutes.[52-55] With longer periods of complete cerebral ischemia, permanent loss of higher cortical functions may be anticipated. Abrupt cessation of blood flow to the brain results in prompt loss of consciousness and pupillary dilatation. These initial changes are frequently accompaned by grand mal seizure activity. While a detailed description of the neurologic changes that occur after cardiac arrest is outside the scope of this chapter, as a practical matter the patient's level of consciousness and pupillary status are the two most important indices of brain function that may be followed easily during the course of CPR. There are a number of reasons, certain of which will be discussed subsequently, why the level of consciousness may not immediately return to normal immediately when adequate cardiopulmonary resuscitation is initiated or spontaneous cardiac activity is restored promptly after cardiac arrest. On the other hand, anyone who has had experience with cardiopulmonary resuscitation, particularly in the coronary care unit setting where resuscitative efforts can be initiated promptly, will have encountered patients who revert to a virtually normal level of consciousness during the application of resuscitative techniques. Since the level of consciousness may not improve immediately, the single most useful and practical sign indicating that blood flow to the brain is sufficient during resuscitative efforts is the resumption of normal pupillary responses. Even the latter, however, may be modified by various factors such as drugs given during cardiopulmonary resuscitation. Thus, the ultimate test of the adequacy of brain blood flow during resuscitation is the subsequent return of higher cortical functions. It is worth emphasizing that while it is the brain's sensitivity to the cessation of blood flow that poses the critical time consideration for resuscitative efforts, it should be possible in virtually all circumstances to restore flow to the brain promptly and effectively in the coronary care unit.

## TECHNIQUES USED DURING CARDIOPULMONARY RESUSCITATION

Optimal performance of cardiopulmonary resuscitation requires a detailed knowledge of a variety of techniques and therapeutic modalities, ranging from basic life support to sophisticated approaches to the treatment of dysrhythmias. In addition, these diverse techniques must be coordinated in such a fashion that the most definitive forms of therapy are recognized and used as early as possible. It is therefore crucial that a precise plan of action be formulated beforehand. Such a plan must recognize the importance and primacy of basic life support, it must achieve maximum efficiency, and it must remain flexible enough to deal with individual patient variation. In this section, we shall discuss, in an individual fashion, the various techniques and therapeutic modalities available and then attempt to synthesize them into an organized approach. As previously, this material will be specifically geared to the coronary care unit setting.

## INDICATIONS FOR CARDIOPULMONARY RESUSCITATION

The first step to be taken before basic life support measures are initiated is to ensure that the patient has indeed suffered circulatory collapse, which will require resuscitative measures. This is rarely a problem in patients who suffer ventricular tachycardia or fibrillation in the coronary care unit. In this situation, it is not necessary to check the arterial pulse but rather to merely ascertain that the electrocardiographic monitor demonstrates one of these malignant rhythm disturbances and that the patient is unresponsive. Occasionally, artifacts may occur during monitoring, which simulate these dysrhythmias. Although the concept is self-evident, it is important to emphasize that if the patient appears normal, one should not initiate resuscitative measures, and the presence of an artifact should be considered. In the case of a bradydysrhythmia, the same guidelines apply. That is, the combination of monitor lead findings and unresponsiveness are sufficient justification to initiate resuscitative measures. It should be kept in mind that vasovagal reactions, which will often revert spontaneously, are not unusual in the coronary care unit setting. Even if a vasovagal reaction is suspected, however, resuscitative measures should be initiated. Such patients will usually respond promptly to appropriate therapy, and resuscitation can then be discontinued quickly. If the patient loses consciousness abruptly and cardiac rhythm does not change, it is prudent to first determine that arterial pulsations are absent or markedly diminished (i.e., that electromechanical dissociation is indeed present) before initiating resuscitative measures, and to be sure that unconsciousness is due to circulatory collapse and not to some other cause. This is best done by checking the carotid pulse, although it is perfectly reasonable to check some other pulse known to be present previously. Occasionally, patients will abruptly develop either rhythm disorders or hemodynamic difficulties that result in major reductions in cardiac output, which are not severe enough to produce complete loss of consciousness. In many circumstances, this type of situation will resolve itself quickly. For instance, patients with ventricular tachycardia, who do not lose consciousness completely, will usually either spontaneously revert to sinus rhythm, degenerate into ventricular fibrillation, or respond to a maneuver such as a chest thump. In instances in which this does not occur, considerable judgment is required as to whether resuscitation should be started or other therapeutic and/or diagnostic maneuvers should be begun. As a general rule, in this situation, it is probably wise to err on the side of initiating resuscitative procedures. Finally, if a prior decision has been made not to resuscitate a patient, it is of utmost importance that this be communicated and understood by all personnel in the coronary care unit.

## BASIC LIFE SUPPORT

Basic life support refers to techniques used for the mechanical maintenance of both circulation and ventilation sufficient to sustain life until such time as the patient can survive without such assistance or it is elected to terminate resuscitative efforts. Although basic life support is not necessarily the first resuscitative technique utilized in the coronary care unit setting as soon as a patient with circulatory collapse is identified, steps should be taken so that basic life support can be instituted promptly. It is of prime importance that basic life support be applied as continuously as possible throughout the course of cardiopulmonary resuscitation, until such time as the patient can spontaneously maintain an adequate cardiac output and ventilation or more advanced life support measures (e.g., endotracheal intubation and mechanical ventilation) have been instituted. (For an excellent detailed discussion of basic life support, the reader is referred to the Supplement to the Journal of the American Medical Association published in 1974 in conjunction with the American Heart Association.[56] An update of this supplement is scheduled for publication in JAMA in the latter half of 1980.)

The so-called "two rescuer" technique will be summarized here because it is assumed that in the coronary care unit setting, at least two individuals will be available for cardiopulmonary resuscitation. The three underlying principles of basic life support (the "ABCs") are (1) *airway,* (2) *breathing,* and (3) *circulation.*[56] These three steps must be carried out in rapid sequence. The first step is to ensure a patent airway (Fig. 31.1). The most commonly employed technique is the head-tilt method, which is simple to perform and effective in almost all cases, particularly in the coronary care unit where situations in which airway obstruction is a primary event are unusual. For this maneuver, the patient must be supine. One hand is placed behind the patient's neck and the other on the forehead. By exerting pressure on the forehead, the patient's head is tilted backward, thus extending the neck and relieving airway obstruction by the tongue. If this maneuver does not open the airway, the jaw thrust technique

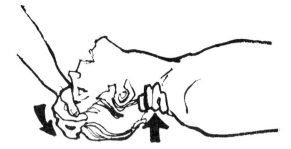

Fig. 31.1 The head-tilt method for ensuring a patent airway during CPR. (Reprinted from the Supplement to Journal of the American Medical Association, February 18, 1974. Copyright 1974, the American Medical Association. Reprinted with permission from the American Heart Association. JAMA 227 [suppl 7]:883–868, 1974.)

can be used. This technique is performed best from a position behind the patient's head. The fingers are placed behind the patient's jaw and used to forcefully displace the mandible forward. At the same time, the head is tilted backward and the thumbs used to retract the lower lip, allowing ventilation through both the nose and the mouth.

On extremely rare occasions a tracheotomy may be necessary to ensure a patent airway in patients who have suffered abrupt circulatory collapse in the coronary care unit. Hence, knowledge of this technique is highly desirable. Once a patent airway is established, the next step is to initiate artifical respiration. Here, the simplest and generally most effective technique is mouth-to-mouth ventilation (Fig. 31.2). With the head maximally tilted by the hand placed behind the neck, the other hand is used to pinch the patient's nostrils while simultaneously continuing to maintain pressure on the forehead to aid in gaining maximum tilt. Artificial ventilation is then initiated by taking a deep breath, making a tight seal around the patient's mouth, and forcibly exhaling into the patient's mouth. It is initially recommended that four rapid lung inflations be performed without full deflation. Subsequently, the lungs should be inflated every 5 seconds and allowed to deflate passively. Adequacy of ventilation is ensured by (1) observing the patient's chest rise and fall, (2) encountering some degree of resistance as the patient's lungs are expanded, and (3)

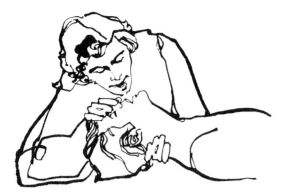

Fig. 31.2 The technique of mouth-to-mouth ventilation during CPR. (Reprinted from the Supplement to Journal of the American Medical Association, February 18, 1974. Copyright 1974, the American Medical Association. Reprinted with permission from the American Heart Association. JAMA 227 [suppl 7]:883–868, 1974.)

feeling air escape during deflation. In an occasional patient, mouth-to-nose ventilation may be more appropriate, usually when the mouth cannot be opened easily, but this form of ventilation is most commonly necessary in noncoronary care settings. While technically not considered a form of basic life support, supplemental techniques for maintaining a patent airway and artificial ventilation are readily and rapidly available in the coronary care unit setting, and personnel should be thoroughly trained in their use. These supplemental techniques involve use of an airway device and a bag-valve-mask system. These offer advantages over mouth-to-mouth ventilation in that supplemental oxygen can and should be delivered easily; in addition, they are more convenient. However, they generally do not provide as large an inspiratory volume as mouth-to-mouth ventilation. For this reason, they must be used carefully, with particular attention paid to achieving a tight seal. A variety of airway devices are available, each of which has advantages and disadvantages. We have favored the combination of S-tubes, because of their simplicity, and an AMBU (Air-Mask-Bag-Unit) bag. The latter may also be connected to an endotracheal tube. If there is any question as to the adequacy of ventilation, supplemental airway and ventilation devices should be abandoned in favor of the more certain mouth-to-mouth technique.

Once artificial ventilation is established, closed-chest cardiac massage (CCCM) should be initiated, as a practical matter immediately after the first rapid lung inflations. Closed-chest cardiac massage, first popularized by Kouwenhoven in 1960,[57] is perhaps the single most important advance in cardiopulmonary resuscitation techniques. It is well-documented that with CCCM, it is usually possible to maintain blood flow sufficient for recovery of cerebral function.[31,57-59] Indeed, it is not unusual for a patient to regain responsiveness when CCCM is initiated even though cardiac rhythm remains completely ineffective. Closed-chest cardiac massage has, in addition, virtually completely displaced open-chest cardiac massage. Although the latter still has a role in certain situations, particularly in the postcardiac surgical patient and in the victim of trauma, there is virtually no indication for open-chest massage in the coronary care unit. It has generally been taught that CCCM is effective because the heart is compressed directly between the sternum and the vertebral column. MacKenzie et al.[58] suggested, in 1964, that the latter may be less important than the changes in intrathoracic pressure that occur during CCCM and more recent work supports this concept. The latter indicates that, in dogs, sternal compression is effective because the resultant increase in intrathoracic pressure produces a pressure gradient between intra- and extrathoracic arteries and veins and thereby produces blood flow.[58a] No pressure gradients are measured within the heart, and, therefore, the heart is viewed merely as a conduit for blood flow. If this work is validated, it is possible that in the future significant changes in the technique of CCCM will emerge. These include the use of techniques such as abdominal binding [58b] and the application of positive airway pressure during sternal compression alternating with negative airway pressure between compressions.[58c]

At the present time, CCCM, as traditionally taught, remains a proven technique that is relatively simple to perform (see Fig. 31.3). The patient should be supine and on a hard surface. For this reason, a board or cafeteria tray should be readily available. There is no reason to wait for the latter before beginning

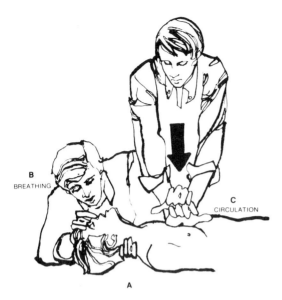

Fig. 31.3 The technique of closed-chest cardiac massage. (Reprinted from the Supplement to Journal of the American Medical Association, February 18, 1974. Copyright 1974, the American Medical Association. Reprinted with permission from the American Heart Association. JAMA 227 [suppl 7]:883–868, 1974.)

CCCM. It is also advantageous to elevate the lower extremities in an effort to improve venous return. The individual performing CCCM should position himself at the side of the patient's chest, facing the individual performing artificial respiration, and first identify a point on the sternum approximately 2 inches above the xiphoid process. The heel of one hand is placed over this point, and the other hand is placed on top of the first hand. With arms held straight and the shoulders directly above the sternum, pressure is then exerted vertically downward in order to depress the sternum about 2 inches. Compression should be continuous and smooth, not jerky, and immediately followed by relaxation, which should be of the same duration as compression. Particular care must be taken to position the heel of the hand over the sternum (not the costochondral junction or ribs) and to avoid compression over the xiphoid, since this may result in hepatic laceration. After the first series of lung inflations, CCCM should be initiated at a rate of 60/min, with ventilation performed after every five compressions. Ventilation should not interrupt the rhythm of CCCM. The two most important guidelines for the performance of adequate basic life support are the presence of a palpable pulse and the status of the pupillary light reflex. The carotid pulse is most ideal and should be checked frequently. Occasionally, this may be technically difficult, in which case the femoral pulses may be easily monitored. Palpable pulses may be misleading in that they may merely reflect the transmission of changes in intrathoracic pressure produced by CCCM. However, the absence of palpable pulses is usually an indication that CCCM is inadequate.

In the coronary care unit setting, the pupils should promptly become reactive to light, although drugs, particularly catecholamines, often result in dilatation. Reactive pupils indicate adequate oxygen delivery to the brain. If pulses cannot be palpated, if the pupils remain nonreactive, or both, the adequacy of basic life support techniques should be questioned. In an occasional patient (for instance, one who has suffered circulatory collapse due to a complication such as left ventricular rupture and resultant cardiac tamponade or massive mitral regurgitation), it may not be possible to maintain adequate basic life support with CCCM. At the present time, although this obviously cannot be known when the patient first sustains circulatory collapse, such complications are essentially untreatable. The inability to perform adequate life support, even though optimal techniques are used, is rarely, if ever, an indication for open-chest cardiac massage *in the coronary care unit setting* because this situation almost always indicates that a currently untreatable complication has occurred.

Once basic life support has been initiated, a decision must often be made as to whether a more definitive airway (i.e., endotracheal intubation or the use of an esophageal obturator airway) should be established. This is obviously not a problem in patients who respond promptly to definitive therapy, such as electrical defibrillation. Although techniques and indications for establishment of a more definitive airway are discussed in a separate chapter, it is important to stress that such techniques must be performed by individuals adept in their use. Attempts at endotracheal intubation by inexperienced personnel are often unsuccessful and result in important interruptions in basic life support. At all times, basic life support must be maintained as continuously as possible until such time as resuscitative efforts are discontinued.

Finally, several mechanical devices to perform CCCM have been designed. These have not been shown to be more effective than CCCM as described above and, therefore, are properly regarded as useful only from a convenience standpoint or when only a limited number of trained personnel are available. These devices are not indicated or necessary in a properly staffed coronary care unit.

## THERAPY OF DYSRHYTHMIAS DURING CARDIOPULMONARY RESUSCITATION

Although the treatment of dysrhythmias in the coronary care unit has been discussed in detail elsewhere in this book, dysrhythmias initiating circulatory collapse or occurring during the course of cardiopulmonary resuscitation merit special attention. While this section will not be concerned with the electrocardiographic diagnosis of rhythm disturbances, in all patients with sudden circulatory collapse in the coronary care unit, a 12-lead electrocardiogram should be attached to the patient as soon as it is feasible to supplement monitor leads in establishing a rhythm diagnosis. However, it is rarely necessary to wait for this information before initiating antidysrhythmic therapy in this particular setting.

### Ventricular Tachycardia and Fibrillation

These are the most common dysrhythmias resulting in circulatory collapse in the coronary care unit, and their treatment may be considered simultaneously. As noted previously, they are usually initiated by a premature ventricular complex, but they may also occur in association with bradycardic rhythm disturbances. In either case, initial treatment is similar.

Several reports have documented the efficacy of the chest thump in reverting ventricular tachycardia and, unusually, ventricular fibrillation.[60-62] The chest thump is performed by delivering a sharp, quick blow to the midsternum with the outer surface of the fist from a distance of 8 to 12 inches. This mechanical stimulus imparts a small electric stimulus to the heart. The chest thump is probably most effective in reverting ventricular tachycardia because it is likely that this rhythm disturbance often has a reentrant mechanism that may be interrupted by small amounts of electrical energy.[61] An example of a successful chest thump is provided in Fig. 31.4. Ventricular fibrillation rarely responds because much larger amounts of energy are required to depolarize both ventricles.[62] Because the chest thump is so easy to perform and requires only a few seconds, in patients with circulatory collapse due to ventricular tachycardia or fibrillation, it is quite reasonable to deliver one chest thump as the initial therapeutic maneuver. If there is no response, further attempts are not warranted and will only delay further therapy.

The most definitive and rapid form of therapy both for ventricular tachycardia and fibrillation is an electric countershock. However, in the

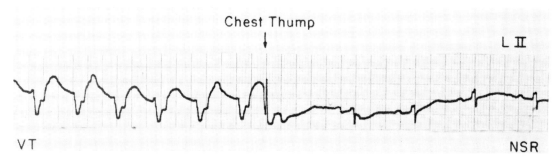

Fig. 31.4 An example of reversion of ventricular tachycardia by a precordial thump. (Pennington JE, Taylor J, Lown B: Chest thump for reverting ventricular tachycardia. N Engl J Med 283:1194, 1970.)

case of ventricular tachycardia it may sometimes be elected to administer an intravenous
bolus of lidocaine, 75 to 100 mg, before attempting electric countershock. Whether or not this
is done is strictly a logistic question. That is,
lidocaine should be administered if it is possible
to do so without delaying the application of
an electric countershock. Lidocaine should not
be administered initially if the rhythm is ventricular fibrillation.

The first report of successful external electrical defibrillation (using an alternating current
device) was that of Zoll et al. in 1956.[63] In
1962, Lown et al.[64] first described a direct current defibrillator, and since that time the advantages of direct over alternating current have
been well-established.[65,66] A large number of
companies manufacture direct current defibrillators. For the coronary care unit setting, in
which ease of transport is not a major consideration, the most desirable defibrillators are those
providing the highest energy levels (usually in
the 400 to 500 watt-sec range), since there is
evidence that larger individuals may require
energy levels in excess of that available from
many commercial defibrillators.[67] Defibrillators
should have the capacity to synchronize their
discharge with the patient's QRS complex.
However, in the case of ventricular fibrillation,
this is obviously unnecessary, and in ventricular
tachycardia, it usually is not justified because
of time considerations. Another occasionally
useful feature of the DC defibrillator in the coronary care unit is the ability to record the patient's electrocardiogram directly from the defibrillator paddles, since it is not unusual for
monitor leads to become detached during the
resuscitative procedures.

There has been some debate about optimal
placement of the defibrillator paddles,[68-70] and
in theory anteroposterior placement may be the
most advantageous.[69] However, as a practical
matter, this appears to be, at best, a marginal
advantage. Therefore, in ventricular fibrillation
and tachycardia, when time is of the essence,
we have favored the simplest approach, that
is, an anterior placement of both paddles. Considerable minor variation in the exact placement
of the two anterior paddles exists in the literature. However, all of the approaches are reason-

able, in that they are likely to include both ventricles in the electric field set up between the
paddles. It is our recommendation that one paddle be placed just to the right of the sternum
at the level of the second and third intercostal
spaces and the other at the level of the fifth
and sixth intercostal spaces, about halfway between the left midclaviclar and anterior axillary
lines. Alternatively, the first paddle may be
placed just below the suprasternal notch. In
our experience, an occasional patient has appeared to respond to minor variations in these
positions. It has been our impression that this
is sometimes related to factors such as heart
size and chest configuration, but there are no
systematic studies of these variables in relation
to paddle position.

If anterior placement is unsuccessful, the anteroposterior approach may be attempted. In
this case, one paddle is placed over the sternum
at the level of the apex of the heart and the
second, in the left infrascapular area (but not
over the vertebral column). Before defibrillation
is actually attempted, a layer of electrode paste
should be applied to each paddle to improve
conductivity and to reduce the chance of burns
to the skin. It is important that the skin under
the paddles be dry and that there be no chance
of a short circuit between the paddles. Alternatively, gauze pads presoaked in electrolyte solution may be used in place of electrode paste.

The most important single factor in determining whether DC countershock will be successful in defibrillating the heart is time.[71-73]
It has been well-shown that after 1 minute of
ventricular fibrillation, chances of success are
significantly reduced. The latter may be related
to a number of factors, including the development of acidosis, which increases the electrical
threshold for successful defibrillation.[74-76] The
other major factor in determining the success
of electrical defibrillation is whether the arrhythmia is primary or secondary, with chances
for success being much greater with a primary
rhythm disturbance.[72,73] It is not known
whether the same time considerations apply for
ventricular tachycardia, but because of the
tendency for this rhythm to degenerate rapidly
into ventricular fibrillation, it is equally important to apply DC countershock rapidly in this

situation. The time between the occurrence of ventricular tachycardia or fibrillation and the first attempt at electric countershock should not be longer than 2 minutes, and preferably less than 1 minute. Thus, as part of the initial automatic and coordinated response to ventricular tachycardia and fibrillation, the defibrillator should be brought to the patient's bedside (if there are no bedside defibrillators in the unit), set up, and charged by previously designated personnel. During these first seconds, the chest thump and basic life support will have been simultaneously initiated, but defibrillation should not be delayed by these maneuvers. Immediately before the defibrillator is discharged, all personnel should be told to move away from the patient's bed. It may also be necessary to turn off certain other electric devices, for instance, electrocardiographic monitors and temporary pacemaker generators, but this will depend on the characteristics of these devices in individual coronary care units.

The mechanism by which DC cardioversion is successful depends on the nature of the rhythm disturbance. Thus, for ventricular fibrillation, one depends on simultaneous depolarization of the entire heart and the subsequent capacity of pacemaker cells to then assume their normal function. This requires large amounts of energy (usually at least 300 watt-sec and sometimes considerably more). Ventricular tachycardia in the setting of ischemic heart disease, at a rate sufficient to cause circulatory collapse, is thought to represent a reentrant rhythm in most cases.[77] As such, it will often respond to much lower energy levels, which need only interrupt a portion of the reentrant pathway.[61,77] Therefore, in patients in whom this rhythm does not result in circulatory collapse and who are to be cardioverted, it is advisable to synchronize to the QRS complex and begin at relatively low energy levels. However, when this rhythm does result in circulatory collapse and time becomes a crucial factor, high energy levels should be used initially and one need not be concerned with synchronization. Thus, for both ventricular fibrillation and tachycardia (when associated with circulatory collapse), the defibrillator should be charged to the highest energy level available.

Brief periods of asystole are common after defibrillation, before the sinus node resumes normal function. If these last longer than a few seconds, basic life support procedures should be immediately reinstituted and the cardiac rhythm checked after a short period of ventilation and CCCM. If the first attempt fails, it is probably worthwhile to attempt defibrillation again as soon as possible. If a second attempt also fails, a number of things may be done to optimize the chances of later success. First, careful attention should be paid to the status of oxygenation and acid-base balance. A blood gas should be obtained as early as possible and arterial $PO_2$ maximized. How this is done will depend on the manner in which the patient is being ventilated. If endotracheal intubation has not yet been performed, it should be considered if an experienced person is available. In addition, if an initial bolus of sodium bicarbonate has not yet been administered (see section below on maintenance of acid-base balance) this should be done. If sufficient time has passed, a second dose may be administered. Although overtreatment with sodium bicarbonate should be avoided, the major consideration at this point is treatment of the cardiac rhythm and, as indicated previously, acidosis may markedly impair the ability to perform defibrillation.

Another consideration is that of "fine" versus "coarse" ventricular fibrillation (Fig. 31.5). For some time it has been recognized that it is more difficult to successfully defibrillate if the fibrillatory waves are of low amplitude (fine) and that the administration of catecholamines may increase their amplitude.[34,35] Unfortunately, there is no well-established quantitative guideline as to what distinguishes coarse from fine ventricular fibrillation. We have empirically considered patients with fibrillatory waves of less than 0.5 mV, using the standard electrocardiogram leads, to be candidates for catecholamine therapy. However, if initial attempts at defibrillation fail, it may well be advisable to use catecholamines, regardless of the height of the fibrillatory waves. In this situation, epinephrine (5 ml of a 1:10,000 solution) may be administered intracardiac or through a central circulatory access site and defibrillation attempted again. The technical aspects of defibrillation should also

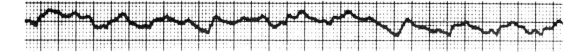

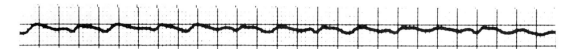

Fig. 31.5 Examples of "coarse" (top) and "fine" (bottom) ventricular fibrillation. (Reprinted by permission from Laiken L, Laiken SL, Karliner JS: Interpretation of Electrocardiograms: A Self-Instructional Approach. Appleton-Century-Crofts, New York, NY, 1978.)

be scrutinized at this point. Thus, the possibility of poor skin contact or short circuits between the paddles should be reviewed and paddle placement varied, with consideration given to changing to an anteroposterior placement. Additionally, the possibility that the defibrillator itself is not functioning properly should be considered, particularly since stimulation of muscle does not necessarily indicate that the maximum energy level is actually being discharged. Since adequate testing of defibrillator output is too time consuming to be performed during cardiopulmonary resuscitation, it is advisable to try another defibrillator if the first few attempts are unsuccessful. Another consideration is whether CCCM is being performed adequately. Occasional patients appear to respond better to defibrillation after a period of CCCM, perhaps because myocardial blood flow has improved. Finally, the question of whether other specific factors may be contributing to difficulty in defibrillation should be considered. Once again, the most important of these is correction of acidosis. Less commonly, factors such as specific electrolyte imbalance or digitalis toxicity may be considered. Once all of these factors have been reviewed and corrected to the fullest extent possible and a reasonable number of attempts at defibrillation have been unsuccessful, a final alternative is the use of bretylium tosylate. This drug will be discussed separately, but it is worth pointing out that it is the only known pharmacologic agent in clinical use that can abolish established ventricular fibrillation.[78-80]

Since it also has considerable toxicity, at present it should probably be reserved as a last measure.

Once successful defibrillation has been accomplished, a number of other rhythm disturbances may occur, which require emergency treatment. As noted previously, brief periods of asystole may follow defibrillation before the sinus node begins functioning. In this case, basic life support is immediately resumed, but it will quickly become apparent that it is no longer required. It is not unusual for asystole to be prolonged or for the heart to resume fibrillating after a period of asystole following successful defibrillation. If the latter occurs, the most rational therapy is the administration of agents that increase the automaticity of supraventricular pacemakers, before defibrillation is attempted again. We have favored atropine sulfate as the first choice in this situation because it has little or no effect on pacemaker tissue below the A-V node. Alternatively, catecholamines (isoproterenol or epinephrine) with predominant beta-agonist properties may be used and are preferred to atropine, if the fibrillatory waves are low in amplitude. If the heart remains asystolic, therapy for asystole, as described subsequently, should be initiated. Another mode of therapy for the patient with asystole is insertion of a transthoracic ventricular pacemaker, if the patient demonstrates a pattern of asystole followed by recurrent fibrillation after DC countershock. The use of electronic pacemakers during cardiopulmonary rescuscitation is discussed in more detail in a separate section (see below). Another commonly encountered rhythm disturbance after defibrillation is a slow idioventricular rhythm, which is usually mechanically ineffective. The approach to this rhythm is also discussed separately.

Successful defibrillation does not necessarily require that normal sinus rhythm be the result. Any cardiac rhythm that provides an adequate cardiac output may be considered a success. The latter applies mainly to a variety of supraventricular tachycardias, for example, atrial fibrillation or junctional tachycardia, which may be seen following defibrillation. These rhythms usually revert spontaneously to sinus rhythm and, if they provide an adequate cardiac output, should not be treated further, at least initially. More important, in the patient who is successfully defibrillated aggressive therapy should be directed toward the prevention of recurrent ventricular fibrillation or tachycardia. It has been our policy that any patient successfully defibrillated receives prophylactic lidocaine immediately afterward and for a period of 24 to 48 hours thereafter. The goal is to abolish ventricular couplets or short runs of ventricular tachycardia not requiring DC cardioversion, and/or suppression of single ventricular premature beats. Ideally, isolated ventricular premature beats should be completely suppressed. However, it may often be necessary to accept less than complete suppression, providing more complex ventricular dysrhythmias do not occur. In this situation, we have generally attempted to suppress isolated ventricular premature beats to a frequency of less than 2 to 3/min. If the patient has not been receiving lidocaine before defibrillation, the usual initial intravenous bolus of 75 to 100 mg should be administered after defibrillation. If the patient does not have ventricular dysrhythmias after defibrillation, the bolus should be followed by an intravenous lidocaine drip at a rate of 2 to 4 mg/min. As many of these patients will have reduced cardiac output, particular care must be taken to avoid subsequent lidocaine toxicity as a result of too rapid an infusion rate. If the patient continues to have ventricular dysrhythmias after an initial lidocaine bolus, the bolus should be repeated. In patients who have received lidocaine before successful defibrillation,

postdefibrillation antidysrhythmic therapy requires considerable judgement and individualized treatment, in particular, a careful review of prior lidocaine therapy and specific factors that might influence blood levels of the drug. In most such patients, it is safe to administer a single additional bolus of lidocaine (50 to 100 mg) in an effort to acutely increase blood levels, but this is not advisable in patients likely to have relatively high blood levels before defibrillation.

If single ventricular premature beats at a rate greater than 2 to 3/min, or more complex ventricular dysrhythmias continue to occur despite lidocaine therapy, we have favored the use of intravenous procainamide as follows. A loading dose of the drug is given at a rate of 100 mg every 5 minutes, either in a continuous infusion or in intermittent doses, until the desired endpoint with respect to dysrhythmia control is reached, and then a continuous infusion at a rate of 2 to 6 mg/min is begun.[81-84] The latter must be reduced if renal insufficiency is present. During the administration of the loading dose, blood pressure must be monitored carefully. Modest declines in blood pressure of 10 to 15 mmHg are the rule when procainamide is administered intravenously. Larger reductions are often an indication to terminate administration of the drug. Additionally, we have also found it useful to carefully monitor the PR interval and the width of the QRS complex during intravenous procainamide administration. Increases in QRS width of up to 15 to 25 percent are often associated with a therapeutic effect. Larger increases are another indication to terminate its administration, especially if ventricular dysrhythmias continue. Procainamide does not appear to widen the QRS as predictably as quinidine, however, and good results are often obtained without a significant change in QRS duration. There is no firm guideline as to how much procainamide should be administered (providing the blood pressure or QRS width endpoints noted previously are not reached) before the drug is considered to be unsuccessful. In our experience and that of others,[83] intravenous procainamide is quite effective and most patients will respond to less than a 1 g loading dose, although we have given as much as 2 g. In this type of patient, it is often necessary to accept a less than ideal endpoint—for instance, the continuance of single ventricular premature beats without more complex or malignant dysrhythmias. However, if the patient who has been successfully defibrillated continues to have malignant ventricular dysrhythmias (particularly recurrent ventricular tachycardia or fibrillation) despite the use of lidocaine and procainamide, we have proceeded to the use of bretylium tosylate or overdrive ventricular pacing. Ventricular pacing during cardiopulmonary resuscitation is discussed separately.

It must also be stressed that careful consideration of any factors contributing to recurrent ventricular dysrhythmias after defibrillation should be undertaken. Most of these are similar to those that should be taken into account in the patient who cannot be successfully defibrillated, i.e., electrolyte and ventilatory status. Thus, for instance, occasional patients who may have reason to be potassium depleted may respond to intravenous potassium even if serum levels are normal; others may improve by increasing arterial $PO_2$. In patients who receive digitalis, the possibility of toxicity should be considered, in which case drug therapy with diphenylhydantoin may be more appropriate than a drug such as procainamide. Other contributory factors may be poorly controlled heart failure and/or active myocardial ischemia or infarction.

## Bradycardic Rhythm Disturbances

Bradycardic rhythm disturbances consist of disorders of impulse initiation, for instance, profound sinus node depression with or without slow escape pacemakers, or of impulse conduction, and are much less common in producing circulatory collapse than ventricular tachycardia or fibrillation. Many bradycardic rhythm disturbances occur in association with major increases in vagal tone [22-27] and thus, when occurring as the primary rhythm disturbance producing circulatory collapse, are frequently rapidly reversible with simple maneuvers. Profound sinus node depression, occurring as a result of increased vagal tone, is usually accompa-

nied by suppression of other supraventricular pacemakers and impaired atrioventricular conduction. On the other hand, complete heart block following anterior myocardial infarction is not associated with increased vagal tone. Regardless of their mechanism of production, the initial approach to primary bradycardic rhythm disturbances resulting in circulatory collapse is similar. This consists of initiation of basic life support (in this situation, it may be particularly useful to elevate the legs) and the administration of intravenous atropine sulfate (1 mg), preferably through a central circulatory access site. If prompt improvement does not occur, a second dose of atropine should be administered. These considerations apply whether the initial rhythm disturbance is ventricular asystole or a slow escape rhythm and, in addition, whether these are encountered as the primary cause of circulatory collapse or during the course of resuscitation from cardiac arrest due to other causes. We have not favored the initial use of beta-stimulating catecholamines in this setting because atropine is often all that is required and catecholamines, such as isoproterenol and epinephrine, have considerable potential for initiating a number of other rhythm disturbances. However, if atropine does not produce prompt improvement, bolus injections of isoproterenol (5 to 15 $\mu$g) or epinephrine (5 ml of $1:10,000$ solution) are indicated, followed by constant infusions, if necessary. These agents in particular should be given through a central access site. If a central site is not immediately available they should be given intracardiac (either through the third or fourth intercostal space to the left of the sternum or at the cardiac apex).

While use of catecholamines will often result in the resumption of a supraventricular rhythm (frequently some form of supraventricular tachycardia), it is also not uncommon for them to accelerate a ventricular escape rhythm to the point of ventricular tachycardia, or to produce ventricular fibrillation. In either case, the dysrhythmia must then be treated as described previously. It is also not unusual for these agents to produce an accelerated idioventricular rhythm, which may or may not be capable of maintaining an adequate cardiac output. Although this rhythm is usually intrinsically unstable, if an adequate cardiac output results, it is best to try and maintain this type of rhythm with infusions of a catecholamine. Under these circumstances, a supraventricular rhythm often appears spontaneously with time, particularly if atrioventricular dissociation was present and the sinus rate increases. Alternatively, if an accelerated idioventricular rhythm with A-V dissociation is present, the catecholamine infusion may be gradually reduced in the hope that conduction of sinus node impulses will begin as the rate of the ventricular pacemaker slows. If this is done, it is also possible that the accelerated idioventricular rate may simply slow without the development of a supraventricular rhythm. The presence of an accelerated idioventricular rhythm sufficient to maintain cardiac output but requiring beta-adrenergic stimulation to provide an adequate rate is one indication for a trial of emergency ventricular pacing if a supraventricular mechanism does not appear, although it may be elected to merely continue support with catecholamines. An accelerated idioventricular rhythm that does not support an adequate cardiac output despite the use of catecholamines may be considered a form of electromechanical dissociation and appropriate therapy, as discussed subsequently, should be initiated. Basic life support and CCCM must, of course, be continued whenever an adequate cardiac output is not being generated.

Patients known to have had complete heart block (Fig. 31.6) resulting in circulatory collapse constitute a somewhat special group. As indicated previously, this rarely occurs in acute inferior wall myocardial infarction. While such unusual patients will commonly respond well to basic life support and atropine, a temporary ventricular pacemaker should be inserted never-theless. This procedure need not be done under emergency conditions as long as there is a good response to atropine. Patients who suffer circulatory collapse as a result of complete heart block in association with acute anterior wall infarction usually will exhibit extensive anterior necrosis, and will generally not respond to atropine. Although an initial bolus of atropine is not an unreasonable measure in such patients, it may be anticipated that beta-adrenergic stimulation will be required as a temporary measure before emergency ventricular pacing is instituted. In this instance, either an initial bolus of isoproterenol or epinephrine, followed by a constant infusion (or simply the latter), should be used in an attempt to produce an accelerated idioventricular rhythm and/or a lesser degree of heart block. Pharmacologic therapy is basically a temporary measure in these circumstances. In any patient with heart block resulting in circulatory collapse, which is not responsive to atropine, emergency ventricular pacing should be instituted. Whether or not a transthoracic or transvenous route is employed will depend on the patient's condition. When the transvenous route is selected, it is best to insert a standard pacemaker catheter under fluoroscopic control. It has been our feeling that if it is impossible to produce an adequate cardiac output by using catecholamines in patients with complete heart block, thereby necessitating the continuance of basic life support measures, a transthoracic pacing approach or a "floating" transvenous pacemaker is indicated. On the other hand, if it is possible to discontinue basic life support as a result of pharmacologic therapy, a transvenous approach, using a standard pacing catheter, is in general more desirable. Further details in regard to electronic pace-

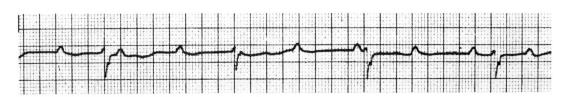

Fig. 31.6 An example of slow idioventricular rhythm with wide QRS complexes, in this case in association with complete heart block as indicated by the presence of regular, independent p waves. (Reprinted by permission from Laiken L, Laiken SL, Karliner JS: Interpretation of Electrocardiograms: A Self-Instructional Approach. Appleton-Century-Crofts, New York, NY, 1978.)

makers during cardiopulmonary resuscitation are provided in a separate section.

Occasional patients with bradycardic rhythm disturbances can be managed temporarily by mechanical stimulation of the heart. This technique seems to be most applicable when initial measures do not result in prompt improvement of a bradycardic rhythm disturbance, and yet the patient is capable of generating an adequate cardiac output when the heart rate is increased. This technique dates to certain examples in the literature in which repeated chest thumps were used to provoke electrical depolarization and effective mechanical activity in patients who were previously asystolic.[85-88] The principle is thus identical to that of the chest thump, except that in this case a regular series of mechanical stimuli are used to produce a small electrical force sufficient to initiate a cardiac contraction. Indeed, a device has been described to do precisely this without the need for repeated chest thumps.[89] While it is likely that a rather small number of patients in the coronary care unit can be managed using this technique, further investigation is warranted in order to define its role. Additionally, it is important to be quite certain that asystole or a very slow escape rhythm is indeed present since repeated mechanical stimulation during ventricular tachycardia may induce ventricular fibrillation.[60] Another technique that should be mentioned for the sake of completeness is the cough maneuver, familiar to anyone who has worked in a cardiac catheterization laboratory. Coughing is remarkably effective in maintaining an adequate cardiac output in patients who are asystolic, and in rare circumstances may be applicable in the coronary care unit.

## Other Dysrhythmias and Special Situations during Cardiopulmonary Resuscitation

It is exceedingly rare for arrhythmias other than ventricular tachycardia and fibrillation and the bradyarrhythmias, mentioned previously, to result in circulatory collapse. A few special circumstances that may occasionally be encountered in the coronary care unit should be mentioned. Thus, patients with preexcitation syndrome may have supraventricular tachycar-

dias (particularly atrial fibrillation) with ventricular rates so rapid that circulatory collapse may occur.[90] Patients with hypertrophic cardiomyopathy and aortic stenosis are susceptible to severe hemodynamic consequences if they develop atrial fibrillation with a rapid ventricular response, although circulatory collapse requiring resuscitation is quite unusual. Additionally, patients with ischemic heart disease, in general, may have profound left ventricular dysfunction in association with supraventricular tachyarrhythmias at rates that would ordinarily be well-tolerated, although once again circulatory collapse requiring resuscitation is most unusual. For these rare examples of supraventricular tachyarrhythmias resulting in circulatory collapse, the treatment is emergency countershock.

Digitalis toxicity also constitutes a special case, although digitalis-toxic arrhythmias, which may result in circulatory collapse, are no different than those discussed in the prior section, i.e., ventricular tachycardia, fibrillation, bradyarrhythmias, or asystole due to heart block. Usually a diagnosis of digitalis toxicity will have been suspected before the patient suffers circulatory collapse based on clinical history and the presence of prior digitalis-toxic arrhythmias. Initial therapy for digitalis-toxic arrhythmias causing circulatory collapse is no different than when these arrhythmias occur in the absence of digitalis. However, when electrical defibrillation is employed, the incidence of malignant arrhythmias after countershock is high if digitalis toxicity is present.[91,92] The risk of postcardioversion arrhythmias in patients receiving digitalis is related to the amount of energy employed. Thus, ventricular tachycardia is one instance in which lower energy levels should be used despite the fact that circulatory collapse has occurred. Kleiger and Lown [92] recommend the use of 25 watt-sec initially, with increases in the energy level if initial countershock is unsuccessful. The use of diphenylhydantoin and/or lidocaine in conjunction with countershock should be considered early for suppression of ventricular dysrhythmias in these patients. Potassium replacement is of course another mainstay of therapy in digitalis toxicity with ventricular dysrhythmias, although care must be taken in administering potassium when heart block is present. Finally, temporary pacing is often required in patients with digitalis toxicity and may be mandatory in patients receiving antiarrhythmic drugs and aggressive potassium replacement because of the potential for increasing A-V block or abolishing escape pacemakers with these forms of therapy.

Hyperkalemia may also occasionally be encountered in the coronary care unit as a primary cause of circulatory collapse, although the effects of hyperkalemia usually appear gradually and do not result in abrupt cardiac arrest. Along with the usual CPR measures, emergency therapy directed specifically to the correction of hyperkalemia (e.g., sodium bicarbonate, calcium, glucose-insulin-potassium infusion) is indicated.

As noted previously, although abrupt circulatory collapse due to arrhythmias is rarely caused by rhythm disturbances other than ventricular tachycardia, fibrillation, or the bradyarrhythmias described previously, virtually any arrhythmia may be encountered during the course of CPR. The approach to these secondary arrhythmias depends on their hemodynamic consequences. If they are adequate to support the circulation, it is judicious to carefully consider whether specific antiarrhythmic therapy is really indicated. If they are not adequate to support the circulation, CPR and antiarrhythmic therapy must be continued. The appearance of asystole or slow idioventricular rhythms unassociated with appreciable mechanical activity during the course of CPR (as opposed to the occurrence of these rhythms as a primary event or immediately after DC countershock) usually indicates a very poor prognosis and an essentially agonal state. While appropriate therapy should be directed toward correction of these rhythm disturbances as they appear, the chances for a successful outcome are slim.

## Emergency Cardiac Pacing during CPR

The most important indication for emergency electronic pacing during CPR is the treatment of bradyarrhythmias in patients in whom there is a reasonable possibility that a normal heart rate will result in an adequate cardiac output. Needless to say, patients with bradyarrhythmias who respond promptly to simple measures, such as the administration of atropine, do not require emergency pacing, although in some of these patients pacing may be subsequently indicated. The most important example of patients who deserve a trial of emergency pacing are those with primary bradyarrhythmias in whom an adequate cardiac output is achieved if the heart rate is increased by pharmacologic means (usually catecholamines), or patients in whom a normal rate cannot be achieved with drugs. It must be stressed that, in patients responsive to drugs, the physician may elect to continue drugs and not resort to pacing, depending on the individual circumstances. Regardless of the actual rhythm, if an adequate heart rate can be restored but the patient still cannot maintain an adequate cardiac output, emergency pacing is rarely indicated. On the other hand, all patients with circulatory collapse known to be due to primary complete heart block with either asystole or slow escape rhythms deserve a trial of emergency pacing, if drug therapy is ineffective. As noted previously, the appearance of asystole or slow ventricular escape rhythms unassociated with mechanical activity during the course of CPR (rather than as the primary event producing cardiac arrest) indicates a very poor prognosis, particularly if pharmacologic therapy does not improve cardiac output. Attempts at emergency transthoracic pacing under these circumstances usually do not produce satisfactory results. Even if pacing can be established, the higher heart rates rarely improve mechanical activity. Therefore, in this situation emergency pacing is rarely warranted.

The choice of a technique for emergency pacing depends on the patient's condition. If it is possible to maintain an adequate cardiac output with pharmacologic therapy, or perhaps with the use of external mechanical stimulation, we have favored a transvenous approach, using a standard pacemaker catheter under fluoroscopic guidance. This approach offers the advantages of a lesser incidence of complications and a high chance of success. On the other hand, if basic life support must be continued or the patient is extremely unstable, either the transthoracic approach or the use of a "floating" pacemaker catheter is indicated. Each of the latter techniques has advantages and disadvantages. A "floating" pacing electrode (either a Killip wire or a balloon-tip catheter), inserted without fluoroscopic guidance, is less traumatic, less likely to result in complications, and basic life support measures need not be interrupted. However, the chances of achieving stable pacing, at least in our own experience, are greater with the transthoracic approach. This is particularly true if cardiac output is inadequate and basic life support must be continued. Therefore, in this circumstance we have generally favored the transthoracic approach, despite the fact that basic life support must be interrupted.

With this approach, a commercially available needle-obturator assembly is passed through the fourth intercostal space just to the left of the sternum, or at the site of the cardiac apex. When the needle is inserted to its full length, the obturator is removed and the needle is gradually withdrawn until blood returns. At this point, the bipolar pacing electrode is inserted through the lumen of the needle, and the needle is removed. Commercially available transthoracic pacing electrodes have a j-shaped tip, constructed in such a way that as the electrode is gradually withdrawn tension should be appreciated when the tip is against the surface of the myocardium of either the left or right ventricle. As a practical matter, this is a rather subtle finding. We have favored attaching the pacing electrode to a temporary pacing generator as soon as it is within the cardiac chamber and initiating pacing at 5 to 10 mA before beginning to withdraw the electrode to the optimal site. With the generator turned on, capture may or may not be apparent. If 100 percent capture is present, the electrode should not be manipulated further, even if high levels of current (up to 5 to 10 mA) are required. If 100 percent capture is not present, the electrode is gradually withdrawn until it occurs. At this point, attempts may be made to reduce the current, but under these circumstances, high current levels are acceptable providing 100 percent capture is present. If it is not possible to achieve capture as the electrode is withdrawn, the approach is

incorrect and either the left or right ventricle has not been entered or the myocardium is incapable of responding to the pacemaker stimulus. The latter is frequently the case in agonal situations. If a second attempt at transthoracic pacing is thought warranted, a different anatomic approach should be attempted.

The complications of transthoracic pacing include myocardial or coronary arterial lacerations, pneumothorax, and infection. Further, as indicated previously, CCCM must be interrupted for a brief period of time. Therefore, transthoracic pacing should be instituted by personnel who can accomplish the technique rapidly. Multiple attempts at pacing, such that CCCM is interrupted for prolonged periods, are not warranted. Under these circumstances, if indications for emergency pacing are clear, passage of a "floating" transvenous pacemaker electrode should be attempted. In the unusual circumstance in which a patient can maintain an adequate cardiac output as a result of pharmacologic therapy, but is felt to be too unstable to allow passage of a standard pacing catheter under fluoroscopic guidance, use of a "floating" pacing electrode is probably the technique of choice. Patients who are successfully paced, using either the transthoracic approach or a "floating" electrode, should have either of these replaced with a standard pacing catheter as soon as this is feasible.

A final indication for emergency pacing in the CPR setting is overdrive suppression of malignant ventricular dysrhythmias. This is most appropriate in the patient with recurrent (rather than refractory) ventricular fibrillation or tachycardia in whom overdrive pacing often succeeds in abolishing ventricular premature beats that initiate more malignant rhythm disturbances. The choice of a technique for emergency pacing will once again depend on the stability of the patient. However, in this instance, a "floating" pacemaker catheter is probably more advisable than the transthoracic approach, if it is not feasible to insert a standard pacemaker catheter under fluoroscopic guidance. When used for overdrive suppression, the pacemaker generator should be set at a rate 10 to 20 beats greater than the patient's intrinsic rate. If adequate dysrhythmia suppression does not occur, the rate may be gradually increased until such time as the higher heart rate is no longer well tolerated. In some patients, overdrive suppression may worsen ventricular dysrhythmias. If this appears to be the case, pacing should be abandoned in favor of other therapeutic modalities.

## MANAGEMENT OF ELECTROMECHANICAL DISSOCIATION

By electromechanical dissociation (EMD) is meant the absence of effective cardiac contraction despite the presence of an adequate heart rate, regardless of the actual cardiac rhythm.

Electromechanical dissociation may occur under one of three circumstances during CPR. It may be the initiating event for circulatory collapse, in which case sinus rhythm will be present initially; it may occur transiently during the course of CPR, as a result of one or more of a number of factors; or it may be an agonal, irreversible phenomenon. In the latter two circumstances, any cardiac rhythm may be present.

The pathogenesis of EMD, occurring as an initiating event for circulatory collapse, has been discussed previously. In patients with ischemic heart disease, EMD implies either an acute structural alteration, such as rupture of the free wall of the left ventricle or rupture of the belly of a papillary muscle, or profound global ischemic dysfunction. Usually it is not possible to reliably distinguish these possibilities if circulatory collapse occurs in a truly abrupt fashion. However, if EMD occurs over a somewhat longer period of time, it may be possible to detect features of cardiac tamponade, which would indicate free wall rupture, or the sudden appearance of a systolic murmur, indicating mitral regurgitation. Although the structural alterations mentioned above are, at present, essentially untreatable, if they are severe enough to result in EMD, there presumably are patients with global ischemia in whom this situation is potentially reversible. Accordingly, although one can anticipate a low chance of success, CPR should be initiated in these patients. If cardiac

tamponade due to free wall rupture, massive mitral regurgitation due to papillary muscle rupture, or irreversible global ischemia is the cause of circulatory collapse, efforts to restore an effective circulation will not be successful.

Basic life support should be initiated in the usual fashion in these patients. Although difficult to document, it has been our impression that an occasional patient with EMD, presumably on the basis of global ischemia, will improve spontaneously as CPR is initiated. If EMD persists despite initial CPR efforts, one of the most effective means of rapidly improving myocardial function is to administer an intravenous bolus of calcium gluconate (10 ml of a 10 percent solution) or calcium chloride (2.5 to 5 ml of a 10 percent solution).[56] Either of these may also be administered directly into the heart in the same dose.[56] Calcium is very rapidly effective and has fewer chronotropic effects and less dysrhythmic potential then beta-stimulatory catecholamines although, as with any positive inotropic agent, it will increase myocardial oxygen demands. Because of these properties, we have favored calcium as the initial pharmacologic therapy for EMD. It must be recognized that the effects of a bolus injection of calcium last for only a few minutes. Therefore, if improvement after calcium does not occur or is not sustained, one must promptly resort to therapy with beta-stimulatory catecholamines. In this circumstance, the ideal agents are those with major positive inotropic effects and relatively little chronotropic and arrhythmogenic potential. Two such agents currently available are dopamine and dobutamine.

Dopamine has been available for several years and most clinicians are now familiar with its use in cardiac failure.[93-95] The drug is given by constant intravenous infusion at a dose of 1 to 5 $\mu$g/kg/min. With larger doses, the drug tends to increase systemic vascular resistance and may result in deleterious effects. Dobutamine is a newer agent with which there is less experience. It has potent inotropic effects, modest effects on heart rate, and apparently insignificant effects on systemic vascular resistance.[95-99] It has been given by constant intravenous infusion in doses ranging from 2.5 to 15 $\mu$g/kg/min. If these agents fail, isoproterenol, which is an even more potent inotropic agent with major chronotropic effects, should be employed.

Another potential therapeutic modality in this setting is the use of intraaortic balloon counterpulsation.[100,101] This approach would be theoretically beneficial in the patient with either acute, massive mitral regurgitation or global ischemia. While there is no published experience with this technique in patients who abruptly develop EMD requiring CPR, it is possible that balloon counterpulsation might save certain of these patients. This would require the capacity to insert an intraaortic balloon, on very short notice, on a round-the-clock basis followed by emergency cardiac catheterization, coronary arteriography, and heart surgery. The extensive commitment of time, money, and personnel required for such an approach is probably not warranted in view of the relatively small numbers of patients who might be saved. However, in a center routinely equipped to use these techniques on an emergency basis, this approach is feasible in patients who abruptly develop EMD and who show some response to more conservative management.

When EMD occurs during the course of CPR, but is not the initiating event, the most effective initial therapy is once again intravenous calcium. As noted previously, EMD will sometimes appear transiently during the course of successful CPR, not infrequently after successful defibrillation. This is likely due to transient myocardial depression as a result of a number of factors, for instance, reduced coronary blood flow, acidosis, or hypoxemia. Careful attention should therefore be directed toward the adequacy of basic life support and the patient's metabolic status. We have been impressed that in patients such as this, bolus injections of calcium sometimes appear to provide a "pump-priming" action. That is, improvement is maintained beyond the point at which calcium's action should have disappeared. Additionally, patients with transient EMD sometimes appear to respond to basic life support and/or improvement in metabolic or ventilatory status. If the above measures are not successful, then once again the use of catecholamines with predominant positive inotropic

effects, such as dopamine or dobutamine, is indicated. Electromechanical dissociation, occurring as an agonal state, may respond transiently to the above measures, but soon reverts to a situation in which effective mechanical activity is lost despite appropriate therapy.

## USE OF DRUGS DURING CPR

The use of certain drugs for specific indications during CPR has been discussed in previous sections. In this section, an attempt will be made to provide a more inclusive listing of drugs and indications, and a more general overview. Virtually all drugs used during CPR will be administered intravenously. Therefore, it is worthwhile to first briefly consider the question of intravenous access site. All patients admitted to the coronary care unit should, of course, have a peripheral intravenous cannula. Thus, intravenous access should be available immediately if CPR is required. If initial CPR efforts are successful in restoring effective cardiac activity, there is no need for an additional intravenous access site. However, if resuscitation efforts are more prolonged, a central intravenous access site should be established as soon as possible, if one has not been previously available. This provides assurance that cardioactive drugs will reach the central circulation in a predictable fashion. The choice of a site will depend on individual circumstances and the experience of personnel performing CPR. We have favored either the internal or external jugular vein because of relative ease of access and low complication rates, particularly in comparison to the subclavian approach. Insertion of a central intravenous line from a peripheral vein is often uncertain and unnecessarily time-consuming during CPR.

### Sodium Bicarbonate

The use of sodium bicarbonate to correct the metabolic acidosis accompanying circulatory collapse has undergone considerable revision in recent years. It is well-established that acidosis both impairs cardiac function [43-46] and reduces the ventricular fibrillation threshold.[102,103]

Thus, the need for appropriate correction of acidosis remains unquestioned. However, more recent work indicates that overaggressive administration of sodium bicarbonate may worsen the patient's status in several ways.[42,104] Perhaps the most important detrimental effect of sodium bicarbonate administered to excess is lowering of the cerebrospinal fluid pH and subsequent worsening of the patient's mental status.[105,106] The mechanism by which cerebrospinal fluid pH is paradoxically lowered is thought to be related to the fact that the blood-brain barrier is relatively impermeable to bicarbonate ion but freely permeable to carbon dioxide. The latter is generated when sodium bicarbonate is administered and, in turn, generates hydrogen ions after it crosses the blood-brain barrier. This situation is therefore quite comparable to the adverse central nervous system effects observed after metabolic acidosis is corrected too rapidly in patients with diabetic ketoacidosis. Additionally, it has been suggested that a similar effect occurs in the myocardium, resulting in lowering of intracellular pH and further impairment of myocardial function.[107] Hyperosmolal states, which may be accentuated by sodium bicarbonate, are also frequently encountered after prolonged periods of CPR.[42,108] Finally, in theory, sodium bicarbonate, by increasing the affinity of hemoglobin for oxygen, may adversely influence tissue oxygenation.[108]

With respect to the quantitative need for sodium bicarbonate to correct acidosis, Bishop and Weisfeldt[42] have shown that when patients suffering cardiac arrest were not previously acidotic, maintenance of adequate ventilation alone is remarkably effective in controlling arterial pH, although metabolic acidosis progressively appears.

With the above considerations in mind, the 1973 National Conference on Cardiopulmonary Resuscitation (CPR) and Emergency Cardiac Care (ECC)[56] reduced the recommended doses of sodium bicarbonate to be used during CPR. Current recommendations are as follows: if ventricular fibrillation or tachycardia is present, DC countershock should be attempted before sodium bicarbonate is administered. The same principle applies for bradycardic rhythm disturbance, i.e., sodium bicarbonate should not be administered unless initial measures are unsuccessful. If sodium bicarbonate is necessary, it should be administered in an initial dose of 1 mEq/kg by either bolus injection or infusion over a 10-minute period. Once effective cardiac activity is restored, no further sodium bicarbonate need be administered. If initial defibrillation is ineffective, countershock should be attempted again after sodium bicarbonate has been administered. A second dose of sodium bicarbonate may be given, preceding a third attempt at defibrillation if necessary. Subsequent use of sodium bicarbonate during prolonged CPR should be governed by serial arterial blood gas samples rather than by any fixed formula, with care being taken to avoid metabolic alkalosis. Catecholamines combined with sodium bicarbonate often help to improve the chance of reverting ventricular fibrillation or converting asystole to ventricular fibrillation, which may then be treated with countershock. Finally, the importance of adequate ventilation in maintaining blood pH and reducing the necessity for sodium bicarbonate cannot be overemphasized.

## Catecholamies

Catecholamines may be used to treat dysrhythmias and/or increase cardiac output during CPR. Both of these indications and doses of the drugs have been discussed in some detail previously. Catecholamines with major beta-stimulatory and positive chronotropic effects, such as epinephrine or isoproterenol, effectively increase the amplitude of ventricular fibrillatory waves and thereby improve the chance of successful DC cardioversion, particularly when they are administered in conjunction with appropriate doses of sodium bicarbonate. In addition, as noted previously, these agents are also useful in increasing the rate of slow escape pacemakers and in improving atrioventricular conduction. Because of their beta-stimulatory effects, these drugs also improve mechanical activity and cardiac output. However, catecholamines with major chronotropic effects have considerable arrhythmogenic potential. Thus, it is not unusual for various types of supraventricular arrhythmias or ventricular tachycardia or fibrillation to develop when these drugs are used. If catecholamines are to be used primarily to increase cardiac output (i.e., not to increase heart rate), it is advisable to administer agents that retain their major beta-stimulatory inotropic effects but have modest chronotropic effects in order to reduce the chance of catecholamine-induced dysrhythmias. Two such agents, which are currently available, are dopamine and dobutamine. The detailed clinical pharmacology of these agents is discussed in other chapters.

The major indications for the use of these catecholamines during CPR are the treatment of EMD and the presence of residual myocardial depression after effective cardiac rhythm has been restored. Unlike isoproterenol or epinephrine, which often are given as bolus injections followed by a constant infusion, dopamine and dobutamine should be administered by constant infusion and dosage titrated until a desired effect is obtained. It should be remembered that at doses greater than 5 $\mu$g/kg/min, the systemic vasoconstrictive properties of dopamine become relatively more important, and much of the therapeutic advantage of the drug is lost. There is rarely an indication during CPR in coronary care unit patients for catecholamines with predominantly alpha-adrenergic properties, such as norepinephrine or phenylephrine. While these drugs may increase arterial pressure, they reduce cardiac output because of their relative lack of positive inotropic effects and major vasoconstrictive properties, and should therefore be avoided.

## Antiarrhythmic Agents

The use of antiarrhythmic drugs during CPR has been discussed in considerable detail previously. In the setting of CPR, such agents should be used virtually exclusively for the treatment of ventricular arrhythmias. As indicated previously, the major role for antiarrhythmic drugs is in the prevention of recurrent malignant ventricular arrhythmias and, at times, as an initial form of therapy for ventricular tachycardia. The two criteria most pertinent for the use of antiarrhythmic agents during CPR are (1) drug effectiveness and (2) the ability to administer

the drug rapidly and safely by the intravenous route. Long-term antiarrhythmic drug toxicity, for example procainamide-induced systemic lupus erythematosus or disopyramide-induced anticholinergic effects, are not important considerations in this setting. As indicated previously, the most widely used agent is lidocaine because it best satisfies these two criteria. Other agents with antiarrhythmic properties currently available, and which meet these criteria to a greater or lesser extent, are procainamide, disopyramide, bretylium tosylate, propranolol, and diphenylhydantoin. In the setting of CPR, these agents are virtually uniformly second-line drugs to be used if lidocaine is ineffective. As indicated previously, we have considered procainamide to be the most optimal of these second-line agents. Published experience indicates that the drug is effective in this setting.[82,83] Its disadvantages in comparison with lidocaine are the fact that it cannot be administered to a therapeutic level as rapidly, and it fairly routinely causes some degree of hypotension when given rapidly by the intravenous route.[81-84] Disopyramide, which has electrophysiologic properties similar to those of procainamide and quinidine,[109-111] has also been used intravenously for ventricular arrhythmias during myocardial infarction.[112] However, this drug may be more of a myocardial depressant than procainamide[109,113,114] and should not supplant procainamide as the first of these second-line agents. (Dysopyramide is not available for i.v. use in the U.S.A.)

Propranolol can be administered rapidly by the intravenous route but has rather limited effectiveness in the treatment of ventricular dysrhythmias in general. In the CPR setting in particular, it should be avoided because of its myocardial depressant properties. Diphenylhydantoin can also be given rapidly. This drug's efficacy in the treatment of ventricular dysrhythmias has been somewhat disappointing, however, except for the special case of digitalis toxicity, and therefore is rarely indicated during CPR.[115] Bretylium tosylate is a ganglionic-blocking agent whose mechanism of action as an antidysrhythmic drug is not entirely certain.[116-119] It is an extremely effective drug, however, and is the only agent available that can terminate established ventricular fibrillation.[78-80,120-123] For the latter reasons, it has a definite place during CPR. Because it may also be quite toxic (most importantly causing major hypotension and nausea and vomiting), this drug should be reserved for situations in which neither lidocaine nor procainamide successfully abolishes recurrent malignant dysrhythmias or for patients with ventricular fibrillation refractory to DC cardioversion. Under these circumstances, bretylium tosylate may be a life-saving drug. Bretylium tosylate is given in a dose of 5 mg/kg as an intravenous bolus. If it is effective, patients may then be maintained with either a constant intravenous infusion or intramuscular injections at 6 to 8 hour intervals. It should be noted that the effects of bretylium tosylate may take some time to be manifest. Therefore, in patients with refractory ventricular fibrillation, CPR should be maintained for 30 to 45 minutes after an initial bolus of the drug is administered. Further attempts at electrical defibrillation should be made during this time.

### Atropine Sulfate

As discussed previously, atropine is indicated in the treatment of a number of bradycardic rhythm disturbances during CPR, particularly if heart block is present or an increase in vagal tone is thought to be an initiating event for cardiac arrest. In the CPR setting, atropine should be given in an initial dose of 1 mg followed by a second dose, if necessary. The use of atropine should not delay any other therapeutic modalities, since many of the bradyarrhythmias in which a trial of the drug is indicated will not respond satisfactorily. It is also worth noting that during CPR the drug should not be given slowly but rather administered as a bolus injection.

### Positive Inotropic Agents

By far, the two most common agents used for their positive inotropic effects during CPR are calcium and catecholamines, both of which may be used to treat EMD or lesser degrees of myocardial depression during CPR. It is worth reiterating the transient nature of the effects of intravenous bolus injections of calcium and the advantages of catecholamines such as dopamine and dobutamine, which have relatively modest chronotropic effects, when the goal of therapy is purely increased mechanical performance.

There is rarely an indication for the use of digitalis glycosides as positive inotropic agents during CPR. First, digitalis glycosides have rather modest positive inotropic effects compared to calcium or catecholamines. Second, in order to be effective in the CPR setting, a large intravenous dose of a rapidly acting agent would have to be administered. When given in this fashion, digitalis glycosides result in significant systemic vasoconstriction and an increase in arterial pressure, which may act to increase ventricular afterload and impair myocardial shortening.[124-126] Third, it would be anticipated that patients undergoing CPR would be particularly susceptible to digitalis toxicity because of rapidly occurring changes in acid-base balance, electrolytes, and respiratory function.

Another agent with positive inotropic properties, which may occasionally be used during CPR, is glucagon. Despite initially encouraging reports in which glucagon was used for the treatment of severe heart failure,[127] there has been relatively little further interest in the drug as a positive inotropic agent. Glucagon has never been subjected to clinical testing during CPR. Nonetheless, it may be worth attempting glucagon therapy in patients with EMD unresponsive to other agents. Glucagon has been administered as an intravenous bolus of 3 to 5 mg, or as a constant infusion at a dosage of 1 to 4 mg/hr.

## MONITORING THE EFFECTIVENESS OF CPR

The two most basic parameters to be followed during CPR are pupillary status and adequacy of pulses. As noted previously, pupils should become reactive to light reasonably promptly as CPR is instituted, providing the patient has been attended to properly. They may, however, dilate due to a number of drugs, especially catecholamines. The light reflex should be checked frequently during CPR. Correctly performed CCCM should produce easily palpable carotid, brachial, or femoral pulses. The carotid pulse is the most optimal to monitor, but it may be more practical to palpate the femoral or brachial pulse.

In patients with arterial cannulae in place at the time of cardiac arrest, it should be possible to produce an intraarterial systolic pressure of at least 80 to 90 mmHg with each closed chest compression. In patients undergoing prolonged CPR, it is often advisable to insert a systemic arterial cannula, both to monitor blood pressure and to obtain blood for gas analysis. Arterial blood gases should be measured frequently in any patient who does not respond promptly to initial resuscitative measures. For this reason, equipment for performing arterial blood gas determinations should be located in close proximity to the coronary care unit. The arterial $PO_2$ and $PCO_2$ are of course the best indices of adequacy of ventilation. In addition, as discussed previously, frequent pH determinations are the best guide to the use of sodium bicarbonate. While many patients undergoing CPR may subsequently require more sophisticated forms of monitoring after cardiac activity has been restored, there is no need for anything further than frequent assessment of pupillary status and the adequacy of CCCM, arterial blood gas measurements, and, of course, electrocardiographic monitoring to satisfactorily monitor the progress of CPR.

## ORGANIZATION OF CPR

### In the Coronary Care Unit

Optimal performance of CPR in the coronary care unit requires a well-rehearsed plan of action, both from the standpoint of therapeutic maneuvers and the role of various personnel. All nursing staff must be carefully trained in the initial assessment of the patient suffering abrupt circulatory collapse, particularly with regard to the recognition and identification of life-threatening dysrhythmias. Further, nursing staff must be equipped to handle the initial ther-

apy of these dysrhythmias and to begin CPR techniques in an integrated, predetermined fashion. Adequate staffing of the coronary care unit should allow two to three nursing personnel to be available for the initial phase of CPR. Once the patient with cardiac arrest or circulatory collapse is identified, a team of previously identified individuals with specific responsibilities should be alerted immediately. This team should include one physician who will have responsibility for overall management of resuscitative efforts. In hospitals with house staff physicians, it is often helpful to include one or two other physicians on the team to help in general management. The team should also include an individual who is expert in endotracheal intubation, a respiratory therapist, and an individual who is responsible for bringing a 12-lead ECG machine to the bedside, connecting it to the patient, and running the machine during CPR. In most hospitals, previously identified nursing personnel will be responsible for bringing the "crash cart" containing all necessary drugs and equipment and for preparing the defibrillator. Subsequently, these same individuals will be responsible for preparing drugs and keeping a continuous record of all therapeutic modalities employed. It is also important that at least one physician member of the team be thoroughly conversant with various means of intravenous access, including cutdowns, if necessary, and other techniques that might be required, such as intracardiac injections, transthoracic pacing, and tracheostomy.

A flow sheet for CPR, which we believe to be relatively simple and flexible and which is specifically designed for the coronary care unit setting, is presented in Fig. 31.7. This schema is predicated on the prompt recognition of various patterns of circulatory collapse in the coronary care unit and the immediate application of techniques appropriate for their management.

### Outside of the Coronary Care Unit

Coronary and other special intensive care units provide an environment in which the chances for successful CPR are maximal. In other settings, both in and outside of the hospi-

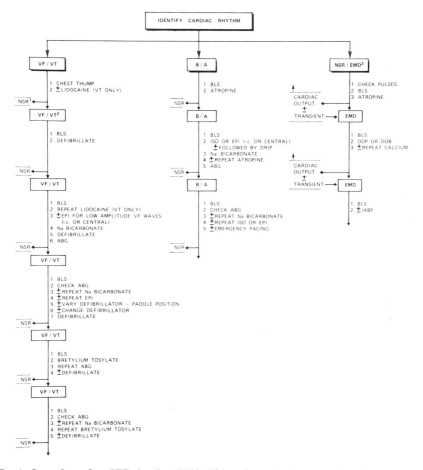

Fig. 31.7 A flow sheet for CPR in the CCU. This schema is by necessity simplified and may be subject to modification in individual cases. During the course of CPR, patients may of course change from one of the three main groups to another. ± indicates a technique or intervention which should be considered but used only if felt to be indicated. Numbers do not necessarily indicate actual order of interventions. Drug doses are indicated in the text.

[1] NSR = either normal sinus rhythm or any rhythm sufficient to support the circulation.

[2] Implies continued VF or VT rather than recurrent VF or VT. Treatment of the latter is discussed in the text.

[3] EMD is considered to be present regardless of the cardiac rhythm if the rate would ordinarily be rapid enough to support the circulation.

Abbreviations: VT = ventricular tachycardia; VF = ventricular fibrillation; NSR = normal sinus rhythm; BLS = basic life support; ABG = arterial blood gas; iso = isoproterenol; epi = epinephrine; dop = dopamine; dob = dobutamine; B/A = bradycardia or asystole; EMD = electromechanical dissociation; i.c. = intracardiac; IABP = intraaortic balloon counterpulsation.

tal, various elements present in the coronary care unit will be missing, at least initially. Some of the more important differences between CPR inside and outside of the intensive care setting are as follows: (1) many instances of cardiac arrest outside of the special care unit are unwitnessed. Therefore, a decision must be made as to whether CPR should be initiated at all by quickly assessing the presence or absence of advanced postmortem changes, such as rigor mortis and dependent pooling of blood. In the case of unwitnessed cardiac arrest, the same principles of CPR, which have been discussed previously, apply. Thus, basic life support should be initiated, but in this case without attempting a precordial thump, since the time considerations of unwitnessed cardiac arrest make the chance of success of this maneuver highly unlikely. (2) Virtually all such instances of cardiac arrest outside of the special care unit will be unmonitored, from an electrocardiographic standpoint. In cases of witnessed, unmonitored cardiac arrest, an initial precordial thump *is* indicated. Another pertinent technique, whether or not cardiac arrest is witnessed, is the use of blind electrical defibrillation without prior knowledge of the cardiac rhythm. Again, this appears to be indicated, since it is not likely to cause significant harm in this situation and obviously may be lifesaving. A third major difference between the special care unit setting and most others is that CPR will often have to be performed by one individual. In this circumstance, the single rescuer technique [56] in which artificial respiration and CCCM are alternated, must be used. Finally, outside of the special care unit, individuals performing CPR must have the ability to be flexible and use available resources as effectively as possible.

Recent years have seen a dramatic increase in the education of the general public in CPR techniques. This movement, along with continued interest in telemetered mobile coronary care units staffed by paramedics, constitutes what may prove to be the most important advance in CPR since the introduction of CCCM and early coronary care unit experience indicating the effectiveness of CPR.

## COMPLICATIONS AND SEQUELAE OF CPR

In a discussion of the complications of CPR, it is often difficult to separate postresuscitative phenomena, which are the result of periods of organ anoxia and ischemia, from true complications of the techniques of CPR. Thus, for instance, a wide variety of neurologic sequelae may occur after periods of cerebral anoxia, which are obviously of great importance but which should not be considered complications of CPR. On the other hand, CPR itself may occasionally cause central nervous system dam-

age. In this section, an attempt will be made to deal with both true complications of CPR and with certain postresuscitative sequelae, which do not necessarily result from CPR itself.

The specific complications of CPR are predominantly traumatic. Perhaps the most common complication is the occurrence of rib fractures. The latter may result from excessively vigorous CCCM or may occur unavoidably in elderly patients subjected to CCCM. In some series, the incidence of rib fractures has been greater than 50 percent.[128] Among other traumatic complications of CCCM and defibrillation are gastroesophageal, pulmonary, and hepatic lacerations (particularly if CCCM is performed too close to the xiphoid process); defibrillation burns (which are usually avoidable); fractures of the sternum, vertebral bodies, and scapula; bone marrow and fat emboli; and spinal cord damage.[128] Mouth-to-mouth ventilation and endotracheal intubation are associated with another group of complications, most important of which are gastric dilatation and tension pneumothorax. The latter may also occur as a result of CCCM. Both gastric dilatation and tension pneumothorax are important to emphasize because they are readily correctable, often not recognized, and can cause major difficulties during resuscitation.[128]

Significant cardiac complications of CCCM are quite unusual but occasionally rupture or laceration of various chambers may occur.[128] If strongly suspected, this may constitute one of the few indications for pericardiocentesis and/or open-chest cardiac massage in the coronary care unit setting. Repeated defibrillation may cause superficial burns to the surface of the heart, but these and other direct effects of countershock probably do not have significant consequences from the standpoint of cardiac performance.[66,129] Serum enzyme elevations (most importantly, creatine kinase) are routine after CPR, but appear to be noncardiac and predominantly of skeletal muscle origin.[130] Intracardiac drug injections also entail a risk of myocardial or coronary arterial laceration. Any of the drugs used during CPR may have undesirable effects, which have been alluded to previously and which are often unavoidable. One of the most important to keep in mind is lidocaine toxicity, since the latter results predominantly in central nervous system effects and frequently causes grand mal seizures.

In most patients who do not recover central nervous system function promptly after cardiac activity is restored successfully, the cause is cerebral anoxia. However, another cause of prolonged periods of depressed central nervous system function after resuscitation is the hyperosmolar state that frequently occurs following lengthy efforts.[42,108] As indicated previously, the excessive use of sodium bicarbonate may contribute to the latter state and may also be a factor in prolonged postresuscitative coma by virtue of the production of paradoxical central nervous system acidosis.[105,106]

As opposed to specific complications of resuscitative measures, certain problems may arise after resuscitation, which are intrinsic to the sudden loss of consciousness and variable periods of reduced or absent organ perfusion. While a detailed consideration of the neurologic complications of cerebral anoxia is beyond the scope of this chapter, suffice it to say that a myriad of postresuscitative neurologic syndromes may appear, indicating varying degrees and types of central nervous system damage. The latter may result not just from generalized anoxia but, in addition, from regional anoxia in specific areas of the central nervous system in patients with preexisting cerebrovascular disease. Seizures of varying types are a particularly common problem, which frequently occur at the time of circulatory collapse or in the postresuscitative period. Intravenous diazepam, which has virtually no effect on the cardiovascular system, is often particularly helpful if seizure activity is interfering with resuscitative efforts.

Aspiration of gastric contents occurs very commonly at the time of circulatory collapse or during CPR and is frequently unavoidable. If aspiration is known or strongly suspected to have occurred, we have considered this an indication for postresuscitation antibiotics, regardless of whether pneumonia is subsequently detected. Pneumonia, in general, is a common problem in the postresuscitation period and should be treated aggressively.

Another relatively common problem in the postresuscitation period, particularly if resuscitation is prolonged, is acute tubular necrosis. There are several potential mechanisms for oliguria following CPR, especially if heart failure is present and cardiac output is low. An element of acute tubular necrosis may often be unrecognized as a result.

Finally, a variety of psychiatric sequalae may be anticipated in the postresuscitation period. These are discussed in a separate chapter.

The complications and sequelae of CPR discussed above by no means constitute a complete list. The reader is referred to the reference list for a more extensive consideration of this area. A particularly complete discussion in one source may be found in Cardiac Arrest and Resuscitation edited by H.E. Stephenson, Jr.[131]

## TERMINATION OF CPR

There is no totally satisfactory answer to the question, When should resuscitation be stopped? Indeed, the philosophic, legal, and medical considerations of this issue dictate that there will often be situations in which the answers are far less than satisfactory. With these problems in mind, current recommendations are as follows: [56] (1) patients who have been deeply comatose, without spontaneous respiration, and who have fixed and dilated pupils for 15 to 30 minutes or longer despite CPR may be considered to have suffered brain death and resuscitative measures may be discontinued; (2) patients with continuing absence of ventricular electrocardiographic activity after 10 minutes of CPR, including drug therapy, may be considered to have suffered cardiac death and again, resuscitative measures may be discontinued; and (3) patients who have only occasional spontaneous ventricular depolarizations unassociated with mechanical activity after 10 minutes of CPR should probably be classed with the latter group. The implication of the latter recommendations is that in patients with refractory primary ventricular fibrillation, resuscitative efforts should be continued until electrical silence appears and is present for at least 10 minutes.

A few other considerations apply. If the patient has a personal physician, he or she should be called and/or be present and should agree with the decision to terminate resuscitation. If at all possible, the patient's family should understand and agree to termination of resuscitation. Finally, although not really applicable to the area of coronary care, there have been occasional reports of remarkable recoveries in children after periods of apparent brain death. Resuscitative efforts should therefore be continued for longer periods in the case of a child.

## CPR TRAINING AND MAINTENANCE OF EXPERTISE

The performance of optimal CPR in the coronary care unit requires that all personnel involved in its performance undergo initial training and retraining on a continuing basis. Such training is best carried out as part of an organized, inservice program. The precise organization of such a program is a matter of individual preference, but major input from, and cooperation between, the cardiology, pulmonary, anesthesiology, and nursing services is desirable.

The Joint Commission on the Accreditation of Hospitals (JCAH) currently recommends that all personnel who work with patients in special care units, including physicians, nurses, and ancillary service personnel, receive training in basic life support. The American Heart Association training program in basic life support provides an excellent means whereby standardized training and certification may be provided. In order to provide such training as part of an inservice effort, a qualified American Heart Association CPR instructor must be available to certify personnel at the end of such training.

Coronary care unit nursing personnel require more advanced training, which should at the very least include, in addition to basic life support, recognition of life-threatening dysrhythmias, indications for and techniques of defibrillation, the use of drugs during CPR, and the use of airways and bag-mask-valve devices for ventilation. Again, the American Heart Association has organized standardized programs of training in advanced life support, which may be used for inservice education and also offer tangible recognition for successful completion of training. Because these more advanced techniques are constantly undergoing revision and reexamination and because local factors may modify the use of certain of these techniques, standardized training programs in advanced life support must be updated as necessary. It is particularly advisable that these programs be administered as an inservice function, which is readily susceptible to change as techniques are modified, and that rigorous proof of mastery of these techniques be required.

Unfortunately, training of physicians in basic and advanced resuscitative techniques has, in the past, been one of the less standardized aspects of coronary care. Current JCAH guidelines, which require minimum levels of physician training, are changing this situation rapidly. It is highly advisable that all physicians receive more than minimum levels of training, however, and that this training begin in medical school with required coursework that deals with the theoretic and practical aspects of CPR in a sophisticated fashion. Both housestaff and attending level physicians who work in the coronary care unit must receive training in these areas and be able to demonstrate continued proficiency. An optimal inservice training program for nurses and physicians working in the coronary care unit should include some mechanism for at least annual review of CPR techniques and recertification. Additionally, such a program should include organized and regular educational experiences in which coronary care unit personnel may be exposed to individuals who are expert in the various aspects of CPR. The latter will provide a regular opportunity to review basic principles and to become acquainted with new developments. In our own coronary care unit, we have utilized cardiologists, pulmonary specialists, anesthesiologists, hospital pharmacists, and nurse-education specialists as part of an ongoing series of lectures and seminars to accomplish this goal.

Inservice training in CPR is markedly facilitated by the use of "dummy" devices that allow the trainee to practice CPR with immediate feedback. An example of the use of such a device, the Resusci-Anni, is provided in Figure 31.8. As shown, the trainee can determine how effectively he or she is performing mouth-to-

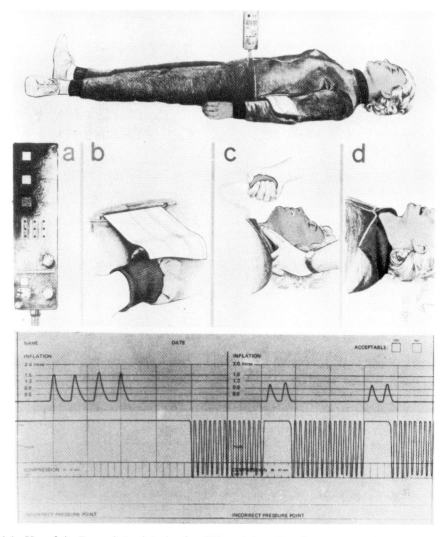

Fig. 31.8  Use of the Resusci-Anni device for CPR training. (Reprinted by permission of the American Heart Association, Inc. from Berkebile PE, et al. In: Proceedings of the National Conference on Standards for Cardiopulmonary Resuscitation (CPR) and Emergency Cardiac Care (ECC). 1975, p. 21.)

mouth resuscitation and CCCM. In addition, such devices can be used to simulate dysrhythmias and test appropriate responses. We have found such a device to be an invaluable aid in the teaching of CPR.

## REFERENCES

1. Lown B: In: Cardiac Pacing and Cardioversion. Meltzer LE, Kitchell JR, editors. The Charles Press, Philadelphia, 1967, p 77.
2. Pantridge JF, Geddes S: A mobile intensive-care unit in the management of myocardial infarction. Lancet 2:271–273, 1967.
3. Lawrie DM, Higgins MR, Godman MJ, et al: Ventricular fibrillation complicating acute myocardial infarction. Lancet 2:523–528, 1968.
4. McNeilly RH, Pemberton J: Duration of heart attack in 998 fatal cases of coronary artery disease and its relation to possible cardiac resuscitation. Br Med J 3:139–142, 1968.
5. Fabricius-Bierre N, Astvad K, Kjaerulff J: Cardiac arrest following acute myocardial infarction. Acta Med Scand 195:261–265, 1974.
6. Lie K, Wellens H, Downar E, et al: Observations on patients with primary ventricular fibril-

lation complicating acute myocardial infarction. Circulation 52:755–759, 1975.

7. Conley MJ, McNeer JF, Leek L, et al: Cardiac arrest complicating acute myocardial infarction: Predictability and prognosis. Am J Cardiol 39:7–12, 1977.

8. Cobb LA, Conn RD, Samson WE, et al: Prehospital coronary care: The role of a rapid response mobile intensive coronary care system. Circulation 43 (suppl II):139, 1971.

9. Baum RS, Alvarez III H, Cobb LA: Survival after resuscitation from out-of-hospital ventricular fibrillation. Circulation 50:1231–1235, 1974.

10. Cobb LA, Baum RB, Alvarez III HA, et al: Resuscitation from out-of-hospital ventricular fibrillation: 4 year follow-up. Circulation 52 (suppl III):223–235, 1975.

11. Meltzer LE, Kitchell JR: The incidence of arrhythmias associated with acute myocardial infarction. Prog Cardiovasc Dis 9:50–63, 1966.

12. Lawrie DM, Greenwood TW, Goddard M, et al: A coronary care unit in the routine management of acute myocardial infarction. Lancet 2:109–114, 1967.

13. Pentecost BL, Mayne NMC: Results of a general hospital coronary care service. Br Med J 1:830–833, 1968.

14. Church G, Bierh RO: Intensive coronary care—a practical system for a small hospital without house staff. N Eng J Med 281:1155–1159, 1969.

15. Dhurander RW, MacMillan RL, Brown KWG: Primary ventricular fibrillation complicating acute myocardial infarction. Am J Cardiol 27:347–351, 1971.

16. Cohen DB, Doctor L, Pick A: The significance of atrioventricular block complicating acute myocardial infarction. Am Heart J 55:215–219, 1958.

17. Epstein EJ, Coulshed N, McKendricks CS, et al: Artificial pacing by electrode catheter for heart block or asystole complicating acute myocardial infarction. Br Heart J 28:546–556, 1966.

18. Friedberg CK, Cohen H, Donoso E: Advanced heart block as a complication of acute myocardial infarction: Role of pacemaker therapy. Prog Cardiovasc Dis 10:466–481, 1968.

19. Lassers BW, Julian DG: Artificial pacing in management of complete heart block complicating myocardial infarction. Br Med J 2:142–146, 1968.

20. McNally EM, Benchimol A: Medical and physiologic considerations in the use of artificial cardiac pacing: I. Am Heart J 75:380–398, 1968.

21. Beregovich J, Fenig S, Lassers J: Management of acute myocardial infarction complicated by advanced atrioventricular block: Role of artificial pacing. Am J Cardiol 23:54–56, 1969.

22. Constantin L: Extracardiac factors contributing to hypotension during coronary occlusion. Am J Cardiol 11:205–217, 1963.

23. George M, Greenwood TW: Relation between bradycardia and the site of myocardial infarction. Lancet 2:739–740, 1967.

24. Adgey AAJ, Geodes GS, Mulholland HC, et al: Incidence, significance and management of early bradyarrhythmias complicating acute myocardial infarction. Lancet 2:1097–1101, 1968.

25. Gregory JJ, Grace WJ: The management of sinus bradycardia, nodal rhythms and heart block for the prevention of cardiac arrest in acute myocardial infarction. Prog Cardiovasc Dis 10:505–517, 1968.

26. Rotman M, Wagner GS, Wallace AG: Bradyarrhythmias in acute myocardial infarction. Circulation 45:703–722, 1972.

27. Corr PB, Gillis RA: Role of the vagus nerves in the cardiovascular changes induced by coronary occlusion. Circulation 49:86–97, 1974.

28. Come PC, Pitt B: Nitroglycerine-induced severe hypotension and bradycardia in patients with acute myocardial infarction. Circulation 54:624–628, 1976.

29. Raizes G, Wagner GS, Hackel DB: Instantaneous nonarrhythmic cardiac death in acute myocardial infarction. Am J Cardiol 39:1–6, 1977.

30. London RE, London SB: Rupture of the heart. A critical analysis of 47 consecutive autopsy cases. Circulation 31:202–208, 1965.

31. Meurs AAH, Vos AK, Verhey JB, et al: Electrocardiogram in ventricular rupture after myocardial infarction. Br Heart J 32:232–235, 1970.

32. Robinson JS, Stannard NM, Long M: Ruptured papillary muscle after acute myocardial infarction. Am Heart J 70:233–238, 1965.

33. Negovskii VA: In: Cardiac Arrest and Resuscitation. Stephenson HE Jr, editor. CV Mosby, St Louis, 1974, pp 3–15.

34. Gordon AS: In: Textbook of Coronary Care. Meltzer LE, Dunning AJ, editors. The Charles Press Publishers, Philadelphia, 1972.

35. Stephenson HE Jr: In: Cardiac Arrest and Resuscitation. Stephenson HE Jr, editor. CV Mosby, St Louis, 1974, pp 475–492.

36. Han J, Garcia de Jalon P, Moe GK: Adrenergic effects on ventricular vulnerability. Circ Res 14:516–524, 1964.

37. Valori C, Thomas M, Shillingford J: Free noradrenaline and adrenaline excretion in relation to clinical syndromes following myocardial infarction. Am J Cardiol 20:605–617, 1967.

38. Januszewicz W, Sznajderman M, Wocial B, et al: Urinary excretion of free norepinephrine and free epinephrine in patients with acute myocardial infarction in relation to its clinical course. Am Heart J 76:345–352, 1968.

39. Jewitt DE, Mercer CJ, Reid D, et al: Free noradrenaline and adrenaline excretion in relation to the development of cardiac arrhythmias and heart failure in patients with acute myocardial infarction. Lancet 1:635–641, 1969.

40. Maroko PR, Kjekshus JK, Sobel BE, et al: Factors influencing infarct size following experimental coronary occlusion. Circulation 43:67–82, 1971.

41. Richardson DW, Wasserman AJ, Patterson JL: General and regional circulatory responses to change in blood pH and carbon dioxide tension. J Clin Invest 40:31–43, 1961.

42. Bishop RL, Weisfeldt ML: Sodium bicarbonate administration during cardiac arrest. JAMA 235:505–509, 1976.

43. Opie LH: Effect of extracellular pH on function and metabolism of isolated perfused rat heart. Am J Physiol 209:1075–1080, 1965.

44. Vaughn-Williams EM, White JM: Chemosensitivity of cardiac muscle. J Physiol (London) 189:119–137, 1967.

45. Caress DL, Kissack AS, Slovian AJ, et al: The effect of respiratory and metabolic acidosis on myocardial contractility. J Thorac Cardiovasc Surg 56:571–577, 1968.

46. Cingolani HE, Mattiazzi AR, Blesa ES, et al: Contractility in isolated mammalian heart muscle after acid-base changes. Circ Res 26:269–278, 1970.

47. Schmidt CF: In: The Cerebral Circulation in Health and Disease. Charles C Thomas, Springfield, Ill, 1950.

48. Honig CL, Tenney SM: Determinants of the circulatory response to hypoxia and hypercapnia. Am Heart J 53:687–698, 1957.

49. Korner PI, Edwards AW: The immediate effects of acute hypoxia on the heart rate, arterial pressure, cardiac output and ventilation in the unanesthetized rabbit. Q J Exp Physiol 45:113–122, 1960.

50. Green HD, Wegria R: Effects of asphyxia, anoxia and myocardial ischemia on the coronary circulation. Am J Physiol 135:271–280, 1942.

51. Fishman AP, Fritts HW Jr, Cournand A: Effects of acute hypoxia and exercise on the pulmonary circulation. Circulation 22:204–215, 1960.

52. Cantu RC, Ames A III, Dixon J, et al: Reversability of experimental cerebrovascular obstruction induced by complete ischemia. J Neurosurg 31:429–431, 1969.

53. Hossmann KA, Olsson Y: Suppression and recovery of neuronal function in transient cerebral ischemia. Brain Res 22:313–325, 1970.

54. Miller JR, Myers RE: Neurological effects of systemic circulatory arrest in the monkey. Neurology 20:715–724, 1970.

55. Stephenson, HE Jr: In: Cardiac Arrest and Resuscitation. Stephenson HE Jr, editor. CV Mosby, St Louis, 1974, pp 687–707.

56. Standards for cardiopulmonary resuscitation (CPR) and emergency cardiac care (ECC). JAMA 227 (suppl 7):833–868, 1974.

57. Kouwenhoven WB, Jude JR, Knickerbocker GG: Closed-chest cardiac massage. JAMA 173:1064–1067, 1960.

58. MacKenzie GJ, Taylor SH, McDonald AH, et al: Haemodynamic effects of external cardiac compression. Lancet 1:1342–1345, 1964.

58a. Rudikoff MT, Maughan WL, Effron M, Frend P, Weisfeldt ML: Mechanisms of blood flow during cardiopulmonary resuscitation. Circulation 61:345–352, 1980.

58b. Chandra N, Snyder L, Weisfeldt ML: Abdominal binding during CPR in man. Circulation 59–60 (suppl II):45, 1979.

58c. Chandra N, Cohen JM, Tsitlik J, et al: Negative airway pressure between compressions augments carotid flow during CPR. Circulation 59–60 (suppl II):46, 1979.

59. Falsetti HI, Greene DG: Technique of compression in closed-chest cardiac massage. JAMA 200:793–796, 1967.

60. Bornemann C, Scherf D: Paroxysmal ventricular tachycardia abolished by a blow on the precordium. Dis Chest 56:83–84, 1969.

61. Pennington JE, Taylor J, Lown B: Chest thump for reverting ventricular tachycardia. N Engl J Med 283:1192–1195, 1970.

62. Barrett JS: Letter to the editor. N Engl J Med 284:393, 1971.

63. Zoll PM, Linenthal AJ, Gibson W, et al: Treatment of unexpected cardiac arrest by external

electrical stimulation of the heart. N Engl J Med 254:541–546, 1956.

64. Lown B, Amarasingham R, Neuman J: New method for terminating cardiac arrhythmias. Use of synchronized capacitor discharge. JAMA 182:548–555, 1962.

65. Lown B, Neuman J, Amarasingham R, et al: Comparison of alternating current with direct current electroshock across the closed chest. Am J Cardiol 10:223–233, 1962.

66. Stephenson HE Jr: In: Cardiac Arrest and Resuscitation. Stephenson HE Jr, editor. CV Mosby, St Louis, 1974, pp 336–343.

67. Tacker WA Jr, Gulioto FM, Giuliani E, et al: Energy dosage for human trans-chest electrical ventricular defibrillation. N Engl J Med 290:214–215, 1974.

68. Kouwenhoven WB, Jude JR, Knickerbocker GG, et al: Closed chest defibrillation of the heart. Surgery 42:550–561, 1957.

69. Lown B, Kleiger R, Wolff G: The technique of cardioversion. Am Heart J 67:282–284, 1964.

70. Nachlass MM, Bix HH, Mower MM, et al: Observations on defibrillators, defibrillation and synchronized countershocks. Prog Cardiovasc Dis 9:64–89, 1966.

71. DeSanctis RW, Block P, Hutter AM Jr: Tachyarrhythmias in myocardial infarction. Circulation 45:681–702, 1972.

72. Lawrie D: In: Acute Myocardial Infarction. Julian DG, Oliver MF, editors. E and S Livingstone, Edinburgh, 1968.

73. Pentecost BL: Coronary artery disease. Management of the acute episode. Br Med J 1:93–95, 1971.

74. Stewart JSS, Stewart WK, Gillies H Cr: Cardiac arrest and acidosis. Lancet 2:964–967, 1962.

75. Harder K, MacKenzie IL, Ledingham MCA: Spontaneous reversion of ventricular fibrillation. Lancet 2:1140–1142, 1963.

76. Wada J: In: Cardiac Arrest and Resuscitation. Stephenson HE Jr, editor. CV Mosby, St Louis, 1974, pp 344–347.

77. El-Sherif N, Scherlag BJ, Lazarra R: Electrode catheter recordings during malignant ventricular arrhythmia following experimental acute myocardial ischemia. Circulation 51:1003–1014, 1975.

78. Bacaner MB: Bretylium tosylate for suppression of induced ventricular fibrillation. Am J Cardiol 17:528–534, 1966.

79. Bacaner MB: Quantitative comparison of bretylium with other antifibrillatory drugs. Am J Cardiol 21:504–512, 1968.

80. Bacaner MB: Treatment of ventricular fibrillation and other acute arrhythmias with bretylium tosylate. Am J Cardiol 21:530–543, 1968.

81. Koch-Weser J, Klein S: Procaine amide dosage schedules, plasma concentration and clinical effects. JAMA 215:1454–1460, 1971.

82. Miller RR, Lies J, Hilliard G, et al: Comparative hemodynamic effects of procaine amide and lidocaine in patients with acute myocardial infarction. Am J Cardiol 29:281, 1972.

83. Giardina EG, Heissentbuttel RH, Bigger JT: Intermittent intravenous procaine amide to treat ventricular arrhythmia. Correlation of plasma concentration with effect on arrhythmia, electrocardiogram and blood pressure. Ann Intern Med 78:183–193, 1973.

84. Jawad-Kanber G, Sherrod TR: Effect of loading dose of procaine amide on left ventricular performance in man. Chest 66:269–272, 1974.

85. Roberts B, Schnabel T Jr, Ravdin IS: Multiple episodes of cardiac arrest. JAMA 154:581–584, 1954.

86. Don Michael TA, Stanford RL: Precordial percussion in cardiac asystole. Lancet 1:699, 1963.

87. Semple T, Al Badran RH, Boyes BE: Physical stimulation of the heart. Br Med J 1:224, 1968.

88. Wild JB, Grover JD: The fist as an external cardiac pacemaker. Lancet 2:436–437, 1970.

89. Zoll PM, Belgard AH, Weintraub MJ, et al: External mechanical cardiac stimulation. N Engl J Med 294:1274–1275, 1976.

90. Yahini JH, Zahavi I, Neufeld HN: Paroxysmal atrial fibrillation in Wolff-Parkinson-White syndrome simulating ventricular tachycardia. Am J Cardiol 14:248–254, 1964.

91. Katz MJ, Zitnik RS: Direct current shock and lidocaine in the treatment of digitalis-induced ventricular tachycardia. Am J Cardiol 18:552–556, 1966.

92. Kleiger R, Lown B: Cardioversion and digitalis. II. Clinical studies. Circulation 33:878–887, 1966.

93. Rosenblum R, Tai AR, Lawson D: Dopamine in man: Cardiorenal hemodynamics in normotensive patients with heart disease. J Pharmacol Exp Ther 183:256–263, 1972.

94. Holzer J, Karliner JS, O'Rourke RA, et al: Effectiveness of dopamine in patients with cardiogenic shock. Am J Cardiol 32:79–84, 1973.

95. Goldberg LI, Hsieh Y, Resnekov L: Newer catecholamines for treatment of heart failure and shock: An update on dopamine and a first look at dobutamine. Prog Cardiovasc Dis 19:327–340, 1977.

96. Jewitt D, Mitchell A, Birkhead J, et al: Clinical cardiovascular pharmacology of dobutamine, a selective inotropic catecholamine. Lancet 2:363–367, 1974.

97. Beregovich J, Bianchi C, D'Angelo R, et al: Hemodynamic effects of a new inotropic agent (dobutamine) in chronic cardiac failure. Br Heart J 37:629–634, 1975.

98. Bush CA, Webel J, Leier MD: Treatment of end-stage cardiac failure with dobutamine. Am J Cardiol 37:125, 1976.

99. Loeb HS, Bredakis J, Gunnar RM: Superiority of dobutamine over dopamine for augmentation of cardiac output in patients with chronic low output cardiac failure. Circulation 55:375–381, 1977.

100. Powell WJ Jr, Daggett WM, Magro AE, et al: Effects of intraaortic balloon counterpulsation on cardiac performance, oxygen consumption, and coronary blood flow in dogs. Circ Res 26:753–764, 1970.

101. Mundth ED, Yurchak PM, Buckley MJ, et al: Circulatory assistance and emergency direct coronary-artery surgery for shock complicating acute myocardial infarction. N Engl J Med 283:1382–1384, 1970.

102. Gerst PH, Fleming WH, Malm JR: Increased susceptibility of the heart to ventricular fibrillation during metabolic acidosis. Circ Res 19:63–70, 1966.

103. Wada J: In: Cardiac Arrest and Resuscitation. Stephenson HE Jr, editor. CV Mosby, St Louis, 1974, pp 783–795.

104. Editorial, Sodium bicarbonate in cardiac arrest. Lancet 1:946–947, 1976.

105. Posner JB, Plum F: Spinal-fluid pH and neurologic symptoms in systemic acidosis. N Engl J Med 277:605–613, 1967.

106. Berenyi KJ, Wolk M, Killip T: Cerebrospinal fluid acidosis complicating therapy of experimental cardiopulmonary arrest. Circulation 52:319–324, 1975.

107. Clancy RL, Cingolani HE, Taylor RR, et al: Influence of sodium bicarbonate on myocardial performance. Am J Physiol 212:917–923, 1967.

108. Mattar JA, Weil MH, Shubin H, et al: Cardiac Arrest in the critically ill. II. Hyperosmolal states following cardiac arrest. Am J Med 56:162–168, 1974.

109. Befeler B, Castellanos A Jr, Wells DE, et al: Electrophysiologic effects of the antiarrhythmic agent disopyramide phosphate. Am J Cardiol 35:282–287, 1975.

110. Kus T, Sasyniuk BI: Electrophysiological action of disopyramide phosphate on canine ventricular muscle and Purkinje fiber. Circ Res 37:844–854, 1975.

111. Danilo P Jr, Rosen MR: Cardiac effects of disopyramide. Am Heart J 92:532–536, 1976.

112. Vismara LA, ZaKanddin V, Miller RR, et al: Efficacy of disopyramide phosphate in the treatment of refractory ventricular tachycardia. Am J Cardiol 39:1027–1034, 1977.

113. Mathur P: Cardiovascular effects of a newer antiarrhythmic agent, disopyramide phosphate. Am Heart J 84:764–770, 1972.

114. Willis PW: The hemodynamic effects of Norpace II. Angiology 26:102–110, 1975.

115. Mercer EN, Osborne JA: The current status of diphenlhydantoin in heart disease. Ann Intern Med 67:1084–1107, 1967.

116. Bacaner M, Schreinemachers D: Bretylium tosylate for suppression of ventricular fibrillation after experimental myocardial infarction. Nature 220:494–496, 1968.

117. Wit AL, Steiner C, Damato AN: Electrophysiologic effects of bretylium tosylate on single fibers of the canine specialized conducting system and ventricle. J Pharmacol Exp Ther 173:344–356, 1970.

118. Bigger JT Jr, Jaffe CC: The effect of bretylium tosylate on the electrophysiologic properties of ventricular muscle and Purkinje fibers. Am J Cardiol 27:82–92, 1971.

119. Sasyniuk BI, Cardinal R, Levy P: Comparison of the effects of bretylium on electrophysiological properties of normal Purkinje fibers and those surviving acute myocardial infarction. Fed Proc 34:775, 1975.

120. Terry G, Vellani CW, Higgins MR, et al: Bretylium tosylate in treatment of refractory ventricular arrhythmias complicating myocardial infarction. Br Heart J 32:21–25, 1970.

121. Bernstein JG, Koch-Weser J: Effectiveness of bretylium tosylate against refractory ventricular arrhythmias. Circulation 45:1024–1034, 1972.

122. Sanna G, Arcidiacono R: Chemical ventricular defibrillation of the human heart with bretylium tosylate. Am J Cardiol 32:982–987, 1973.

123. Holder DA, Sniderman AD, Fraser G, et al: Experience with bretylium tosylate by a hospital cardiac arrest team. Circulation 55:541–544, 1977.

124. Ross J Jr, Waldhausen JA, Braunwald E: Studies on digitalis: I. Direct effects on peripheral vascular resistance. J Clin Invest 39:930–936, 1960.

125. Mason DT, Braunwald E: Studies on digitalis:

X. Effects of ouabain on forearm vascular resistance and venous tone in normal subjects and in patients in heart failure. J Clin Invest 43:532–543, 1964.

126. Cohn JN, Tristani FE, Khatri IM: Cardiac and peripheral vascular effects of digitalis in clinical cardiogenic shock. Am Heart J 78:318–330, 1969.

127. Parmley WW, Sonnenblick EH: Glucagon: A new agent in cardiac therapy. Am J Cardiol 27:298–303, 1971.

128. Stephenson HE Jr: In: Cardiac Arrest and Resuscitation. Stephenson HE Jr, editor. CV Mosby, St Louis, 1974, pp 717–736.

129. Pansegrau DG, Abboud FM: Hemodynamic effects of ventricular defibrillation. J Clin Invest 49:282–297, 1970.

130. Ehsani A, Ewy GA, Sobel BE: Effects of electrical countershock on serum creatine phophokinase isoenzyme activity. Am J Cardiol 37:12–18, 1976.

131. Stephenson HE Jr: In: Cardiac Arrest and Resuscitation. Stephenson HE Jr, editor. CV Mosby, St Louis, 1974, pp 681–765.

# 32 Mechanical Respiratory Support: With Special Emphasis on Tracheal Intubation

## Jonathan L. Benumof, M.D.

## CAUSES OF HYPOXEMIA FOLLOWING ACUTE MYOCARDIAL INFARCTION

### Decreased Cardiac Output

Assuming a constant tissue oxygen consumption, a decrease in the cardiac output necessitates that the peripheral tissues extract more oxygen per unit blood volume. This extraction will result in a decrease in the oxygen content of the mixed venous blood. Mixed venous blood with decreased oxygen content will then pass through whatever right-to-left transpulmonary shunt pathways exist, inevitably mix with oxygenated end-pulmonary capillary blood (blood perfusing ventilated alveoli), and decrease the oxygen content of arterial blood. Thus, a decrease in the cardiac output primarily decreases the oxygen content of venous blood and then secondarily decreases the oxygen content of arterial blood.

Figure 32.1 shows these relationships quantitatively for several different intrapulmonary shunts.[1] Notice that for a given decrease in the cardiac output the larger the intrapulmonary shunt (carrying more venous blood with less than normal oxygen content), the greater is the decrease in the oxygen content of arterial blood. Increased oxygen extraction, as may occur with excessive sympathetic nervous system activity, hyperthermia, or shivering, will also primarily decrease the oxygen content of venous blood

and secondarily decrease the oxygen content of arterial blood and thereby contribute to impaired oxygenation of arterial blood.[2] Cardiac arrest is a special circumstance of Figure 32.1 where the cardiac output is zero.

### Pulmonary Edema

The effect of pulmonary edema on arterial oxygenation can best be understood in terms of the relationship between the functional residual capacity (the volume of lung that exists at the end of a normal exhalation) and the closing volume of the lung. As lung volume de-

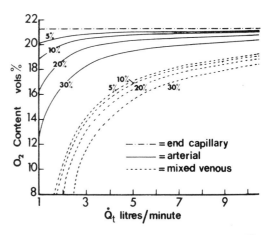

Fig. 32.1 Effect of changes in cardiac output ($\dot{Q}_t$) on the $O_2$ content of end pulmonary capillary, arterial, and mixed venous blood. (After Kelman GF et al: Br J Anaesth 39:450–458, 1967).

creases during expiration towards residual volume, small airways (0.5 to 0.9 mm in diameter) show a progressive tendency to close, whereas larger airways remain patent.[3] Airway closure occurs first in the dependent lung regions, since the distending transpulmonary pressure is less and the volume change during expiration is greater. In the presence of lung disease, when the closing volume of some airways is greater than the whole of the tidal volume, this circumstance is equivalent to atelectasis; if the closing volume of some airways lies within the tidal volume, this circumstance indicates a low ventilation to perfusion region; if the closing volume of the lung is below the whole of tidal respiration, then no airways are closed at any time during tidal respiration and this is a normal circumstance (Fig. 32.2).

There is now good evidence to indicate that peribronchial pulmonary edema can cause an acute increase in airway closure, while at the same time perialveolar interstitial edema can cause an acute decrease in the functional residual capacity.[4-6] The movement of the functional residual capacity down and the closing

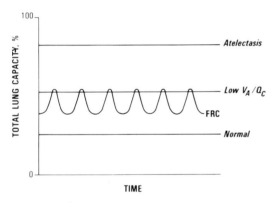

Fig. 32.2 The *relationship* between the *functional residual capacity* (FRC) (which is the percent of total lung capacity, Y axis) that exists at the end of exhalation (the level of each trough of the sine wave tidal volume) and the *closing capacity* of the lung (three different closing capacities are indicated by the three different straight lines). See text for explanation of why the three different relationships of functional residual capacity to closing capacity depicted result in ventilation-to-perfusion relationships that are normal, low, or associated with atelectasis.

volume up will create regions both of low ventilation to perfusion ratios and atelectasis. Intraalveolar edema fluid will additionally cause alveolar collapse and atelectasis. All of these changes result in stiff, noncompliant lungs for which the work of breathing may be excessive. Hypoxic pulmonary vasoconstriction can minimize the venous admixture from areas where the ventilation to perfusion ratio is low and from atelectatic regions.

## Pulmonary Hypertension and Vasodilator Drug Therapy: Inhibition of Hypoxic Pulmonary Vasoconstriction

Decreased regional alveolar partial pressure of oxygen causes regional pulmonary vasoconstriction. The regional hypoxic pulmonary vasoconstriction diverts blood flow from underventilated or nonventilated regions of the lung to better ventilated regions of the lung and thereby minimizes venous admixture and protects the arterial partial pressure of oxygen ($P_aO_2$). It has been clearly shown that, since the pulmonary vasculature is poorly endowed with smooth muscle, small increases in pulmonary vascular pressure greatly inhibit hypoxic pulmonary vasoconstriction.[7] Pulmonary hypertension is a common and often necessary sequel of acute myocardial infarction and left ventricular failure.

Vasodilator drug infusion (sodium nitroprusside, nitroglycerin) has been used to decrease left ventricular afterload in patients with acute myocardial infarction and those with low cardiac output states.[8-11] All of the subjects in these human studies could be presumed to have a hypoxic lung compartment (and, therefore, preexisting hypoxic pulmonary vasoconstriction) by virtue of either old age [12] or pulmonary edema.[4-6] Vasodilator drug infusion in these patients [8-11] caused an increase in transpulmonary shunt and a decrease in pulmonary artery pressure, pulmonary vascular resistance and $P_aO_2$. All of these changes are compatible with the hypothesis that vasodilator drug infusion inhibits hypoxic pulmonary vasoconstriction. Indeed, there is a plethora of experimental evidence to support that conclusion.[13]

Hypoventilation (see below)

## CAUSES OF HYPERCAPNIA FOLLOWING ACUTE MYOCARDIAL INFARCTION

### Increases in the Work of Breathing

In marginal patients, increases in the work of breathing can cause $CO_2$ retention (see pulmonary edema above).

### Hypoventilation Due to Airway Obstruction [14]

Following acute myocardial infarction, patients may hypoventilate due to depressed central nervous system function and/or, as stated above, inability to do the work of breathing with lungs that have increased airway secretions, bronchiolar wall edema, and pulmonary edema. In the majority of these instances, the cause of hypoventilation is airway obstruction. Total airway obstruction is characterized by a lack of breath sounds, which may be coupled with continuing, sometimes strenuous, but ineffectual efforts at breathing. Excessive diaphragmatic activity causes abdominal movements and chest retraction, but these do not represent movement of air. Checking for air movement can be done by listening continuously with a stethoscope over the chest or trachea.

Partial airway obstruction is characterized by: (1) diminished tidal exchange with diminished breath sounds; (2) retraction of the chest with inspiration which prolongs the inspiratory phase; (3) excessive diaphragmatic activity; (4) discrepancy between the movement of a breathing bag and the chest; and (5) various characteristic sounds to be described below.

Partial obstruction caused by the tongue causes a rough, irregular, stuttery noise frequently associated with "stertorous" respiration, whereas laryngospasm may cause a high-pitched whistle or squeak. Partial obstruction by the lips is most noticeable during expiration and is accompanied by a low-pitched, rough,

fluttery sound. Pharyngeal secretions cause a gurgling, bubbling noise.

Lower airway obstruction is characterized by: (1) diminished tidal change; (2) excessive intercostal and diaphragmatic activity; (3) active inspiration and expiration during spontaneous respiration; and most importantly, (4) adventitious breath sounds consisting of rales, rhonchi, or wheezing. The breathing bag classically empties and refills slowly, and moderate changes in compliance can be detected in the feel of the breathing bag.

Partial obstruction at the trachea due to foreign materials and secretions produces a "rattly" or "sloshy" noise. Endobronchial intubation will cause absent breath sounds in the contralateral lung, and this lung will not expand during inspiration. Bronchiolar secretions cause rhonchi, and bronchiolar constriction causes wheezing rales. Alveolar obstruction may be associated with all types of adventitious sounds.

## CLINICAL INDICATIONS FOR INTUBATION OF THE TRACHEA

In the absence of frank cardiopulmonary arrest, the decision to intubate the trachea should be based on both quantitative [15] and qualitative objective criteria.

### Quantitative Objective Criteria (See Table 32.1)

### Qualitative Objective Criteria

**Trends.** Equally important as the "numbers" in Table 32.1 is the *trend* of these numbers. For example, progressively increasing $P_aCO_2$ from a normal $P_aCO_2$ in a patient without previous lung disease is more important than an already or normally high $P_aCO_2$ in a patient with emphysema (see below).

**Preacute Myocardial Infarction Data.** These data permit assessment of the severity of the present illness in relation to the patient's usual status. This assessment, particularly in patients with chronic obstructive pulmonary disease (COPD), will influence the decision to intubate.

Table 32.1 Quantitative Criteria Objective (Indications) for Tracheal Intubation

|  |  | Acceptable Range | Chest PT, Oxygen, Close Monitoring Possible Intubation | Probable Intubation and/or Ventilation Necessary |
|---|---|---|---|---|
| Mechanical | Respiratory rate | 12–20 | 25–35 | >35 |
|  | Vital capacity ml/kg | 65–75 | <65 >15 | <15 |
|  | Inspiratory force, cm $H_2O$ | 100–50 | <50 >25 | <25 |
| Oxygenation | A-a$DO_2$, mm Hg<br>room air<br>$F_IO_2 = 1.0$ | <38<br><100 | >38 >55<br>>100 <450 | >55<br>>450 |
|  | $PaO_2$, mm Hg<br>room air<br>$F_IO_2 = 1.0$ | >72<br>>400 | <72 >55<br><400 >200 | <55<br><200 |
| Ventilation | $\dot{V}_D/\dot{V}_T$ | 0.3–0.4 | 0.4–0.6 | >0.6 |
|  | $PaCO_2$, mm Hg | 35–45 | 45–60 | >60 |

PT = physical therapy; A-a$DO_2$ = alveolar-arterial partial pressure of oxygen difference; $PaO_2$ and $PaCO_2$ = arterial partial pressure of oxygen and carbon dioxide, respectively; $F_IO_2$ = inspired concentration of oxygen; $\dot{V}_D/\dot{V}_T$ = dead space to tidal volume ratio.
(Pontpoppidan H, Geffin B, Lowenstein E: Acute respiratory failure in the adult [second of three parts]. N Engl J Med 287:743–752, 1972.)

For example, a $P_aO_2 = 50$ torr and $P_aCO_2 = 65$ torr might be normal for a COPD patient, but these same values would indicate a marked degree of respiratory embarrassment for a previously normal patient.

**X-ray.** Review of the chest radiograph may reveal readily reversible pathology (pneumothorax, diuretic-responsive pulmonary edema) that would obviate the need (as dictated by the "numbers") for intubation. The trend in changes in the x-ray findings is important also.

**Cardiovascular and Fluid Balance Data.** Consideration should be given to the contribution of the cardiac output and fluid balance to impaired gas exchange. Pharmacologic and intravascular volume manipulation of the cardiac output and urinary output is often quickly possible.

**Sensorium.** Comatose patients may not have protective reflexes that prevent aspiration of regurgitated material; as noted above, they may also have obstructed airways. Changes in sensorium generally occur very slowly, but in selected patients expected changes may be a factor in the decision to intubate.

## INTUBATION OF THE TRACHEA[16-18]

Following myocardial infarction, tracheal intubation may be necessary at any time. During different clinical circumstances, varying degrees of speed of accomplishment of tracheal intubation are required. For example, dysrhythmias may cause sudden cardiopulmonary arrest. Subsequent to the initial myocardial insult, slowly but progressively developing left ventricular failure may cause pulmonary hypertension and edema leading to the onset of respiratory failure. Finally, late in a patient's clinical course, infection in edematous and atelectatic regions of the lung may cause slowly developing pneumonia and respiratory embarrassment. The anatomic route and method of tracheal intubation are usually dictated by the urgency of the clinical situation. In general, urgent intubations require oral intubation, and semielective intubations are compatible with both oral and nasal intubation. The discussion of oral intubation assumes that the indications are urgent and obvious: for example, the patient has suffered a cardiac arrest, or is profoundly hypoxic (blue), or has agonal or markedly obstructed and distressed respirations. The discussion of nasal intubation assumes that the indications are progressive but not immediately life threatening: for example, the blood gas values are deteriorating or respirations are becoming uncomfortably labored and the vital capacity is decreasing.

## Oral Intubation

**Pre-laryngoscopy Maneuvers.** Suctioning the pharynx may be necessary at any time, but it is often the first necessary therapeutic intervention, since regurgitation of gastric contents frequently follows acute myocardial infarction. The regurgitation may be passive due to external cardiac compression or active due to splanchnic hypoperfusion. A curved, clear, hard plastic suction catheter should be used.

From the moment a resuscitator begins laryngoscopy to the initiation of positive pressure ventilation via tracheal tube, a finite period of time must pass. The duration of this period is directly proportional to the degree of difficulty (often increased by external cardiac compression) and inversely proportional to the skill of the intubationist. Since even skilled intubationists may require 30 sec to 1 min for this period, preoxygenation with 100 percent $O_2$ ventilation via face mask with a large tidal volume for a minute is indicated. However, a note of caution must be mentioned. First, positive-pressure mask ventilation may be inadequate due to mask leak or glottic obstruction or some combination of both. The assessment of the adequacy of ventilation in the urgent clinical situation is a matter of experience and medical judgment. In certain instances of poor mask mechanical ventilation with no spontaneous ventilation it is possible for the $P_aO_2$ actually to decrease during attempts to preoxygenate. With regard to mechanical ventilatory properties, anesthesiologists have found the esophageal obturator airway to be inferior to the black rubber mask-oropharyngeal airway system.[19]

The *correct head position* for laryngoscopy is important. The head must be flexed at the neck and extended at the junction of the spine and the skull (atlantooccipital joint). This position of the head is commonly called the "sniff"

position. The upper airway is maximally patent in this position and is the reason why long distance runners instinctively assume this head posture.

In the sniff position, the airway is also the straightest. The oral, pharyngeal, and tracheal anatomic planes must be considered in tracheal intubation (Fig. 32.3). In the normal nonsniff position (Fig. 32.3A) the oral plane passes along the mouth and is intersected at 90° by the pharyngeal plane. The tracheal plane (Fig. 32.3A) ordinarily lies between the oral plane and the pharyngeal plane. Flexion of the neck brings the pharyngeal plane more into alignment with the tracheal plane. Extension of the head decreases the angle between the oral plane and the other two planes. At best, the three planes can be manipulated so that they nearly coincide. Then, it is almost a straight line which an endotracheal tube must traverse through the oral plane into the pharyngeal plane and then

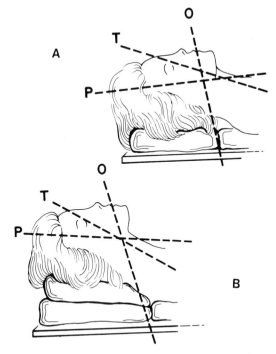

Fig. 32.3 *(A)* The oral (O), pharyngeal (P), and tracheal (T) planes of the upper airway with one pillow under the head. *(B)* Flexion of the neck on the chest and extension of the head on the neck bring the three planes (ideally) to a point where they coincide (lower drawing, with two pillows under the head).

through the vocal cords into the trachea. Thus, the same positioning movements that make the airway largest also make the airway straightest. The correct position is most easily obtained by placing the head on an elevated cushion support (Fig. 32.3*B*), which flexes the neck, and then extending the head by moving the chin up and back.

In barrel-chested and obese patients and large-breasted female patients, it may be difficult to insert the blade of a laryngoscope correctly into the mouth and avoid interruption of this procedure by anterior chest wall obstruction to movement of the handle of the laryngoscope. In these patients, further initial skull-spine extension (atlantooccipital joint) or 90° rotation of the laryngoscope to the right will permit easier introduction of the blade of the laryngoscope into the mouth and avoid anterior chest wall obstruction to movement of the handle of the laryngoscope.

**Laryngoscopy.** The laryngoscope handle is held in the left hand. In order to open the mouth widely, the thumb of the right hand presses down (caudad) on the lower molar teeth and the index finger of the right hand presses up (cephalad) on the upper molar teeth (Fig. 32.4). The laryngoscope blade tip is inserted at the right side of the mouth (Fig. 32.5*A*). The blade is advanced forward to the base of the tongue and swept centrally toward the midline so that the tongue is completely kept to the left side of the laryngoscope blade (and the mouth) (Fig. 32.6*A*). Many unsuccessful or difficult intubations are due to the fact that the tongue flops over the blade onto the right side, thus establishing a narrow "tunnel" through which subsequent attempts to visualize the vocal cords and to pass the endotracheal tube are made with obscured vision (Fig. 32.6*B*). All of the tongue must be to the left of the blade (Fig. 32.6*A*). After the blade has been applied to the base of the tongue, the laryngoscope is lifted to expose the epiglottis (Figs. 32.5*C* and *D*). Hereafter, the left wrist of the operator should remain straight, all lifting being done by the left shoulder and arm. If the laryngoscopist follows a natural inclination to rotate and flex the wrist, thereby raising the laryngoscope like a lever whose fulcrum is the upper incisor or gum, bro-

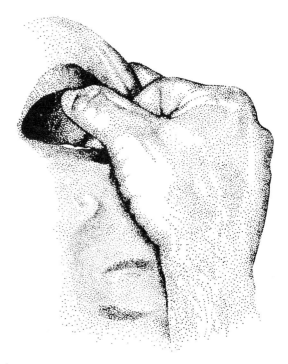

Fig. 32.4  To maximally open the mouth of a patient, the thumb should press caudad on the lowermost posterior molar teeth and the index finger should press cephalad on the uppermost posterior molar teeth.

ken teeth or gum bleeding are likely to result. With the patient in the sniff position, the direction of force necessary to lift the mandible and tongue and thereby expose the glottis is along an approximately 45° straight line above an imaginary line from the patient's head to feet. Careful study of Figs. 32.3, 32.5 and 32.6 will make this consideration obvious. If the blade is curved (Mackintosh), the tip should be placed in the vallecula (space between the base of the tongue and epiglottis) (Fig. 32.5*B* and *D*); if the blade is straight (Miller), the tip should extend just behind (posterior to) the epiglottis (Fig. 32.5*C*). In either case, lifting up as described above will cause first the arytenoid cartilage and then, with favorable anatomy, the glottic opening and vocal cords to come into view (Fig. 32.6*A*).

If either blade has been directed off the midline to the right or advanced too far, the opening of the esophagus will be visualized rather than the glottic aperture. The two openings are differentiated as follows: (1) the esophagus is lo-

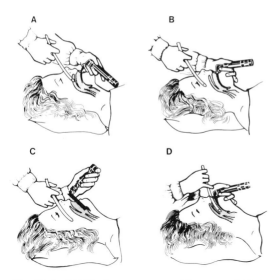

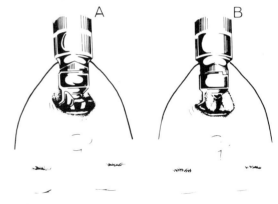

Fig. 32.6 *(A)* Correct view of larynx as seen by laryngologist with the tongue kept completely off to the left side of the mouth by the phalange on the laryngoscope blade.
*(B)* Failure to trap tongue on the left side of the mouth by the phalange of the laryngoscope blade results in a tongue that flops on both sides of the laryngoscope blade, causing a poor, obstructed, narrow tunnel view of the practically unvisualized larynx.

Fig. 32.5 *(A)* The laryngoscope with a curved blade (Mackintosh) is inserted at the right side of the mouth along the base of the tongue and is advanced until . . .
*(B)* The tip of the blade engages in the valleculae (space between the base of the tongue and epiglottis).
*(C)* If a straight blade (Miller) is used, the tip of the blade should be advanced until it is just posterior to (under) the epiglottis.
*(D)* in either case *(B* or *C)* *(B* is represented here), when the laryngoscope is pulled forward at a 45° angle away from the longitudinal plane of the body, the glottic opening enlarges and comes into view.

cated to the right of the midline and posteriorly; (2) the esophageal opening is round and puckered with no structures around it; (3) the glottis is triangular; (4) the glottis is located in the midline; (5) the glottis contains the prominent knobs of the arytenoids posteriorly; and (6) the vocal cords and dark cavity of the trachea can be seen beyond the glottis.

A common error in performing laryngoscopy is getting too close to the objects being viewed. In the properly positioned patient with the vocal cords exposed, the mouth is only 6 to 8 inches from the cords. This is barely the distance that most people require to focus their eyes on a close object. Yet the beginner at intubation is often seen with one eye virtually in the patient's mouth, as if taking aim with a shotgun. This close distance compromises vision, which is better at a slightly greater distance, and denies the advantage of depth perception, which depends greatly on the use of both eyes.

**Tracheal Intubation.** The actual insertion of the tracheal tube is usually easy once the vocal cords are exposed (and the tongue is out of the way) Fig. 32.5*D*, Fig. 32.6*A*). The endotracheal tube used should be a clear plastic one which is tissue implantable (has the printed marking Z79) and has a large volume low pressure cuff on it. The tip of the endotracheal tube should be introduced into the right corner of the mouth and passed along an axis which intersects the line of the laryngoscope blade at the glottis. In that way, the tube does not interrupt the view of the vocal cords. The common error of trying to use the laryngoscope blade as a guide, under which the tube is passed, violates this principle and is a significant source of difficulty for the inexperienced operator. The tube tip is passed through the cords stopping just after the tube cuff disappears from sight.

I use a stylette in the endotracheal tube whenever a curved laryngoscope blade is used because the glottic opening can be unexpectedly anterior and, therefore, unvisualized. In this case, in order to intubate the trachea the tube must pass along but to the right of the curved route made by the blade. (See "The Difficult Intubation" later in this chapter.) When intubation speed is important, an endotracheal tube should always contain a stylette. The reason for this recommendation is that if the larynx is anterior (expectedly or unexpectedly) no time will be lost in locating and then placing a stylette in an endotracheal tube. This is an avoidable delay that can only harm the patient. A stylette should be malleable and well lubricated. Occasionally, a curved endotracheal tube containing a stylette will impinge on the anterior tracheal wall as it is being pushed in. Under these circumstances, the stylette should be withdrawn when the endotracheal tube is past the vocal cords. This will permit the endotracheal tube to regain its inherent flexibility and allow further passage caudad.

The laryngoscope is removed from the mouth with the left hand. The tube should be secured by one hand (continuously until the tube is taped) and the cuff of the tube should be blown up until a slight resistance to further movement of the plunger is felt. The tube should then be connected to a source of ventilation and 100 percent $O_2$ administered. The symmetry of ventilation should be ascertained by observing equal expansion of both hemethoraces and by stethoscopic examination for breath sounds throughout both peripheral lung fields. However, hearing uniform breath sounds throughout all lung fields does not guarantee that the tube does not lie in a main stem bronchus (if so, almost always the right main stem); if there is any question, one should retract the tube about one cm at a time and reexamine the breath sounds. A simpler and yet more definitive way of determining the location of the tube in the trachea and of preventing endobronchial intubation is to inflate and deflate the cuff rapidly while palpating the neck externally just above the sternal notch. If the tube is properly placed, inflation of the cuff can be felt and one can be reasonably certain (more certain than by listening to the chest) that there has not been inadvertent endobronchial placement of the tip of the tube. It is always advisable to confirm endotracheal tube position by chest radiograph; ideally the tip of the tube should be at the clavicular level. If breath sounds cannot be heard and/or no chest movement occurs, pull the tube out, ventilate the patient with a

mask and bag system several times with 100 percent $O_2$, and reattempt tracheal intubation again after inspecting the tube for plugs. Changes in the curvature of the endotracheal tube, need for anterior tracheal pressure, and positioning of the head need to be coordinated.

After the tracheal tube is in place and symmetrical ventilation is assured, the marking of the endotracheal tube at the level of the lower teeth must be noted. There are three reasons why this is important. First, during taping of the tube to the face, anxious beginners have a tendency to unwittingly advance the tube further into the trachea. Second, the patient may cough or make retching movements postintubation and, unless the tube has been continuously secured, the patient may self-extubate the tracheal tube. Movement of the initial marking outward facilitates this diagnosis. Third, following intubation of the trachea and the initiation of positive-pressure ventilation, if the left chest suddenly stops moving or no left chest breath sounds can be heard, there are two likely causes which the mark of the tube at the teeth can help differentiate between: (1) the tube has advanced into the right mainstem bronchus, causing left lung atelectasis; or (2) a left pneumothorax, possibly under tension, has developed. If the tube had been marked when ventilation was normal bilaterally, and this mark subsequently advanced into the patient's mouth, bronchial intubation would be much more likely than pneumothorax, whereas the converse would be true if the mark were stationary. Similar considerations apply to apparent absent ventilation of the right lung.

After the mark of the tube at the lower teeth level has been noted, the tube should be taped in place. This is important not only for the prevention of accidental extubation but also to minimize tube movement within the airway. Figure 32.7 suggests two different ways to tape the tube in place. Application of tincture of benzoin to the skin before the tape is applied will help provide a stronger bond between the tape and the skin. In cases of prolonged intubation, changing the tape and reapplying it to a new area on the face every two days will help prevent maceration of the skin. A very secure method of fastening an orotracheal tube is to

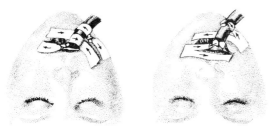

Fig. 32.7  Two different methods of taping the endotracheal tube in place.

wire the tube to a tooth. Adhesive tape is wrapped around the tube at the level of the lower incisor teeth. Stainless steel wire (25 to 28 gauge) is passed around a lower incisor tooth and twisted around the tape on the tube. A bite block, rolled gauze, or oral airway should be placed between the teeth to prevent the patient from biting down and occluding the lumen of an oral tube. Finally, the mouth and pharynx should be suctioned, and the tube cuff should be fully deflated during peak positive-pressure inspiration and then reinflated to a just seal volume during the next few peak positive-pressure inspirations.

## Nasal Intubation

Since many of the instructions for oral intubation apply equally to nasal intubation, they will not be repeated in their entirety. Positioning the patient, preoxygenation, laryngoscopy technique, correct depth of tube insertion, and marking and securing the tube are the same for either method. Nasal intubation is contraindicated in any patient with abnormal (>10 sec above control) clotting times.

**Blind Nasal Intubation.** Candidates for this procedure *must be* breathing spontaneously. If conscious and cooperative, the patient should be asked to judge which nasal passage is larger, by alternately occluding each nostril and determining the ease of breathing through the open one. The larger nostril should be sprayed with a vasoconstrictor drug to further increase its patency and to prevent or minimize bleeding from nasal mucosal trauma. The conscious patient undergoing blind nasal intubation will also require anesthetization of the nose, pharynx, larynx, or trachea, or any combination of these,

as dictated by the urgency of the clinical situation (see Table 32.2).

Several notes of caution must be appended to the methods outlined in Table 32.2. Instillation of a vasoconstrictor into the nostril may potentially cause systemic vasoconstriction and hypertension and cardiac dyshythmias. Increases in afterload may cause an increase in myocardial oxygen consumption and, therefore, possibly cause infarct extension. Similarly, inadequate anesthesia in an awake, anxious, hypertensive patient could also result in infarct extension. Above all, just as the urgency of the clinical situation dictates the route of intubation, the particular combination of the above anesthesia methods is also dictated by the urgency of the clinical situation and may range from no topical anesthesia for a spontaneously

**Table 32.2  Blind Nasal Intubation**

*Methods of Vasoconstriction*

1. Application of 2 ml of 10% cocaine or 4 ml of 5% cocaine by cotton swab, atomizer spray, or 26-gauge needle spray.
2. Application of 1.0 ml of 1.0% phenylephrine in 3 ml of saline or 2% lidocaine (resultant solution is 4 ml of 0.25% phenylephrine) by cotton swab, atomizer spray, or 26-gauge needle spray.
3. Application of 1:200,000 solution of epinephrine in 2% lidocaine.

*Methods of Anesthesia for the Nose*

1. Application of 2 ml of 10% cocaine or 4 ml of 5% cocaine by cotton swab, atomizer spray, or 26-gauge needle spray.
2. Application of 2% lidocaine solution by cotton swab, atomizer spray, or 26-gauge needle spray.
3. Application of 2% lidocaine ointment·by coating a rubber nasopharyngeal airway.

*Methods of Anesthesia for the Pharynx*

1. Gargle 30 ml of 4% viscous lidocaine for one minute.
2. Spray 2% lidocaine on tongue. Slowly advance laryngoscope along tongue spraying 2% lidocaine ahead of the blade.

*Methods of anesthesia for the Larynx and Trachea*

1. Spray 4% lidocaine on larynx and in trachea as the blade engages the vallecular space.
2. Perform transtracheal block through cricothyroid membrane with 4 ml of 4% lidocaine.
3. Perform superior laryngeal nerve block with 2 ml of 2% lidocaine bilaterally.

breathing but unconscious or comatose patient to use of just less than toxic doses of cocaine and 4 percent lidocaine (do not exceed 200 mg of each) or of 2 percent lidocaine (do not exceed 500 mg) for an awake, anxious patient who is in obvious respiratory distress. A few minutes' wait is necessary before any topically applied anesthetic is clinically effective. Finally, consideration should be given to the future need for fiberoptic bronchoscopy. An 8-mm tube is necessary for fiberoptic bronchoscopy and occasionally the nares of some patients will not permit introduction of this size tube.

The clear, plastic, low-pressure/high-volume cuff nasotracheal tube should be well lubricated with local anesthetic jelly or ointment. The tube should be guided slowly but firmly into the nasal passage, going up from the nostril (to avoid the large inferior turbinate), then backward and down into the nasopharynx, in a pathway which may be visualized as an inverted "U." As the tube passes through the nose into the nasopharynx, it must turn downward to pass through to the oropharynx. While making this turn, it may impact against the posterior nasopharyngeal wall and resist any attempt to push it further. The tube should be pulled back a short distance and the patient's head should be extended further to facilitate attempts to pass this point smoothly and atraumatically. If this is not done and the tube is forced, the mucosal covering of the posterior nasopharyngeal wall may be torn open, and the tube may be passed into the submucosal tissues. If the tube cannot be passed, one should try either the other nostril, use a smaller tube, or resort to oral intubation.

Once the tube is in the oropharynx, the tip of the tube must be aligned with the glottic opening. This is best done by listening to the volume and quality of sound of air moving through the tube. This is why it is necessary to have the patient breathing spontaneously and, if possible, deeply when attempting a blind nasal intubation. When the tip of the tube is directly in front of the glottic opening, a large volume of air can be best heard and felt. One then times the advance of the tube into the glottic opening with an inspiration. The tube is advanced quickly and with a full motion,

not gently and slowly. Timing is critical because the vocal cords are open at inspiration. Entrance of the tube is determined by a continuation of the air movement through the tube, by a cough, or by vigorous bucking.

If the tip of the tube is excessively anterior, posterior, or lateral to the glottic opening, it will not enter this orifice. Lateral tip location, as indicated by bulging soft tissue in the lateral neck, can be corrected in either direction by twirling or rotating the adaptor of the tube at the nose. Alternatively, this problem can be identified by noting rotation of a curved adaptor, whose curve coincides with that of the tube, away from the midline. Anterior tip location, as indicated by bulging soft tissue under the mandible, can be corrected by flexion of the head or by picking up (anterior displacement) the larynx and trachea externally. Posterior tip location almost always means esophageal intubation and is indicated by loss of breath sounds heard or felt from the tube. Posterior tip location can be corrected by extending the patient's head, which will cause the tip of the tube to become more anterior in relation to the larynx. Posterior direction can also be corrected by using a ring tube (Endotrol). A ring tube has a cord which runs from the anterior surface of the tip of the tube up the length of the tube to a ring on the proximal end of the tube. Pulling on the ring causes anterior bending of the tip of the tube. Finally, posterior tip location can be corrected by pushing the larynx down (posterior displacement), which will cause the larynx to become more posterior in relation to the tip of the tube.

## Direct Vision Nasal Intubation

Even the most adept intubationist will encounter patients in whom he cannot blindly pass a nasal tube. Either a reasonably small tube will not pass the hypopharynx or excessive anterior, posterior, or lateral tube tip location cannot be corrected by the procedures described above. With the exception of the first problem, it is then necessary to look, via laryngoscopy, at the spatial relationship between the tip of the tube and the larynx. The laryngoscopy for nasal intubation is identical to that described for oral intubation. The procedures described above for correction of the anterior, posterior, and lateral malpositions are repeated more precisely under direct vision compared to blind attempts and result in success more readily. Since one hand must hold the laryngoscope and another may be necessary for head or larynx manipulation, an assistant is necessary to push the tube into the larynx when the appropriate elements are lined up correctly. Additionally, if the tube is in the midline but too posterior, and this is not correctable by extension of the head, the tube must be grasped in the pharynx with a (Magill) forceps (Fig. 32.8) and directed anteriorly through the vocal cords. The advantage of the design of these forceps is that, when the grasping ends are in the axis of the tracheal tube, the handle is at a right angle to the outside of the right side of the mouth. Thus, the intubationist can have the larynx exposed by the laryngoscope held in the left hand, the tube in full view, and a means of manipulating the tube by the forceps held in the right hand away from the line of sight. At this point, an assistant is

again necessary to advance the proximal end when directed by the intubationist so that the intubationist is free to guide the tube without having to pull it along by the Magill forceps.

In some patients, as the tube enters the trachea, the tube's anterior curvature may direct it against the anterior tracheal wall and interfere with passage past this point. To resolve this difficulty, the head must be lifted (flexed) slowly as the tube is advanced. A nasotracheal tube should be advanced only until the cuff is entirely below the vocal cords. A nasotracheal tube can be additionally secured by a suture through the wall of the tube and the nasal septum. The tube's correct placement must be verified as in any intubation, but this is particularly critical in blind nasal intubations because the tube is not actually observed to enter the larynx. If nasal bleeding occurs, it is probably wise to leave the tube in place to act as a tampon. If the bleeding is severe, the tube can be retracted and the cuff inflated to act as a better tampon.

## THE DIFFICULT INTUBATION

There are two general causes of a difficult intubation. First, a struggling, bucking, retching patient can make any tracheal intubation difficult. Under these circumstances, it may be necessary to either paralyze the patient with d-tubocurarine 3 mg i.v. followed by succinyldicholine 100 mg i.v. or to sedate the patient with repeated small doses of diazepam (5 to 10 mg i.v.) or pentothal (50 to 100 mg i.v.) or narcotics (fentanyl ½ to 1 ml, meperidine 10 to 20 mg, morphine 2 mg).

Second, on an anatomic basis, a difficult intubation, especially by the oral route, can be anticipated if: (1) the patient's neck is thick and short; (2) the tissue from mandible to sternum is in a straight line (fullness); (3) the jaw recedes ("Andy Gump" type); (4) the upper teeth override; (5) the lateral oral opening is narrow (small mouth); (6) the patient can open the mouth only slightly; (7) the teeth are "buck" type or some are loose; (8) the mobility of the neck is limited by arthritis, cervical tumor, cer-

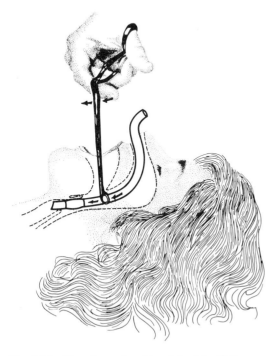

Fig. 32.8 View from the side of the Magill forceps grasping the nasotracheal tube in the axis of the nasotracheal tube.

vical fusion, cervical fracture and/or dislocation; and (9) contraction scars of the neck are present.

The number of fingers that can be placed between the inside of the mandible and the hyoid bone appears to correlate well with the expected view of the larynx (how anterior the larynx is). For a 70-kg, 5'8" male, two-finger placement suggests the arytenoids can be seen. Progressively more than two fingers means progressively more of the vocal cords will be seen until, when in excess of three fingers, all of the vocal cords will be seen. When progressively less than two fingers fit between the inside of the mandible and the hyoid bone, all that will be seen is the arytenoids and then only the epiglottis.

There are three nonsurgical solutions to the difficult intubation. The first two are: (1) blind intubation and (2) blind oral intubation (only epiglottis visualized during laryngoscopy). Skilled intubationists are considerably adept and successful in making a carefully curved styletted orotracheal tube (which often appears like a "hockey stick") blindly poke around the curvature of the epiglottis until the tip of the tube is felt to "fall" into the glottic opening. This is one of the arts of medicine, and only experience will make one skillful.

The third is the use of fiberoptic laryngoscopy. I prefer to perform fiberoptic laryngoscopy with a fiberoptic bronchoscope because the bronchoscope has a suction port which the laryngoscope lacks. This is an important difference because secretions will cloud the view seen through fiberoptics.

The fiberoptic scope consists of a flexible portion containing the fiberoptics for the viewing system eyepiece and a light source. A knob or switch on the handle controls deflection of the instrument's tip. Repeated use is required before one becomes adept at handling this instrument, but, with experience, interpretation of the visual images seen through the fiberoptic viewing system becomes easier. A good practice is to use the flexible scope for several "routine" intubations before trying it on a difficult case.

The flexible fiberoptic scope can be passed through the mouth, but it is easier to direct if inserted nasally through a partially passed naso-

tracheal tube. In addition, the danger of ruining the delicate flexible portion by clenching of the patient's teeth is avoided by introducing the scope through the nose. The same anesthetic considerations apply as for nasotracheal intubation. Rubber nasotracheal tubes should be avoided, for their internal surfaces are not smooth enough to allow easy removal of the scope once the tube is in place.

A light coating of lubricant should be applied to the flexible portion of the scope. Care should be taken not to get lubricant on the end of the instrument or else the viewing system will become coated. The fiberoptic instrument is inserted through a partially passed nasotracheal tube through the nasopharynx and oropharynx until the epiglottis is seen. At this point, it is usually necessary to deflect the tip of the scope (by the control on the handle) so that the tip of the scope may pass underneath the epiglottis and allow the vocal cords to be visualized. After introducing the fiberoptic scope about 5 cm beyond the vocal cords, the tracheal tube is advanced until it reaches the tip of the scope in the trachea. While one hand holds the tracheal tube in place, the fiberoptic scope is removed. Securing the tube and confirmation of position is the same as for nasotracheal intubation. Thus, in essence, the fiberoptic scope functions as a stylette, guiding the tracheal tube into the trachea.

## INTUBATION EQUIPMENT AND PERSONNEL REQUIREMENTS

Based on the foregoing discussion, Table 32.3 lists the materials for intubation that should be present and immediately available.

The personnel requirements differ slightly, depending on the urgency of the clinical situation. If the clinical situation is very urgent, only personnel who, on the basis of prior experience, can reasonably be expected to intubate quickly and efficiently should perform the procedure. This is not a teaching situation, and cardiopulmonary resuscitation of patients should not be interrupted in order to let inexperienced individuals attempt intubation. If the intubation is elective or semielective, then this may be con-

**Table 32.3  Equipment for Tracheal Intubation**

1. Suction apparatus should be turned on and hard plastic suction catheter attached.
2. $O_2$ source should be turned on and attached to a self-inflating ventilation bag.
3. Small, medium, large black rubber masks must be present.
4. 7, 8, 9 mm orotracheal tubes
5. 7, 8, 9 mm nasotracheal tubes
6. Malleable stylette
7. 3-way stopcock connected to 10 ml syringe
8. 4% lidocaine jelly and ointment
9. Laryngoscope handle
10. #3 and #4 Miller blades
11. #3 and #4 Mackintosh blades
12. Magill forceps
13. 4% lidocaine multi-dose and 2 ampules of phenylephrine
14. Atomizer
15. Small, medium and large oral and nasal airways
16. Tongue blades
17. Tincture of benzoin
18. Adhesive and umbilical tape
19. Relaxants
20. Syringes and needles

sidered a teaching situation, but the intubation should be performed only under the supervision of an experienced physician and only if the patient is reasonably stable. In general, if a previously untrained individual practices on and can efficiently orally intubate a Resusci-Anne mannikin, my teaching experience indicates that approximately a 60 percent success rate can be expected with orotracheal intubation in patients. This success rate is, of course, far less than the close to 100 percent rate for experienced individuals.

## MECHANICAL VENTILATION OF THE INTUBATED PATIENT

The recent introduction of positive end-expiratory pressure (PEEP) and intermittent mandatory ventilation (IMV) of a spontaneously breathing patient, along with an increased understanding of the toxicity of unnecessarily high concentrations of inspired oxygen ($F_IO_2$), have changed the clinical management of patients whose lungs are ventilated mechanically. The following briefly describes current practice of mechanical ventilation, weaning, and extubation.[20-22]

As soon as the trachea of a critically ill patient is intubated, controlled mechanical ventilation is initiated with a tidal volume of 12 ml/kg of body weight, an IMV respiratory rate of 10 to 12 breaths/min, with or without spontaneous breathing by the patient, and an $F_IO_2$ of 1.0. IMV used in this way is a ventilation modality. PEEP is progressively added (range 0 to 20 torr) until the arterial partial pressure of oxygen ($P_aO_2$) is normal for that patient (usually 80 to 90 torr) with an $F_IO_2$ less than 0.5 (oxygen toxicity has not been described below this level). Use of fiberoptic bronchoscopy, chest physical therapy, coughing routine, hourly turning of the patient, frequent suctioning, incentive spirometry, and, in selected patients, diuretics, colloid infusion and inotropic drugs generally allow the physician to decrease the PEEP to less than 10 torr with continued maintenance of an adequate $P_aO_2$ with a low $F_IO_2$ (less than 0.5). When the PEEP is less than 10 torr and the patient has an adequate $P_aO_2$ with a low $F_IO_2$, the patient is a candidate for weaning from mechanical ventilation. Weaning is accomplished by a progressive decrease in the IMV rate. The rapidity by which the IMV can be reduced is dictated by and is directly proportional to the patient's vital capacity (VC) and maximum inspiratory force (MIF). As the IMV rate is decreased, the patient is monitored by VC, MIF, and the spontaneous respiratory rate (SRR) and arterial partial pressure of carbon dioxide ($P_aCO_2$). The x-ray film of the chest is critically examined when the $P_aO_2$ is adequate, the $F_IO_2$ is less than 0.5, the PEEP is approximately 5 torr, VC is greater than 10 ml/kg of body weight, MIF is greater than $-20$ torr, IMV is less than or equal to 1/min, SRR is less than 20/min, and $P_aCO_2$ is approximately 40 torr. If the x-ray findings are reasonably equivalent to the premorbid x-ray findings, or if they are rapidly improving and no new changes have appeared (such as infiltrates or pneumothorax), the patient's trachea then is extubated and oxygen is administered via nasal prongs or plastic mask. It must be emphasized that, throughout this entire mechanical ventilation and weaning period, analgesics and sedatives must be administered and titrated so that the patient is comfortable, not bucking on the endotracheal tube, and is without active expiration.

The logic of this approach is that, first, the patient's lungs are required to function as an efficient gas exchange organ as indicated by an adequate or reasonable $P_aO_2$, with an $F_IO_2$ less than 0.5, and a PEEP level of less than 10 torr; second, that the patient can sustain this gas exchange without respirator aid as indicated by an adequate or reasonable VC, MIF, SRR, $P_aCO_2$ on a low IMV; and third, that no new complicating factor has occurred as indicated by lack of new findings and by resolution of old findings on the chest x-ray film.

## EXTUBATION OF THE TRACHEA

Prior to extubation of the trachea, the pharynx and nasogastric tube (if present) should be suctioned. Extubation of the trachea should be accomplished by inflating the patient's lungs with 30 cm $H_2O$ pressure, holding the pressure constant while the endotracheal tube cuff is rapidly deflated, and then immediately pulling the tube out. This insures that the first event following extubation is a forceful expiration (due to the elastic recoil of the chest wall) which will blow out any material lodged on top of the endotracheal tube cuff.

## COMPLICATIONS OF MECHANICAL RESPIRATORY SUPPORT

The complications of mechanical respiratory support can be divided into those due to tracheal intubation (Table 32.4) and those due to mechanical ventilation (Table 32.5).[23,24]

Although the list in Tables 32.4 and 32.5 of possible complications of mechanical respiratory support appears formidable, all are individually infrequent to rare events and, more importantly, most are avoidable. Proper technique and adequate anesthesia should make the actual insertion of the endotracheal tube uncomplicated. Adequate sedation, using a just seal volume of air in the endotracheal tube cuff, frequent suctioning and turning of the patient will render the presence of an endotracheal tube be-

**Table 32.4   Complications of Tracheal Intubation**

### During Intubation

1. Trauma to the cervical spinal column, nose, teeth, lips, tongue, larynx and trachea
2. Aspiration (blood, tooth, laryngoscope bulb, gastric bulb, gastric contents and partial dentures)
3. Esophageal intubation
4. Endobronchial intubation
5. Reflexes
   a. Sympathetic (hypertension, tachycardia, myocardial ischemia)
   b. Vagal (hypotension, bradycardia, cardiac arrest)

### With Endotracheal Tube in Place

1. Bronchospasm
2. Tracheomalacia
3. Tracheal perforation (by cuff, by tip of the tube)
4. Inadequate secretion removal (possible obstruction of the tube)
5. Trauma to all areas of contact (exacerbated by patient movement)
6. Excessive inflation of cuff causing tube lumen narrowing
7. Ruptured cuff

### During Extubation

1. Trauma to glottis by persistent inflated cuff
2. Aspiration of supraendotracheal tube cuff secretions
3. Laryngospasm
4. Respiratory obstruction by immediate edema of any part of the airway previously in contact with the endotracheal tube

### After Extubation

1. Sore throat, dysphagia
2. Aphonia
3. Paralysis of the hypoglossal and/or lingual nerves
4. Vocal cord paralysis
5. Ulceration, inflammation, infection, edema of any part of the airway previously in contact with the endotracheal tube
6. Laryngeal granulomas and polyps
7. Laryngotracheal membranes and webs
8. Tracheal stenosis

(Blanc VF, Tremblay NAG: The complications of tracheal intubation: A new classification with a review of the literature. Anesth Analg 53:202–213, 1974.)

nign. However, it is not possible to know about or eliminate pressure on the tissues in all areas of contact. The volume of air in the endotracheal tube cuff should be checked for a minimum volume ("just") seal limit one hour after each inspired oxygen concentration change and

**Table 32.5  Complications of Mechanical Ventilation**

*Complications Attributable to Operation of the Ventilator*

1. Machine failure or disconnect
2. Alarm failure
3. Alarms not turned on
4. Inadequate humidification
5. Excessive inspired oxygen concentration

*Medical Complications of Positive Pressure Breathing*

1. Inadequate positive pressure breathing-alveolar hypoventilation
2. Excessive positive pressure breathing-alveolar hyperventilation
3. Massive gastric distension
4. Pneumothorax, pneumomediastinum
5. Atelectasis
6. Pneumonia
7. Hypotension and decreased cardiac output
8. Increased ventilatory dead space
9. ADH secretion and water retention

ADH = antidiuretic hormone
(Zwillich CW, Pierson DJ, Creagh CE, Sutton FD, Schatz E, Petty TL: Complications of assisted ventilation: A prospective study of 354 consecutive episodes, Am J Med 57:161–170, 1974.)

only after the mouth has been suctioned. The endotracheal tube should be suctioned whenever breath sounds indicate the presence of tracheal or bronchial secretions.

# REFERENCES

1. Kelman GF, Nunn JF, Prys-Roberts C, Greenbaum R: The Influence of the cardiac output on arterial oxygenation: A theoretical study. Br J Anaesth 39:450–458, 1967.
2. Prys-Roberts C: The metabolic regulation of circulatory transport. Section II, Chapter 2. Scientific Foundations of Anaesthesia. Edited by Scurr C, Feldman S. F.A. Davis Company, Philadelphia, 1970.
3. Burger EJ Jr, Macklem P: Airway closure: Demonstration by breathing 100% $O_2$ at low lung volumes and by $N_2$ washout. J Appl Physiol 25:139–148, 1968.
4. Hales CA, Kazemi H: Small airways function in myocardial infarction. N Engl J Med 290:761–768, 1974.
5. Harken AH, O'Conner NE: The influence of clinically undetectable edema on small airway closure in the dog. Ann Surg 184:183–188, 1976.
6. Biddle TL, Yu PN, Hodges M, Chance JA, et al: Hypoxemia and lung water in acute myocardial infarction. Am Heart J 92:692–699, 1976.
7. Benumof JL, Wahrenbrock EA: Blunted hypoxic pulmonary vasoconstriction by increased lung vascular pressures. J Appl Physiol 38:846–850, 1975.
8. Mookherjee S, Warner R, Keighley J, et al: Worsening of ventilation perfusion relationship in the face of hemodynamic improvement during nitroprusside infusion. (Abstract) Am J Cardiol 39:282, 1977.
9. Chatterjee K, Parmley WW, Ganz W, et al: Hemodynamic and metabolic responses to vasodilator therapy in acute myocardial infarction. Circulation 48:1183–1193, 1973.
10. Berkowitz C, McKeever L, Croke RP, Jacobs WA, Loeb HS, Gunnar RM: Comparative responses to dobutamine and nitroprusside in patients with low output cardiac failure. Circulation 56:918–924, 1977.
11. Palmer RF, Lasseter KC: Drug therapy: Sodium nitroprusside. N Engl J Med 292:294–297, 1975.
12. Campbell EJ, Lefrak SS: How aging affects the structure and function of the respiratory system. Geriatrics 33:68–74, 1978.
13. Benumof JL: Hypoxic pulmonary vasoconstriction and sodium nitroprusside infusion. (Editorial) Anesthesiology 50(1):65–66, 1979.
14. Benumof JL: Monitoring respiratory function during anesthesia. In Monitoring During Anesthesia. Chapter 3. Edited by Saidman LJ, Smith NT. John Wiley and Sons, New York, 1978.
15. Pontpoppidan H, Geffin B, Lowenstein E: Acute respiratory failure in the adult (second of three parts). N Engl J Med 287:743–752, 1972.
16. Dripps RD, Eckenhoff JE, Vandam LD: Intubation of the trachea. In: Introduction to Anesthesia. Fourth edition. W. B. Saunders, Philadelphia, 1972.
17. Cullen SC, Larson CP Jr: Management of the airways. In: Essentials of Anesthetic Practice. Year-Book Medical Publishers, Chicago, 1974.
18. Applebaum EL, Bruce DL: Tracheal Intubation. Saunders, Philadelphia, 1976.
19. Bryson TK, Benumof JL, Ward CF: The esophageal obturator airway: A clinical comparison to mask-oral airway ventilation. Chest 74:537–539, 1978.
20. Benumof JL: Update on mechanical ventilation. An epitome. West J Med 128:147, 1978.
21. Downs JB, Klein EF Jr, Desautels D, et al: Inter-

mittent mandatory ventilation: A new approach
to weaning patients from mechanical ventilators.
Chest 64:331–335, 1973.

22. Powers SR Jr, Mannal R, Neclerio M, et al:
Physiologic consequences of positive end-expiratory pressure (PEEP) ventilation. Ann Surg
178:265–272, 1973.

23. Blanc VF, Tremblay NAG: The complications

of tracheal intubation: A new classification with
a review of the literature. Anesth Analg 53:202–
213, 1974.

24. Zwillich CW, Pierson DJ, Creagh CE, Sutton
FD, Schatz E, Petty TL: Complications of assisted ventilation: A prospective study of 354
consecutive episodes. Am J Med 57:161–170,
1974.

# 33 | *Pharmacology of Analgesics, Tranquilizers, Sedatives, and Hypnotic Drugs*

*S. Craig Risch, M.D.*
*David S. Janowsky, M.D.*

## INTRODUCTION

Psychotropic medications account for approximately 20 percent of all prescriptions in this country, and at least 10 percent of the American population at present use psychotropic medications by prescription.[1] These facts, together with the widespread illicit use of various psychoactive drugs (narcotics, psychostimulants, and central nervous system depressants), make it likely that the internist and cardiologist may encounter many patients with cardiovascular disease who are also using, either by prescription or surreptitiously, a variety of psychoactive agents. The practicing clinician must be alert to this possibility and be well-informed as to the cardiovascular side effects of psychoactive agents, as well as to numerous potential drug interactions. This would seem particularly critical for the Coronary Care Unit (CCU) practitioner.

Consequently, we have reviewed the pharmacology of the major classes of psychoactive agents: opiates (morphine, meperidine, codeine, pentazocine, methadone, and heroin); major tranquilizers (phenothiazines, thioxanthines, butyrophenones, and reserpine); antidepressants (tricyclic antidepressants and monoamine oxidase inhibitors); minor tranquilizers, sedatives, and hypnotics (benzodiazepines and barbiturates); the antimanic agent lithium carbonate; and anticholinergic agents used to antagonize the extra-pyramidal side effects of the antipsy-

chotic drugs, focusing on their intrinsic cardiotoxicity, cardiovascular side effects, and potential drug interactions. Generally, each group of drugs will be discussed under the following headings: (1) psychiatric indications, (2) proposed psychobiologic mechanism of action, (3) effects of these agents on cardiovascular function, and (4) potential beneficial and adverse cardiovascular drug interactions. Recommendations will be made as to the management of patients with acute myocardial infarction who are already receiving psychotropic medications; the management of patients who have overdosed on psychotropic medications; and the potential therapeutic use of psychotropic agents in acute myocardial infarction and cardiovascular disease.

## ANALGESICS

Opiates (morphine, meperidine, codeine, pentazocine, heroin, methadone)

An understanding of the pharmacology, cardiovascular side effects, and drug interactions of the narcotic analgesics may be important to the coronary care unit practitioner in three major areas: (1) the proper management of pain secondary to acute myocardial infarction (AMI); (2) the management of narcotic overdoses; and (3) the management of cardiovascular complications in the withdrawing heroin addict or an addict on methadone maintenance.

The pertinent pharmacologic properties of opiate analgesics will be reviewed, including their cardiovascular side effects; effects on other organ systems, which, in turn, may adversely influence an injured cardiovascular system; and drug interactions pertinent to the management of AMI. The major narcotic analgesics useful in the management of pain secondary to AMI will then be compared and contrasted. Finally, recommendations will be made as to the recognition and treatment of narcotic abuse and overdose.

*Morphine.* This narcotic is the active analgesic component of opium and the oldest and most throughly studied analgesic. No other analgesic is superior to morphine in relieving pain of cardiac origin,[2-4] and at equal analgesic doses, other narcotic analgesics appear to offer no advantages over morphine in the degree of respiratory depression,[3,4] hemodynamic effects,[2-4] or incidence of nausea and vomiting.[2,4] In fact, other narcotic analgesics may possess adverse hemodynamic side effects, making them less desirable than morphine in the management of pain in AMI,[4,5] as will be discussed below.

**Indications.** Narcotic analgesics have proved useful in the management: (1) of pain, both acute and chronic; (2) of dypsnea secondary to acute left ventricular heart failure and pulmonary edema; (3) of cough and diarrhea suppression; (4) of anesthesia; and (5) in the symptomatic management of opiate withdrawal in narcotic addicts.

**Mechanism of Action.** Despite a great deal of investigation, the mechanisms by which narcotics exert their analgesic and other actions remain unknown. Opiates produce analgesia, sedation, euphoria or dysphoria, mental confusion, respiratory depression, increased cardiac index with decreased systemic vascular resistance and postural hypotension, urinary retention and constipation, cough suppression, nausea and vomiting, diaphoresis, hyperglycemia, miosis, antidiuresis, and systemic release of histamine.[2-4] Opiates presumably mediate these diverse effects by acting in complex ways at various levels of the organism, including directly on target tissues in peripheral organ systems, and at various levels in the peripheral

nervous system, the spinal cord, and throughout the brain.[2] Opiates effect the release of a variety of central nervous system transmitters, including acetylcholine,[6] norepinephrine, dopamine, and serotonin.[6] Although the literature is still controversial, it appears that a reduction of central nervous system norepinephrine at the $\alpha$-receptor, but not at the $\beta$-receptor, potentiates morphine-induced respiratory depression,[7,8] and that a selective depletion of central nervous system serotonin may reduce morphine-induced respiratory depression.[8] Similarly, a reduction in central nervous system norepinephrine, at the level of the receptor, may potentiate morphine-induced analgesia.[7] These interactions may be important in understanding drug interactions between opiate analgesics and various psychotropic medications, which also are believed to influence brain levels of the above central nervous system neurotransmitters.

**Effects of Opiate Analgesics on Cardiovascular Function.** In the normal supine patient, therapeutic analgesic doses of morphine (10 to 15 mg IM), or equal analgesic doses of other narcotics, have no significant adverse effect on heart rate and rhythm, or cardiac output.[2,3] In fact, with higher doses morphine may actually increase coronary blood flow.[9] These findings have been exploited in the anesthetic management of patients with aortic valve disease undergoing open heart surgery, where large doses of intravenous morphine, 1.5 to 3.0 mg/kg, resulted in significant increases in cardiac index, stroke index, central venous pressure, and pulmonary artery pressure, and a significant decrease in systemic vascular resistance, allowing the safe operative management of patients with minimal circulatory reserve.[10] However, therapeutic analgesic doses of morphine and other narcotics may produce significant peripheral vasodilation, presumably through histamine release, which may precipitate severe orthostatic hypotension,[2-4] particularly pronounced in patients with AMI.[11] Similarly, patients with a preexisting diminished circulating blood volume may be particularly sensitive to the hypotensive and syncopal effects of narcotic analgesics,[2,3] and the use of narcotics for anesthesia or analgesia during operations may necessitate additional fluid and blood requirements.[12] Because morphine as well as equivalent analgesic doses of related narcotics (meperidine, codeine, and methadone), have been thought to cause systemic vascular venous pooling of blood and possibly a subsequent decreased return of blood to an already failing cardiovascular system, many investigators [13,14] have recommended the use of pentazocine for analgesia in AMI, reporting that its use in equianalgesic doses to morphine is relatively free from hypotension or systemic vascular venous pooling of blood. It should be recognized, however, that the evidence that morphine produces a "pharmacologic phlebotomy" in man is scanty.[14a,14b,14c] Moreover, other investigators [5,15] have reported that pentazocine, in patients with myocardial infarction, is associated with a significant increase in systemic arterial pressure, total peripheral resistance, left ventricular end-diastolic pressure, mean pulmonary artery pressure, and cardiac work, which may also further compromise a failing cardiovascular system. Consequently, most authors [4] recommend the use of morphine sulfate to a cumulative dose of 10 to 15 mg IM or IV, or meperidine to a cumulative dose of 75 mg IM, in the initial management of pain in AMI, although pentazocine may be used judiciously in hypotensive patients.[13,14] Incidentally, one investigator,[14] in a study comparing the analgesic efficacy of the major narcotic analgesics in AMI, reported that heroin was superior to all other narcotic analgesics; it induced little circulatory lability, and did not produce a significantly greater incidence of adverse side effects. However, at present, heroin is not commercially available in the United States.

**Effects of Opiate Analgesics on Respiration.** The respiratory depressant effects of narcotic analgesics may be of greater relevance to the CCU practitioner than the relatively mild effects on the cardiovascular system, discussed above. Therapeutic analgesic doses of morphine in man depress all phases of respiratory activity (rate, minute volume, and tidal exchange).[2-4] Even therapeutic doses of a narcotic analgesic may result in irregular or periodic breathing.[2] Narcotic analgesics effect these changes in respiration, both by depressing pontine and medullary centers, regulating respiratory rhythmicity,

and by diminishing the sensitivity of respiratory chemoreceptors to increases in carbon dioxide tension.[2-4] As these changes occur as early as 7 minutes after intravenous administration, or 30 minutes after intramuscular administration, the patient must be observed carefully during this period.[2] Respiratory depression may last up to 5 hours after the administration of a therapeutic analgesic dose of narcotic. When the various narcotic analgesics are given in equianalgesic doses, there are no significant differences in the degree of respiratory depression induced by each.[2,4] When the sensitivity of respiratory chemoreceptors to carbon dioxide tension is decreased, a patient sedated with narcotic analgesics may respond only to hypoxic stimulation, so that the concurrent use of oxygen therapy may result in apnea. Nevertheless, all patients with AMI who are given narcotic analgesics should also receive supplemental oxygen therapy, and be observed carefully for the development of apnea. This may be particularly relevant to the management of narcotic overdosage, as will be discussed below.

**Interactions Between Narcotic Analgesics and Other Medications**

1. *Opiates and Pentazocine.* Pentazocine has both opiate agonistic and opiate antagonistic activity. In patients tolerant to opiates, the use of pentazocine may reduce opiate analgesia, or even precipitate opiate withdrawal.[16] However, pentazocine does *not* similarly antagonize opiate respiratory depression.

2. *Narcotic Analgesics and Phenothiazines.* Generally the phenothiazines exert additive or synergistic effects with narcotic analgesics.[17,18] The depth of meperidine, morphine, and other narcotic-induced analgesia is increased in the presence of some phenothiazine antipsychotic agents, although this effect may simply be an additive rather than a synergistic one.[17] Among the phenothiazines, promethazine appears to be antianalgesic, and several other phenothiazines (perphenazine, prochlorperazine, fluphenazine, trifluperazine) appear to possess slight antianalgesic properties.[19] *Note: even though these agents may be antianalgesic, nevertheless their sedative, hypotensive, and respiratory depressant effects may be additive or synergistic.* In rodents and in man, the respiratory depressant effects

of narcotic analgesics are enhanced by the presence of phenothiazines, probably through a synergistic interaction.[18] The sedative-hypnotic effects of meperidine and promethazine are additive.[17] Similarly, narcotic and antipsychotic drug-induced hypotension may combine to produce dramatic hypotensive episodes.[19] The mechanism by which phenothiazines potentiate the effects of narcotic analgesics is uncertain. In summary, phenothiazines generally reduce narcotic requirements. However, significant respiratory depression and hypotension can occur in patients who are given therapeutic doses of a narcotic while receiving maintenance doses of antipsychotic drugs.[17,18,19]

3. *Narcotic Analgesics and Reserpine.* The data on reserpine-morphine interactions in animals are difficult to evaluate. Potentiation of analgesia is apparent in some species, such as rats and rabbits. Depending on the test system employed, reserpine may potentiate or antagonise morphine analgesia in mice.[20,21] The ability of reserpine to alter the effects of narcotic analgesics has not been well-studied in man. Hence, the importance of a narcotic analgesic-reserpine interaction is uncertain.

4. *Narcotic Analgesics and Tricyclic Antidepressants.* Although little human data exist to support the contention that tricyclic antidepressants augment the analgesic and other effects of narcotic analgesics, imipramine and amitriptyline are known to potentiate morphine analgesia in mice, and to increase meperidine-induced respiratory depression.[22] One investigator[23] reports that amitriptyline, 10 mg, and meperidine, 50 mg, given together were more effective as a preanaesthetic medication in reducing anxiety and apprehension than either agent given alone. He reports that the combination did not produce more adverse effects or longer anaesthesia or recovery time than meperidine alone. However, these results must be interpreted with caution, as this was a single dose of amitriptyline, 10 mg, whereas most patients receiving antidepressant medications have been receiving the medication for a period of time in doses of 150 to 300 mg/day. In light of the evidence in animals,[22] we would suggest using lower doses of narcotics in patients on tricyclic antidepressants.

5. *Narcotic Analgesics and Monoamine Oxidase Inhibitors.* Monoamine oxidase (MAO) inhibitors have been reported to interact with meperidine,[24] producing a syndrome of agitation, excitement, restlessness, hypertension, headache, rigidity, convulsions, and hyperpyrexia. A similar reaction has been reported between phenelzine (a monoamine oxidase inhibitor) and dextromethorphan.[25] Although, to date, there have been no reported interactions between morphine and MAO inhibitors in humans,[26] several studies in mice have demonstrated that pretreatment with an MAO inhibitor increased mortality, not only from meperidine but from morphine, pentazocine, and phenazocine as well.[27] Although the precise mechanism of these interactions is uncertain, based on animal experiments, several authors[27] have postulated that the interaction may be mediated by elevated levels of serotonin in the brain.

If these medications are inadvertently given together, and the above described syndrome occurs, several authors[24] have recommended treatment with prednisolone hemisuccinate, 25 mg intravenously, together with control of excessive arterial blood pressure and other supportive measures.

Narcotic analgesics, particularly meperidine, have also been reported to interact with MAO inhibitors to cause coma, hypotension, and respiratory depression, apparently a potentiation by MAO inhibitors of primary narcotic effects. This interaction appears to be mediated by the inhibition of narcotic metabolism in the liver by the action of MAO inhibitors on enzymes other than monoamine oxidase, leading to increased brain levels of free narcotic. Treatment is primarily supportive, using the narcotic antagonist naloxone.[28] Additionally, acidification of urine with lysine or arginine hydrochloride, or sodium biphosphate intravenously, and the production of a large urine volume, have been used to hasten meperidine excretion.[29] This procedure, in a patient with AMI, must be performed with careful attention to fluid replacement.

One-quarter to one-fifth of the usual narcotic dose should be given to patients receiving MAO inhibitors, who, for whatever reason, must receive a narcotic. However, the patient must be observed carefully over the next 15 to 20 minutes for any changes in vital signs or level of consciousness. Churchill-Davidson [30] and Evans-Prosser [31] have described "sensitivity tests," using small incremental injections of morphine (or meperidine), at hourly intervals, while carefully observing the patient for signs of adverse reactions. However, as the response to meperidine in patients receiving MAO inhibitors is extremely unpredictable it should be avoided, and reduced doses of morphine should be used if a narcotic is necessary.

6. *Meperidine and Benzodiazepine.* Dundee et al.[32] have reported that diazepam, 10 mg, and meperidine, 100 mg intravenously, before anesthesia produced significantly more hypotension and tachycardia than did meperidine, 100 mg alone, given intravenously. Therefore caution should be used in giving these medications together.

7. *Meperidine and Anticholinesterases.* Although there have been no reports of interactions between anticholinesterases and meperidine in man, it has been reported that physostigmine can inhibit the hydrolytic catabolism of meperidine in rat liver in vitro.[33] Thus, it is possible that anticholinesterases could potentiate the primary narcotic effects of meperidine.

8. *Morphine and Propranolol.* Morphine has been reported to potentiate cardiovascular β-blockade produced by propranolol in mice,[34] with extreme bradycardia and cardiac arrest, within minutes after the combination was administered, whereas there were no deaths when either medication was given alone. However, Slogoff et al.[35] report the morphine has an additive, but not a synergistic, effect on the β-blocking activity of propranolol in dogs. Although there are no studies of the interaction between morphine and propranolol in man, the above results would suggest caution in the use of these two medications together.

9. *Morphine and Dopamine.* In α-adrenergically (phenoxybenzamine) blocked anesthetized cats, morphine, 15 to 30 mg/kg IV, reversed the vasodepressor response of dopamine to a pressor response in the intact animals; in doses of 2 to 6 mg intraarterially, morphine significantly reduced canine renal vasodilator responses to intrarenal arterial dopamine.[36] The clinical significance of these results is unknown, but they suggest the careful use of morphine in patients in shock receiving dopamine.

**Recognition and Management of Narcotic Overdose.** Narcotic overdose may occur accidentally in the opiate abuser or addict; it may occur as a suicide attempt; or it may be iatrogenic, the result of administering a miscalculated dose or "therapeutic" doses to a patient in shock, which, though initially poorly absorbed, are excessively absorbed as normal circulation is restored.

A patient sustaining an overdose of narcotic may first be seen stuporous, asleep, or in profound coma; may exhibit depressed respiration, occasionally to the point of coma; or may appear cyanotic, with flaccid muscle tone (the tongue may fall back and obstruct the airway). The pupils are miotic, unless profound hypoxia has led to mydriasis. If coma is prolonged and untreated, shock with hypotension, renal failure, and seizures may occur.

Coma, miosis, and depressed respiration or apnea suggest narcotic overdose; needle tracts among addicts, or rapid toxicologic analysis of blood, urine, and gastric contents may support or confirm the diagnosis.

An adequate airway must be established immediately, initially with hyperextension of the neck and oropharyngeal intubation coupled to an Ambu bag attached to high flow 100 percent oxygen. Nasotracheal suction should be used to clear any aspirated gastric contents, and arterial blood gases should be checked frequently. Pulmonary edema (best detected by a "stat" chest X-ray examination) should be managed by intermittent positive-pressure ventilation.

After an intravenous line is secured, naloxone (Narcan) may be given intravenously in an initial dose of 0.4 to 0.8 mg, repeated, if necessary, every 20 to 30 minutes. A poor respiratory response to naloxone suggests the presence of nonopiate respiratory depressants (e.g., alcohol, barbiturates, etc.). Naloxone is preferred to nalorphine or levallorphan, as the latter agents possess opiate agonistic as well as antagonistic properties, and their use in a patient overdosed on ethanol or barbiturates may further depress respiration. Respiratory depression due to an overdose of opiate usually responds within minutes to the administration of naloxone; however, the antagonistic effects of naloxone may last only 1 to 4 hours, and repeated doses may be necessary, especially if the overdose was due to a long-acting opiate, such as methadone. On the other hand, naloxone must be used sparingly in the opiate-dependent patient, so as not to precipitate acute opiate withdrawal. Naloxone is indicated in the management of respiratory depression due to all opiates, both semisynthetic and synthetic narcotics, including pentazocine and cyclazocine.

Narcotic overdose among addicts may be complicated by a variety of serious medical problems. As noted above, pulmonary edema occurs frequently and may be best detected by a stat chest radiograph (physical examination is unreliable) and is managed by intermittent positive-pressure ventilation, high-flow oxygen therapy, and diuretics. Pneumonia, which may occur from the aspiration of gastric contents, is best treated by obtaining blood and sputum cultures, and administering a penicillinase-resistant penicillin parenterally, as staphylococci are frequently incriminated. Infective endocarditis has been estimated to occur in up to 9 percent of all general hospital admissions of heroin users [37] and may be complicated by pulmonary and systemic embolization. Similarly, pulmonary hypertension [38] and necrotizing angiitis [39] are frequent among parenteral drug abusers. A variety of electrocardiographic changes have been described among heroin abusers. Lipski et al.[40] report the frequent occurrence of bradycardia as well as conduction, depolarization, and repolarization abnormalities on the electrocardiograms of 75 asymptomatic (free of demonstrable cardiac, renal, or pulmonary disease) parenteral drug abusers admitted to a methadone maintenance program. Electrocardiographic abnormalities were found in up to 66 percent, with QT prolongation in up to 34 percent, prominent U waves in up to 32 percent, and bradydysrhythmias in up to 32 percent. Similarly, Duberstein and Kaufman [41] report a 25 percent incidence of atrial arrhythmias or conduction disturbances among 149 heroin abusers. Stimmel [42] notes that quinine, frequently mixed with heroin, alters the electrocardiogram in the same manner as quinidine, although a greater dose is required to produce the same effect. He concludes that the ECG abnormalities and sudden deaths among heroin addicts may frequently be related to adulterants in the injected mixture, rather than to the heroin per se. However, Weller and Perry [43] report several instances of bizarre cardiac and neurologic reactions in healthy addicts receiving uncontaminated parenteral narcotics, cocaine, or both.

In summary, narcotic overdosage frequently presents with coma, apnea, and miosis. Respiratory depression and coma may be safely managed by ensuring a patent airway, respiratory assistance, the intravenous administration of 0.4 to 0.8 mg of naloxone, and careful follow-up observation of the patient's need for additional doses of naloxone or, conversely, the development of opiate withdrawal symptoms. However, a variety of concurrent serious medical problems, including pneumonia, pulmonary edema, pulmonary hypertension, infective endocarditis, necrotizing angiitis, and a variety of cardiac rate and rhythm disturbances occur frequently in parenteral drug abusers and may further complicate their medical management.

**Management of Opiate Withdrawal Symptoms.** As discussed above, the injudicious use of naloxone in the management of narcotic overdose in an opiate-dependent subject may precipitate severe opiate withdrawal symptoms. Additionally, patients who receive opiates over a long period of time, either surreptitiously or iatrogenically, may experience opiate withdrawal symptoms when given analgesics with mixed opiate agonist and antagonist properties (e.g., pentazocine). Opiate dependence should always be recognized if it is iatrogenic. In the narcotic abuser, opiate addiction may be suspected by the presence of multiple needle tracts, or by unusual tolerance to the analgesic properties of standard therapeutic doses of narcotic analgesics.

Patients physically addicted to heroin, morphine, meperidine, or similar narcotics usually begin experiencing withdrawal symptoms 8 to 12 hours after their last injection, with peak withdrawal symptoms occurring at 24 to 36 hours. Withdrawal symptoms may be arbitrarily divided into four levels of severity ranging from mild to severe. Level 1 (mild) presents with lacrimation, rhinorrhea, diaphoresis, restlessness, and insomnia. Level 2 progresses to dilated pupils, piloerection, muscle twitching, myalgias, arthralgias, and abdominal cramping. Level 3 is characterized by tachycardia, hypertension, tachypnea, fever, anorexia, nausea, and extreme restlessness. Level 4 (severe) progresses to diarrhea, vomiting, dehydration, hyperglycemia, and hypotension. Opiate withdrawal should be managed with the oral administration of methadone whenever possible. A patient presenting in Level 1 withdrawal can usually be managed by the oral administration of 5 mg of methadone, followed by 5 to 10 mg 12 hours later. Level 2 withdrawal generally requires an initial dose of 10 mg of methadone followed by an additional 10 mg 12 hours later. Patients in Level 3 or 4 withdrawal generally require a parenteral dose of 10 mg of morphine concurrent with the first oral dose of methadone. Level 3 withdrawal requires an oral dose of 15 mg of methadone with a follow-up dose of 15 mg 12 hours later. Level 4 withdrawal is treated with an initial oral dose of methadone, 20 mg, and an additional dose of 20 mg 12 hours later. After the first 24 hours, methadone may be withdrawn at the rate of 5 mg per day. Supplemental doses of 10 mg of parenteral morphine may be given whenever Level 2, 3, or 4 withdrawal signs and symptoms appear.

Patients may also be managed by the oral administration of 10 mg methadone as needed to keep the patient above Level 2 withdrawal for 24 to 36 hours (patients rarely require more than 30 mg methadone per day) and then methadone may be tapered by 10 mg per day.

*Concurrent sedative-hypnotic addiction must always be suspected,* is often detected on initial stat toxicology screening of blood and urine, and, if present, must be managed concurrently.

Gold et al.[44] recently reported that clonidine is remarkably effective in managing opiate withdrawal. The authors hypothesize that opiate withdrawal is mediated by increased activity of noradrenergic neurons in the nucleus locus coeruleus. Locus coeruleus activity is believed to be regulated both by $\alpha_2$-adrenergic and opiate receptors. Clonidine, an $\alpha_2$-noradrenergic re-

ceptor agonist, is believed to have no affinity for opiate receptors,[44] and is believed to eliminate opiate withdrawal symptoms by augmenting $\alpha_2$-receptor mediated inhibition of locus coeruleus noradrenergic activity. Gold et al.[44] report that clonidine, 5 $\mu$g/kg orally, twice daily in a double-blind, placebo-controlled study, eliminated signs and symptoms of heroin and methadone withdrawal within 90 minutes in 12 subjects. Patients were continued on the same dosage, as outpatients, for 1 week, and 2-week follow-up revealed no signs of opiate withdrawal nor any adverse side effects other than occasional episodes of "sluggishness" and "a sleep continuity disturbance." Although these results are preliminary and require further study, it would appear that clonidine may soon be the drug of choice in managing opiate withdrawal.

## MAJOR TRANQUILIZERS

### Antipsychotic Medications

Phenothiazines, thioxanthines, and butyrophenones are useful in the management of psychotic symptomalogy secondary to schizophrenia, mania, and some forms of delirium and dementia. It is theorized that the antipsychotic efficacy of these medications is related to central dopaminergic receptor blockade[45] and all commercially available products appear equiefficacious in this regard. However, side effects among medications vary markedly, and the therapeutic selection of an antipsychotic agent is usually based on expected beneficial and adverse side effects. For example, chlorpromazine and thioridazine possess marked anticholinergic and antiadrenergic actions, and often elicit hypotension, sedation, and a variety of anticholinergic symptoms. Antidopaminergic side effects, such as extrapyramidal symptoms, occur infrequently, presumably because of their concurrent anticholinergic activity. Therefore, their sedative side effects may be exploited in the early management of an acutely agitated psychotic state, or their use may be desirable in patients extremely sensitive to extrapyramidal side effects. On the other hand, fluphenazine, trifluperazine, haloperidol, and butaperazine are much less sedating and have less anticholinergic activity, but frequently elicit extrapyramidal side effects. Therefore, they are often selected in the management of ambulatory, chronically psychotic patients where sedation and anticholinergic side effects are undesirable. However, the addition, at least initially, of an antiparkinsonian agent (benzotrophine, trihexyphenidyl, diphenhydramine, and so on) is frequently necessary to reduce extrapyramidal reactions. Nevertheless, all of the antipsychotic agents possess, to a greater or lesser degree, all of the above side effects. Chlorpromazine, an aliphatic phenothiazine, will be discussed, and where pharmacologic properties of other antipsychotic agents differ markedly, they will be noted.

Chlorpromazine acts at numerous levels of the organism to affect a wide variety of psychologic and behavioral events. It also affects the physiologic function of many organ systems, as well as numerous neurotransmitter systems at various levels throughout the nervous system. As discussed above, it is theorized that antipsychotic efficacy is mediated by dopamine blockade, presumably in the limbic system.[45] However, chlorpromazine may, directly or indirectly also mediate changes in central nervous system norepinephrine, serotonin, acetylcholine,[46] and possibly $\gamma$-aminobutyric acid and endorphins as well. Chlorpromazine has a variety of autonomic and endocrinologic actions, as well as effects on brain stem, striatal, limbic, and cortical processes.[46] Chlorpromazine's effects on the autonomic nervous system are complex. Chlorpromazine possesses peripheral cholinergic blocking activity, $\alpha$-adrenergic blocking activity, adrenergic activity, antihistaminic, and antitryptaminergic activities.[46] Anticholinergic activity may result in blurred vision, dry mouth, decreased gastric motility, constipation, and urinary retention. $\alpha$-Adrenergic blocking activity may block the effect of $\alpha$-agonist pressors, and reverse the effect of pressor amines, such as epinephrine, that have both $\alpha$- and $\beta$-agonist activity. Adrenergic activity, caused when the reuptake of epinephrine and norepinephrine is blocked, may result in decreased tissue but increased circulating levels of these catechol-

amines. Chlorpromazine disrupts neurotransmitter function in the hypothalamus, resulting in a diminished release of gonadotrophins, corticotrophin, growth hormone, and an increased release of prolactin.[46] Furthermore, this agent may disrupt temperature and appetite regulatory mechanisms[46] and depress hypothalamic and brain stem vasomotor regulatory centers, resulting in a centrally mediated fall in blood pressure.[46] Chlorpromazine acts on the medullary chemoreceptor trigger zone to reduce centrally mediated nausea and emesis.[46] It has been theorized that chlorpromazine may stimulate filtering mechanisms in the reticular formation of the brain stem, selectively reducing the inflow of stimuli into the brain.[46] This effect may account for the efficacy of neuroleptics in some types of delirium and dementia where environmental stimuli may "overload" an impaired central nervous system. Chlorpromazine's ability to produce dopamine receptor blockade in the striatal system is believed to result in a state of relative cholinergic dominance. This sequence is similar to the presumed pathophysiology of Parkinson's disease, resulting in a variety of "extrapyramidal reactions" such as akathesia, akinesia, and acute dystonic reactions. It is to be noted that these reactions are less common with chlorpromazine than with other neuroleptics (piperazine, phenothiazines and butyrophenones), which are agents with less anticholinergic activity. Finally, chlorpromazine may act at higher cortical levels to produce the "neuroleptic syndrome" characterized by psychomotor slowing, affective indifference, and emotional quieting, as well as EEG slowing and a lowering of the seizure threshold.[46]

## Effects of Major Tranquilizers on the Cardiovascular System

The neuroleptics may act directly and indirectly at a variety of levels of the cardiovascular system, and these actions may be additive, synergistic, or antagonistic. Furthermore these effects may vary with the class and dosage of neuroleptic agent.

**Direct Myocardial Depressant Effects.** The chronic administration of phenothiazines has been associated with the development of cardiomegaly, congestive heart failure, and refractory dysrhythmias.[47] Phenothiazines are believed to induce lesions in intramyocardial arterioles secondary to the accumulation of acid mucopolysaccharides.[48] Phenothiazines decrease cell membrane ionic permeability [49] and, consequently, diminish myocardial contractility [50] and alter repolarization.[51] Additionally, phenothiazines may chelate such cofactors as calcium, magnesium, and zinc to further disrupt cardiac enzymatic activity.[42] Chlorpromazine inhibits the reuptake of epinephrine and norepinephrine into cardiac cells,[52] resulting in increased circulating levels and decreased tissue levels of these compounds. These various direct myocardial depressant effects may combine to produce a variety of electrocardiographic changes, as well as cardiac conduction defects and arrhythmias.

**Electrocardiographic Changes.** Ban and St. Jean [53] report the prospective induction of "benign" and "nonspecific" changes in the electrocardiograms of psychiatric patients without cardiovascular pathology by all three classes of phenothiazine antipsychotic agents. Increased Q-T intervals and T wave alterations (blunting and notching) as well as changes in the appearance of U waves often followed the administration of therapeutic doses of phenothiazines. They were most common with the piperadine derivatives (thioridazine), less common with the aliphatic derivatives (chlorpromazine), and least common with the piperazine deravitives (trifluoperazine). Backman and Elosuo [54] also report the prospective induction of depressed T waves, increased Q-T duration, lowered S-T segments, and slight changes in AV conduction in patients receiving chlorpromazine, 150 mg/day for at least 1 week. Similarly, a retrospective study by Huston and Bell [51] demonstrated characteristic T wave changes in patients receiving therapeutic doses of chlorpromazine and thioridazine (again more frequent with thioridazine) and concluded that these changes were not related to the duration of medication. Kelly et al.[55] report a quinidine-like effect on the ECG of patients receiving thioridazine. However, unlike the effects produced by quinidine, these T wave changes may be corrected by isosorbide dinitrate or potassium salts.[56] The ECG changes induced by phenothiazines usually disappear when the neuroleptic agent is discontinued.[51] The same ECG changes may be produced by phenothiazines in isolated animal heart preparations,[57] suggesting that these effects are due to a direct myocardial depressant effect, rather than to autonomic or central nervous system regulatory disturbances. The other major classes of antipsychotic agents (thioxanthines, indole derivatives, and butyrophenones) produce similar ECG changes, although much less frequently than do the aliphatic or piperadine phenothiazine derivatives.[58]

**Cardiac Arrhythmias and Sudden Death.** Although uncommon, there are reports in the literature of serious conduction disturbances, cardiac arrhythmias, and sudden death associated with the use of phenothiazines. Such reports are usually retrospective and difficult to interpret, as patients frequently may have had preexisting cardiovascular pathology and often were receiving other cardioactive medications. Nevertheless, some authors report an increase in the incidence of sudden death among psychiatric patients since phenothiazines were introduced into psychiatric practice,[59] although others[60] could not find such an association. Even if sudden death syndrome among psychiatric patients is more common since the introduction of phenothiazines and is directly attributable to these drugs (neither of these assumptions have, by any means, been proven), the mechanisms by which phenothiazines might cause sudden death syndrome are not clear. The relatively "benign" changes in ECG tracings due to phenothiazines described above (prolongation of the Q-T interval, nonspecific T wave changes) might assume a more sinister significance in patients with concurrent cardiac disease. For example, otherwise benign and infrequent ventricular premature contractions, in the presence of a prolonged Q-T interval, may proceed to potentially fatal ventricular fibrillation. Alternatively, phenothiazine effects on coronary circulation and systemic blood pressure (described below) might further compromise an ischemic heart. Aspiration of food or gastric contents, and possibly asphyxiation via central mechanisms, have been implicated at autopsy in some cases of sudden death attributed to phenothiazines.[61] Nevertheless, some cases of sudden death in young, healthy individuals appear to be directly related to cardiac arrhythmias resulting from chlorpromazine [62] and thioridazine [63] therapy (usually heart block and ventricular arrhythmias). In summary, it appears that all antipsychotic agents have a direct myocardial depressant effect (particularly piperadine and aliphatic phenothiazines) usually manifested by benign ECG changes, i.e., prolongation of Q-T interval and nonspecific T wave changes. However, in some apparently healthy individuals, and particularly in patients with preexisting cardiovascular pathology, these agents may alter conduction time and induce serious and potentially fatal ventricular arrhythmias. In rare instances, these myocardial depressant effects may combine with phenothiazine-induced alterations in blood pressure, respiration, and autonomic function to produce a poorly understood sudden death syndrome.

**Neuroleptic Effects on Coronary and Systemic Circulation.** Although it is generally accepted clinically that neuroleptics may cause hypotension, particularly orthostatic hypotension, there are few well-controlled studies in the literature investigating this phenomenon. Several authors [64] report that oral administration of chlorpromazine, 50 to 200 mg/day, over 12 hours to 60 days, caused no appreciable changes in systolic blood pressure in psychiatric patients. However, doses of 25 to 50 mg of chlorpromazine, given intramuscularly or intravenously,[65] or larger doses (up to 750 mg/day) given orally, depress systolic pressure significantly (10 to 40 mmHg). Even when there are no alterations in systolic blood pressure, chlorpromazine frequently produces orthostatic hypotension,[64] which may be particularly prominent and dangerous in patients with depleted intravascular volume or an otherwise compromised cardiovascular system.

Although all neuroleptics may cause orthostatic alterations in blood pressure, these changes are more frequent and severe with aliphatic and piperadine phenothiazines (chlorpromazine and thioridazine).[66] In addition, hospitalized psychiatric patients,[67] even when free of psychotropic medications for up to 6 weeks, appear to have a greater incidence of circulatory lability than a normal control population.

Phenothiazines may produce hypotension by acting at various levels of the blood pressure regulatory systems. Chlorpromazine acts centrally to inhibit vasomotor centers,[68] as well as peripherally to depress cardiovascular reflexes, such as pressor responses to carotid occlusion and vagal stimulation.[69] In addition, neuroleptics produce peripheral α-adrenergic blockade [46] and may have a local vasodilator effect. Patients receiving long-term phenothiazine therapy may have elevated resting and exercise pulse rates, and a diminished exercise-induced cardiac output,[70] presumably a result of increased plasma levels of norepinephrine and concurrent α-adrenergic blockade induced by chlorpromazine.[71] These effects may culminate in myocardial infarction [48] or sudden death as described above.[72] In addition, because chlorpromazine has peripheral α- but not β-antagonistic effects, the use of epinephrine in patients receiving chlorpromazine may result in severe hypotension.[73] Phenothiazine-induced hypotension and shock should be managed with volume replacement and pure α-agonists only. For the same reasons, patients with pheochromocytomas may experience severe hypotension if given neuroleptics.[74]

There are very few studies on the effect of chlorpromazine on the coronary circulation, and there is little agreement among the existing studies. Courvoisier et al.[73] and Melville,[75] working with animal heart preparations, report an increase in cardiac output and coronary blood flow, respectively, when chlorpromazine was administered in high concentrations. However, in both studies there was an overall depression in cardiac activity. Another investigator [76] reports that large doses of chlorpromazine, 5 to 20 mg/kg, administered to animal heart-lung preparations resulted in an increase in coronary blood flow without affecting cardiac output, although another study [77] reports no changes in coronary blood flow or cardiac output when chlorpromazine was administered to dog preparations. Finally, Kaverina,[9] recording coronary vessel outflow in anesthetized cats, reports that chlorpromazine, 1 mg/kg, produced a 15 percent increase in volume and rate of coronary blood flow concomitant with a 30 percent fall in blood pressure; at 2 mg/kg there was a 22 percent increase in coronary blood flow but a 64 percent reduction in blood pressure. It appears from these studies that chlorpromazine may increase coronary blood flow by local spasmolytic properties, but that concurrent systemic hypotension may partially negate this action.

## The Therapeutic Use of Antipsychotic Medications in Acute Myocardial Infarction

Despite the cardiac depressant and hypotensive effects of neuroleptics reviewed above, numerous investigators [78,79] report the therapeutic efficacy of neuroleptics in the management of AMI. Lal and Bahl [78] report that 50 patients with AMI were treated with phenergan IM, every 8 hours, and triflupromazine 10 to 20 mg/day or chlorpromazine, 25 to 50 mg IM per day, for 3 days. The patients were then switched to oral promethazine, 25 mg three times daily. They report that these patients, when compared to 50 patients receiving standard anticoagulant therapy, had comparable outcomes, with the neuroleptic group having a lower incidence of arrythmias and cardiac failure. Elkayam et al. [79] report that the intravenous administration of chloropromazine to 12 patients with AMI and pump failure resulted in significant reductions in systemic vascular resistance (28.4 percent), an increased cardiac index (23.0 percent), and a decline in mean pulmonary capillary wedge pressure (38.2 percent). Heart rate and mean stroke work index as well as the transmyocardial pressure gradient did not change. Elkayam et al. report an overall decrease in myocardial demand for oxygen, and conclude: "Intravenous administration of chlorpromazine proved to be of benefit in patients with moderate to severe congestive heart failure and cardiogenic shock." Chlorpromazine was administered by intravenous bolus in increments of 2.5 mg every 5 minutes until mean arterial blood pressure decreased 20 mmHg, or pulmonary capillary wedge pressure fell significantly. The total dose of chlorpromazine averaged 12.5 mg, range 2.5 to 27.5 mg.

Pratt [80] reports the successful induction of "twilight sleep" (patient appears to be sleeping but is able to talk, eat, and respond immediately) in patients with AMI using haloperidol 5 mg IM every 4 to 6 hours, for 24 to 48 hours postinfarction. He reports great therapeutic benefit with no decline in blood pressure or other adverse side effects.

Riss et al. [81] reports the successful use of dehydrobenzperidol, 5 mg IM every 4 hours for 5 days to successfully prevent the recurrence of ventricular tachycardia and fibrillation in four patients with AMI. The arrythmias had previously been resistent to adequate trials of the commonly used antiarrhythmic agents, procaineamide and lidocaine. No adverse side effects were noted.

Numerous investigators [82] report the successful use of chlorpromazine in the treatment of cardiogenic shock, secondary to AMI, open-heart surgery, or pulmonary embolism. In cardiogenic shock, the fall in blood pressure is often associated with reflex vasoconstriction and subsequent poor tissue perfusion. In these patients, chlorpromazine's spasmolytic effect dilates resistance and capacitance vessels so that adequate tissue perfusion resumes. In most cases, cardiac output did not decline, and often improved. Chlorpromazine was administered intravenously in doses of 2.5 to 5 mg every 5 minutes to total doses of 25 mg. Similarly, Murphy et al. [83] report that chlorpromazine induces renal vasodilation and decreases vascular resistance in normotensive or hypotensive dogs, and is successful in combating hemorrhagic hypotension, if given early enough. The use of chlorpromazine to treat shock in volume depleted patients must be accompanied by blood transfusions or fluid replacement to prevent systemic blood pressure from deteriorating.

Kovach [84] reports the successful management of hypertensive crises in 36 patients with the intravenous administration of 5 mg of droperidol. Arterial blood pressures ranged from 180/110 to 260/160 mm Hg, and all patients were symptomatic, with headache, dizziness, nausea, and disorientation. The author reports: "The drug (droperidol) applied in 5 mg intravenous doses significantly decreased the systolic and diastolic blood pressure 10 to 30 minutes following administration and moderated or relieved the characteristic clinical symptoms of the patients. In the majority of cases the acute state could be controlled."

Finally, numerous investigators report the antiarrhythmic action of some phenothiazines.[73,85,86] The phenothiazines appear to be effective in both supraventricular [85] and ventricular [86] arrhythmias. The mechanism by which some phenothiazines may correct various arrhythmias is unknown, but it appears to be related to the N-substituted phenothiazine side chain, with various substitutions effecting greater or lesser potency against a variety of different types of supraventricular and ventricular arrhythmias.[85,86] To date, most of these studies have been carried out in experimental animal preparations and the clinical utility of phenothiazines in the management of cardiac arrythmias awaits further experimentation.

Although the above-described studies document the potential utility of neuroleptics in the management of a variety of cardiac disturbances (AMI, cardiogenic shock, hypertensive crises, and supraventricular and ventricular arrythmias), these initial reports of therapeutic efficacy must be tempered by other literature (described above) reporting a variety of adverse cardiac effects associated with neuroleptics (ECG changes, disturbances in cardiac conduction, hypotension, arrhythmias, and sudden death).[87] Furthermore, we are aware of no prospectively controlled studies demonstrating greater therapeutic benefit from neuroleptics than from the standard, accepted therapeutic modalities. Until such studies demonstrate the superiority of neuroleptic agents in the management of cardiac disturbances, we would urge great caution in their use in preference to standard coronary care in AMI and other cardiac crises.

## Interactions of Neuroleptics with Other Cardiac Medications

1. *Antipsychotics/Narcotic Analgesics.* The phenothiazines exert an additive and/or synergistic effect with narcotic analgesics [17,18] and may produce dramatic episodes of hypotension and respiratory depression.[19] (See Interactions of Narcotic Analgesics with other Medications, Part 2.)

2. *Antipsychotics/Central Nervous System Depressants (Sedatives, Hypnotics, Barbiturates).* In animal experiments,[88] as well as studies in humans,[89] antipsychotic drugs increase barbiturate and sedative-hypnotic sleep time and respiratory depression and decrease the narcosis threshold. For example, Dripps et al.[89] report that in the anesthetic management of 50 patients, chlorpromazine prolonged thiopental sleep time and subsequently reduced the thiopental requirement by 60 percent. Consequently, lower doses of barbiturates or sedative-hypnotics should be used when a patient is receiving antipsychotic medications.

3. *Antipsychotics/Sympathomimetic Drugs.* As discussed above, antipsychotic medications have central and peripheral antiadrenergic and antidopaminergic actions, and thus may interact with a variety of pressor agents. Antipsychotic agents may reduce or block the pressor effects of norepinephrine and other $\alpha$-adrenergic agonists. However, because antipsychotics may act at a variety of sites within the cardiovascular system, these effects may not always be predictable. For example, dogs pretreated with chlorpromazine have an enhanced pressor response to norepinephrine, an effect attributed to the depressant effect of chlorpromazine on baroreceptor reflexes.[90] Conversely, antipsychotics may reverse the pressor effects of agents with both $\alpha$- and $\beta$-agonist activities, by blocking the $\alpha$ effects, thereby leading to a predominance of $\beta$-adrenergic effects. For example, in animals the combination of chlorpromazine and epinephrine leads to significant hypotension,[90] while in man [91] the combination may cause vasodilation and severe hypotension. If paradoxic $\beta$-adrenergic activation occurs in individuals receiving antipsychotic drugs, fluid replacement and a $\beta$-adrenergic blocking agent, such as propranolol, are indicated. Similarly, intravenous dopamine is commonly used as a vasoactive agent in the management of shock, and, theoretically, dopamine pressor action could be decreased or blocked by the concurrent administration of neuroleptics.

4. *Antipsychotics/Anticholinergic Drugs.* Neuroleptics, particularly the aliphatic (chlorpromazine) and piperidine phenothiazines (thioridazine), possess inherent anticholinergic activity, and these effects may be additive with other anticholinergic drugs, such as antiparkinsonian or anticholinergic cardiac medications, such as atropine or scopolamine. The elderly are particularly sensitive to anticholinergic effects, and phenothiazines, either alone or in combination with other anticholinergic agents, may precipitate peripheral (adynamic ileus, glaucoma, and urinary retention) as well as central (confusion, fever, delirium, and agitation) anticholinergic toxicity.[92] Utilization of non-centrally-acting anticholinergic drugs, such as methscopolamine, may reduce the risk of central anticholinergic syndrome.[93] Should adverse anticholinergic symptoms develop, intravenous neostigmine may reduce or block peripheral anticholinergic symptoms, and physostigmine will act centrally as well as peripherally.

5. *Antipsychotics/Adrenolytic Agents.* Antipsychotic drugs intensify the effects of $\alpha$-adrenergic blocking agents, such as phentolamine, and may lead to the development of severe hypotension.

6. *Phenothiazines/Quinidine.* As discussed above, phenothiazines, particularly thioridazine, possess quinidine-like myocardial depressant effects. Concurrent use of phenothiazines and quinidine may lead to additive myocardial depression, and quinidine should be administered in reduced doses or when possible, avoided altogether.

7. *Phenothiazines/Antidysrythmia Agents (Propranolol, Diphenylhydantoin).* Phenothiazines decrease metabolism and thereby increase plasma levels of propranolol[94] and diphenylhydantoin.[95] Consequently, reduced doses may be indicated to prevent toxicity.

8. *Neuroleptics/Oral Anticoagulants.* Phenothiazines administered together with oral anticoagulants may produce an increased hypoprothrombinemic effect.[95] Conversely, haloperidol may lower the anticoagulant effect of oral anticoagulants through enzyme induction.[95]

9. *Phenothiazines/Thiazide Diuretics.* Combined use of phenothiazines and thiazide diuretics may result in severe hypotension.[96] In addition, diuretic-induced hypokalemia may enhance thioridazine-induced cardiac toxicity.[91]

10. *Phenothiazines/Digoxin.* Phenothiazines decrease gastric motility and may thereby increase the absorption of digoxin and other substances, potentially leading to toxicity.[95]

11. *Phenothiazines/Guanethidine.* Chlorpromazine (but not the antipsychotic agent molindone) may antagonize the antihypertensive action of guanethidine, probably by inhibiting its uptake.[91]

12. *Neuroleptics/Methyldopa.* Phenothiazines may potentiate the hypotensive effects of methyldopa.[98] Conversely, methyldopa may potentiate the effects of haloperidol, leading to toxicity.[91]

### Rauwolfia Alkaloids (Reserpine)

Prior to the introduction of chlorpromazine and other dopamine receptor-blocking antipsychotics in the early 1950s, reserpine was widely used as an effective antischizophrenic and antimanic agent.[99] However, with the development of chlorpromazine and related antipsychotic agents, which proved more efficacious and have fewer depressant, hypotensive, and cholinomimetic side effects, reserpine became clinically obsolete, although it continues to be used occasionally in internal medicine as an effective antihypertensive agent. More recently, the serious side effects of the newer antipsychotic agents (phenothiazines, butyrophenones, thioxanthines) have become clinically apparent. In particular, tardive dyskinesia, a syndrome of frequently irreversible choreoathetoid tongue, body, and extremity movements, is associated with long-term use of dopamine receptor-blocking antipsychotic agents. Since reserpine seldom if ever causes tardive dyskinesia, reserpine may regain its former popularity as an antipsychotic agent in psychiatry, particularly in chronically psychotic populations, who appear at greatest risk for the development of this seriously disfiguring and disabling syndrome. In addition, preliminary studies[100] suggest that in chronically ill psychotic patients resistant to the usual dopamine receptor-blocking antipsychotic agents, the addition of reserpine may result in greater therapeutic benefit than either agent used alone. Finally, some psychopharmacologic authorities have suggested that in patients who already are suffering from tardive dyskinesia, reserpine may help to ameliorate the syndrome, or prevent its progression. Consequently, it appears that reserpine may regain some of its former popularity in the psychopharmacologic management of seriously disturbed psychotic patients, and its pertinent pharmacology will be reviewed below.

As discussed for other psychotropic agents, reserpine's pharmacologic properties are complex, reflecting its actions at numerous levels and sites. Resperine's antipsychotic action is presumably mediated by its depletion of intraneuronally bound dopamine, via interference with catecholamine reuptake into synaptic vesicles, allowing its degradation by intraneuronal cytoplasmic monoamine oxidase. However, this effect is not specific for dopamine, and depletion of serotonin and other catecholamines such as norepinephrine appears responsible for the ability of reserpine to produce serious depression in some subjects. Goodwin et al.[101] report that up to 6 percent of patients receiving reserpine may develop serious depression, requiring hospitalization or electroconvulsive therapy, and as many as 58 percent of patients with a previous history of depressive episodes may develop clinically significant depression while receiving reserpine.[102] This depletion of central and peripheral stores of catecholamines also appears responsible for reserpine's numerous other side effects to be described below. It is not yet clear whether catecholamine depletion, per se, accounts for the state of parasympathetic predominance produced by reserpine (drowsiness, nightmares, excessive salivation, nasal congestion, increased gastric secretion, cutaneous vasodilation, nausea, and diarrhea), or whether, reserpine has additional intrinsic cholinomimetic properties.[46]

Reserpine produces the characteristic "neuroleptic syndrome" of indifference to environmental stimuli, ptosis, a tendency to sleep, but with easy arousability, unaccompanied by ataxia or disequilibrium.[46] As with other neuroleptics, extrapyramidal effects may occur with prolonged administration of high doses of reserpine,[46] although these reactions are much less frequent than with the dopamine receptor-blocking neuroleptics.

Large doses of reserpine may lower body temperature, result in central respiratory depression (decreased respiratory rate, depth, and minute volume) and ultimately lead to coma and death.[46]

As with other neuroleptics, reserpine may cause numerous disturbances in hypothalamic regulatory centers, inhibiting the ovarian cycle and menstruation and depressing fertility in women. In men, reserpine in large doses may cause feminization and impair sexual function.[46]

**Effects of Reserpine on the Cardiovascular System.** Reserpine causes numerous cardiovascular disturbances, including hypotension, both supine and orthostatic, bradycardia, a reduction or inhibition of pressor responses (i.e., carotid artery occlusion), and a reduction in cardiac output and systemic resistance.[103] Reserpine may also produce edema, and in susceptible individuals, it may precipitate frank heart failure.[46]

Reserpine acts both centrally and peripherally to competitively antagonize ATP-Mg$^{++}$ dependent uptake of catecholamines into synaptic vesicles, allowing their degradation by monamine oxidase.[103] This effect appears to be irreversible,[104] presumably accounting for reserpine's very long duration of action. Administered chronically in doses of less than 1 mg, reserpine has been demonstrated to severely reduce the norepinephrine content of the human myocardium.[105] This effect, along with reserpine's capacity to cause fluid retention, may account for its ability to aggravate congestive heart failure in patients with already compromised cardiac reserve.[106] Administered intraarterially, reserpine causes systemic vasodilation, as well as a reduction in cardiac output. These effects presumably account for the supine and orthostatic hypotension observed with the administration of this drug. With long-term therapy, however, cardiac output returns to pretreatment levels, but systemic resistance remains reduced.[107]

By preventing the reuptake of catecholamines into synaptic vesicles, reserpine may initially enhance the pressor effects of indirectly acting sympathomimetic amines; however, with long-term use, as the free catecholamines are degraded by monoamine oxidase and synaptic vesicles are consequently depleted, the response to indirectly acting sympathomimetics may be dramatically reduced.[107] Through similar mechanisms, a catecholamine receptor denervation hypersensitivity may develop with chronic administration of reserpine, and responses to direct acting $\alpha$-adrenergic agonists may be dramatically and dangerously enhanced.[106] Consequently, although direct-acting sympathomimetics are the drugs of choice in managing dangerous reserpine-induced hypotensive episodes, they should initially be given cautiously in reduced doses.

**Interactions of Reserpine with Cardiac Medications.**

1. *Reserpine/Digitalis Glycosides.* Although reserpine and digitalis glycosides are frequently used together with no apparent ill effects, cardiac arrhythmias (atrial tachycardia, ventricular bigeminy and tachycardia, and atrial fibrillation) as well as bradycardia and a decreased inotropic effect have been reported to result from their interaction.[108] Although the mechanism of this interaction is unknown, reserpine's release of catecholamines is suspected; consequently, large doses of reserpine should be avoided in digitalized patients.[108]

2. *Reserpine/Indirect Acting Sympathomimetics.* As discussed above, chronic treatment with reserpine may deplete synaptic vesicle catecholamine stores, and diminish pressor responses to indirect-acting sympathomimetics.[109] Consequently, indirect-acting pressor amines (e.g., metaraminol, ephedrine, amphetamine, tyramine, mephentermine, propadrine, and methylphenidate) should not be used to control serious reserpine-induced hypotensive episodes.

3. *Reserpine/Direct Acting Sympathomimetics.* As discussed above, chronic treatment with reserpine may result in a state of receptor denervation hypersensitivity, and the use of directly

acting sympathomimetics (dopamine, phenylephrine, norepinephrine, and epinephrine) may result in an enhanced and potentially dangerous pressor response,[106,109] Therefore, although directly acting pressor amines are preferred in the management of reserpine-induced hypotension, they should be used cautiously in reduced dosages.

4. *Reserpine/Narcotic Analgesics.* Reserpine's interactions with narcotic analgesics in man have not been well studied. In animals, such as rats and rabbits, reserpine appears to potentiate the effects of narcotic analgesics, whereas, in mice, depending on the test system employed, reserpine may either potentiate or antagonise morphine analgesia.[20,21] Until these interactions are better understood in humans, reserpinized subjects should initially receive reduced doses of narcotic analgesics.

5. *Reserpine/Thiazide Diuretics.* Reserpine may augment diuretic efficacy,[110] and reserpinized subjects may require reduced dosages of thiazide diuretics.

6. *Reserpine/Anticholinesterases.* In rats, reserpine pretreatment increases the lethality of sublethal doses of physostigmine and neostigmine, an effect prevented by the prior administration of anticholinergic agents.[111] Although these interactions have not yet been reported in humans, it would appear that anticholinesterases should be administered cautiously in reserpinized subjects.

7. *Reserpine/Barbiturates.* Animal studies have demonstrated that reserpine increased barbiturate sleeping time in small rodents,[88] and that it may increase sleeping time and sedation in man.[112] Although the administration of barbiturates to reserpinized subjects has resulted in hazardous reactions during anesthesia,[112] cardiovascular complications have not yet been reported.

8. *Reserpine–Monoamine Oxidase Inhibitors.* In patients receiving monoamine oxidase inhibitors, the addition of reserpine may result in psychomotor excitement and hypertension.[113] Therefore, reserpine should be avoided in patients receiving monoamine oxidase inhibitors. Conversely, in patients on long-term reserpine therapy, monoamine oxidase inhibitors would

have reduced therapeutic benefit secondary to a reduction in catecholamine stores, although this has not been studied in humans.

## ANTIDEPRESSANTS

### Tricyclic Antidepressants

The tricyclic antidepressants (imipramine, desimipramine, amitriptyline, nortriptyline, protriptyline, and doxepin) are used in the management of a variety of psychiatric disorders. Their efficacy in the treatment of severe depressions is well established, and they have also proved useful in the management of chronic pain, phobic anxiety, and a variety of psychosomatic disorders. No tricyclic antidepressant appears to be more efficacious than any other when they are administered in sufficient doses and adequate blood levels are achieved. Their widespread use (in 1972 they accounted for 14 percent of the leading 200 medications, about 20 million prescriptions a year[114]) along with the increased incidence of depression in the older age groups, makes their interface with cardiovascular disease very likely. Furthermore, they are being used more and more frequently by depressed patients as a means of suicide, and their severe cardiovascular toxicity in toxic amounts frequently requires continuous monitoring in the coronary care unit, as will be discussed below. Even when administered in therapeutic doses, they have significant cardiovascular effects, which are particularly dangerous in patients with preexisting cardiovascular pathology. Numerous potentially dangerous drug interactions have been documented, particularly with agents frequently used in cardiology. For these reasons, a coronary care unit practitioner must be particularly knowlegable about the pharmacology of the tricyclic antidepressants.

Tricyclic antidepressants block the reuptake of norepinephrine and/or serotonin (but not dopamine) in presynaptic nerve endings, thereby increasing central and peripheral adrenergic tone. Although this hypothesis is not yet proven, many investigators believe that this action may be responsible for the antidepressant activity of this class of drugs. Most tricyclic

antidepressants also possess significant anticholinergic effects, which may also play a role in alleviating depression. These anticholinergic and catecholamine uptake-blocking properties, mechanistically implicated in their antidepressant efficacy, also appear largely responsible for their autonomic side effects (blurred vision, dry mouth, urinary hesitancy or retention, constipation, tachycardia, orthostatic hypotension) as well as some direct cardiovascular toxicity and numerous drug interactions to be discussed.

**Effects of Tricyclic Antidepressants on the Cardiovascular System.** Therapeutic doses of the tricyclic antidepressants to apparently healthy patients free of cardiovascular disease have been implicated in almost every variety of cardiovascular disturbance. Reversible and apparently benign ECG changes (prolongation of the Q-T interval and flattening or inversion of the T wave) have been frequently reported.[115] Sinus and supraventricular tachycardia, atrial fibrillation,[116] and ventricular tachycardia[117] as well as bundle-branch block and other intraventricular conduction disturbances[118] also have been reported to occur with therapeutic doses of the tricyclic antidepressants in patients allegedly free of heart disease. These drugs have been demonstrated to depress cardiovascular reflexes (carotid occlusion reflex, the Bezold-Jarisch reflex, and a variety of postural responses),[46,119] which may have clinical significance in patients with preexisting cardiovascular disease. Finally, reports of chronic myocarditis[120] and subendocardial bundle branch and papillary muscle arteriolar and capillary lesions,[121] as well as myocardial infarction, congestive heart failure,[122] and sudden unexpected deaths[123] have all been associated with therapeutic doses of tricyclic antidepressants in apparently healthy individuals. Nevertheless, there is considerable controversy among investigators[124,125] as to whether therapeutic doses of the tricyclic antidepressants in patients without significant cardiovascular disease can really cause serious cardiovascular effects. Almost all of the above reports are retrospective and implicate the tricyclic antidepressants in an associational rather than a causal manner. To date, there have been few well-designed prospective clinical studies of the effects of these drugs on human cardiovascular pathophysiology.

*Animal Studies.* Several investigators [124] have established that therapeutic doses (2 to 4 mg/kg) of amitriptyline, administered intravenously to normotensive dogs, produces few if any ECG changes, although in higher doses (5 to 8 mg/kg), extrasystoles, widened QRS complexes, depression of S-T segments, and T wave flattening or inversion are common. In hypertensive dogs, therapeutic doses (2.5 mg/kg) produced marked ECG changes and incipient cardiac failure. These findings add credence to clinical reports that patients with hypertension or other cardiovascular diseases are much more susceptible to the cardiotoxic effects of tricyclic antidepressants.

In isolated animal heart preparations, a dose-dependent reduction in myocardial contractility and heart rate [126] as well as a significant reduction in cardiac output, at doses of 5 mg/kg (supratherapeutic),[119] has been demonstrated for the tricyclic antidepressants.

At higher doses (10 mg/kg) the tricyclic antidepressants have been shown to prolong both intraatrial and intraventricular conduction time, as well as to produce disturbances of ventricular repolarization.[127]

Paul et al.[128] summarize these findings, concluding that in animals the tricyclics appear to have two primary cardiotoxic actions: (1) a low-dose effect, which acts primarily on peripheral autonomic structures influencing heart rate, and (2) a high-dose effect, which acts directly on the myocardium.

*Clinical Studies.* As summarized above, a wide variety of cardiovascular disturbances have been associated with therapeutic doses of the tricyclic antidepressants in apparently healthy individuals. However, until recently, few well-controlled prospective studies have examined the effects of tricyclic antidepressants on cardiovascular pathophysiology. These more recent findings will be discussed.

Several well-controlled prospective studies of patients free of cardiovascular disease have demonstrated that therapeutic levels of nortriptyline frequently produce a significant increase in the PR interval of ECG tracings.[129] Likewise, in an elegant study employing 24-hour ECG

recordings [130] and high-speed, high-fidelity ECG recordings,[131] Bigger et al.[125] report that therapeutic blood levels of imipramine significantly increase mean heart rate as well as PR, QRS, and Q-T intervals. As discussed by Bigger et al.,[125] partial or complete AV block can result from anatomic lesions or drug effects in either the atrioventricular node or, more distally, in the bundle of His and upper bundle branches, and conduction defects in these different areas have different prognostic and therapeutic implications. Vohra et al.[132] recorded intracardiac electrograms [133] to determine the anatomic site of conduction disturbance resulting from tricyclic antidepressants (nortriptyline). They were able to discriminate the "A-H" interval (conduction time across the A-V node) from the "H-V" interval (the time from activation of the bundle of His to activation of ordinary ventricular muscle) of the standard PR interval. All patients with prolonged PR intervals (42 percent) had the conduction defect in the H-V interval with normal A-H conduction. Thus the ability of tricyclic antidepressants to prolong the PR, QRS, and QT intervals in the ECG, and the H-V interval in the His bundle electrogram resembles the cardiac effects of Type I cardiac antiarrhythmic drugs, quinidine, procainamide, and disopyramide.[125] Of importance was that all patients with prolonged conduction times, although they were receiving standard therapeutic doses of nortriptyline, had plasma nortriptyline levels outside the therapeutic window limits for nortriptyline efficacy. Thus, these individual variations in antidepressant drug metabolism further illustrate the clinical utility of monitoring plasma levels of tricyclic antidepressants, as reviewed elsewhere.[134,135]

In apparent agreement with the above-described animal studies,[119,126] the few existing human experiments [125,136] suggest that therapeutic doses of tricyclic antidepressants cause a slight, but significant, decrease in myocardial contractility.

Although therapeutic doses of tricyclic antidepressants have little or no effect on supine blood pressure, significant postural hypotension (both systolic and diastolic) occurs frequently,[125] and may be particularly severe in elderly patients and in those with preexisting cardiovascular pathology. Although clinical experience has demonstrated that the symptoms of postural hypotension usually abate with the continued administration of a tricyclic antidepressant, the actual orthostatic hypotension does not.[125] Thus, patients with cardiovascular pathology remain at risk for hypotensive episodes despite an apparent abatement of symptoms. The mechanism of tricyclic antidepressant-induced orthostatic hypotension has not yet been elucidated, and may involve the above-described depression of cardiovascular reflexes, reduction of myocardial contractility, or unknown central and/or peripheral adrenergic or cholinergic effects.

**Cardiovascular Effects of Toxic Doses of Tricyclic Antidepressants and Management of Overdoses.** Toxic concentrations of the tricyclic antidepressants may produce severe CNS and respiratory depression; neuromuscular dysfunction, including myoclonus and pseudoseizures; and cardiovascular disturbances, such as sinus tachycardia, atrioventricular and intraventricular conduction disturbances, ventricular arrhythmias, and collapse of supine blood pressure, presumably secondary to depressed myocardial contractility and peripheral arterial and venous vasodilation.[125]

The adrenergic and anticholinergic activity of tricyclics appear responsible for the sinus tachycardia that frequently accompanies tricyclic overdose, although sinus bradycardia has also been observed.[125] Tricyclic depression of the H-V interval or intraventricular conduction system, discussed above, may result in second-degree or third-degree AV block and bundle branch block, and secondarily in ventricular premature contractions, ventricular tachycardia, and ventricular fibrillation.[125] These disturbances in cardiac conduction, along with collapse of blood pressure, and severe CNS and respiratory depression frequently culminate in death without proper management in a coronary intensive care unit. Any serious tricyclic overdose *requires* admission and continuous cardiac monitoring for at least 48 hours. Forced diuresis and hemo- or peritoneal dialysis have proved ineffective in removing tricyclic antidepressants from the body [137] due to the high lipid solubility of these drugs and plasma protein binding. However, gastric lavage and nasogastric administration of activated charcoal is useful, if performed early enough before the drug is completely absorbed.

Respiratory depression is usually severe, and intubation and the use of a respirator are usually required.

As discussed by Bigger et al.,[125] atrioventricular conduction disturbances secondary to tricyclic antidepressant toxicity are distal to the AV node, so pharmacologic attempts to improve conduction through the AV node with atropine or catecholamines have proved fruitless. Therefore, if atrioventricular blockade is serious enough, the only viable option is to insert an artificial pacemaker in the right ventricle. In their experience, intraventricular conduction defects are usually not severe enough to require specific therapy. However, if severe intraventricular conduction disturbances occur and are felt to be contributing to the ventricular arrhythmias, Bigger et al. recommend molar sodium lactate as for quinidine toxicity.

Similarly, ventricular arrhythmias may be managed with sodium lactate, ventricular pacemaking, and electrical defibrillation; continuous electrocardiographic monitoring is therefore a requirement. They caution that Type I antiarrythmic drugs (quinidine, procainamide) are contraindicated, as their effects on the heart are similar to the tricyclics themselves, and further advise against the use of propranolol, as it may further depress myocardial contractility. They report that there has not been enough clinical experience with lidocaine in tricyclic-induced ventricular arrhythmias to support its routine use as with other types of ventricular arrhythmias. Nevertheless, both lidocaine and propranolol have been used safely and effectively.[137a] If a transvenous pacemaker is in place, overdrive pacing may be tried to treat ventricular arrhythmias. Overdrive pacing may also permit the use of antiarrhythmic agents such as lidocaine without fear of producing advanced A-V block.

As discussed above, circulatory collapse is common with overdoses of the tricyclic antidepressants, and Bigger et al.[125] recommend a pulmonary arterial catheter be inserted routinely and arterial blood gases, pulmonary arterial pressure, pulmonary artery wedge pressure, as well as cardiac output, monitored continuously. If the pulmonary artery wedge pressure is low, they recommend volume expansion. If the wedge pressure exceeds 18 mmHg in the presence of decreased cardiac output and peripheral resistance, they report success with a dopamine drip to increase cardiac contractility.

The anticholinergic properties of the tricyclic antidepressants in toxic doses may result in CNS depression and an atropine-like anticholinergic delirium, characterized by agitation, confusion, disorientation and pseudoseizures concurrent with hyperthermia, dry skin, tachycardia, dilated pupils, decreased bowel sounds, and urinary retention. These symptoms may be managed with the intramuscular or intravenous administration of physostigmine, 1 to 2 mg every 30 minutes as needed. As the half-life of the tricyclic antidepressants (24 to 48 hours) greatly exceeds that of physostigmine, the patient may need repeated doses and must be monitored frequently for recurrence of the above symptoms.

Bigger et al.[125] caution against the misdiagnosis of tricyclic-induced pseudoseizures (myoclonic jerks and chorioathetoid movements without concomitant EEG seizure activity) as true seizures, because diazepam or barbiturates, when used to treat pseudoseizures, may produce further CNS and respiratory depression. Pseudoseizures from tricyclic poisoning may be successfully diagnosed and managed with physostigmine, as described above.

Although some investigators [128,138] report that some tricyclic antidepressants (doxepin) or the new tetracyclic maprotiline may have less cardiotoxicity than others (protriptyline, imipramine, amitriptyline), these reports require further study and substantiation. The relative newness of these drugs and, possibly, their lower bioavailability may account for the lower incidence of cardiotoxicity reported with these agents.

In summary, tricyclic poisoning may result in serious CNS depression, including an anticholinergic syndrome and delirium, respiratory collapse, circulatory collapse, neuromuscular dysfunction, and cardiovascular disturbances, including atrioventricular and intraventricular conduction disturbances and serious ventricular arrhythmias. Inadequately managed, tricyclic poisoning is frequently fatal; significant overdoses always require admission to the coronary care unit for respiratory and circulatory monitoring and support, as well as for continuous ECG monitoring. Conduction disturbances and ventricular arrhythmias may require artificial ventricular pacemaking as well as other supportive management. Arrhythmias may occur up to 2 to 3 days after ingestion, and the patient should not be discharged or transferred to a psychiatric service prematurely. Doses of 1,000 mg are usually clinically serious and doses of 2,000 mg frequently fatal. However, in patients with idiosyncratic tricyclic metabolism, or in the elderly patients with preexisting cardiovascular pathology, much smaller doses (even therapeutic doses) have proved fatal.

**Antiarrhythmic Effects of Tricyclic Antidepressants.** Because many tricyclic antidepressants have quinidine-like effects on the cardiovascular system, Bigger et al.[125] and others have postulated that these drugs might be useful antiarrhythmic agents. They suggest that the long elimination half-life of the tricyclics would offer advantages in that fewer doses would be required and therefore compliance would be greater than with the more commonly used antiarrhythmic agents, which have much shorter half-lives. In fact, Bigger et al. report [125] several patients in whom preexisting ventricular premature contractions either disappeared or were reduced in frequency during the first week of imipramine therapy. The antiarrhythmic effect of the drug proved to be unrelated to patient improvement or recovery from depression, however; the arrhythmias recurred when, after the depression lifted, the tricyclics were discontinued. The doses employed were the same as those used for standard antidepressant therapy.

To date, the use of antidepressants as antiarrhythmics is experimental and clearly not recommended clinically. However, their systematic investigation in the treatment of arrhythmias is warranted.

**Interactions of the Tricyclic Antidepressants (TCA) with Cardiac Medications.**

1. *TCA/Digoxin.* Animal studies have demonstrated an increased lethality of digoxin in

rats pretreated acutely or chronically with large doses of TCAs.[139] However, interactions between these agents have not yet been reported in man.

2. *TCA/Direct Acting Sympathomimetic Amines (Norepinephrine, Epinephrine, and Phenylephrine).* The tricyclic antidepressants may increase, two- to tenfold, the pressor response of injected, direct-acting sympathomimetic amines, such as norepinephrine, epinephrine, and phenylephrine.[140-142] Hyperthermia, sweating, hypertensive crisis, severe headache, cerebrovascular accident, and death have been reported. In fact, this interaction has occurred clinically in dental patients on tricyclic antidepressants after they were given a local anesthetic containing norepinephrine as a vasoconstrictor.[142] The hypertensive crises presumably result from the amine reuptake blocking properties of the tricyclic antidepressants,[140] or, alternatively, it has been proposed that tricyclics may induce postsynaptic receptor hypersensitivity.[141] Should these hypertensive crises develop, they can be successfully managed with an $\alpha$-adrenergic blocking agent, such as phentolamine and/or with a vasodilator, such as sodium nitroprusside. If the patient is hyperpyrexic, cooling measures may be necessary.

The synthetic vasoconstrictor felypressin (2-phenylalanine, 8-lysine vasopressin) does not interact adversely with tricyclic antidepressants and might be employed if a direct-acting sympathomimetic amine is necessary. Unfortunately, felypressin is not yet available in the United States.

3. *TCA/Indirect Acting Sympathomimetic Amines: (tyramine, phenethylamine, ephedrine, metaraminol, amphetamine, methylphenidate).* Tricyclic antidepressants may *block or potentiate* the pressor effects of indirect-acting sympathomimetics, or those with both direct- and indirect-acting sympathomimetic properties. By blocking the uptake of indirect-acting sympathomimetics, TCAs may block their pharmacologic action.[95] However, if the indirect-acting sympathomimetics have already gained access to the presynaptic neuron, the tricyclic agent will potentiate and prolong their action by preventing the reuptake of released sympathomi-

metic. Furthermore, tricyclic antidepressants and the stimulant amphetamines and methylphenidate compete for the same liver metabolic enzymes, and may thereby further potentiate both their toxicities. Amphetamine abuse in patients on tricyclic antidepressant therapy may be fatal,[143] although evidence for this interaction is only circumstantial (associational).

4. *TCA/Phenothiazines.* The hypotensive and anticholinergic properties of these two groups of drugs may be additive. Furthermore, the phentothiazines can inhibit the metabolic inactivation of the tricyclics[91] which may be significant in mixed overdoses of both of these agents.

5. *TCA/Anticholinergics.* As the tricyclics have anticholinergic activity, they may potentiate both the central and peripheral effects of other anticholinergic agents,[91] and induce the central anticholinergic syndrome described above. This interaction is particularly likely in the elderly, and noncentrally acting anticholinergic agents should be employed when feasible.[93]

6. *TCA/Narcotic Analgesics.* In animal studies, tricyclic antidepressants potentiate morphine analgesia and increase meperidine-induced respiratory depression.[22] Clinical reports of these interactions are lacking; however, mixed overdoses of TCAs and narcotics may potentiate their relative toxicities, and lower doses of meperidine are probably initially indicated in patients receiving tricyclic antidepressants.

7. *TCA/Sedative Hypnotics (Barbiturates, Benzodiazepines, Meprobamate).* Tricyclic antidepressants potentiate the CNS and respiratory depressant effects of barbiturates and related sedative-hypnotics[91] and increased tricyclic antidepressant lethality occurs in the presence of a barbiturate, and vice-versa.

8. *TCA/Propranolol.* Tricyclic antidepressants may antagonize the cardiovascular effects of propranolol, a drug that has been used successfully to help manage the cardiotoxicity associated with tricyclic antidepressant drugs in man.[144] However, as noted above, propranolol may also further reduce the depressed myocardial contractility that occurs secondary to tricyclic toxicity.

9. *TCA/Oral Anticoagulants: (Bishydroxy-coumarin, Sodium Warfarin).* TCAs inhibit the metabolism of oral anticoagulants, increasing their serum levels and prolonging their half-life by as much as 300 percent.[145] This can cause excessive anticoagulation, so that prothrombin levels need to be checked periodically.

10. *TCA/Antihypertensive Agents (Guanethidine, Bethanidine, Debrisoquine, Clonidine).* The antihypertensive effects of these agents appear to depend, at least partially, on their uptake into the peripheral sympathetic nerve terminal via the amine pump, which is responsible for the reuptake of norepinephrine into the nerve terminal. TCAs act peripherally to block the reuptake of norepinephrine and the above antihypertensive agents, thereby diminishing significantly their antihypertensive efficacy.[146] Therefore blood pressure control may be lost when a TCA regimen is introduced to patients on long-term antihypertensive therapy. The rate at which the antagonism develops depends on the antihypertensive drug's duration of action, occurring within hours for bethanidine or desbrisoquine, but over several days for guanethidine. Conversely, in patients receiving TCA therapy, the efficacy of these antihypertensive agents in controlling hypertensive crises is diminished. Reserpine, $\alpha$-methyldopa, and propranolol do not appear to have significant peripheral interactions with TCAs. However, they may have central interactions, resulting in loss of blood pressure control or CNS toxicity. Furthermore, reserpine, $\alpha$-methyldopa, and propranolol have all been reported to cause significant depressive episodes, so that they would be poor choices in patients already receiving therapy for depression. Interactions between tricyclic antidepressants and diuretics are not significant per se, but their hypertensive effects may be additive. Therefore, few good choices remain although, with the proper precautions and monitoring, any of the above agents may be used. Diuretic therapy, plus propranolol or $\alpha$-methyldopa, if necessary, would probably be the best choices, although careful monitoring for hypotension or exacerberation of depression is indicated.

Alternatively, in patients who have been receiving TCA therapy and whose blood pressure has been stabilized on guanethidine, bethanidine, debrisoquine, or clonidine, the sudden withdrawal of TCA may result in serious hypotension, because the action of the antihypertensive agent is no longer antagonized.

## Monoamine Oxidase (MAO) Inhibitors

Before the tricyclic antidepressants were developed and marketed, the monoamine oxidase inhibitors were widely used as effective antidepressants. Although they have been largely replaced by the TCAs, they are still used in some areas of psychiatric practice. As medicolegal sanctions against electroconvulsive therapy increase, MAO inhibitors are regaining some of their former popularity, particularly in patients unresponsive to TCAs. In fact, one study [147] has demonstrated that patients unresponsive to TCAs are more likely to respond to MAO inhibitor therapy than to electroconvulsive therapy (ECT). Similarly, recent reviews have suggested that TCAs and MAO inhibitors may be safely combined in the therapeutic management of depressive illness refractory to tricyclic antidepressants.[148] Currently, in the United States, only two MAO inhibitors, tranylcypromine and phenelzine, are approved for the treatment of depression. Another, pargyline, is approved as an antihypertensive agent. However, many other MAO inhibitors are in use outside the United States and may offer advantages over those currently available. For example, it is now known that there are several forms of monoamine oxidase, including MAO-A and MAO-B. These different types of MAO exist in differing proportions throughout the body and have different substrate specificities. Clorgyline is felt to be a selective inhibitor of MAO-A,[149] whereas deprenil appears selective for MAO-B. The clinical relevance of these findings is apparent in that early reports [150] suggest that selective inhibition of MAO-B may have significant antidepressant efficacy without causing serious hypertensive crises in combination with ingested tyramine, a complication of other MAO inhibitors that has always made them difficult to use safely. This is a relatively recent area of investigation, and appears extremely complex, but it seems that MAO inhibitors may be gaining a new popularity in psychiatric practice.

**Mechanism of Action.** The MAO inhibitors are believed to relieve depressive symptoms by inhibiting monoamine oxidase, a major intraneuronal enzyme involved in the oxidative deamination of serotonin, norepinephrine, and dopamine. As discussed above, the catecholamine hypothesis postulates that depression results from a relative deficiency of catecholamines in certain areas of the CNS, and that MAO inhibitors are effective in relieving depression by allowing the repletion of monoamine stores in the brain.

Monoamine oxidase is widely distributed throughout the body, including the brain, liver, heart, and gastrointestinal tract. It may also inhibit other enzymes, particularly hepatic microsomal enzymes. These factors account for the complex and multitudinous drug interactions that occur with MAO inhibitors, and account for their inherent dangers.

**Effect of MAO Inhibitors on the Cardiovascular System.** Little is known about the effects of MAO inhibitors on the cardiovascular system, partially due to the paucity of studies and, in part, due to the complexity of the results from the existing literature. In isolated papillary cat muscle, some MAO inhibitors (iproniazid) were demonstrated to have a negative inotropic effect, whereas others (phenelzine) had a significant positive inotropic effect.[151] Tranylcypromine (and perhaps phenelzine) may also have an amphetamine-like effect independent of MAO inhibition. Hypertensive episodes, with headache and tachycardia, have occurred in patients at doses of tranylcypromine insufficient to significantly inhibit monoamine oxidase.[152] Adding further to the complexity are the unusually wide differences in amounts and specificities of MAO across animal species, and the opposite effects of MAO inhibitors on the cardiovascular system of different animal species.[153] It would appear that different MAO inhibitors have widely differing effects on the myocardium, and that at least some MAO inhibitors have a direct effect on the myocardium in addition to their effect on MAO.[128]

Several investigators [154] have reported that MAO inhibitors have a direct coronary vasodilator effect in the isolated animal heart preparation, but only in large doses, and this effect is slight. Others [155] were unable to correlate this effect with MAO inhibition. If clinical doses of MAO inhibitors have a significant effect on coronary circulation, it would appear to be slight, and incompletely understood.

The MAO inhibitors cause a variety of autonomic (anticholinergic) side effects, including orthostatic hypotension, dry mouth, blurred vision, constipation, urinary retention, and occasionally dizziness. MAO inhibitors produce hypotension by preventing the normal breakdown of tyramine by MAO, allowing its $\beta$-hydroxylation to form octopamine, which is stored intraneuronally replacing norepinephrine, thus acting as a "false transmitter" with very little pressor response.

**Therapeutic Uses of MAO Inhibitors in Cardiology.** Because of the potential for multitudinous severe cardiotoxic drug interactions to be described below, the MAO inhibitors have limited, if any, usefulness in routine cardiologic practice.

There have been numerous reports of the ability of MAO inhibitors to relieve angina pectoris.[156] However, many other studies have failed to demonstrate any superiority of MAO inhibitors over placebo in this regard.[157] If MAO inhibitors do have any antianginal effect, which is far from clear, the mechanism is unknown and has been postulated to vary among analgesic effects, CNS stimulation, ganglionic blockade, an oxygen-sparing effect, and coronary dilatation. At present, the usefulness of MAO inhibitors in the therapy of angina seems suspect at best.

There are numerous reports of the usefulness of MAO inhibitors in combination with tyramine in the treatment of severe cases of idiopathic (neurogenic) hypotension refractory to other pharmacologic management.[158] This treatment exploits the ability of MAO inhibitors to markedly potentiate the tyramine pressor response, which accounts for the dangerous hypertensive crises in normal populations. This would appear to be a legitimate, although limited, use of MAO inhibitors, requiring great caution and used only in otherwise refractory cases.

### Interactions of the Monoamine Oxidase Inhibitors with Cardiac Medications.

1. *MAO Inhibitors/Sympathomimetic Amines.* The ability of MAO inhibitors to interact with sympathomimetic agents to produce a dangerous and potentially lethal "hypertensive crisis" is their most widely known (and feared) drug interaction. Patients on MAO inhibitors who ingest large doses of tyramine in their diet, or who receive a sympathomimetic medication, may experience a "sympathetic storm" or hypertensive crisis characterized by precipitous hypertension, throbbing occipital headache, sweating, tachycardia, and hyperpyrexia, all of which may potentially lead to rupture of intracranial vessels and death.[29,159] Indirectly acting sympathomimetics are more likely to produce this reaction than direct acting sympathomimetics, because MAO inhibitors act primarily intraneuronally, and indirect-acting sympathomimetics produce their pressor effect through the release of intraneuronal monoamines. Thus, amphetamine, metamphetamine, methylphenidate, tyramine, mephentermine, metaraminol, ephedrine, and phenylpropanolamine, all of which release norepinephrine and dopamine from bound intraneuronal stores, are most likely to interact with MAO inhibitors to cause hypertensive crises.[141] Through a similar mechanism, the acute administration of reserpine to patients pretreated with an MAO inhibitor may lead to a hypertensive crisis, because reserpine depletes intracellular catecholamines by causing their release from bound stores.[160] Levodopa, a dopamine precursor, has been reported to interact with MAO inhibitors to produce a hypertensive crisis.[161] Interestingly, the MAO inhibitors have been reported to prolong and potentiate the pressor effects of dopamine, but not norepinephrine, on the contractile force of the heart.

Direct-acting sympathomimetics, such as norepinephrine and epinephrine, appear less likely to interact with MAO inhibitors to precipitate hypertensive crises.[141] Although anecdotal reports exist indicating that these agents have interacted with MAO inhibitors to produce hypertension,[162] controlled studies have demonstrated only mild hypertensive effects when these agents are used together.[141] This lack of a reaction reflects the fact that exogenous, directly acting sympathomimetic amines do not flood the intracellular site of the MAO inhibitors with monoamines (as do the indirect-acting sympathomimetics). Additionally, the direct-acting sympathomimetics may be degraded via an alternative route, the extracellular enzyme, catechol-o-methyltransferase. The hypertensive reactions that occur in subjects on MAO inhibitors receiving direct-acting sympathomimetics probably reflect a "denervation hypersensitivity" caused by the administration of the MAO inhibitor.

In summary, indirectly acting sympathomimetics are much more likely to precipitate a hypertensive crisis in patients receiving MAO inhibitors than direct-acting sympathomimetics, although both have occurred. If pressor amines are necessary in a patient receiving chronic MAO inhibitor therapy, low doses of directly acting amines, such as norepinephrine, are preferable to indirectly acting amines. Should a hypertensive crisis occur, an $\alpha$-adrenergic blocking agent, such as phentolamine, a vasodilator, such as nitroprusside, or both may be used.[141,159] Cooling may be necessary to alleviate hyperpyrexia. Cardiac arrhythmias, should they occur, may be managed with a $\beta$-blocker, such as propranolol. However, one must institute $\alpha$-blockade before administering $\beta$-adrenergic blocking agents, to prevent further hypertension from unopposed $\alpha$-adrenergic activity.

2. *MAO Inhibitors/Narcotic Analgesics.* MAO inhibitors have been noted to interact clinically with meperidine[24] or dextromethorphan[25] to produce a syndrome of agitation, restlessness, hypertension, headache, rigidity, convulsions, and hyperpyrexia (similar to the "hypertensive crises" discussed above). A similar reaction between MAO inhibitors and morphine, pentazocine, and phenazocine has been noted in animal studies,[27] but not clinically.[26] (See above for the presumed mecha-

nism, prevention, and management of these reactions.)

3. *MAO Inhibitors-Sedative/Hypnotics.* MAO inhibitors have been demonstrated to augment barbiturate and sedative-hypnotic effects in animals and in man.[163] The presumed mechanism by which this interaction occurs is MAO inhibition of liver microsomal enzymes involved in barbiturate detoxification. Experimentally, a combination of an MAO inhibitor and a barbiturate leads to an increased sleep time, increased duration of anesthesia, and an increased mortality rate in animals. Similar effects have been noted in man.[163] Consequently, in a patient pretreated with an MAO inhibitor, lower doses of barbiturates and sedative-hypnotics should be used.

4. *MAO Inhibitors/Guanethidine.* Guanethidine, when given to patients on MAO inhibitor therapy, has precipitated severe hypotensive as well as hypertensive reactions,[95,146] and this combination is contraindicated.

5. *MAO Inhibitors/α-Methyldopa.* The combination of MAO inhibitor and α-methyldopa can lead to CNS excitement and hypertension, in animals[164] and in man.[146]

6. *MAO Inhibitors/Propranolol.* Propranolol, given in association with MAO inhibitor has caused hypertensive crises, presumably by β-adrenergic receptor blockade, and resultant imbalanced activation of α-adrenergic receptors.[165]

7. *MAO Inhibitors/Thiazide Diuretics.* Hypotension, presumably additive, has been reported[166] with the combination of MAO inhibitors and thiazide diuretics.

8. *MAO Inhibitors/Anticholinergics.* MAO inhibitors have been reported to significantly increase the anticholinergic effects of atropine.[167]

9. *MAO Inhibitors/Oral Anticoagulants.* MAO inhibitors may have an intrinsic anticoagulant effect, and thereby may potentiate the effect of oral anticoagulants.[95]

10. *MAO Inhibitors/Hydralazine.* Hypotension, probably additive, has been observed when hydralazine was given in combination with MAO inhibitor therapy.[95] MAO inhibitors may inhibit the hepatic microsomes that metabolize hydralazine, and they may have an intrinsic vasodilating effect as well.[95]

11. *MAO Inhibitors/Digoxin.* Phenelzine has significantly potentiated digoxin toxicity in animals,[168] but this has not yet been reported in man. However, caution is urged.

12. *MAO Inhibitors/Droperidol.* One patient, receiving a large dose of droperidol, an anesthetic drug very similar to haloperidol, in combination with MAO inhibition therapy developed severe cardiovascular depression lasting 36 hours.[169] Similar reactions with other neuroleptics have been observed.[95]

13. *MAO Inhibitors/Chloral Hydrate.* MAO inhibitors may prolong and potentiate the CNS depressant effects of chloral hydrate[95] and this combination should be avoided.

## LITHIUM CARBONATE (LiCO₃)

In 1949 Cade[170] first reported the effectiveness of lithium in the treatment of mania, and the drug has been used for this indication since the early 1960s. Recent studies have demonstrated the usefulness of lithium in the prevention of recurrent depressions, both unipolar and bipolar types.[171] At the present time, lithium therapy has been advocated in greater than 30 other disorders, both psychiatric and nonpsychiatric, ranging from alcoholism and thyrotoxicosis to Huntington's chorea, ulcerative colitis, and granulocytopenia.[172]

Chemically, lithium is a monovalent cation, the lightest of the alkali metals and in the same group of elements in the periodic table as sodium and potassium. It generally occurs in nature as a salt (lithium carbonate, lithium chloride), rather than as a free element. The ion has no known physiologic role.[171] Approximately 95 percent of ingested lithium is excreted by the kidneys, complete excretion requiring 10 to 14 days in both acute and chronic therapy.

At the cellular level, lithium acts as an imperfect substitute for $Na^+$. It moves intracellularly during depolarization, but is extruded from the cell at a rate only 10 percent of that of $Na^+$. Lithium, therefore, accumulates within the cell, and may affect processes dependent on the movement of monovalent cations.[173] Many studies have dealt with the effects of lithium on amine metabolism in the brain. Lithium inhibits the release of norepinephrine and serotonin, increases the reuptake of norepinephrine, and possibly increases the synthesis and turnover rate of serotonin. There appears to be little effect on dopaminergic systems. Lithium also inhibits the activation of adenylate cyclase in the CNS of experimental animals. Furthermore, lithium may inhibit the synthesis and release of acetylcholine, and may alter the metabolism of amino acids thought to be synaptic neurotransmitters, including glutamate and γ-aminobutyric acid. It is not known at this time, which, if any of these actions are involved in its multiple therapeutic effects.[172,173]

Because the use of lithium is becoming increasingly widespread in psychiatry and medicine, and it has numerous actions throughout the body, the CCU practioner may expect to encounter an increasing number of patients on lithium therapy, as well as a variety of complex adverse cardiovascular toxicities and drug interactions.

## Effect of Lithium on the Cardiovascular System

At the cellular level, lithium may affect the heart in several ways. It may replace sodium during the generation of an action potential, but is extruded at only 10 percent of the rate of sodium, and may therefore accumulate in the cardiac muscle cell. By a similar mechanism, lithium may also replace potassium intracellularly. These changes in intracellular-extracellular electrolyte concentrations could theoretically affect myocardial contraction and repolarization, as well as cardiac conduction. Additionally, the above described effects of lithium on catecholamines could further influence cardiac performance.

Most investigators believe that therapeutic concentrations of lithium (0.8 to 1.5 mEq/l) in an individual free of cardiovascular pathology have only benign and reversible effects

on the cardiovascular system. Numerous investigators [174,175] have demonstrated that therapeutic levels of lithium in individuals free of cardiovascular pathology reliably produce T wave flattening or inversion (and occasionally U waves) in ECG tracings. These changes were, in all cases, benign and could be reversed by withdrawing lithium therapy. These changes may reflect the replacement of intracellular potassium by lithium. However, they occur in the presence of normal serum potassium levels and independently of high or low sodium intake.[174] Similarly, in an elegant prospective study, Tilkian et al.[175] report that therapeutic levels of lithium did not adversely affect cardiac functioning in 10 patients undergoing ECG monitoring during treadmill testing.

Despite the apparent safety of therapeutic levels of lithium on the cardiovascular system in controlled prospective trials, a number of case reports have associated lithium therapy with reversible interference of sinus node [176] and atrioventricular conduction.[177] Similarly, in the prospective study of Tilkian et al.,[175] lithium was found to decrease the frequency of preexisting premature atrial contractions. It may decrease the frequency of paroxysmal supraventricular tachyarrhythmias, and ventricular arrhythmias may occur or be aggravated. Tangedahl and Gau [178] reported premature ventricular contractions in a 46-year-old patient with a normal exercise tolerance test and no known history of cardiovascular pathology. These abnormalities occured at therapeutic lithium levels and disappeared when the drug was withdrawn.

Lithium has been reported to cause edema and to precipitate or aggravate congestive heart failure, which effects disappeared when the dose was reduced or therapy was withdrawn.[179] Additionally, there have been several reports of diffuse myocarditis and death in several individuals undergoing lithium therapy with apparently normal serum lithium levels.[180] Therapeutic levels of lithium carbonate do not appear to alter blood pressure.

In summary, therapeutic levels of lithium consistently cause benign and reversible T wave changes in the ECGs of individuals without cardiovascular pathology. Rare case reports, however, have associated supraventricular arrhythmias and ventricular premature contractions with lithium therapy, so it cannot be presumed to be completely benign. Therefore, baseline and serial ECGs are indicated when lithium therapy is given to individuals with suspected or overt cardiovascular pathology.

### The Effect of Toxic Levels of Lithium on the Cardiovascular System

Moderately toxic levels of lithium (4.5 to 8.2 mEq/1) have caused ST depression [181] and QT prolongation, [182] reversing as the drug was excreted and levels fell to therapeutic concentrations. Higher levels have been associated with arrhythmias, circulatory failure, coma, and death.[173]

**Diagnosis and Management of Lithium Toxicity.** Lithium toxicity or poisoning, generally seen at serum levels exceeding 1.5 to 2.0 mEq/l, although at much lower levels in some individuals, has an enormous range and variety of clinical manifestations, reflecting its complex effects throughout the body. A lithium toxicity checklist developed by Shopsin and Gershon [173] includes: (1) gastrointestinal symptoms—anorexia, nausea, vomiting, diarrhea, constipation, dryness of mouth, and metallic taste; (2) neuromuscular symptoms and signs—general muscle weakness, ataxia, tremor, muscle hyperirritability (fasciculations, twitching, and clonic movements of whole limbs), choreoathetoid movements, and hyperactive deep tendon reflexes; (3) central nervous system—anesthesia of the skin, incontinence of urine and feces, slurred speech, blurring of vision, dizziness, vertigo, epileptiform seizures, and EEG changes; (4) mental symptoms—difficulty concentrating, slowing of thought, confusion, somnolence, restlessness-disturbed behavior, stupor and coma; (5) cardiovascular system—arrhythmias, fall in blood pressure, ECG changes, peripheral circulatory failure, and circulatory collapse; and (6) miscellaneous—polyuria, polydipsia, glycosuria, general fatigue, lethargy and drowsiness, dehydration, skin rash, weight loss or gain, alopecia, and angioneurotic edema.

There is no specific antidote for lithium poisoning, and treatment is supportive while attempts are made to eliminate the drug from the system. Severe cases require admission to the intensive care unit, and either continuous or serial ECG monitoring. Obviously, the drug should be discontinued at once, and studies [173] have demonstrated that serum lithium levels may drop 50 percent every 1 to 2 days after lithium therapy is discontinued. As discussed by Gershon and Shopsin,[173] supportive therapy is basically that used in barbiturate poisoning and includes lavage to eliminate significant amounts of lithium left in the stomach, correction of fluid and electrolyte blance, and regulation of kidney function, as well as routine ECG monitoring, blood pressure and respiration support, and infection prophylaxis.

Additionally, osmotic diuresis, alkalinization of the urine, administration of aminophylline, urea, mannitol and institution of hemodialysis, alone or in combination, have all proved useful in increasing the excretion of lithium.[173] Patients recovering from lithium poisoning rarely suffer permanent sequelae, even in severe cases.

**Interaction of Lithium with Cardiovascular Medications**

1. *Lithium-Thiazide Diuretics (Sodium).* Administration of thiazide diuretics or restriction of sodium may precipitate lithium toxicity in individuals with previously therapeutic levels of lithium. Sodium depletion increases the retention of lithium ion at the proximal tubule of the kidney, and a low sodium diet or a thiazide diuretic, may thereby induce lithium poisoning.[183] Diuretics that deplete both sodium and potassium, such as thiazides, ethacrynic acid, and furosemide, appear to be more hazardous in this regard than do those with a potassium-sparing effect, such as spironolactone and triamterene.[184] On the other hand, osmotic diuretics, such as mannitol, may increase the excretion of lithium.

2. *Lithium-Sedative-Hypnotics.* Supratherapeutic levels of lithium (2.2 to 3.4 mEq/l) have been reported to markedly potentiate sedative-hypnotics (barbiturate, benzodiazepine) sleep time, both in animals [185] and in man.[186] However, therapeutic levels of lithium (0.8 to 1.5 mEq/l) do not appear to have this effect.

3. *Lithium-Hydroxyzine.* Hydroxyzine may potentiate lithium's effects on cardiac repolarization [187] and precipitate cardiovascular toxicity.

4. *Lithium-Methyldopa.* Hypertension as well as lithium toxicity has been reported with the concomitant use of these two drugs.[188]

## SEDATIVE-HYPNOTICS, MINOR TRANQUILIZERS

The sedative-hypnotics and minor tranquilizers comprise a wide variety of chemically unrelated group of drugs that include the barbiturates, benzodiazepines, meprobamate, methaqualone, glutethimide, methyprylon, chloral hydrate, methapyririline, and scopolamine. These medications regularly induce sedation and sleep in small doses, and may induce anesthesia in larger doses. They have applications in the psychopharmacologic management of anxiety states, minor depressive illnesses, and a variety of psychosomatic disorders. In addition, they have widespread indications throughout medical practice in the management of numerous nonpsychiatric disorders, particularly in cardiology in the treatment of acute myocardial infarction, essential hypertension, and a variety of arrhythmias. Indeed, the benzodiazepines alone constitute by far the most widely prescribed drugs in medical practice.[189] In addition, they probably constitue the most widely abused medications in our society today, and habituation and even addiction are becoming increasingly frequent problems.

Although the sedative-hypnotics and minor tranquilizers have been widely used in general medicine for decades, the mechanism by which they exert their antianxiety and sedative effects has yet to be understood. They affect virtually every organ system at every level throughout the body by their actions on membrane permeability, enzymatic activity, and a variety of neurotransmitters throughout the peripheral and central nervous systems. Although a number of hypotheses exist to explain their numerous effects, none appears to have much validity or been able to withstand new experimental findings.

## Effects of Hypnotics, Sedatives, and Minor Tranquilizers on the Cardiovascular System

The benzodiazepines appear to have different therapeutic indications and a much greater margin of safety than do the barbiturates and other sedative-hypnotics. The barbiturates may be considered the prototype of most minor tranquilizers and sedative-hypnotics, with the exception of the benzodiazepines. Despite early enthustiac reports, many other sedative-hypnotics, such as glutethimide (Doriden), methyprylon, and methaqualone (Quaalude) have similar CNS, respiratory, and cardiovascular toxicities as do the barbiturates, but differences, when present, will be noted.

The barbiturates and other sedative-hypnotics, when used at therapeutic doses as antianxiety agents or hypnotics, have little or no demonstrable effect on cardiovascular function.[128,190] When given intravenously in larger doses as anesthetics, however, there may be a slight fall in mean arterial blood pressure, although in many patients blood pressure may be unchanged or even increased.[42,190] Barbiturates depress the medullary vasomotor center, but have little or no effect on baroreceptors and autonomic regulatory mechanisms.[42,190] A pronounced hypotensive response may be observed in previously hypertensive patients, or in those with congestive heart failure or in hypovolemic shock.[190]

Generally, however, intravenous anesthetic doses of barbiturates decrease cardiac output, and secondarily increase total peripheral resistance and heart rate,[190] although in healthy patients this is rarely of clinical significance.

In contrast, toxic doses of barbiturates and other sedative-hypnotics (except benzodiazepines) regularly produce severe and dangerous CNS, respiratory, and cardiovascular depression.[42,190] Hypotension and negative chronotropism are the rule, and are often fatal unless quickly and agressively treated.

## Management of Acute Barbiturate Poisoning

Severe poisoning may occur at approximately 10 times the hypnotic dose, unless alcohol or other depressant drugs are also present, in which case the lethal dose may be considerably lower. Short-acting barbiturates are generally more toxic than the longer-acting barbiturates, and fatal blood levels of 1 mg/100 ml and 6 mg/100 ml, respectively, have been recorded.[190]

Moderate intoxication resembles alcoholic inebriation, and in severe intoxication the patient may be comatose with flaccidity, loss of reflexes, and positive Babinski signs.[190] Respiratory depression is the rule, and is frequently severe; hypoxia and respiratory acidosis often develop. Pupils are initially miotic and reactive, but hypoxia may result in paralytic mydriasis.[190] Severe hypotension may ensue secondary to depression of medullary vasomotor centers, and to a direct depressant effect of barbiturates on the myocardium, sympathetic ganglia, and vascular smooth muscle, compounded by hypoxia.[190] Consequently, a shock-like syndrome may develop with a weak and rapid pulse, severe hypotension, and hypothermia; respiratory complications and renal failure may develop.[190]

Barbiturate poisoning is extremely dangerous, and even when handled appropriately by experienced personnel a 2 to 5 percent mortality rate may be expected.[190]

As with lithium poisoning, there is no specific antidote for barbiturate or other sedative-hypnotic poisoning; treatment is generally supportive, while attempts are made to eliminate the drug from the system.

If the patient is still conscious, emesis by apomorphine or syrup of ipecac, may eliminate any unabsorbed drug. Similarly, the oral administration of activated charcoal may be useful. In a comatose patient, gastric lavage may be attempted, although this must be done carefully to prevent the patient from aspirating the lavage fluid.

Attention must be immediately focused on support of vital functions, such as maintenance of respiration, body temperature, circulation, and renal function, as well as electrolyte and acid-base balance.

Respiratory support may vary from the insertion of an oropharyngeal airway or endotracheal tube, to tracheotomy or an artificial respirator, depending on the patient's state of consciousness and respiratory status. Supple-

mental oxygen should be administered, and there should be careful attention to pulmonary toilet to prevent atelectasis or pneumonia. Daily chest radiographs and broncoscopy may be necessary.

Hypotension and shock may be managed by supplemental blood or other parenteral fluids, along with careful monitoring of hematocrit, electrolytes, and acid-base balance. Even with supplemental fluids, vasopressor agents (norepinephrine or dopamine) and digitalis may be necessary to support the circulation and maintain renal perfusion.

Renal function must be monitored frequently. If renal function is adequate, alkalinization of the urine and forced diuresis may be used to hasten excretion, particularly of the longer-acting barbiturates. If renal failure occurs, hemodialysis may significantly hasten (10 to 45 times) the elimination of longer-acting barbiturates. A lipid containing dialysate may improve the removal of shorter-acting barbiturates.[190]

The above method of managing barbiturate poisoning,[190] evolved from the "Scandinavian Method" of Clemmensen and Nilsson[191] and has reduced mortality from upwards of 40 percent in some centers to around the 2 to 5 percent seen today.

Despite early enthustiac reports about their relative safety, most other sedative hypnotics (except the benzodiazepines) have proved to have CNS, respiratory, and cardiovascular depressant effects that are almost as severe as the barbiturates, and poisoning from glutethimide (Doriden),[42] methyprylon,[190] and metaqualone (Quaalude)[42] appears clinically similar (both in presentation and prognosis) to that of the barbiturates.

## Effects of the Benzodiazepines on the Cardiovascular System

The benzodiazepines have proved much safer and clinically more useful than other sedative-hypnotics. Numerous clinical studies have demonstrated that the benzodiazepines (diazepam, chlordiazepoxide, flurazepam, nitrazepam, oxazepam, and so on), probably alone among currently available sedative hypnotics, have little or no cardiovascular toxicity. Large doses of benzodiazepines, including major overdoses, have essentially no clinically significant cardiotoxic effects in normal subjects,[192] and the same holds true for subjects with a variety of significant cardiovascular pathologies.[193] Similarly, although the benzodiazepines have significant CNS and respiratory depressant effects, they occur less frequently, and are much less severe than those of the barbiturates and other sedative hypnotics.[192] Intravenous doses of diazepam (15 mg or 0.2 mg/kg) and equivalent doses of other benzodiazepines have been shown to produce no clinically significant respiratory depression[192] in normal subjects, in contrast to equivalent doses of other sedative-hypnotics. However, there are several case reports of respiratory failure precipitated by benzodiazepines in subjects with chronic obstructive pulmonary disease with $CO_2$ retention.[192] Therefore these patients must be carefully monitored for this interaction. Nevertheless, the benzodiazepines are still much safer sedative-hypnotics in these patients than equivalent doses of barbiturates or narcotics.[192]

Two cases of ectopic ventricular activity associated with the use of diazepam in cardioversion have been reported,[194] although most authorities doubt the causal association of diazepam in these cases.[192] In contrast, the benzodiazepines have proved useful in the management of a variety of otherwise refractory arrhythmias.

**Therapeutic Uses of the Benzodiazepines in Cardiology.** Due to their greater safety as well as their greater therapeutic efficacy, the benzodiazepines have largely replaced the barbiturates and other sedative-hypnotics in clinical cardiology.

**Cardioversion, Angiography and Cardiac Catheterization.** As reviewed by Greenblatt and Shader[192] numerous investigators have demonstrated the safety and efficacy of diazepam as a sedative-hypnotic prior to direct current cardioversion.[195] Diazepam has proved as effective as thiopental in this regard, and appears to be associated with a decreased frequency of ventricular extrasystoles compared with thiopental.[196]

As described by Greenblatt and Shader,[192] in elective cardioversion digitalis is withheld

for at least 24 hours and replaced by quinidine sulfate, 200 mg orally, every 6 hours. Diazepam is then administered intravenously at a rate of 5 mg/min until dysarthria occurs. The usual effective dose is 10 to 20 mg, and cardioversion may then be performed with the patient in a light sleep and amnesic for the event. Recovery is within minutes to a few hours.

Diazepam has been demonstrated to be equally safe and effective in coronary angiography and cardiac catheterization.[192]

**Management of Refractory Arrhythmias.** There are several case reports in the literature attesting to the usefulness of benzodiazepines in the management of otherwise refractory atrial[197] and ventricular[197] arrhythmias. Diazepam has been reported to have an intrinsic antiarrhythmic effect, as well as an ability to potentiate the antiarrhythmic effects of lidocaine.[198] Nevertheless, these agents are not routinely employed as primary antiarrhythmic therapy. Also, the benzodiazepines have been reported to be ineffective against digitalis-induced arrhythmias.[197]

**Sedative, Antianxiety Effects in Acute Myocardial Infarction.** Several investigators have reported the usefulness of benzodiazepines (diazepam, 15 mg orally three times daily; chlordiazepoxide, 10 mg as needed, up to 100 mg/day for relieving stress and pain), citing analgesic requirements and cardiovascular complications in the early management of acute myocardial infarction.[199,200] The benzodiazepines proved superior to equivalent doses of barbiturates in double-blind comparisons.[199] One study[200] reports a greatly reduced excretion of catecholamines with diazepam during early phases of acute myocardial infarction, suggesting that diazepam lowered the stress reaction. Free fatty acid and cortisol levels were not significantly changed with diazepam.

**Ischemic Heart Disease.** Animal[201] and human[202] studies have demonstrated diazepam-induced coronary artery vasodilation and an increase in coronary blood flow, while other human studies have shown that intravenous diazepam may produce direct arterial vasodilation,[203] thereby improving cardiac function. Both direct local systemic vasodilatory effects and central gamminoergic mechanisms appear to be involved.[203] The clinical utility, if any, of these observations await further study.

**Benzodiazepines in the Management of Essential Hypertension.** Benzodiazepines have been repeatedly shown to be entirely ineffective in the management of essential hypertension,[204] although they continue to be widely used by physicians for this purpose.[205] One study demonstrated that patients in a hypertension clinic with psychologic complaints were much more likely to be prescribed benzodiazepines than patients without such complaints. However, contrary to prevailing evidence, these patients appeared to benefit by the benzodiazepines with a significant reduction in blood pressure (6.7 mmHg diastolic), leaving this issue unresolved.[205] In general, it appears that the benzodiazepines are no more effective than a placebo in reducing hypertension.[204]

### Interactions of the Minor Tranquilizers, and Sedative-Hypnotics with Cardiovascular Medications

1. *Enzyme Induction or Inhibition:* The barbiturates, and to a lesser extent, other sedative-hypnotics and minor tranquilizers, are notorious for their ability, with chronic use, to stimulate the production and activity of the hepatic microsomal enzymes involved in the metabolic degradation of a great number of medications.[95,190] Consequently, the therapeutic efficacy of any medication metabolized by hepatic microsomal enzymes may be reduced with the long-term administration of barbiturates or other sedative-hypnotics. This may have particular clinical relevance with cardiac medications such as oral anticoagulants or diphenylhydantoin, requiring a readjustment of dosage.

Conversely, the acute administration of barbiturates or other sedative-hypnotics may potentiate the therapeutic activity or precipitate the toxicity of virtually any agent metabolized by the hepatic microsomes, as the barbiturates or other sedative-hypnotics will compete stoichiometrically for the enzymatic degradation of that agent.

2. *Chloral Hydrate.* Chloral hydrate is metabolized to trichloracetic acid, which may in turn displace acidic proteins from serum pro-

teins, thereby reducing their half-life and increasing their free blood level. Conversely, although chloral hydrate, itself, does not appear to be metabolized by the hepatic microsomal enzymes, nevertheless, it may induce the accelerated metabolism of a large number of drugs (including dicumarol and warfarin) and may dangerously lower their therapeutic efficacy.[190]

3. *Interaction of Minor Tranquilizers or Sedative-Hypnotics with other CNS Depressants.* As noted above, the minor tranquilizers and sedative-hypnotics may dangerously (fatally) potentiate the toxicity of virtually any other CNS depressant (particularly other minor tranquilizers and sedative-hypnotics, as well as alcohol and narcotics) and significantly reduced doses of these agents are initially indicated. Benzodiazepines are least potent in this regard.

4. *Chloral Hydrate-i.v. Furosemide.* These two agents should not be used concurrently, as they have precipitated agitation, diaphoresis, and hypertension when given together.[206]

## CONCLUSIONS

The psychotropic medications have significant cardiovascular toxicities, and these drugs may also interact adversely with a variety of cardiac and noncardiac medications. This is particularly likely given the increasingly widespread use of psychotropic medications throughout general medical practice today. These interactions are of particular concern to the CCU practiner, who is dealing with patients generally in the older age groups (and thus more susceptible to psychotropic drug toxicities) and who are already in serious cardiovascular distress. Pertinent psychotropic drug cardiotoxicities and drug interactions have been reviewed, as well as potential therapeutic applications of the psychotropic medications in coronary care practice.

## REFERENCES

1. Perry HJ, Bolter MD, Mellinger GD, Cisin IU, Manheimer DJ: National patterns of psychotherapeutic drug use. Arch Gen Psychiatry 28:729–783, 1973.

2. Jaffe JH, Martin WR: Narcotic analgesics and antagonists. In: The Pharmacological Basis of Therapeutics. 5th ed. Goodman LS, Gilman A, editors. MacMillan, New York 1975, pp 245–283.

3. Vandam LD; Drug therapy: analgetic drugs— the potent analgetics. N Engl J Med 286:249–253, 1972.

4. Kerr F, Donald KW: Editorial. Analgesia in myocardial infarction. Br Heart J 36:117–121, 1974.

5. Jewitt PE, Maurer BJ, Hubner PJ: Increased pulmonary arterial pressures after pentazocine in myocardial infarction. Br Med J 1:795–796, 1970.

6. Lees GM, Kosterlitz HW, Waterfield AA: Characteristics of morphine-sensitive release of neurotransmitter substances. In: Agonist and Antagonist Actions of Narcotic Analgesic Drugs. Kesterlitz HW, Collier HOJ, Villarreal JE, editors. University Park Press, Baltimore, 1973, pp 142–152.

7. Cicero TJ: Effects of alpha-adrenergic blocking agents on narcotic-induced analgesia. Arch Int Pharmacodyn Ther 208:5–13, 1974.

8. Florez S, Delgado G, Armigc SA: Adrenergic and serotonergic mechanisms in morphine-induced respiratory depression. Psychopharmacologia 24:258–274, 1972.

9. Kaverina NV: Pharmacology of the Coronary Circulation. Pergamon Press, New York, 1965, pp 118–152.

10. Lowenstein E, Hollowell P, Levine FH, Daggett WM, Austen WG, Laver MB: Cardiovascular response to large doses of intravenous morphine in men. N Engl J Med 281:1389–1393, 1969.

11. Thomas M, Malmerona R, Fillmore S, Shillingford J: Haemodynamic effects of morphine in patients with acute myocardial infarction. Br Heart J 27:863–875, 1965.

12. Stanley TH, Gray NH, Stanford W, Armstrong R: The effects of high dose morphine on fluid and blood requirements in open-heart operations. Anesthesiology 38(6):536–541, 1973.

13. Maurer B, Murneghan D, Hickey N, Mulcahy R: Pentazocine in the relief of acute cardiac pain. Acta Cardiol (Brux) 25:153–164, 1970.

14. Nagle RE, Pilcher J: Respiratory and circulatory effects of pentazocine—review of analgesics used after myocardial infarction. Br Heart J 34:244–251, 1972.

14a. Zelis R, Mansour EJ, Capone RJ, Mason DT: The cardiovascular effects of morphine. The peripheral capacitance and resistance vessels in human subjects. J Clin Invest 54:1247–1258, 1974.

14b. Vismara LA, Leaman DM, Zelis R: The effects of morphine on venous tone in patients with acute pulmonary edema. Circulation 54:335–337, 1976.

14c. Ryan WF, Henning H, Karliner JS: Effects of morphine on left ventricular dimensions and function in patients with previous myocardial infarction. Clin Cardiol 2:417–423, 1979.

15. Alderman EL, Barry WH, Graham AF, Harrison DC: Hemodynamic effects of morphine and pentazocine differ in cardiac patients. N Engl J Med 287:623–627, 1972.

16. Beaver WT, Wallenstein SL, Heude RW, Rogers A: A comparison of the analgesic effects of pentazocine and morphine in patients with cancer. Clin Pharmacol Ther 7:740–751, 1966.

17. Keets AS, Telford J, Kurosu Y: Potentiation of meperidine by promethazine. Anesthesiology 22:34–41, 1961.

18. Lambertson CJ, Wendel H, Longenhager JB: The separate and combined respiratory effects of chlorpromazine and meperidine in normal men controlled at 46 mmHg alveolar $pCO_2$. J Pharmacol Exp Ther 131:381–393, 1961.

19. Dundee JW, Nichell RM, Moore J: Clinical studies of induction agents. x: the effects of phenothiazine premedication on thiopentone anesthesia. Br J Anaesth 36:106–109, 1964.

20. Matilla MJ, Soarnivaara L: Potentiation with indomethacin of the morphine analgesia in mice and rabbits. Ann Med Exp Fenn 45:360–362, 1977.

21. Tabojnikova M, Kovalcik V: On the mechanism of the inhibiting effect of reserpine on morphine. Activ Nerv Sup 9:317–319, 1967.

22. Griffin JP, O'Arcy PF: A manual of adverse drug interactions. John Wright and Sons, Bristol, 1975.

23. Torneth FJ: Controlled comparison of amitriptyline and meperidine as preanesthetic treatment. Anesth Analg 50:761–768, 1971.

24. Shee JC: Dangerous potentiation of pethidine by iproniazid and its treatment. Br Med J 2:507–509, 1960.

25. Rivers N, Horner B: Possible lethal reaction between nardil and dextromethorphan. Can Med Assoc J 103:85, 1970.

26. Jounela AJ: Influence of monamine oxidase inhibitors on the cardiovascular action of some analgesics. Ann Med Exp Biol Fenn 48:249–260, 1970.

27. Rogers KJ, Thornton JA: Interaction between monoamine oxidase inhibitors and narcotic analgesics in mice. Br J Pharmacol 36:470–480, 1969.

28. Vigran IM: Dangerous potentiation of meperidine hydorchloride by pargyline hydrochloride. JAMA 187:954, 1964.

29. Editorial: Analgesics and monoamine oxidase inhibitors. Br Med J 4:284, 1967.

30. Churchill-Davidson HC: Anaesthesia and monoamine oxidase inhibitors. Br Med J 1:520, 1965.

31. Evans-Prosser CD: The use of pethioline and morphine in the presence of monoamine oxidase inhibitors. Br J Anaesth 40:279–282, 1968.

32. Dundee JW, Haslett WH, Keilty SR, Pandit SK: Studies of drugs given before anaesthesia. xx diazepam-containing mixtures. Br J Anaesth 42:143–150, 1970.

33. Bernhein F, Bernhein MLC: The hydrolysis of demerol by liver in vitro. Anesthesiology 22:34, 1945.

34. Murmann W, Almirante L, Sarcani-Guelfi M: Effects of hexobarbitone, ether, morphine and urethene upon the acute toxicity of propranolol and D-(—)-INPEA. J Pharm Pharmacol 18:692–694, 1966.

35. Slogoff S, Keats AS, Hibbs CW, Edmonds CH, Bragg DA: Failure of general anaesthesia to potentiate propranolol activity. Anesthesiology 47:504–508, 1977.

36. Dressler WE, D'Alonzo G, Rossi GV, Orzechowsky RF: Modification of certain vascular responses to dopamine by morphine. Eur J Pharmacol 28:108–113, 1974.

37. Stimmel B, Donoso E, Hack S: A comparison of infective endocarditis in drug addicts and nondrug users. Am J Cardiol 32:924–929, 1973.

38. Hopkins GB: Pulmonary angiothrombotic granulomatosis in drug offenders. JAMA 221:909–912, 1972.

39. Rumbongh CL, Bergeron RT, Fang H, et al: Cerebral angiographic changes in the drug abuse patient. Radiology 101:335–344, 1971.

40. Lipski J, Stimmel B, Donoso E: The effect of heroin and multiple drug abuse on the electrocardiogram. Am Heart J 86:663–668, 1973.

41. Duberstein JL, Kaufman DM: A clinical study of an epidemic of heroin intoxication—heroin induced pulmonary edema. Am J Med 51:704, 1971.

42. Stimmel B: The effects of mood-altering drugs on the heart. In: Drugs in Cardiology, Part I. Donoso, E, editor. Stretton Intercontinental

43. Medical Book Corporation, New York, 1975, pp 203–234.

43. Weller M, Perry RH: Unusual cardiac and neurological reaction to narcotics (Letter). Lancet 2:799–801, 1973.

44. Gold MS, Redmond DE, Kleber HD: Noradrenergic hyperactivity in opiate withdrawal supported by clonidine reversal of opiate withdrawal. Am J Psychiatry 136:1, 100–103, 1979.

45. Snyder SH: The dopamine hypothesis of schizophrenia. Am J Psychiatry 133:197–202, 1976.

46. Byck R: Drugs and the treatment of psychiatric disorders. In: The Pharmacological Basis of Therapeutics. 5th ed. Goodwin LS, Gilman A, editors. MacMillan, New York, 1975, pp 152–200.

47. Alexander CS: Cardiotoxic effects of phenothiazines and related drugs. Circulation 38:1014–1015, 1968.

48. Richardson HL, Graupner KI, Richardson ME: Intramyocardial lesions in patients dying suddenly and unexpectedly. JAMA 195:254–260, 1966.

49. Landmark K: Changes in rat atrial action potentials induced by promazine and thioridazane. Acta Pharmacol Toxicol 30:465–479, 1971.

50. Langer GA: Ion fluxes in cardiac excitation and contractions and their relation to myocardial contractility. Physiol Rev 48:708–757, 1968.

51. Huston JR, Bell GE: The effect of thioridazine hydrochloride and chlorpromazine on the electrocardiogram. JAMA 198:16–20, 1966.

52. Axelrod J, Hertting GL, Potter L: Effect of drugs on the uptake and release of $H^3$-norepinephrine in the rat heart. Nature 194:297, 1962.

53. Ban TA, St Jean A: The effect of phenothiazines on the electrocardiogram. Can Med Assoc J 91:537–540, 1964.

54. Backman H, Elosuo R: Electrocardiographic findings in connection with clinical trial of chlorpromazine with particular reference to T-wave changes and the duration of ventricular activity. Ann Mod Intern Fenn 53:1–8, 1964.

55. Kelly GH, Fay JE, Laverty SG: Thioridazine hydrochloride (Mellaril): Its effects on the electrocardiogram and a report of two fatalities with electrocardiographic abnormalities. Can Med Assoc J 89:546, 1963.

56. Alexander CS, Shadir R, Grinspoon L: Electrocardiographic effects of thioridazine hydrochloride. Circulation (suppl III) 34:43, 1966.

57. Landmark K, Glomstein A, Qye I: The effect

of thioridazine and promazine on the isolated contracting rat heart. Acta Pharmacol Toxicol 27:173–182, 1969.

58. Goldstein BJ, Clyde OJ, Caldwell JM: Clinical efficacy of the butyrophenones as antipsychotic agents. In: Psychopharmacology, A Review of Progress. Efron, DH editor. Public Health Service Publication No. 1836, U.S. Government Printing Office Washington, D.C., 1968, pp 1085–1091.

59. Richardson ML, Graupner KD, Richardson ME: Intramyocardial lesions in patients dying suddenly and unexpectedly. JAMA 195:254–260, 1966.

60. Brill M, Patton RE: Clinical-statistical analysis of population changes in New York State mental hospitals since the introduction of psychotropic drugs. Am J Psychiatry 119:20–33, 1962.

61. Leestma SE, Koenig KL: Sudden death and phenothiazine. Arch Gen Psychiatry 18:137–148, 1968.

62. Aherwedker SJ, Efendigil MC, Coulshed N: Chlorpromazine therapy and associated acute disturbances of cardiac rhythm. Br Heart J 36:1251–1252, 1964.

63. Giles TO, Modlin RV: Death associated with ventricular arrhythmia and thioridazine hydrochloride. JAMA 205:108–110, 1968.

64. Korol B, Lang WJ, Brown ML, Gershon S: Effects of chronic chlorpromazine administration on systemic arterial pressure in schizophrenic patients: relationship of body position to blood pressure. Clin Pharmacol Ther 6:587–591, 1965.

65. Bourgeois-Govardin M, Nowill WK, Margolis G, Stephen CR: Chlorpromazine: a laboratory and clinical investigation. Anesthesiology 16:829–847, 1955.

66. National Institute of Mental Health, Psychopharmacology Service Center for Collaborative Study Group: Phenothiazine treatment in acute schizophrenia. Arch Gen Psychiatry 10:246–261, 1964.

67. Bishop MP, Mason LB, Gallant DM: Blood pressure abnormalities in schizophrenic patients. Curr Ther Res 10:315–322, 1968.

68. Crimson C: Chlorpromazine and imipramine: Parallel studies in animals. Psychopharmacol Bull 4:9–15, 1967.

69. Dosgupta SR, Werner G: Inhibition of hypothalamic, medullary and reflex vasomotor responses by chlorpromazine. Br J Pharmacol 9:389–39, 1954.

70. Carlson C, Dencker SJ, Grimby G, Haggendal J: Circulatory studies during exercise in mentally disordered patients. I. Effects of large doses of chlorpromazine. Acta Med Scand 184:499–509, 1968.

71. Carlsson C, Dencker SJ, Grimby G, Haggendal J, Johnson G: Effects on hemodynamics and plasma noradrenaline levels in man on long term treatment with imipramine, haloperidol and chlorpromazine. Eur J Clin Pharmacol 3:163, 1971.

72. Hollister LE, Kosek JC: Sudden death during treatment with phenothiazine derivatives. JAMA 192:1035–1038, 1965.

73. Courveisier S, Fournel J, Ducrot R, Kolsky M, Koetschet P: Pharmacodynamic properties of 3-chloro-10-(3-demethyliminiopropyl) phenothiazine Hll (RP 4560). Arch Int Pharmacodyn 92:305–361, 1953.

74. Lund-Johansen P: Shock after administration of phenothiazines in patients with pheochromocytoma. Acta Med Scand 172:525, 1962.

75. Melville KI: Observations on the adrenergic blocking and anti-fibrillatory actions of chlorpromazine. Fed Proc 13:386–387, 1954.

76. Witzleb E, Budde H: Zur wirkung von phenothiazin-derivaten anf die dynamik und energetik des wurmbluter-herzens. Arch Intern Pharmacodyn 104:33–41, 1955.

77. Maxwell GM, Rowe GG, Castillo C, Schuster B, White DH, Crumpton CW: Hemodynamic effect of chlorpromazine including studies of cardiac work and coronary blood flow. Anesthesiology 1964–71, 1958.

78. Lal HB and Bahl AL: Treatment of myocardial infarction with phenothiazine derivatives. J Assoc Physicians Index 15:69–72, 1967.

79. Elkayam U, Rotmensch HH, Terdiman R, Geller E, Laniado S: Hemodynamic effects of chlorpromazine in patients with acute myocardial infaction and pump failure. Chest 72:623–627, 1977.

80. Pratt IT: Twilight sleep after infarction. Br Med J 3:475–476, 1971.

81.. Riss E, Hemli S, Abinader E: Neuroleptanalgesia in the treatment of acute myocardial infarction. Isr J Med Sci 5:747–749, 1969.

82. Gulotta SJ: Chlorpromazine in the treatment of cardiogenic shock. Am Heart J 80:570–573, 1970.

83. Murphy GP, Benson DW, Schirmer KA: Renal response to chlorpromazine in hemorrhagic hypotension: hemodynamic and metabolic changes and adrenolytic effects in dogs. Ann Surg 164:867–876, 1966.

84. Kovach G: The effect of droperidol in hypertensive crises. Ther Hung 25:126–128, 1977.

85. Singh KP, Sharma VN: 10-N substituted phenothiazine derivatives in auricular arrhythmias. Arch Int Pharmacodyn Ther 177:168–178, 1969.

86. Singh KP, Sharma VN: Chemical constitution and drug action of N-substituted phenothiazine in ventricular ectopic tachycardia. Jap J Pharmacol 20:173–178, 1970.

87. Canero R, Wilder R: A mechanism of sudden death in chlorpromazine therapy. Am J Psychiatry 127:368–371, 1970.

88. Richards AB, Forney RB, Hughes FW: Enhancement of the depressant action of hexobarbitol by tranquilizers in mice. Life Sci 4:1019–1024, 1965.

89. Dripps RD, Vandam LD, Pierce EC, Oesh SR, Lurie AA: The use of chlorpromazine in anesthesia and surgery. Ann Surg 142:775–785, 1955.

90. Eggers GN, Corssen G, Allen C: Comparison of vasopressor responses in the presence of phenothiazine derivatives. Anesthesiology 20:261–267, 1959.

91. Thornton WE, Pray BJ: Combination drug therapy in psychopharmacology. J Clin Pharmacol 15:511–517, 1975.

92. El-Yousef MK, Janowsky DS, Davis JM, Sekerke HJ: Reversal of antiparkinsonian drug toxicity by physostigmine: a controlled study. Am J Psychiatry 130:141–145, 1973.

93. Janowsky DS, Janowsky EC: Methscopolamine as a pre-anesthetic medication. (Letter to the Editor) Can Anaesth Soc J 23:334–335, 1976.

94. Vestal RE, Kornhauser DM, Hollified JW, Shand DG: Inhibition of propranolol metabolism by chlorpromazine. Clin Pharmacol Ther 25:19–24, 1979.

95. Gaultieri CT, Powell SF: Psychoactive drug interactions. J Clin Psychiatry 39:720–729, 1978.

96. Cluff LE, Petrie JC: Clinical effects of interactions between drugs. American Elsevier, New York, 1974.

97. Janowsky DS, El-Yousef MK, Davis MJ, Fann WE: Antagonism of guanethidine by chlorpromazine. Am J Psychiatry 130:808–812, 1973.

98. Chouinard G, Pinard G, Prenoveau Y, Tetreault L: Alpha methyldopa-chlorpromazine interaction in schizophrenic patients. Curr Ther Res 15:60–72, 1973.

99. Barsa JA, Klint NS: Treatment of two hundred disturbed psychotics with resperine. JAMA 158:110–113, 1955.

100. Bacher NM, Lewis HA: Addition of reserpine to antipsychotic medication in refractory chronic schizophrenic outpatients. Am J Psychiatry 135:488–489, 1978.

101. Goodwin FK, Ebert MH, Bunney WE Jr: Mental effects of reserpine in man: a review. In: Psychiatric Complications of Medical Drugs. Shader RI, editor. Raven Press, New York, 1972, pp 25–47.

102. Quetsch RM, Achor RWP, Litin EM, et al: Depressive reactions in hypertensive patients. A comprehensive study of those treated with rauwolfia and those receiving no specific antihypertensive treatment. Circulation 19:366–375, 1959.

103. Nickerson M and Collier B: Drugs inhibiting adrenergic nerves and structures innovated by them. In: The Pharmacological Basis of Therapeutics (5th edition), Goodman CS, Gilman A, editors. MacMillan, New York, 1975, pp 557–559.

104. Haggendal D, Dahlstrom A: The recovery of the capacity for uptake-retention of $^3$H-noradrenaline in rat adrenergic nerves after reserpine. J Pharm Pharmacol 24:565–574, 1972.

105. Chidsey CA, Braunwald E, Morrow AG, Mason DT: Myocardial norepinephrine concentration in man—effects of reserpine and of congestive heart failure. N Engl J Med 269:653–658, 1963.

106. Braunwald E, Chidsey CA, Harrison DC, Gaffney TE, Kahler RL: Studies on the function of the adrenergic nerve endings in the heart. Circulation 28:958–969, 1963.

107. Reusch CS: The cardiorenal hemodynamic effects of antihypertensive therapy with reserpine. Am Heart J 64:643–649, 1962.

108. Hansten PD: Drug Interactions. 3rd ed. Philadelphia, Lea and Febiger, 1976.

109. Gelder MG, Vane JR: Interaction of the effects of tryamine, amphetamine and reserpine in man. Psychopharmacology 3:231–241, 1962.

110. Cohen MS: Therapeutic drug interactions. Drug Information Center, University of Wisconsin Medical Center, Madison, Wisconsin, pp 199–200, 1970.

111. Janowsky DS, Pechnick R, Janowsky EC: Lethal effects of reserpine plus physostigmine and neostigmine in mice. Clin Exp Pharmacol Physiol 3:483–486, 1976.

112. Ominsky AJ, Wollman H: Hazards of general anesthesia in the reserpinized patient. Anesthesiology 30:443–446, 1969.

113. Goldberg, CI: Monoamine oxidase inhibitors—adverse reactions and possible mechanisms. JAMA 190:456, 1964.

114. Blackwell B: Psychotropics in use today. JAMA 225:1637–1641, 1973.

115. Seraf KR, Klein DF, Gittleman-Klein R, Groff S: Imipramine side effects in children. Psychopharmacology 37:265–274, 1974.

116. Moorehead CN, Knox SJ: Imipramine-induced auricular fibrillation. Am J Psychiatry 122:216–217, 1965.

117. Scollins MJ, Robinson DS, Nies A: Cardiotoxicity of amitriptyline. Lancet 2:1202, 1972.

118. Kantor SJ, Bigger JT Jr, Glassman AH, Macken DL, Perel JM: Imipramine-induced heart block. A longitudinal case study. JAMA 231:1364–1366, 1975.

119. Sigg EB, Osborne M, Korol B: Cardiovascular effects of imipramine. J Pharmacol Exp Ther 141:237–243, 1963.

120. Gwynne JF: Tricyclic antidepressants and heart disease. NZ Med J 74:414–415, 1971.

121. Richardson HL, Graupner KI, Richardson ME: Intramyocardial lesions in patients dying suddenly and unexpectedly. JAMA 195:254–260, 1966.

122. Kristiansen ES: Cardiac complications during treatment with imipramine (tofranil). Acta Psychiatr Neurol Scand 36:427–442, 1961.

123. Moir DC: Tricyclic antidepressants and cardiac diseases. Am Heart J 86:841–842, 1973.

124. Cairneross KD, Gershon S: A pharmacological basis for the cardiovascular complications of imipramine medication. Med J Aust 2:372–375, 1962.

125. Bigger JT Jr, Kantor SJ, Glassman AH, Perel JM: Cardiovascular effects of tricyclic antidepressant drugs. In: Psychopharmacology: A Generation of Progress. Lipton MA, DiMassio A, Killan KF, editors. Raven Press, New York, 1978, pp 1033–1046.

126. Greeff K, Wagner J: Cardiodepressive und dokal-anaesthetisike wirkirngen der thynoleptica. Arzneim-Forsch 19:1662–1664, 1969.

127. Baum T, Shropshire AT, Rouls G, Goukman M: Antidepressants in cardiac conduction; iprindole and imipramine. Eur J Pharmacol 13:289–291, 1971.

128. Paul SM, Gallant D, Mielke DH: Cardiotoxicity: clinical implications. In: Psychotherapeutic Drugs—Part I. Usdin E, Forrest I, editors. New York, 1976.

129. Burrows GD, Vohra J, Dumovic P, et al: Proceedings of the 10th congress collegium internationale neuropsychopharma-coloqium. Pergamon Press, London, 1977.

130. Florenz MK, Rolnitzky LM, Bigger JT Jr: Computers in Cardiology Conference. EEE Computer Society, Long Beach, Calif., 1974, pp 145–150.

131. Heissenbuttel RH, Bigger JT Jr: The effect of oral quinidine on intraventricular conduction in man: Correlation of plasma quinidine with changes in QRS duration. Am Heart J 80:453–462, 1970.

132. Vohra J, Burrows GD, Hunt D, Sloman G: The effect of toxic and therapeutic doses of tricyclic antidepressant drugs on intracardiac conduction. Eur J Cardiol 3:219–227, 1975.

133. Scherlag BJ, Lau SH, Helfent RH, Berkowitz WD, Stein E, Domato AN: Catheter technique for recording His bundle activity in man. Circulation 39:13–18, 1969.

134. Risch SC, Huey LY, Janowsky DS: Plasma levels of tricyclic antidepressants and clinical efficacy: review of the literature—part I. J Clin Psychiatry 40:4–16, 1979.

135. Risch SC, Huey LY, Janowsky DS: Plasma levels of tricyclic antidepressants and clinical efficacy: review of the literature—part II. J Clin Psychiatry 40:58–69, 1979.

136. Muller V, Burckhardt D: Die wirkung tri-und tetrazyklischer antidepressiva auf herz und kreislauf. Schwei Med Wochenschr 104:1911–1913, 1974.

137. Hall R: Tricyclic antidepressant tranquilizers. Bull U.S. Department of Health, Education and Welfare, May–June, 1970.

137a. Hollister LE: Tricyclic antidepressants. N Engl J Med 299:1168–1172, 1978.

138. Weinberger DR: Tricyclic choice for ill elderly patients (Letter). Am J Psychiatry 134:1048–1049, 1977.

139. Attree T, Sawyer P, Turnbull MJ: Interaction between digoxin and tricyclic antidepressants in the rat. Eur J Pharmacol 19(2):294–296, 1972.

140. Svedmyr N: The influence of a tricyclic antidepressive agent (protriptyline) on some of the circulatory effects of noradrenaline and adrenaline in man. Life Sci 7:77–84, 1968.

141. Boakes AJ, Laurence DR, Teoh PC, Barar FSK, Benadikter LT: Interactions between sympathomimetic amines and antidepressant agents. Br Med J 1:311–315, 1973.

142. Verrill PJ: Adverse reactions to local anaesthetics and vasoconstrictor drugs. Practitioner 218:380–387, 1975.

143. Raisfeld IH: Cardiovascular complications of antidepressant therapy. Am Heart J 83:129, 1972.

144. Vohro J: Cardiovascular abnormalities following tricyclic antidepressant drug overdosage. Drugs 7:323–325 1974.

145. Vesell ES, Passananti T, Greene FE: Impairment of drug metabolism in man by allopurinol and nortriptyline. N Engl J Med 283:1484–1488, 1970.

146. Cocco G, Ague C: Interactions between cardioactive drugs and antidepressants. Eur J Clin Pharmacol 11:389–393, 1977.

147. Hamilton M: Drug resistant depressives: Response to ect. Pharmakopsychiat/Neuro-Psychopharmakol 7:205–206, 1974.

148. Schuckit M, Robbins E, Feighner J: Tricyclic antidepressants and monamine oxidase inhibitors. Arch Gen Psychiatry 24:509, 1971.

149. Johnston JP: Some observations upon a new inhibitor of monoamine oxidase in brain tissue. Biochem Pharmacol 17:1285–1297, 1968.

150. Varga E, Tringer L: Clinical trial of a new type promptly acting psychoenergetic agent (phenyl-isopropyl-methyl-propenyl-HCl, "e-250"). Acta Med Acad Sci Hung 23:289–295, 1967.

151. Lee WC, Shin YH, Shideman FE: Cardiac activities of several monamine oxidase inhibitors. J Pharmacol Exp Ther 133:180–185, 1961.

152. Cooper AJ, Magnus RV, Rose MJ: Hypertensive syndrome with tranylcypromine medication. Lancet 1:527–534, 1964.

153. Goldberg ND, Shideman FE: Species differences in the cardiac effects of monoamine oxidase inhibitor. J Pharmacol Exp Ther 136:142, 1962.

154. Chavlier R: Coronary Vasodilators. Pergamon Press, New York, 1961.

155. Zbinden G: Theoretic background of therapy with monoamine oxidase inhibitors in cardiology. Am J Cardiol 6:1121–1124, 1960.

156. Östör E: Effect of noredal on angina pectoris. Ther Hung 16:121–122, 1968.

157. Fisch S: Antianginal drugs: V. monamine oxidase (MAO) inhibitors. Am Heart J 71:837–838, 1966.

158. Davies B, Bannister R, Sever P: Pressor amines and monoamine oxidase inhibitors for treatment of postural hypotension in autonomic failure. Limitations and hazards. Lancet 1:172–175, 1978.

159. Raskin A: Adverse reactions to phenelzine. Results of a nine hospital depression study. J Clin Pharmacol 12:22–25, 1972.

160. Davies TS: Monoamine oxidase inhibitors and ranwolfia compounds. Br Med J 2:739, 1960.

161. Teyehenne PF, Caine DB, Lewis PJ, Findley LJ: Interactions of levodopa with oxidase and 1-aromatic amine acid decarboxylase. Clin Pharmacol Ther 18:273–278, 1975.

162. Horwitz D, Goldberg LI, Sjoerdsma A: Increased blood pressure responses to dopamine and norepinephrine produced by monoamine oxidase inhibitors in man. J Lab Clin Med 56:747–753, 1960.

163. Domino E, Sullivan TS, Luby ED: Barbiturate intoxication in a patient treated with a MAO inhibitor. Am J Psychiatry 118:941–943, 1962.

164. Van Rossum JM: Potential danger of monoamine oxidase inhibitors and α-methyldopa. Lancet 1:950, 1963.

165. Frieden J: Propranolol as an anti-arrhythmic agent. Am Heart J 75:283–285, 1967.

166. Moser M: Experience with isocarboxazid. JAMA 176:276, 1961.

167. Sjoquist F: Psychotropic drugs (2): interaction between monoamine oxidase (MAOI) inhibitors and other substances. Proc R Soc Med 58:967–978, 1965.

168. Bohrman JS, Thompson EB: Cardiovascular effects of digoxin-phenelzine interactions in rabbits. J Pharm Sci 62(11):1876–1878, 1973.

169. Penlinglon GN: Droperidol and monoamine oxidase inhibitors. Br Med J 1:483–484, 1966.

170. Cade JFJ: Lithium salts in the treatment of psychotic excitement. Med J Aust 10:349–352, 1949.

171. Davis JM, Janowsky DS, El-Yousef-MK: The use of lithium in clinical psychiatry. Psychiatr Ann 3:78–89, 1973.

172. Greist JH, Jefferson JW, Combs AM, Schou M and Thomas A: The lithium librarian. Arch Gen Psychiatry 34:456–459, 1977.

173. Gerson S, Shopsin B: Lithium, Its Role in Psychiatric Research and Treatment. Plenum Press, New York-London, 1976.

174. Demers RG, Heninger GR: Electrocardiographic T-wave changes during lithium carbonate treatment. JAMA 218:381, 1971.

175. Tilkian AG, Schroeder JS, Kao J: Effect of lithium on cardiovascular performance: report on extended ambulatory monitoring and exercise testing before and during lithium therapy. Am J Cardiol 38:701–708, 1976.

176. Wilson JR, Kraus ES, Bailes MM, et al: Reversible sinus node abnormalities due to lithium carbonate therapy. N Engl J Med 294:1223–1224, 1976.

177. Jaffe CM: First-degree atrioventricular block during lithium carbonate treatment. Am J Psychiatry 134:88–89, 1977.

178. Tangedahl TN, Gan GT: Myocardial irritability associated with lithium carbonate therapy. N Engl J Med 287:867–868, 1972.

179. Stancer HC, Kivi R: Lithium carbonate and oedema. Lancet 2:985, 1971.

180. Swedberg K, Winblad B: Heart failure as a complication of lithium treatment. Acta Med Scand 196:279–280, 1974.

181. Verbov JL, Phillips JD, Fife DG: A case of lithium intoxication. Postgrad Med 41:190, 1965.

182. Horowitz LC, Fisher GN: Acute lithium intoxication. N Engl J Med 281:1369, 1969.

183. Macfie AL: Lithium poisoning precipitated by diuretics. Br Med J 1:516, 1975.

184. Ascione FJ: Lithium with diuretics. Drug Ther 7:53–54, 1977.

185. Mannisto PT, Saarnivaara L: Effect of lithium and rubiduim on the sleeping time caused by various intravenous anaesthetics in the mouse. Br J Anaesth 48:185–189, 1976.

186. Jephcott G, Keny RJ: Lithium, an anesthetic risk. Br J Anaesth 46:389–390, 1974.

187. Hollister LE: Hydroxyzine hydrochloride, possible adverse cardiac interactions Psychopharmacol Commun 1:61–65, 1975.

188. Byrd GJ: Methyldopa and lithium carbonate: suspected interaction (Letter). JAMA 233:320, 1975.

189. Blackwell B: Psychotropic drugs in use today: The role of diazepam in medical practice. JAMA 225:1637, 1973.

190. Harvey SC: Hypnotics and sedatives. In: The Pharmacological Basis of Therapeutics. Goodman LS, Gilman A, editors. MacMillan, New York, 1975, pp 102–136.

191. Clemmesen C, Nilsson E: Therapeutic trends in the treatment of barbiturate poisoning. Clin Pharmacol Ther 2:220–229, 1961.

192. Greenblatt DJ, Shader RI: Benzodiazepines in Clinical Practice. Raven Press, New York, 1974.

193. Rao S, Sherbaniuk RW, Prasad K, Lee SVK, Spronte BJ: Cardiopulmonary effects of diazepam. Clin Pharmacol Ther 14:182–189, 1973.

194. Barrett JS, Hey EB: Ventricular arrhythmias associated with the use of diazepam for cardioversion. JAMA 214:1323–1324, 1970.

195. Somers V, Gunstone RF, Patel AK, D'Arbela PG: Intravenous diazepam for direct current cardioversion. Br Med J 4:13–15, 1971.

196. Muenster JJ, Rosenberg MS, Carleton RA, Graettinger JJ: Comparison between diazepam and sodium thiopental during DC countershock. JAMA 199:758–760, 1967.

197. Spracklen FHN, Chambers RJ, Schrire V: Value of diazepam ("Valium") in treatment of cardiac arrhythmias. Br Heart J 32:827–832, 1970.

198. Dunbar RW, Boettner RB, Haley JV, Hall VE, Morrow DH: The effect of diazepam on the antiarrhythmic response to lidocaine. Anesth Analg 50:685–692, 1971.

199. Benson WH: Comparative evaluation of diazepam (Valium) and phenobarbital for the relief of anxiety-related symptoms in patients hospitalized for acute myocardial infarction. J Med Assoc Ga 60:276–278, 1971.

200. Melson M, Andreassen P, Nelson H, Hansen T, Grendahl H, Hilleskid LK: Diazepam in acute myocardial infarction—clinical effects on catecholamines, free fatty acids and cortisol. Br Heart J 38:804–810, 1976.

201. Abel RM, Reis RL, Staroscik RN: The pharmacological basis of coronary and systemic vasodilator actions of diazepam (Valium). Br J Pharmacol 39:261–274, 1970.

202. Ikram H, Rubin AP, Jewkes RF: Effect of diazepam on myocardial blood flow of patients with and without coronary artery disease. Br Heart J 35:626–630, 1973.

203. Bolme P, Fuxe K: Possible involvement of GABA mechanisms in central cardiovascular and respiratory control. Studies on the interaction between diazepam, picrotoxin and clonidine. Med Biol 55:301–309, 1977.

204. Medical Letter: Diazepam (Valium) in hypertension. Med Lett Drug Ther 16:96, 1974.

205. Whitehead WE, Blackwell B, Robinson A: Why psysicians prescribe benzodiazepines in essential hypertension: a phase IV study. Biol Psychiatry 12:597–601, 1977.

206. Malach M, Berman V: Furosemide and chloral hydrate. Adverse drug reaction. JAMA 232:638–639, 1975.

# 34 | Psychiatric Problems in Patients with Acute Myocardial Infarction

## Ned H. Cassem, M.D.

Newspaper headlines recently acclaimed a 55-year-old man who had had chest pain for about one year. A stress test given by his cardiologist was found to be markedly abnormal. Angiography revealed obstruction in three coronary arteries—greater than 95 percent in two and about 75 percent in the other. Coronary bypass surgery was recommended. The patient refused. Instead, he decided to diet, lost 37 pounds, and began an exercise program. Subsequently, he ran in a number of marathons—first the Honolulu marathon and later, in 90-plus degree heat, the Boston marathon. So, concluded the newspaper item: "Man defies Doctors and Medical Science." What few know is that, during the Honolulu marathon, this man developed chest pain that persisted for 6 hours. Even so, on the very next day he began training for a subsequent marathon. When he returned to his cardiologist for a follow-up examination, the ECG revealed that he had sustained a myocardial infarction. Undaunted by the news, he continues to train for future marathons. What if *no* follow-up ECG had been taken? What if he had stopped running in Honolulu and had it taken then? In the first case, you might say that medical science had been defied, and, in the second case, vindicated. Yet there seems to remain some truth in both. At the very least, this case illustrated that psychological reactions to heart disease can be more astonishing and dramatic than those of the cardiovascular system itself. Studies of Massachusetts General Hospital coronary patients have, since 1967, focused on the psychological consequences of myocardial infarction (MI).[1-5] Some of the basic reactions are outlined below.

## DELAY DURING THE PREHOSPITAL PHASE

The prehospital phase of acute myocardial infarction—i.e., the time between symptom onset (usually chest pain) and the arrival of the infarcting patient to an emergency room—can be dissected into three phases: decision time (from symptom onset to the decision to seek medical help), physician time (time with a doctor prior to starting for the emergency facility), and transportation time. Studies over the past decade [6-13] have shown that the most crucial of these phases is the patient's decision time, since death from acute myocardial infarction is most likely to occur in the minutes immediately following the onset of symptoms. The decade of investigative exploration has also shown that, despite public education efforts to encourage prompt response to chest pain and reduce the delay of the infarcting patient, patient decision time remains remarkably constant at 3 to 6 hours in duration.

Schroeder et al.[13] studied the delay of 211 patients consecutively admitted to their coronary care unit (CCU) with suspected myocardial infarction, carefully demarcating the delay

Table 34.1  Precoronary Care Delay Times *

| Final Diagnosis | Decision | Physician | Transportation | Unaccounted | Total † |
|---|---|---|---|---|---|
| Noncardiac pain | 240 ± 297 (93) | 66 ± 64 (40) | 11 ± 6 (10) | 61 ± 29 (13) | 331 ± 336 (178) |
| Myocardial infarction ruled out | 328 ± 618 (90) | 156 ± 364 (39) | 14 ± 9 (12) | 52 ± 15 (30) | 447 ± 639 (270) |
| Inhospital myocardial infarction | 312 ± 821 (60) | 202 ± 467 (32) | 16 ± 16 (11) | 140 ± 96 (18) | 529 ± 1179 (138) |
| Acute transmural myocardial infarction | 247 ± 365 (59) | 278 ± 597 (33) | 12 ± 6 (11) | 31 ± 46 (20) | 418 ± 572 (127) |
| Acute subendocardial myocardial infarction | 447 ± 483 (260) | 42 ± 16 (33) | 77 ± 203 (16) | 147 ± 38 (73) | 692 ± 511 (478) |
| Total group | 307 ± 575 (90) | 180 ± 436 (38) | 17 ± 49 (12) | 66 ± 19 (26) | 456 ± 703 (210) |

* Delay times in minutes. Mean ± standard deviation (median).
† Does not include emergency room delay.
(Schroeder JS, Lamb IH, Hu M: The pre-hospital course of patients with chest pain. Am J Med 64:742–748, 1978.)

time spent in each of the aforementioned phases. Table 34.1 reproduces their results. A fundamental lesson of these data is that, once a decision has been made to get a patient to the emergency facility, transporting him there is done with laudable swiftness—11 to 16 minutes for all patients in the Schroeder study except those with subendocardial infarcts. The physician-induced delay in this study is greater than that of other studies.[2,6,11] As in all studies, the time spent by the patient making up his mind to seek help is the largest contributor to delay and clearly the largest obstacle to reducing potentially fatal procrastination after the onset of acute coronary symptoms. Even those patients with transmural infarcts delayed for a median of 59 minutes (mean 247), but their patient counterparts who infarcted in the hospital did no better (median 60 minutes, mean 312), despite their already having the entire hospital and its facilities literally within reach.

This indomitable human trait of procrastination in the face of symptoms remains poorly understood, and clearly quite complicated. Of particular concern is the fact that medical knowledge does not affect patient delay.[12] Factors associated with increased delay were: presence of known heart disease, stable angina, or progressive unstable angina;[13] recent physician consultation;[12] displacement of symptoms to another organ system, especially the gastrointestinal system;[2] and disbelief that the heart

was involved.[13] Factors tending to reduce procrastination were: greater severity of pain;[2,12] impatience;[10,12] being away from home when symptoms began;[9] and being influenced by others.[2] Patients often took action in the form of self-treatment (antacid, for example),[2,9] and, although consultation with another lay person could prolong appropriate action about half the time, those patients who consulted no one had longer delay times.[2,11] Sjögren et al. discuss the complicated factors in a multivariate analysis of patients' delay behavior.[12] Until coronary symptoms are better understood by the public, reduction of patient decision time to seek help for such symptoms is not likely to occur.

## EMOTIONAL PROBLEMS IN THE ACUTE PHASE OF MI

Of all the potentially emotional features of coronary artery disease, none is more significant than its capacity to kill its owner. The major threat, then, is death. One could argue that the fatal implications of myocardial infarction are not known by the patient with a routine, stable MI. But the physician has no way of knowing what the individual's experiences with heart disease have been and what conditioned fears lurk in his mind. Blacher[14] has underlined the universality of fears about the heart.

## Emotional Reactions of the CCU Staff

Even if the patient is spared knowledge of all possible complications of myocardial infarction, the CCU staff (both doctors and nurses) are not. Their reactions to the development of a potentially fatal complication like cardiogenic shock are an important feature of the CCU experience. Using an Atmosphere Assessment Scale (AAS)[15] to assess unit morale, reactions of the CCU staff were documented during the terminal days of a balloon-dependent shock patient (Fig. 34.1). Four subscales are depicted: harmony (unit feels harmonious, together, etc.); depression (unit feels blue, depressed, sad, etc.); anxiety (unit feels tense, etc.); and conflict (unit feels in conflict, hostile, etc.). Scores were recorded as a 34-year-old man with inoperable triple-vessel disease and ineffective ventricular function approached death. After his first episode of ventricular tachycardia, the depression scores of the CCU staff rose steadily until his death. Despite the significant elevation in feelings of despondency, the feeling of harmonious group action was unaffected, if not enhanced. Harmony scores reflect the sense among the nurses of smooth interpersonal cooperation and mutual support. Caring for a patient who faces a tragic outcome is of its nature likely to make a staff nurse feel despondent, but this feeling

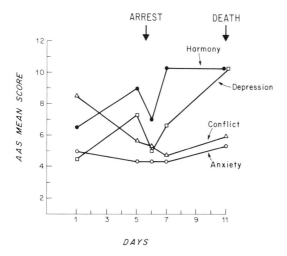

Fig. 34.1   Morale scores of CCU nursing staff associated with the approaching death of an intraaortic balloon pump-dependent, inoperable patient. (Am Operating Room Nurses J 20:79–92, 1974.)

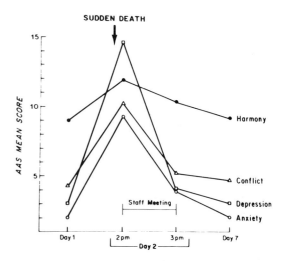

Fig. 34.2   Morale scores of CCU nursing staff after a sudden death on morning rounds, with assessments before and after a staff meeting. (Am Operating Room Nurses J 20:79–92, 1974.)

need in no way disrupt the harmonious performance of duty. In fact, such challenges can stimulate the staffs to work together more effectively.

Death—even when it is expected, as in the case illustrated in Figure 34.1—exacts its emotional toll from all concerned. When it makes a sudden unexpected appearance, the psychological consequences are even more intense. Figure 34.2 illustrates the AAS scores following the sudden cardiac arrest of a 51-year-old man admitted on the preceding night with a routine inferior MI. He arrested during CCU morning rounds. Resuscitation efforts failed, and later postmortem examination confirmed ventricular rupture. All subscale scores, taken 5 hours later, were the highest recorded for a 15-month period. The value of a 45-minute staff meeting in reducing anxiety, depressions and conflict scores among the staff is also demonstrated.

## Patient Anxiety and Depression

In order to assess the incidence of psychological difficulties in acute coronary patients, we surveyed a 15-month period in the Massachusetts General Hospital Coronary Care Unit.[4] Of 445 patients admitted during that time, 145 (33 percent) were referred for psychiatric consultation. The reasons for consultation are pre-

**Table 34.2  Reasons Prompting Psychiatric Consultation in 150 Consecutive Patient Consultations from the MGH CCU**

| Problem Specified | Number of Times |
|---|---|
| Anxiety | 47 |
| Depression | 44 |
| Management of behavior | 30 |
| Hostility | 12 |
| Delirium | 11 |
| Functional contribution to symptoms | 8 |
| Family intervention | 7 |
| Sleep disturbances | 6 |
| Medication advice | 5 |

(Cassem NII, Hackett TP: Psychiatric consultation in a coronary care unit. Ann Intern Med 75:9–14, 1971.)

sented in Table 34.2. The most frequently reported difficulties were anxiety and depression. Management-of-behavior consultations were prompted when patients wanted to sign out or were acting out dependency conflicts by whining, demanding, or aggressively rejecting therapeutic limitations. In order to summarize the complex set of emotional reactions a normal individual might have to a myocardial infarction, we took careful note of the timing of the consultations (most for anxiety occurred on day 1 or 2, those for signing out on day 2, and those for depression on days 3–5) and constructed Figure 34.3. The typical patient is anxious when he is admitted to the CCU. At this point, the patient is preoccupied with death or death's heralds—recurrence of pain or shortness of breath, a sense of imminent danger or doom, or simply the intimidation of the un-

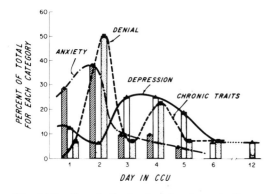

Fig. 34.3  Hypothetical schedule of onset of emotional and behavioral reactions of a CCU patient. (Ann Intern Med 75:9–14, 1971.)

known. As the patient feels better, denial becomes mobilized. He may find it hard to believe that he really had a heart attack. If the damage is unconfirmed, he may protest his detention in the unit and insist on returning to important business obligations. By day 3 or 4, however, the implications of his cardiac injury begin to take the shape of a specific concern. As he becomes more cognizant of his true condition, despondency sets in. The more devastating the effects of the infarct, the more profound the depression is likely to be. (This is expanded below.) If he also has premorbid abrasive personality traits, especially those centering on dependency or passivity, he may, after a "civil interval," start irritating or perplexing the staff by his behavior. Provocative behavior usually begins around day 4, when the immediate threat to life seems to have passed.[4] It has been our experience that hostile, disruptive behavior in a CCU patient on day 1 is almost always due to anxiety and subsides as the sense of security increases. Patients who become difficult after the threat is over usually remain so, reverting to life patterns characterizing behavior styles prior to CCU admission.

Many emotional reactions stem from the basic threat of death, as has been mentioned above. One 45-year-old psychoanalyst eloquently described his own anxiety: "I continue to regard myself as living under the sword of Damocles, but as the years go by I also begin to see how neurotic and damaging such an attitude is. I do not believe I will ever totally adapt to it and begin to think that perhaps, in essence, worrying about my heart becomes a way of life for me. As each year goes by I damn myself for all the unnecessary concern I've had, and yet I face the coming year with new doubts— a vicious circle which gets me nowhere! I cannot tell you why I feel my pulse or dread the prospect of surgery except to relate it to a basic fear of death and viewing the heart as a symbolic fountain of life, a fear and a symbolic meaning which I believe are present in all men."[16]

Anxiety is produced by the "number one" threat of coronary disease: death. But if anxiety is the commonest feeling of coronary patients, depression ranks a very close second. The second major threat faced by the coronary patient is that to his self-esteem. One might say, in fact, that a myocardial infarction (or even a close call with it) produces an ego infarction.[5] Even while in the CCU, a patient begins to ruminate about all that his heart attack has done to him: his job is in danger, earning power is lost, he is getting old and falling apart; he won't be able to drive, exercise, satisfy his wife sexually; intercourse, smoking, eating, drinking—all may be forbidden. Even if he survives the heart attack, most of life's pleasures have been forfeited. Such thoughts are the content of the "homecoming depression" experienced by many patients after leaving the hospital. Again, psychoanalyst Abram depicts this poignantly: "I feel the agony of living with heart disease. Denial, the most prevalent defense mechanisms used by patients with somatic illness, seems lacking in me. I see the worst and dread heart surgery and death from one day to the next. Do I wish such a course and do I protest too much? My middle age leaves me depressed. I wonder what I have missed in life, what I could have done, what I have accomplished, how I have failed and what is left. Do I dread death for fear of annihilation and nothingness or do I dread it for the separation from loved ones and the loss I will inflict on them? I suspect both." [16]

## SLEEP DISTURBANCES AFTER AMI

Increased jeopardy to the heart during sleep, a common conviction of anxious patients at bedtime, is a longstanding topic in medical literature.[17] In 1923 MacWilliams reported the association of disturbed sleep, angina, and death peaking around 5 to 6 A.M.—i.e., in the last third of the night when rapid eye movement (REM) sleep is the most pronounced.[18] Samuel Levine [19] and Paul D. White [20] both noted the relatively high frequency of angina and myocardial infarction in sleep. With the advent of nighttime EEG recordings, it became known that recurrent nocturnal angina occurs during periods of REM sleep.[21-23] Broughton and Baron [17] point out that this association is thought to be due to the markedly altered blood

pressure during REM sleep. This is characterized both by an overall increase in pressure and by an increased variability. In non-REM sleep, the variability in blood pressure is much less, prompting Moruzzi [24] to introduce the distinction between transient, brief "phasic" events in sleep and more sustained "tonic" events. Perhaps the phasic events of transient fluctuations in blood pressure and heart rate that occur during REM sleep could be related to the onset of nocturnal angina. Kales and Kales [25] also proposed that, as the amount of REM sleep and the intensity of its phasic events increase during the recovery (or "rebound") period following REM-suppressant drugs, this time could be dangerous for patients with ischemic heart disease.

Broughton and Baron [17] studied 12 patients with confirmed MIs. They recorded the patients' nocturnal sleep patterns, in the intensive care unit and subsequently on the ward, for up to 13 days after infarction, and contrasted the recordings to those of 12 age-matched laboratory controls. In general, although they found that severe insomnia was uncommon, there was a marked disruption of normal sleep patterns, with greater wakefulness, low REM sleep percent, long REM latency, fewer REM periods, more awakenings, more stage shifts, and decreased sleep efficiency. The usual circadian variation in heart rate was absent. Eight to 10 hours were spent in estimated unrecorded daytime sleep. In a study of four patients after AMI, Karacan et al.[26] reported similar findings, but with a total absence of Stage 3 and Stage 4 sleep. As the patients studied by Broughton and Baron recovered, the striking fragmentation of biological rhythms decreased, daytime sleep decreased, and nocturnal wakefulness decreased, while REM sleep increased. Slow-wave sleep frequency exceeded normal over postinfarction nights 3 to 9, and the sleep pattern renormalized by postinfarction night 9. No changes occurred with transfer out of the intensive care unit. The altered sleep patterns were mainly attributed to the infarction itself. Twelve nocturnal anginal attacks occurred during the study period. Ten of these began in non-REM sleep and two in REM periods without particularly intense phasic activity. Thus, postinfarction angina, which occurs largely during non-REM sleep, appears to be different from angina occurring in the absence of infarction, which usually occurs during REM sleep. Most attacks (10/12) occurred on postinfarction nights 4 and 5, suggesting that undetermined factors produce a secondary period of heightened risk at this time. A more recent study of 42 coronary patients by Dohno et al.[27] confirmed the findings of a general disruption of sleep patterns in acute postinfarction patients. Patients in a semiprivate setting had no less fragmentation of sleep patterns than those in the open-ward setting, and the authors concluded that the most significant variable associated with sleep pattern disturbance was the severity of the infarction. Hence, much remains to be learned about the relationship between the heart and the sleeping brain, although in most patients a stable relationship appears to be restored a week to ten days after myocardial infarction.

## PATTERNS OF PATIENT ADAPTATION

What are some of the coping strategies used by cardiac patients to counteract the threats to life and self-esteem? The commonest is denial. For example, Croog et al.[28] interviewed a large number of postcoronary patients who had been explicitly told they had had a heart attack. Yet three weeks after infarction, one of five stated that, according to his physician, he had not had a heart attack. It has been estimated that, at the time of discharge after myocardial infarction, one-third of patients have no understanding whatsoever of the pathophysiology of myocardial infarction. This does not appear to be due to a lack of intelligence, but to the natural process by which persons protect themselves from thinking about the threatening implications of disease.

A second style of coping is seen in the patients who, like the marathon runner in the initial example, simply overdo it. We have all known patients who have refused to comply with most or all of the medical limitations placed on them, and some of them seem to escape unscathed; On the other hand, some do not. Not long after

the popularity of jogging became widespread in 1968, reports of jogging fatalities appeared in the literature.[29,30]

A third response for the patient is to quit altogether. Having a heart attack, after all, is an honorable way to retire from the traumas of daily life. Much of the early psychoanalytic literature stressed the importance of fear of competition in the etiology of heart disease, theorizing that an infarction might intervene to remove the individual from the need to face hostile rivals (surrogates for the parent of the same sex).[31]

A fourth reaction to myocardial infarction is the development of cardiac neurosis. Whether labeled as a special case of anxiety neurosis (usually present in some form prior to MI) or as malignant hypochondriasis, its manifestations are well known to the practitioner. A patient I have seen, a cardiologist, did fairly well after an initial myocardial infarction, but repeated angina brought him back for a triple saphenous vein bypass operation. Subsequent to that, after a period of three years, he became, in his own words, "a basket case." He was often seen lying in bed with his stethoscope placed over his heart, feeling for a liver edge, or inspecting his legs for the development of pedal edema. Despite the reminder that his pedal edema was unilateral and therefore on the basis of venous obstruction, neither his medical knowledge nor his physician's reassurance brought him relief from worry. A course of electroshock therapy helped him for a few months, but he then became convinced he had carcinoid syndrome and colonic cancer. When his depression was again relieved, rumination about minor symptoms continued to fill his daytime hours. As this case illustrates, cardiac neurosis is extremely resistant to treatment; recovery is very slow, at best.

## INFLUENCE OF THE BRAIN ON THE HEART: VENTRICULAR ECTOPIC ACTIVITY AND SUDDEN DEATH

When John Hunter, who had stress-induced angina for 20 years, said that his fate lay "in the hands of any rascal who chooses to annoy and tease me," he accurately foretold his death, which occurred during a board meeting of St. Joseph's Hospital.[32] Since then, anecdotal support for the heart's vulnerability to emotional stress has abounded. In 1955 Jarvinen reported seven cases of sudden death that occurred in postmyocardial infarction patients as doctors conducted ward rounds.[33] In 1962 Horan and Venables[34] documented by ECG an attack of ventricular fibrillation (VF) in a 6-year-old Maltese girl, the result of a deliberately induced emotional upset—the threat of making her walk downstairs, to which she had particular aversion. Engel[35] collected 170 case reports of sudden death occurring in the wake of strong emotion—mostly negative experiences like death of a loved one or loss of self-esteem, but including some reports where the occasion was one of success or rejoicing. Perhaps the most carefully studied case of emotion-related ventricular fibrillation was that by Lown et al,[36] who reported a 39-year-old man with normal coronary arteries who sustained cardiac arrest after wrestling with his two teenage daughters. Although his exercise tolerance test was essentially normal, in the CCU he demonstrated malignant ventricular ectopic activity associated with emotional upset and on the sixth night during sleep suffered a second episode of VF.

Despite the extensive "folklore" about the mind's effect on the heart, most treatments of cardiac patients emphasize the heart rather than the brain as the target for therapy. In their extensive review, Lown, Verrier and Rabinowitz[37] issued this challenge:

> For too long the heart and vasculature have been deemed a self-contained system. Arrhythmias have been related to anatomic derangements within the myocardium and have been treated by altering one or another property of cardiac excitability. Resolution of the problem of sudden death requires that the central nervous system be restored to its premier integrating role in cardiac function.

The physiologic mechanisms mediating the integrating role of the central nervous system (CNS) on the heart have been increasingly clarified over the past half century. Reviewing in 1966 the emotional and sensory stress factors in myocardial pathology, Raab[38] confirmed the accuracy of his nearly 30-year insistence[39] on the preeminence of the sympathetic nervous system in the brain-heart relationship. The foundations of modern understanding were laid by Karplus and Kreidl's 1911 report[40] demonstrating connections between the central nervous and peripheral sympathetic systems and Cannon's classic studies[41] published in 1920 showing activation of the latter by emotional and sensory stimuli. The next crucial step illuminating the pathophysiology of this relationship was von Euler's 1946 demonstration of norepinephrine as the intramyocardially liberated neurotransmitter of the sympathetic nervous system.[42]

Study of sudden death has been crucial in the search for CNS-cardiac connections because of repeated demonstrations that it does not require far advanced coronary artery disease as a prerequisite, but is the result of VF, which can be reversed and prevented.[37] The detailed review of animal and human data pertinent to the CNS-cardiac connections in sudden death by Lown et al[37] is summarized below.

Although the precise mechanisms by which the brain alters myocardial susceptibility to VF remain uncertain, the posterior hypothalamus is an important cardiac neuroregulatory center transmitting impulses from cortical areas to the heart via the reticular formation. CNS stimulation does not ordinarily produce VF in the normal heart, but often does so in the presence of myocardial ischemia. An intact vagus and both stellate ganglia appear to be necessary for this to occur. Substantial evidence suggests that increased sympathetic nervous system activity lowers the heart's threshold to VF and that this is the result of direct action of norepinephrine at localized myocardial sites. Furthermore, in the balance of sympathetic innervation to the heart, the left stellate ganglion (whose fibers project to the posterior ventricular wall) appears dominant over the right in its ability, when stimulated, to lower the vulnerable period threshold. Also, animals with right stellate ganglion ablation are more vulnerable, suggesting an increased danger of VF in the presence of unopposed or enhanced stimulation of the left sympathetic system. Moss and Schwartz[43] have reviewed data on the idiopathic long QT syndrome in humans, suggesting that it results from an imbalance of cardiac sympathetic innervation due to left-sided dominance. Moreover, this syndrome has been suppressed clinically by blockade of the left stellate ganglion.[44] Lown et al.[37] also review extensive evidence that suggests that the vagus exerts an important action which is indirect—namely, it opposes the effects of heightened adrenergic tone.

It becomes clear that any psychological stress that augments a patient's sympathetic tone could alter cardiac excitability and, in the presence of myocardial ischemia, lead to sudden death. In 1949 the Cornell group in Harold Wolff's laboratory published detailed demonstrations of the association between emotionally charged life situations and extra systoles.[45] Further detailed documentation of this association is presented by Lown et al.[36,37]

Patients who live with chronic psychological stress have also been identified as having a higher risk of sudden death. Greene et al.[46] inspected information available on 26 patients who died suddenly in an industrial population of 44,000. The majority, all men, had been depressed for a week up to several months prior to death, which occurred in a setting of acute arousal stemming from increased activity, anxiety, or anger. Bruhn et al.[47] found that individuals characterized by the "Sisyphus reaction," a joyless striving in work and living patterns, were significantly more likely to die of myocardial infarction or sudden death. Increased arousal, uncertainty, and powerlessness are common descriptive features of the setting for sudden death.[35,48,49] So accepted has this brain-heart connection become that the precipitation of sudden death by emotional arousal can provide legal grounds for homicide.[50]

## BEYOND THE BRAIN: ENVIRONMENTAL STRESS AND CORONARY ARTERY DISEASE

Brain-heart connections through the sympathetic nervous system make the danger of suddenly aroused anxiety or anger a plausible threat to the equilibrium of ventricular activity, but the modern use of the word "stress" encompasses a far wider scope than what goes on in a person's mind. Rosch,[51] noting that a report by Selye was the sole article on stress in 1950, estimated that close to 10,000 articles on this topic were written in 1978. Russek and Russek [52] graphically portray the dilemma of stressed modern man by saying: "Since his appearance on this planet, homo sapiens has spent some 3 and ¾ million years in the forest, 10,000 years on the farm, and only 300 years in the factory." Because adaptation of a species to a changing environment usually requires at least 100,000 years, the existence of "stress" should be no surprise. Two basic questions, however, are: How can stress be operationally defined, and, once so defined, can it be shown to be atherogenic?

Epidemiologic study of Japanese men living in Japan, Hawaii, and California showed that the incidence of coronary heart disease (CHD) in samples of 45- to 68-year-old men was lowest in Japan, where it was 50 percent less than that observed in Hawaii, and highest in California, where it was nearly 50 percent greater than that in Hawaii.[53] When 3,809 Japanese-Americans in California were classified according to the degree to which they retained a traditional Japanese culture, the most traditional group showed a CHD prevalence as low as that observed in Japan. The group most acculturated to Western society had a three- to five-fold excess in CHD prevalence, a difference which could not be accounted for by differences in the major coronary risk factors.[54]

In their recent comment on the role of emotional stress in the development of heart disease, Buell and Eliot noted that traditional risk factors are absent in more than half of the newly encountered cases of coronary artery disease.[55] Jenkins undertook an extensive critical review of the evidence supporting psychosocial risk factors for coronary artery disease. Inspecting 12 studies of sociologic indices associated with CHD in several countries and cultures, he concluded that early in the process of urbanization higher socioeconomic groups appear to be at greater risk, whereas at the end of the process lower socioeconomic groups were at more risk. Although early studies suggested that social mobility and status incongruity were significantly related to CHD, new evidence has clouded their association, and they may be valid predictors only in certain times or settings, or when other variables are present. Although efforts to relate neuroticism, life dissatisfaction, and life change have produced some provocative studies, the data remain unconvincing. A finding by Keys [57] that a rise in diastolic blood pressure during the cold pressor test was the strongest single predictor of future CHD has been confirmed by Thomas and Greenstreet.[58] Among all categories of psychosocial variables reviewed, Jenkins [56] found evidence for an association with CHD strongest for the coronary prone behavior pattern.

## Coronary-Prone (Type A) Behavior

Before 1900 William Osler described the typical coronary patient as "a keen and ambitious man, the indicator of whose engines is always set at full speed ahead." [59] The greatest contribution toward a manageable formulation of the coronary-prone behavior pattern has come from the work of Drs. Meyer Friedman and Ray Rosenman.[60] Friedman describes the pattern as "a characteristic action-emotion complex which is exhibited by those individuals who are engaged in a relatively *chronic struggle* to obtain an *unlimited* number of *poorly defined* things from their environment in the *shortest period of time* and, if necessary, against the opposing efforts of other things or persons in this same environment." [61] The definition includes all or some of the following overt, intense features: striving for achievement, competitiveness, easily provoked impatience, time urgency, abruptness of gesture and speech, hyperalert posture, overcommitment to vocation or profession, and excesses of drive and hostility.[62] Jenkins,[56] in a review of 24 studies (8 prospective and 16 cross-sectional and retrospective) attempting to relate some aspect of the Type A behavior pattern to some manifestation of CHD, found that only 1 of the 24 studies had negative results and 2 had equivocal results. Moreover, the studies associated the Type A behavior pattern with the development of both angina and myocardial infarction.

The coronary-prone behavior pattern is often mislabeled a "personality" pattern, which erroneously implies some inborn character structure or psychiatric diagnosis. Although Theorell et al.[63] found evidence for genetic influence in two measures of Type A behavior applied to a series of twins, the constellation is still most clearly portrayed as an overt style of reacting which can be measured. Two standardized methods for measuring Type A behavior exist: the standardized clinical interview [64] and a self-administered computer-scored questionnaire known as the Jenkins Activity Survey (JAS).[65] The reliability of both methods has been demonstrated.

The Western Collaborative Group (WCG) Study is a prospective study of a cohort of more than 3000 employed men, aged 39 to 59 years, in which all were defined according to Type A behavior interview measures. (The last 2600 men of the study received both the interview and the JAS questionnaire.) At the completion of an 8.5-year follow-up, risk of coronary heart disease was studied with the use of a multiple-risk model.[66] The incidence of CHD showed a highly significant association with behavior pattern, serum cholesterol level, cigarette smoking, and systolic blood pressure. The strong relationship of the Type A behavior pattern to the incidence of CHD was independent of interrelations of the behavior pattern with any other risk factor. Using a Framingham study equation to predict CHD risk in their own sample, the authors of the WCG study found the results highly correlated with their own risk factor predictions.[67] The observed number of CHD events in the WCG study was not significantly different from the expected number of events derived from the Framingham study equation, after correction for length of follow-up. The authors estimated that removal of the excess risk associated with Type A behavior would correspond to a 31 percent reduction of CHD incidence in the WCG study.

What is the relationship of coronary prone (Type A) behavior to the anatomic extent of disease in the coronary vessels? Six years after the beginning of the WCG study, Friedman et al.[68] were able to examine at autopsy 51 of the 82 men who had died. The Type A subjects among these 51 individuals exhibited, irrespective of the actual cause of death, severe coronary atherosclerosis 6 times more frequently than the Type B subjects in the same autopsy sample. More recently, four studies using either the clinical interview or the JAS questionnaire or both have studied the relationship of the Type A scores to the extent of CHD as judged by coronary angiography.[69-72] With the exception of Blumenthal et al.,[71] who used ≥ 75 percent narrowing, all studies defined vessel disease as ≥ 50 percent narrowing. Two studies measured Type A behavior only by the JAS questionnaire,[69,72] one only by the interview,[70] and one by both.[71] Only the study of Dimsdale et al.[72] (using the JAS questionnaire) showed entirely negative results. Blumenthal et al.[71] were unable to find a positive relationship between the JAS questionnaire measurement of Type A behavior and the extent of CHD, but interview ratings significantly predicted the presence and extent of CHD. Likewise, the studies of Zyzanski et al.,[69] using the JAS questionnaire, and Frank et al.,[70] using the interview, found that those patients who scored higher for Type A behavior had significantly more extensive CHD on angiography, and that this association was independent of other risk factors. In short, the evidence that this behavior constellation makes a significant contribution to the development of CHD is overwhelming.

How the central nervous system translates this network of psychosocial stress into the relentless, accelerated atherosclerotic changes in coronary vessels is unknown. Kones [73] recently argued that plasma catecholamines are the culprit, but this has yet to be studied in patients with Type A behavior.

## INTERVENTIONS

What sorts of interventions are available to reduce anxiety and prevent or contain extension of the ego infarction incurred in the wake of damage to the heart?

### CCU and Post-CCU Phase

While anxiety is accepted as a normal component of a patient's reaction to acute myocardial infarction, the increased sympathetic arousal is not only uncomfortable but potentially hazardous. Because of the nature of CNS control of sympathetic cardiac innervation, emotional arousal should be minimized. Therefore, we routinely prescribe mild 'round-the-clock sedation, usually a benzodiazepine. If the patient demonstrates panic that is unresponsive to benzodiazepines or appears to impair rationality or judgment, we switch to haloperidol, aiming for swift sedation (e.g., 2 to 10 mg parenterally or orally q. ½ to 1 hr) followed by the swiftest dose reduction consonant with symptom control, culminating in one nighttime maintenance dose every 24 hours.

Panic is often obvious, but the subtler signs of its presence include mute withdrawal, hostility, or uncooperativeness, particularly when present on the first day or two in the CCU, or after a new complication or relapse. Delirium is more likely to occur later, although premonitory signs often herald its coming. Both physicians and nurses should be alert for an episode of mild nocturnal confusion, muteness, restlessness, and emergence of suspicious or paranoid remarks. The usual story, unfortunately in retrospect, is that these signs preceded the night on which the patient became combative, pulled out his arterial line and Foley catheter, seriously jeopardized his already damaged myocardium, and created several hours of havoc for the staff and covering physician. Prevention by administration of an antipsychotic drug is much preferred, and, since the brain is more vulnerable to delirium at night, an antipsychotic drug should be given before the patient prepares for his (already fragmented) night's sleep. We prefer haloperidol for emergencies and administer it intravenously.[74]

If the milder symptoms are noted early, any high-potency (i.e., low-dose) antipsychotic drug administered orally at bedtime will be effective—e.g., trifluoperazine (Stelazine) 2 to 5 mg, fluphenazine (Prolixin) 1 to 5 mg, thiothixene (Navane) 2 to 5 mg or perphenazine (Trilafon) 4 to 10 mg. The α-adrenergic blocking properties of the lower potency (high dose) antipsychotics, such as chlorpromazine (Thorazine) or thioridazine (Mellaril), make them less safe for unstable cardiac patients because of the possible reduction in total peripheral resistance and consequent hypotension.

When should psychiatric consultation be requested for the coronary patient in the CCU or during the post-CCU phase? A representative list would include the following situations: panic states; confusional states; angina consistently related either to emotional stresses beyond the patient's control or to chronic emotional conflict; myocardial infarction precipitated by an unresolved marital, family, or work conflict; uncontrolled or unstable psychiatric illness independent of CHD; depression with endogenous features (disturbance of sleep, appetite, pleasure, energy, motor arousal, ability to concentrate) or any depressed state that retards recovery; any mental or emotional state (anger, dependency, denial, etc.) that appears to be an obstacle to treatment or recovery; symptoms that appear to have some emotional etiology, especially where this is of diagnostic or therapeutic significance (such as atypical chest pain in a patient with single-vessel disease); and those patients who appear to be using the myocardial infarction to justify escaping life.

## Posthospital Phase

**Mobilization and Discharge Advice.** Our work suggests that the most beneficial antidote to both anxiety and depression is early and progressive mobilization. Many patients feel overwhelmed by a sense of physical weakness on returning home, and most attribute this to extensive damage to the heart. Typical was the 39-year-old teacher who recovered smoothly until reaching home. "I felt great in the hospital. No matter what anybody told me, I pictured myself breaking records in getting back to work. But the first week home I could hardly walk the length of the house without feeling exhausted. I felt like a cooked goose, like I was done for." In a follow-up study of coronary patients, we learned that weakness was the single most distressing symptom reported.[3] This symptom is almost surely due to muscle atrophy and the systemic effects of immobilization. Physicians forget too easily that bed rest is a disease in itself, promoting venous stasis, orthostatic hypotension, a progressive increase in

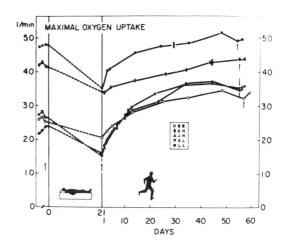

Fig. 34.4  Maximal oxygen uptake before and after three weeks of bed rest in five healthy college students. (Circulation 38 (suppl. no. 7):1, 1968.)

resting heart rate, a loss of about 10 to 15 percent of strength per week of bed rest, and a reduction of about 20 to 25 percent in maximal oxygen uptake capacity.[75] These data are portrayed in Figure 34.4. Three of the subjects represented in Figure 34.4 had sedentary lifestyles, while the other two were trained athletes. After being tested in the laboratory, all were placed on 3 weeks of bed rest, exactly as previously required of an MI patient in many hospitals. After their MI regimen, they were returned to the laboratory for testing. It took the three sedentary individuals 8, 10, and 13 days to regain their pre-bedrest $MVO_2$ levels, while it took the two athletes 28 and 43 days to reach their original capacities. Unaware of muscle atrophy, postmyocardial infarction patients regularly ascribe physical weakness to a damaged heart. Early mobilization programs represent an effective method to counter both the physical and psychological damages of immobilization. Progress has been greatly assisted by the definition and use of the metabolic equivalent (met). One met is defined as the energy expenditure per kg per min of the average 70-kg individual sitting quietly in a chair. This amounts to about 1.4 cal per min or 3.5 to 4 ml of $O_2$ per min. Tables 34.3 to 34.6 provide lists of activities which have been assigned measurements in mets. It is of interest, for example, to notice in Table 34.3 that using a bedpan requires one third again as much energy as using a bedside commode. If one follows this particular level of energy expenditure—4 mets—through the other tables, one sees that using a bedpan is equivalent to wheeling a 115-lb wheelbarrow at 2.5 mph (Table 34.4), beating carpets—the most strenuous of housework activities—(Table 34.5), or swimming 20 yd per min, (Table 34.6). More extensive lists of activities with their metabolic equivalents are readily available.

**Table 34.3  Energy Expenditure for Self-Care Activities for a 70-kg Man**

| Activity | Mets |
| --- | --- |
| Rest, supine | 1 |
| Sitting | 1 |
| Standing, relaxed | 1 |
| Eating | 1 |
| Conversation | 1 |
| Dressing, undressing | 2 |
| Washing hands, face | 2 |
| Bedside commode | 3 |
| Walking, 2.5 mph | 3 |
| Showering | 3.5 |
| Using bedpan | 4 |
| Walking downstairs | 4.5 |
| Walking, 3.5 mph | 5.5 |
| Propulsion, wheelchair | 2 |
| Ambulation with braces and crutches | 6.5 |

Taken from Exercise Equivalents, Colorado Heart Association, Denver, Colorado.

**Table 34.4  Energy Expenditure for Industrial Activities**

| Activity | Mets |
| --- | --- |
| Watch repairing | 1.5 |
| Armature winding | 2.0 |
| Radio assembly | 2.5 |
| Sewing at machine | 2.5 |
| Bricklaying | 3.5 |
| Plastering | 3.5 |
| Tractor ploughing | 3.5 |
| Wheeling barrow, 115 lb, 2.5 mph | 4.0 |
| Horse ploughing | 5.0 |
| Carpentry | 5.5 |
| Mowing lawn by hand | 6.5 |
| Felling trees | 6.5 |
| Shoveling | 7.0 |
| Ascending stairs, 17-lb load, 27 ft per min | 7.5 |
| Planing | 7.5 |
| Tending furnace | 8.5 |
| Ascending stairs, 22-lb load, 54 ft per min | 13.5 |

Taken from Exercise Equivalents, Colorado Heart Association, Denver, Colorado.

**Table 34.5  Energy Expenditure for Housework Activities**

| Activity | Mets |
| --- | --- |
| Hand sewing | 1 |
| Sweeping floor | 1.5 |
| Machine sewing | 1.5 |
| Polishing furniture | 2 |
| Peeling potatoes | 2.5 |
| Scrubbing, standing | 2.5 |
| Washing small clothes | 2.5 |
| Kneading dough | 2.5 |
| Scrubbing floors | 3 |
| Cleaning windows | 3 |
| Making beds | 3 |
| Ironing, standing | 3.5 |
| Mopping | 3.5 |
| Wringing by hand | 3.5 |
| Hanging wash | 3.5 |
| Beating carpets | 4 |

Taken from Exercise Equivalents, Colorado Heart Association, Denver, Colorado.

**Table 34.6  Energy Expenditure for Recreational Activities**

| Activity | Mets |
| --- | --- |
| Painting, sitting | 1.5 |
| Playing piano | 2 |
| Driving car | 2 |
| Canoeing, 2.5 mph | 2.5 |
| Horseback riding, slow | 2.5 |
| Volley ball | 2.5 |
| Bowling | 3.5 |
| Cycling, 5.5 mph | 3.5 |
| Golfing | 4 |
| Swimming, 20 yd per min | 4 |
| Dancing | 4.5 |
| Gardening | 4.5 |
| Tennis | 6 |
| Trotting horse | 6.5 |
| Spading | 7 |
| Skiing | 8 |
| Squash | 8.5 |
| Cycling, 13 mph | 9 |

Taken from Exercise Equivalents, Colorado Heart Association, Denver, Colorado.

Hellerstein [76] indicates that champion athletes can perform at about 20 mets and healthy untrained young men at about 12 mets. Average middle-aged men three months or more after an uncomplicated MI are capable of performing at a level of 8 to 9 mets. This includes running at 5.5 mph, cycling at 13 mph, skiing at 4 mph, noncompetitive squash and handball, fencing, and "vigorous" basketball. If less than ordinary activity produces symptoms in the postmyocardial infarction patient, then his capacity is closer to 4 mets. Even though such a patient's performance is clearly impaired, his capacity includes the following: swimming the breast stroke at 20 yd per min, cycling at 5.5 mph, walking up a 5 percent incline at 3 mph, raking leaves, and playing ping pong, golf (carrying his own clubs), badminton, or tennis doubles. These are quantitated capacities, carefully computed. These are far more concrete than statements like "Use your own judgment" or "Do it in moderation." We believe, for example, that it would do a patient great good to have an entire list of activities with their metabolic equivalents. One could then say to the patient, for example, at an appropriate point in his convalescence, "I now move you to a level of activity of about 4 to 5 mets. You will find at this level all the activities that your heart is physically capable of doing. The activities you enjoy are the best. Remember that getting emotionally upset or very competitive during activity greatly increases the energy cost to your heart. If you cannot do some of these things without getting all worked up, you will have to ease off; only you can judge that. But you should know that now your heart is physically capable of 4 to 5 mets." In the foregoing statement, vagueness is allowed to remain but it is placed in the realm of emotions. This is the part of himself that the patient not only understands better than anyone else but is usually conscious of. Emotional self-control is a fair request of the patient, for, although he cannot be expected to detect a rise in his pulmonary capillary wedge pressure, the rising of his gorge on the tennis court is another matter entirely—one which he must become accountable for and attempt to control.

Use of behavioral techniques may be very helpful in returning patients to normal sexual activity and predischarge sexual counseling may be of considerable benefit.[76a] Sexual intercourse can usually be regarded as an energy expenditure of from 4 to 6 mets, but emotional factors can drive this level much higher. Reminding the patient and his spouse that return to sexual activity is normally accompanied by anxiety for both partners, the physician can helpfully inquire how much they judge this subjective factor to be. If it worries either person, techniques of sexual therapy can be suggested which are far less physically demanding than coitus. For example, the couple may wish to initiate resumption of sexual activity by mutual pleasuring techniques, such as gentle body massage, with avoidance of intercourse. In some cases the progression may need to be spelled out— e.g., mutual massage avoiding genital areas, then massage including genital areas, then resumption of normal foreplay short of coitus, and finally to accustomed patterns of intercourse.

Tables are available that permit the practitioner to use a modified step or treadmill test in the office to determine at what level of mets an exercise prescription can be written. Figure 34.5 shows comparable energy expenditures for the more commonly used step and treadmill tests and relates them to clinical status and functional class.[77] When a patient is tested by one of these methods, the level of energy expenditure that is safe for him can then be used to specify activities he can safely pursue in his current stage of rehabilitation. In a disease where there are so many *don'ts* in the instructions at the time of hospital discharge, this approach has the advantage of providing something for the patient to *do*.

Other forms of intervention can also be extremely helpful in reversing the psychological impact of myocardial infarction. Relaxation techniques of all kinds have great potential for minimizing stress factors that commonly contribute to the development of coronary artery disease and infarction.

## MANAGING STRESS

How can "stress" be managed in the patient's life? One can reasonably divide this into two parts: (1) the "stress" that is acute and episodic, producing acute emotional arousal, and (2) stress that is more chronic and habitual, possibly resulting in coronary-prone (Type A) behavior patterns.

The physician, noting in the cardiac history those situations which the patient identified as

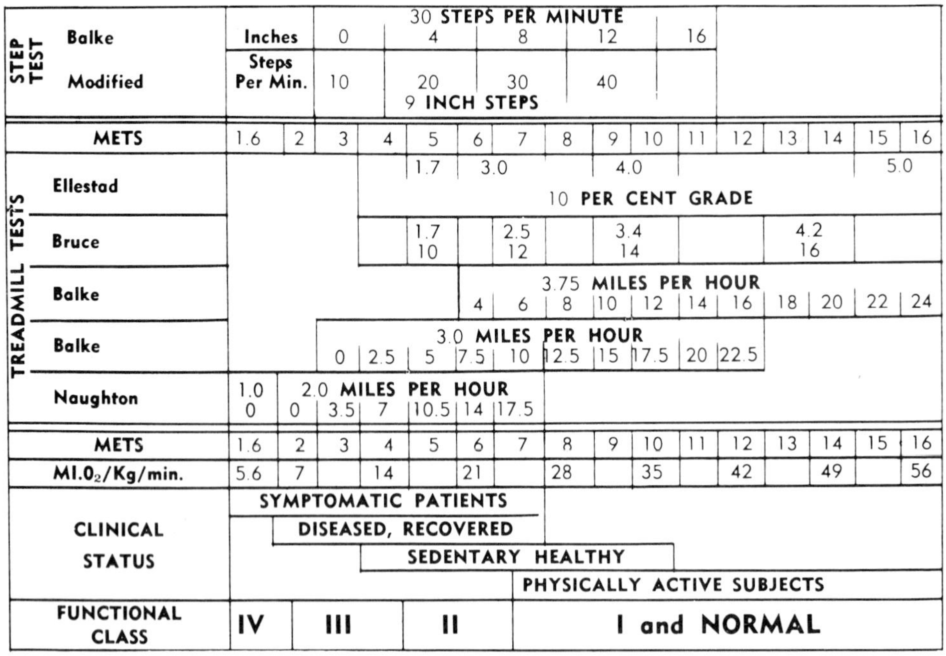

| STEP TEST | Balke | Inches | 30 STEPS PER MINUTE: 0 | 4 | 8 | 12 | 16 |
| | Modified | Steps Per Min. | 10 | 20 | 30 | 40 (9 INCH STEPS) |

| METS | 1.6 | 2 | 3 | 4 | 5 | 6 | 7 | 8 | 9 | 10 | 11 | 12 | 13 | 14 | 15 | 16 |

| TREADMILL TESTS | | | | |
|---|---|---|---|---|
| Ellestad | 1.7 | 3.0 | 4.0 | 5.0 — 10 PER CENT GRADE |
| Bruce | 1.7 / 10 | 2.5 / 12 | 3.4 / 14 | 4.2 / 16 |
| Balke | 3.75 MILES PER HOUR: 4 | 6 | 8 | 10 | 12 | 14 | 16 | 18 | 20 | 22 | 24 |
| Balke | 3.0 MILES PER HOUR: 0 | 2.5 | 5 | 7.5 | 10 | 12.5 | 15 | 17.5 | 20 | 22.5 |
| Naughton | 1.0 / 0 ; 2.0 MILES PER HOUR: 0 | 3.5 | 7 | 10.5 | 14 | 17.5 |

| METS | 1.6 | 2 | 3 | 4 | 5 | 6 | 7 | 8 | 9 | 10 | 11 | 12 | 13 | 14 | 15 | 16 |
| Ml.O$_2$/Kg/min. | 5.6 | 7 | | 14 | | 21 | | 28 | | 35 | | 42 | | 49 | | 56 |

| CLINICAL STATUS |
|---|
| SYMPTOMATIC PATIENTS |
| DISEASED, RECOVERED |
| SEDENTARY HEALTHY |
| PHYSICALLY ACTIVE SUBJECTS |

| FUNCTIONAL CLASS | IV | III | II | I and NORMAL |

Fig. 34.5 Energy expenditures for the more commonly used step and treadmill tests in relation to clinical status and functional class. (Tennessee Affiliate, American Heart Association, Physicians Handbook, 2nd ed., 1972.)

sources of stress, particularly if they were the prelude for anginal attacks or the current MI, can make them the target of therapeutic intervention. If a specific family or marital conflict, no matter how chronic, figured prominently, psychiatric consultation should be requested for its specific mitigation or resolution. If the patient is easily aroused emotionally—i.e., made anxious and/or angry—these situations can be made the target of relaxation exercises. Such exercises include: hypnosis, meditation, biofeedback (using $\alpha$-waves or EMG tracings), or self-hypnosis. When biofeedback is used, a patient is shown a continuous tracing of his own EEG or the electromyogram voltage of his temporalis muscles and instructed to increase $\alpha$-wave production in the first instance or reduce voltage in the second. As this is done, progressive relaxation occurs. The other relaxation techniques require the subject to concentrate on slow, deep breathing and the progressive voluntary relaxation of individual muscle groups. In addition, some instruction may be added to occupy the subject's conscious attention. The object may be a tranquil scene meant to fully absorb atten-

tion and imagination, such as a remote beach scene. Or the object may be a simple "mantra"—a phrase or number to be repeated over and over, such as "one," "krishna," or "The Lord is one," until the subject's consciousness is entirely empty except for the mantra. Once the patient has learned by one of these methods to achieve a relaxed state, he is encouraged either to resort to it when he feels pressured or to utilize the relaxation exercise regularly—e.g., twice daily—so that he might become more relaxed in general. Even prior to hospital discharge, the patient can be instructed to think of the situations in which he feels stressed, threatened, or about to explode. He may then employ the relaxation technique so that the stressful pattern is disrupted. It is of interest to note a study by Davidson et al.[78] on the effects of deep muscle relaxation therapy on cardiac parameters (BP, HR, and indices of myocardial contractility) and sympathetic activity in six postsurgical cardiac patients (five bypass, one valve replacement) with surgically implanted tantalum myocardial markers. Davidson et al. found that relaxation produced decreases in plasma norepinephrine and that these decreases were related to simultaneous decreases in BP, HR, and ventricular dimensions. Therefore, one can hope that these relaxation exercises are accurately aimed at the mechanism that makes the heart vulnerable to ventricular ectopic activity and sudden death.

Eliot and Forker have suggested that $\beta$-adrenergic blockade with propranolol can be helpful for persons whose excessive sympathetic nervous system activity leaves them more vulnerable to the development of coronary artery disease and myocardial infarction.[79] Most commonly, these individuals respond to stressful situations with tachycardia and excessive sweating.

**Behavior Modification.** Can Type A behavior be changed? The importance of the question is underlined by the finding of Jenkins et al.[80] that, among men surviving their first MI, there is a stronger association between Type A score and risk of recurrent MI. It therefore makes sense to change this behavior, if possible, even after an infarction has already occurred. In a pilot comparison of 10 patients and 10 controls, Suinn et al.[81] used two behavior modification programs—anxiety management training, and visuomotor behavioral rehearsal. Anxiety management training trains patients to recognize the physiological signs of stress in themselves and then focuses on eliminating them. Visuomotor behavioral rehearsal trains patients to form new behavior patterns by practicing them. Of the treated patients, 83 percent believed that the program led to substantial improvements in their reactions to stress, and to major changes in their lifestyle. Rosenman and Friedman[82] themselves describe their detailed program of Type A behavior modification, which is aimed at two features of the behavior pattern: the sense of time urgency and the enhanced aggressiveness or hostility of Type A individuals. Treated in groups, the patients are exposed to two strategies, the effort to change their philogophy of behaving and a series of guided exercises to reengineer their habits and daily routines. An effort is made to convince the group that their excessive sense of time urgency has been destructive to their careers and advancement. They are then urged through self-analysis to reflect more on the past and past accomplishments, assess their level of creative energy, evaluate their capacity for flexibility, catalogue their intellectual, emotional, and spiritual potentials, acknowledge their hostility and identify its sources, and take stock of their capacity for affection, friendship, and moral integrity.

In addition to this reorientation, patients are then put through exercises directed at changing patterns. Tapes and group feedback are enlisted to help them see their explosive, intense voice patterns, how they interrupt a speaker before he can finish, etc. Patients are drilled to decelerate their rate of walking, talking, and eating and to take up or resume avocational activities. Self-reward-and-punishment systems are constructed (e.g., going a week without exploding at another driver is rewarded by buying oneself a bottle of rare wine; racing through an intersection is punished by turning right at the next corner, stopping for a full minute, and circling the block to cross the intersection again). Relaxation methods mentioned earlier are liberally used as well. Data on results of this treatment approach will soon be available.

Rahe et al. randomly assigned 44 post-MI patients to group therapy or control status and followed them for 4 years.[83] Patients who received group therapy had significantly less follow-up coronary morbidity (insufficiency, reinfarction, or bypass surgery) and mortality. Neither group meaningfully altered traditional risk factors (body weight, smoking, cholesterol), and the educational information about CHD taught to the group therapy patients was forgotten over follow-up. But the group therapy patients successfully altered selected coronary-prone behaviors (overwork and sense of time urgency).

Much work remains to be done before the rehabilitation process is understood and the effects of our interventions demonstrated. Most patients treated with exercise programs or relaxation techniques report subjective benefit, but this may well be due to the natural reconstructive processes of the body itself. Perhaps nothing benefits the physician so much as patience with the process, for treatment must still be individualized. We will continue to see the occasional person who seems rehabilitation-resistant for decades, yet is coping as best he can. However, most patients recover quite well from their acute cardiac illnesses. Utilization of methods outlined in this chapter may help to make these recoveries more rapid.

# REFERENCES

1. Hackett TP, Cassem NH, Wishnie HA: The coronary care unit: An appraisal of its psychological hazards. N Engl J Med 279:1365–1370, 1968.
2. Hackett TP, Cassem NH: Factors contributing to delay in responding to the signs and symptoms of acute myocardial infarction. Amer J Cardiol 24:651–658, 1969.
3. Wishnie HA, Hackett TP, Cassem NH: Psychological hazards of convalescence following myocardial infarction. J Amer Med Assoc 215:1292–1296, 1971.
4. Cassem NH, Hackett TP: Psychiatric consultation in a coronary care unit. Ann Intern Med 75:9–14, 1971.
5. Cassem NH, Hackett TP: Psychological rehabilitation of myocardial infarction patients in the acute phase. Heart & Lung 2:382–388, (May–June), 1973.
6. Moss AJ, Wynar B, Goldstein S: Delay in hospitalization during the acute coronary period. Amer J Cardiol 24:659–665, 1969.
7. Tjoe SL, Luria MH: Delays in reaching the cardiac care unit: An analysis. Chest 61:617–621, 1972.
8. Simon AB, Feinleib M, Thompson HK: Components of delay in the pre-hospital phase of acute myocardial infarction. Am J Cardiol 30:476–482, 1972.
9. Erhardt LR, Sjogren A, Sawe U, Theorell T: Prehospital phase of patients admitted to a coronary care unit. Acta Med Scand 196:41–46, 1974.
10. Theorell T, Erhardt R, Lind E, Sjogren A, Sawe U: Selected psychosocial variables in the delay of reaching the coronary care unit. Acta Med Scand 198:315–317, 1975.
11. Gillum RF, Feinleib M, Margolis JR, Fabsitz RR, Brasch RC: Delay in the pre-hospital phase of acute myocardial infarction. Arch Int Med 136:649–654, 1976.
12. Sjogren A, Erhardt LR, Theorell T: Circumstances around the onset of a myocardial infarction. Acta Med Scand 205:287–292, 1979.
13. Schroeder JS, Lamb IH, Hu M: The pre-hospital course of patients with chest pain. Am J Med 64:742–748, 1978.
14. Blacher R: The hidden psychosis following open heart surgery. JAMA 222:305–308, 1972.
15. Cassem NH: What is behind our masks? Am Operating Room Nurses J 20:79–92, 1974.
16. Abram HS: Emotional aspects of heart disease: A personal narrative. Presented at Nashville Cardiovascular Society, Dec. 11, 1975.
17. Broughton R, Baron R: Sleep patterns in the intensive care unit and on the ward after acute myocardial infarction. Electroencephalogr Clin Neurophysiol 45:348–360, 1978.
18. MacWilliams AJ, Blood pressure and heart action in sleep and dreams: Their relationship to hemorrhage, angina and sudden death. Brit Med J 2:1195–1200, 1923.
19. Levine SA: Clinical Heart Disease. Saunders, Philadelphia, p. 816, 1951.
20. White PD, Heart Disease. MacMillan, New York, p. 87, 1964.
21. Knowlin BJ, Troyer WG, Collins WS, Silverman G, Nicholas CR, McIntosh HD, Estes EH, Bogdonoff MD: The association of nocturnal angina with dreaming. Ann Int Med 63:1040–1046, 1965.
22. Murao S, Harumi K, Katayama S, Mashima S, Shimomura K, Murayama M, Matsuo H, Yamamoto H, Kato R, Chen C: All-night polygraphic studies of nocturnal angina pectoris. Jpn Heart J 13:295–306, 1972.
23. King MJ, Zir LM, Kaltman AJ, Fox AC: Variant angina associated with angiographically demonstrated coronary artery spasm in REM sleep. Am J Med Science 265:419–422, 1973.
24. Moruzzi G: General discussion. In M Jouvet (ed.), Aspects Anatomofonctionnels de la Physiologie du Sommeil, CNRS, Paris, 639–640, 1965.
25. Kales A, Kales J: Evaluation, diagnosis and treatment of clinical conditions related to sleep. JAMA 213:2229–2232, 1970.
26. Karacan I, Green JR, Taylor WJ, Williams JC, Eliot RS, Williams RL, Thornby JI, Salis PJ: Sleep in post-myocardial infarction patients. In R.S. Eliot (ed.), Stress and the Heart, Futura Publications, New York, 1974, pp. 163–195.
27. Dohno S, Paskewitz DA, Lynch JJ, Gimbel KS, Thomas SA: Some aspects of sleep disturbance in coronary patients. Perceptual and Motor Skills 48:199–205, 1979.
28. Croog SH, Shapiro DS, Levine S: Denial among male heart patients. Psychosom Med 33:385, 1971.
29. Cantwell JD, Fletcher GF: Cardiac complications while jogging. J Am Med Assoc 210:130, 1969.

30. Resnekov L: Jogging and coronary artery disease. J Am Med Assoc 210:126, 1969.

31. Menninger KA, Menninger WMC: Psychoanalytic observations in cardiac disorders. Am Heart J 11:10–23, 1936.

32. Home E: A short account of the author's life. In Hunter J (ed), A Treatise on the Blood, Inflammation and Gunshot Wounds. T Bradford, Philadelphia, 1976, p. i.

33. Jarvinen KAJ: Can ward rounds be a danger to patients with myocardial infarction? Brit Med J 1:318–320, 1955.

34. Horan M, Venables AW: Paroxysmal tachycardia with episodic unconsciousness. Arch Dis Child 37:82–85, 1962.

35. Engel GL, Sudden and rapid death during psychologic stress. Folklore or folk wisdom? Ann Intern Med 74:771–782, 1971.

36. Lown B, Tempe JV, Reich P et al: Basis for recurring ventricular fibrillation in the absence of coronary heart disease and its management. N Engl J Med 294:623–629, 1976.

37. Lown B, Verrier RL, Rabinowitz SH: Neural and psychologic mechanisms and the problem of sudden cardiac death. Am J Cardiol 39:890–902, 1977.

38. Raab W: Emotional and sensory stress factors in myocardial pathology. Am Heart J 72:538–564, 1966.

39. Raab W: Nebennieren und angina pectoris. Arch Kreislaufforsch 1:255, 1937 (cited in reference 7).

40. Karplus JP, Kreidl A: Gehirn und sympathicus, Pflugers Arch Ges Physiol 143:109, 1911 (cited in reference 7).

41. Cannon WB: Bodily Changes in Pain, Hunger, Fear and Rage. Appleton-Century, New York, 1920.

42. von Euler US: A specific sympathiomimetic ergone in adrenergic nerve fibers (sympathin) and its relation to adrenalin and noradrenalin. Acta Physiol Scand 12:73, 1946.

43. Moss AJ, Schwartz PJ: Sudden death and the idiopathic long QT syndrome. Am J Med 66: 6–7, 1979.

44. Moss AJ, McDonald J: Unilateral cervicothoracic sympathetic ganglionectomy for the treatment of long Q-T interval syndrome. N Engl J Med 285:903, 1971.

45. Stephenson IP, Duncan CH, Wolf S, Ripley HS, Wolff HG: Life situations, emotions, and extrasystoles. Psychosom Med 11:257–272, 1949.

46. Greene WA, Goldstein S, Moss AJ: Psychosocial aspects of sudden death. Arch Int Med 129:725–731, 1972.

47. Bruhn JG, Paredes A, Adsett CA, Wolf S: Psychological predictors of sudden death in myocardial infarction. J Psychosom Res 18:187–191, 1974.

48. Dimsdale JE, Emotional causes of sudden death. Am J Psychiatry 134:1361–1366, 1977.

49. Engel GL: Psychologic stress, vasodepressor (vasovagal) syncope, and sudden death. Ann Intern Med 89:403–412, 1978.

50. Davis JH: Can sudden cardiac death be murder? J Forensic Science 23:384–387, 1978.

51. Rosch PJ: Stress and illness. JAMA: 242:427–428, 1979.

52. Russek HI, Russek LG: Is emotional stress an etiologic factor in coronary heart disease? Psychosomatics 17:63–67, 1976.

53. Marmot MG, Syme SL: Acculturation and coronary heart disease in Japanese-Americans. Am J Epidemiology 104:225–247, 1976.

54. Robertson TL, et al: Epidemiologic studies of coronary heart disease and stroke in Japanese men living in Japan, Hawaii and California. Am J Cardiol 39:239–243, 1977.

55. Buell JC, Eliot RS: The role of emotional stress in the development of heart disease. JAMA 242:365–368, 1979.

56. Jenkins CD: Recent evidence supporting psychologic and social risk factors for coronary disease. N Engl J Med 294:987–994, 1033–1038, 1976.

57. Keys A, Taylor HL, Blackburn H et al: Mortality in coronary heart disease among men studied for 23 years. Arch Intern Med 128:201–214, 1971.

58. Thomas CB, Greenstreet RL: Psychobiological characteristics in youth as predictors of five disease states: suicide, mental illness, hypertension, coronary heart disease and tumor. John Hopkins Med J 132:16–43, 1973.

59. Osler W: Lectures on angina pectoris and allied states. NY Med J 4:224, 1896.

60. Friedman M, Rosenman RH: Association of specific overt behavior pattern with blood and cardiovascular findings: blood cholesterol level, blood clotting time, incidence of arcus senilis and clinical coronary artery disease. JAMA 169:1286–1296, 1959.

61. Friedman M: Pathogenesis of Coronary Artery Disease. New York, McGraw-Hill, 1969.

62. Jenkins CD, Zyzanski SJ, Rosenman RH: Coronary-prone behavior: one pattern or several? Psychosom Med 40:25–43, 1978.

63. Theorell T, DeFaire U, Schalling D, Adamson U, Askevold F: Personality traits and psychophysiological reactions to a stressful interview

in twins with varying degrees of coronary heart disease. J Psychosom Res 23:89–99, 1979.

64. Rosenman RH, Friedman M, Straus R et al: A predictive study of coronary heart disease: The Western Collaborative Group Study. JAMA 189:15–22, 1964.

65. Jenkins CD, Rosenman RH, Friedman M: Development of an objective psychological test for the determination of the coronary-prone behavior pattern in employed men. J Chronic Dis 20:371–379, 1967.

66. Rosenman RH, Brand RJ, Sholtz RI, Friedman M: Multivariate prediction of coronary heart disease during 8.5 year follow-up in the Western Collaborative Group Study. Am J Cardiol 37:903–910, 1976.

67. Brand RJ, Rosenman RH, Sholtz RI, Friedman M: Multivariate prediction of coronary heart disease in the Western Collaborative Group Study compared to the findings of the Framingham Study. Circulation 53:348–355, 1976.

68. Friedman M, Rosenman RH, Straus R, Wurm M, Kositchek R: The relationship of behavior pattern A to the state of the coronary vasculature. Am J Med 44:525–537, 1968.

69. Zyzanski SJ, Jenkins CD, Ryan TJ, Flessas A, Everst M: Psychological correlates of coronary angiographic findings. Arch Intern Med 136:1234–1237, 1976.

70. Frank KA, Heller SS, Kornfeld DS, Sporn AA, Weiss MB: Type A behavior pattern in coronary angiographic findings. JAMA 240:761–763, 1978.

71. Blumenthal JA, Williams RB, Cong Y et al: Type A behavior pattern and coronary atherosclerosis. Circulation 58:634–639, 1978.

72. Dimsdale JE, Hutter AM, Gilbert J, Hackett TP, Block PC, Catanzano DM: Predicting results of coronary angiography. Am Heart J 98:281–286, 1979.

73. Kones RJ: Emotional stress, plasma catecholamines, cardiac risk factors, and atherosclerosis. Angiology. 30:327–336, 1979.

74. Cassem NH, Hackett TP: The setting of intensive care. In Hackett, Cassem (eds.), Massachusetts General Hospital Handbook of General Hospital Psychiatry, St. Louis, CV Mosby, 1978, pp. 319–341.

75. Saltin B, Blomqvist G, Mitchell JH et al.: Response to exercise after bedrest and after training. Circulation 38 (suppl VII):1, 1968.

76. Hellerstein HK: Rehabilitation of the postinfarction patient. Hosp Pract 7:45, 1972.

76a. McLane M, Krop H, Mehta J: Psychosexual adjustment and counseling after myocardial infarction. Ann Int Med 92:514–519, 1980.

77. Tennessee Heart Association: Physician's Handbook for Evaluation of Cardiovascular and Physical Fitness, 2nd ed., Nashville, Tenn, 1972.

78. Davidson DM, Winchester MA, Taylor CB, Alderman EA, Ingel NB: Effects of relaxation therapy on cardiac performance and sympathetic activity in patients with organic heart disease. Psychosom Med 41:303–309, 1979.

79. Eliot RS, Forker AD: Emotional stress and cardiac disease. J Am Med Assoc 236:2325–2326, 1976.

80. Jenkins CD, Zyzanski SJ, Rosenman RH: Risk of a new myocardial infarction in middle-aged men with manifest coronary heart disease. Circulation 53:342–355, 1976.

81. Suinn RM, Brock L, Edie CA: Behavior therapy for type A patients. Am J Cardiol 36:269, 1975.

82. Rosenman RH, Friedman M: Modifying type A behaviour pattern. J Psychosom Res 21:323–331, 1977.

83. Rahe RH, Ward HW, Hayes V: Brief group therapy in myocardial infarction rehabilitation: Three- to four-year follow-up of a controlled trial. Psychosom Med 41:229–242, 1979.

# 35 | Pulmonary Problems in the CCU

*Roger G. Spragg, M.D.*
*Kenneth M. Moser, M.D.*

## CHRONIC OBSTRUCTIVE PULMONARY DISEASE

In patients admitted to the coronary care unit, the presence of chronic obstructive pulmonary disease (COPD) may complicate management in several different ways. First, an exacerbation or complication of COPD may *mimic* acute cardiac disease. Second, certain physiologic consequences of COPD—in exacerbation, particularly—can *induce* cardiac dysfunction. Third, COPD can obscure the presence of cardiac disease by interfering with standard clinical and laboratory approaches to cardiac diagnosis.

Before exploring the specifics of each of these potential management problems, let us explore the major pulmonary and hemodynamic consequences of COPD.

In "pure" *chronic bronchitis,* the central anatomic problem is narrowing of the airways due to edema of the bronchial wall and the presence of excess secretions in the bronchial lumen.[1-3] Physiologically, this translates into an increased resistance to airflow during both inspiration and expiration, and, therefore, a substantial increase in the work of breathing. Because the airway narrowing is not uniform, the distribution of ventilation within the lungs is uneven, leading to ventilation/perfusion abnormalities. Thus, some areas receive excessive ventilation; some, not enough.[4] This maldistribution impairs pulmonary gas exchange, resulting initially in alveolar (and, therefore, arterial) hypoxemia. In

acute exacerbations of chronic bronchitis, all of these derangements worsen. Gas exchange becomes even more markedly impaired with the development of alveolar and arterial *hypercapnia* as well as hypoxemia. This acute rise in arterial $PaCO_2$ leads to systemic acidosis.

These events have significant hemodynamic consequences. Alveolar hypoxia and hypercapnia both serve to *constrict* the resistance vessels in the lung, as does acidosis of the mixed venous blood. Thus, pulmonary arterial hypertension results.[5] In stable chronic bronchitis, in which only modest alveolar and arterial hypoxia are present, the elevation in pulmonary artery pressure also is quite modest.[6] However, in exacerbation, with significant reduction in $PaO_2$, and elevation of $PaCO_2$ and acidosis, a substantial degree of pulmonary hypertension can develop acutely and lead to the rapid onset of right ventricular failure. The propensity for the chronic bronchitic to follow this sequence is expressed in the clinical description of such patients as "blue bloaters"; i.e., they are cyanotic with dependent edema due to acute right ventricular failure.[7] Thus, pulmonary hypertension (and right ventricular failure) are inevitable concomitants of exacerbations of chronic bronchitis.

In "pure" *emphysema,* the anatomic problem is destruction of alveolar walls; the airways, per se, are not involved.[3] The major result of this lesion is a loss of lung elasticity or lung "recoil." Normally, inspiration is an active event: a negative pleural pressure is generated by inspiratory muscle contraction (chiefly that of the diaphragm), and the lungs are inflated. However, *expiration* normally is a *passive* event. The inspiratory muscles relax, the elastic lungs "recoil," and air is expelled. In emphysema, elastic recoil is diminished; therefore, energy must be expended to achieve expiration. Thus, the energy cost of breathing is increased. Furthermore, active expiration is associated with a more positive pleural pressure than is normally present; this tends to compress the airways during expiration, further increasing the work of breathing. Gas exchange also may be impaired in emphysema, due to an *uneven* distribution of alveolar destruction and loss of lung elasticity. The consequence is the development of ventilation/perfusion disturbances. However, these result in only modest alterations in arterial $PaCO_2$ and $PaO_2$, for two reasons: (1) These patients tend to maintain a high level of minute ventilation; and (2) Capillary loss obviously accompanies alveolar destruction, thus minimizing the extent of ventilation/perfusion mismatch.[8]

Therefore, hemodynamic alterations are modest in the patient with emphysema until parenchymal loss is very severe. Then mild pulmonary hypertension appears due to loss of vascular bed.[6-9] However, ultimately most patients with emphysema develop respiratory failure—that is, an inability to maintain normal gas exchange. Alveolar and arterial hypoxia and hypercapnia occur—with the same effects on the resistance vessels in the lung as described previously. Respiratory failure most commonly occurs because of either infection or the sedative effects of drugs. With recovery from exacerbation, and return of gas exchange toward normal, pulmonary hypertension also abates.[6]

*Asthma,* the third of the chronic obstructive lung diseases, is best considered as a state in which the tracheobronchial tree is hyperreactive to various stimuli. The stimuli may include irritant gases (e.g., "smog"), cold air, specific allergens, or the products of inflammation. The hyperreactivity includes three elements: constriction of bronchial smooth muscle, mucosal edema, and production of secretions. All three of these responses serve to narrow the bronchi (and perhaps obstruct them in the case of secretions). As might be expected, the pulmonary and gas exchange consequences are the same as those described for chronic bronchitis. However, the bronchial narrowing and obstruction are characteristically episodic ("attacks"), and lung function may be totally normal between episodes. If the attack is severe enough, acute respiratory failure may occur, leading to acute pulmonary hypertension and right ventricular failure.

These are the basic events in the "pure" forms of COPD. While such "pure" entities do exist in some patients, most commonly there is some mixture of the abnormalities described. A large group of patients exists with dominant chronic bronchitis, but some element of emphysema; and many of these patients also have some hyperreactivity of the airways. Likewise, many dominantly emphysematous patients have a degree of chronic bronchitis.

How do these facts relate to the management of patients admitted to the CCU? As stated at the outset, they can lead to diagnostic and management problems in three ways: mimicking primary cardiac problems, inducing them, or obscuring their presence. It should be noted that many patients with significant COPD go unrecognized for years. Therefore, most are *not* admitted to a CCU wearing a "label" stamped "COPD is present here, beware diagnostic confusion." But even were such a label present, diagnostic problems would (and do) occur.

## MIMICKING INTRINSIC CARDIAC DISEASE

The dominant complaint of patients with COPD is *dyspnea*. Patients admitted to the CCU with acute left ventricular (LV) failure share this symptom; and, in fact, patients with COPD often are treated initially for LV failure.

There are some historical clues which may aid in the differential diagnosis. Patients with COPD usually complain of dyspnea with *effort.* They are without dyspnea at rest and rarely complain of paroxysmal nocturnal dyspnea. (However, some COPD patients do have dyspnea during sleep which is due to a worsening of bronchoconstriction. Usually, effort dyspnea has been present previously.) Unfortunately, an exacerbation of COPD (due to a viral or other infection, or some exposure provoking bronchospasm) can present with acute dyspnea, and the patient may then be more dyspneic while recumbent than while sitting.

Physical examination may also be misleading.[10,11] Patients with COPD, particularly in exacerbation, often have bibasilar rales and rhonchi due to secretions in airways. Thoracic configuration may be helpful if the patient has advanced emphysema with a "barrel-shaped chest;" however, many patients with COPD do *not* have an increased antero-posterior diameter, and older patients with LV failure may have a kyphosis suggesting (falsely) that lung hyperinflation is present. A better indication of COPD is marked limitation of diaphragmatic descent. Hyperresonance to percussion may also provide a clue.

Cardiac examination also may be deceptive in patients with COPD. Cardiac auscultation may be difficult because of damping of heart sounds and murmurs by lung hyperinflation and the presence of adventitial sounds. A third heart sound may be present (indicating right, not left, ventricular failure). Accentuation of the pulmonary closure sound may be present, but this does not distinguish pulmonary hypertension due to LV failure from that resulting from the pulmonary anatomic-pathophysiologic events that occur in COPD. The same is true of other physical findings such as hepatomegaly, peripheral edema, jugular venous distension, and cyanosis.

Laboratory studies may be of value. The chest radiograph may disclose hyperinflation of the lungs, low and flat diaphragms, and an increase in the retrosternal air space. Further, it may *fail* to disclose the upward shift in pulmonary perfusion characteristic of pulmonary *venous* hypertension. However, peribronchial inflammation in COPD may be interpreted as pulmonary "vascular" congestion. Examination of the cardiac silhouette may be helpful in showing either the "small" heart associated with lung hyperinflation or the classic upward "rounding" of the left border indicative of right ventricular enlargement.

Arterial blood gas analysis will disclose hypoxemia in COPD, but this also occurs with acute LV failure.[12] As noted below, hypercapnia may occur with LV failure, although it does signify that significant lung disease also is present. Metabolic acidosis can occur with either right ventricular (RV) or LV failure if the cardiac output becomes inadequate.

An hematocrit determination may disclose erythrocytosis in COPD patients who have been chronically hypoxemic; and the white blood cell count may be increased if infection is present. But both these abnormalities may be absent despite an exacerbation of COPD.

The electrocardiogram may be of differential value in that the classical findings of an acute myocardial infarction are absent in COPD. However, COPD in exacerbation can be associated with a variety of dysrhythmias; low voltage due to lung hyperinflation may render the EKG difficult to interpret; cardiac rotation may suggest a loss of anterior forces in the precordial leads; and nonspecific ST-T changes are common. In a recent study, we found the ECG to be of no value in distinguishing between COPD patients with and without LV failure.[10]

Thus, in summary, the patient with COPD in exacerbation can closely mimic the patient with LV failure due to myocardial injury or disease. Sudden onset of dyspnea in a patient who demonstrates pulmonary rales, a third heart sound, peripheral edema, and cyanosis often leads the physician away from the correct diagnosis, particularly in the older patient with a vague history of chest discomfort. This ability of COPD to mimic LV failure is important because, as will be noted below, good treatment for the latter may be bad treatment for the former.

## CARDIAC DYSFUNCTION AS A CONSEQUENCE OF COPD

As has been discussed above, pulmonary hypertension, right ventricular dilatation, hypertrophy, and failure are all common in severe, chronic COPD; and rapid accentuation of pulmonary hypertension and RV dysfunction can occur acutely when alveolar hypoxia and/or hypercapnia develop. Dysrhythmias of virtually any type also may develop in these patients, leading to further hemodynamic compromise.[13] Dysrhythmias seem chiefly related to hypoxemia, although acidosis and catecholamine release related to these events also may play a role.

But beyond these well-documented events, there is the question of whether left ventricular performance is altered in patients with chronic obstructive lung disease.[10,11,14-16] There is no doubt that left ventricular dysfunction occurs in patients who have left ventricular *disease* as well as COPD; e.g., systemic hypertension, myocardial infarction, or myocarditis. But there is controversy as to whether COPD, per se, can cause alterations of LV performance. Definitive answers are not yet available. Some studies have suggested that hypoxemia and acidosis can adversely affect LV performance; and, of course, arterial hypoxemia may compromise myocardial oxygenation. Less clear is whether RV hypertrophy and dilatation, due to lung disease, can adversely affect LV performance. Data available to date suggest that there may be mild changes in LV pressure-volume characteristics secondary to RV hypertrophy-dilatation, but that left ventricular ejection fraction is not altered.[14-17]

In summary, then, RV dysfunction and dysrhythmias are common in COPD. Also, hypoxemia and acidosis associated with COPD (especially in exacerbation) may induce LV dysfunction in patients with latent or overt LV disease; and, in cases of severe hypoxemia/acidosis, perhaps in patients without intrinsic myocardial disease. But COPD per se, even when it leads to significant RV hypertrophy and dilatation, does not appear to compromise LV performance in a clinically significant way.

## ABILITY OF COPD TO OBSCURE LV FAILURE

Patients with COPD are subject to the development of left ventricular failure from all of the usual causes, including myocardial infarction. Just as an exacerbation of COPD may be misinterpreted as an episode of LV failure, so may the onset of LV failure be misinterpreted as an exacerbation of COPD[10-12]—and for the same reasons cited above. Hyperinflation and adventitious lung sounds may render cardiac auscultation and percussion difficult; the murmurs of mitral or aortic valvular disease may be difficult to hear or may be atypical. An audible third heart sound may be of right or left ventricular origin. Jugular venous distension and other indicators of right ventricular failure may have a primary right ventricular (COPD) origin or be secondary to left ventricular failure. Finally, patients with lung disease may have chest discomfort which suggests angina or coronary insufficiency. In our own investigations, we have found that some 15 percent of patients with significant COPD who present with increasing dyspnea prove to have left ventricular failure.[10,11,16]

## DISTINGUISHING COPD FROM LV FAILURE

There is one final point worth noting in this context; namely, that LV failure can *induce* respiratory failure in the patient with COPD. Specifically, the pulmonary mechanical alterations promoted by interstitial and alveolar edema may, by further compromising the respiratory apparatus, lead to frank respiratory failure (hypercapnia, acidosis, and hypoxemia). Thus, we have come full circle in this discussion—from COPD in exacerbation masquerading as LV failure, to LV failure masquerading as an exacerbation of COPD.

These considerations make it clear that the patient with COPD who complains of sudden or increasing dyspnea presents a significant challenge in differential diagnosis in the CCU. Equally evident is that this diagnostic challenge is not easily met. The first step toward resolution is the recognition of this fact; the second is vigilance regarding the presence of COPD in patients admitted to the CCU. There is a tendency (understandable) to think "cardiac" first in patients admitted to the CCU and "pulmonary" first in patients admitted to the Respiratory ICU. A high index of suspicion is the best safeguard against diagnostic error in both locations.

However, even armed with such suspicion, the differential diagnostic task is not easy. Our own investigations have indicated that an accurate differential diagnosis often is *not* possible despite careful history taking and physical examination, and detailed review of standard laboratory tests.[10,11] Thus, the only definitive way out of this diagnostic dilemma is the use of techniques which directly or indirectly assess left ventricular performance. Unfortunately, one of the simplest approaches—measurement of systolic time intervals—is worthless in the COPD patient.[11,18,19] However, three other methods have been shown to be useful: right heart catheterization with a balloon tip catheter, echocardiographic assessment of left ventricular function, and radionuclide assessment of left (and right) ventricular performance.[9–11,15–17] It has now been shown that each of these approaches can resolve the question: is left ventricular dysfunction present in the patient with COPD? Local access and expertise often will dictate which of the techniques is most widely applied in a given CCU. We have moved from right heart catheterization to echocardiography and, more recently, chiefly to radionuclide methods because we have a portable scintillation camera and other supporting personnel and facilities that make this approach readily accessible. But the central fact is that one of these methods should be applied if the differential diagnosis is to be made accurately.

## THERAPEUTIC IMPLICATIONS

Considering the complexities of the differential diagnosis, a reasonable question is, "What harm would be done by making a mistake and treating empirically? Specifically, what harm would result from treating all COPD patients with increasing dyspnea as if they had left ventricular failure—and vice versa?"

Aside from the desire for academic "purity," there are substantive reasons for not taking this approach. Let us first examine the consequences of treating COPD in exacerbation as LV failure. The classical treatment for acute LV failure

would include digitalization, diuresis, sedation, and, perhaps, supplementary oxygen. All of these are potential "negatives" in the management of COPD in exacerbation.

Digitalis is of no proven benefit in the patient with RV failure due to COPD (in the absence of atrial dysrhythmias). Furthermore, the risk of inducing dysrhythmias with digitalis in the COPD patient appears to be enhanced by the presence of hypoxemia and, perhaps, by acidosis.[20,21] Thus, digitalis is of equivocal value—and potential hazard—in these patients.

Diuresis is relatively contraindicated in such patients, in whom drying of secretions is to be avoided. Thus, withholding fluid or inducing a diuresis, or both, are potential negatives in COPD in exacerbation.

Sedation is a clear negative, even though patients with COPD in exacerbation may be anxious or agitated. The reason is that no sedative (especially morphine) is devoid of respiratory depressant qualities—and any central respiratory depression in the COPD patient may worsen or provoke respiratory failure.

A similar hazard accompanies oxygen use. Oxygen must be given cautiously to the patient with COPD who has chronic hypercapnia. In such patients, oxygen doses that are perfectly safe in the patient with cardiogenic pulmonary edema (2 to 4 l/min) may promote serious respiratory depression with worsening hypercapnia and acidosis.

There is one commonly used drug which may be beneficial despite diagnostic error: aminophylline. The bronchodilator and respiratory stimulant attributes of aminophylline are useful in treating most COPD patients—and its diuretic effects are useful in treating the cardiac failure patient. Further, by reducing RV afterload, aminophylline may improve RV performance.[22] However, this agent may increase heart rate unacceptably in the patient with acute myocardial infarction. Of course, special hazard is posed to the COPD patient by propanolol or other β-blocking drugs. The bronchospastic potential of these agents in patients with airways disease is now widely appreciated.

Thus, standard therapy for LV failure presents several real and potential hazards for the patient who actually has COPD in exacerbation. But an even greater negative is what is *not* done. Assumption that LV failure is present leads to neglect of those modalities which the COPD patient needs most: bronchial cleansing maneuvers, bronchodilatation, careful monitoring of gas exchange, treatment of pulmonary infection, and, perhaps, assisted ventilation. These basic interventions also constitute the best treatment for RV failure secondary to respiratory failure because they improve pulmonary gas exchange and relieve pulmonary arterial constriction.

Thus, treating COPD in exacerbation as if it were LV failure is fraught with hazards of commission and omission.

A similar scenario attaches to the reverse: neglecting LV failure in the patient with COPD. The most effective regimen of respiratory care will not help the patient with LV failure. This patient needs digitalization and the other elements of a vigorous cardiac regimen. Furthermore, the use of large doses of corticosteroids and/or of sympathomimetics with mixed $\beta_1$ and $\beta_2$ agonist effects—often used with good effect in COPD—are relatively contraindicated in most patients with cardiogenic pulmonary edema. Corticosteroids may worsen fluid retention; isoproterenol may provide undesirable chronotropic and dysrhythmic effects. So-called "more pure" $\beta_2$ agonist drugs such as terbutaline also have $\beta_1$ agonist effects that may not be desirable in the face of left ventricular failure.

## CONCLUSIONS

The differentiation of "deteriorating" COPD from left ventricular failure in the patient with coexistent COPD is a common problem in the CCU. Accurate differentiation is important because of the therapeutic implications. Pulmonary artery catheterization and echocardiographic or radionuclide assessment of ventricular function are available to make this differential—and often are required because of the nondiagnostic nature of clinical assessment and standard laboratory technics. A high index of suspicion, and recognition of the often con-fusing nature of this differential, are the best safeguards against diagnostic and therapeutic error.

## PULMONARY EMBOLISM

Pulmonary embolism arises in two contexts among patients admitted to or residing in CCUs: (1) most commonly, as a complication of deep venous thrombosis of the lower extremities; and (2) rarely, as a complication of right atrial or ventricular mural thrombosis.

Clinically, the need to consider pulmonary embolism appears at two points in time in the CCU: (1) on admission as part of the differential diagnosis; (2) during the course of admission for a known cardiac disorder (e.g., myocardial infarction).

**On Admission.** The myriad of presentations of pulmonary embolism include a number that mimic acute, primary cardiac disorders. Severe, nonpleuritic substernal chest pain can follow embolism of extensive degree (but rarely embolism involving one lobe or less). This pain, somehow induced by acute pulmonary hypertension, is usually associated with severe dyspnea, diaphoresis, anxiety, and tachycardia and/or atrial or ventricular dysrhythmias.[23,24,25] The chest radiograph is usually within normal limits, because infarction is rare and, if present, requires 24 hours or more to achieve radiographic expression. For the same reasons, hemoptysis is uncommon. The electrocardiogram most commonly discloses a tachycardia and nondiagnostic ST and T wave changes. Most patients do not have clinically obvious venous thrombosis (< 50 percent). Therefore, many such patients are admitted to the CCU to rule out myocardial infarction and hours to days may elapse before pulmonary embolism is diagnosed.

Syncope, on occasion associated with a dysrhythmia, is another less common presenting complaint. This event can suggest a primary cardiac disorder, particularly since dyspnea often persists after recovery from syncope. Finally, dyspnea or syncope on effort are often complaints of patients who have suffered and survived massive (but clinically inapparent) major embolism weeks or months before.[26]

The second context in which embolism is encountered on admission to the CCU is among patients with *known* cardiac disease who undergo unexplained clinical deterioration: particularly dysrhythmia, worsening of dyspnea, and/or evidence of pulmonary edema or syncope. Pulmonary embolism is always a candidate to explain such deterioration.

**During Admission.** It is now well established, from studies utilizing radio-labeled fibrinogen leg scanning, that deep venous thrombosis is a common consequence of myocardial infarction—occurring in 17 to 22 percent of patients.[27-29] This is not surprising, in view of the stasis induced by the immobility (bed rest) in the early stages of management. It is likely, though not established, that venous thrombosis is especially common in the patient with other risk factors in addition to infarction—e.g., left ventricular failure, obesity, varicosities, or prior history of thromboembolism. While any patient with venous thrombosis is at potential risk of embolism, it is becoming clear that the risk of clinically significant embolism is quite low with thrombi limited to the calf veins but is substantially higher with thrombi involving veins above the knee.[27-30] Unfortunately, the incidence of embolism (and lethal embolism) is not yet well established in patients with myocardial infarction, though the embolic risk is substantially less than that of deep venous thrombosis.[27-29] Also not well established is the incidence of mural thrombus in infarction and of embolic risk from this site.

Patients admitted to the CCU with cardiac disease other than infarction also are at significant risk of deep venous thrombosis and embolism; but virtually no solid incidence data are available in this patient group (e.g., those with left and/or right ventricular failure due to such diverse entities as hypertensive cardiac disease, myocardiopathy, coronary artery disease, valvular disease and congenital cyanotic and acyanotic heart diseases). What is clear is that these patients are at increased embolic risk (vis-a-vis the normal population) and that a frequent cause for deterioration in a previously stable patient is embolism.

**Diagnostic Approach.** In the patient who presents to the CCU with an acute syndrome that mimics cardiac disease, pulmonary embolism should be in the differential diagnosis. As data accumulate from clinical and laboratory tests which cast doubt on the cardiac diagnosis (e.g., myocardial infarction), a perfusion lung scan should be obtained. Mobile cameras are now available to perform this study at the bedside in many institutions and, even when they are not, a strong suspicion warrants movement of the patient to obtain the study. A negative perfusion scan rules out the diagnosis.[23,31] If a positive scan is obtained, this may suffice as a diagnostic test, depending upon the sum of the other data available and the safety of anticoagulant therapy. If a higher degree of diagnostic specificity is desired, a ventilation scan[32] is the next logical step (if available), and pulmonary angiography is reserved for those in whom the highest degree of diagnostic certitude is required.[33,34] Other diagnostic procedures—such as radiofibrinogen leg scanning or impedance phlebography—may add useful information by identifying the embolic source in the legs.[35-38]

This same diagnostic sequence is useful in patients with previously "stable" cardiac disease who are admitted because of sudden deterioration in clinical status.

A different approach is now available to *monitor* patients admitted to the CCU *without* embolism but at risk of developing it (e.g., the patient with myocardial infarction). This approach consists of using radiolabelled fibrinogen leg scanning and impedance phlebography serially to detect the onset of deep venous thrombosis.[35-38] Such monitoring is an alternative to prophylactic anticoagulation (see below). Because venous thrombosis so often escapes clinical detection, *clinical* monitoring (e.g., daily leg examination), is not an adequate alternative.

**Therapy.** "Full-dose" heparin is the drug of choice in virtually all patients in whom the diagnosis of embolism is seriously entertained or established.[39] If the diagnosis is considered strongly, heparinization should *not* await laboratory confirmation unless relative contraindications to heparin therapy exist.

The "best" regimen for heparin administration and the ideal method(s) for monitoring that regimen are not established. These controversies have recently been reviewed elsewhere, as have been supportive measures that may be useful in major embolism.[40,41]

When to use thrombolytic agents in pulmonary embolism also is an unresolved issue.[25] At best, their toxic/therapeutic ratio is such that they should be reserved for the patient with serious cardiopulmonary compromise due to embolism.

The drug of choice for treating deep venous thrombosis also is heparin, with the same choices (and controversies) regarding regimen and monitoring. There is question as to whether thrombi limited to the calf merit therapy, in view of their low embolic risk; but firm data do not yet exist which warrant withholding of therapy. There is no controversy about "above knee" thrombi. They should be treated.

What about the patient admitted to the CCU without venous thrombosis who is "at risk" of this complication (e.g., patients with myocardial infarction)? Two major alternatives now exist: (1) monitor patients with radio-labeled fibrinogen and impedance phlebography, treating those who become positive; (2) place all such patients on "mini-dose heparin" (5000 units subcutaneously every 12 hours). The risk involved in mini-dose heparin therapy is modest indeed,[42,43] except in patients with known contraindications to anticoagulant drugs (e.g., severe hypertension, or bleeding diathesis). Parenthetically, the risk of hemorrhagic pericarditis during mini-dose heparin therapy in patients with myocardial infarction seems to be extremely low.[27-29] As better data become available regarding the incidence of deep venous thrombosis, embolism and fatal embolism in subgroups of patients with cardiac disease, indications for both monitoring and prophylaxis will become more discrete. At the moment, no "hard and fast" mandates exist.

As to prophylactic alternatives to mini-dose heparin, no major ones currently exist.[40] Warfarin is probably effective but more cumbersome (and probably more hazardous); dextran is not established as efficacious, nor is it a wise choice in patients with cardiac disease; and antiplatelet agents (e.g., aspirin) have not been shown to be effective.

## THE ADULT RESPIRATORY DISTRESS SYNDROME (ARDS)

The occurrence of the adult respiratory distress syndrome in patients within a CCU is an uncommon, though by no means rare, event. However, it is important to recognize this form of noncardiogenic pulmonary edema and to distinguish it from cardiogenic edema of the lungs. Also, patients with ARDS may develop hypoxic myocardial injury because of the primary failure in gas exchange. Care of these patients requires minute-to-minute attention to details of mechanical ventilation, fluid balance, and cardiac function and may be both disruptive and difficult in an environment unused to their presence.

It has become apparent to clinicians that insults to the pulmonary parenchyma of diverse nature may have rather similar acute clinical, physiologic, and histologic consequences, and it has become convenient to recognize these consequences as a syndrome termed the adult respiratory distress syndrome. The similar responses to pulmonary injuries related to such events as aspiration or systemic sepsis have made the creation of a "syndrome" useful.

Certain elements are uniformly seen when observing a patient with ARDS. A well-defined and discrete clinical event is frequently recognized which precedes and is felt to be the cause of the eventual pulmonary injury. Following this event there is often an interval of apparent normal pulmonary function. However, the rapid onset and progression of pulmonary dysfunction quickly terminate this interval. Patients become dyspneic, and hypoxemia quickly appears. The lungs become increasingly stiff, and diffuse infiltrates become apparent on the chest radiographs. In the absence of appropriate intervention, death may occur within hours.[44]

A large number of insults have been reported to have an etiologic relationship to the adult respiratory distress syndrome.[45] Cardiogenic, hemorrhagic, and septic shock states have all been reported in association with this injury. Bacterial, fungal and viral infections as well as parasitic and mycoplasma infections have been reported to result in ARDS. Exposure to inhaled, ingested, or parenteral toxins may also produce this syndrome. Among those drugs or toxins reported to cause ARDS are heroin, methadone, propoxyphene, colchicine, and oxygen.

Multiple immunologic reactions including anaphylaxis and allergic alveolar reactions to inhaled materials may also cause diffuse pulmonary injury. Certain hematologic insults, including disseminated intravascular coagulation and multiple transfusions; trauma causing either direct contusion of the lung or the syndrome of fat embolism; and central nervous system diseases of multiple etiologies have also been related to the onset of ARDS. Finally, both aspiration of gastric contents and certain metabolic aberrations such as uremia and pancreatitis may cause ARDS.

It is thus apparent that, while the uncomplicated patient with myocardial infarction has little reason to develop ARDS, the patient with complicating pathologic conditions such as trauma, infection, adverse drug reaction, or aspiration may be at risk for the development of this form of noncardiogenic pulmonary edema.

At the present time the pathophysiologic mechanisms which trigger this injury are unknown. Because of the similar characteristics seen despite the different cause of events, it is tempting to think that there may be final common pathways mediating the injury. The final pathways appear to include an increase in permeability of the pulmonary capillaries to water and plasma proteins, and this may be a constant feature in the adult respiratory distress syndrome.[46] It appears, at times, that this increased permeability is not limited to capillary endothelial surfaces within the lung but is also seen throughout the body.

Although the diagnosis of ARDS rests on clinical and physiologic observations, lung tissue is frequently available for examination following either transbronchial or open biopsy or at postmortem examination. Gross edema and, frequently, hemorrhage of the lungs are evident. Microscopic examination shows leakage of erythrocytes into interstitial and alveolar spaces. The alveolar septa and peribronchial areas are edematous. Plasma and red cells are present in alveolar and interstitial areas. Pro-

teinaceous material and cellular debris are often seen filling alveoli, and large portions of the lung may show alveolar collapse. Type I pneumocytes are lost and replaced by Type II pneumocytes. Frequently, hyaline membranes are seen lining damaged alveolar ducts and alveoli.[47,48]

Physiologic changes in patients with ARDS are both profound and dramatic. The consequence of increased leak of the capillary membrane with loss of fluid into the pulmonary parenchyma is that the lung becomes markedly stiffer—that is, compliance of the lung falls. This becomes evident in the intubated patient as greater and greater pressures are required to produce the same degree of pulmonary inflation with the mechanical ventilator. In the nonintubated patient, an increased work of breathing occurs and may be perceived as dyspnea. Secondly, the functional residual capacity (the volume of air in the lungs at the end of a passive expiration) decreases because of the increased recoil of the lungs. The oxygen tension in arterial blood falls, and the difference between the oxygen tension in alveolar gas and that in arterial blood increases. This is due predominantly to the shunting of venous blood through nonventilated regions of the lung. However, regions of very low ventilation which may continue to be perfused also contribute to this widened alveolar-arterial oxygen gradient. Finally, there may be an impairment of oxygen diffusion across the greatly thickened alveolar membranes. Thus, shunt, ventilation-perfusion mismatch, and perhaps also a diffusion abnormality, can contribute to the marked hypoxemia.[49-50]

Several factors may cause an increase in the resistance to blood flow through the pulmonary vasculature. As hypoxemia develops, reactive vasoconstriction narrows the cross-sectional area of the pulmonary vascular bed. There is some suggestion that aggregates of circulating platelets and white cells may occur and cause obstruction of pulmonary capillaries.[51] Additionally, release of mediators from platelets within the lung may cause pulmonary vasoconstriction and an increase in pulmonary artery pressure.[52] The increase in pulmonary vascular resistance, which is uniformly seen in severe cases of ARDS, may cause failure of the right ventricle.[53]

Physical examination of the patient with ARDS often shows a tachypneic, cyanotic individual with a rapid heartbeat. Chest examination is often remarkable for the absence of rales, rhonchi, or wheezes. This finding is consistent with the presence of edema fluid largely confined to interstitial spaces rather than in airways. Routine studies obtained from the clinical chemistry and hematology laboratories are nondiagnostic. Arterial blood gas analysis establishes the presence of profound hypoxemia. The chest x-ray film often shows a diffuse haziness which may or may not be uniform. No specific electrocardiographic changes are associated with ARDS.

In considering the differential diagnosis of this syndrome, one must think particularly of local infectious processes within the lung which require specific diagnosis and treatment. The most commonly seen are bacterial pneumonias. In the acutely ill patient with rapidly advancing pulmonary infiltrates, it is now our practice to perform bronchoscopy and obtain brushings from the lower airways in a sterile fashion using the Bartlett catheter. This technique appears to avoid contamination from organisms in the upper airway and to be successful in recovering organisms responsible for the infection.[54] Other diagnostic maneuvers to evaluate the presence of infection include obtaining blood cultures, material for viral cultures, and serum for viral, mycoplasmal, and fungal serologies.

The second point to be considered in the differential diagnosis of this syndrome is whether LV failure is either causing or contributing to the diffuse edema. While determination of the clearance of serum protein into bronchoalveolar fluid might be expected to be relatively high in ARDS and relatively low in cardiogenic pulmonary edema,[55] samples for such measurements are frequently unavailable. The protein content of edema fluid reflects the relative presence or absence of a leak of serum proteins seen in ARDS or cardiogenic pulmonary edema, respectively.

Studies in our institution have attempted to evaluate the success of noninvasive methods diagnosing LV failure in this setting; it has been our conclusion that, without invasive measurement of pulmonary artery and pulmonary artery wedge pressures, such differentiation is difficult.[56] While radionuclide and echocardiographic techniques may allow noninvasive evaluation of cardiac performance, they do not provide an accurate estimate of pulmonary vascular pressures. For this reason, right heart catheterization is routinely performed in patients who are more than moderately ill with suspected ARDS.

The interpretation of pressure measurements obtained from the balloon tip catheter has been a matter of some discussion. Frequently, these patients require mechanical ventilation at elevated pressures, and there is concern that these pressures may be partially transmitted to the measuring catheter. While one would prefer to measure transmural pressure in order to evaluate as closely as possible forces tending to cause transudation of fluid across the pulmonary vasculature,[57] this measurement is unavailable when one is forced to measure the pressure in vessels relative to atmospheric pressure. Fortunately, it appears from clinical observations that, in patients with severely decreased compliance, little if any of the ventilating pressure is transmitted to the measuring catheter. This has been repeatedly demonstrated by measuring pressures on sequential cardiac cycles as high ventilating pressures are abruptly discontinued and then reinstituted. Changes of less than 1 or 2 mmHg are the rule.[58] Thus, if one sees elevated pulmonary artery wedge pressures in the patient with ARDS, this is consistent with LV failure. Additionally, with the thermal dilution cardiac output catheter in place, one has the capability of measuring cardiac output and obtaining mixed venous blood for analysis.

The cornerstone of treatment of a patient with ARDS is, first, to rule out the presence of "treatable" causes of the disease process. Secondly, one attempts to maintain an arterial oxygen tension sufficient to support life. Thirdly, meticulous attention is directed to the details involved in avoidng potentially fatal complications.

Both local and systemic infections are potentially treatable causes of the adult respiratory distress syndrome. It is our practice to institute antibiotic coverage based on the results of the gram stain of material obtained from the lower airway. If this examination is not helpful, broad spectrum antibiotic coverage is instituted until culture results are available. In the immunocompromised patient, a very aggressive approach to the diagnosis of infection is fully warranted and may only be possible in the early hours of the patient's disease. Such an approach may involve not only the routine collection of blood, sputum, and urine cultures, but the early performance of invasive procedures to obtain brushings from both the distal airways and pulmonary tissue for examination.[59] Fungi or pneumocystis carinii may sometimes be discovered only in this fashion.

Additionally, allergic alveolitis, which may be suggested by an appropriate exposure history, is a second potentially treatable cause of ARDS and may respond dramatically to the use of intravenous corticosteroids.

The maintenance of an adequate arterial oxygen tension requires careful fluid and ventilator management. The adequacy of the cardiac output (C.O.) for supplying systemic oxygen needs may be evaluated by measuring the difference between arterial and venous oxygen content, $(A-\bar{V})\ DO_2$. This value, expressed in cc $O_2$/100 ml, when multiplied by the cardiac output in liters, equals systemic oxygen consumption $(\dot{M}O_2)$:

$$(A-\bar{V})\ DO_2 \times C.O. \times 10 = \dot{M}O_2$$

Accurate measurements of blood oxygen content are best made directly, (for example, on the Lex-$O_2$-Con by Lexington Laboratories) rather than by measuring gas tensions and assuming a normal oxyhemoglobin dissociation curve. Noting an $(A-\bar{V})\ DO_2$ above 5.5 cc $O_2$/100 ml suggests that the cardiac output is inadequate relative to the systemic needs. This may indicate either a need for interventions designed to raise cardiac output or strategies designed to lower $\dot{M}O_2$—for example, sedation or cooling.

There is some evidence now from several centers that the traditional concepts of oxygen delivery may not be completely valid in the setting of the adult respiratory distress syndrome. Under conditions of adequate cardiac output, increasing oxygen delivery (the product of arterial $O_2$ content and cardiac output) should not result in an increased oxygen consumption. However, in a number of patients with ARDS who had a normal $(A-\bar{V})\ DO_2$, oxygen uptake increased as oxygen delivery was increased. Thus, the usefulness of the $(A-\bar{V})\ DO_2$ to evaluate the adequacy of cardiac output in patients with ARDS has been brought into question.[60]

The Starling equation, which describes the balance between hydrostatic and oncotic forces acting across the capillary membrane, predicts the net flux of fluid into or out of the lung.[61] The therapeutic goal which one sets is to minimize the hydrostatic forces that contribute to extravasation of fluid across the pulmonary capillary membrane while maintaining adequate perfusion. Therefore, repeated determinations of cardiac output as the pulmonary artery wedge pressure is lowered by inducing volume loss are necessary to determine the minimum pressures which are consistent with an adequate cardiac output and adequate oxygen delivery.

The blood colloid osmotic pressure is another factor which is readily accessible to measurement and which may affect fluid flux in the lung. While the accurate determination of this factor is gaining in popularity, it has yet to be shown that alterations in colloid osmotic pressure in the setting of ARDS are of therapeutic benefit.[62]

The use of positive end-expiratory pressure (PEEP) has been well-demonstrated to increase the functional residual capacity and the arterial oxygen content in patients with ARDS.[63] It is possible to apply PEEP during continuous mechanical ventilation or during intermittent mandatory ventilation. In this latter mode, the patient is delivered a prescribed number of mechanical breaths per minute but has the ability to breathe spontaneously at other times. Positive airways pressures up to 60 or more cm of water have been used; however it is uncommon in most centers for the value of PEEP to be more than 18 to 22 cm of water. Even the use of these levels of pressure is commonly associated with a decrement in cardiac output.[64] The reasons for this are poorly understood but may involve multiple mechanisms.[65-66] The presence of an increase in the mean intrathoracic pressure may result in a significant "back pressure," causing a decrease in venous return to the right side of the heart. The increase in airway pressure may result in compression of the pulmonary vasculature, which may be either a passive phenomenon or an active phenomenon mediated through reflex mechanisms. This increased resistance may also limit cardiac output.

Thirdly, failure of the right ventricle may induce volume and compliance changes in the left ventricle which may contribute to diminishing cardiac output. As the right heart fails, the interventricular septum may be displaced, compromising the volume of the left ventricle. Also, if the pericardial compliance is low, an increase in right ventricular volume will limit left ventricular volume. A fourth consideration, which has been suggested by certain workers, is the effect of humoral depressors of myocardial function independent of other etiologies. Finally, there is indication from the animal laboratory that the use of PEEP may cause pulmonary distension and traction on the left atrium by the pulmonary veins. A decrease in left atrial volume with resulting increase in left atrial and pulmonary capillary pressures may be an additional hemodynamic effect of PEEP.

Whatever the possible etiologies, PEEP frequently does cause a decrease in cardiac output. Thus, the use of PEEP may be associated with both the bad news of a decreased cardiac output and the good news of an increased arterial oxygen content. The product of these two values, oxygen content and cardiac output, is termed oxygen delivery. It is expressed as the amount of oxygen per minute that is being delivered from the left ventricle to the systemic circulation, and it is an excellent indicator of the effectiveness of mechanical ventilation. In the absence of the ability to determine this value, either inadequate or overly high values of positive end-expiratory pressure may be applied with no indication to the physician of the error.

Recently, a cooperative NIH study has shown that the mortality in patients with ARDS requiring intubation and ventilation with at least 50 percent oxygen for 24 hours approaches 70 percent. Mortality increases as complications occur. These most commonly are thrombocytopenia, renal failure, sepsis, hypotension, pneumothorax, and gastrointestinal bleeding.[67] As the number of complications experienced by any one patient increases, his potential for mortality increases proportionately.

The pathogenetic mechanisms that result in the diffuse pulmonary injury seen in ARDS are currently the focus of numerous investigations. In the coming years, additional information should be available which should help guide not only the diagnosis but also the therapy and the prevention of the adult respiratory disease syndrome.

## SPECIFIC PULMONARY CONSEQUENCES OF ACUTE MYOCARDIAL INFARCTION

Patients experiencing acute myocardial infarction may develop several pulmonary consequences of that event. These may include dyspnea, an impaired ability to oxygenate pulmonary arterial blood, and alterations in static lung volumes.

The physiologic causes of dyspnea—the subjective sensation of being "short of breath"—are poorly understood. Alterations in arterial blood gas tensions sensed by the carotid body or by central nervous system chemoreceptors may provide one input to the sensation of dyspnea. A second input may come from stretch receptors within lung parenchyma. An increase in interstitial fluid within the lung, as may be seen with an increment in pulmonary capillary pressures following a myocardial infarction, may stimulate these receptors to fire transmitting impulses centrally via the vagus nerve.[68] Experimentally, induction of edema in dogs with alloxan has allowed identification of specific nerve axons with these properties.[69]

That oxygenation may be impaired following a myocardial infarction is well established.[70,71,72] The observed fall in the partial pressure of oxygen in arterial blood ($PaO_2$) is directly proportional to the degree of heart failure—measured either by clinical class or by quantitative pulmonary artery wedge pressure. Patients in clinical Class I (no evidence of heart failure) or with a mean wedge pressure less than 12 mmHg may show no evidence of impaired oxygenation. However, as clinical evaluation of heart failure worsens—Classes II, III, and IV—or as the wedge pressure becomes higher, ability to oxygenate blood falls proportionately.

What are the mechanisms that might explain this impairment of oxygenation? They include shunt, mismatch of ventilation and perfusion, and diffusion impairment in the transfer of gas.

In differentiating between shunt and ventilation/perfusion mismatch, the response to 100 percent oxygen breathing and the influence of changes in venous oxygen content on arterial oxygen content are valuable.

When areas of the lung are underventilated relative to the blood perfusing them, hypoxemia develops and is correctable with 100 percent oxygen. In addition, when poorly ventilated areas of the lung exist, a patient given 100 percent oxygen to breathe will show a prolonged washout of nitrogen. In contrast, when shunt is the major cause of hypoxemia, breathing 100 percent oxygen has little effect on the $PO_2$ of arterial blood. Because blood passing alveoli is almost fully saturated when room air is breathed, 100 percent oxygen breathing adds little more oxygen. When this blood mixes with shunted blood, the saturation falls. Consequently, arterial $PO_2$ in the presence of a substantial shunt is raised only minimally by breathing 100 percent $O_2$.

Venous oxygen content may fall under conditions of decreased cardiac output, anemia, or increased peripheral oxygen extraction. When venous—and also shunted—$PO_2$ is low, arterial $PO_2$ will fall when a substantial shunt is present. Such a fall may also occur when ventilation/perfusion mismatch is present. Failure of the arterial $PO_2$ to fall with a fall in mixed venous $PO_2$, however, suggests the absence of a significant shunt.

Several observations in patients with myocardial infarction suggest that of these two mechanisms, shunt and ventilation/perfusion mismatch, the latter is of more importance. First, administration of oxygen frequently is helpful in raising the $PaO_2$. Secondly, the cardiac index (and hence the venous $PO_2$) shows no correlation with the $PaO_2$.[70] Additionally, patients

with myocardial infarction and hypoxemia show prolongation of nitrogen wash-out.[73]

The precise mechanisms whereby increased pulmonary capillary pressures and increased extravascular lung water cause mismatch of ventilation and perfusion is unclear. It has been suggested that the function of small airways within the lung may be affected by this increase in extravascular water, resulting in a transiently increased closing volume following myocardial infarction.[74] When areas of the lung are "closed" to ventilation during part of the respiratory cycle, regional diminution of ventilation relative to perfusion may occur and cause hypoxemia. Such "closure" during ventilation has been demonstrated to be due to a fall in functional residual capacity as well as to a rise in the closing volume.[75]

Diffusion impairment in gas transfer from alveolus to capillary blood might be suspected in the face of edema, and might cause a fall in $PaO_2$. Although it is difficult to rule out this mechanism as contributing to the observed hypoxemia, measurements of the diffusing capacity of the lung for carbon monoxide have shown only minimal changes in patients with hypoxemia accompanying myocardial infarction.[70]

In addition to the relative hypoxemia seen following myocardial infarction, predictable changes in lung mechanics also occur. Vital capacity, total lung capacity, and residual volume all have been shown to decrease following acute myocardial infarction with return to normal in follow-up studies.[75] Multiple factors are most likely responsible for these reductions in lung volumes. Gas trapping within the lung may increase the noncommunicating air space and cause an apparent reduction in functional residual capacity and total lung capacity when measured by methods other than plethysmography or chest radiography. Studies have demonstrated that the reduction in vital capacity in patients with heart disease correlates with a fall in pulmonary compliance.[76] Additionally, studies in dogs have suggested that as pulmonary vascular engorgement occurs a reduction in outward recoil of the chest wall is seen.[77] Because these two forces—pulmonary compliance and recoil of the chest wall—help to determine the lung volumes in question, alterations in these volumes are likely to be explained by changes in compliance and chest wall recoil.

Investigations of dynamic pulmonary function have shown no evidence of increased large airway obstruction following myocardial infarction. However, changes consistent with an increase in small airways resistance at reduced lung volumes are seen.[78]

## Use of Mechanical Ventilation

The physician caring for patients who have sustained a myocardial infarction must be familiar with the techniques for controlling the airway and supplying mechanical ventilation. In the presence of a cardiopulmonary arrest, severe pulmonary edema, or acute respiratory failure complicating a myocardial infarction, it may be necessary to place an endotracheal tube using correct techniques.[79] With an endotracheal tube in place, functions of the upper airway are no longer possible, and it is necessary to insure that gas ventilating the patient is appropriately warmed and humidified. While nebulization of water droplets may be desirable to help mobilize pulmonary secretions, it should be kept in mind that large quantities of water may be inadvertently administered to a patient in this fashion.[80]

If mechanical ventilation is required, two distinct kinds of ventilators are available. The pressure-cycled ventilator forces air into a patient at a specified flow rate until a given pressure is achieved. Thus, the volume of gas delivered to the patient is dependent upon the patient's pulmonary compliance. In a setting where the pulmonary compliance may change drastically—as in developing congestive heart failure—the tidal volume achieved at a given pressure setting will also change significantly. Thus, a volume-cycled ventilator is frequently used in the care of critically ill patients with cardiopulmonary disease. This device delivers a preset volume to the patient at a prescribed flow rate, producing whatever pressure is necessary. To avoid extraordinarily high pressures, a pressure "pop off" is mandatory so that a pressure limit may be set, above which no further volume is delivered to the patient. The variety of settings

on the volume-cycled ventilator allow the operator to set the inspiratory flow rate and the time of inspiration, thus defining the inspired volume.

Inspiratory flow rate and inspired volume are variables which must be suited to the clinical situation. It has become customary to use tidal volumes somewhat in excess of those seen during spontaneous ventilation. Ventilation with volumes on the order of 8 to 12 cc/kg appears to avoid the development of progressive atelectasis.[81] However, in the face of a decreased pulmonary compliance, the use of large volumes may be distinctly unpleasant to the alert patient and may cause considerable agitation and hyperventilation. In such cases, a downward adjustment of the tidal volume is necessary.

The choice of an inspiratory flow rate is also based upon the particular clinical situation. In the presence of emphysema when airways obstruction is predominantly expiratory in nature, it is frequently advisable to increase inspiratory flow rate and allow a longer time for expiration. When airways obstruction is present during both inspiration and expiration, as in patients with asthma or chronic bronchitis, inspiration and expiration are more usually set in a 1:2 ratio. It must be stressed that appropriate ventilatory settings can be made only when the patient's pathology is understood and frequently must be readjusted after noting the clinical and physiologic effects.

A major effect of mechanical ventilation is altered gas exchange. The product of respiratory frequency and the tidal volume delivered is termed the minute ventilation. As minute ventilation increases, the amount of carbon dioxide removed from the blood is increased and $PaCO_2$ falls. Only by measuring arterial blood gases and knowing the $PaCO_2$ can the adequacy of mechanical ventilatory support be assessed. In a similar fashion, arterial oxygen tension must be measured to evaluate the adequacy of the inspired oxygen content.

Patients who generate spontaneous breaths have in the past been treated with the "assist" mode of ventilation wherein a spontaneous breath triggers the ventilator to deliver a preset tidal volume. More recently, the use of intermittent mandatory ventilation (IMV) has increased both patient comfort and the appropriateness of minute ventilation. With the use of intermittent mandatory ventilation, the patient is able to take voluntary breaths of a volume determined by the patient between mandatory ventilator breaths. The number of ventilator breaths delivered per minute can be gradually decreased, providing a convenient method for weaning difficult patients from the ventilator.[82]

It is clear from the foregoing discussion that the care of patients critically ill with cardiopulmonary disease requires the accurate determination of arterial blood gases. The reliability of arterial blood gas determinations depends upon the use of specially trained personnel for performing determinations and a strict quality control program.[83]

# REFERENCES

1. Reid L: Pathology of chronic bronchitis. Lancet 1:275–278, 1954.
2. Reid L: Measurement of the bronchial mucous gland layer: a diagnostic yardstick in chronic bronchitis. Thorax 15:132–141, 1960.
3. Thurlbeck WM: Chronic airflow obstruction in lung disease. W.B. Saunders Co., Philadelphia, 1976.
4. Wagner PD, Dantzker R, Dueck R, Clausen JL, West JB: Ventilation/perfusion inequality in chronic obstructive pulmonary disease. J Clin Invest 59:203–216, 1977.
5. Bergofsky EH: Active control of the normal pulmonary circulation in Pulmonary Vascular Disease, Moser KM, Ed, Marcel Dekker, New York, 1979, pp 233–277.
6. Wertzenblum E, Loiseau A, Hirth C, Nierhom R, Rasaholinjanahary J: Course of pulmonary hemodynamics in patients with chronic obstructive pulmonary disease. Chest 75:656–662, 1979.
7. Bishop JM: Cardiovascular complications of chronic bronchitis and emphysema. Med Clin North America 57:771–780, 1973.
8. Heath D, Smith P: Pulmonary vascular disease secondary to lung disease in Pulmonary Vascular Disease, Moser KM, Ed. Marcel Dekker, New York, 1979, pp 387–426.
9. Boushy SF, North LB: Hemodynamic changes in chronic obstructive pulmonary disease. Chest 72:565–570, 1977.
10. Kline LE, Crawford MH, MacDonald WJ, Schelbert H, O'Rourke R, Moser K: Noninvasive assessment of left ventricular performance in patients with chronic obstructive pulmonary disease. Chest 77:558, 1977.
11. Unger K, Shaw D, Karliner JS, et al: Evaluation of left ventricular function in acutely ill patients with chronic obstructive lung disease. Chest 68:135, 1975.
12. Rosenow EC III, Harrison CE: Congestive heart failure masquerading as primary pulmonary disease. Chest, 58:28–36, 1970.
13. Holford FD, Mithoefer JC: Cardiac arrhythmias in hospitalized patients with chronic obstructive pulmonary disease. Am Rev Resp Dis 108:879, 1973.
14. Bahler RC: Does increased work of the right ventricle diminish left ventricular function? Chest 72:551, 1977.
15. Steele P, Ellis JH, Van Dyke D, Sutton F, Creagh E, Davies H: Left ventricular ejection fraction in severe chronic obstructive airway disease. Am J Med 59:21–27, 1975.
16. Slutsky RA, Ackerman W, Karliner JS, Ashburn WL, Moser KM: Right and left ventricular dysfunction in patients with chronic obstructive lung disease: assessment by first-pass radionuclide angiography. Am J Med 68:197–205, 1980.
17. Berger H, Matthay R, Lake J, Marshall R, Gottschalk A, Zaret B: Assessment of cardiac performance with quantitative radionuclide angiography: right ventricular ejection fraction with reference to findings in chronic obstructive lung disease. Am J Cardiol 41:897–902, 1978.
18. Alpert J, Rickman F, Howe J, Dexter L, Dalen J: Alterations of systolic time intervals in right ventricular failure. Circulation 50:1205–1211, 1974.
19. Alpert J, Crawford M, Karliner J, O'Rourke R: STI in COPD (letter to editor). Circulation 52:354, 1975.
20. Green LH, Smith TW: The use of digitalis in patients with pulmonary disease. Ann Intern Med 87:459, 1977.
21. Morrison J, Killip T: Hypoxemia and digitalis toxicity in patients with chronic lung disease. Circulation 44 (suppl 11) :11, 1971.
22. Matthay RQ, Berger HJ, Loke J, Gottschalk A, Zaret BL: Effects of aminophylline upon right and left ventricular performance in chronic obstructive pulmonary disease. Am J Med 65:903–910, 1978.
23. Moser KM: Pulmonary Embolism. Am Rev Resp Dis 115:829–852, 1977.

24. Miller GAH, Sutton GC: Acute massive pulmonary embolism. Clinical and hemodynamic findings in 23 patients studied by cardiac catheterization and pulmonary arteriography. Brit Heart J 32:518–523, 1970.

25. The Urokinase-pulmonary embolism trial: A national cooperative study. Circulation, 47:Suppl. II, 1973.

26. Moser KM, Braunwald NS: Successful surgical intervention in severe chronic thromboembolic pulmonary hypertension. Chest 64:29–35, 1973.

27. Gallus DS, Hirsh J, Tuttle RJ, Trebilcock R, O'Brien S, Carroll JJ, Minden JH, Hudecki SM: Small subcutaneous doses of heparin in prevention of venous thrombosis. N Engl J Med 288:545–551, 1973.

28. Wray R, Maurer R, Shillingford J: Prophylactic anticoagulation in the prevention of calf-vein thrombosis after myocardial infarction. N Engl J Med 228:815–817, 1973.

29. Warlow C, Beattie AG, Terry G, Ogston D, Kenmure ACF, Douglas AS: A double-blind trial of low doses of subcutaneous heparin in the prevention of deep vein thrombosis after myocardial infarction. Lancet 2:934–936, 1973.

30. LeMoine R, Moser KM: Does a "safe" form of lower extremity venous thrombosis exist? Clin Res 26:136A, 1978.

31. Alderson PO, Doppman JL, Diamond SS, Mendenhall KG, Barron EL, Girton M: Ventilation-perfusion lung imaging and selective pulmonary angiography in dogs with experimental pulmonary embolism. J Nucl Med 19:164–171, 1978.

32. De Nardo GL, Goodman R, Rovisini R, Dietrich DA: The ventilatory lung scan in the diagnosis of pulmonary embolism. N Engl J Med 282:1334–1338, 1970.

33. Stein PD, O'Connor JR, Dalen JE, Pur-Shahriani FG, et al: The angiographic diagnosis of acute pulmonary embolism: evaluation of criteria. Am Heart J 73:730, 1967.

34. Bookstein JJ, Silver TM: The angiographic differential diagnosis of acute pulmonary embolism Radiology 110:25–33, 1974.

35. Hull R, Taylor DW, Hirsh J, Sackett DL, Pomeroy P, Turpie AGG, Walker P: Impedance plethysmography: the relationship between venous filling and sensitivity and specificity for proximal vein thrombosis. Circulation 58:898–902, 1978.

36. Hull R, Hirsh J, Sackett DC, et al: Combined use of leg scanning and impedance plethysmography in suspected venous thrombosis. N Engl J Med 296:1497, 1977.

37. Moser KM, Brach BB, Dolan GF: Clinically suspected deep venous thrombosis: A comparison of venography, impedance plethysmography and radiolabelled fibrinogen. JAMA 237:2195, 1977.

38. Kakkar VV, Howe CT, Flanc C, Clark MB: Natural history of operative deep vein thrombosis. Lancet 2:230, 1969.

39. Genton E: Guidelines for heparin therapy. Ann Intern Med 80:77, 1974.

40. Moser KM: Pulmonary Embolism, Current therapy. W.B. Saunders, Co., Philadelphia, 1978 (pp 134–140).

41. Prophylactic therapy of deep vein thrombosis and pulmonary embolism. DHEW Publication No. (NIH) 76–866, 1976.

42. Kakkar VV, Corrigan TP, Fossard DP: Prevention of postoperative embolism by low dose heparin: an international multicenter trial. Lancet 2:45, 1975.

43. Council on Thrombosis, American Heart Association. Prevention of venous thromboembolism in surgical patients by low dose heparin. Circulation 55:423A–426A, 1977.

44. Hopewell PC, Murray JF: The adult respiratory distress syndrome. Ann Rev Med 27:343–356, 1976.

45. Wilson RS, Pontoppidan H: Acute respiratory failure: Diagnostic and therapeutic criteria. Crit Care Med 2:293–304, 1974.

46. Robin ED, Carey LC, Grenvik A, Glauser F, Gaudio R: Capillary leak syndrome with pulmonary edema. Arch Intern Med 130:66–71, 1972.

47. Martin AM Jr, Simmons RL, Heisterkamp CA III: Respiratory insufficiency in combat casualties: I. Pathologic changes in the lungs of patients dying of wounds. Ann Surg 170:30–38, 1969.

48. Bachofen J, Weibel ER: Basic pattern of tissue repair in human lungs following unspecified injury. Chest 65:145–195, 1974.

49. Lamy M, Fallat RJ, Koeniger E, Dietrich H, Ratliff J, Eberhart RC, Tucker HJ, Hill JD: Pathologic features and mechanisms of hypoxemia in adult respiratory distress syndrome. Am Rev Resp Dis 114:267–284, 1976.

50. Wagner PD, Laravuso RB, Ahl RR, West JB: Distributions of ventilation-perfusion ratios in acute respiratory failure. Chest 65:325–355, 1974.

51. Blaisdell FW: Pathophysiology of the respiratory distress syndrome. Arch Surg 108:44–49, 1974.

52. Rodegren K, McAslon C: Circulatory and ventilatory effects of induced platelet aggregates and

their inhibition by acetylsalicylic acid. Acta Anaesth Scand 16:76–84, 1972.

53. Zapol WM, Snider MJ: Pulmonary hypertension in severe acute respiratory failure. N Engl J Med 296:476–480, 1977.

54. Wimberley N, Foling LJ, Bartlett JG: A fiberoptic bronchoscopy technique to obtain uncontaminated lower airway secretions for bacterial culture. Am Rev Resp Dis 119:337–343, 1979.

55. Anderson RR, Holliday RL, Driedger AA, Lefcoe M, Reid B, Sibbold WJ: Documentation of pulmonary capillary permeability in the adult respiratory distress syndrome accompanying human sepsis. Am Rev Resp Dis 119:869–877, 1979.

56. Unger KM, Shibel EM, Moser KM: Detection of left ventricular failure in patients with adult respiratory distress syndrome. Chest 67:8–13, 1975.

57. Orist JH, Pontoppidan H, Wislon RS, Lowenstein E, Lauer MB: Hemodynamic responses to mechanical ventilation with PEEP. Anesthesiology 42:45–55, 1975.

58. Berryhill RE, Benumof JL: PEEP-induced discrepancy between pulmonary arterial wedge pressure and left atrial pressure. Anesthesiology 51:303–308, 1979.

59. Poe RH, Utell MJ, Israel RH, Hall WJ, Eshleman JD: Sensitivity and specificity of the nonspecific transbronchial lung biopsy. Am Rev Resp Dis 119:25–31, 1979.

60. Danek SJ, Weg JG, Dantzger D: The dependence of oxygen consumption on oxygen delivery in patients with adult respiratory distress syndrome. Am Rev Resp Dis 119, (suppl) p. 104, 1979.

61. Starling EH: On the absorbtion of fluids from the connective tissue spaces. J Physiol London 19:312–326, 1896.

62. Morissette MD: Colloid osmotic pressure: Its measurement and clinical value. Can Med Assoc J 116:897–900, 1977.

63. Falke KJ, Pontoppidan H, Kumar A: Ventilation with end-expiratory pressure in acute lung disease. J Clin Invest 51:2315–2323, 1972.

64. Suter PM, Fairley HB, Isenberg MD: Optimum end-expiratory airway pressure in patients with acute pulmonary failure. N Engl J Med 292:284–289, 1975.

65. Scharf SM, Caldini P, Ingram RH Jr: Cardiovascular effects of increasing airway pressure in the dog. Am J Physiol 232:H35–H43, 1977.

66. Cassidy SS, Eschenbacher WL, Robertson CH Jr, Nixon JV, Blomquist G, Johnson RL: Cardio-

vascular effects of positive-pressure ventilation in normal subjects. J Appl Physiol: Respirat Environ Exercise Physiol 47:453–461, 1979.

67. Hill RN, Shibel EM, Spragg RG, Moser KM: Adult respiratory distress syndrome: Early predictors of morality. Trans Am Soc Artif Int Organs 21:199–203, 1975.

68. Rapaport E: Dyspnea: Pathophysiology and differential diagnosis. Prog in Cardiovasc Dis 13:532–540, 1971.

69. Glogowska M, Widdicombe JG: The role of vagal reflexes in experimental lung oedema, bronchoconstriction, and inhalation of halothane. Resp Physiol 18:116–128, 1973.

70. Valencia A, Burgess JH: Arterial hypoxemia following acute myocardial infarction. Circulation 40:641–652, 1969.

71. Fillmore SJ, Shapiro M, Killip T: Arterial oxygen tension in acute myocardial infarction. Serial analysis of clinical state and blood gas changes. Am Heart J 79:620, 1970.

72. Fillmore SJ, Guimaraes AC, Scheidt SS, Killipp T III: Blood gas changes and pulmonary hemodynamics following acute myocardial infarction. Circulation 45:583–591, 1972.

73. Pain MCF, Stannard M, Sloman G: Disturbances of pulmonary function after acute myocardial infarction. Br Med J 2:591–594, 1967.

74. Hales CA, Kazemi H: Small-airways function in myocardial infarction. N Engl J Med 290:761–765, 1975.

75. Gray BA, Hyde RW, Hodges M, Yu PN: Alterations in lung volume and pulmonary function in relation to hemodynamic changes in acute myocardial infarction. Circulation 59:551–559, 1979.

76. Frank NR, Lyons HA, Siebens AA, Nealon TF: Pulmonary compliance in patients with cardiac disease. Am J Med 22:516–523, 1957.

77. Gray BA, McCaffree DR, Sivak ED, McCurdy HT: Effect of pulmonary vascular engorgement on respiratory mechanics in the dog. J Appl Physiol 45:119–125, 1978.

78. Interiano B, Hyde RW, Hodges M, Yu PN: Interrelation between alterations in pulmonary mechanics and hemodynamics in acute myocardial infarction. J Clin Invest 52:1994–2002, 1973.

79. Salem MR, Mathrubnutham M, Bennett EJ: Difficult intubation. N Engl J Med 295:879–881, 1976.

80. Mercer TT, Goddard RF, Flores RL: Output characteristics of three ultrasonic nebulizers. Ann Allergy 26:18–27, 1968.

81. Hedley-White, J, Pontoppidan H, Laver MB,

Hallowell P, Bendixen HH: Arterial oxygenation during hypothermia. Anesth 26:595–602, 1965.

82. Downs JB, Perkins HM, Modell JH: Intermittent mandatory ventilation. Arch Surg 109:519–523, 1974.

83. Mohler J: Quality control for blood gas determination in standards for clinical pulmonary function testing: Equipment, methods, normals. Jack L. Clausen, ed., California Thoracic Society, 1980.

# 36 | *Precoronary Care*

*Dennis L. Costello, M. D.*

Coronary artery disease-related mortality continues to be the leading cause of death in the United States today. Numerous investigators had reported a 30 to 40 percent in-hospital mortality rate from acute myocardial infarction prior to the development of modern technology and specialized coronary care facilities.[1-4] The appearance of certain arrhythmias in the early phases of infarction was noted to be a poor prognostic indicator in these early studies.[3,9-12] With the development of electrical cardioversion,[5-6] cardiac pacing capability,[7-8] and the widespread utilization of antiarrhythmic agents, the means became available to prevent and treat potentially lethal arrhythmias in the setting of acute myocardial infarction (AMI). Such therapeutic advances were ineffective in reducing hospital mortality rates without the concomitant ability to rapidly identify patients with potentially dangerous arrhythmias. The detection of such rhythm disturbances required the hospitalization of critically ill patients in a centralized unit where constant electrocardiographic monitoring could be accomplished. This unit required staffing by experienced personnel trained in arrhythmia detection and capable of instituting prompt therapy.

With the widespread utilization of this specialized coronary care unit approach to the in-hospital treatment of acute myocardial infarction, investigators noted an approximate 50 percent reduction in the in-hospital mortality from acute myocardial infarction.[14-19] These early

data suggested that the decrease in mortality could be attributed to early aggressive treatment of cardiac arrhythmias with little additional improvement in survival in patients with severe heart failure and shock.[16,17,20]

Thus, it has been generally accepted that the utilization of the coronary care unit will reduce the mortality in acute myocardial infarction among those patients admitted to the hospital. The majority of deaths from myocardial infarction, however, occur soon after the onset of symptoms (Fig. 36.1). Various studies have reported a 40 to 60 percent mortality within the first hour of the onset of symptoms.[21-26] The average interval between the onset of myocardial infarction and admission to the coronary care unit has been variously reported to be 5 to 8 hours or longer.[23,25] Thus, it may be concluded that the majority of deaths from acute myocardial infarction occur prior to the patient's receiving intensive care therapy. Prompted by these initial reports of the incidence of morbidity and mortality in the first few hours of acute infarction, Pantridge and Geddes [27] initiated the concept of the mobile intensive care unit in Belfast, Northern Ireland in 1966. This mobile unit was expressly designed to reduce the interval between the onset of signs and symptoms of acute infarction and the institution of intensive care monitoring and treatment.

In May 1966, a conference on cardiopulmonary resuscitation sponsored by the National

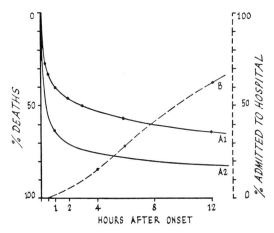

Fig. 36.1 Composite figure compiled from data by McNeilly and Pemberton [23] (A₁), Bainton and Peterson [21] (A₂), and McDonald [117] (B), describing the percentage of death from acute myocardial infarction occurring within the first hours after the onset of symptoms. Curve A₁ describes a 40 percent incidence of death within the first hours among patients of all ages. Among men of middle age or less (A₂), 63 percent of deaths occur within the first hours. As indicated by Curve B, only 16 percent of patients reached the hospital within 4 hours, and the median time for arrival was greater than 8 hours. (Pantridge and Adgey: The prehospital phase of acute myocardial infarction. In Textbook of Coronary Care. Meltzer LE and Dunning AJ, editors, Charles Press Publishers, Inc., Bowie, Md., 1972.)

Academy of Sciences–National Research Council recommended guidelines for the training of medical, allied health, and professional paramedical personnel in cardiopulmonary resuscitation according to the standards set by the American Heart Association.[28]

Community-wide integrated systems of emergency mobile units and hospital coronary care units were developed. Fixed life-support units were equipped in offices, industries, and stadiums where large numbers of persons congregated. Extensive public and professional educational programs have been undertaken in numerous communities to inform both physicians and the public of the available emergency facilities and to train the public and physicians in basic and advanced life-support systems.

Subsequently, the National Conference on Standards for Cardiopulmonary Resuscitation and Emergency Cardiac Care was convened under the auspices of the American Heart Association and the National Academy of Sciences–National Research Council in 1973.[29] The goal of the conference was to establish a new set of standards for basic life support, advanced life support, life-support units, and medical-legal aspects of cardiopulmonary resuscitation and emergency cardiac care to satisfy the national need for an effective community-wide stratified system of emergency cardiac care.[30]

## SYMPTOMS OF ACUTE MYOCARDIAL INFARCTION

### Premonitory Symptoms

The clinical manifestations of acute infarction are classically thought to appear abruptly. Prior to the onset of the acute event, however, many patients, with careful questioning, will describe a prodromal phase of the acute infarction (Fig. 36.2). Goldstein et al.[39] and Simon et al.[32] have suggested that there is a 44 to 70 percent incidence of premonitory symptoms in the weeks prior to infarction. Chest pain described as constricting, squeezing, or crushing in nature may be described with increasing frequency in the days or weeks prior to the acute

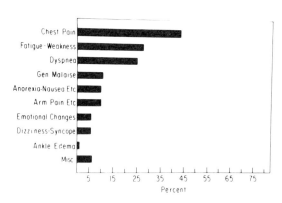

Fig. 36.2 Frequency and distribution of symptoms in the days or weeks prior to the acute event among 160 patients admitted with acute myocardial infarction. 70 percent noted one or more symptoms in the prodromal period. (Simon AB et al: Components of delay in the pre-hospital phase of acute myocardial infarction. Am J Cardiol 30:476–482, 1972 with permission of the publishers.)

event. This "preinfarction angina" may occur with less and less exertion or may occur at rest or nocturnally. The pain is typically substernal, and the choking quality occasionally prompts the patient to describe the feeling as shortness of breath. This discomfort may radiate to either arm or shoulder, although more commonly it radiates to the inner aspect of the left arm; also, it may radiate to the neck or lower jaw or to the mid-epigastric region. The pain gradually increases in intensity and then gradually subsides, usually lasting no more than 5 to 10 minutes.

In addition to chest pain, patients may describe muscle weakness, excessive fatigability, effort intolerance, or vague mid-epigastric distress or "indigestion." Such prodromal symptoms have been noted in more than one-half of patients with acute myocardial infarction.[31-32] In general, the symptoms will occur for periods lasting from less than one week to as long as a month. Local Heart Associations, through extensive use of radio, television, and newspaper, have attempted to educate the public with regard to these signs and symptoms of coronary heart disease (CHD). The combination of increasing public awareness of cardiovascular health and such patient education programs may prove to increase the number of patients seeking medical assistance during the prodromal phase.

## Presenting Symptoms

Prolonged chest pain of a squeezing or constricting nature is the most common symptom of acute infarction. Moss et al.[34] noted that pain in the chest or chest and arms was recognized to be the presenting symptom in over 84 percent of the patients. The pain is similar in quality to angina pectoris but much more severe and usually lasts longer than 20 minutes. Associated symptoms of nausea, diaphoresis, or shortness of breath may be present. Syncope may occur in the presence of advanced degrees of heart block, sinus bradycardia, or tachyarrhythmias. A small percentage of patients may experience an asymptomatic, "silent" myocardial infarction.[42]

## FACTORS CONTRIBUTING TO DELAY DURING THE PREHOSPITAL PHASE OF AMI

As indicated earlier, most deaths due to acute myocardial infarction occur within the first few hours of the onset of symptoms. To further reduce this mortality rate, a significant reduction in the time interval between the onset of symptoms and the initiation of intensive care therapy is required. Numerous studies have attempted to define the variables that result in delay in hospital admission.[31-41]

### Decision Time

The "decision time" has been defined as the interval between the onset of symptoms and the patient's decision to seek medical help (Fig. 36.3). This decision-making process initially requires recognition on the part of the patient of the seriousness of the symptoms and realization of the need for medical help. Simon et al.[32] noted that 53 percent of the patients with acute infarction seek lay advice within the first 15 minutes and 70 percent within the first 60 minutes of the onset of symptoms.[22] Moss et al.[34] have noted that the shortest decision times and hospital arrival times occur when the patient himself rather than a spouse or friend makes the decision to seek hospital care. The presence of previous angina or previous myocardial infarction has had variable effects on the length of the "decision time." [32,39,41] Patient indecision in the prehospital period may also reflect denial or rationalization of a life-threatening illness.[43-45] Other factors contributing to delay in the decision-making process include the occurrence of pain on weekends or during daylight hours [34] or at various times during the day,[33,46] or a history of recent increase in the frequency of angina.[32]

### Physician Consultation

Once a patient has decided to seek medical attention, the next significant delay in establishing intensive cardiac care relates to the method of seeking medical assistance. Several studies

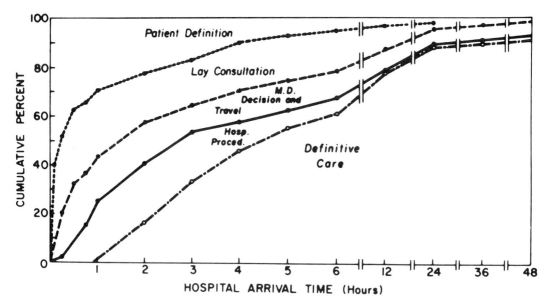

Fig. 36.3  Cumulative curves of the various components of the time delay in receiving definitive care in patients with acute myocardial infarction. The median time for hospital arrival was greater than 4 hours (solid line). (Simon AB et al: Components of delay in the pre-hospital phase of acute myocardial infarction. Am J Cardiol 30:476–482, 1972 with permission of the publishers.)

have reported only a 16 to 26 percent incidence in the number of patients going directly to the hospital without seeking prior medical advice.[32,40]

The delay encountered by the patient consulting his physician is directly related to the attitude of the physician. Those patients who were instructed to go immediately to the hospital had a median hospital arrival time similar to those patients who went to the hospital at once without seeking prior medical advice. Considerable physician-induced delay occurred when the physician's recommendations included an office visit, a house call, a trial of medication, or a cardiovascular consultation. A 40 to 60 percent incidence of such physician-induced delay has been reported [32,47,48] among those patients seeking outpatient medical advice.

## Transportation Delay

Delay in receiving intensive care monitoring may also occur after the decision to seek medical assistance is made. Although patients in both urban and suburban communities in the United States commonly live within 5 to 10 miles of the nearest hospital, delays of one hour or more in travel time are common. In spite of significant symptoms, patients may complete their activities, continue working, or wash and change clothes prior to their departure. This nontherapeutic behavior occurs more commonly in patients with a history of angina and those who had been experiencing less severe symptoms in the recent past. This delay is less common in patients with the abrupt onset of severe complaints without premonitory symptoms.

In the United States, the private automobile is still a primary method of transportation for patients with acute infarction.[49] Prolongation in arrival time may be due to traffic congestion, inadequate directions, or automobile breakdown. Patients whose symptoms occur away from the home may even drive many miles to be hospitalized closer to home. Considerable use of the private automobile still occurs in cities with well-publicized municipal ambulance and mobile intensive care unit services. This problem may reflect the public's association of ambulance service more commonly with traumatic, obstetric, or hemorrhagic emergencies.

## Hospital Delay

The emergency room and admitting area have been noted to be additional sources of delay of treatment of acute myocardial infarction. In one study, only 22 percent of patients with acute infarction were transferred to the intensive care unit within 30 minutes of arrival to the hospital.[32] Administrative procedures required for emergency treatment and hospital admission are obvious sources of delay. Emergency room diagnostic evaluation by the physician and bed preparation in the intensive care unit may also contribute to delay in reaching the intensive care unit.

## SUMMARY

Delay in receiving medical treatment following symptoms of acute infarction is a most important potentially reversible factor contributing to the immediate mortality from the acute event. An intensive community effort is required to alert both the medical profession and the general public to the prodromal symptoms of acute infarction. The public should be made aware of the emergency medical resources available in the community and the need for electrocardiographic monitoring and antiarrhythmic therapy in the early stages of acute infarction.

As more communities develop the capability of providing this immediate, on-the-scene intensive care therapy, the value of bystander-initiated cardiopulmonary resuscitation will become more important.

## LIFE-SUPPORT STATIONS

A life-support station is a medical care facility designed to provide immediate intensive care therapy including electrocardiographic monitoring, defibrillation capability, and intravenous medications to the patient with symptoms of an acute coronary event. The aim of this emergency care program is to significantly reduce the time interval between the initial coronary event and admission to a coronary care unit environment—the so-called prehospital phase of acute myocardial infarction.

The facility may consist of a mobile intensive care unit or a fixed life-support facility located in an area of high population density such as an industrial park or an athletic stadium. The unit is staffed by specialized physicians, nurses, or paramedical personnel thoroughly trained in cardiopulmonary resuscitation and advanced life support including electrocardiographic interpretation and defibrillation. The major functions of such units include: (1) immediate screening and monitoring of patients with acute infarction soon after the acute event; (2) prevention and treatment of cardiac arrhythmias; (3) cardiopulmonary resuscitation including ventricular defibrillation; and (4) stabilization of the patient and transportation directly to the hospital coronary care unit.[50]

## Mobile Coronary Care Units

Pantridge and Geddes initiated the first mobile coronary care unit in Belfast in 1966 [27] with the goal of delivering immediate intensive care to patients with suspected myocardial infarction. The early effectiveness of the mobile unit in treating ventricular fibrillation either at the site of the event or during transportation to the hospital prompted the institution of similar pilot programs in New York,[51,52] Los Angeles,[53] Charlottesville,[54] Seattle,[55] Miami,[56] and Columbus.[59]

Mobile units are utilized extensively in the United States today, yet there may be considerable variability in different communities, depending on financial resources as well as the availability of facilities and personnel. Mobile units have been established in conjunction with hospital emergency departments,[51,52,54] fire department rescue services,[53,55] and county police departments.[57] Units may be stationed at fire stations or near hospital emergency rooms. With a fully integrated communication network (Fig. 36.4), the unit can respond to cardiac emergency calls directed to the police or fire department emergency telephone number, the hospital emergency room, or general ambulance services.

The initial mobile units were stationed in

## SEATTLE MI/CCU SYSTEM

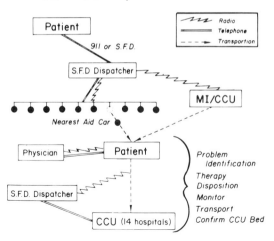

Fig. 36.4 The Seattle system of mobile intensive/coronary care unit, Medic I, is designed to utilize paramedical personnel for delivery of near-physician level, out-of-hospital care. Primary care vehicles are dispatched by the Seattle fire department with the aim of providing basic life support within 3 minutes of the call for assistance. Mobile intensive care units are dispatched simultaneously when life-threatening emergencies are suspected. (Reproduced from Proceedings of the National Conference on Standards for Cardiopulmonary Resuscitation (CPR) and Emergency Cardiac Care, 1975, with permission of the American Heart Association.)

proximity to hospital emergency rooms and staffed by hospital-based physicians.[27,51,52] As the need to reduce the emergency unit response time became apparent, many communities increased the number of mobile units and stationed the units in strategically located fire stations, staffed by specially trained paramedical personnel. In many such programs, the mobile unit staff is in constant radio communication with hospital-based physicians trained in emergency medical care. Continuous telemetry has been employed to transmit vital electrocardiographic data to the hospital physician.[56-58]

Depending on individual resources, some communities have instituted a two-tiered system of basic and advanced life support (basic life support consisting of cardiopulmonary resuscitation). In Seattle, strategically located rescue units or fire department engine companies are dispatched with each emergency call to provide a 2- to 5-minute response time for each

patient.[55] A mobile intensive care unit is simultaneously dispatched in life-threatening situations or following medical evaluation by paramedics assigned to the primary rescue unit. In other communities, hospital or private ambulance services are staffed by trained paramedical personnel, and these units are prepared to provide mobile intensive care therapy during each call for assistance.[60-64] In still other communities, all hospital, fire department, or private ambulances are fully equipped as mobile intensive care units. These units are staffed by emergency medical technicians certified in advanced life support and respond to all emergency calls for assistance [59-65] (Fig. 36.5). All of these varied systems have had some success in the common goal of reducing out-of-hospital morbidity and mortality from acute myocardial infarction.

**Mobile CCU Standards and Equipment.** The mobile coronary care unit should be strategically stationed and capable of immediately transporting equipment, drugs, and trained personnel to the site of a life-threatening emer-

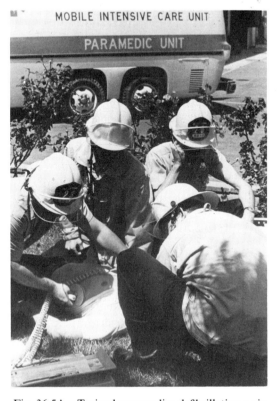

Fig. 36.5A Trained paramedics defibrillating a victim of "sudden death."

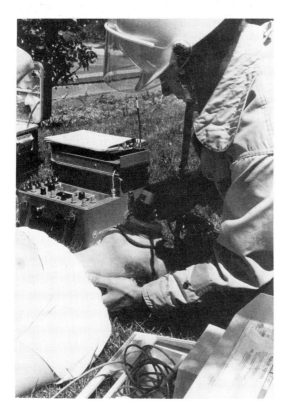

Fig. 36.5B Oxygen being administered following out-of-hospital resuscitation.

gency. The unit should be part of an integrated system of emergency medical care including police and fire departments, rescue units, and private ambulance services with the goal of supplying basic life support (cardiopulmonary resuscitation) within 4 minutes and advanced life support within 10 minutes of the call for assistance.[70]

The unit must be equipped with a mobile battery-operated monitor-defibrillator. Such immediate continuous electrocardiographic monitoring is imperative in the critically ill patient. The unit must be additionally equipped with the means of maintaining an intravenous fluid lifeline. Endotracheal and esophageal intubation capability is also necessary (Table 36.1). Pharmacologic agents including antiarrhythmic and pressor agents must be available (Table 36.2).

Finally, a two-way communication network is necessary for communication between the mobile unit and police and fire dispatch coordi-

nators. The mobile unit must also have the capability to communicate the patient's impending arrival time and condition to the hospital emergency room or intensive care unit. A communications network is imperative for physi-

Table 36.1  Mobile Unit Life-Support Equipment

*Ventilatory Support*

1. Oxygen Supply: minimum of two cylinders with reducing valve and flowmeter capable of delivering 15 l/min with mask and reservoir bag and accumulator
2. Bag-Valve-Mask: capable of administering 100 percent oxygen by use of oxygen reservoir tubing
3. Adequate oxygen reserve
4. Mask for mouth-to-mask ventilation
5. Esophageal obturator airway
6. Oropharyngeal airway
7. Nasopharyngeal airway
8. Nasogastric tube
9. Laryngoscope with straight and curved blades—adult, child, and infant size
10. Inflation syringe and clamp or one-way valve
11. Magill forceps for foreign body removal
12. Portable suction and catheters including #6 to #16 and Yankauer-type suction tips
13. Cricothyreotomy and tracheostomy set
14. Transtracheal jet ventilation set
15. Pleural drainage tubes, underwater seal or vacuum chest bottles

*Circulatory Support*

1. Portable DC defibrillator-monitor with ECG electrode-defibrillator paddles
2. Venous infusion sets—microdrip and regular
3. Indwelling venous catheters with 14- to 22-gauge needles
4. Central venous catheter
5. Intravenous solutions—5 percent dextrose in water, lactated Ringer's solution in plastic bags
6. Pressure intravenous infusors
7. Antishock trousers (optional)
8. Cut-down tray
9. Sterile gloves
10. Urinary catheters (with closed-volume urinary systems)
11. Assorted syringes, needles, stopcocks, venous extension tubing
12. Intracardiac needles
13. Tourniquets, adhesive tape, disposable razor
14. Portable demand pacemaker
15. Transthoracic pacing wires
16. Intracardiac pacing catheter

**Table 36.2 Pharmacologic Agents—Advanced Life Support Unit**

*Essential Drugs*
  Sodium bicarbonate (prefilled syringes, 50 ml ampules, 500 ml 5% bottles)
  Epinephrine (prefilled syringes)
  Atropine sulfate (prefilled syringes)
  Lidocaine (prefilled syringes)
  Morphine sulfate
  Calcium chloride

*Useful Drugs*
  Aminophylline
  Bretylium tosylate
  Dexamethasone
  Digoxin
  Diphenhydramine hydrochloride
  Dopamine
  Diazoxide
  Ethacrynic acid
  Furosemide
  Isoproterenol
  Lanatoside C
  Meperidine hydrochloride
  Metaraminol bitartrate
  Methylprednisolone sodium succinate
  Naloxone
  Nitroglycerin
  Norepinephrine
  Phenylephrine
  Potassium chloride
  Propranolol hydrochloride
  Procainamide hydrochloride
  Quinidine
  Succinylcholine chloride
  Tubocurarine chloride

cian consultation. Telemetry electrocardiogram transmission has proved valuable in many emergency care systems.[56-58]

**Mobile CCU Personnel.** The initial pilot programs of mobile intensive care utilized physicians and hospital staff nurses to treat the out-of hospital sequellae of acute myocardial infarction. Subsequent programs have demonstrated the safety and effectiveness of a paramedic-staffed unit.[53-56,73,74] The use of paramedical personnel rather than physicians in telemetry-equipped mobile units has enabled more units to be strategically located in high population density areas distant from the hospital emergency room. Under such a system, a single in-hospital physician need only be available for radio and telemetry consultation, thus allowing for more efficient utilization of physician manpower.

Paramedics typically undergo a rigorous six-month, one thousand-hour course in emergency medical care before certification.[73,75] The San Diego County Paramedic Curriculum[73] includes 250 hours of physician-directed and -instructed lectures, 200 hours of clinical experience at the training hospital, and 500 hours of field internship under the supervision of senior paramedics (Table 36.3).

Paramedical trainees undergo near physician-level training in cardiopulmonary resuscitation, electrocardiographic interpretation, and dysrhythmia detection. They receive extensive clinical and didactic instruction in cardiac defibrillation, tracheal and esophageal intubation, intravenous lifeline initiation and maintenance, and medical pharmacology (Table 36.3). The well-trained paramedic can effectively treat cardiac, respiratory, neurologic, obstetric, and traumatic emergencies (Fig. 36.6).

### Fixed Life-Support Units

In addition to mobile intensive care capability, the need exists to provide intensive care services in areas where large numbers of persons congregate or in areas where cardiopulmonary emergencies could be anticipated. Fixed life-support units capable of intensive care monitoring and resuscitation have been organized in football stadiums,[66-68] sports arenas, convention centers, industrial parks,[69] office buildings, airports, and railway stations. These units should be located in a highly visible and accessible area of the complex with easy access to ambulance service. Employees such as ushers and security guards should be aware of the location of the unit, and rapid communication between employees in distant areas of the complex and the life-support unit personnel is necessary. The fixed life-support unit should have sufficient mobile capability to provide immediate cardiac resuscitation to the patient experiencing sudden cardiac arrest in these distant areas. Ideally, some employees should be certified in cardiopulmonary resuscitation techniques in order to initiate resuscitation prior to the arrival of the

Table 36.3   1978 Paramedic curriculum—San Diego County Paramedic Service

| Class Title | Time (Hours) | Class Title | Time (Hours) |
|---|---|---|---|
| Abdominal and Genitourinary Emergencies | 2 | Injection Technique—Intramuscular and Subcutaneous | 3 |
| Allergy and Anaphylaxis | 1.5 | Injection Technique—IV | 6 |
| Ambulance Procedure | 2 | IV Theory and Fluid Regulation | 1.5 |
| Anatomy and Physiology, General Review | 2.5 | Legal Aspects | 2 |
| Anatomy and Physiology of the Heart and Circulatory System | 2.5 | MAST Suit | 1 |
| | | Mathematics of Drugs and Solutions | 1.5 |
| Arrhythmias: Introduction to Electrophysiology | 2.5 | Medical Ethics | .5 |
| Arrhythmias: Introduction to Interpretation | 1.5 | Medical Terminology and Abbreviations | 2 |
| Arrhythmias: Sinus and Atrial | 2.5 | Monitoring the EKG | 1 |
| Arrhythmias: A-V Conduction Disturbances | 2 | Multiple Trauma | 1.5 |
| Arrhythmias: Ventricular | 2 | Nasogastric Intubation | 1 |
| Arrhythmias, Treatment of | 2.5 | Near-Drowning | 1.5 |
| Arrhythmias: Complex | 2.5 | Neurological Disorders | 2.5 |
| Aseptic Technique | 1 | Neurological Trauma | 2.5 |
| Assisted Ventilation | 2.5 | Obstetrical and Gynecological Emergencies | 2.5 |
| Bandaging and Splinting | 2.5 | Obstructed Airway | 1 |
| Bleeding and Control of Hemorrhage | 1.5 | Orthopedic Emergencies | 3 |
| Burns | 1.5 | Patient Assessment: Introduction | 5 |
| Cadaver Lab | 2.5 | Patient Assessment | 2 |
| Cardiogenic Shock | 1 | Pediatric Emergencies | 2.5 |
| Carotid Sinus Massage | .5 | Pharmacology | 15.5 |
| Case Presentations (General Review) | 3 | Poisoning | 1.5 |
| Chest Auscultation | 2 | Preservation of Evidence and Crowd Control | .5 |
| Chest Pain: Differential Diagnosis of | 2 | Psychosocial Concerns | 1.5 |
| Clinical Evaluations and Expectations | 1 | Public Relations | 1 |
| Communicable Diseases | 1.5 | Radio Format Communications | 1.5 |
| Congestive Heart Failure/Pulmonary Edema | 1.5 | Radio Man Role and Demonstration | 2 |
| Continuing Education | 1 | Respiratory Disorders | 2.5 |
| Coronary Artery Disease | 2 | Respiratory Trauma | 2 |
| Coronary Observation Radio | 1.5 | Rotating Tourniquets | 1 |
| Defibrillation and Cardioversion | 2.5 | Shock: Introduction | 2.5 |
| Diabetes | 1.5 | Simulations | |
| Dog Lab | 3 | Introduction | .5 |
| Drug Abuse and Overdose | 1.5 | Didactic | 16 |
| Emergency Eye Care | 1.5 | Clinical | 6 |
| Environmental Emergencies | 1.5 | Smoke and Gas Inhalation | 1 |
| Esophageal Airway | 1 | Tracheal Suctioning | 1 |
| Extrication | 4 | Triage | 1 |
| Facial Injuries | 1 | Troubleshooting the Defibrillator/Oscilloscope | 1 |
| Field Expectations and Evaluation | 1 | Unconscious Patient | 2 |
| Forms | 1 | Visual Interpretations | 2.5 |
| Injection Technique—External Jugular | 1 | Vital Signs | 2 |
| Injection Technique—Intracardiac | 1 | Quizzes | 35 |
| | | Review Sessions | 35 |

life-support unit staff in cases of sudden cardiac arrest. Finally, the fixed life-support unit should have communication capability with other emergency agencies in order to facilitate the

transfer of the patient to the hospital intensive care unit.

The hospital emergency room is an additional obvious setting for a fixed life-support unit. The

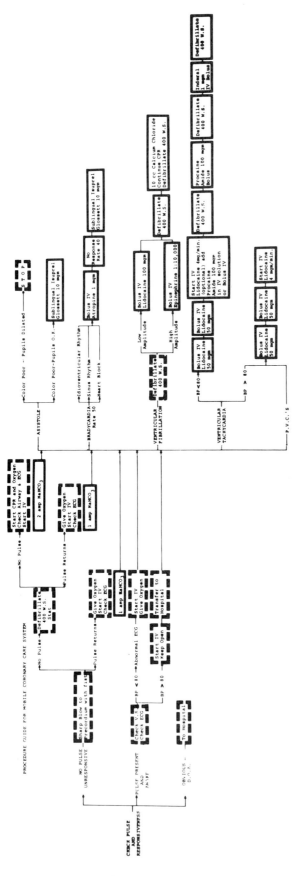

Fig. 36.6  Procedure guide for the mobile coronary care personnel designed by the Heart Association of Upstate New York. Open-hatched rectangles define procedures that may be initiated without physician's orders. Closed rectangles include actions and pharmacologic agents requiring verbal orders from the emergency room physician. Limitations of non-physician-initiated therapy may vary in different communities. (Reproduced from the Proceedings of the National Conference on Standards for Cardiopulmonary Resuscitation (CPR) and Emergency Cardiac Care, 1975, with permission of the American Heart Association.)

emergency room should be equipped to immediately provide cardiopulmonary resuscitation, including tracheal intubation and cardiac defibrillation. As has been emphasized earlier in this chapter, the emergency room is potentially a significant source of delay in providing intensive care treatment, both in the identification of the cardiac patient and in the transfer of the patient to the intensive care unit.

Emergency room personnel should initially screen the presenting complaints of the patient seeking emergency medical assistance prior to emergency room registration. Those patients with signs or symptoms of a possible cardiovascular nature should be monitored immediately. Such monitoring should always precede any administrative procedures or further physician evaluation. Sudden cardiac arrest among patients sitting in the waiting area of the hospital emergency room is an all too frequent occurrence in the busy emergency room setting.

Transfer of the appropriate patient to the coronary care unit should occur promptly upon stabilization of the patient's condition. Medical personnel trained in cardiopulmonary resuscitation, such as a physician or coronary care unit nurse, should accompany the patient in the transfer. The patient should be connected to a mobile battery-operated monitor-defibrillator, and appropriate medications such as lidocaine and atropine should be immediately available for rapid intravenous administration during transfer.

## RESULTS OF PREHOSPITAL EMERGENCY CARE

Greater than 50 percent of all deaths from acute myocardial infarction occur within the first 4 hours after onset of symptoms,[13,82,23,76] and a substantial percentage of these deaths occurs within the first hour.[76] Frequently these deaths result from rhythm disturbances such as ventricular fibrillation, asystole, or complete heart block, all of which are potentially reversible with prompt prehospital care.[27,77-81] These rhythm disturbances have been shown to increase during movement or transportation,[78-79] and numerous studies have suggested a 10 to 20 percent incidence of sudden cardiac death during routine ambulance transportation of the patient with an acute infarction [23,39,84,85] (Table 36.4).

These data suggest that the widespread application of immediate mobile coronary care in the first few hours of acute infarction may have an important impact in reducing prehospital cardiac death. Early reports by Pantridge and others [54,91] indicated a 3 to 36 percent incidence of sudden prehospital cardiac arrest among all patients with acute infarction receiving prehospital coronary care. Among patients with sudden cardiac arrest as a presenting symptom, approximately one-third were successfully resuscitated by mobile unit paramedics.[92,93] Cardiac arrest in other patients may have possibly been prevented by prompt use of lidocaine and atropine before and during transport. Among those patients presenting with cardiac arrest in whom basic resuscitative efforts were begun within 5 minutes, fully 50 to 87 percent eventually recovered to be discharged from the hospital.[78,84,86-90,92,93] Thus, an integrated mobile rescue system may successfully contribute to the reduction of prehospital mortality from myocardial infarction and sudden cardiac arrest.

## BRADYARRHYTHMIAS IN ACUTE MYOCARDIAL INFARCTION

Bradyarrhythmias—including sinus bradycardia, sinus arrest, high degrees of atrioventricular block, or junctional rhythm—have commonly been observed in the early stages of acute infarction.[80-81,96,102-104] Numerous groups have reported a 16 to 27 percent incidence of such bradyarrhythmias.[80,96] The precipitating causes of these bradyarrhythmias may include autonomic disturbances [81] or ischemic injury to the sinus and atrioventricular nodal tissue.[99] Such bradyarrhythmias may dispose the patient to more serious ventricular arrhythmias and hypotension.[81] Atropine administration may afford transient improvement of both blood pressure and ventricular ectopy in the setting of significant bradycardia.[102] However, recurrent ischemia or ventricular fibrillation have been

Table 36.4  Coronary Death in Ambulance

| Community | Ambulance Death | All Prehospital Coronary Death | Percentage of Prehospital Death |
|---|---|---|---|
| Baltimore (84)* | 23 | 148 | 15.5 |
| Belfast (23) | 109 | 596 | 18.3 |
| Charlottesville (85) | 83 | 478 | 17.4 |
| Montgomery County, Maryland (86) | 11 | 127 | 8.7 |

* Numbers in parentheses refer to references.

observed following atropine administration in the early phases of acute infarction.[105-107]

In a small group of patients, Warren and Lewis [102] noted a substantial mortality rate in untreated patients with both bradycardia and hypotension. The judicious use of atropine in this setting was associated with no untoward affects. In addition, in only 12 percent of these patients did spontaneous remission of the bradycardia occur, and recurrence of such bradycardia was commonly seen in the treated group.

In summary, bradycardia is a frequent complication of acute infarction and may be associated with hypotension or recurrent ventricular arrhythmias. The judicious use of atropine in doses of 0.5 to 1.0 mgm intravenously may be indicated for treatment of bradycardia associated with hypotension or ventricular ectopy. Recurrence of bradycardia following hospitalization is frequent and may require further therapy.

## SUDDEN CARDIAC DEATH

Sudden cardiac death may be defined as the sudden collapse and expiration of a previously well-appearing person within minutes to one hour after the onset of symptoms. Most patients who experience sudden cardiac death have a history of cardiovascular disease including systemic hypertension, angina pectoris, or previous myocardial infarction.[95,96,98-100,108] Cigarette smoking, electrocardiographic evidence of left ventricular hypertrophy, and obesity may also predispose to sudden cardiac death.[108]

Many of these patients experience chest pain or dyspnea in the weeks preceding the sudden event, although new or changing patterns of chest pain or dyspnea are frequently absent.[96] Recent physician consultation is common in this group of patients.[86-96] Liberthson et al.[96] noted that, in one-half of the victims of sudden cardiac death in their series, collapse was instantaneous with no definable precipitating cause. Others in this group had noted new or changing patterns of chest pain or dyspnea minutes to hours prior to the collapse.[96] These patients might have benefited from the availability of mobile rescue units and educational programs designed to reduce prehospital delay.

### Results of Prehospital Resuscitation

Ventricular fibrillation is commonly the initial rhythm noted by rescue units among victims of sudden cardiac collapse. The survival rate of these patients is directly related to bystander-initiated cardiopulmonary resuscitation and the response time of the rescue units. Thompson et al.,[109] reporting on the Seattle experience, where the average rescue unit response time is 3 minutes, noted a 43 percent hospital-to-home discharge rate among patients who had received bystander-initiated cardiopulmonary resuscitation. Among patients for whom resuscitation was delayed until the arrival of the rescue units, only 21 percent survived to be discharged home. Improved survival was largely due to a reduction in subsequent hospital mortality from shock and anoxic encephalopathy rather than to a higher rate of initially effective resuscitation.

Lund and Skulberg [110] reported a 36 percent survival among patients with bystander-initiated resuscitation in contrast to an 8 percent survival rate among patients initially resuscitated by a rescue unit whose average response time was 8 minutes.

## Pathophysiologic Profiles in Sudden Cardiac Death

Various autopsy studies [93,98-100,108,111] have noted approximately an 80 percent incidence of atherosclerotic disease in all patients in the 35 to 64 age group experiencing sudden cardiac death. Acute coronary thrombosis or disruption of the intimal lining of the coronary vessels have been variably reported to be present in 13 to 58 percent of reported cases of sudden death.[84,96,100,111,114] The presence of early histologic changes in the myocardium has been noted in 10 to 47 percent of these autopsy cases.[84,96,100,114,115] Such standard histologic examination will generally underestimate the prevalence of infarction, since death may occur prior to the evolution of these microscopically evident alterations in myocardial structure.

Angiographic studies in patients successfully resuscitated from out-of-hospital ventricular fibrillation have demonstrated the presence of widespread coronary artery stenosis in the majority of cases [101] (Fig. 36.7). The distribution

of these coronary artery stenoses varies, and extensive three-vessel disease is commonly present. Considerable ventricular asynergy and pulmonary congestion have also been noted in the majority of survivors.

## Prognosis Among Patients Successfully Resuscitated

As noted previously, the immediate prognosis among patients with out-of-hospital ventricular fibrillation is directly related to the interval from the witnessed collapse until defibrillation. Liberthson et al.[97] also noted the prognostic importance of postdefibrillation heart rate and rhythm on short-term survival (Fig. 36.8). Those patients with postdefibrillation rapid atrial fibrillation or sinus tachycardia had significantly improved survival as compared to those patients who demonstrated postdefibrillation junctional or idioventricular rhythm. Recurrent in-hospital ventricular fibrillation, severe congestive heart failure, and cardiogenic shock portend a poorer in-hospital survival rate.[97]

Weaver et al.[101] and Schaffer et al.[116] noted

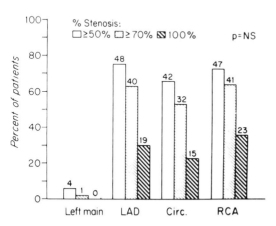

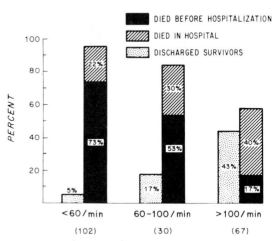

Fig. 36.7 Distribution of angiographic coronary artery stenosis among survivors of out-of-hospital ventricular fibrillation. Only 4 of 64 patients did not exhibit 70 percent stenosis in at least one major artery. (Reproduced from Weaver et al: Angiographic findings and prognostic indicators in patients resuscitated from sudden cardiac death. Circulation 54:895–900, 1976, with permission of the American Heart Association.)

Fig. 36.8 Prognostic implications of post-defibrillation heart rate. Sinus tachycardia (>100) and rapid atrial fibrillation were the most common findings on the post-defibrillation electrocardiogram among discharged survivors of out-of-hospital ventricular fibrillation. (Reproduced from Liberthson RR et al: Pre-hospital ventricular fibrillation. New England Journal of Medicine, with permission of the publisher.) (N Engl J Med 291:317–321, 1979.)

a 26 percent incidence of recurrent ventricular fibrillation in the months following hospital discharge. More extensive evidence of left ventricular dysfunction, triple-vessel coronary artery disease, and congestive heart failure was noted in this subgroup of patients with recurrent ventricular fibrillation.

## SUMMARY

The majority of deaths from acute myocardial infarction occur prior to admission to the hospital and frequently within the first hour of the onset of symptoms. Bradyarrhythmias and ventricular tachyarrhythmias are potentially lethal in the early hours of acute infarction. A community-wide integrated system of patient education, bystander-initiated cardiopulmonary resuscitation, and mobile and fixed life-support stations may significantly reduce out-of-hospital mortality from acute myocardial infarction.

## REFERENCES

1. Master AM, Dack S, Jaffe HL: Age, sex and hypertension in myocardial infarction due to coronary occlusion. Arch Intern Med 64:767, 1939.
2. Billings FT, Kalstone BM, Spencer JL, Ball CT, McNeely GR: Prognosis of acute myocardial infarction. Am J Med 7:356, 1949.
3. Rosenbaum FF, Levine SA: Prognostic value of various clinical and electrocardiographic features of acute myocardial infarction. Immediate Prognosis. Arch Intern Med 68:913, 1941.
4. Harnagel EE, Jelink VV, Andonian AA, Ulrich CW: Survival in acute myocardial infarction. Factors observed in 318 patients. California Medicine 90:264,1959.
5. Beck CS, Pritchard WD, Feil H: Ventricular fibrillation of long duration abolished by electric shock. JAMA 135:985, 1947.
6. Zoll PM, Linenthal AJ, Gibson W, Paul MH, Norman LR: Termination of ventricular fibrillation in man by externally applied electric countershock. N Eng J Med 254:272, 1952.
7. Zoll PM: Resuscitation of the heart in ventricular standstill by external electric stimulation. N Eng J Med 247:768, 1952.
8. Hunter AL, Insall JN: Myocardial infarction in young adults. Brit Med J 1:1282, 1959.
9. Master AM, Dack S, Jaffe HL: Disturbances of rate and rhythm in acute coronary artery thrombosis. Ann Intern Med 11:735, 1937.
10. Mintz SS, Katz LN: Recent myocardial infarction. Arch Intern Med 80:205, 1947.
11. Smith FJ, Denham RM: Myocardial infarction: A study of the acute phase in 920 patients. Am J Med Sciences 221:508, 1951.
12. Johnson CC, Miner PF: The occurrence of arrhythmias in acute myocardial infarction. Dis Chest 33:414, 1958.
13. Stillerman R, Aldrich RF, McCormack RC, Crampton RS: Coronary artery disease death in a community before and after the advent of hospital coronary care units. Circulation 42 (suppl III):202, 1970.
14. Goble AJ, Sloman G, Robinson JS: Mortality reduction in a coronary care unit. Brit Med J 1:1005, 1966.
15. Grace WJ: Mortality rates from acute myocardial infarction: What are we talking about? Am J Cardiol 24:651, 1969.
16. Lown B, Fakhro AM, Hood WB, Jr, Thorn GW: The coronary care unit. New Perspectives and directions. JAMA 199:188, 1967.
17. Killip T, Kimball JT: Treatment of myocardial infarction in a coronary care unit. A two year experience with 250 patients. Am J Cardiol 20:457, 1967.
18. Sloman G, Stannard M, Goble AJ: Coronary care unit: A review of 300 patients monitored since 1963. Am Heart J 75:140, 1968.
19. Thomas M, Jewitt DE, Shillingford JP: Analysis of 150 patients with acute myocardial infarction admitted to an intensive care and study unit. Brit Med J 1:787, 1968.
20. Scheidt S, Ascheim R, Killip T: Shock after acute myocardial infarction. Am J Cardiol 26:556, 1970.
21. Bainton CR, Petersen DR: Death from coronary heart disease in persons fifty years of age and younger; community-wide study. N Eng J Med 268:569, 1965.
22. Kannel WR, Barry P, Dawber T: Immediate mortality in coronary heart disease. Framingham Study. 4th World Congress Cardiology Proc 3:176, 1963.
23. McNeilly RH, Pemberton J: Duration of last attack in 998 fatal cases of coronary artery disease and its relation to possible cardiac resuscitation. Brit Med J 3:139, 1968.
24. Yoon P, Watts R: A mobile coronary care unit:

An evaluation for its need. Ann Intern Med 73:61, 1970.

25. Moss AJ, Wynar B, Goldstein S: Delay in hospitalization during the acute coronary period. Am J Cardiol 24:659, 1969.

26. Soffer A: Only one third reach the hospital. Dis Chest 55:272, 1969.

27. Pantridge JF, Geddes JS: A mobile intensive care unit in the management of myocardial infarction. Lancet 2:271, 1967.

28. Cardiopulmonary resuscitation: Statement by the Ad Hoc Committee on Cardiopulmonary Resuscitation of the Division of Medical Sciences, National Academy of Sciences-National Research Council. JAMA 198:373, 1966.

29. Proceedings of the National Conference of Standards for Cardiopulmonary Resuscitation and Emergency Cardiac Care. American Heart Association and National Academy of Science. Washington DC, May 1973.

30. Standards for cardiopulmonary resuscitation and emergency cardiac care. JAMA (suppl) 227:Feb 18, 1974.

31. Solomon HA, Edwards AL, Killip T: Prodromata in acute myocardial infarction. Circulation 40:463, 1969.

32. Simon AB, Feinleib M, Thompson HK Jr: Components of delay in the prehospital phase of acute myocardial infarction. Am J Cardiol 30:476, 1972.

33. Armstrong A, Duncan B, Oliver MF, et al: Natural history of acute coronary heart attacks. A community study. Brit Heart J 34:67, 1972.

34. Moss AJ, Wynar B, Goldstein S: Delay in hospitalization during the acute coronary period. Am J Cardiol 24:659, 1969.

35. Moss AJ, Goldstein S: The pre-hospital phase of acute myocardial infarction. Circulation 41:737, 1970.

36. Levine HJ: Pre-hospital management of acute myocardial infarction. Am J Cardiol 24:826, 1969.

37. Pantridge JF: Pre-hospital coronary care. Brit Heart J 36:233, 1974.

38. Smyllie HC, Taylor MP, Cuninghame-Green RA: Acute myocardial infarction in Doncaster: Delays in admission and survival. Brit Med J 1:34, 1972.

39. Goldstein S, Moss AJ, Greene W: Sudden death in acute myocardial infarction. Relationship to factors affecting delay in hospitalization. Arch Intern Med 129:720, 1972.

40. Erhardt LR, Sjögren A, Sawe U, et al: Pre-hospital phase of patients admitted to a coronary care unit. Acta Med Scand 196:41, 1974.

41. Gilchrist NC: Factors affecting admission to a coronary care unit. Brit Med J 4:153, 1971.

42. Margolis JR, Kannel WS, Feinleib M: Clinical features of unrecognized myocardial infarction-silent and symptomatic eighteen year follow-up. The Framingham study. Am J Cardiol 32:1, 1973.

43. Olin HS, Hackett TP: Denial of pain in acute myocardial infarction. JAMA 190:977, 1964.

44. Hackett TP, Cassem NH: Factors contributing to delay in responding to the signs and symptoms of acute myocardial infarction. Am J Cardiol 25:651, 1969.

45. Yu PN: Pre-hospital care of acute myocardial infarction. Circulation 45:189, 1972.

46. Barber JM, Boyle D, Walsh MJ, et al: Delay times in acute ischemic heart disease. Brit Heart J 35:861, 1973.

47. Whipple GH: Physician-induced treatment delays in the pre-CCU period. Proceedings of the national conference on standards for cardiopulmonary resuscitation and emergency cardiac care. Amer Heart Assoc 139, 1973.

48. Kamaryt P, Minarik J, Miklis P: Total delay between first appearance of symptoms and hospitalization of patients with acute myocardial infarction. Cor et Vasa 14:1, 1972.

49. Oscherwitz M, Edlavitch SA, Greenough K: Patient and system delay in pre-hospital coronary care. Proceedings of the National Conference on standards for cardiopulmonary resuscitation and emergency cardiac care. Amer Heart Assoc, 1972.

50. Yu PN: Life support stations. Arch Intern Med 134:234, 1974.

51. Grace WJ: The mobile coronary care unit and the intermediate coronary care unit in the total systems approach to coronary care. Chest 58:363, 1970.

52. Grace WJ, Chadbourn JA: The mobile coronary care unit. Dis Chest 55:452, 1969.

53. Lewis AJ, Ailshie G, Criley JM: Pre-hospital cardiac care in a paramedical mobile intensive care unit. West J Med 117:1, 1972.

54. Crampton RS, Aldrich RF, Gascho JA, et al: Reduction of pre-hospital, ambulance and community coronary death rates by the community-wide emergency cardiac care system. Am J Med 58:151, 1975.

55. Cobb LA, Alvarez H: Medic I: The Seattle system for the management of out-of-hospital emergencies: National conference on standards for cardiopulmonary resuscitation and emer-

gency cardiac care. Amer Heart Assoc p 179, 1973.

56. Nagel EL, Hirschman JC, Nussenfeld SR: Telemetry-medical command in coronary and other mobile emergency care systems. JAMA 214:332, 1970.

57. Lambrew CT, Schuchman WL, Cannon TH: Emergency medical transport systems: Use of ECG telemetry. Chest 63:477, 1973.

58. Uhley HN: Electrocardiographic telemetry from ambulances. A practical approach to mobile coronary care units. Am Heart J 80:838, 1970.

59. Lewis RP: The Columbus experience with mobile emergency care. National conference on standards for cardiopulmonary resuscitation and emergency cardiac care. Amer Heart Assoc p 217, 1973.

60. Crampton RS, Aldrich RF, Stillerman R, et al: Reduction of community mortality from coronary artery disease after initiation of pre-hospital cardiopulmonary resuscitation and emergency cardiac care. National conference on standards for cardiopulmonary resuscitation and emergency cardiac care. Amer Heart Assoc p 193, 1973.

61. Rose LB, Press E: The Oregon coronary ambulance project: An experiment in independent performance by emergency medical technicians. National conference on standards for cardiopulmonary resuscitation and emergency cardiac care. Amer Heart Assoc p 197, 1973.

62. Duggan JJ, Barrett MC: A community approach to coronary care. National conference on standards for cardiopulmonary resuscitation and emergency cardiac care. Amer Heart Assoc p 185, 1973.

63. Carveth SW, Olson DC, Bechtel J: An emergency care system-Lincoln mobile heart team. National conference on standards for cardiopulmonary resuscitation and emergency cardiac care. Amer Heart Assoc, p 201, 1973.

64. Grace WJ, Chadbourn JA: Mobile coronary care unit: National conference on standards for cardiopulmonary resuscitation and emergency cardiac care. Amer Heart Assoc p 209, 1973.

65. Swanson LW, Rosenfeld WC, Jorde A: Resume of mobile coronary care unit service in Mason City, Iowa. National conference on standards for cardiopulmonary resuscitation and emergency cardiac care. Amer Heart Assoc p 211, 1973.

66. Graf WS, Polin SS, Paegal BL: Emergency cardiac care in Los Angeles. National conference on standards for cardiopulmonary resuscitation and emergency cardiac care. Amer Heart Assoc p 221, 1973.

67. Carveth SW: Cardiac resuscitation program at the Nebraska football stadium. Dis Chest 53:8, 1968.

68. Carveth SW, Reese HE: The spectator's heart. Nebraska State Medical Journal 55:610, 1970.

69. Easley RM, Moss AJ: Fixed life support station in an industrial location. National conference on standards for cardiopulmonary resuscitation and emergency cardiac care. Amer Heart Assoc p 167, 1973.

70. Kassanoff I, Whaley W, Walter WH, et al: Stadium coronary care, a concept in emergency health care delivery. JAMA 221:397, 1972.

71. Carveth SW: Eight year experience with a stadium-based mobile coronary care unit. Heart and Lung 3:770, 1974.

72. Pantridge JF, Adgey AJ: Pre-hospital coronary care: The mobile coronary care unit. Am J Cardiol 24:666–673, 1969.

73. Standards for emergency cardiac care in advanced life support units. Amer Heart Assoc, April 9, 1976.

74. Alvarez H, Miller RH, Cobb LA: Medic I: The Seattle advanced paramedic training program. National conference of standards for cardiopulmonary resuscitation and emergency cardiac care. Am Heart Assoc p 43, 1973.

75. DeLeo BC: Training of rescue squads in endotracheal intubation. National conference of standards for cardiopulmonary resuscitation and emergency cardiac care. Amer Heart Assoc p 39, 1973.

76. San Diego County mobile intensive care paramedic curriculum. April 1978.

77. Gordon T, Kannel WB: Premature mortality from coronary heart disease. JAMA 215:1617, 1971.

78. Pantridge JF: Mobile coronary care. Chest 58:229, 1970.

79. Adgey AA, Nelson PG, Scott ME: Management of ventricular fibrillation outside the hospital. Lancet 1:1169, 1969.

80. Adgey AA, Geddes JS, Mulholland HC: Incidence, significance and management of early bradyarrhythmia complicating acute myocardial infarction. Lancet 2:1097, 1968.

81. Webb SW, Adgey AA, Pantridge JF: Autonomic disturbance at onset of acute myocardial infarction. Brit Med J 3:89, 1972.

82. Adgey AAJ, Allen JD, Geddes JS et al: Acute

phase of myocardial infarction. Lancet 2:501, 1971.

83. Aldrich RF, Stillerman R, McCormack RC, et al: Sudden coronary artery disease death in community and the prospective role of mobile coronary care. Circulation 42 (Suppl III):83, 1970.

84. Kuller L, Cooper M, Perper J: Epidemiology of sudden death. Archives Int Med 129:714, 1972.

85. Crampton RS, Aldrich RF, Stillerman R, et al: The influence of prehospital emergency cardiac care upon mortality from coronary artery disease. Paramed J 6:13, 1974.

86. Simom AB, Alonzo MA: Sudden death in non-hospitalized cardiac patients. Arch Intern Med 132:163, 1973.

87. Kernohan RJ, McCucken RB: Mobile intensive care in myocardial infarction. Brit Med J 3:178, 1968.

88. Gearty GF, Hickey N, Bourke GJ et al: Pre-hospital coronary care services. Brit Med J 3:33, 1971.

89. Rose LB, Press E: Cardiac defibrillation by ambulance attendants. JAMA 219, 63, 1972.

90. White NM, Parker WS, Binning RA, et al: Mobile coronary care provided by ambulance personnel. Brit Med J 3:618, 1973.

91. Lewis RP, Warren JV: Factors determining mortality in the prehospital phase of acute myocardial infarction. Am J Cardiol 33:152, 1974.

92. Webb SW: Mobile coronary care. Lancet:559, 1974.

93. Cobb LA, Baum RS, Alvarez H: Resuscitation from out-of-hospital ventricular fibrillation: 4 year follow-up. Circulation 51–52 (suppl III):223, 1975.

94. Nagel EL, Liberthson RR, Hirschman JC, et al: Emergency care. Circulation (Suppl III) 51–52:216, 1975.

95. Friedman GD, Klatsky AL, Siegelaub AB: Predictions of sudden cardiac death. Circulation (Suppl III) 51–52:164, 1975.

96. Liberthson RR, Nagel EL, Hirschman JC, et al: Pathophysiologic observation in pre-hospital ventricular fibrillation and sudden cardiac death. Circulation 49:790, 1974.

97. Liberthson RR, Nagel EL, Hirschman JC, et al: Pre-hospital ventricular defibrillation: Prognosis and follow-up. N Eng J Med 291:317, 1974.

98. Kuller L, Perper J, Cooper M: Demographic characteristics and trends in atherosclerotic heart disease mortality: Sudden death and myo-cardial infarction. Circulation 51, 52 (suppl III):1, 1975.

99. Perper JA, Kuller LH, Cooper M: Atherosclerosis of coronary arteries in sudden unexpected deaths. Circulation 51, 52 (suppl III):27, 1975.

100. Spain DM, Brodness VA, Mohr C: Coronary atherosclerosis as a cause of unexpected and unexplained death. Autopsy study from 1949–1959. JAMA 174:384, 1960.

101. Weaver DG, Lorch GS, Alvarez HA: Angiographic findings and prognostic indicators in patients resuscitated from sudden cardiac death. Circulation 54:895, 1976.

102. Warren JV, Lewis RP: Beneficial effects of atropine in the prehospital phase of coronary care. Am J Cardiol 37:68, 1976.

103. Grauer LE, Gershen BJ, Orlando MM, Epstein SE: Bradycardia and its complications in the pre-hospital phase of acute myocardial infarction. Am J Cardiol 32:607, 1973.

104. Iseri LT, Humphrey SB, Siner EJ: Pre-hospital brady-asystolic cardiac arrest. Ann Int Med 88:741, 1978.

105. Massumi RA, Mason DT, Amsterdam EA, et al: Ventricular fibrillation and tachycardia after intravenous atropine for treatment of bradycardias. N Eng J Med 287:336, 1972.

106. Zipes DP, Knoebel SB: Rapid rate-dependent ventricular ectopy. Adverse responses to atropine-induced rate increase. Chest 62:255, 1972.

107. Richman S: Adverse effect of atropine during myocardial infarction: Enhancement of ischemia following intravenously administered atropine. JAMA 228:1414, 1974.

108. Kannel WB, Doyle JT, McNamara PM, Quickenton P, Gordon T: Precursors of sudden coronary death. Factors related to the incidence of sudden death. Circulation 51:606, 1975.

109. Thompson RG, Hallstrom AP, Cobb LA: Bystander-initiated cardiopulmonary resuscitation in the management of ventricular fibrillation. Ann Intern Med 90:737, 1979.

110. Lund I, Skulberg A: Cardiopulmonary resuscitation by lay people. Lancet 2:702, 1976.

111. Kuller L: Sudden death in arteriosclerotic heart disease. Am J Cardiol 24:617, 1969.

112. Crawford T, Dexter D, Teare RD: Coronary artery pathology in sudden death from myocardial ischemia. Lancet 1:181, 1961.

113. Lie JT, Oxman HA, Titus JL: Morphologic evidence for myocardial ischemia in sudden unexpected death from coronary heart disease. Circulation 44 (suppl II):142, 1971.

114. Baroldi G: Myocardial infarction and sudden coronary heart death in relation to coronary occlusion and collateral circulation. Am Heart J 71:826, 1966.

115. Scott RF, Briggs TS: Pathologic findings in prehospital deaths due to coronary arteriosclerosis. Am J Cardiol 29:782, 1972.

116. Schaffer WA and Cobb LA: Recurrent ventricular fibrillation and modes of death in survivors of out-of-hospital ventricular fibrillation. N Eng J Med 292:259, 1975.

117. MacDonald EL: Coronary care units, the London Hospital, in Acute Myocardial Infarction: University of Edinburgh Symposium, p 29, editors DG Julian and MF Oliver. E and S Livingston, Edinburgh.

# 37 | *Intermediate Coronary Care and Predischarge Evaluation*

## *Dennis L. Costello, M.D.*

The development of the Coronary Care Unit approach to the treatment of acute myocardial infarction has contributed to the significant reduction of in-hospital mortality during the initial few days following the acute event.[1-5] This reduction of in-hospital mortality has been attributed to the prompt detection and effective prevention and treatment of potentially lethal arrhythmias. Only slight improvement in survival among patients with cardiogenic shock following infarction has been observed.[6-7]

The observation of a significant mortality rate during the later in-hospital phase following acute infarction prompted Gotsman and Schrire [8] to propose the establishment of an Intermediate Coronary Care Unit for continued and progressive cardiac care following discharge from the Intensive Care Unit. Grace and Yarvote [9] noted that 30 percent of the in-hospital mortality from acute infarction occurred following discharge from the Intensive Care Unit. Many of these deaths occurred suddenly and unexpectedly. Accordingly, they instituted the Intermediate CCU with the goal of reducing the incidence of sudden death following discharge from the CCU.

## DESIGN OF THE INTERMEDIATE CCU

The Intermediate CCU is designed to provide the cardiac patient with continued cardiac monitoring and skilled cardiovascular nursing assistance following discharge from the CCU.

Theoretically, the institution of the concept of continued cardiac care would provide for reduction in the frequency of cardiac arrests by early detection and prophylactic therapy of potentially dangerous arrhythmias. The success rate of cardiac resuscitation would be increased due to prompt recognition and skilled treatment by specialized cardiovascular personnel. Progressive ambulation would be monitored by telemetry, and patients at low or high risk for recurrent arrhythmias late in their hospital course would be identified. Such early recognition would provide for possible early discharge among low-risk patients and accordingly decrease hospital costs and increase bed availability. The presence of such a unit would also provide the possibility of early transfer of uncomplicated patients from the CCU, and thus improve the utilization of intensive care unit beds.

The unit should be composed of private and semiprivate rooms in proximity to a centralized nursing station equipped with a central telemetry console (Fig. 37.1). The ideal number of beds and monitoring units is dependent on the size of the particular hospital and the prevalence of coronary artery disease in the population. The unit should possess sufficient telemetry capability to insure monitoring of all high-risk patients following discharge from the CCU.

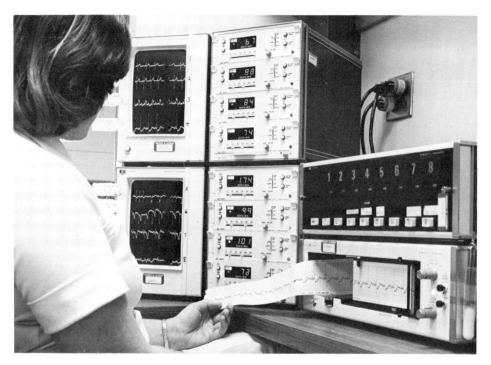

Fig. 37.1 A telemetry console, located in a ward nursing area. Up to eight patients can be monitored by the nurse, who is able to recognize arrhythmias and initiate emergency care. The unit is staffed around-the-clock and patients are monitored during both bed rest and ambulation.

Such telemetry capability would insure more efficient utilization of CCU beds.

The individual beds in the intermediate care unit should be equipped with oxygen, suctioning equipment, bag-valve-mask means of artificial ventilation, and other equipment and drugs vital for delivering cardiopulmonary resuscitation (see Ch. 31). A portable defibrillator should be located in the immediate proximity for emergency use among these patients who have a higher risk than the general in-hospital population for experiencing cardiac arrest.

Each bed in the unit should be hard-wired for continuous bedside monitoring of all non-ambulatory patients. Remote telemetry units should be available for distant monitoring of all ambulatory patients and such equipment may also be used for monitoring of patients confined to bed if the above-mentioned hard-wire capability is not available.

Each room should be spacious, with windows and exposure to external stimuli such as radio and television. Frequently, the coronary patient has just spent a considerable number of days in the windowless, timeless environment of the CCU. Normalization of the hospital environment is valuable in the psychological as well as physical rehabilitation of the patient with perhaps newly diagnosed coronary artery disease.

A unit of this kind should be located in geographic proximity to the CCU and ideally should share medical, nursing, and paramedical personnel. Such a sharing of personnel insures a level of professional expertise comparable to that found in the CCU and provides for continuity of medical care during the period of progressive ambulation. If such sharing is not feasible in the individual hospital, the intermediate unit nursing and paramedical staff should be skilled in the recognition of arrhythmias and should appreciate the goals and risks attendant upon progressive rehabilitation following acute infarction.

## IN-HOSPITAL AMBULATION AND DISCHARGE

Prior to 1952, patients with uncomplicated but definite myocardial infarction were frequently placed at bed rest for 4 to 8 weeks following the acute event.[10] Such treatment was presumably based on pathologic studies demonstrating the time course of myocardial scar formation.[11] Proponents of this approach suggested that early physical activity might conceivably increase the risk of ventricular rupture, aneurysm formation, or recurrent infarction.

Such prolonged bed rest increases the risk of thromboembolic events [12] and contributes to generalized and cardiovascular physical deconditioning.[13] A shorter period of immobilization might also decrease the patient's emotional and psychological disability following the acute event and speed the process of physical and psychological rehabilitation. In addition, a hospital stay of this length today would have severe economic disadvantages both for the patient and the health care system in general, and would expand the need for hospital beds in the community.

Levine and Lown [14] in 1952 first demonstrated that patients with uncomplicated infarction could safely be mobilized to a chair by the third hospital day. Others [15-18] during the 1950s and 1960s advocated reduction in bed rest to 2 to 3 weeks. Naughton et al.[19] in 1969 again suggested the currently employed method of bed-to-chair on the third day in uncomplicated infarction. Such broad divergence of opinion regarding bed rest had resulted in a wide variety of physician practices in the 1970s. Duke [20] in 1971 noted that an average of 7 to 15 days of bed rest was still common among all patients admitted to one community hospital. Today, the recommendation of bed-to-chair in 3 days as first proposed by Levine and Lown has finally been widely accepted in patients with uncomplicated infarction.

This slowly evolving change in the time frame of ambulation following infarction has also influenced opinion and practice regarding the optimal period for in-hospital recuperation from acute infarction. Gilchrist [21] in the late 1950s suggested that the majority of patients were ready for discharge following 4 weeks of hospitalization. Hutter et al.,[22] Harper et al.,[23] and Royston [24] observed no additional benefit from more than a 2-week hospital stay among a selected group of patients with uncomplicated infarction. Lown and Sidel [25] recognized that hospitalization was clearly indicated in the United States following acute infarction to provide pharmacologic and electrical means of correcting potentially lethal arrhythmias. They suggested, however, that patients exhibiting no complications in the first week derived no special medical benefit by remaining in the hospital beyond the tenth to twelfth day. They additionally concluded that such a decrease in hospitalization time would have a significant economic impact on the cost of medical care and that this decrease in length of hospitalization would result in more effective utilization of acute care beds.

Concurrent with Lown's work, Mather and colleagues, [26-27] reporting from England where home care of acute infarction is not uncommon, reported no difference in survival among normotensive patients with acute infarction treated at home or in hospital intensive care units.

Proponents of Mather's approach argue that death from acute infarction is most common in the first hour,[28] long before hospital admission, and that the act of transportation itself may increase the risk of arrhythmias.[29] Thus, they argue that those uncomplicated patients reaching the CCU hours after the acute event may be at less risk for experiencing a fatal arrhythmia and thus may be safely treated at home.

Although Mather's work has raised questions of experimental design, randomization, and response time for seeking assistance, Hill et al.[30] and Collings et al.[31] more recently have supported this view. They argue that, in a select population with uncomplicated infarction, who have suitable home circumstances and continuity of general practitioner care, hospital admission might not confer any significant improvement in short-term survival.

In the United States today, most physicians support Lown's view that "the major problem is not whether to hospitalize but how to expedite such hospitalization." [25] The length of hospitalization following acute infarction is frequently determined by the accepted practice in the institution or community. Wenger et al.,[32] reporting the results of an extensive nation-wide survey in 1970, noted that 95 percent of all practicing physicians who participated in the survey reported that they routinely hospitalized patients with uncomplicated infarction and that the median hospital stay for these patients was 21 days. McNeer et al.[41] identified a group of 265 patients with acute infarction who experienced no serious complications through the fourth hospital day. Such patients experienced no further in-hospital complications or mortality. On the basis of these data, they suggested a prospective clinical trial of early discharge in uncomplicated patients. To date, the in-hospital management of uncomplicated myocardial infarction continues to be based on local practice and physician preference.

## IN-HOSPITAL MORTALITY FOLLOWING DISCHARGE FROM THE CCU

Patients experiencing myocardial infarction continue to be at risk for death in the weeks following discharge from the CCU. Grace and Yarvote [9] and others [33-36] have reported that 28 to 34 percent of all in-hospital deaths following acute infarction occur following discharge from the CCU. Many of these deaths result from progressive heart failure and cardiogenic shock. Sudden and unexpected death, however, may result from massive pulmonary embolism, electromechanical dissociation,[37] or an abrupt arrhythmia. Thompson and Sloman [34] reported that a majority of recently infarcted patients with late in-hospital sudden cardiac arrest experienced ventricular fibrillation (VF). Others [38-40] indicate that 36 to 57 percent of patients with late ventricular fibrillation survive to be discharged, and 41 percent of hospital survivors of late ventricular fibrillation may be expected to live 5 years.[40] Thus, continuous monitoring following CCU discharge may afford considera-

ble long-term benefit among these selected patients at risk for developing the late in-hospital occurrence of ventricular fibrillation.

## HIGH-RISK GROUPS FOR LATE IN-HOSPITAL VF

As noted above, patients with acute myocardial infarction continue to be at risk for sudden cardiac death following discharge from the CCU. Early identification of those patients at risk for late ventricular arrhythmias and sudden death would be extremely valuable in individualizing patient-management decisions in the later phases of in-hospital recovery. Thus, decisions regarding ambulation, monitoring, predischarge exercise testing, and discharge medication and plans for early angiography or rehabilitation might vary with the relative risk of further complications. Resnekov [33] notes that patients with extensive anterior wall infarction, and those patients developing congestive heart failure, fascicular block, or persistent ventricular arrhythmias are at particular risks for late in-hospital sudden death. Graboys [35] observed that persistent sinus tachycardia beyond the second hospital day (without evidence of significant left ventricular dysfunction), recurrent VF, new onset atrial fibrillation, intraventricular or atrioventricular conduction disturbances, and anterior location of infarction were factors common to the sudden death group. Although CCU monitoring revealed that frequent ventricular premature beats and ventricular tachycardia were more common in patients with late sudden death, the results were not statistically significant.

Thompson and Sloman [34] also noted a significant incidence of late in-hospital sudden death among those CCU patients demonstrating anterior wall infarction, persistent sinus tachycardia, frequent ventricular arrhythmias, and LV failure. Bornheimer et al.[36] suggested that ventricular ectopy detected in the CCU was more frequent in patients with extensive infarction and congestive heart failure. Others [37-40] thought that patients with extensive infarction and congestive heart failure were at increased risk of sudden death independent of the degree of ventricular ectopy. McNeer et al.,[41] in a study of 522 consecutive patients with acute infarction, noted that the only patients who were at risk for sudden in-hospital cardiac death were those who experienced one of the following complications by the fourth day: ventricular tachycardia or fibrillation, second- or third-degree heart block, pulmonary edema, cardiogenic shock, persistent sinus tachycardia or hypotension, atrial flutter or fibrillation, and infarction extensions. Patients who experienced none of these complications through the fourth CCU day experienced neither late in-hospital sudden deaths nor appearance of these serious complications during the latter phases of hospital recovery. In addition, signs such as first degree A-V block, sinus tachycardia, intraventricular conduction disturbances, frequent premature ventricular contractions despite lidocaine therapy, and third heart sounds were more prevalent in the high-risk group than in those patients without major CCU complications.[41]

## Fascicular Block

Right or left bundle branch block complicates myocardial infarction in 5–11 percent of cases.[44,45,54] The in-hospital mortality among patients developing such an abnormality has variously been reported to be between 36 and 70 percent.[42-54] Lie et al.[42] observed that 6 percent of patients experienced anteroseptal infarction complicated by transient or persistent right or left bundle branch block. Of patients with such conduction abnormalities, 36 percent sustained late in-hospital VF. Subsequent angiography revealed that patients with fascicular block sustained extensive infarctions with severe LV dysfunction and aneurysm formation.[43] From these data, Lie et al. concluded that patients with transient or persistent bundle branch block following anteroseptal infarction warranted long-term in-hospital monitoring and vigorous antiarrhythmic therapy.

Scheinman and Brenman[44] also recognized that the development of fascicular block in the midst of acute infarction had considerable in-hospital prognostic importance. They noted a two-fold increase in congestive heart failure and death among patients developing fascicular block. Most of these deaths resulted from severe LV dysfunction rather than progressive conduction disturbances and thus were not readily preventable by pacemaker implantation.

Others have confirmed that the in-hospital mortality among patients with new bundle branch block complicating acute infarction ranged from 36 to 70 percent.[45-51] Progression to complete heart block is common in patients developing bifascicular block such as right bundle branch block and left anterior or posterior hemiblock.[45] Such progression of conduction disturbances may reflect the extent of myocardial and conduction system damage particularly with anterior wall infarctions. Approximately 43 to 55 percent of such patients with bifascicular block will progress to complete heart block.[47-48] In patients in whom left bundle branch block complicates acute infarction, only 17 to 20 percent progress to complete heart block.[54] The progression of right or left bundle branch block to complete heart block defines a subgroup of patients with extensive myocardial damage and increases the likelihood of in-hospital mortality to 75 to 85 percent.[45,47,54]

In most series, patients developing bundle branch block have concomitant severe, refractory LV failure. Many investigators suggest that heart failure, rather than arrhythmias or progressive conduction abnormalities, is the primary factor in the majority of in-hospital deaths. Such investigators conclude that prophylactic pacemaker implantation in this group of patients with bundle branch block affords no improvement in long-term survival. Others have argued that prophylactic permanent pacemaker insertion may significantly alter long-term survival statistics among patients with fascicular block and transient complete heart block.[46-47.]

In summary, 5 to 11 percent of patients with acute infarction develop left or right bundle branch block. A substantial in-hospital mortality of 40 to 60 percent may occur in this group. Particularly ominous associated signs include congestive heart failure and transient or persistent higher degrees of conduction disturbance. Prolonged in-hospital monitoring in a telemetry-equipped Intermediate Care Unit seems advisable in this subgroup of patients. The role of long-term prophylactic pacemaker implantation in patients with conduction disturbances following infarction remains to be determined.

## Ventricular Arrhythmias

Frequent persistent premature ventricular beats occurring during the latter phase of CCU convalescence have been observed to be a significant risk factor for late in-hospital and early posthospital sudden death.[34-36] Early studies indicated that the presence of PVCs on a resting ECG results in a three-fold increase in the risk of sudden death in the general population.[55] Hinkle,[56] employing 6-hour Holter monitor recordings on a random sample of middle-aged men, observed ventricular premature contractions in 62 percent of the recordings. Such arrhythmias were associated with clinical evidence of ischemic heart disease at the time of examination and with an increased risk of subsequent sudden death. Reports from the Coronary Drug Project[57] indicate that survivors of acute infarction in whom one or more premature ventricular beats were noted on a resting ECG had a two-fold increase in 3-year mortality including sudden death. Furthermore, the patients with greater frequency of ectopic beats per resting ECG or pairs or runs of premature beats had an even greater likelihood of late death. Kotler et al.[58] confirmed that, in a small group of victims of sudden cardiac death occurring in the late post-infarction period, 10 of 14 deaths occurred in patients with premature ventricular beats observed on a resting 12-lead ECG prior to the event.

Furthermore, Kotler et al.[58] demonstrated that complex ventricular arrhythmias, including frequent unifocal beats, multifocal beats, or pairs or runs of ventricular beats on ambulatory tape recordings were present in 12 of 14 patients experiencing sudden cardiac death.

The method of identifying and monitoring ventricular arrhythmias in the post-CCU phase of convalescence remains of critical importance. The standard 12-lead ECG is extremely insensitive, since the patient is monitored for only a short period of time while inactive.[59-60] In the initial reports of the Intermediate Care Unit,[9] electrocardiographic rhythm strips were recorded every 4 hours during the late hospital phase in the hope of identifying early impending serious arrhythmias. The development of ambulatory monitoring techniques[60-61] and telemetry[62-63] tremendously advanced our ability to identify ominous arrhythmias in the post-CCU phase of acute infarction.

The sensitivity of early CCU monitoring in predicting late in-hospital ventricular arrhythmias remains unresolved. Thompson and Sloman[34] and Graboys[35] both include persistent complex ventricular arrhythmias observed in the later phases of the CCU period of hospitalization as a risk factor for sudden late in-hospital death. Vismara et al.[64] noted that 35 percent of postinfarction patients had complex ventricular arrhythmias in the CCU and 42 percent had complex ventricular arrhythmias late in the hospital course. In less than one-half of these patients with late ventricular arrhythmias, however, had complex arrhythmias been identified during the CCU phase of monitoring. Moss et al.[60] noted that 6-hour Holter monitoring performed prior to discharge and at 3 weeks following infarction demonstrated a 20 percent incidence of multifocal premature ventricular beats, an 18 percent incidence of ventricular bigeminy or couplets and a 4 percent incidence of transient ventricular tachycardia. Although fully 36 percent of post-infarction patients demonstrated significant ventricular irritability that was not demonstrated during the CCU stay, the prevalence of such arrhythmias was similar to that reported in a random middle-aged male population.[56]

Late ventricular arrhythmias have commonly been observed in patients with severe congestive heart failure,[37-40,65] recurrent ischemia,[65] major wall motion disorders,[66-67] and extensive infarction.[68] Vismara et al. noted that patients with late in-hospital complex ventricular arrhythmias commonly had higher pulmonary wedge pressure and lower cardiac output during the acute phase of the infarction.[64] More extensive ST-segment abnormalities on the discharge ECG were also present in patients with complex ventricular arrhythmias.

Schulze et al.[69] also noted the relationship of complex ventricular arrhythmias with the extent of LV dysfunction. Thirteen of fourteen patients with complex ventricular arrhythmias identified on a 24-hour Holter recording demonstrated significant LV dysfunction with ejection fractions lower than 40 percent by nuclear scanning techniques performed prior to discharge. In a subsequent study, Schulze et al.[70] found that 26 of 45 patients with an ejection fraction below 40 percent demonstrated complex ventricular arrhythmias including multifocal PVCs, bigeminy, couplets, and ventricular tachycardia. Only three of 36 patients with an ejection fraction greater than 40 percent demonstrated such complicated arrhythmias. Eight patients, all with complex ventricular arrhythmias and severe dysfunction, experienced late sudden death following infarction. Recently, Shah et al. reported that a severely reduced LV ejection fraction (<0.30), determined by gated equilibrium radionuclide angiography within the first 24 hours of acute infarction, heralded the onset of irreversible pump failure in 6 patients and intractable ventricular arrhythmias in a seventh.[70a] Thus, the presence of significant LV dyfunction and associated complex ventricular arrhythmias defines a subgroup of patients at risk for late in-hospital complications.

In summary, premature ventricular contractions are common in a middle-aged male population and more frequent among patients with evidence of ischemic heart disease. Arrhythmias occurring during the CCU phase of recovery from acute infarction may not identify patients at risk for later life-threatening ventricular arrhythmias. The standard 12-lead ECG is a poor means of identifying those patients with the late occurrence of complex ventricular arrhythmias. Longer periods of continuous ambulatory monitoring during the later in-hospital phase of recovery may more effectively identify the presence of potentially life-threatening ventricular arrhythmias. Patients with complex ventricular arrhythmias and major left ventricular dysfunction may benefit from prolonged hospitalization in a monitored Intermediate Care Unit and from aggressive utilization of antiarrhythmic agents.

# OTHER ELECTROCARDIOGRAPHIC INDICATORS OF IN-HOSPITAL MORTALITY

Patients with extensive transmural anterior wall infarction and large cardiac enzyme elevations [68] have previously been noted to be at risk for late in-hospital complications and sudden death. The prognostic significance of nontransmural myocardial infarction without Q-wave evolution remains unclear. Patients with nontransmural infarction have typically been thought to have a better short term and long term prognosis than those with transmural infarction.[71-73] Such improved prognosis with nontransmural infarction may reflect the fact that short-term, in-hospital prognosis seems to be determined mainly by the extent of infarction and residual myocardial function. Madias et al.[74] and Rigo et al.,[75] however, found no difference in in-hospital mortality and morbidity between the two types of infarction. Cannom et al.[76] demonstrated that, although there was a slightly greater in-hospital mortality among patients with transmural infarction, the long-term survival was significantly reduced among patients experiencing nontransmural infarction. Typically, such patients with nontransmural infarction have a higher incidence of recurrent angina and recurrent infarction [76] with the concomitant risk of later appearance of lethal ventricular arrhythmias during an ischemic episode.

In addition to the presence or absence of pathologic Q waves, the behavior of any ST segment abnormalities in the first 48 hours may have some prognostic importance. Wilson and Pantridge [77] noted that the resolution of the ST-segment abnormalities is a valuable indicator of the return of electrical stability. Thirty percent of patients with persistent ST-segment displacement had significant late ventricular arrhythmias, as compared to only 5 percent among those patients in whom the ST-segments normalized. Data from the Coronary Drug Project research group have emphasized that persistent ST-segment depression was the most important independent risk predictor of subsequent mortality.[78]

In summary, electrocardiographic changes, including the presence or absence of Q waves and the evolution of ST segment abnormalities, may provide additional data concerning the management of the post-infarction patient following discharge.

## RESULTS OF THE INTERMEDIATE CARE UNIT CONCEPT

As noted previously in this chapter, certain subsets of patients with acute infarction continue to be at risk for recurrent lethal ventricular arrhythmias in the initial weeks following infarction. Although intermediate care units have routinely been established in many institutions, very few controlled trials have been reported and the value of such a unit remains unclear.

Grace[79] attempted to confirm the effectiveness of the Intermediate Care Unit concept by demonstrating an 11 percent post-CCU mortality among 136 acute infarction patients treated in such a unit. These data compared favorably with the 31 percent post-CCU mortality reported from the same institution prior to the initiation of intermediate coronary care.

Reynell,[80] however, reported conflicting data in a randomized trial conducted in England over a 5-year period. Five hundred and twenty patients remained on the Intermediate Care Unit until discharge from the hospital. They were nursed by the same trained staff that serviced the CCU, and resuscitation equipment was immediately available. No long-term electrocardiographic monitoring was performed, however. Patients in the control group were transferred from the intensive care unit to a general medical ward. Forty-four of the intermediate unit patients and 43 patients on the general medical ward (9 percent) died during the late hospital phase of recovery. Resuscitation was initiated on 35 patients in the intermediate care unit and 41 patients on the general ward. The initial success rate of resuscitation in the intermediate unit was 46 percent, as compared to only 22 percent in the general ward. This difference may reflect the resuscitative skill of the intermediate care staff, the immediate availability of resuscitative equipment, or the speed with which victims of sudden cardiac arrest were identified. A similar number of survivors of sudden death in each group, however, eventually recovered sufficiently to be discharged.

From the Reynell study, the impact of the Intermediate Care Unit concept in reducing in-hospital mortality seems to be questionable. Others,[33,81] noting the experimental design and lack of long-term monitoring, have questioned the conclusiveness of Reynell's work.

Weinberg[81] compared survival statistics among 1,361 patients with acute myocardial infarction, including 814 patients treated prior to the establishment of an Intermediate Care Unit and 557 patients managed in such a unit. Analyses of the two groups failed to reveal a reduction in in-hospital mortality after introduction of the Intermediate Care Unit.

Frieden and Cooper reviewed the results of the first 1,917 patients treated in their 22-bed Intermediate Care Unit equipped with continuous electrocardiographic monitoring. Twenty-seven patients (1.4 percent) suffered cardiac arrest and 18 (67 percent) were successfully resuscitated. This low incidence of cardiac arrest, as compared to Reynell's data,[80] suggests that continuous 24-hour monitoring and prompt institution of antiarrhythmic therapy may significantly reduce such complications. Frieden and Cooper additionally noted that the availability of adequately monitored and staffed Intermediate Care Units resulted in an increase of coronary care unit admissions of over 15 percent, thus improving the utilization of the coronary care unit. The monitoring capability resulted in increased patient and physician confidence in early ambulation and thus contributed to an overall reduction in hospital stay by 3 days.

Leak et al.[83] compared in-hospital mortality statistics among patient groups treated on a general ward prior to the institution of an intermediate care unit and patients treated in an intermediate care unit with and without monitoring ability. They concluded that a significant reduction in mortality from 5.1 to 2.6 percent occurred when patients were cared for in a monitored, well-equipped Intermediate Care Unit rather than a general medical floor. The number of arrhythmias detected and successful resuscitations from VF were increased only in a monitored unit.

In summary, Intermediate Care Units were introduced with the goal of reducing late in-hospital mortality from acute infarction. At present, the intermediate care concept is less clearly defined than the coronary care unit concept, and many institutions with coronary care units still do not have intermediate care facilities. Studies purporting to show a reduction of hospital mortality have been inconclusive and suffer from a lack of satisfactory randomization. Evaluations of the intermediate care concept are complicated by the following factors: variable lengths of stay in the CCU prior to transfer; the variable quality of staffing and monitoring capabilities; variability of patient populations in reference to age, sex, and extent and location of infarction; and prevalence of arrhythmias.

In spite of these criticisms, the intermediate care concept has contributed important other benefits in addition to the possible reduction in mortality. Detection and early treatment of arrhythmias have definitely been demonstrated in monitored, well-equipped units. Early ambulation and discharge in the uncomplicated patient can be accomplished with greater confidence and thus reduce both the length of hospital stay and the consequent economic burden on the health care system. More effective utilization of CCU beds can be accomplished when such monitored beds are available. Thus, the coronary care unit stay may be shortened and the number of patients utilizing the coronary care system might be increased without a costly expansion of the size of the coronary care unit.

## POSSIBLE IMPLICATIONS OF INTERMEDIATE CORONARY CARE FOR PREDISCHARGE EVALUATION

Finally, the intermediate care unit is the ideal location for the initiation of patient education, long-term management, and progressive cardiac rehabilitation. Nurses, nutritionists, and social workers working with physicians in a well-organized intermediate care environment provide the coronary patient with information regarding risk factor modification, education, employment, progressive exercise, medications, and warning signs of recurrent coronary disease. Thus, the opportunity for careful observation of the post-infarction patient may in addition permit more effective initiation of risk stratification and future management that may be crucial for the patient's long-term survival.

In this connection, the prognostic value of limited exercise testing prior to hospital discharge was evaluated by Théroux et al.[84] All 210 patients who were entered into the study had been free of chest pain for at least 4 days and none were in overt heart failure. These investigators reported that during a 1-year follow-up period 28 of 43 patients (65 percent) who had chest pain during the test reported angina, as compared with 60 of 167 patients (35 percent) who had no chest pain during the test ($P < 0.001$). The 1-year mortality rates were 2.1 percent in patients without changes in the ST segment during exercise and 27 percent (17 of 64) in those with ST segment depression ($P < 0.001$). Only one patient died suddenly among those without ST segment changes while 10 of 64 (16%) with ST segment depression had sudden death ($P < 0.001$). Davidson and DeBusk also reported that an exercise test 3 weeks after the onset of symptoms contained important prognostic information in uncomplicated patients.[85]

Whether patients with chest pain and/or ST segment depression should undergo early coronary arteriography with a view toward coronary artery revascularization is open to question and must be decided by further study.[86,87] The report of Théroux et al. did not employ objective measures of LV function, such as radionuclide angiography, either at rest or during exercise. Since the degree of LV dysfunction may bear importantly on subsequent mortality, including sudden death, this issue deserves further investigation as a part of risk stratification involving predischarge exercise testing. Thus, currently available information suggests that a rational approach to predischarge evaluation should include ambulatory (Holter) monitoring, assessment of LV function (radionuclide angiography or 2-D echocardiography) and possibly a low level stress test in uncomplicated patients. In some patients the stress test may be delayed for several weeks or not performed at all in the presence of angina pectoris and/or congestive heart failure.

With regard to medical therapy of patients surviving acute myocardial infarction, there has been considerable interest in the use of drugs such as aspirin and sulfinpyrazone. Both of these agents inhibit formation of prostaglandin endoperoxides and thereby of thromboxane $A_2$. Thromboxane $A_2$ causes platelet aggregation leading to vasospasm. It is also thought that platelet aggregation may play an important role in the pathogenesis of atherosclerosis. The potential utility of aspirin has also been underscored by its apparent benefit in men with transient cerebral ischemic attacks. Nevertheless, several trials of prophylactic aspirin therapy following acute myocardial infarction have been dissappointing. As an example, the AMIS (Aspirin Myocardial Infarction Study), a cooperative trial sponsored by the National Heart, Lung and Blood Institute, showed that aspirin, one gm daily, failed to reduce total mortality over a 3-year period.[88] Although the incidence of recurrent nonfatal infarction was lower in patients taking aspirin than in those taking a placebo, this difference was not statistically significant. Despite entrance of patients into the study at 8 weeks to 5 years after infarction, analysis by time-since-infarction made no difference in the results. A subject that deserves further study is whether these results would be altered by prospective identification of high-risk patients by complications (either in the CCU or in an intermediate care unit) or by delineation of depressed LV function and/or an abnormal response to exercise prior to discharge.

Similar considerations apply to the use of sulfinpyrazone. In a randomized, double-blind, multicenter trial comparing sulfinpyrazone (200 mg 4 times a day) with placebo in 1558 patients followed for an average of 16 months beginning 25 to 35 days after uncomplicated myocardial infarction, it was found that there was a marked reduction in sudden death in the sulfinpyrazone group during the second to the seventh month postinfarction (6 vs. 24 in the placebo group,

$P = 0.003$).[89] However, this study was initially designed to ascertain whether sulfinpyrazone would reduce the incidence of reinfarction. Thus, patients were not randomized with regard to LV functional status or severity of arrhythmias; in fact, Holter monitor studies were not carried out, save at a few cooperating institutions, nor were radionuclide ventriculograms or echocardiograms obtained routinely in any of the patients as part of the study. No data were obtained ragarding blood levels of concurrent antiarrhythmic drugs. While the results are highly promising, further validation is required in patients who are at risk as indicated by a complicated hospital course in the CCU or Intermediate Care Unit, abnormal left ventricular function, and/or an abnormal response to exercise stress prior to or shortly after hospital discharge.

# REFERENCES

1. Goble AJ, Sloman G, Robinson JS: Mortality reduction in a coronary care unit. Br Med J 1:1005, 1966.
2. Grace WJ: Mortality rates from acute myocardial infarction—what are we talking about? Am J Cardiol 24:651, 1969.
3. Killip T, Kimball JT: Treatment of myocardial infarction in a coronary care unit. A two year experience with 250 patients. Am J Cardiol 20:457, 1967.
4. Sloman G, Stannard M, Goble AJ: Coronary care unit. A review of 300 patients monitored since 1963. Am Heart J 75:140, 1968.
5. Thomas M, Jewitt DE, Shillingford JP: Analysis of 150 patients with acute myocardial infarction admitted to an intensive care and study unit. Br Med J 1:787, 1968.
6. Scheidt S, Ascheim R, Killip T: Shock after acute myocardial infarction. Am J Cardiol 26:556, 1970.
7. Gunnar RM, Cruz A, Boswell J, et al: Myocardial infarction with shock: Hemodynamic studies and results of therapy. Circulation 33:753, 1966.
8. Gotsman MS and Schrire V: Acute myocardial infarction-an ideal concept of progressive coronary care. South African Medical Journal 42:829, 1968.
9. Grace WJ and Yarvote PM: Acute myocardial

infarction: The course of the illness following discharge from the coronary care unit. Chest 59:15, 1971.

10. Lewis T: Diseases of the Heart. The Macmillan Company, New York, 1937.

11. Mallory GK, White PD, Salcedo-Salgar J: The speed of healing of myocardial infarction: A study of pathological anatomy in seventy-two cases. Am Heart J 18:647, 1939.

12. Sevitts S and Gallagher N: Venous thrombosis and pulmonary embolism. Br J Surg 48:475, 1961.

13. Fareeduddin K and Abelmann WH: Impaired orthostatic tolerance after bed rest in patients with myocardial infarction N Engl J Med 280:345, 1969.

14. Levine SA and Lown B: Armchair treatment of acute coronary thrombosis. JAMA 148:1365, 1952.

15. Irvin CW and Burgess AM: The abuse of bed rest in the treatment of myocardial infarction. NEJM 243:486, 1950.

16. Brummer P, Linko E, Kasenen A: Myocardial infarction treated by early ambulation. Am Heart J 52:269, 1956.

17. Beckwith JR, Kernodle DT, Lehew AE, Wood JE: The management of myocardial infarction with particular reference to the chair treatment. Ann Intern Med 41:1189, 1954.

18. Brummer P, Kallio V, Tala E: Early ambulation in the treatment of myocardial infarction. Acta Med Scand 180:231, 1966.

19. Naughton J, Bruhn J, Lategola MT and Whitsett T: Rehabilitation following myocardial infarction. Am J Med 46:725, 1969.

20. Duke M: Bed rest in acute myocardial infarction—a study of physician practices. Am Heart J 82:486, 1971.

21. Gilchrist AR: Problems in the management of acute myocardial infarction. Br Med J 1:215, 1960.

22. Hutter AM, Sidel VW, Shine KI, DeSanctis RW: Early hospital discharge after myocardial infarction. N Engl J Med 288:1141, 1973.

23. Harper JE, Kekket RJ, et al: Mobilization and discharge from hospital in uncomplicated myocardial infarction. Lancet 2:1331, 1971.

24. Royston GR: Short stay hospital treatment and rapid rehabilitation of cases of myocardial infarction in a district hospital. Brit Heart J 34:526, 1972.

25. Lown B, Sidel VW: Duration of hospital stay following acute myocardial infarction. Am J Cardiol 23:1, 1969.

26. Mather HG, Pearson HG, Read KLQ, et al: Acute myocardial infarction: Home and hospital treatment. Br Med J 3:334, 1971.

27. Mather HG, Morgan DC, Pearson NG et al: Myocardial infarction: a comparison between home and hospital care for patients. Br Med J 1:925, 1976.

28. McNeilly RH and Pemberton J: Duration of the last attack in 998 fatal cases of coronary artery disease and its relation to possible cardiac resuscitation Br Med J 3:139, 1968.

29. Adgey AAJ, Nelson PG, Scott ME: Management of ventricular fibrillation outside the hospital. Lancet 1:1169, 1969.

30. Hill JD, Hampton JR, Mitchell JRA: A randomized trial of home-versus-hospital management for patients with suspected myocardial infarction. Lancet 1:837, 1978.

31. Collings A, Carson P, Hampton J: Home or hospital care for coronary thrombosis. Br Med J 1:1254, 1978.

32. Wenger NK, Hellerstein HK, Blackburn H, Castranova SJ: Uncomplicated myocardial infarction. JAMA 224:511, 1973.

33. Resnekov L: The intermediate care unit—a stage in continued coronary care. Br Heart J 39:357, 1977.

34. Thompson P, Sloman G: Sudden death in hospital after discharge from the coronary care unit. Br Med J 4:136, 1971.

35. Graboys TB: In-hospital sudden death after coronary care unit discharge. Arch Intern Med 135:512, 1975.

36. Bornheimer J, de Guzman M, Haywood LJ: Analysis of in-hospital deaths from myocardial infarction after coronary care unit discharge. Arch Intern Med 135:1035, 1975.

37. Raizes G, Wagner G, Hackel DB: Instantaneous non-arrhythmic cardiac death in acute myocardial infarction. Role of electro-mechanical dissociation. Am J Cardiol 39:1, 1977.

38. Spracklen FHN, Besterman EMM, Everest MS et al: Late ventricular arrhythmias after myocardial infarction. Br Med J 4:364, 1968.

39. Restieaux N, Bray C, Bullard H, et al: 150 patients with cardiac infarction treated in a coronary care unit. Lancet 1:1285, 1967.

40. Wilson C, Adgey AAJ: Survival of patients with late ventricular fibrillation after myocardial infarction. Lancet 2:124, 1974.

41. McNeer JF, Wallace AG, Wagner GS: The course of acute myocardial infarction. Feasibility of early discharge of the uncomplicated patient. Circulation 51:410, 1975.

42. Lie KI, Liem KL, Schuilenburg RM, David GK and Durrer D: Early identification of patients developing late in-hospital ventricular fibrillation after discharge from the coronary care unit. Am J Cardiol 41:674, 1978.

43. Lie KI, Wellens HJJ, Schuilenburg RM et al: Factors influencing prognosis of bundle branch block complicating acute anteroseptal infarction. Circulation 50:935, 1974.

44. Scheinman M and Brenman B: Clinical and anatomic implications of intraventricular conduction blocks in acute myocardial infarction. Circulation 46:753, 1972.

45. Norris RM, Croxson MS: Bundle branch block in acute myocardial infarction. Am Heart J 79:728, 1970.

46. Godman MJ, Lassers BW, Julian DG: Complete bundle branch block complicating acute myocardial infarction. N Engl J Med 288:237, 1970.

47. Waters DD, Mizgala HF: Long term prognosis of patients with incomplete bilateral bundle branch block complicating acute myocardial infarction. Am J Cardiol 34:1, 1974.

48. Col JJ, Weinberg SL: The incidence and mortality of intraventricular conduction defects in acute myocardial infarction. Am J Cardiol 29:344, 1972.

49. Godman MJ, Alpert BA, Julian DG: Bilateral bundle branch block complicating acute myocardial infarction. Lancet 2:345, 1971.

50. Scanlon PJ, Pryor R, Blount SG: Right bundle branch block associated with left superior or inferior hemiblock. Circulation 42:1135, 1970.

51. Lim CH, Toh CCS, Low LP: Atrioventricular and associated intraventricular conduction disturbances in acute myocardial infarction. Br Heart J 33:947, 1971.

52. Fenig S, Lichstein E: Incomplete bilateral bundle branch block and AV block complicating acute anterior wall myocardial infarction. Am Heart J 84:38, 1972.

53. Waugh RA, Wagner GS, Haney TL, et al: Immediate and remote prognostic significance of fascicular block during acute myocardial infarction. Circulation 47:765, 1973.

54. Atkins JM, Leshin SJ, Blomqvist G, Mullins CB: Ventricular conduction blocks and sudden death in acute myocardial infarction. N Engl J Med 288:281, 1973.

55. Chiang BN, Perlman LV, Ostrander LD, Epstein FH: Relationship of premature systoles to coronary heart disease and sudden death in the Tecumseh epidemiology study. Ann Intern Med 70:1159, 1969.

56. Hinkle LE, Carver ST, Stevens M: The frequency of asymptomatic disturbances of cardiac rhythm and conduction in middle-aged men. Am J Cardiol 24:629, 1969.

57. Coronary Drug Project: Prognostic importance of premature beats following myocardial infarction. JAMA 223:1116, 1973.

58. Kotler MN, Tabatznik B, Mower MM, Tominaga S: Prognostic significance of ventricular ectopic beats with respect to sudden death in the late post-infarction period. Circulation 47:959, 1973.

59. Vismara L, Pratt C, Miller R, et al. Correlation of standard electrocardiogram and continuous ambulatory monitoring in detection of ventricular arrhythmias in coronary patients. Circulation 53 and 54 (suppl II):9, 1976.

60. Moss AJ, Schnitzler R, Green R, DeCamilla J: Ventricular arrhythmias three weeks after acute myocardial infarction. Ann Intern Med 75:837, 1971.

61. Harrison DC, Fitzgerald J, Winkle RA: Ambulatory ECGs to diagnose and treat cardiac arrhythmias. N Engl J Med 294:373, 1976.

62. Gorfinkel HJ, Kercher L, Lindsay J: Electrocardiographic radiotelemetry in the early recuperative period of acute myocardial infarction. Chest 69:158, 1976.

63. Lindsay J and Gorfinkel HJ: Arrhythmias in the post CCU phase of myocardial infarction. Chest 72:571, 1977.

64. Vismara LA, DeMaria AN, Hughes, JL et al: Evaluation of arrhythmias in the late hospital phase of acute myocardial infarction compared to coronary care unit ectopy. Br Heart J 37:598, 1975.

65. Vismara LA, Hughes JL, Mason DT, et al: Identification of predisposing factors to ventricular arrhythmias in the late hospital phase of acute myocardial infarction. Am J Cardiol 33:175, 1974.

66. Sharma SD, Ballantyne F, Goldstein S: The relationship of ventricular asynergy in coronary artery disease to ventricular premature beats. Chest 66:358, 1974.

67. Hans J: Mechanism of ventricular arrhythmias associated with myocardial infarction. Am J Cardiol 24:800, 1969.

68. Roberts R, Husain A, Ambos D, Oliver GC, Cop Jr. JR, Sobel BE: Relation between infarct size and ventricular arrhythmia. Br Heart J 37:1169, 1975.

69. Schulze RA, Rouleau J, Rigo P, et al: Ventricular arrhythmias in the late hospital phase of acute

myocardial infarction. Relation to left ventricular function detected by gated cardiac blood pool-scanning. Circulation 52:1006, 1975.

70. Schulze RA, Strauss HW, Pitt B: Sudden death in the year following myocardial infarction. Am J Med 62:192, 1977.

70a. Shah PK, Pichler M, Berman DS, Singh BN, Swan HJC: Left ventricular ejection fraction determined by radionuclide ventriculography in early stages of first transmural myocardial infarction. Relation to short-term prognosis. Am J Cardiol 45:542, 1980.

71. Scheinman MM, Abbott JA: Clinical significance of transmural versus nontransmural electrocardiographic changes in patients with acute myocardial infarction. Am J Med 55:602, 1973.

72. Mahony C, Aronin N, Wagner C: The excellent short and long term prognosis of patients with subendocardial infarction (Abstr) Am J Cardiol 41:407, 1978.

73. Edson JN: Subendocardial myocardial infarction. Am Heart J 60:323, 1960.

74. Madias JE, Chahine RA, Gorlin R, Blacklow DJ: A comparison of transmural and nontransmural acute myocardial infarction. Circulation 49:498, 1974.

75. Rigo P, Murray M, Taylor DR, et al: Hemodynamics and prognostic findings in patients with transmural and non-transmural infarction. Circulation 51:1064, 1975.

76. Cannom DS, Levy W, Cohen LS: The short and long term prognosis of patients with transmural and non-transmural myocardial infarction. Am J Med 61:452, 1976.

77. Wilson C and Pantridge JF: ST-segment displacement and early hospital discharge in acute myocardial infarction. Lancet 2:1284, 1973.

78. Coronary Drug Project Research Group: The prognostic importance of the electrocardiogram after myocardial infarction. Ann Intern Med 77:677, 1972.

79. Grace WJ: Intermediate coronary care units revised. Chest 67:510, 1975.

80. Reynell PC: Intermediate coronary care—a controlled trial Br Heart J 37:166, 1975.

81. Weinberg SL: Intermediate coronary care—observations on the validity of the concept. Chest 73:154, 1978.

82. Frieden J and Cooper JA: The role of the intermediate cardiac care unit. JAMA 235:816, 1976.

83. Leak D and Eydt JE: An assessment of intermediate coronary care. Arch Intern Med 138:1780, 1978.

84. Théroux P, Waters DD, Halphen C, Debaisieux JC, Mizgala HF: Prognostic value of exercise testing soon after myocardial infarction. N Engl J Med 301:341, 1979.

85. Davidson DM and DeBusk RF: Prognostic value of a single exercise test 3 weeks after uncomplicated myocardial infarction. Circulation 61:236, 1980.

86. Turner JD, Rogers WJ, Mantle JA, Rackley CE, Russell Jr. RO: Coronary angiography soon after myocardial infarction. Chest 77:58, 1980.

87. Rahimtoola SH: Coronary arteriography in asymptomatic patients after myocardial infarction. The need to distinguish between clinical investigation and clinical care. Chest 77:53, 1980.

88. Aspirin Myocardial Infarction Study Research Group: A randomized, controlled trial of aspirin in persons recovered from myocardial infarction. JAMA 243:661, 1980.

89. The Anturane Reinfarction Trial Research Group. Sulfinpyrazone in the prevention of sudden death after myocardial infarction. N Engl J of Med 302:250, 1980.

# 38 | Rehabilitation and Exercise Early After Acute Myocardial Infarction

*Victor F. Froelicher, M.D.*
*M. D. McKirnan, Ph.D.*

## EARLY AMBULATION

Prior to 1960, patients with acute myocardial infarction were thought to require prolonged restriction of their physical activity. Patients were often kept at strict bed rest for two months, with all activities performed by nursing personnel. The concern was that physical activity would lead to ventricular aneurysm formation, cardiac rupture, congestive heart failure, dysrhythmias, reinfarction, or sudden death as listed in Table 38.1. Hospitalization could last for 3 to 4 months with limitation of activities for at least one year. This approach was based on pathologic studies indicating that at least 6 weeks were required for necrotic myocardium to form a firm scar [1] and on the increased incidence of cardiac rupture reported among patients who infarcted in mental hospitals where bed rest could not be enforced.[2]

A "revolutionary approach" to treatment occurred in the 1940s when Levine recommended "chair treatment" for the postinfarction patient.[3] Levine emphasized the benefit of the sitting versus supine position for increasing peripheral venous pooling and decreasing preload on the myocardium. Such a reduction should theoretically lead to a decrease in resting left ventricular wall tension and, hence, to a reduction in myocardial oxygen demand. Dock agreed with this approach stressing the risk of thrombosis and pulmonary embolism and further recommended the use of the bedside commode in order to avoid the Valsalva maneuver.[4] The Valsalva maneuver, which is common when an individual strains with a bowel movement, can lead to deleterious elevations of systemic blood pressure early after infarction. The potential disadvantages of prolonged bed rest are listed in Table 38.2. Physiological studies

Table 38.1 Hypothetical Risks of Early Ambulation After Acute Myocardial Infarction

Dysrhythmias
Congestive heart failure
Left ventricular aneurysm
Cardiac rupture
Reinfarction
Sudden death

Table 38.2 The Potential Disadvantages of Prolonged Bed Rest

Orthostatic hypotension
Venous thrombosis
Reduced lung volume
Pulmonary emboli
Atelectasis; pneumonia
Metabolic alterations
Musculoskeletal problems

have documented the hemodynamic alterations caused by deconditioning.[5] After a prolonged bed rest, tachycardia and hypotension are common upon standing. This is most likely due to alterations of vasomotor reflexes and to hypovolemia that occurs with bed rest. It is now recommended that postinfarction patients begin the activities listed in Table 38.3 and outlined in Appendix 3 as soon as possible in the CCU.

In 1961 Cain and colleagues reported the use of a progressive activity program for acute infarction patients.[6] This report had difficulty getting published because it was considered to be a dangerous approach. They reported 335 patients with uncomplicated myocardial infarction who were at least 15 days postinfarction. The patients had been restricted to bed, chair, and commode. The ECG was monitored after the patient performed activities including climbing stairs and walking up a grade. They concluded that ECG monitoring of early activity was a more reliable means of ascertaining the presence of coronary insufficiency than physical signs or symptoms. Cain and colleagues tried to explain that they were not advising early ambulation for all patients, but only for those who responded favorably.

In 1964 Torkelson reported his results in ten patients with uncomplicated myocardial infarction.[7] On the sixth week of his in-hospital rehabilitation program, a low-level treadmill test was performed using 1.7 mph at a 10 percent grade. Torkelson concluded that the treadmill test was a valuable procedure for the documentation of the specific exercise response of patients recovering from an acute myocardial infarction. He felt that consideration of the response to a treadmill test made possible proper progression of an exercise program.

Most of the later publications failed to indicate the need for ECG monitoring as part of progressive ambulation. Instead, generalized statements as to the activities on each postinfarction day have been made for all patients, rather than individualizing activity progression. Recently, Sivarajan, Bruce, and colleagues [8] have returned to the approach of Cain and Torkelson. They reported 12 patients with acute myocardial infarction whose symptoms, signs, and hemodynamic and ECG responses during and after three activities were assessed. These activities included sitting upright, walking to the toilet, and walking on a treadmill. These activities were studied at 3, 6, and 10 days, respectively, after infarction. They concluded that successful performance of these three activities provided useful criteria for discharge of the patient with myocardial infarction. At this time, these researchers are conducting a controlled early rehabilitation study in the Seattle community using these techniques. If a patient has an abnormal response, such as a systolic blood pressure drop, severe chest pain, marked ST changes, or dysrhythmias, his or her progressive ambulation program and discharge from the hospital are delayed until the responses are acceptable. This approach is very attractive and possibly constitutes optimal care of the postinfarction patient.

## COMPLICATED VS. UNCOMPLICATED MI

It is well known that morbidity and mortality in postinfarction patients who have complicated courses are much higher than in those with uncomplicated infarcts.[9] The criteria for a complicated infarct are listed in Table 38.4. Certainly early ambulation is not appropriate for the patient with a complicated infarct. The progressive ambulation program should be delayed until such individuals reach an uncomplicated status, and even then progressive ambulation should be slower. The following controlled studies of patients with uncomplicated infarction have demonstrated that the risks of early ambulation are minimal and that progressive mobilization during the early stages of acute myocardial infarction is recommended.

**Table 38.3  Physical Activities in the Coronary Care Unit**

Self care

Active and passive arm and leg movement

Postural changes

Chair

Bedside commode

**Table 38.4    Criteria for A Complicated Myocardial Infarction**

Continued cardiac ischemia (pain, late enzyme rise)

Left ventricular failure (congestive heart failure, new murmurs, x-ray changes)

Shock (blood pressure drop, pallor, oliguria)

Important cardiac dysrhythmias (PVCs greater than 6/min, atrial fibrillation)

Conduction disturbances (bundle branch block, A-V block, hemiblock)

Severe pleurisy or pericarditis

Complicating illnesses

Marked creatine kinase rise without a noncardiac explanation

## CONTROLLED STUDIES OF EARLY MOBILIZATION AND HOSPITAL DISCHARGE

Hayes and colleagues studied 189 patients with uncomplicated myocardial infarction selected at random for early or late mobilization and discharge from the hospital.[10] Patients were admitted to the study after 48 hours in a coronary care unit if they were free of pain and showed no evidence of heart failure or significant dysrhythmias. One group of patients was mobilized immediately and discharged home after a total of 9 days in the hospital; the second group was mobilized on the ninth day and discharged on the sixteenth day. Out-patient assessment was carried out 6 weeks after admission. No significant differences were observed between the groups in terms of morbidity or mortality, as reflected by the incidence of recurrent chest pain or myocardial infarction, heart failure, dysrhythmia, or venous thrombosis detected either clinically or by radionuclide scanning.

In a strictly randomized, controlled study, Bloch and colleagues studied the effects of early mobilization after uncomplicated myocardial infarction.[11] One-hundred and fifty-four patients under 70 years of age who were hospitalized for an acute myocardial infarction and had no complications on day one or day two were randomly assigned to two treatment groups. In the early mobilization group, patients were treated by a physiotherapist with a progressive activity program beginning on day 2 or 3 after infarction. In the control group, the patients underwent the traditional hospital regimen of strict bed rest for 3 weeks or more. The mean duration of hospitalization was 21 days for active patients and 33 days for the control group. The follow-up period ranged from 6 to 20 months with an average of 11 months. There were no significant differences between the two groups with regard to hospital or follow-up mortality, rate of reinfarction, dysrhythmias, heart failure, angina pectoris, ventricular aneurysm, or the results of an exercise test. On follow-up examination there was actually greater disability in the control than in the active group.

## SUBENDOCARDIAL VS. TRANSMURAL MI

Recently there has been some controversy over the relative long-term risk of subendocardial versus transmural myocardial infarction.[12,13] Some of this difficulty has been due to terminology. Traditionally, an infarct with evolving Q waves on the ECG has been called transmural and considered large, while an infarct with only ST and T wave changes has been called subendocardial and considered small. Estimation of the severity of a myocardial infarct requires consideration of clinical findings and other test results besides the ECG in order to judge a patient's risk and infarct size. The presence of Q waves does not assure that transmural myocardial infarction has occurred, as transmural infarction can produce only ST and T wave changes. [14] The severity of an infarct should be judged by clinical findings, hemodynamic monitoring, the level of creatine kinase (CK) elevation, and the presence of congestive heart failure and/or shock. The concept that a subendocardial infarct is incomplete and unstable while a transmural infarct is stable is probably not the case. The first studies of prognosis mixed patients with previous myocardial infarctions, while recent studies have separated those with a first infarction exhibiting ST and T wave changes and have found that their prognosis is relatively good.

## EXERCISE TESTING EARLY AFTER MI

It is desirable to submit patients with recent acute infarction to an exercise test to optimize their progression through hospitalization and discharge. The test can be performed to determine the possible risk of the patient during physical activities. It is certainly better that adverse reactions be observed in controlled circumstances. The exercise test can be used to demonstrate the patient's reactions to exercise so that work capacity and limiting factors are known at the time of discharge. This provides a safer basis for advising a patient's activity level and return to work. The exercise test can demonstrate to the patient, as well as to his relatives and employer, how his capacity for physical performance was affected by his infarction. It can also have a therapeutic effect by making a patient less anxious about daily physical activities. The exercise test can be the first step in cardiac rehabilitation.

The benefit/risk ratio of this procedure can be improved by a number of considerations. Although maximal testing has been reported, we still feel that a heart rate limited test is indicated until 2 months after infarction. Arbitrarily, a heart rate limit of 140 is used for patients under 40 and 130 for patients over 40. Also, we use conservative clinical indications for stopping the test. The exercise test should not be ordered without the patient's primary physician involved in its performance. It is important that the physician who knows the patient be there at the test and interact with the patient. The current status of the exercise test in the management of acute infarction patients is outlined in Table 38.5. The protocol used

**Table 38.5   The Use of Exercise Testing as Part of Cardiac Rehabilitation**

1. To prescribe progressive in-hospital activity

2. The discharge exercise test, 6 to 8 weeks post infarction exercise test, and the follow-up exercise test which are performed in order to:
   a. Prescribe exercise
   b. Give reassurance
   c. Predict risk and severity of coronary disease
   d. Determine type of exercise program
   e. Triage to cardiac catheterization, surgery, medical treatment or exercise

at University Hospital, University of California, San Diego is described in the Appendix.

Atterhog and colleagues reported the electrocardiographic response to exercise at varying periods after an anterior myocardial infarction.[15] Three weeks after infarction, 10 of their 12 patients exhibited an exercise-induced rise in ST segments in anterior precordial leads over the infarcted areas. This ECG response decreased over the following months, and some subjects had exercise-induced ST segment depression. The ST segment elevation was interpreted as a sign of ischemia in the infarcted zone, and the rate at which this resolved was thought to have prognostic significance.

The results of treadmill testing in 100 patients 3 weeks after acute infarction were reported by Ericsson and colleagues.[16] Premature ventricular contractions were recorded in three patients immediately before the test and in 19 patients during and/or after the test. It was concluded that the treadmill test proved to be a sensitive method for demonstrating arrythmias in patients with recent infarctions. Ibsen and colleagues reported the results of a maximal bicycle test in the third week after acute myocardial infarction in 209 patients.[17] They concluded that an exercise test was safe in such patients, that it was an objective measure of physical work capacity, and that it demonstrated the reaction to physical activity. They felt that because it was a maximal test it gave a better basis for advising return to a normal life and was of great psychological importance to the patient.

Granath and colleagues performed exercise tests at 3 and 9 weeks after acute myocardial infarction in 205 patients and followed them for 2 to 5 years.[18] The appearance of tachycardia at low workloads and major ventricular dysrhythmias or anginal complaints during these early exercise tests was followed by significantly increased mortality. Exercise-induced premature ventricular contractions proved to be of higher prognostic significance than those recorded at rest. They found that early exercise tests were valuable for evaluating the reponse to antiarrhythmic agents. Wohl and colleagues studied 50 patients after acute myocardial infarction.[19] They found that, in stable patients, there was an early improvement of the relationship between myocardial oxygen supply and demand as detected by ST segment changes. There was a delayed improvement of functional capacity associated with increased stroke volume and cardiac output. The early improvement was noted in a study done at 3 weeks, and the later studies were done between 3 and 6 months. Markiewicz and colleagues studied 46 men under the age of 70 using treadmill testing at 3, 5, 7, 9, and 11 weeks after myocardial infarction.[20] They concluded that two tests— the one at 3 to 5 weeks and the one at 7 to 11 weeks—appeared to provide most of the information obtained in all five tests performed. In selected low-risk patients who underwent maximal treadmill testing at 3 weeks after infarction, they found that a low heart rate response indicated a poor prognosis.

At a mean of 18 days after admission, Smith and colleagues performed exercise tests to 60 percent of maximal predicted heart rate on 62 of 109 consecutive AMI patients.[21] Exercise testing influenced management in 21 percent of these patients. Therapy with antiarrhythmic agents was started in four patients, the dose of antianginal agents was increased in three patients, and hospitalization was prolonged in four patients. Fourteen patients died after discharge, six of whom had undergone exercise testing. Thirty percent of the patients (6 out of 20) who developed ST segment depression during exercise either died or had another myocardial infarct after discharge from the hospital. This is in contrast to the occurrence of death or reinfarction in only 2 of the 42 patients who did not have ST segment depression during exercise. They concluded that the exercise test is safe and useful for clinical management of MI patients and possibly valuable in predicting coronary events after hospitalization.

Kramer and colleagues reported a retrospective study of 115 consecutive symptomatic patients who had exercise tests, selective coronary angiography, and left ventriculography.[22] Analysis of the false-negative group (normal ECG in patients with coronary heart disease [CHD]) demonstrated more ventriculographic and hemodynamic abnormalities when compared to the true positive responders (i.e., those

with abnormal ECG response and CHD). Five out of six patients with the most serious wall motion disorders in this study were false-negative responders. Among the shortcomings of this study was that the anterior leads were not recorded and ST segment elevation was not considered.

In a retrospective study, Castellanet et al. reported 97 patients with prior transmural myocardial infarction who underwent coronary angiography and treadmill testing.[23] Among patients with previous inferior wall infarction, the ST segment response to the treadmill test had an 87 percent sensitivity (percent with CHD who have an abnormal response) and a 90 percent specificity (percent of those without CHD who have a normal response) in detecting additional significant coronary artery disease. In patients with previous anteroseptal myocardial infarction, the ST segment response showed a sensitivity of 52 percent and a specificity of 90 percent. The presence of Q waves in the precordial leads extending to lead V4 or beyond decreased the sensitivity rate of treadmill testing to 33 percent. A major shortcoming of this study was that only bipolar CM5 was monitored.

In order to determine whether the exercise test might predict multivessel coronary disease and left ventricular aneurysm after myocardial infarction, Weiner and colleagues presented the results of 154 patients with a single documented myocardial infarct who had had both exercise testing (12-lead) and coronary angiography.[24] Patients were studied 2 to 36 months after infarction for the evaluation of symptoms or to estimate their prognosis. The results of this study are shown in Table 38.6. They concluded that: ST segment depression with or without ST elevation predicts multivessel disease; ST elevation alone or a negative exercise test suggests single-vessel disease; and ST elevation with or without ST segment depression predicts a left ventricular aneurysm. Figure 38.1 shows an example of ST depression and Figure 38.2 shows an example of ST elevation from our laboratory.

Paine and colleagues did a similar study of 100 consecutive patients at a median of 4 months after infarction.[25] Multi-lead exercise

Table 38.6 The Results of Exercise Tests and Angiography in 154
Patients with a Single Myocardial Infarct 2 to 36 Months After Their
Infarction Studied Because of Symptoms or for Prognosis

|  | Multivessel Disease | Aneurysm |
|---|---|---|
| 83 with ST depression only | 76% | 31% |
| 22 with elevation and depression | 91% | 68% |
| 19 with elevation only | 21% | 79% |
| 30 with normal ST response | 13% | 40% |

(From the data of Weiner et al: Circulation 58:887, 1978)

testing was performed using a submaximal exercise protocol. Eighty-seven percent of the patients with abnormal ST segment depression had double- or triple-vessel disease. Of the patients with a negative exercise test, 62 percent had only single-vessel disease, 33 percent had double-vessel disease, and 5 percent had triple-vessel disease. Fourteen patients had ST segment elevation during exercise. These patients had a lower ejection fraction and a larger angiographic scar than the other patients. Patients terminating exercise because of symptoms of left ventricular dysfunction (fatigue or dyspnea) showed a mild correlation between the duration of exercise, ejection fraction, and the size of the angiographic scar.

Recently Theroux and colleagues evaluated the prognostic value of exercise testing soon after myocardial infarction.[26] A submaximal treadmill test was performed in 210 consecutive patients one day before hospital discharge after AMI. They had no overt heart failure and had been free of chest pain for four days. One year of follow-up revealed a mortality rate of 2.1 percent vs. 27 percent and a sudden death rate of 0.7 percent vs. 16 percent in those without ST segment depression compared to those with ST segment depression. Angina during the test also predicted those who were going to develop angina during the ensuing year.

Pulido and colleagues studied the relationship between global and regional left ventricular

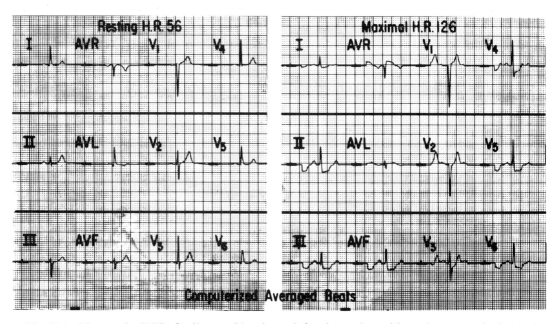

Fig. 38.1 The exercise ECG of a 60-year-old male postinfarction patient with persistent exercise-induced ST-segment depression on repeated tests. He decided against coronary artery bypass surgery because of minimal symptoms and has done well in the UCSD Cardiac Rehabilitation Program.

**Resting H.R. 76**          **Maximal H.R. 140**

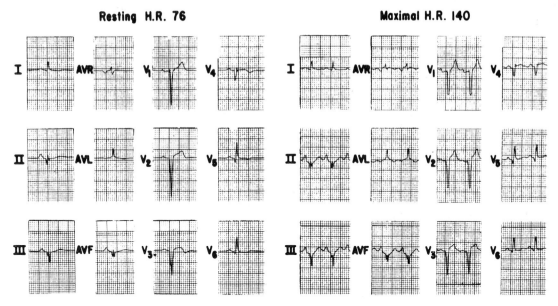

Fig. 38.2   The exercise ECG of a 38-year-old male postinfarction patient who has a large left ventricular apical aneurysm. He shows exercise-induced ST-segment elevation in the anterior leads. He did well in cardiac rehabilitation and has returned to work.

function and the ECG at rest and during sub-maximal supine exercise in 27 patients 2 to 3 weeks after an AMI.[27] Gated equilibrium radionuclide left ventriculograms were obtained during submaximal exercise. Exercise was terminated when the patient's heart rate reached 125/min or if angina, dangerous PVCs, or electrocardiographic evidence of myocardial ischemia developed before this rate was reached. Patients with recent acute anterior myocardial infarction manifested a significant reduction in left ventricular ejection fraction during submaximal exercise. Most of these patients also had segmental wall motion abnormalities at rest. Only 2 of 13 patients with an inferior infarct had segmental wall motion abnormalities during submaximal exercise, and two others had wall motion abnormalities at rest which became more marked during exercise. Of the six patients with infarcts but without Q waves, four had no wall motion abnormalities at rest and in one of these an abnormality developed with exercise. The remaining two patients had wall motion abnormalities at rest and one developed an abnormal ECG response. They concluded that patients with an anterior infarct appeared to have a different functional ventricu-

lar response to submaximal exercise than patients with an inferior infarct or an infarct not exhibiting Q waves. All patients with anterior transmural infarcts had a decreased ejection fraction with exercise, those with inferior infarcts varied but showed a small mean drop as a group, and those with subendocardial infarcts varied but showed a small mean increase as a group.

Although the use of electrocardiographic monitoring of activities after an acute infarction requires additional time and an interested staff, it would appear to be the ideal way of prescribing a safe level of physical activity. An exercise test prior to discharge is important for giving a patient guidelines for exercise at home, reassuring him of his physical status, and determining his risk of complications. An interesting question is whether the predischarge exercise test is therapeutic. The psychological impact of a good performance on the exercise test is impressive. Many patients increase their activity and actually rehabilitate themselves after being encouraged and reassured by their response to this test. In interpreting the exercise test, consideration should be given to the responses listed in Tables 38.7 and 38.8.

**Table 38.7    Exercise-Induced Electrocardiographic Changes Possibly Due to Ischemia or Left Ventricular Dysfunction**

1) QRS changes:
   Transient infarct patterns
   Changes in R-wave amplitude
   Changes in S-wave amplitude
   Axis changes and left anterior hemiblock
   QRS prolongation and bundle branch block
   Spatial magnitude and direction

2) ST segment:
   Depression
   Elevation
   Normalization
   Spatial magnitude and direction

3) U wave inversion

4) Ventricular ectopy

5) Supraventricular ectopy and blocks

6) P wave changes

**Table 38.8    Non-ECG Exercise Test Results to be Considered**

1) Heart rate and blood pressure
2) Functional capacity
3) Symptoms
4) Physical findings
5) Thallium scan
6) Left ventricular imaging for ejection fraction, wall motion abnormalities, volumes

## POSTHOSPITAL CARDIAC REHABILITATION

The goal of rehabilitation is to restore the patient to optimal physiological, psychological, and vocational status and, if possible, to prevent the underlying disease from progressing. The American Heart Association has concluded that over one-half of the survivors of acute myocardial infarction have significant psychologic, physiologic, or sociologic disabilities. The impact of an infarction on risk can be seen from the Göteborg Study summarized in Table 38.9.[28] Approximately one million Americans will have a myocardial infarction this year. Since 65 percent will die, this leaves 350,000 survivors and at least 175,000 individuals in need of rehabilitation. One-third of the individuals placed on Social Security disability during 1977 qualified because of heart disease. There

are many patients disabled by angina pectoris and many asymptomatic individuals at high risk for developing the manifestations of coronary disease.

Exercise training has an important role in cardiac rehabilitation because of documented hemodynamic, physiologic, and symptomatic benefits.[29] However, other behavior modification such as cessation of cigarette smoking and control of hypertension and diet must be included. Exercise training is an expensive therapeutic modality that includes the phases listed in Table 38.10 and carries risks. This is further complicated by the fact that definitive studies on coronary disease patients have not been able to document beneficial effects on morbidity and mortality, or on ischemia and ventricular dysfunction. There is also a need for serial studies, using objective, noninvasive methods, that are concerned with categorizing patients and assessing the effects of exercise on the left ventricle. These could be followed by controlled large studies of cardiac rehabilitation with careful categorization of patients to assess differences in morbidity and mortality. As indicated above,

**Table 38.9    Summary of the Göteborg Acute Myocardial Infarction Study**

1) 5 year follow-up of 300 males less than 55 years of age with their first myocardial infarction

2) Total mortality (in hospital, pre-hospitalization and post-hospitalization = 47%)

3) If first myocardial infarction, 30x risk of morbidity and mortality over the next year compared to age matched general population

4) 2nd year—10x risk

**Table 38.10    The General Activity Phases of Cardiac Rehabilitation (Requiring Modification According to Clinical Judgement and Test Results)**

1) Coronary care unit (early ambulation if uncomplicated)

2) Remainder of hospitalization (about 10cc oxygen/kg/min, or 3 METS)

3) Two to eight weeks post-hospitalization (about 15cc oxygen/kg/min, or 5 METS)

4) Physical reconditioning or exercise training

5) Activity maintenance

such rehabilitation can begin in the CCU in the early postinfarction period.

Inadequately controlled studies of cardiac rehabilitation suggest a decrease in morbidity and mortality for those who adhere to an exercise program, but these findings have not been substantiated by better controlled studies.[30,31] It has not been possible to document definitive changes in myocardial ischemia or cardiac function secondary to exercise training in patients with coronary artery disease. Also, it has not been possible to categorize patients most likely to have long-term physiological benefit from cardiac rehabilitation. It is unlikely that exercise has a direct effect on the atherosclerotic process. However, many studies have documented beneficial changes in hemodynamic measurements and work capacity secondary to an exercise program in patients with coronary disease.[32] These beneficial changes could be due to changes in the peripheral circulation, in the levels of circulating catecholamines, the sympathetic nervous system, and/or skeletal muscle rather than to cardiac alterations.[33,34] Hemodynamic and work capacity changes that occur within several months of training in older subjects are most likely due to noncardiac peripheral changes, and longer periods of training are needed for cardiac alterations to occur.

The use of exercise in the rehabilitation of coronary disease patients would be supported if the cardiac alterations documented in animal studies, including increased myocardial perfusion, myocardial hypertrophy, and improved cardiac function could also be documented in humans. Unfortunately, most of these beneficial changes are most evident in younger animals.[35] The areas to be discussed evaluating the effects of exercise training on the hearts of patients with coronary artery disease include changes in cardiac morphology, coronary atherosclerosis, and cardiovascular hemodynamics.

## Cardiac Morphology and Coronary Angiography

The results of previous studies of exercise training on coronary patients in which cardiac dimensions were assessed by routine chest radiograph have been very variable. This is par-

tially due to age-related factors, but it may also have been due to variability in the techniques. Only one echocardiographic study before and after cardiac rehabilitation attempted to measure changes in left ventricular wall thickness and volumes, but the findings were inconclusive.[36] Certain echocardiographic studies have been able to detect changes in myocardial mass and left ventricular volumes in younger, normal subjects secondary to training.[37,38] However, such changes have not yet been found in older, normal subjects.[39] Coronary angiography before and after exercise training has not demonstrated significant changes in atherosclerotic lesions or collateral vessels.[40,41] One study analyzed left ventriculograms performed before and after 3 months of cardiac rehabilitation and found no changes.[42] However, Sylvester and colleagues have catheterized the largest number of patients (>100) before and after cardiac rehabilitation.[43] They concluded that certain patients show improvement or a decrease in the rate of disease progression as assessed by coronary angiographic anatomy and left ventricular function.

## Cardiovascular Hemodynamics

Bruce and colleagues performed invasive hemodynamic studies in coronary patients who had been in a long-term exercise program.[44] Although all patients had improvement in their exercise capacity and were able to perform at an exercise level satisfactory to them, some of the patients exhibited deterioration of left ventricular function. This study points out the inability to assess cardiac changes by functional alterations even when measured from treadmill testing.

Carter and Amundsen compared infarct size estimated from serum CK elevations to the functional exercise capacity of 22 MI patients.[45] The patients were studied 2.5 to 4.5 months after infarction. Eleven of the 22 entered an exercise program for 3 to 4 months and were subsequently retested on a bicycle ergometer. Prior to this exercise training, a significant correlation was demonstrated between aerobic capacity and estimated infarct size ($r = -0.68$), but the correlation was higher ($r = -0.84$) after training. Infarct size was not a predictor of the capacity of a patient to obtain a training effect. These results suggest that more accurate comparisons of training responses may be made when both infarct size and the time postinfarct are considered.

Sim and Neill studied eight patients with coronary disease and exertional angina pectoris before and after a 3- to 4-month program of physical conditioning.[46] The double product for angina was determined for upright bicycle ergometry and for atrial pacing. The product of heart rate and systolic blood pressure at the exercise angina threshold was higher after conditioning, suggesting that conditioning increased the maximal myocardial oxygen supply during exercise. However, when the angina was induced by atrial pacing, the heart rate, arterial blood pressure, coronary blood flow, and myocardial oxygen consumption at the angina threshold were the same before and after conditioning. Myocardial lactate extraction was still abnormal during pacing, and there were no changes in coronary obstruction or collaterals as judged by coronary angiograms. The increase in anginal threshold during exercise appears to be due to functional adaptation in either myocardial oxygen supply or the relationship between hemodynamic work and myocardial oxygen consumption. The adaptation was limited to exercise and did not occur during atrial pacing. One patient developed ventricular fibrillation and was successfully defibrillated. He had single-vessel disease of the right coronary artery and he did not have a myocardial infarct associated with this event. Pressures and cardiac output at rest, left ventricular volumes, and ejection fractions remained unchanged, as did the coronary angiograms. These findings are a strong argument against a training effect on maximal coronary flow, but it is possible that coronary flow during exercise did increase. An alternate explanation for increased exercise capacity after training is that changes affecting the determinants of myocardial oxygen demand occurred which are not accounted for by the rate-pressure product (e.g., smaller left ventricular volume, less prominent increase in contractile state during exercise).

In ten patients with exertional angina pectoris, Ferguson and colleagues studied the effects of 6 months of bicycle ergometry training on coronary sinus blood flow and left ventricular oxygen consumption.[47] The measurements were made before and after training with the patient in the upright position at rest, during exercise at 400 kpm, during exercise at equivalent heart rates, and during symptom-limited maximal exercise. After training, patients increased their physical work capacity by 18 percent at the same submaximal heart rate of approximately 114/min. Coronary blood flow, myocardial oxygen consumption, and the pressure-rate product were not significantly different, despite this increase in workload. Symptom-limited maximal exercise capacity increased by 43 percent with training but the above measurements were also not significantly different after training. At an equivalent workload of approximately 400 kpm, heart rate, coronary sinus blood flow, and pressure rate product were significantly lower after training. The post-training increase in exercise tolerance in patients with angina pectoris did not depend upon an augmented myocardial oxygen delivery, but was related to a reduction in coronary flow requirement for a given workload.

Two recent preliminary studies have utilized radionuclide left ventricular angiography to study the effects of training. Rerych and colleagues reported an increase in end-diastolic volume both at rest and during erect maximal bicycle exercise after training in normals.[48] Wallace and colleagues reported the results of exercise training in 12 patients with symptomatic, documented coronary disease.[49] End-diastolic volume and stroke volume increased at rest and during exercise. Ejection fraction did not deteriorate at maximal exercise, despite higher heart rate, blood pressure, and end-diastolic volume. We have found mixed ejection fraction responses but some patients improve their thallium-201 scans and ejection fraction responses after training.

## Cardiovascular Complications During Cardiac Rehabilitation

Haskell surveyed 30 cardiac rehabilitation programs in North America using a questionnaire to assess major cardiovascular complications.[50] Only centers performing medically supervised cardiac exercise classes were included. This survey included approximately 14,000 patients for 1.6 million exercise hours. Complications were classified as fatal or nonfatal, including cardiopulmonary arrest, myocardial infarction, and others. Of 50 cardiopulmonary resuscitations, eight resulted in death; of seven myocardial infarctions, two resulted in death. Exercise programs resulted in four other fatalities occurring after hospitalization, including pulmonary embolization and pulmonary edema. There was one nonfatal event per 35,000 patients. The complication rates were lower in ECG-monitored programs and in data reported since 1970. The current programs reported a 4 percent annual mortality rate during exercise, which is a rate not different from that expected in such patients. These data support the recommendation that, in a medical situation where an exercise program can be prescribed and supervised, certain screened, selected cardiac patients can exercise safely. The Georgia Baptist Program in Atlanta reported a ventricular fibrillation rate of 1 in 13,000 gymnasium hours;[51] the Toronto program reported 1 in 15,000 gymnasium hours;[52] and the CAPRI Program in Seattle reported the highest rate of 1 in 6,000 exercise hours.[53] All of the 15 such patients reported by the CAPRI group were successfully resuscitated. Eleven had angiography, which showed single-vessel disease in four and multivessel disease in seven. These studies are summarized in Table 38.11.

Fletcher and Cantwell reported five coronary disease patients resuscitated after experiencing ventricular fibrillation during an exercise program.[54] Multivessel coronary disease that could be treated with bypass surgery was present in four of these patients. Cardiopulmonary resuscitation was required unexpectedly and unpredictably anytime from 2 to 48 months after being in the exercise program. These two experienced cardiologists are now reluctant to "graduate" patients to exercise without medical supervision. Shephard and Kavanagh also agree that the potential victim of a cardiac arrest during exercise training cannot be identified.[55] Even trained patients should avoid excessive

**Table 38.11  Data Regarding the Safety of Cardiac Rehabilitation Programs**

1) *A Summary of Haskell's Survey*
—30 medically supervised cardiac rehabilitation programs
—Cardiovascular complications by questionnaire classified as non-fatal or fatal including cardiac arrest, myocardial infarction, and "other"
—14,000 patients, 1.6 million exercise hours
—50 events requiring cardiopulmonary resuscitation (CPR) with 8 deaths directly related, for 1 CPR/32,000 exercise hours leading to 2 deaths—four other fatalities
—One non-fatal complication/35,000 patient hours
—One fatal complication/116,000 patient hours
—Complications lower 1) in ECG monitored classes; 2) Since 1970
—There was a 4% annualized mortality rate during exercise classes (i.e., no increase of risk over coronary patients not in rehabilitation)

2) *Individual Programs*
Capri—1 CPR/6,000 exercise hours
Georgia Baptist—1 CPR/13,000 exercise hours
Toronto—1 CPR/25,000 exercise hours

and unusual exertion, particularly when associated with competition and emotional excitement. Patients should also learn to recognize dysrhythmias and angina, and should moderate their activity if they sense ischemic prodromes, tension, or depression.

## SUMMARY

Early ambulation for the uncomplicated myocardial infarction patient has been found to be very safe. In fact, the debilitating effects of bed rest provide very strong support for its use. The benefit/risk ratio of exercise testing soon after infarction has been excellent. Although maximal testing has been safely carried out within 3 weeks of the acute event, it seems more prudent to postpone maximal testing until 2 months after infarction, by which time tissue repair and scar formation should be complete. Arbitrarily, early exercise testing before 2 months should observe the following recommendations: heart rate limits of 140 and 130 for patients under 40 and over 40, respectively; conservative clinical indications for stopping; and the primary physician's involvement in testing. Benefits of early exercise evaluations in-

**Table 38.12   The Benefits of Cardiac Rehabilitation Possibly Include the Following**

Fewer complications than bed rest

Better psychological adjustment

Improved cardiovascular function due to peripheral (and cardiac?) changes

Return to employment

Favorable influence on re-infarction

Behavior modification favorably affecting risk

clude: optimal activity progression in-hospital; triaging of patients; prediction of risk and severity of disease; prescribing exercise; and patient reassurance.

The potential benefits of cardiac rehabilitation are listed in Table 38.12. Exercise training provides an important intervention in posthospital rehabilitation. Documented benefits include hemodynamic, physiologic, and symptomatic improvement; however, risk factor modification certainly must also be emphasized. Controlled studies have failed to demonstrate any decrease in morbidity and mortality in patients adhering to an exercise program. Furthermore, the hemodynamic and physiologic improvements that have been attributed to peripheral adaptations and central changes in myocardial perfusion or ventricular function have not been consistently documented. However, a medically supervised cardiac rehabilitation program places the patient at no increased risk, and the qualitative improvement experienced by many patients strongly supports its use.

## REFERENCES

1. Mallory GK, White PD, and Salcedo-Salgar J: The speed of healing of myocardial infarction: a study of the pathologic anatomy in seventy-two cases. Am Heart J 18:647, 1939.
2. Jetter WW, White PD: Rupture of the heart in patients in mental institutions. Ann Intern Med 21:783, 1944.
3. Levine SA, Lown B: The "chair" treatment of acute coronary thrombosis. Trans Assoc Am Physicians 64:316, 1951.
4. Dock W: The evil sequelae of complete bed rest. JAMA 125:1083, 1944.
5. Saltin B, Blomqvist G, Mitchell JH et al: Response to exercise after bed rest and training. Circulation 37 (suppl 7):1, 1968.
6. Cain HD, Frasher WG, Stivelman R: Graded activity program for safe return to self-care after myocardial infarction. JAMA 177:111, 1961.
7. Torkelson LO: Rehabilitation of the patient with acute myocardial infarction. J Chronic Dis 17:685, 1964.
8. Sivarajan ES, Snydsman A, Smith B et al: Low-level treadmill testing of 41 patients with acute myocardial infarction prior to discharge from the hospital. Clin Stud Crit Care 6:975, 1977.
9. Froelicher VF: Review of epidemiology in clinical cardiology. Aviat Space Environ Med 48 (7):659, 1977.
10. Hayes MJ, Morris GK, Hampton JR: Comparison of mobilization after two and nine days in uncomplicated myocardial infarction. Br Med J 3:10, 1974.
11. Bloch A, Maeder J, Haissly J et al: Early mobilization after myocardial infarction. Am J Cardiol 34:152, 1974.
12. Cannom DS, Levy W, Cohen LS: The short and long term prognosis of patients with transmural and nontransmural myocardial infarction. Am J Med 61:452, 1976.
13. Szklo M, Goldbert R, Kennedy HL, Tonascia JA: Survival of patients with nontransmural myocardial infarction: A population-based study. Am J Cardiol 42:648, 1978.
14. Roberts WC, Gardin JM: Location of myocardial infarcts: A confusion of terms and definitions. Am J Cardiol 42:868, 1978.
15. Atterhog JH, Ekelung LG, Kaijser L: Electrocardiographic abnormalities during exercise 3 weeks to 18 months after anterior myocardial infarction. Br Heart J 33:871, 1971.
16. Ericsson M, Granath A, Ohlsen P et al: Arrhythmias and symptoms during treadmill testing three weeks after myocardial infarction in 100 patients. Br Heart J 35:787, 1973.
17. Ibsen H, Kholler E, Styperek J, Pedersen A: Routine exercise ECG three weeks after acute myocardial infarction. Acta Med Scand 198:463, 1975.
18. Granath A, Sodermark T, Winge T et al: Early work load tests for evaluation of long-term prognosis of acute myocardial infarction. Br Heart J 39:758, 1977.
19. Wohl AJ, Lewis HR, Campbell W et al: Cardiovascular function during early recovery from acute myocardial infarction. Circulation 56:931, 1977.

20. Markiewicz W, Houston N, DeBusk RF: Exercise testing soon after myocardial infarction. Circulation 56:26, 1977.

21. Smith JW, Dennis CA, Gassmann RN et al: Exercise testing three weeks after myocardial infarction. Chest 75:1, 1979.

22. Kramer N, Susmano AAA, Shekelle RB: The "false negative" treadmill exercise test and left ventricular dysfunction. Circulation 57:763, 1978.

23. Castellanet MJ, Greenberg PS, Ellestad MH: Comparison of S-T segment changes on exercise testing with angiographic findings in patients with prior myocardial infarction. Am J Cardiol 42:29, 1978.

24. Weiner DA, McCabe C, Klein MD, Ryan TJ: ST segment changes post-infarction: Predictive value for multivessel coronary disease and left ventricular aneurysm. Circulation 58:887, 1978.

25. Paine TD, Dye LE, Roitman DI et al: Relation of graded exercise test findings after myocardial infarction to extent of coronary artery disease and left ventricular dysfunction. Am J Cardiol 42:716, 1978.

26. Theroux P, Waters D, Halphen C, Debaisieux J, Mizgatz H: Prognostic value of exercise testing soon after myocardial infarction. N Engl J Med 301:341, 1979.

27. Pulido JI, Doss J, Twieg D et al: Submaximal exercise testing after acute myocardial infarction: Myocardial scintigraphic and electrocardiographic observations. Am J Cardiol 42:19, 1978.

28. Vedin A, Wilhelmsen L, Wedel H, Pettersson B, Wilhelmsson C, Elmfeldt D, Tibblin G: Prediction of cardiovascular deaths and non-fatal reinfarctions after myocardial infarction. Acta Med Scand 201:309, 1977.

29. Kallio V: Results of rehabilitation in coronary patients. Adv Cardiol 24:153, 1978.

30. Wilhelmsen L, San H, Elmfeldt D et al: A controlled trial of physical training after myocardial infarction. Prev Med 4:491, 1975.

31. Palastsi I: Feasibility of physical training after myocardial infarction and its effect on return to work, morbidity and mortality. Acta Med Scand suppl 599, 1976.

32. Froelicher VF: The hemodynamic effects of physical-conditioning in healthy young, and middle-aged individuals, and in coronary heart disease patients. Exercise Testing and Exercise Training in Coronary Heart Disease, edited by Naughton and Hellerstein, New York, Academic Press, Inc., 1973, pp. 63–77.

33. Clausen JP: Circulatory adjustments to dynamic exercise and effect of physical training in normal subjects and in patients with coronary artery disease. Prog Cardiovasc Dis 18:459, 1976.

34. Rousseau MF, Brasseur LA, Detry JR: Hemodynamic determinants of maximal oxygen intake in patients with healed myocardial infarction: Influence of physical training. Circulation 48:943, 1973.

35. Froelicher VF: Animal studies of the effect of chronic exercise on the heart and atherosclerosis. A Review. Am Heart J 84:496, 1972.

36. Frick MH, Katila M, Sjogren AL: Cardiac function and physical training after myocardial infarction. Coronary Heart Disease and Physical Fitness, edited by Larson OA, Mamlborg O, Baltimore, Maryland, Univ. Park Press, 1971.

37. DeMaria AN, Neumann A, Lee G, Fowler W, Mason DT: Alterations in ventricular mass and performance induced by exercise training in man evaluated by echocardiography. Circulation 57:237, 1978.

38. Stein RA, Michielli D, Fox EL, Krasnow N: Continuous ventricular dimensions in man during supine exercise and recovery. Am J Cardiol 41:655, 1978.

39. Ferguson FJ, Petitclerc R, Choquette G et al: Effect of physical training on treadmill exercise capacity, collateral circulation and progression of coronary disease. Am J Cardiol 34:764, 1974.

40. Conner J, LcCamera F, Swanick E et al: Effects of exercise on coronary collaterization-angiographic studies of six patients in a supervised exercise program. Medicine and Science in Sports 8:145, 1976.

41. Kennedy CC, Spiekerman RE, Linsay MI et al: One-year graduated exercise program for men with angina pectoris. Mayo Clin Proc 51:231, 1976.

42. Letac B, Cribier A, Desplanches JF: A study of LV function in coronary patients before and after physical training. Circulation 56:375, 1977.

43. Selvester R, Camp J, Sanmarco M: Effects of exercise training or progression of documented coronary arteriosclerosis. The Marathon: Physiological, Medical, Epidemiological and Psychological Studies, edited by Milvy P, New York, Academy of Sciences, 1977, pp. 495–508.

44. Bruce RA, Kusumi F, Frederick R: Differences in cardiac function with prolonged physical training for cardiac rehabilitation. Am J Cardiol 40:597, 1977.

45. Carter CL, Amundsen LR: Infarct size and exercise capacity after myocardial infarction. J Appl Phys 42:786, 1977.

46. Sim DN, Neill WA: Investigation of the physio-

logical basis for increased exercise threshold for angina pectoris after physical conditioning. J Clin Invest 54:763, 1974.

47. Ferguson RJ, Cote P, Gauthier P, Bauirassa MG: Changes in exercise coronary sinus blood flow with training in patients with angina pectoris. Circulation 58:41, 1978.

48. Rerych SK, Scholz PM, Sabiston DC, Jones RH: Effects of training on left ventricular function in normal subjects: A longitudinal study. Circulation 57 & 58 (suppl II):7, 1978.

49. Wallace AG, Rerych SK, Jones RH, Goodrich JK: Effects of exercise training on ventricular function in coronary disease. Circulation 57 & 58 (suppl II):197, 1978.

50. Haskell WL: Cardiovascular complications dur-

ing exercise training of cardiac patients. Circulation 57:920, 1978.

51. Cantwell JD, Fletcher GF: Instant electrocardiography: Use in cardiac exercise programs. Circulation 50:962, 1974.

52. Shephard RJ, Kavanagh T: Predicting the exercise catastrophe in the "Post-Coronary" patient. Can Fam Physician 24:614, 1978.

53. Mead WF, Pyfer HR, Trombold JC, Frederick RC: Successful resuscitation of near simultaneous cases of cardiac arrest with a review of fifteen cases occurring during supervised exercise. Circulation 53:187, 1976.

54. Fletcher GF, Cantwell JD: Ventricular fibrillation in a medically supervised cardiac exercise program. JAMA 238:2627, 1977.

# Appendix 1: Do's and Don'ts Regarding Postinfarction Exercise

*DO:*

Exercise regularly, daily or every other day, since regularity is the key to improvement and a decrease in fatigue.

Warm up with moderate, rhythmic activity before moving to more vigorous exercise.

Taper off following exercise using decreased activity and walking; do a "cool down."

Learn to take your heart rate by feeling the pulse at your wrist or neck.

Get a good pair of shoes to exercise in—shoes especially made for running which have thick soles and heels.

Adjust your exercise intensity and duration to the climatic conditions. Be careful of hot and especially humid conditions as well as cold.

*DON'T:*

Exercise when you are ill or have a fever or a serious infection.

Exercise within 2 hours following a full meal, or longer if you feel full.

Drink coffee, tea, or cola drinks (containing caffeine) before exercising.

Smoke before exercising (or ever).

Start exercise with arm work (push-ups, pull-ups, weight lifting); these increase blood pressure more than leg work.

Take a hot shower, sauna, steam bath, jaccuzzi, or whirlpool following exercise.

Wear heavy clothing or plastic or rubber suits when exercising; these cause a dangerous heat accumulation.

Hold your breath and strain during exercise; breathe regularly and through the mouth.

# Appendix 2: Warning Symptoms for Coronary Heart Disease Patients (UCSD Cardiac Rehabilitation Program)

1. These symptoms suggest that your activity progression is too fast. Slow down to an activity level that avoids these:

   Chest pain or discomfort during or following activity

   Palpitations or awareness of pounding or irregular heart beat during or following activity

   Shortness of breath: if more than you would expect for the particular activity

   A pulse rate greater than * until your first visit or 4 weeks after discharge; or an increase of 16 to 20 beats per minute over resting heart rate for any activity

   Unusual or excessive fatigue during or at the end of the day

2. Seek *IMMEDIATE* medical attention if you notice:

   Severe substernal chest pain, pressure, or tightness not relieved by rest or nitroglycerin (pain may radiate to neck, arms, jaw)

   Fainting or black-out spell

3. Call your physician within 24 hours if you notice:

   Recent onset of shortness of breath or an increase in shortness of breath

   Awakening at night because of shortness of breath

   A need to sleep on more pillows than before

   An unexplained episode of dizziness or light-headedness

   The onset of chest pain (angina pectoris) or a change in chest pain pattern (more frequent, more severe, or new occurrence at night or at rest)

   Palpitations, or awareness of a pounding or irregular heart beat

   An unexplained episode of weakness and sweating

---

* Individualized for each patient as determined by physician.

# Appendix 3: Example of Progressive Inpatient Exercises Post-Myocardial Infarction

| Exercise | Ward Activity | Date/Day Post AMI/MD |
|---|---|---|
| STEP 1 | 1. Feeding self with bed rolled up. Trunk and arms supported<br>2. Complete bed bath by nurse. If able, patient allowed to wash face and genital area, do oral hygiene.<br>3. Use of bedside commode. | |
| STEP 2 | 1. Armchair rest 20 minutes twice daily, not during or immediately following meals.<br>2. Complete bed bath by the nurse. Patient allowed to wash face and genital area, do oral hygiene.<br>3. Feeding self with bed up. Trunk and arms supported.<br>4. Use of bedside commode.<br>5. May read with trunk and arms supported. | |
| STEP 3 | 1. Feeding self in armchair with support of arms.<br>2. Armchair rest with meals and at bedtime 20 minutes.<br>3. Partial bed bath by the nurse. Patient allowed to wash front of upper torso, do oral hygiene.<br>4. Use of bedside commode. | |
| STEP 4 | 1. Feeding self in armchair with support of arms.<br>2. Armchair rest with meals and at bedtime.<br>3. Partial bed bath by the nurse. Patient allowed to wash front of upper torso, do oral hygiene.<br>4. Bedside commode.<br>5. May read with trunk and arms supported. | |
| STEP 5 | 1. Sitting ad lib.<br>2. Walking in room twice daily with assistance.<br>3. Bathroom privileges with assistance.<br>4. Bed bath with minimal assistance. Patient allowed to shave and comb hair. | |
| STEP 6 | 1. Walking to bathroom ad lib.<br>2. Washing, sitting down at sink, with supervision. | |
| STEP 7 | 1. Bathing in tub; must have assistance getting in and out of tub. If tub is out of room, patient must ride in wheelchair.<br>2. May walk one length of hall twice daily with assistance. | |
| STEP 8 | 1. Same as above. | |
| STEP 9 | 1. Walking to waiting room twice daily. May stay for 5 to 10 minutes if tolerated. | |
| STEP 10 | 1. Walking to waiting room twice daily. May stay 10 to 20 minutes if tolerated. | |
| STEP 11 | 1. Same as above. | |
| STEP 12 | 1. Walking to waiting room ad lib. | |
| STEP 13 | 1. Self dressing in street clothes for half a day. | |

# Appendix 4: Example of a Treadmill Protocol Used Predischarge After A Myocardial Infarction (UCSD Medical Center—University Hospital)

The test is stopped arbitrarily at a heart rate of 130/min for individuals over 40 and at 140/min for younger individuals. The patient is told to stop if he or she feels badly or develops ischemic chest pain as assessed by his or her physician; (1) develops more than 0.15 mv of ST segment elevation or depression; (2) exhibits serious dysrhythmias; or (3) has a 20 mmHg or more drop in systolic blood pressure. We are conservative during the predischarge test and may stop because the patient just looks poorly or gets cold and clammy.

| Stage | Grade | Speed | Duration |
|-------|-------|-------|----------|
| 1 | 0% | 1.0, 1.5, or 2.0 mph adjusted to patient's stride | 3 minutes |
| 2A | 0% | 3.3 mph if the patient's stride permits | 2 to 3 minutes |
| 2B | 0% | 0.5 mph or more speed increments to maximal comfortable walking speed up to 3.3 mph | |
| 3 | 5% | same speed | 2 to 3 minutes |
| 4 | 10% | same speed | 2 to 3 minutes |
| 5 | 15% | same speed | 2 to 3 minutes |

# 39 | *Surgical Approach to Unstable Angina and Acute Myocardial Infarction*

## *Joe R. Utley, M.D.*

Myocardial oxygen demand in excess of oxygen supply results in myocardial ischemia, which may produce a wide spectrum of clinical manifestations depending on duration, severity, and anatomic location. Ischemia without cell death or infarction may cause the pain of angina pectoris, cardiac arrhythmias, or sudden cardiac death. More severe ischemia resulting in cell death or myocardial infarction may be followed by a variety of life-threatening complications, including arrhythmias, congestive failure, cardiogenic shock, acute and chronic ventricular aneurysms, false ventricular aneurysms, ventricular septal defect, papillary muscle dysfunction or rupture, and cardiac rupture. The syndrome of unstable angina, which is intermediate in severity between stable angina and myocardial infarction, may proceed to myocardial infarction and other life-threatening complications. As aortocoronary bypass grafting has become an effective treatment of chronic stable angina, its usefulness in the management of unstable angina and myocardial infarction has been better understood in recent years. Medical management of unstable angina and myocardial infarction is directed principally toward decreasing myocardial oxygen demand by controlling the main determinants of myocardial oxygen consumption: contractility, systolic pressure (wall tension), and heart rate. As a means of increasing myocardial oxygen supply, coronary artery bypass grafting has obvious theoretical advantages. The role of this form of

surgical treatment has been established by comparing the early and late complications and mortality in subgroups of patients with unstable angina and myocardial infarction treated medically and surgically. Subgrouping of patients allows one to rationally select the intervention that will offer the patient the best chance of survival and relief of symptoms. In this complicated group of patients, meticulous medical and surgical care is essential.

## UNSTABLE ANGINA

Unstable angina is defined as a syndrome with clinical manifestations intermediate between chronic stable angina and myocardial infarction. Other terms used to describe this syndrome include preinfarction angina, intermediate syndrome, crescendo angina, and acute coronary insufficiency. Patients with Prinzmetal angina, or variant angina often are included in the classification of unstable angina. The anginal pain in this syndrome is characterized by (1) recent onset (within 1 month); (2) changing or increasing severity of exertional angina; and (3) angina at rest. Unstable angina is further defined as protracted pain lasting up to 20 to 30 minutes, which is not readily relieved by nitroglycerin. During the pain of unstable angina, ECG abnormalities, which return to normal with relief of pain, are commonly observed. These abnormalities are usually ST depression or elevation with or without T wave inversion. Premature ventricular contractions may also accompany the pain. An essential part of the definition of unstable angina is the lack of elevation of serum enzyme activity of myocardial origin and the absence of ECG evidence of recent subendocardial or transmural infarction.

Patients who develop angina of increasing severity in the presence of chronic angina are more difficult to control medically and have a greater mortality.[1] During the chest pain of angina pectoris, tachycardia and hypertension are common, while clinical signs of left ventricular failure develop in 35 percent of patients with unstable angina.[2] The distribution of coronary disease in patients with unstable angina is similar to that of patients with stable angina: no coronary disease in 10 percent; single-vessel disease in 30 percent; double-vessel disease in 30 percent; and triple-vessel disease in 30 percent. Among those patients with coronary artery disease, approximately 15 percent have involvement of the left main coronary artery in addition. Abnormalities of the left ventriculogram increase in frequency and severity with the number of vessels involved. Patients with unstable angina and single-vessel disease have poor collateral development.[3]

Patients with unstable angina can be classified into subgroups, based on their response to therapy, severity of coronary disease, left ventricular function, presence of arrythmias, and other associated abnormalities, including hypertension, and left ventricular hypertrophy. This subgrouping of patients has proved important in selecting medical or surgical therapy and in timing interventions, including cardiac catheterization and coronary artery bypass grafting.

## Medical Therapy

Medical therapy of unstable angina, includes bed rest, sedation (morphine, diazepam), $\beta$-blockade with propranolol, vasodilator therapy (nitroglycerin, long-acting nitrates, and nitroprusside), and treatment of hypertension and arrhythmias. Patients with unstable angina who become stable with in-hospital medical therapy usually have coronary arteriography to determine the severity of coronary disease and the status of ventricular function, as prognostic factors.

Mortality with medical treatment is greater with three-vessel disease, congestive heart failure, and ejection fraction less than 0.50.[4] The 10-year survival is 20 percent in patients with frequent in-hospital pain, ECG changes with pain, and prior stable angina, compared to 50 percent in other patients.[5] Coronary artery bypass grafting is usually recommended in patients who respond to medical therapy and who have left main coronary artery disease; three-vessel disease; abnormalities in ventricular contraction, which are potentially reversible; severe ST and T wave abnormalities; arrhythmias; a history of chronic stable angina; and who are young and have no associated diseases.

## Failure to Respond to Medical Treatment

More urgent surgical intervention is recommended in patients who fail to respond to medical therapy. Such failure places them in a group that has a 35 percent risk of infarction at 3 months and a death rate of 43 percent at 1 year and 73 percent at 5 years.[6]

Patients who fail to respond to medical therapy should have frequent ECGs and serum enzyme determinations to detect possible myocardial infarction. Surgical risks are reduced if myocardial infarction is excluded by isoenzyme estimations.[7] Technetium–99$^m$ pyrophosphate scans are positive in 35 percent of patients with unstable angina, who do not have elevated serum isoenzyme levels of cardiac origin.[6]

Patients with medically uncontrolled unstable angina frequently have severe three-vessel disease or left main coronary artery disease, and they may have global but reversible depression of left ventricular function. Emergency surgery is frequently necessary in patients with severe coronary disease.

**Results.** The risk of emergency coronary artery bypass grafting for medically uncontrolled unstable angina is greater (5 percent mortality) than for medically controlled unstable or stable angina (1 percent mortality). A few patients (6 percent) are not suitable candidates for coronary artery bypass grafting.[8]

Prospective randomized studies of unstable angina show no difference in early mortality or the rate of infarction between medical and surgical groups.[9,10] In one study, patients with left ventricular hypertrophy and hypertension, who failed to respond to therapy had a greater risk of mortality when treated surgically than other patients.[11] One-third of patients treated medically cross over to surgical therapy in most series. The nonrandomized series show increased survival and a decreased rate of infarction in surgically treated groups.[12,13]

Late studies show better symptomatic and functional results in surgical than in medical patients, a finding that clearly justifies elective or semielective operations in patients who respond to medical therapy.[9,14-18] An 84 percent survival rate at 43 months in operated patients is better than that reported in medical series.[18] Other series have reported no early or late mortality with surgical therapy.[15]

There has been no comparative study of surgical and medical therapy in the high-risk subgroups of patients with unstable angina unresponsive to medical therapy. In the future, such a study may be increasingly difficult to mount because of the current preference for surgical therapy in patients who do not respond to medical treatment.

One of the important contributions of the randomized series is that they have indicated that the excellent results of medical therapy allow the operation to be done on an elective basis. The results of semielective coronary artery bypass grafting in these patients has been better than when the operation is done as an emergency. Emergency bypass grafting should be employed only for patients who do not respond to medical therapy or who have a myocardial infarct during or after cardiac catheterization.

## Ventricular Arrhythmias

Patients with ventricular arrhythmias and unstable angina may require coronary artery bypass grafting primarily for their arrhythmias. The decision to operate and the type of operation depends on the anatomy of the coronary arteries, left ventricular function, and whether a left ventricular aneurysm is present. Patients with a chronic ventricular aneurysm may develop intractable ventricular arrhythmias associated with unstable angina, which responds well to aneurysm resection and coronary bypass grafting to the noninfarcted myocardium. Patients with ischemia without recent or old infarction may be relieved of their ventricular arrhythmias by coronary artery bypass grafting. Occasionally, patients with distal vessel disease unsuitable for bypass grafting may have severe ventricular arrhythmias with unstable angina, which resolve with the development of a small, localized, spontaneous infarction.

## Surgical Therapy of Variant or Prinzmetal Angina

The syndrome of variant angina pectoris, described by Prinzmetal, is an unstable form of angina pectoris with chest pain at rest and concomitant electrocardiographic ST segment elevation. The chest pain of variant angina tends to occur at the same time every day, often in the early morning hours, awakening the patient from sleep. The episodes of chest pain may be accompanied by a variety of rhythm abnormalities, including various degrees of atrioventricular block, ventricular ectopic activity, episodes of ventricular tachycardia, or ventricular fibrillation. In contrast to typical angina pectoris, variant angina is not accompanied by an increase in the left ventricular pressure-time index. Therefore, these episodes of variant angina are not precipitated by an increase in myocardial oxygen demand but by a reduction in myocardial oxygen supply due to coronary artery spasm, causing transmural ischemia rather than subendocardial ischemia. The ST segment elevation in the appropriate ECG leads is a reflection of the transmural ischemia.

These patients may have a variety of patterns of coronary artery anatomy. There may be single- or multiple-vessel obstruction due to atherosclerosis. Many have coronary artery spasm associated with atherosclerosis. In others, spasm is the only obstructive process in coronary arteries otherwise free of atherosclerotic disease.

It may be necessary to manage the preoperative period in patients with spasm differently than in those with typical angina pectoris. $\beta$-adrenergic blockade may not be beneficial in these patients because it leaves $\alpha$-adrenergic coronary vasoconstriction unopposed. Coronary vasodilators, such as verapamil and nifedipine may be extremely useful in these patients. The indications for surgical therapy in variant angina are similar to those in typical angina and are principally for the relief of pain and control of arrhythmias. The benefit of surgical therapy in variant angina is less than in typical angina. Collected results from the literature show 9 percent mortality, 13 percent perioperative infarction, 80 percent graft patency, and only 56 percent good results following coronary bypass grafting for variant angina.[19] In general, the results have been better in patients with predominant atherosclerotic disease and poor when obstruction is primarily due to spasm.[5,20]

The role of the autonomic nervous system in coronary spasm has important surgical implications. A recent report describes excellent results in two patients with coronary spasm treated by surgical removal of the periaortic and pretracheal autonomic nerves and ganglia, as well as saphenous vein grafting.[19]

## ACUTE MYOCARDIAL INFARCTION

Approximately 1.3 million myocardial infarctions occur in the United States each year. The prehospital mortality is 50 percent, and another 10 to 15 percent, of infarct victims are dead in 1 year.

The decision to intervene surgically in patients with acute myocardial infarction is a complex one. Among the factors that influence the decision to perform a surgical procedure are: (1) the interval from infarction to the time of the operation, (2) the size of the infarction, and (3) the complications of infarction observed in the patient. Among the complications of myocardial infarction which may require surgical therapy are (1) continued unstable angina pectoris and impending extension of infarction (2) acute left ventricular power failure, (3) rupture of the ventricular septum, (4) papillary muscle dysfunction or rupture producing mitral insuffi-

ciency, (5) left ventricular aneurysm, (6) cardiac rupture, and (7) ventricular arrhythmias.

There appears to be a "golden period" during the first 4 to 6 hours following the onset of myocardial infarction, during which myocardial revascularization can be performed with low mortality and with the benefit of preserving myocardial function. During the period from 6 hours to 1 week, however, the risk of myocardial revascularization is high. During this period, reperfusion of infarcted myocardium may cause further myocardial damage. It has been shown experimentally and clinically that reperfusion of an acute infarction may convert the pale infarct to a hemorrhagic infarction with extension of myocardial damage and hemodynamic deterioration. In addition to the development of hemorrhagic infarction following reperfusion, there may be deterioration of mitochondrial function and deposition of calcium compounds in the myocardium as well.[21] Further, a "no-flow phenomenon" may occur due to swelling of vascular endothelium in the infarcted area so that revascularization is not accompanied by reperfusion of this tissue.

The timing of myocardial revascularization following infarction is most important. Coronary occlusion resulting in myocardial infarction, which occurs during the course of cardiac catheterization, has been treated surgically within 6 hours with low mortality. Coronary occlusion during coronary angiography occurs in 0.3 to 0.9 percent of patients.[22] Occlusion of the right coronary artery, which accompanies cardiac catheterization, is a relatively benign event and is usually not accompanied by life-threatening infarction, arrhythmia, or power failure.[23] In contrast, occlusion of a branch of the left coronary artery, particularly the left anterior descending branch, accompanying cardiac catheterization, has a much higher mortality and much higher risk of transmural infarction, arrhythmia, and power failure.[22,23] The risk of myocardial revascularization in patients who infarct during or immediately after cardiac catherization is acceptably low if the revascularization can be performed in less than 4 to 6 hours following the onset of the infarction.[24-31] Patients whose infarction develops during catheterization should be taken immediately from the catheterization laboratory to the operating room, and myocardial revascularization performed. Similarly, if the patient develops an acute infarction during hospitalization, following cardiac catheterization, consideration should be given to emergency aortocoronary bypass grafting within the first few hours following infarction. Patients in whom infarction begins outside the hospital, or before coronary angiography, usually cannot be studied and operated upon before the end of the "golden period." One report shows excellent results of immediate coronary arteriography and revascularization of patients who proved to have infarction.[32] One must proceed with immediate coronary arteriography in patients with acute ischemia syndromes before the diagnosis is made by serum enzyme elevation in order to accomplish revascularization before the end of the "golden period." The majority of centers do not advocate this approach, but recommend early medical management without immediate coronary angiography.

The decision to intervene surgically following the 6-hour "golden period" following infarction is a more difficult one. One group reported a 38 percent mortality following coronary revascularization during the first 7 days following infarction, 16.4 percent between 8 and 30 days following infarction, and 5.8 percent mortality after 30 days following infarction.[33]

Factors other than the interval from infarction to revascularization are important to the outcome of surgical therapy in patients operated on 6 hours to 7 days following infarction. The group at Massachusetts General Hospital performed myocardial revascularization on a series of patients with cardiogenic shock complicating acute myocardial infarction. Three of seven patients survived. The survivors had smaller infarcts than those who did not survive.[34] A recent study found that the status of left ventricular function was a better determinant of survival than the interval between infarction and revascularization.[35,27] Thus it would appear that mortality during this high-risk interval (6 hours to 7 days) was lower in patients with well-preserved left ventricular function than in patients with severe left ventricular dysfunction.[36] The Mayo Clinic group found a 3.6 percent mortality for early myocardial revascularization following subendocardial

myocardial infarction in patients with a wide range of left ventricular function (e.g., ejection fraction ranging from 32 to 76 percent).[37] A comparison of results of coronary artery bypass grafting in stable angina, unstable angina, and after subendocardial infarction showed no significant differences in graft patency, improvement in left ventricular function, and symptomatic improvement. There were no early or late deaths in this study.[38]

It is important for the surgeon to assess the extent of myocardial infarction when considering revascularization during the first week following infarction. Patients with a small infarction, who continue to have unstable angina and impending extension of the infarction, will have more favorable results from revascularization than do patients with larger infarctions. Patients with large infarctions, in addition to having continued unstable angina, may also have ventricular power failure, acute left ventricular aneurysm, ventricular septal defect, or papillary muscle rupture.

## Acute Infarction Followed by Unstable Angina or Impending Extension

These patients should be managed initially with maximal medical measures to control the unstable angina. Serial CK isoenzyme determinations, ECGs, and $^{99m}$technetium pyrophosphate scans should be performed. Taken together, the ECG changes, serial enzyme levels, and $^{99m}$technetium pyrophosphate scans are the best indices of the extent of myocardial necrosis. The $^{99m}$technetium pyrophosphate scan may be positive in unstable angina without serum enzyme elevation. The ECG changes during episodes of unstable angina may provide some indication of the extent of jeopardized myocardium that is ischemic but not infarcted. The patients with the greatest benefit-to-risk ratio for myocardial revascularization are those with small infarctions who have evidence of impending massive extension. In such a patient, the ECG shows stable changes of the small infarction with intermittent changes suggesting a much larger area of ischemia, including transient Q waves during periods of pain and ischemia. These patients frequently have severe global depression of left ventricular function, and three-vessel coronary artery disease at the time of cardiac catheterization. Under these conditions, particularly if this is the patient's first myocardial infarction, the abnormalities of ventricular function may return almost to normal following coronary artery bypass grafting. The medical treatment of these patients should be similar to those with unstable angina without infarction. The use of nitroglycerin, chronic vasodilators, propranolol, and morphine is essential. The success of revascularization depends on avoiding extension of the infarction prior to the revascularization of the ischemic area. These patients should undergo complete cardiac catheterization, including left ventriculography and coronary angiography.

## Acute Infarction and Left Ventricular Power Failure

Patients who develop left ventricular power failure following myocardial infarction usually have greater than 40 percent of the left ventricle infarcted. Three-vessel coronary artery disease is usually present and the remaining noninfarcted myocardium frequently exhibits depressed function due to ischemia. Intraaortic balloon counterpulsation has been used in these patients to decrease left ventricular afterload, improve cardiac output, and increase coronary diastolic perfusion pressure. Numerous studies have shown that intraaortic balloon counterpulsation has a beneficial effect on the hemodynamic status of these patients.[39,40,41] If the patient continues to have left ventricular power failure without arrhythmias, impending extension, ventricular septal defect, ventricular aneurysm, mitral insufficiency, or cardiac rupture, the possible benefit of surgical therapy is small. In 27 such patients, 19 were benefited by balloon counterpulsation; 9 were weaned from balloon counterpulsation, but only 3 survived to be discharged from the hospital. Ten patients became balloon dependent and 8 of the 10 underwent cardiac catheterization; 4 were found to be inoperable, and of 4 who were operated on, only 1 survived to leave the hospital. An ejection fraction below 30 percent was a poor prognostic sign in this group of patients. Two

patients with inferior myocardial infarctions and an ejection fraction above 30 percent, were weaned from balloon support and survived hospitalization.[41] The mortality following myocardial revascularization for left ventricular power failure complicating acute infarction has been high (40 to 100 percent).[34,36,41,42] The results of balloon counterpulsation in these patients without myocardial revascularization also have been poor.[41] However, one group from the Netherlands reported 56 percent survival for 3 months following balloon-pumping without cardiac surgery.[40] In general, surgical therapy is not advantageous in left ventricular power failure following large myocardial infarctions in the absence of ventricular septal defect, papillary muscle disruption, or recurrent ventricular arrhythmias.

## Postinfarction Rupture of the Ventricular Septum

Acute rupture of the ventricular septum occurs in 1 to 2 percent of all patients with myocardial infarction. It usually occurs during the first week following infarction, but can occur as late as 6 weeks after the event. The incidence is probably increased by hypertension or by too vigorous ambulation following myocardial infarction. Acute rupture of the ventricular septum is usually associated with heart failure and the appearance of a new precordial systolic murmur. Bedside diagnosis may be made with the Swan-Ganz balloon-float catheter. An increase in oxygen saturation at the level of the right ventricle is indicative of a ventricular septal defect. The diagnosis is further supported by the absence of a large V-wave in the pulmonary wedge pressure tracing due to mitral insufficiency resulting from papillary muscle disruption. Bedside diagnosis is important in the seriously ill patient because of the increased risks of cardiac catheterization and coronary angiography in unstable patients with septal rupture and left ventricular failure.[43] Patients may have both ventricular septal rupture and papillary muscle dysfunction or rupture, but this combination is rare. Once the diagnosis is confirmed, the patient's hemodynamic status may improve with intraaortic balloon counterpulsation or afterload reduction.[44] With the Swan-Ganz catheter in place, the pulmonic to systemic blood flow ratio and the pulmonary wedge pressure may be measured to determine the effect of afterload reduction. A significant decrease in pulmonary to systemic blood flow ratio as well as narrowing of the systemic arteriovenous oxygen difference accompanies balloon counterpulsation.

Twenty-four percent of patients with ventricular septal rupture die the first day following rupture. There is a 65 percent mortality at 2 weeks, an 87 percent mortality at 2 months, and a 90 percent mortality at 1 year.[43] The mortality of surgical closure is related to the interval between rupture and operation. Tabulated mortality from reported series was 70 percent for repairs undertaken less than 6 weeks following rupture, and 35 percent for repairs performed more than 6 weeks following rupture.[45] One series reported a 9 percent 1-year survival if repairs were undertaken less than 6 weeks following rupture. The results of earlier repair have improved in recent years, and one recent report shows three of three patients surviving early operation.

Septal rupture following myocardial infarction is virtually always associated with obstruction of the left anterior ascending coronary artery. This vessel supplies the anterior two-thirds of the ventricular septum. Infarction of the adjacent left ventricular wall is usually present. In 35 percent of patients, left ventricular aneurysm is associated with septal rupture.[35,46-48] Ruptures located in the posterior position of the septum associated with an inferior or diaphramatic infarction may occur in one-third of the cases.[45] Septal rupture associated with inferior infarction carries a worse prognosis.[48a]

Thirty-six percent of patients with postinfarction septal rupture have associated abnormalities of atrioventricular conduction.[49] The percent of left ventricle infarcted, the size of the ventricular septal defect, the function and volume of the noninfarcted myocardium, and the presence of associated mechanical abnormalities, such as left ventricular aneurysm and papillary muscle dysfunction or rupture, are all important factors in determining the patient's survival.[50-53] Ventricular septal rupture is always associated with a transmural myocardial infarction, but has not been associated with subendocardial infarction.

Patients who are in cardiac failure or cardiogenic shock refractory to medical therapy early after septal rupture should be operated upon immediately following the diagnosis made by a right-sided catheter study.[54] Because of the high risks of left ventriculography and coronary angiography in these patients, operation may be undertaken without catheterizing the left side of the heart. The operative risk is high, but mortality with medical therapy in this group of patients is virtually 100 percent.

Patients who respond well to afterload reduction, however, may be treated medically for 6 weeks or more and then undergo conventional cardiac catheterization, including left ventriculography and coronary angiography. They may be operated upon semielectively with more favorable results.[50,52,55] Obviously, a major factor in the outcome of any individual patient will be those factors that contribute to hemodynamic deterioration at the time of ventricular septal rupture. Patients who remain stable and can be operated upon after 6 weeks will have a lower operative mortality (20 percent) than those whose hemodynamic status requires closure early after septal rupture (50 percent mortality). A significant advantage of the 6 weeks delay following infarction is the improved character of myocardial tissue. The left ventricular muscle is very friable following infarction, and there are often technical difficulties in accomplishing satisfactory repair of the septum and ventricular walls when operation is undertaken early. Histologic study shows that fibrosis increases with time after infarction. At 8 weeks or more following infarction, sufficient fibrous tissue is present to allow better repair of the ventricular septum and ventricular wall.[46]

Intraaortic balloon counterpulsation may be instituted as an emergency procedure to allow safer transition through the operation and early postoperative period. This procedure is not helpful during a longer waiting period (6 weeks). Delay for 6 weeks may be recommended only in patients who respond to medical afterload reduction without balloon counterpulsation.

## Mitral Insufficiency Due to Papillary Muscle Rupture

Mitral insufficiency due to reversible papillary muscle dysfunction is common with myocardial infarction. Rupture of this muscle is usually a catastrophic hemodynamic event complicating myocardial infarction. Rupture most commonly is associated with disruption of the posterior papillary muscle, which is supplied by a dominant right coronary or dominant circumflex coronary artery, via the posterior descending coronary artery. Rupture of the anterior papillary muscle is much less common. Virtually all patients have three-vessel coronary arterial disease and left ventricular abnormalities.[56] Papillary muscle rupture usually follows transmural infarction but may complicate subendocardial infarction. Within 1 hour of the onset of the rupture, 18 percent of patients die, 52 percent are dead within 24 hours, and 80 percent succumb within 2 weeks following disruption of the papillary muscle.[57] The degree of left ventricular impairment, the volume of infarcted left ventricle, and the function of noninfarcted left ventricle are very important determinants of survival following papillary muscle disruption. The outcome of an acute rupture depends on the degree to which the muscle is disrupted and the status of left ventricular function.[58] If the entire trunk of the papillary muscle is disrupted, the patient will usually die immediately. If only one head of the papillary muscle is disrupted, the patient may survive with cardiac failure, providing left ventricular function is good. If partial rupture is accompanied by impairment of left ventricular function, early death will usually occur. In one series there were only five patients with papillary muscle rupture among 24 who were operated upon for mitral insufficiency associated with coronary artery disease.[59]

Mitral insufficiency complicating myocardial infarction may be transient and reversible. With papillary muscle dysfunction, afterload reduction may improve cardiac output. Mitral valve replacement is rarely required during the early postinfarction period for papillary muscle dysfunction.

Rupture of the papillary muscle is such a life-threatening event that mitral valve replacement is necessary for most patients to avoid death from low cardiac output. The results of mitral valve replacement depend on the status of left ventricular function. In one series, two of five patients survived.[60] Overall survival is 40 percent following mitral valve replacement and coronary bypass grafting for papillary muscle dysfunction.[6]

## Ventricular Aneurysms

The incidence of ventricular aneurysms following myocardial infarction is about 15 percent. The indications for surgical therapy of left ventricular aneurysms following myocardial infarction depend on the complications produced by the aneurysm, the position of the left ventricular aneurysm, the associated abnormalities, and the acute or chronic nature of the aneurysm. In general, left ventricular aneurysms may be anterior or posterior, acute or chronic, and may be true or false.

Acute left ventricular aneurysm may be a cause for sudden left ventricular power failure following myocardial infarction. If 20 to 25 percent of the left ventricular wall is inactivated by any mechanism, the degree of shortening required of the remainder of the ventricle exceeds its physiologic limits and cardiac enlargement (Starling mechanism) must develop to maintain stroke volume.[61] During the time required for enlargement, depression of cardiac output accompanies infarction of this magnitude.

In these patients, the left anterior descending coronary artery is usually obstructed. The aneurysm is usually in the anterior and lateral ventricular walls. The probability that resection will benefit the patient is greatest if the power failure is due to a first myocardial infarction, rather than when an aneurysm follows multiple myocardial infarctions. One series reported that four of five patients survived resection of an acute ventricular aneurysm 11 to 63 days after infarction. In collected series the survival following resection of acute left ventricular aneurysm is 40 percent.[6] Results are, in part, related to the amount of left ventricle that must be excised, improvement usually being obtained with excision of 25 to 30 percent of the left ventricle. Survival is poor following excision of more than 35 percent of the left ventricle early after acute infarction.[62]

**Chronic Left Ventricular Aneurysms.** Chronic left ventricular aneurysm may produce intractable arrhythmia, systemic emboli, advanced congestive failure, and severe angina pectoris. In the absence of these complications, operation is usually not recommended. The risk of left ventricular aneurysm resection is related to the function of the remaining myocardium. With good myocardial function, resection of chronic aneurysm carries a low risk.

Most left ventricular aneurysms are anterior, and are associated with complete occlusion of the left anterior descending coronary artery. Posterior ventricular aneurysms are secondary to occlusion of a dominant right coronary artery, and are most commonly accompanied by congestive heart failure or arrhythmias.

In resecting posterior ventricular aneurysms, one must be careful to inspect the posterior papillary muscle because it is frequently infarcted, producing mitral insufficiency.

**False Aneurysm.** False aneurysms of the left ventricle are due to containment of left ventricular rupture by the pericardium. When the left ventricular rupture is delayed for several days or weeks, pericardial adhesions around the site of the infarction may contain the blood at the site of rupture. The diagnosis of left ventricular false aneurysm is rarely made prior to angiography. The typical angiographic appearance of a false aneurysm of the left ventricle is a sharply defined aneurysm with a narrow neck and a large sac. False aneurysms of the left ventricle are prone to rupture, and are therefore life-threatening. If the diagnosis of false aneurysm is made angiographically, this is an absolute indication for surgical repair.

## Cardiac Rupture

Rupture of the heart occurs in 3 to 24 percent of deaths from myocardial infarction. It is more common in women and in hypertensive and ambulating patients. Rupture of the heart is more frequent after the first than after subsequent infarctions, and usually occurs during the first postinfarction week. It may be apical, basal, anterior, lateral, or posterior, and can occur after both large and small infarctions.[7,41,63,64] The histologic dating of the myocardial infarction in patients with cardiac rupture often suggests that infarction may be older than the duration of chest pain. Prior to the onset of cardiac rupture, patients frequently complain of chest pain of pericardial origin. The terminal event may be sudden, refractory electromechanical dissociation in patients who have had no previous hemodynamic difficulties. In other patients, the onset of symptoms may be gradual with persistent or recurrent pericardial chest pain, and evidence of increasing pericardial tamponade. In these patients there is a period from one to three hours during which symptoms develop slowly before electromechanical dissociation occurs. In one report of three patients who were operated for sudden cardiac rupture, two survived.[17] In a collected series, six of 20 patients survived exploration for acute cardiac rupture.[33]

## Arrhythmias

Atrial and ventricular arrhythmias are common after myocardial infarction. Atrial arrhythmias are best treated medically. Most ventricular arrhythmias respond to lidocaine, procainamide, propranolol, overdrive pacing, and cardioversion. Occasionally patients with acute myocardial ischemia, with or without infarction, have life threatening ventricular arrhythmias despite medical therapy.[65] In these patients the role of surgical therapy is still poorly defined. The exact electrophysiology of ectopic ventricular arrhythmias in ischemic heart disease remains controversial. Ischemic myocardium may be the site of reentrant activity due to local reexcitation caused by the potential difference between ischemic and normal tissue, resulting in the development of a "circus" reentry phenomenon. Enhanced automaticity of the specialized conduction fibers has also been proposed as a possible explanation. Ischemic myocardium has a lowered fibrillatory threshold. Coronary bypass grafting has been effective in controlling exercise-induced arrhythmias,[25] although this observation was not confirmed in a randomized trial.[66] Myocardial revascularization has been shown to diminish the 24-month mortality in patients surviving unexpected ventricular fibrillation.[67] Vismara et al.[65] found a 6 percent incidence of sudden death in coronary artery patients treated surgically, compared to 24 percent in medically treated patients.

Many reports demonstrating effective surgical therapy of ventricular arrhythmias following myocardial infarction have described resection of a ventricular aneurysm as an essential part of the therapy.[66,68,69] More recently, control of ventricular arrhythmias has been accomplished with coronary artery bypass grafting without ventricular resection.[51,70,71] The Stanford group reviewed their experience and found that best results followed myocardial resection more than 1 month after infarction in patients with good ventricular function.[72] The Massachusetts General Hospital experience also suggested that results are best if operation is performed more than 1 month following infarction.[73]

Recent studies have emphasized the importance of ventricular mapping in the surgical management of patients with ventricular arrhythmias.[74,75] The Loyola University group found 33 percent early and 27 percent late mortality in patients with drug-resistant ventricular tachyarrhythmias who were not mapped.[74] In 5 patients who were mapped, 1 died early and 4 were long-term survivors without late death. The use of mapping to identify and excise the site of early activation in three other patients with coronary disease or cardiomyopathy has been successful.[75] In another report, four patients with ventricular tachycardia were studied with His bundle electrograms and programmed electrical stimulation.[76] The studies indicated a reentry mechanism occurring in the left bundle branches. Two patients underwent surgical section of the anterior radiation of the left bundle branch. One patient died. Both patients had complicated pathology requiring saphenous vein bypass grafting with either aneurysm resection or mitral valve replacement.

The interruption of the anterior fascicle of the left bundle of the Purkinje system or incision of the endocardium are new techniques whose indications and efficacy are not proven.

## SURGICAL CONSIDERATIONS

The goal of surgical therapy in coronary artery disease is to totally relieve ischemia, with complete myocardial revascularization, without mortality or myocardial damage accompanying the procedure. This is accomplished by adhering to the principles of acute coronary care preoperatively, correctly evaluating the pathophysiology of the patient's coronary circulation, performing the operation meticulously with complete preservation of myocardial function, and precise postoperative care. The operation must correct valve dysfunction, close sites of intracardiac shunting, remove dyskinetic segments of the ventricle, relieve myocardial ischemia, and leave an adequate-size ventricular chamber with good contractile function and without perioperative infarction or reperfusion injury.

### Evaluation of Cardiac Catheterization and Coronary Angiography

The status of the patient's intravascular volume may be assessed by the cardiac index and filling pressure. With depressed cardiac index ($< 2.0$ $1/min/m^2$) and low left ventricular end-diastolic pressure ($< 12$ mm/Hg), volume should be replaced with either blood, plasma, or physiologic saline before the induction of anesthesia. In patients with depressed cardiac index ($< 2.0$ $1/min/m^2$) and a very high left ventricular end-disastolic pressure ($> 25$ mmHg) with pulmonary congestion and edema, careful diuresis (furosemide 10 to 20 mg IV) should be given with careful monitoring of cardiac index, pulmonary wedge pressure, and systemic arteriovenous oxygen difference (Swan-Ganz catheter) and arterial blood gas tensions. The principal acute risk of a high left ventricular filling pressure ($> 30$ mmHg) is that it will occasionally cause a further depression of cardiac output, possibly by further restricting subendocardial blood flow. Diuresis is rarely necessary in preparing a patient for surgery with lesser elevations of left ventricular end-diastolic pressure (15 to 25 mmHg).

The coronary angiogram shows the distribution of obstructive lesions in the coronary arteries. The surgeon should decide from the angiogram which vessels it is most important to bypass. Large vessels with proximal lesions supplying a large portion of the left ventricle have the highest priority for revascularization. These are usually the left main, left anterior descending (LAD), and dominant right or circumflex arteries. In order to bypass these essential arteries, the surgeon may have to perform added maneuvers, such as dissection for an intramyocardial circumflex or LAD vessel, or perform an endoarterectomy to totally revascularize the right coronary artery. From the angiogram, the surgeon should also determine which arteries may be bypassed if favorable anatomy is found at operation. These are usually secondary branches of the LAD, circumflex, and right coronary arteries, including the diagonal branches, ramus intermedius, obtuse marginals, posterior descending and posterior ventricular branches of the right coronary artery. The decision to bypass these vessels depends on operative determination of their size, accessibility, freedom from disease, and presence of scar or infarction in their distribution.

The coronary angiogram may alert the surgeon to the possibility of totally occluded secondary branches, which are not visualized on the angiogram but which are easily bypassable at operation. One should suspect such vessels if there is a large area of left ventricular myocardium without visible coronary arteries but without evidence of recent or old infarction. This situation most commonly occurs when the diagonal, obtuse marginal, ramus intermedius, posterior descending, or posterior ventricular branches are totally occluded at their origin. Even though the distal vessels do not visualize angiographically, they are frequently patent and bypassable. The opportunity to bypass such vessels is more easily missed than with the totally occluded nonvisualized main trunk of vessels such as the LAD, circumflex, or right coronary arteries.

Assessment of the left ventriculogram should ideally allow one to determine the distribution of dyskinesis and its correlation with the coronary lesions; the age and/or reversibility of the dyskinetic area; and the potential benefit of ventricular resection or plication for paradoxical segments. Often the left ventriculogram does not permit one to make such a complete assessment. Nevertheless, the preoperative ventriculogram is essential in evaluating ventricular abnormalities observed at the time of operation.

From the coronary angiogram and the ventriculogram, one should make a tentative determination of the precariousness of the bypassable lesions. This determination, along with myocardial temperature mapping at the operating table, may influence the sequence of vessels grafted and the technique of myocardial protection.

### Intraaortic Balloon Pump: Unstable Angina

Intraaortic balloon pumping (IABP) has been shown to be very effective in relieving the pain of unstable angina. With current medical therapy, particularly with the use of high dose propranolol therapy and its continuation until the operation, IABP is rarely required. The possible indications for IABP are: [77] frequent episodes of anginal pain lasting more than 30 minutes despite therapy for greater than 4 days, history of hypertension, left ventricular end-diastolic pressure more than 18 mmHg, and unfavorable coronary anatomy for complete myocardial revascularization. Relative indications for IABP are: angina at rest with ECG changes, left main coronary disease, left ventricular hypertrophy, and left ventricular dysfunction (ejection fraction less than 30 percent).

The value of IABP is greatest in those patients who become increasingly unstable during the most stressful periods of their management, including cardiac catheterization, induction of anesthesia, and prebypass period in the operating room. With presently employed anesthetic and surgical techniques, preoperative IABP for unstable angina is rarely indicated.

**Myocardial Infarction.** In the presence of myocardial infarction IABP has been recommended to prevent extension and preserve myocardium; for left ventricular power failure; for ventricular septal rupture, mitral insufficiency, and acute ventricular aneurysm; and for ventricular arrhythmias unresponsive to conventional therapy. In these very ill patients, the indication for IABP varies greatly among major medical centers. Our policy is to employ $\beta$-adrenergic blockade and afterload reduction in these patients. We do not employ IABP unless a corrective surgical procedure is contemplated. The most common indication for IABP in our experience has been in patients who cannot be weaned from cardiopulmonary bypass. Half the patients requiring IABP after cardiac surgery have survived to be discharged from the hospital.

## Drugs

**Propranolol.** Earlier it was believed that operating while the patient was on full propranolol dosage caused a high incidence of poor ventricular contractility and low cardiac output postoperatively. Since the risk of increasing ischemia and myocardial infarction during propranolol withdrawal has been recognized, recent experience has shown that it is safe to operate on the patient while on full doses of this agent. Patients operated on while on full propranolol dosage have a stable, slow heart rate without hypertension in contrast to the frequent episodes of tachycardia and hypertension in patients not on propranolol. Our recent practice has been to begin propranolol in unstable patients undergoing coronary artery bypass grafting not already on this drug.

**Digoxin.** Patients with poor left ventricular function and congestive failure need not have digoxin discontinued preoperatively. With present techniques of avoiding hypokalemia, the risk of digitalis toxicity after cardiopulmonary bypass is low.

**Antiplatelet Drugs.** Increasing numbers of patients have been placed on acetylsalicylic acid (aspirin). Patients with a variety of musculoskeletal conditions are frequently placed on indomethacin. These drugs have profound effects on platelet function, which may cause a severe coagulopathy after cardiopulmonary bypass so that multiple blood and platelet transfusions are required. Antiplatelet drugs, including aspirin and indomethacin, should be discontinued

when the possibility of coronary artery bypass grafting is foreseen in a patient with unstable angina. Propranolol also decreases platelet adhesiveness and may contribute to postoperative bleeding, but, as indicated above, this agent should be continued.

## Discussion with the Patient

In the unstable patient, the day preceeding surgery is a time of great risk for developing myocardial infarction. Discussions with the patient by the surgeon, anesthesiologist, nurses, and other medical staff should be to inform him of the operation and its benefits, risks, and consequences without causing undue anxiety. Because of the fear of death that most patients with angina pectoris experience with their chest pain, it is not helpful and may even be deleterious to dwell on the serious life-threatening aspects of their disease. The surgeon should inform the patient of the nature of the disease and the possible consequences with and without surgical therapy, including the risk of death, complications, and disability. A member of the patient's family, usually the spouse, should be similarly informed. Once the patient and family have decided to go forth with surgical therapy following their discussion with the surgeon, cardiologists, and other physicians, further discussion of risks, and seriousness of the situation, unless at the patient's request, are often detrimental to him. Repeated review of risks by many members of the team in an attempt to insure informed consent may produce heightened anxiety in the patient and even progression of unstable angina to infarction.

Preoperative teaching by a member of the postoperative intensive care unit nursing staff is an important step toward relieving the patient's anxiety. Preoperative preparation and shaving should be performed the night before the operation. Patients should receive sleeping medication the night before surgery. The morning of surgery, the patient should be transported to the operating room with minimal disturbance. Family members are encouraged to visit the patient on the evening prior to surgery rather than on the morning of the operation.

## OPERATIVE MANAGEMENT

### Preparation

The period before cardiopulmonary bypass is begun is a very precarious time, during which the patient with unstable angina may progress to myocardial infarction.

Preparations in the operating room suite should be carried out quietly and efficiently. A left radial artery catheter and a Swan-Ganz catheter, via the right internal jugular vein, are inserted using local anesthesia after one or two peripheral intravenous lines are placed. Induction of anesthesia is begun, and when the patient is ready for endotracheal intubation, the urinary catheter and rectal and esophageal temperature probes are placed.

After the patient is prepped and draped, a two-team approach is used for harvesting the saphenous vein and for simultaneous sternotomy. In patients with three-vessel disease, the saphenous vein is harvested from the ankle to the groin. After the pericardium is opened heparin is given before purse-string sutures are placed for cannulation. The activated clotting time (ACT) is determined after the heparin has circulated for 5 minutes. Additional heparin is given before cannulation to achieve an ACT greater than 300 seconds. The ascending aorta is usually cannulated for arterial inflow. Femoral artery cannulation is performed for repeat operations and in the presence of severe calcification, atherosclerosis or medial necrosis of the ascending aorta without occlusive iliac or femoral disease. With use of cardioplegia for myocardial preservation, we prefer to use two venous lines with caval tapes or caval clamps to minimize cooling of the septum by venous blood and to allow harvesting the cardioplegia solution through the pulmonary artery vent catheter.

Before cardiopulmonary bypass is begun, 500 or 1000 ml of the patient's blood is drawn from the venous line, as volume is infused through the arterial line. The pump oxygenator is primed with lactated Ringer's solution containing 50 mg glucose and 44 mg sodium bicarbonate per liter. Cardiopulmonary bypass is begun slowly to prevent hypotension. When flow reaches 2.5/l/min/m², ventilation is stopped, the pulmonary artery is vented with a catheter, and the caval slings are tightened. The water bath temperature is lowered to 26° to 30°C. A purse string suture is placed in the ascending aorta at the site of cardioplegia infusion.

During this period of complete cardiopulmonary bypass before cardioplegia infusion, the coronary vessels are inspected. Diseased, small, or intramyocardial vessels may be difficult to find after blood is washed out by cardioplegia. The bypassable vessels from the preoperative angiogram are inspected. Bypassable vessels not identified on the angiogram are noted. The distribution of disease within the bypassable vessels is determined, and sites suitable for bypass are marked with an incision in the epicardium. From the distribution of the angiographic obstructions and the position of the bypassable vessels, a plan for the saphenous vein grafts is made. Three separate proximal anastomoses are usually performed for separate grafts to the LAD, circumflex, and right coronary arteries, respectively. We frequently perform sequential grafts to different branches of a major vessel, such as LAD and diagonal branches, posterior ventricular, posterior descending, and main trunk of the right coronary artery or multiple obtuse marginal branches (Fig. 39.1). Patients with three-vessel disease usually receive three to seven distal anastomoses. Our goal is to perform as many grafts as necessary to achieve complete revascularization within 60 to 90 minutes of cardioplegic ischemia. Each anastomosis takes 8 to 15 minutes. In patients with three-vessel disease whose main circumflex and right main arteries are not suitable for bypass, grafts to the posterior descending and obtuse marginal branches are done sequentially with one vein graft. Usually only one, and never more than two, side-to-side anastomoses are performed to each vein graft.

**Suture Technique.** A routine suture technique for proximal and distal anastomosis for aortocoronary vein bypass grafting is continuous 5–0, 6–0, or 7–0 Proline. The size Proline is chosen according to the character of the arterial wall and size of the vessel. Heavier suture is used for thicker walled and larger diameter vessels. The technique we use is a continuous

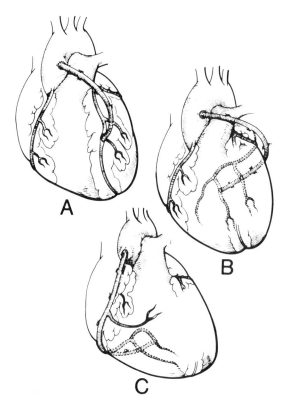

Fig. 39.1 The most common types of sequential vein bypass grafting. *(A)* End-to-side to left anterior descending and side-to-side to diagonal branch. *(B)* End-to-side and side-to-side anastomoses to obtuse marginal branches of circumflex. *(C)* End-to-side to posterior ventricular branch of right coronary artery and side-to-side to posterior descending branch. Each graft supplies branches of one major coronary artery.

suture around the anastomosis with no mattressing of the suture at any point. This has the advantage of producing no invagination of vein into artery and no constriction at the site of mattressing. It does require, however, that during a portion of the anastomosis the needle be passed from outside to inside on the artery, and from inside to outside on the vein. In dealing with coronary vessels without atherosclerotic disease at the site of arteriotomy, stripping-up of intima has not been a problem with this technique. Occasionally, however, passing the needle from outside to inside on the artery must be avoided in coronary vessels because of the presence of atheromatous material, particularly calcified plaque (Fig. 39.2).

With the sequential grafting technique, orientation of the vein in relation to the longitudinal direction of the artery is very important. With either longitudinal or transverse venotomy, the vein can be oriented in virtually any direction relative to the artery. One must be careful, in planning the sequential anastomoses, that the correct orientation of the vein to artery is achieved at each anastomosis to avoid kinking after the next sequential anastomosis is performed. With small veins, the length of the arteriotomy must be limited. This is particularly true with transverse venotomy. If the arteriotomy is more than half the diameter of the vein, a transverse venotomy will cause the vein to constrict at the site of the side-to-side anastomosis. We prefer longitudinal venotomy, which splays the vein over the arteriotomy and avoids any constriction at the side-to-side anastomosis. Great care must be taken to avoid kinking,

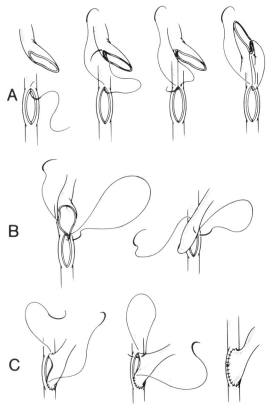

Fig. 39.2 Suture technique of vein grafting without mattressing, continuous over and over suture. Multiple close bites are taken to avoid "pursestring" effect. The suture is passed outside to inside on the artery if there is not mural sclerosis or calcification.

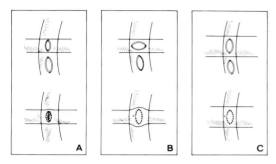

Fig. 39.3 The vein size and direction of venotomy may cause obstruction of vein graft. *(A)* The narrow vein and transverse venotomy produces obstruction of the vein when sutured to a longer arteriotomy. *(B)* The preferred technique is longitudinal venotomy which splays the vein over the arteriotomy avoiding obstruction. *(C)* Transverse venotomy may be used with small arteriotomy and large vein.

twisting, tension, stretching, or redundancy between sequential anastomoses and between the proximal aortic and the distal coronary anastomosis. The veins should be inspected repeatedly between anastomoses and before closure of the stenotomy to assure that kinking and twisting has not occurred (Fig. 39.3).

## Myocardial Protection

Techniques employed for coronary bypass grafting include local coronary artery occlusion in the beating working heart without cardiopulmonary bypass. This has limited applicability and is used by a minority of surgeons. It does not permit anastomosis to posterior vessels. Local occlusion of coronary arteries with the heart fibrillating and perfused has been a safe technique, but retraction and exposure are often more difficult than with myocardial ischemia. Intermittent aortic clamping with periodic reperfusion is a popular technique. Perfusion at colder temperatures (20° to 28°C) usually precludes defibrillating the heart during reperfusion. Reperfusion is more uniform in the warm beating heart, but ischemia without injury is more easily achieved at lower temperatures. As multiple (four to seven) distal anastomoses have become more common, we have chosen a single period of myocardial ischemia, protecting the myocardium by infusing a cold cardioplegic solution through the coronary circulation.

The important ingredients of cardioplegic solutions are that they be cold (5°C), buffered, alkaline (pH 7.8), and hyperosmotic (380 mOsmol), with substrate (5 percent glucose) and depolarizing agent (KCl, 20 mEq/1).

Infusion is begun through a cannula in the ascending aorta as the aorta is clamped to assure aortic valve closure; 1000 ml of the cardioplegic solution is infused rapidly and the aorta is palpated to assess perfusion pressure. The heart is examined for signs of distention. Electrical and mechanical silence with a cold, soft myocardium are signs of effective cardioplegia. The left ventricle is carefully palpated to determine its softness. Cold (5°C) saline is dripped into the pericardium throughout the period of aortic clamping.

After the initial infusion of cardioplegia, the temperature of the anterior, lateral, and posterior regions of the left ventricle is determined. The temperature of the myocardium is usually less than 20°C, and, occasionally, is below 10°C. Temperatures above 20°C are frequently found in areas of fibrosis, old or recent infarction, and areas of severe coronary obstruction. Failure of myocardial cooling by cardioplegia, in a region with viable muscle, may be an indication to perform the vein graft to that region first and then achieve cooling by injecting 50 to 100 ml of cold cardioplegia solution through the vein graft. We have found this effective in dealing with inadequately cooled myocardium.

After each one or two distal anastomoses, 250 ml of cold cardioplegia solution are injected into the aortic root. More frequent infusion of cardioplegia solution is warranted, with warming or evidence of electrical or mechanical activity.

After the distal vein graft anastomoses are performed, the aortic clamp is removed and the heart reperfused. Rewarming is begun and defibrillation is attempted at 30°C. If this is unsuccessful, lidocaine, 50 to 100 mg, is injected intravenously. During the period of reperfusion, while the proximal anastomoses are being done, it is best for the heart to be beating, nonworking, and have left ventricular decompression and perfusion pressure greater than 75 mmHg.

After the proximal anastomoses are completed with a partial occlusion clamp, a stable rhythm is established. After cardioplegia, occasionally use of atrial or ventricular pacing wires is necessary to achieve a stable rhythm, before cardiopulmonary bypass is discontinued.

Other considerations important in myocardial protection before and after cardioplegia are avoidance of ventricular fibrillation, particularly in the hypertrophied heart, and avoidance of ventricular distention. Embolization of air or atheromatous material into the vein grafts should be prevented by continuously aspirating the aorta as cardiopulmonary bypass is discontinued. Repeated defibrillation may produce myocardial necrosis.

All anastomoses are inspected for hemostasis, and cardiopulmonary bypass is discontinued while radial artery pressure and pulmonary artery pressure are monitored. Pulmonary artery diastolic pressures are maintained at 14 to 18 mmHg early after bypass. If contractility is depressed, calcium chloride is given (200 mg intravenously). Low cardiac output is treated by monitoring filling pressures, inotropic drugs (dopamine, epinephrine), and afterload reduction (nitroprusside). In occasional patients with a severely depressed cardiac output, the combination of epinephrine and nitroprusside has been particularly efficacious, allowing afterload and contractility to be adjusted independently. Intraaortic balloon pumping has been used rarely with the cardioplegic technic of myocardial preservation.

## Ventricular Venting

There are several goals of left ventricular venting. Overdistention of the left ventricle may cause stretching and weakening of the sarcomeres and impair postoperative contractility. Distention may create high subendocardial intramyocardial pressure and interfere with coronary flow, delivery of cardioplegia solution, and myocardial cooling. Entry of warm blood into the left ventricle may warm the subendocardium and decrease its protection from ischemia. The distended heart is firm, rigid, and difficult to retract to expose posterior coronary vessels for anastomosis.

The left ventricle may be vented directly by placing a catheter into the chamber through the apex, through the left atrial appendage, through the right superior pulmonary vein, or through the superior approach to the left atrium between the aorta and superior vein cava. One may vent the left ventricle indirectly by placing a catheter in the pulmonary artery. This accomplishes all the goals of venting in the majority of patients, if the ventricle is compressed intermittently during cardioplegia. If ventricular distention is observed after cardioplegia infusion, the catheter in the ascending aorta may be disconnected from the cardioplegia line and placed on cardiotomy suction, which effectively vents the left ventricle through the aortic valve. This avenue of venting is easier, has less chance of introducing air into the left ventricle, and is quicker and safer to close than other direct sites of left ventricular venting (Fig. 39.4)

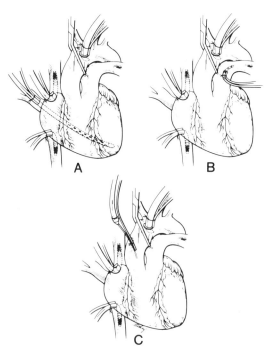

Fig. 39.4  Three commonly used techniques of left ventricular venting during aortic clamping. *(A)* The left ventricle is vented by a catheter placed through the right superior pulmonary vein across the mitral valve. *(B)* The left ventricle is vented indirectly by a catheter in the pulmonary artery. *(C)* The cardioplegia catheter in the aorta is placed on suction to vent the left ventricle and dry the coronary arteriotomy.

## Techniques of Cardiopulmonary Bypass

Hypothermic hemodilution cardiopulmonary bypass, employing a bubble oxygenator and roller pump, has proved to be very safe for conventional cardiac surgery. Most coronary artery bypass procedures requiring multiple distal anastomoses with ventricular resection or valve replacement can be performed in 2 to 3 hours of cardiopulmonary bypass. Hemodilution is important in reversing the hyperviscosity that accompanies hypothermia, which diminishes total body and organ oxygen consumption as well as blood flow requirements. With hypothermia, for each period of cardiopulmonary bypass, a smaller volume of blood must be pumped and oxygenated, producing lesser degrees of hemolysis and mechanical trauma to blood components. Furthermore, the use of clear electrolyte solutions for priming the oxygenator has diminished the need for whole blood, and also has diminished total blood requirements for cardiac procedures, making operations safe without blood transfusion for members of the religious sect known as Jehovah's Witnesses. In addition to meticulous surgical technique, other interventions may decrease homologous blood requirements. Five hundred to 1000 ml of the patient's own blood, drawn before cardiopulmonary bypass is started, may be stored. This blood is then reinfused after cardiopulmonary bypass is discontinued and constitutes a "fresh" autotransfusion rich in coagulation factors. Secondly, all of the red cells of the oxygenator are returned to the patient. These may be infused slowly after cardiopulmonary bypass is discontinued, during a period of diuresis that may be increased by intravenous furosemide (20 to 40 mg). To avoid overloading the patient, the technique of concentrating red blood cells (Haemonetics Cellsaver) may be used to avoid the infusion of excess salt-containing solution. After cardiopulmonary bypass is discontinued, the blood shed into the wound may be harvested into an autotransfusion apparatus and returned to the patient, if blood availability is low or if the patient's religious beliefs preclude the use of blood transfusion. After one venous line and the arterial line are removed, the remainder of the pump oxygenator prime may be infused through the remaining line. During this time, protamine may be administered to reverse heparin anticoagulation and hemostasis may be obtained throughout the wound with suture and coagulation techniques.

### Perfusion Pressure

Preoperatively, the patient is examined carefully for evidence of occlusive vascular disease. The brain is the organ system at greatest risk of ischemic complication from occlusive vascular disease during cardiopulmonary bypass. Therefore, in the patient with transient ischemic attacks the internal carotid artery should be evaluated by noninvasive procedures or by carotid angiography to determine whether carotid endarterectomy should be performed with coronary artery bypass grafting. When carotid stenosis is present, perfusion pressure must be maintained at higher levels during cardiopulmonary bypass. We try to maintain blood pressure above 90 mmHg in the presence of carotid artery stenosis. In its absence, however, we lower perfusion pressure during the period of cold ischemic cardioplegia to diminish the noncoronary collateral flow to the distal coronary bed and thereby lessen the degree of bleeding from the distal arteriotomies, washout of cardioplegia, and myocardial warming. After the distal coronary artery anastomosis has been performed, and during the time of proximal anastomosis when the partial occlusion clamp is applied to the ascending aorta, a high perfusion pressure must be achieved in order to assure high coronary perfusion pressure during the reperfusion. Perfusion pressure is a major determinant of recovery of myocardial function during reperfusion.

**Pacing.** We routinely leave atrial and ventricular pacing wires in place postoperatively. Atrial pacing wires have the advantage of allowing one to record the atrial electrogram directly, which is very helpful in the diagnosis of supraventricular tachycardia and may aid in the control of supraventricular arrhythmias by rapid overdrive atrial pacing. Ventricular pacing wires may also be used for sequential atrioventricular pacing as well as for ventricular pacing in the presence of abnormal atrioventricular conduction. We have found the incidence of abnormalities in atrioventricular conduction to be greater following cardioplegic techniques of myocardial preservation. However, these abnormalities are usually transient.

## Surgical Technique for Complications of Myocardial Infarction

**Coronary Bypass Grafting.** The operation should be conducted in a fashion similar to that for unstable angina pectoris. It may be better not to revascularize an occluded vessel that supplies an area of transmural infarction, if the area of infarction is well localized and in the distribution of a secondary coronary artery branch. All major vessels to functioning myocardium should be bypassed, however.[39] The result of revascularization in this group of patients appears to be improved with modern techniques of cardiopulmonary bypass and cold ischemic cardioplegic myocardial preservation.

**Ventricular Septal Defect.** The principles of surgical repair of acute septal rupture following myocardial infarction include (1) complete repair of the septal rupture without residual ventricular septal defects, (2) preservation of quantity and function of viable ventricular muscle, and (3) bypass of obstructive lesions of the coronary arteries to viable ventricular muscle. Operations are performed with complete cardiopulmonary bypass, using previously described techniques of myocardial preservation with cold cardioplegia. The area of infarction of the adjacent left ventricle can often be identified by inspecting the surface of the heart after the sternotomy is performed. Palpation of the right ventricular cavity through the right atrial appendage and tricuspid valve may help to define the location of the ventricular septal defect.[78] If adjacent portions of the left ventricle are infarcted, the cardiotomy is performed in the infarct. Such infarctions are usually near the apex, and incision through the infarcted left ventricle reveals the ruptured ventricular septum near the apex of the infarcted left ventricle. Although repair by direct suture has been reported, most patients require patch closure or buttressing with free wall of the right and left ventricle

to close the defect. The decision to use a patch in closing the ventricular septum often depends on the amount of septum infarcted and the effect of suturing the viable margin of the left ventricular wall to the margin of the septum. Small defects with fibrous margins may be closed with a single layer patch placed on the left ventricular side of the defect. Larger defects require a double-layered patch technique with a layer of Teflon felt material on the left and right ventricular sides of the defect.[79] These are fastened in place with mattress sutures through the ventricular septum. The reconstruction may be completed by using strips of Teflon felt material, suturing left ventricular septum and right ventricle. If the right ventricle is not infarcted, the left ventricle may be sutured directly to the margin of the ventricular septum (Figs. 39.5 and 39.6).

The left ventricular approach through the infarct is preferable for anterior defects. More posterior defects, however, may be entered through the posterior wall of the right

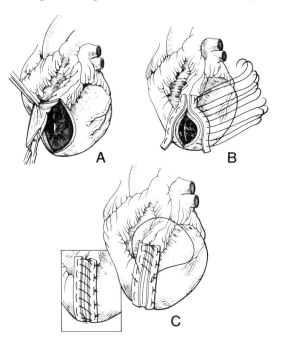

Fig. 39.5  Repair of ventricular septal defect and infarctectomy is shown. *(A)* The infarct is excised. showing the ventricular septal defect. *(B)* Sutures are placed over pledgets through ventricular wall and ventricular septum. *(C)* The interrupted sutures are oversewn with continuous sutures.

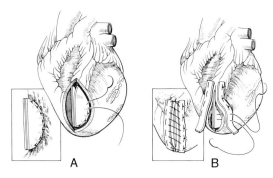

Fig. 39.6  *(A)* Repair of ventricular septal defect with double layer of Teflon felt material employed because of deficient septal tissue. *(B)* Closure of ventriculotomy similar to Fig. 39.5.

ventricle.[78] The principles of repair are similar to those described for those anterior defects. In posterior defects and inferior infarctions, the posterior papillary muscle is frequently necrotic and mitral valve replacement may be performed through the left ventriculotomy.

Coronary bypass grafts to obstructed vessels of the viable left ventricular myocardium should be performed. In patients who have not had coronary angiography, local clues to coronary artery obstruction of the coronary vessels may be used to identify vessels for revascularization. In the process of closing an anterior ventricular septal defect, the region of the left anterior descending coronary artery will usually be obliterated. Coronary grafts are frequently placed in the right and circumflex coronary arteries. Intraaortic balloon counterpulsation is frequently useful in these patients to decrease afterload, improve coronary flow, and increase cardiac output.

**Ventricular Aneurysm.** When excising an acute infarct or aneurysm, care must be taken to preserve an adequate volume of left ventricular muscle and cavity. Survival is not likely if more than 35 percent of the left ventricle is excised. Tests for determining viability of ventricular muscle include electrograms and staining with vital dyes. The gross appearance of the infarcted and viable myocardium usually makes the margin of the acute aneurysm easily distinguishable.

One should be careful to avoid mobilization or dissection of the aneurysm before cardiopul-

monary bypass. The aorta should be clamped before the aneurysm is exposed to avoid embolization from the aneurysm. After the infarct is excised, the ventricle is closed with heavy mattress sutures of 0-Dacron passed through strips of Teflon felt on either side of the ventriculotomy. These sutures are all placed and then gently but firmly tied to avoid tearing the fragile myocardium.

**Chronic Aneurysms.** The surgical principles are similar to those employed for acute left ventricular aneurysms. The aneurysm is entered near its center and any thrombus is removed from the left ventricular wall, leaving 1 cm of fibrous tissue behind to allow for a strong suture closure of the left ventricular aneurysm. The papillary muscles of the mitral valve are carefully avoided. Care must be taken not to create a small left ventricular chamber that would limit diastolic volume. Mitral insufficiency commonly accompanies left ventricular aneurysm, and when the aneurysm is open, the papillary muscles and the mitral valve mechanism must be inspected carefully to determine whether the resection alone will correct the mitral insufficiency. The mitral valve can be replaced through the ventriculotomy at the site of aneurysm excision. The aneurysm is closed with two layers over Teflon felt as described above.

**False Aneurysm.** When operating on a left ventricular false aneurysm, the surgeon should expose the aorta and right atrium before the aneurysm is manipulated. If it is manipulated before cannulation and cardiopulmonary bypass, entry into a false aneurysm may lead to a life-threatening hemorrhage. After cardiopulmonary bypass is instituted, the aorta should be clamped and cardioplegia infused before the aneurysm is dissected. It can be closed in the usual fashion, using a row of horizontal interrupted sutures over Teflon felt followed by a more superficial row of running sutures.

**Cardiac Rupture.** The heart may be sutured at the site of rupture without cardiopulmonary bypass. The cardiac ruptures in patients treated successfully with surgical closure have usually been in the anterior portion of the left ventricle. The thin-walled apical portion of the left ventricle appears to be the area most susceptible to cardiac rupture.

**Ventricular Arrhythmias.** All bypassable diseased vessels should be revascularized. The need for complete revascularization may be greater in patients whose indication for operation is ventricular arrhythmia. Ventricular aneurysms should be resected and areas of dyskinesis plicated. In patients with ventricular arrhythmia, there is a rationale for plication of small areas of dyskinesis that would otherwise be left alone. The focus of early excitation is usually in the dyskinetic area or on its border. Mapping techniques are useful for precisely localizing the focus of early depolarization.

**Perioperative Infarction.** Myocardial injury may occur preoperatively, intraoperatively, or postoperatively. Serial serum CK isoenzyme determinations have demonstrated that the period prior to cardiopulmonary bypass is a time of increased risk of infarction. Prevention of infarction during this period depends principally on anesthetic technique. The use of propranolol, morphine, nitroglycerin, and nitroprusside to control heart rate, preload and afterload are important aspects of anesthetic management. The duration of the preoperative period should be minimized by expeditious placement of monitoring catheters, induction, prepping, draping, and sternotomy. Ideally, the length of time from entry into the operating room to institution of cardiopulmonary bypass should be 60 to 90 minutes. The interventions likely to cause hypertension, hypotension, or tachycardia are endotracheal intubation, skin incision, and manipulation of the heart. The heart is not manipulated until cardiopulmonary bypass is begun.

Prevention of myocardial injury during myocardial ischemia depends on myocardial temperature, duration of ischemia, and absence of electric or mechanical activity. Perioperative infarction occurs more commonly with severe three-vessel disease, and diffuse disease requiring longer periods of ischemia for revascularization. Coronary obstruction, which is not amenable to bypass, also contributes to perioperative injury.

After cardiopulmonary bypass, injury may occur during periods of hypertension or tachycardia if unbypassed coronary obstruction is present. Early vein graft occlusion, emboliza-tion of air, or atheromatous debris to the vein grafts or coronary arteries may cause perioperative myocardial injury. Kinking, twisting, or tension on vein grafts are other causes of injury.

The frequency and severity of myocardial injury depend on the technique used to detect injury and the distribution of the injury. New Q waves on the ECG are the most reliable indicators of perioperative transmural infarction.[26] In our experience, new Q waves occur in 10 percent of patients. A rise in CK isoenzyme levels is the most sensitive indicator of myocardial injury and may be positive with a few grams of myocardial necrosis. Such a rise occurs in 50 to 90 percent of patients.[80] Different techniques used for measuring CK isoenzymes are one cause for variability in the rate of positivity between different groups. The $^{99m}$technetium pyrophosphate scan is useful in detecting localized myocardial injury but may be negative with significant diffuse injury. The incidence of positive $^{99m}$technetium pyrophosphate scans is greater than new Q waves but less than the incidence of elevated CK isoenzyme levels.[49]

The consequences of perioperative infarction depend on its effect on left ventricular function and the tendency to produce arrythmias. The natural history of perioperative infarction is in general more benign than spontaneously occurring myocardial infarction.

## Postoperative Management

Preoperative, intraoperative, and postoperative care of the cardiac surgery patient depends on preventing, correcting, and treating dysfunction related to the heart, lungs, kidneys, and blood clotting mechanisms, and on avoiding infection.

**Cardiac Function.** Clinical signs of low cardiac output should be monitored postoperatively. Important clinical signs include assessment of the contour and amplitude of the pedal pulses as well as the color and temperature of the fingers, toes, and nail beds. Other signs of organ perfusion are adequacy of urine output, responsiveness to diuretics, and cerebral function. In the postanesthesia period, an alert patient aware of his surroundings and with good urine output, strong pedal pulses, and pink fingers and toes will rarely have severe cardiac dysfunction.

Systolic blood pressure should be maintained between 100 to 130 mmHg following coronary artery bypass grafting. Blood pressure below 100 mmHg may be a sign of low cardiac output or low systemic vascular resistance. Systolic blood pressures above 130 mmHg may decrease stroke volume, increase myocardial oxygen demand, and cause bleeding from aortic suture lines, including the proximal vein graft anastomosis. Nitroprusside infusion is employed at a controlled rate, using an intravenous pump to regulate systolic pressure. Cardiac output determinations are essential to evaluate systemic vascular resistance with low, normal, or high arterial pressure. Hypertension treated with nitroprusside in the early postoperative period usually results in an increased stroke volume. When stroke volume is depressed with low, normal, or high arterial pressure, nitroprusside may similarly increase stroke volume. Serial cardiac output determinations, and calculations of systemic vascular resistance are essential for determining the effect of nitroprusside on systemic vascular resistance and stroke volume. We have noted a correlation between decreases in systemic vascular resistance with warming of peripheral tissue, including fingers and feet, and an increase in the volume and upstroke of pedal pulses with nitroprusside.

With a systolic pressure below 90 mmHg and a depressed cardiac output unresponsive to nitroprusside, an inotropic drug may be used. Although most patients will receive digoxin, an intravenous drip of an adrenergic drug is preferred in the early postoperative period. We usually begin with low-dose dopamine (2 to 5 $\mu$g/kg/min). Patients who fail to respond to increasing doses of dopamine may respond to other drugs, such as epinephrine or isoproterenol. We prefer dopamine in the presence of supraventricular or ventricular tachyarrhythmias. Isoproterenol may worsen or produce supraventricular or ventricular dysrythmias. Dopamine has a specific advantage in that it dilates the renal vessels in low doses and may increase urine output when oliguria is secondary to low cardiac output. In some patients in whom cardiac output is severely depressed, we have used a combination of epinephrine and nitroprusside. This combination has the advantage of allowing independent adjustments in contractility and afterload.

Hypotension following coronary artery bypass grafting is not only an important sign of low cardiac output, but also may have an adverse effect on coronary blood flow because as diastolic pressure diminishes, perfusion through the vein grafts falls and leads to myocardial ischemia or vein graft thrombosis. Patients with low systemic vascular resistance, good cardiac output, but low perfusion pressure may be benefited by systemic vasoconstriction, with phenylephrine given as an intravenous bolus.

Maintenance of an elevated left ventricular filling pressure is important in the early postoperative period following coronary artery bypass grafting, particularly if left ventricular function is depressed. Most of the interventions during cardiopulmonary bypass, including hemodilution, hypothermia, and ischemia, result in diminished left ventricular compliance. A higher filling pressure is necessary to achieve satisfactory left ventricular diastolic filling in the presence of diminished compliance. Left ventricular filling pressure is usually estimated by monitoring pulmonary artery diastolic pressure, pulmonary wedge pressure, or left atrial pressure. Whole blood or packed cells are used to increase both blood volume and left ventricular filling pressure until the hematocrit reaches 40 percent. With the hematocrit at 40 percent or above, plasma, fresh frozen plasma, or Plasmanate may be used to increase left ventricular filling pressure. Serial determinations of cardiac output at different filling pressures may help in deciding the optimal filling pressure or the peak of the Starling curve in a particular patient. The short-term risk of high left ventricular filling pressure is mainly related to lung function. Patients whose poor left ventricular function requires a left ventricular filling pressure above 22 mmHg for several days may have accumulation of interstitial fluid in other parts of the body. However, if oxygenation remains satisfactory, there is no life-threatening consequence. Positive pressure ventilation, positive end-expiratory pressure, and continuous positive airway pressure may be helpful in limiting the degree of interstitial pulmonary edema in the presence of high left ventricular filling pressures. In patients who are bleeding postoperatively, filling pressures should also be kept high, because if cardiac tamponade develops, high ventricular pressures are necessary to prevent low cardiac output. Myocardial depression following coronary artery saphenous vein bypass grafting usually is transient. Stroke volume and cardiac output improve as filling pressure falls during the first 6 to 24 hours postoperatively.

**Arrhythmias.** Postoperatively, arrhythmias may produce decreases in cardiac output, increases in myocardial oxygen demand, or predispose to ventricular fibrillation. Following coronary bypass grafting, patients are particularly susceptible to the effects of rapid supraventricular tachyarrhythmias, which cause sudden increases in myocardial oxygen demand. Supraventricular tachyarrhythmias following coronary bypass grafting are dangerous, if accompanied by rapid ventricular response. If the tachyarrhythmia is accompanied by decreasing cardiac output, falling blood pressure, anginal pain, or electrocardiographic signs of myocardial ischemia, it should be treated very quickly by DC cardioversion. If the arrhythmia is not associated with a deleterious effect, it may be managed medically. An atrial electrogram recorded from the atrial pacing wires, as well as the conventional electrocardiogram, will usually differentiate atrial flutter, atrial fibrillation, and sinus tachycardia. With atrial fibrillation, the patient is begun on digoxin, which is repeated using intravenous doses (0.125 to 0.25 mg every 4 to 6 hours) until the ventricular response is below 100 beats per minute. Propranolol, 0.5 to 1.0 mg intravenously, every 30 minutes to 2 hours, may be given to further diminish the ventricular response in the presence of atrial fibrillation. Digoxin and propranolol will usually bring the ventricular response into a satisfactory range in patients with atrial fibrillation. Quinidine 200 mg every 4 to 6 hours may be begun to achieve stable rhythm control. Frequently, patients will revert spontaneously to normal sinus rhythm or may require later DC cardioversion.

Patients with atrial flutter may be converted by rapid atrial pacing, achieved by stimulating the atrial pacing electrodes with an external pulse generator. They should also be started on digoxin, 0.125 to 0.25 mg every 4 to 6 hours intravenously until fully digitalized. Propranolol may also be of benefit in controlling the response of atrial flutter. If the ventricular response is rapid or persistent, despite the above-described measures, DC cardioversion should be employed before full digitalization is achieved.

Ventricular premature beats should be treated vigorously, if frequent, (greater than 6 per minute), multifocal, repetitive, or associated with deterioration in blood pressure or cardiac output. Fifty to 100 mg of lidocaine is given intravenously, followed by an intravenous lidocaine drip. Most ventricular arrhythmias can be controlled with lidocaine bolus and infusion. If the ventricular arrhythmias are associated with a slow, spontaneous ventricular rhythm, pacing via the atrial or ventricular electrodes to increase the ventricular rate may suppress the premature ventricular contractions. Propranolol, 0.5 to 1.0 mg intravenously every 30 minutes to 3 hours, may also decrease the frequency and malignancy of premature ventricular contractions. Occasionally, rhythms unresponsive to the above measures may require intravenous procainamide. In occasional patients, with significant depression of left ventricular function, lidocaine, procainamide, or propranolol will depress the cardiac output. In such patients, ventricular premature contractions sometimes must be tolerated to avoid depression of cardiac output.

The onset of atrial premature contractions often heralds the development of atrial fibrillation or flutter. We begin digoxin in doses of 0.25 mg every 6 to 8 hours, if frequent atrial premature contractions occur, until full digitalization is achieved. In the presence of recurring arrhythmias, frequent monitoring of serum potassium, arterial blood gases, and cardiac function is necessary.

When these methods for control of arrhythmias postoperatively are employed, ventricular fibrillation is rare following aortocoronary saphenous vein bypass grafting. In addition to malignant forms of ventricular premature contractions, inotropic drugs and hypokalemia may be significant predisposing factors to ventricular fibrillation in the postcoronary artery bypass patient.

**Pulmonary Function.** With present techniques of cardiopulmonary bypass and respiratory care, the most important risk factor for postoperative respiratory failure is preoperative pulmonary function. It is unusual for respiratory failure to occur in a patient without preoperative lung dysfunction. We no longer consider abnormal pulmonary function a contraindication to aortocoronary saphenous vein bypass grafting, but do consider diminished pulmonary function a risk factor. The risk of operation appears to be increased in patients with preoperative pulmonary dysfunction, as indicated by a low arterial $PO_2$ or obstructive airways disease. Many factors are important in achieving a low incidence of postoperative pulmonary dysfunction.

These include the use of hypothermic hemodilution cardiopulmonary bypass. Less use of homologous blood transfusion, decompression of the left ventricle and pulmonary circulation during cardiopulmonary bypass by pulmonary artery venting, sternotomy incision, placing of intrapleural chest tubes postoperatively in patients with lung dysfunction, and better techniques of respiratory care, including positive end-expiratory pressure, continuous positive airway pressure, and intermittent mandatory ventilation, are important in preventing and correcting postoperative pulmonary dysfunction.

Poor oxygenation is a more common manifestation of pulmonary dysfunction postoperatively than is $CO_2$ retention. Arterial $PO_2$ levels above 75 mmHg insure that sufficient oxygen is being delivered to the myocardium. The inspired oxygen concentration ($FiO_2$) is diminished to 40 to 50 percent soon after the patient arrives in the postoperative intensive care unit. If blood gas analysis shows poor oxygenation with this level of inspired oxygen concentration, tidal volume is increased and positive end-expiratory pressure is added. We usually begin with a tidal volume of 10 to 12 cc/kg and increase this to 15 to 17 cc/kg. If poor oxygenation does require adding positive end-expiratory pres-

sure, one should monitor its effects on systemic arterial pressure, cardiac output, pulmonary artery pressure, and pulmonary wedge pressure. It is frequently necessary to increase filling pressure to avoid diminished cardiac output with positive end-expiratory pressure. Oxygenation can usually be maintained at satisfactory levels with $FiO_2$ concentrations of 40 to 60 percent and positive end-expiratory pressures up to 10 cm of water with volume ventilation.

We observe the left ventricular filling pressures closely and keep this pressure at the lowest level consistent with satisfactory cardiac output. In the presence of lung failure, diuretics may be used to lower left ventricular filling pressure, and fluid intake should be limited to 1000 ml/m²/day. As respiratory function improves, the positive end-expiratory pressure may be progressively lowered. Inspired oxygen concentration is diminished to 40 percent or less. The patient may then be begun on intermittent mandatory ventilation (IMV), beginning at rates of 10 to 15 ventilations per minute. The patient is allowed to breathe on his own between mandatory ventilations. The rate of the intermittent mandatory ventilation is progressively diminished. The patient should have periods of spontaneous breathing on inspired oxygen concentrations of 40 percent or less before extubation. Occasionally, there may be a question of whether the patient will tolerate extubation and a "trial" of extubation must be used. In such patients, the oxygenation usually will improve after the endotracheal tube is removed and the patient is able to cough and clear his secretions.

Retention of $CO_2$ is not as common as hypocarbia during controlled ventilation, but both must be avoided. The $PCO_2$ may be adjusted by altering respiratory rate, tidal volume, and dead space. Dead space may be altered by increasing positive end-expiratory pressure or by adding dead space to the ventilator. Hypocarbia and the accompanying respiratory alkalosis often leads to brisk kaluresis and predisposes to ventricular arrhythmias as well as cerebral vasoconstriction. Frequently, high tidal volumes and respiratory rates are necessary for adequate oxygenation, but these may lead to significant hypocarbia and respiratory alkalosis, which are best treated by adding dead space to the ventilator.

**Renal Function.** Satisfactory renal function is essential during the recovery period following aortocoronary saphenous vein bypass grafting to excrete the excess interstitial fluid following hemodilution cardiopulmonary bypass. Most patients gain 1 to 5 kg following cardiopulmonary bypass. The trauma of the pump oxygenator and cardiotomy suction causes the release of hemoglobin into plasma. Hemoglobin is filtered at the glomerulus and high urine output is necessary to avoid hemoglobin precipitation in the renal tubules. If hemoglobinuria is noted, the urine pH should be checked and alkaline urine achieved by infusion of bicarbonate. Maintaining high urine output with diuretics diminishes the incidence and severity of renal failure after cardiopulmonary bypass.[74,82] With a drop in urine output below 1 ml/kg/hr, furosemide, 20 to 40 mg intravenously, is given. If patients do not respond to furosemide, mannitol 25 g is infused over 30 minutes. If diuresis does not develop after both furosemide and mannitol, dopamine is occasionally indicated to improve cardiac function and produce renal vasodilation. Transient renal failure, following aortocoronary saphenous vein bypass grafting, is usually related to preexisting renal disease or poor cardiac performance postoperatively.[83] Renal failure seldom requires hemodialysis or peritoneal dialysis following aortocoronary saphenous vein bypass grafting.

**Hemostatic Mechanisms.** Use of the pump oxygenator causes abnormalities of the coagulation mechanism due to destruction and consumption of coagulation components during cardiopulmonary bypass. Complete heparinization is necessary to prevent intravascular coagulation and consumption of coagulation components on the foreign surfaces of the pump oxygenator. The activated clotting time (ACT) is the best method for monitoring heparin dosage. Heparin is given in a dose adequate to achieve an ACT above 300 seconds. The initial dose of 3 mg/kg often must be augmented by additional heparin to achieve an ACT of greater than 300 seconds. Following cardiopulmonary bypass, protamine is used to reverse the effect of heparin. If coagulopathy persists despite protamine, fresh frozen plasma and platelets are given. Preoperative medications may suppress platelet function (acetylsalicylic acid, propranolol, indomethacin). Adequate numbers of platelets after cardiopulmonary bypass are not an indicator of adequate platelet function. Coagulopathy is best managed by infusion of fresh frozen plasma and platelet transfusion. Control of systolic blood pressure and hypertension is important in avoiding delayed bleeding from the aortic anastomoses.

**Potassium Management Perioperatively.** Hypothermic hemodilution cardiopulmonary bypass frequently causes a decrease in serum potassium. The mechanisms for this are diuresis, hemodilution, and shift of potassium intracellularly. Hyperkalemic cardioplegic solutions add a potassium load during cardiopulmonary bypass and may result in hyperkalemia, especially with diabetes mellitus or propranolol therapy. Propranolol appears to block the epinephrine mediated intracellular shifts of potassium and may cause postoperative hyperkalemia. Hyperkalemia at the time of discontinuing cardiopulmonary bypass is an infrequent problem but can be treated effectively with sodium bicarbonate, calcium chloride, diuresis (furosemide), glucose, and insulin. Hypokalemia is a more common problem. Infusions of potassium chloride, 10 to 40 mEq, are given during cardiopulmonary bypass for serum potassium levels less than 4 mEq/l. Following cardiopulmonary bypass, we maintain potassium levels between 4 and 5 mEq/l. This is achieved by hourly infusions of potassium chloride, 10 to 15 mEq/hr, when the serum potassium is below 4 mEq/l. These infusions are not continued for more than 3 hours unless the potassium is rechecked, especially if the patient has low cardiac output. Patients with low cardiac output or low urine output are prone to develop hyperkalemia rapidly and repeated infusion of potassium should be avoided. Maintenance of serum potassium between 4 and 5 mEq/l has been associated with a lower incidence of ventricular arrhythmias postoperatively.

**Infection.** Patients undergoing aortocoronary saphenous vein bypass are particularly susceptible to infection, and a wide variety of measures must be instituted to avoid infection in these patients. It is important to adopt the premise that the patient is not infected at the beginning of the operation and therefore it is due to faulty technique if the patient acquires infection during the course of his surgical therapy.

The number of bacteria introduced into such a patient must be small. This is achieved by avoiding the introduction of bacteria, including skin bacteria, at the time of operation. Plastic drapes are used in the area of all skin incisions, including the skin incision in the leg, for harvesting the saphenous vein. During the operation meticulous surgical technique must be observed. Unnecessary visitors to the operating room are avoided; gowns, gloves, and instruments are changed with any suspicion of contamination during the operative procedure; and antibiotics are used in every patient. We prefer cephalosporin 1 g every 6 hours. This antibiotic is given in a dose of 3.0 g when the patient arrives in the operating room and 3.0 g are added to the pump oxygenator. After cardiopulmonary bypass is discontinued, the sternotomy wound and pericardium are irrigated with a solution of kanamycin, 500 mg/l. This solution is used repeatedly throughout the wound closure to irrigate the pericardium, sternum, and subcutaneous tissue. Intravenous antibiotics (cephalosporin) are continued for 2 days postoperatively and oral antibiotics for a total of 5 days postoperatively.

Special care is used to avoid introducing organisms into the tracheobronchial tree. Sterile disposable nonreactive endotracheal tubes are used. Sterile suctioning of endotracheal tubes is important to avoid contamination in the operating room and in the intensive care unit. Sterile disposable suction catheters and gloves are used in suctioning the endotracheal tube.

The postoperative intensive care unit is kept free of patients with infection. No infected patients are admitted to the unit, and if cardiac patients acquire infection during their postoperative care, they are transferred to another intensive care unit.

Cardiac surgery patients have a high susceptibility to infection for many reasons. The operations are often prolonged (greater than 4 hours), which is a risk factor in acquired operating room infection. The cardiotomy suction of the pump oxygenator draws room air directly into the patient's blood. Thus, air contamination in the operating room may pass directly in the blood stream through the cardiotomy suction. No contaminated procedures should be performed in the operating room used for cardiopulmonary bypass. The presence of an intravascular prosthesis, and other prosthetic materials in the wound, make it particularly susceptible to infection. Wound infection is usually accompanied by a significant risk of mortality as well as high morbidity. Sternotomy wound infection is difficult to clear because of infected bone and foreign material in the wound. Patients undergoing cardiopulmonary bypass have depression of humoral and cellular immune functions with increased susceptibility to infection. Using the above techniques, we have had only one sternotomy wound infection in over 1000 cardiopulmonary bypass procedures.

## REFERENCES

1. Krauss K, Hutter A, De Sanctis R: Acute coronary insufficiency. Arch Intern Med 129:808, 1972.
2. Fischl S, Herman M, Gorlin R: The intermediate coronary syndrome. Clinical, angiographic, and therapeutic aspects. N Eng J Med 288:1183, 1973.
3. Lawson R, Chapman R, Wood J, et al: Acute coronary insufficiency. An urgent surgical condition. Br Heart J 37:1053, 1975.
4. Scanlon P, Nemickas R, Moran J, et al: Accelerated angina pectoris. Clinical, hemodynamic, arteriographic, and therapeutic experience in 85 patients. Circulation 47:19, 1973.
5. Gaasch W, Lufschanowski R, Leachman R, et al: Surgical management of Prinzmetal's variant angina. Chest 66:614, 1974.
6. Cohn L: The Treatment of Acute Myocardial Ischemia. An Integrated Medical/Surgical Approach. Futura, Mount Kisco, NY, 1979.
7. London R, London S: Rupture of the heart. A critical analysis of 47 consecutive autopsy cases. Circulation 31:202, 1965.
8. Hultgren H, Pfeifer J, Angell W, et al: Unstable angina: comparison of medical and surgical management. Am J Cardiol 39:734, 1977.
9. Bertoloasi C, Tronge J, Carreno C, et al: Unstable angina-prospective and randomized study

of its evolution, with and without surgery. Am J Cardiol 33:201, 1974.

10. Seldon R, Neill W, Ritzmann L, et al: Medical versus surgical therapy for acute coronary insufficiency. A randomized study. N Engl J Med, 293:1329, 1975.

11. Wiles J, Peduzzi P, Hammond G, et al: Preoperative predictors of operative mortality for coronary bypass grafting in patients with unstable angina pectoris. Am J Cardiol, 39:939, 1977.

12. Berk G, Kaplitt M, Padmanabham V: Management of preinfarction angina. Evaluation and comparison of medical versus surgical therapy in 43 patients. J Thorac Cardiovasc Surg 71:110, 1976.

13. Matloff J, Sustaita H, Chatterjee K, Chaux A, Marcus H, Swan H: The rationale for surgery in preinfarction angina. J Thorac Cardiovasc Surg 69:73, 1975.

14. Bender H, Fisher D, Faulkner S, et al: Unstable coronary disease. Comparison of medical and surgical treatment. Ann Thorac Surg, 19:521, 1975.

15. Bolooki H, Sommer L, Kaiser G: Long-term follow-up in patients receiving emergency revascularization for intermediate coronary syndrome. J Thorac Cardiovasc Surg 68:90, 1974.

16. Boncheck L, Rahimtoola S, Anderson R: Late results following emergency saphenous vein bypass grafting for unstable angina. Circulation 50:972, 1974.

17. Cobbs B, Hatcher C, Robinson P: Cardiac rupture. JAMA 233:532, 1973.

18. Schroeder J, Lamb I, Hum M, et al: Coronary bypass surgery for unstable angina pectoris. Long-term survival and function. JAMA 237: 2609, 1977.

19. Grondin C, Limet R: Sympathetic denervation in association with coronary artery grafting in patients with Prinzmetal's angina. Ann Thorac Surg 23:111, 1977.

20. Nordstrom L, Lillehei J, Adicoff A, et al: Coronary artery surgery for recurrent ventricular arrhythmias in patients with variant angina. Am Heart J, 89:236, 1975.

21. Montoya A, Mulet J, Pifarre R, et al: Hemorrhagic infarct following myocardial revascularization. J Thorac Cardiovasc Surg 75:206, 1978.

22. Guss S, Zir L, Garrison H, et al: Coronary occlusion during coronary angiography. Circulation 52:1063, 1975.

23. Takara T, Pifarre R, Wuerflein R, et al: Acute coronary occlusion following coronary arteriography: Mechanisms and surgical relief. Surgery 72:1018, 1972.

24. Bolooki H, Kotler M, Lottenberg L, et al: Myocardial revascularization after acute infarction. Am J Cardiol, 36:395, 1975.

25. Cheanvechai C, Effler D, Loop F: Emergency myocardial revascularization. Am J Cardiol 32:901, 1973.

26. Espihoza J, Lipski J, Litwak R, et al: New Q waves after coronary bypass surgery for angina pectoris. Am J Cardiol 33:221, 1974.

27. Jones E, Douglas J, Craver J, et al: Results of coronary revascularization in patients with recent myocardial infarction. Circulation (suppl III) 55:189, 1977.

28. Loop F, Cheanvechai C, Sheldon W, et al: Early myocardial revascularization during acute myocardial infarction. Chest 66:478, 1974.

29. Mills N, Ochsner J, Bower PJ, et al: Coronary artery bypass for acute myocardial infarction. Southern Med J 68:1475, 1975.

30. Pifarre R, Spinazzola A, Nemeckas R: Emergency aortocoronary bypass for acute myocardiol infarction. Arch Surg 103:525, 1971.

31. Reul G, Morris G, Howell J, et al: Emergency coronary artery bypass grafts in the treatment of myocardial infarction. Circulation (suppl III) 47:177, 1973.

32. Berg R, Kendall R, Duvoisin G: Acute myocardial infarction. A surgical emergency. J Thorac Cardiovasc Surg 70:432, 1975.

33. Schechter D: Inventory of surgical operation for cardiac structural sequels of myocardial infarction. NY State J Med 50:120, 1975.

34. Mundth E, Buckley M, Leinbach R, et al: Myocardial revascularization for the treatment of cardiogenic shock complicating acute myocardial infarction. Surgery 70:78, 1971.

35. Javid H, Hunter J, Najafi H, et al: Left ventricular approach for the repair of ventricular septal perforation and infarctectomy. J. Thorac Cardiovasc Surg 63:14, 1972.

36. Keon W, Bedard P, Shankar K, et al: Experience with emergency aortocoronary bypass grafts in the presence of acute myocardial infarction. Circulation (suppl III) 47:151, 1973.

37. Madigan N, Rutherford B, Barnhorst D, et al: Early saphenous vein grafting after subendocardial infarction: Immediate surgical results and late prognosis. Circulation (suppl II) 53:36, 1976.

38. Aintablian A, Hamby R, Weiss D, et al: Results of aortocoronary bypass grafting in patients with subendocardial infarction. Late follow-up. Am J Cardiol 42:183, 1979.

39. Daggett W, Buckley M, Mundth E, et al: The role of infarctectomy in the surgical treatment of myocardial infarction. Am Heart J 84:723, 1972.

40. Hagemeijer F, Laird J, Haalebos M, et al: Effectiveness of intraaortic balloon pumping without cardiac surgery for patients with severe heart failure secondary to a recent myocardial infarction. Am J Cardiol 40:951, 1977.

41. Kendall R, DeWood M: Postinfarction cardiac rupture: surgical success and review of the literature. Ann Thorac Surg 25:311, 1978.

42. Cohn L, Lamberti J, Lesch M, et al: Intra-aortic balloon counterpulsation and coronary revascularization for left ventricular power failure. Eur Surg Res, 6:129, 1974.

43. Kaplan M, Harris C, Kay et al: Postinfarctional ventricular septal rupture. Clinical approach and surgical results. Chest 6:734, 1976.

44. Gold H, Leinbach R, Sanders C, et al: Intraaortic balloon pumping for ventricular septal defect or mitral regurgitation complicating acute myocardial infarction. Circulation 47:1191, 1973.

45. Giuliani E, Danielson G, Pluth J, et al: Postinfarction ventricular septal rupture. Surgical considerations and results. Circulation 49:455, 1974.

46. DeWeese J, Moss A, Yu P: Infarctectomy and closure of ventricular septal rupture following myocardial infarction. Circulation (suppl I) 14:97, 1972.

47. Freeny P, Schattenberg T, Danielson G, et al: Ventricular septal defect and ventricular aneurysm secondary to acute myocardial infarction. Report of four cases with successful surgical treatment. Circulation 43:360, 1971.

48. Selzer A, Gerbode F, Kerth W: Clinical, hemodynamic, and surgical considerations of rupture of the ventricular septum after myocardial infarction. Am Heart J 78:598, 1969.

48a. Graham A, Stinson E, Daily P, et al: Ventricular septal defects after myocardial infarction. Early operative treatment. JAMA 225:708, 1973.

49. Young D, Utley J, Damron J, et al: Results and patterns of perioperative myocardial infarction. J Thorac Cardiovasc Surg 76:528, 1978.

50. Donahoo J, Brawley R, Taylor D, et al: Factors influencing survival following postinfarction ventricular septal defects. Ann Thorac Surg 19:648, 1975.

51. Ecker R, Mullins C, Crammer J, et al: Control of intractable ventricular tachycardia by coronary revascularization. Circulation 44:666, 1971.

52. Hill JD, Lary D, Kerth W, et al: Acquired ventricular septal defects. Evolution of an operation, surgical technique, and results. J Thorac Cardiovasc Surg 70:440, 1975.

53. Lufschanowski R, Angelini P, Del Rio C, et al: Ventricular septal rupture, secondary to myocardial infarction. Chest 65:89, 1974.

54. Miller R, Iben A, Amsterdam E, et al: Successful immediate repair of acquired ventricular septal defect (VSD) and survival in patients with acute myocardial infarction (AMI) shock using a new double patch technique. Circulation (suppl IV) 7:54, 1973.

55. Kitamura S, Mendez A, Kay J: Ventricular septal defects following myocardial infarction. Experience with surgical repair through a left ventriculotomy and review of literature. J Thorac Cardiovasc Surg 61:186, 1971.

56. Shelburne J, Rubinstein D, Gorlin R: A reappraisal of papillary muscle dysfunction. Correlative clinical and angiographic study. Am J Med 46:862, 1969.

57. DeBusk R, Harrison D: The clinical spectrum of papillary muscle disease. N Eng J Med 281:1458, 1969.

58. Morrow A, Cohen L, Roberts W, et al: Severe mitral regurgitation following acute myocardial infarction and ruptured papillary muscle. Hemodynamic findings and results of operative treatment in four patients. Circulation (suppl II) 37:124, 1968.

59. Najafi H, Javid H, Hunter J, et al: Mitral insufficiency secondary to coronary heart disease. Ann Thorac Surg 20:529, 1975.

60. Austen WG, Sokol D, DeSanctis R, et al: Surgical treatment of papillary-muscle rupture complicating myocardial infarction. N Eng J Med 278:1137, 1968.

61. Klein M, Herman M, Gorlin R: A hemodynamic study of left ventricular aneurysm. Circulation 35:614, 1976.

62. Cohn L, Gorlin R, Herman M, et al: Aorta-coronary bypass for acute coronary occlusion. J Thorac Cardiovasc Surg 64:503, 1972.

63. O'Rourke M: Subacute heart rupture following myocardial infarction. Clinical features of a correctable condition. Lancet 2:124, 1973.

64. Van Tassel R, Edwards J: Rupture of heart complicating myocardial infarction. Analysis of 40 cases including nine examples of left ventricular or false aneurysm. Chest 61:104, 1972.

65. Vismara L, Miller R, Price J, et al: Improved longevity due to reduction of sudden death by aortocoronary bypass in coronary atherosclerosis. Prospective evaluation of medical versus sur-

gical therapy in matched patients with multivessel disease. Am J Cardiol 39:919, 1977.

66. Thind G, Blakemore W, Zinsser H: Ventricular aneurysmectomy for the treatment of recurrent ventricular tachyarrhythmia. Am J Cardiol 27:690, 1971.

67. Myerburg R, Ghahramani A, Mallon S, et al: Coronary revascularization in patients surviving unexpected ventricular fibrillation. Circulation (suppl III) 51:219, 1975.

68. Barry W, Alderman E, Daily P, et al: Diagnosis and treatment of a case of recurrent ventricular tachycardia. Am Heart J 84:235, 1972.

69. Magidson O: Resection of postmyocardial infarction ventricular aneurysms for cardiac arrhythmias. Chest 56:211, 1969.

70. Alexander S, Makar Y, Ellis H Jr: Recurrent ventricular fibrillation. Treatment by emergency aortocoronary saphenous vein bypass. JAMA 228:70, 1974.

71. Nakhjavan F, Morse D, Nichols H, et al: Emergency aortocoronary bypass. Treatment of ventricular tachycardia due to ischemic heart disease. JAMA 216:2138, 1971.

72. Ricks W, Winkle R, Shumway N, et al: Surgical management of life-threatening ventricular arrhythmias in patients with coronary artery disease. Circulation 56:38, 1977.

73. Mundth E, Buckley M, DeSanctis R, et al: Surgical treatment of ventricular irritability. J Thorac Cardiovasc Surg 66:943, 1973.

74. Moran JM, Talano J, Euler D, et al: Refractory ventricular arrhythmia: The role of intraoperative electrophysiological study. Surgery 82:809, 1977.

75. Wittig J, Boineau J: Surgical treatment of ventricular arrhythmias using epicardial, transmural, and endocardial mapping. Ann Thorac Surg, 20:117, 1975.

76. Spurell RA, Sowton E, Deucher DC: Ventricular tachycardia in four patients evaluated by programmed electrical stimulation of heart and treated in two patients by surgical division of anterior radiation of left bundle-branch. Br Heart J 35:1014, 1973.

77. Bolooki H, Vargas A: Myocardial revascularization after acute myocardial infarction. Arch Surg 111:1216, 1976.

78. Schumacher H: Suggestions concerning operative management of postinfarction septal defects. J Thorac Cardiovasc Surg 64:452, 1972.

79. Iben A, Pupello D, Stinson E, et al: Surgical treatment of postinfarction ventricular septal defects. Ann Thorac surg 8:252, 1969.

80. Righetti A, Crawford M, O'Rourke R, et al: Detection of perioperative myocardial damage after coronary artery bypass graft surgery. Circulation 55:173, 1977.

81. Peters R, Brimm J, Utley J: Predicting the need for prolonged ventilatory support in adult cardiac patients. J. Thorac Cardiovasc Surg 77:175, 1979.

82. Engelman R, Gouge T, Smith S, et al: The effect of diuretics on renal hemodynamics during cardiopulmonary bypass. J Surg Res 16:268, 1974.

83. McLeish K, Luft F, Kleft S: Factors effecting prognosis in acute renal failure following cardiac operations. Surg Gynecol Obstet 145:28, 1977.

## SUGGESTED READINGS

Bolooki H (Ed): Clinical Application of Intra-Aortic Balloon Pump. Futura, Mount Kisco, NY, 1977.

Bryson A, Parisi A, Schechter E, Wolfson S: Life-threatening ventricular arrhythmias induced by exercise. Cessation after coronary bypass surgery. Am J Cardiol 32:998, 1973.

Cohn L (Ed): The Treatment of Acute Myocardial Ischemia. An Integrated Medical/Surgical Approach. Future, Mount Kisco, NY, 1979.

Dawson J, Hall R, Hallman G, Cooley D: Mortality in patients undergoing coronary artery bypass surgery after myocardial infarction. Am J Cardiol 33:483, 1974.

Donoso E, Lipski J (Eds): Acute Myocardial Infarction. Vol 4. Stratton Intercontinental Medical Book Corporation, New York, 1978.

Favaloro R, Effler D, Cheanvechai C: Acute coronary insufficiency (impending myocardial infarction and myocardial infarction). Surgical treatment by saphenous vein graft technique. Am J Cardiol, 28:598, 1971.

Gazes P, Mobley E, Faris H, Duncan R, Humphries G: Preinfarction (unstable) angina—A prospective study—ten year follow-up. Circulation 48:331, 1973.

Gunnar R, Loeb H, Rahimtoola S (Eds): Shock in Myocardial Infarction. Grune and Stratton, New York, 1974.

Ludbrook P, Klein M, Mimbs J, Gafford F, Gillespie T, Weldon C, Roberts R: Reduction of perioperative risk in patients with unstable angina exclusion of infarction with CPK isoenzymes. Circulation (suppl II) 51:118, 1975.

Mary DA, Pakrashi BC, Ionescu M: Papillary muscle rupture following myocardial infarction. Thorax 28:390, 1973.

Miller C, Cannon D, Fogarty T, Schroeder J, Daily P, Harrison D: Saphenous vein coronary artery bypass in patients with "preinfarction angina." Circulation 47:234, 1973.

Nuutinen L, Hollmén A: The effect of prophylactic use of furosemide on renal function during open heart surgery. Ann Chir Gynaecol 65:258, 1976.

Rahimtoola S (Ed): Coronary Bypass Surgery. FA Davis, Philadelphia, 1977.

Sobel B: Coronary revascularization during evolving myocardial infarction—the need for caution. Circulation 50:867, 1974.

Tilkian A, Pfeifer J, Barry W, Lipton M, Hultgren H: The effect of coronary bypass surgery on exercise-induced ventricular arrhythmias. Am Heart J 92:707, 1976.

Webb W, Parker F, Neville J, Hanson L: Acute mechanical complications of coronary arterial disease. Surgical correction. Arch Surg 1109:251, 1974.

Willerson J, Curry G, Watson J, Leshin S, Ecker R, Mullins C, Platt M, Sugg WL: Intraaortic balloon counterpulsation in patients in cardiogenic shock, medically refractory left ventricular failure and/or recurrent ventricular tachycardia. Am J Med 58:183, 1975.

Vlodaver Z, Edwards J: Rupture of ventricular septum or papillary muscle complicating myocardial infarction. Circulation 55:815, 1977

# 40 | *Drug Interactions*

*Roy V. Ditchey, M.D.*
*Robert T. Weibert, Pharm.D.*

Multiple-drug therapy is a common and often necessary part of the management of patients with cardiovascular disease. The median number of drugs administered to cardiac patients on an acute medical service is 12, with nearly all patients receiving five or more drugs.[1] This stems both from the treatment of coexistent medical problems and from attempts to increase beneficial or decrease untoward effects in comparison to single-drug therapy.

Two or more drugs given concurrently may act independently, interact in such a way as to alter the expected effect of one or both drugs, or lead to new or unexpected reactions. Many drug interactions in a coronary care unit are planned to increase the effectiveness of pharmacotherapy or minimize the adverse effects of a necessary drug. For example, the combined use of a positive inotropic agent and a vasodilator may be more efficacious in the treatment of a patient with low cardiac output than either drug alone; likewise, the use of two antidysrhythmic agents in moderate doses may allow effective dysrhythmia control without causing the side effects seen with higher doses of single agents. These useful drug interactions are an important part of cardiovascular therapeutics and can generally be anticipated from a knowledge of the major pharmacologic effects of the individual agents involved. Such predictable interactions will not be considered further in this section.

Unfortunately, adverse drug interactions are also common and may be responsible for an inadequate therapeutic response or unexpected toxicity. The incidence of adverse drug reactions increases with both the number of concurrently administered drugs and the severity of the underlying illness.[2] Thus, the critical-care physician and nurse must be familiar with potential drug interactions, as well as the pharmacology and toxicity of individual agents.

Although the number of theoretically possible drug interactions is large, many are of little clinical significance. Furthermore, drugs that interact adversely can often be used safely together if dosages are adjusted appropriately. Safe and effective multiple-drug therapy depends on an understanding of the general mechanisms of drug interaction and an awareness of interactions of proven clinical importance.

## MECHANISMS OF DRUG INTERACTIONS

The ultimate pharmacologic effect of any drug depends on many factors, including dosage, absorption, metabolism, excretion, albumin and tissue binding, transport to the site of drug action, receptor binding, and tissue sensitivity.[1] Drug interactions may alter any of these variables, and many cardiovascular drugs interact with other agents by more than one mechanism. Potential sites of interaction are shown schematically in Fig. 40.1.

Most cardiovascular drugs are weak acids

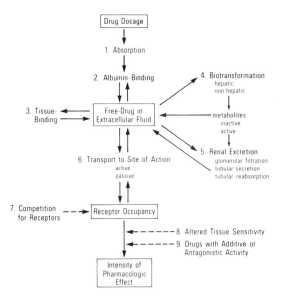

Fig. 40.1 Potential sites for drug interactions. (Modified with permission from Koch-Weser J: Drug interations in cardiovascular therapy. Am Heart J 90:93, 1975.)

or bases, absorbed primarily in the nonionized state. Drugs that change gastrointestinal pH can affect the subsequent absorption of many other agents, as can drug-induced alterations in mucosal function or intraluminal physicochemical binding. Drugs that alter gastrointestinal perfusion or mucosal edema in patients with decreased cardiac output and congestive heart failure may similarly affect the bioavailability of other orally-administered medications. Incompletely absorbed drugs are particularly susceptible to changes in rate and completeness of gastrointestinal absorption, and additional factors such as the time relationship between doses may further alter the nature of any observed interaction. Although parenterally administered medications are often assumed to be fully absorbed, the rate of absorption of intramuscularly or subcutaneously administered drugs may be significantly altered by agents that influence local tissue perfusion.

Many cardiovascular drugs are highly protein bound and may demonstrate altered activity because they have been displaced from their albumin-binding sites by other drugs. Protein displacement leads to a transient rise in the serum concentration of free drug, increasing the drug's availability for pharmacologic action, as well as its metabolism and excretion. However, within 1 to 2 weeks a new steady state is reached in which total and protein-bound drug concentrations are decreased and free drug concentration is unchanged. Therefore, the clinical importance of displacement interactions is limited to highly bound drugs in which a transient increase in the availability of free drug is capable of producing serious toxicity. The coumarin anticoagulants are the drugs most commonly involved in significant protein-displacement interactions.

Similar competition between two or more drugs for tissue-binding sites may also occur. The clinical significance of this type of adverse interaction is less well established, although preliminary evidence suggests that this may be an important factor in a recently recognized interaction between digoxin and quinidine.

Many drugs are transformed by hepatic microsomal enzymes into more readily excretable metabolites. Such products may be pharmacologically inactive, fully active, or even more active than the parent compound. A drug's ultimate effect can thus be readily influenced by interactions that alter its rate of metabolic degradation. One drug may induce enzymes that accelerate the metabolism of another, lowering its serum concentration and diminishing its pharmacologic effects. Conversely, discontinuing such a drug could lead to decreased enzymatic activity, slowed biotransformation, increased serum concentration, and, possibly, even toxic effects. Similar interactions may occur as a result of competition for the same microsomal enzyme system or even direct enzyme inhibition.

In patients with congestive heart failure, drugs that improve cardiac output and hepatic blood flow may indirectly affect the metabolism of other drugs that depend on delivery to hepatic microsomes for their subsequent degradation. Similarly, hemodynamic interventions may influence the fate of drugs primarily dependent on renal excretion for their elimination. Diminished renal blood flow and glomerular filtration rate significantly impair renal clearance of a wide variety of cardiovascular drugs eliminated by this mechanism.

Other determinants of renal drug excretion may also be subject to pharmacologic alterations. Drugs that change the pH of urine can importantly alter the passive reabsorption of weakly acidic or basic cardiovascular drugs. Osmotic or natriuretic diuresis, by increasing urine volume, may lower the intraluminal concentration of a variety of agents and thereby decrease their passive reabsorption. Alternatively, drugs that are actively secreted or reabsorbed may compete with other drugs for renal tubular transport systems.

Delivery of a drug to its ultimate site of action may be further influenced by other drugs that inhibit or compete with membrane transport systems, or alter factors that affect passive diffusion (such as intracellular or extracellular pH). Further competition for final receptor sites, interference with secondary compounds that act as mediators of a drug's effect, and altered tissue sensitivity are other important means of interaction capable of altering a given drug's ultimate pharmacologic effect.

In summary, although the major pharmacologic actions of cardiovascular drugs are predictable, many of these drugs also have additional, less specific effects that can lead to unexpected interactions. These are commonly indirect effects that alter the pharmacokinetics of absorption, distribution, metabolism, tissue interaction, or excretion. A working knowledge of clinically important interactions of this type is essential to the safe and effective use of multiple-drug therapy. The remainder of this chapter will focus on important interactions involving drugs commonly used in cardiac patients.

## INTERACTIONS INVOLVING PRIMARY CARDIOVASCULAR DRUGS

### Digitalis

The digitalis glycosides are among the most widely used of all cardiovascular drugs. Unfortunately, their therapeutic index is small and digitalis toxicity is common. A variety of other agents compound this clinical problem by altering either the pharmacokinetics of the various digitalis preparations or myocardial sensitivity to their effects.

The pharmacokinetics and metabolic fate of the major cardiac glycosides differ considerably. Digitoxin is a nonpolar molecule, which is well absorbed, highly protein bound, and dependent on hepatic metabolism for biotransformation into inactive metabolites. Digoxin, on the other hand, is a polar molecule that is incompletely absorbed, less highly protein bound, and dependent on renal excretion for its elimination, either unchanged or as an active metabolite. These essential differences allow for the variable susceptibility of these agents to interactions with other drugs.

The bioavailability of oral digoxin can be influenced by a variety of other agents. Anticholinergic drugs, which slow gastrointestinal motility (e.g., propantheline), have been shown to increase the absorption of digoxin by allowing greater time for its dissolution and contact with the intestinal mucosa.[3] However, these effects may be important only when tablets with a substandard dissolution rate are used.[4] The usual brief duration of therapy with potent anticholinergic agents (e.g., atropine) in the coronary care unit further limits the clinical significance of this interaction; and, although minor anticholinergic effects are a common attribute of a variety of cardiovascular and other drugs, clinically important potentiation of digoxin absorption by these agents has not been demonstrated. Similarly, although cathartics may potentially reduce digoxin absorption by decreasing intestinal transit time, any clinical importance of this effect due to laxatives in common use remains to be established.

A variety of antacids and antidiarrheal agents have been shown to significantly reduce the absorption of oral digoxin by mechanisms that have not been fully established. Although high degrees of physical adsorption of digoxin to magnesium trisilicate and kaolin-pectin have been demonstrated, only modest adsorption to magnesium and aluminum hydroxide occurs.[5] Furthermore, these agents have variable effects on intestinal transit time. Yet quantitatively similar interference with digoxin absorption has been observed with all four preparations.[5] These effects can be minimized by administering digoxin at least 1 hour prior to any of the other agents.

Activated charcoal, cholestyramine, and colestipol are capable of intraluminal binding with digoxin and may significantly alter its absorption.[6,7] However, the extent of these interactions depends on factors such as relative dosages and dosage intervals. For example, cholestyramine decreases peak and steady state serum glycoside levels when given concomitantly with oral digoxin, with higher doses causing greater effects. The same doses given 8 hours before or after digoxin, however, do not change glycoside pharmacokinetics significantly from the control.[6] A similar interaction occurs between cholestyramine and digitoxin, causing important interference with both primary absorption and enterohepatic circulation.[8] Because digitoxin is completely absorbed under normal conditions, other drugs that reduce digoxin absorption generally have little effect on digitoxin bioavailability.

Neomycin inhibits both the rate and extent of digoxin absorption.[9] These effects are not due to intraluminal binding, although the precise mechanism of interaction is uncertain. Acute interference with cell membrane function and more profound mucosal injury with prolonged usage have been postulated.[9] Similarly, both p-aminosalicyclic acid and sulfasalazine have been observed to cause clinically significant interference with digoxin absorption, and altered mucosal function has again been postulated.[6,10] Chronic phenytoin administration has also been shown to reduce serum levels of digoxin without altering its half-life.[11] The basis for this interaction has not been firmly established, although the presumed mechanism involves impaired digoxin absorption.

A variety of drugs are capable of competing with cardiac glycosides for protein-binding sites, depending on their concentrations and relative affinities for serum albumin. Of these, phenylbutazone and its derivatives are the most important. Still others may alter glycoside protein binding indirectly. For example, heparin induces the release of free fatty acids, which in turn cause displacement of digitoxin and digoxin from albumin-binding sites.[12] However, digoxin is not highly protein bound, and the

distribution of digitoxin is such that only 6 to 7 percent of the drug is present in the serum; thus, although highly protein bound, displaced digitoxin must equilibrate with large total body stores, causing little change in tissue concentration. Ultimately, displacement of either digoxin or digitoxin from serum albumin by other drugs is of little clinical significance.

In contrast, a potentially important adverse interaction between digoxin and quinidine has recently been described.[13-15] The addition of quinidine therapy in patients on maintenance doses of digoxin has been shown to significantly elevate serum digoxin levels in most patients. Initial observations suggest that the incidence of clinical digitalis toxicity resulting from this interaction may be very high.[13] Although the mechanism of this effect has not been firmly established, quinidine has been shown to reduce the number of digitalis-binding sites on cell membranes.[16] This finding and the results of limited kinetic studies suggest that the observed rise in serum digoxin concentration results from displacement of digoxin from tissue-binding sites by quinidine.

Although digoxin is primarily excreted unchanged in the urine, digitoxin is largely dependent upon hepatic metabolism for inactivation; a number of drugs may, therefore, significantly alter digitoxin pharmacokinetics by interfering with this process of biotransformation. Concurrent therapy with phenylbutazone, phenytoin, spironolactone, or phenobarbital results in a marked decrease in serum digitoxin concentration.[8,17] Although phenobarbital also increases the formation of relatively polar metabolites of digitoxin (including active compounds such as digoxin), the overall effect is a decrease in steady state glycoside activity. A variety of other drugs (including antihistamines, oral hypoglycemics, and uricosuric agents) are also known to induce hepatic enzymes which increase their own metabolism as well as that of other drugs. Although such an effect on digitoxin metabolism has not been demonstrated with these agents, the possibility of this type of interaction should be considered when known enzyme-inducing drugs are given to patients receiving maintenance digitoxin.

Digoxin is predominantly eliminated through

the kidneys. This is accomplished equally by glomerular filtration and tubular secretion,[18] and any alteration of either of these mechanisms may potentially interfere with digoxin excretion. Spironolactone (and probably triamterene) inhibit digoxin secretion, leading to diminished digoxin clearance.[18] Spironolactone also cross-reacts with antibodies used in some digoxin radioimmunoassays,[19,20] so that interpretation of serum digoxin concentrations may be difficult when large doses of spironolactone are given concurrently. Hypokalemia also decreases digoxin clearance,[21] an effect that may contribute to the risk of digitalis toxicity in this setting. In the absence of hypokalemia, other more proximally-active diuretics, such as furosemide, do not alter digoxin clearance, even when glomerular filtration rate is reduced.[22-25] This probably reflects a concomitant redistribution of renal blood flow and an increase in digoxin secretion.[24]

Since the cardiac glycosides depend on hepatic biotransformation and renal excretion for their elimination, drugs that alter hepatic or renal blood flow may significantly influence effective digitalis levels. Pharmacologic interventions that improve hepatic congestion and cardiac output in hemodynamically compromised patients can reasonably be expected to increase glycoside clearance. Although the clinical importance of these effects has not been firmly established, a variety of positive inotropic and vasodilating agents in common use can dramatically alter cardiac output and distribution of blood flow. The potential effects of these alterations on digitalis pharmacokinetics should be anticipated and serum glycoside levels used to guide adjustments in dosage.

The association between hypokalemia and digitalis toxicity is well known. Digitalis acts by inhibiting membrane Na-K-ATPase, an effect potentiated by potassium depletion; diuretic-induced changes in potassium balance are undoubtedly the most important drug interaction involving digitalis. This relationship is widely appreciated, and close attention to serum potassium levels during digitalis therapy is standard practice. However, considerable total body potassium depletion can occur in the absence of overt hypokalemia [26] and may contrib-

ute to digitalis-induced dysrhythmias.[27] Although technically difficult to document, this possibility must be considered whenever digitalis toxicity occurs during diuretic therapy. Furthermore, potassium itself may interact adversely with digitalis under certain circumstances. By further impairing atrioventricular conduction, potassium replacement in digitalis-toxic patients may lead to high-grade atrioventricular block. This is an important consideration in the management of digitalis toxicity.

Although potassium is the foremost electrolyte influencing myocardial sensitivity to the cardiac glycosides, changes in serum magnesium and calcium may occasionally be of clinical importance as well. Hypomagnesemia potentiates digitalis inhibition of membrane Na-K-ATPase and may contribute to the development of digitalis toxicity. Diuretic therapy is an important cause of hypomagnesemia, although routine magnesium replacement is not necessary. This type of interaction should be considered and serum magnesium concentration determined in patients with evidence of digitalis excess. Hypercalcemia increases and hypocalcemia decreases the effect of digitalis on the heart. Although adverse drug interactions with digitalis due to altered serum calcium concentration have not been described, calcium-chelating agents, such as ethylenediamine tetraacetic acid (EDTA), have been used experimentally to transiently reverse digitalis toxicity.[28]

The cardiac effects of digitalis can also be potentiated by depolarizing muscle relaxants. Major conduction abnormalities and dysrhythmias, including ventricular tachycardia and fibrillation, have been observed following administration of succinylcholine to fully digitalized patients and experimental animals.[29,30] Furthermore, immediate improvement has been demonstrated following the subsequent administration of d-tubocurare.[29] Nondepolarizing muscle relaxants (such as d-tubocurare) compete with both acetycholine and succinylocholine for receptor sites at myoneural junctions and, possibly, in other tissues as well. It is of further interest that digitalis, acetylcholine, and succinylcholine all lead to a decrease in intramyocardial potassium concentration. However, the

**Table 40.1  Drug Interactions Involving Digitalis Glycosides**

| Drug Interaction | Effect | Mechanism | Clinical Significance | Comments |
|---|---|---|---|---|
| Digitalis with: | | | | |
| Antacids (magnesium hydroxide, magnesium trisilicate, aluminum hydroxide) | Decreased serum digoxin level | Decreased absorption of digoxin by uncertain mechanisms | Moderate | No known effect on digitoxin absorption |
| Barbiturates | Decreased serum digitoxin level | Accelerated hepatic biotransformation | Moderate | Important only during chronic barbiturate therapy; no effect on digoxin elimination |
| Bretylium | Aggravation of dysrhythmias due to digitalis toxicity | Initial catecholamine release by bretylium | Major | Alternative antiarrhythmic agents should be used in treatment of digitalis toxicity |
| Cholestyramine | Decreased serum digoxin and digitoxin levels | Decreased absorption due to intraluminal physicochemical binding | Major | Minimized by separating administration by several hours |
| Ethacrynic acid | Increased tissue sensitivity to digitalis | Potassium and magnesium depletion potentiates inhibition of Na-K-ATPase | Major | May have total body potassium deficit with normal serum potassium |
| Furosemide | Increased tissue sensitivity to digitalis | Potassium and magnesium depletion potentiates inhibition of Na-K-ATPase | Major | May have total body potassium deficit with normal serum potassium |
| Kaolin-pectin | Decreased serum digoxin level | Decreased absorption of digoxin by uncertain mechanisms | Moderate | No known effect on digitoxin absorption |
| Phenylbutazone | Decreased serum digitoxin level | Accelerated hepatic biotransformation | Moderate | Important only during chronic phenylbutazone therapy; no effect on digoxin elimination |

**Table 40.1** (Continued)

| Drug Interaction | Effect | Mechanism | Clinical Significance | Comments |
|---|---|---|---|---|
| Phenytoin | Decreased serum digoxin and digitoxin levels | Decreased absorption of digoxin by uncertain mechanisms; accelerated hepatic biotransformation of digitoxin | Moderate | Important only during chronic phenytoin therapy |
| Quinidine | Increased serum digoxin levels | Displacement from tissue binding sites; other mechanisms may also be involved | Probably major | Only recently described; effect on serum digitoxin concentration has not yet been established |
| Reserpine | Possible potentiation of digitalis toxicity | Unknown | Unestablished | Isolated case reports only |
| Spironolactone | Increased serum digoxin level; decreased serum digitoxin level | Impaired renal tubular secretion of digoxin; accelerated hepatic biotransformation of digitoxin | Moderate | May also interfere with digoxin radioimmunoassay |
| Succinylcholine | Apparent increased tissue sensitivity to digitalis | Unknown | Unestablished | May cause arrhythmias during anesthesia induction (incidence unknown); reversible with d-tubocurare |
| Thiazide diuretics | Increased tissue sensitivity to digitalis | Potassium and magnesium depletion potentiates inhibition of Na-K-ATPase | Major | May have total body potassium deficit with normal serum potassium |
| Triamterene | Increased serum digoxin level | Impaired renal tubular secretion of digoxin | Unestablished | Similar to spironolactone experimentally; no known effects on digitoxin metabolism |

precise mechanism of interaction of these drugs has not been established.

Hyperthyroidism is known to impair the clinical effectiveness of digitalis preparations. Although attempts to investigate the mechanism by which this occurs have yielded conflicting and inconclusive results, return to a euthyroid state could potentially precipitate digitalis toxicity if dosages were not adjusted appropriately. The possibility of this type of interaction should be anticipated when antithyroid drugs are given to hyperthyroid patients receiving large doses of any digitalis preparation.

Finally, reserpine has been reported to potentiate digitalis toxicity by an unknown mechanism, not entirely due to initial catecholamine release.[31,32] Although the importance and nature of this interaction have not been firmly established, some caution is probably warranted if reserpine therapy is to be instituted in a digitalized patient.

Clinically important drug interactions involving digitalis are summarized in Table 40.1. Since the magnitude of most such interactions cannot be reliably predicted, serum glycoside levels should be used to guide adjustments in digitalis dosage whenever therapy with any drug capable of altering glycoside pharmacokinetics is initiated. Additional caution is warranted when drugs that alter myocardial sensitivity to digitalis are employed.

## Antiarrhythmic Agents

Antiarrhythmic drugs are often used in combination for the treatment of serious ventricular arrhythmias. This approach frequently produces greater therapeutic and fewer adverse effects than higher doses of single agents. However, electrophysiologic interactions are complex and combined antiarrhythmic activity is not always predictable. Furthermore, certain toxic effects may be fully additive. Knowledge of the pharmacology and toxicity of individual agents, and careful attention to serum drug concentrations and clinical parameters are, therefore, essential to the successful use of combination antiarrhythmic therapy. This problem has been discussed more thoroughly in previous chapters, and the potential adverse effects of such planned interactions will be mentioned here only briefly; interactions between antidysrhythmic agents and other types of drugs will be discussed in more detail.

**Lidocaine.** Lidocaine is generally administered intravenously and depends on hepatic biotransformation for its inactivation. Drugs that induce hepatic microsomal enzymes (e.g., phenobarbital and others), may accelerate the metabolism of lidocaine and lower its effective serum concentration.[33] Lidocaine pharmacokinetics can also be importantly influenced by drug interventions that alter cardiac output and hepatic blood flow. The volume of distribution of lidocaine is decreased in congestive heart failure and its rate of clearance is reduced when hepatic blood flow falls. Drugs that increase or decrease hepatic perfusion may thus cause similar directional changes in lidocaine clearance and inversely affect serum drug levels.[34,35] These effects should be anticipated, and serum lidocaine concentrations used to guide therapy in severely compromised patients, particularly when hemodynamic parameters are altered by positive inotropic or vasodilating drugs. Serum lidocaine concentrations are also useful when enzyme-inducing drugs are used concomitantly.

Lidocaine and other local anesthetic agents are capable of potentiating the effects of both depolarizing and nondepolarizing muscle relaxants,[36,37] although doses required are generally at or above the upper limit of those used clinically. The mechanism of these interactions is uncertain, although both direct effects on the myoneural junction and the freeing of succinylcholine or d-tubocurare from protein-binding sites have been postulated.[36,37] The combined use of these agents in usual doses is generally safe, although the possibility of more intense and prolonged muscle relaxation must be anticipated.

**Quinidine.** Concomitantly administered antacids decrease the rate but not the extent of oral quinidine absorption. This effect is therefore of no importance during chronic quinidine therapy. Likewise, although drugs that alter hepatic microsomal enzyme activity may influence the kinetics of quinidine degradation, these effects are rarely clinically important. Furthermore, drug elimination is grossly normal in patients with chronic congestive heart failure,[38] and altered pharmacokinetics in patients with more acutely compromised cardiac output and hepatic blood flow are of no proven clinical significance.

Under certain circumstances, however, drug interactions can cause appreciable changes in serum quinidine concentrations. Although inactivation by hepatic biotransformation is of primary importance in determining the intensity and duration of its effects, quinidine also depends, to some extent, on renal excretion for its elimination. Quinidine is a weak base, and the combined use of drugs that increase urinary pH, such as sodium bicarbonate and acetazolamide, can lead to significantly elevated serum quinidine concentrations.[39] Drugs that decrease urinary pH have opposite effects. These interactions are less important than with procainamide, however, because of the smaller proportion of unchanged drug normally excreted in the urine. It has been suggested that magnesium-containing antacids may cause similar effects through secondary changes in urinary pH;[40] the clinical significance of these changes, however, has not been determined.

A potentially important interaction between digoxin and quinidine was discussed previously along with other digitalis-related drug interactions. Although this combination may significantly elevate serum glycoside levels, no unexpected changes in either quinidine concentration or pharmacologic action have been observed.

Procainamide and disopyramide both have electrophysiologic effects very similar to those of quinidine. Combined therapy with these agents is, therefore, of limited usefulness and may lead to serious depression of intraventricular conduction or contractile function. Combinations of these drugs can occasionally be used, however, to eliminate noncardiac side effects encountered with higher doses of a single agent. Careful monitoring of QRS complex duration and other parameters of myocardial toxicity are mandatory in this situation.

Phenothiazines, butyrophenones, and tricyclic antidepressants likewise have many electrophysiologic properties in common with quinidine. These drugs should, therefore, be used with caution in patients taking quinidine because of potentially additive cardiotoxicity. Furthermore, dysrhythmias resulting from overdosage with these agents should be treated with antidysrhythmics other than quinidine and related compounds.

Myocardial sensitivity to quinidine may be influenced by serum potassium levels. Hypokalemia reduces, and hyperkalemia potentiates, many of the electrophysiologic effects of quinidine.[41] However, the importance of this interaction over the range of serum potassium levels generally encountered clinically has not been firmly established.

Theoretically, the vagolytic properties of quinidine could have additive effects with other anticholinergic drugs. Of greater clinical importance is the fact that quinidine antagonizes the effects of cholinergic agents. The usual doses of drugs such as edrophonium may, therefore, be ineffective in the treatment of supraventricular tachycardia in patients receiving quinidine. Furthermore, quinidine may compromise the effects of neostigmine, edrophonium, and other cholinergic agents in the treatment of myasthenia gravis.

Quinidine also potentiates the neuromuscular blockade of both depolarizing and nondepolarizing muscle relaxants.[42,43] The mechanism by which this occurs is uncertain, although a combination of a curare-like action, cholinesterase inhibition, and direct muscle membrane depression have all been postulated. This potentiation appears to be greater than that observed with lidocaine and other antidysrhythmic agents, and the possibility of both increased and prolonged neuromuscular blockade should be anticipated when these drugs are used in combination.

Finally, quinidine may increase the hypoprothrombinemic effects of oral anticoagulants. Excessive prolongation of the prothrombin time and associated hemorrhage have been observed 6 to 10 days following the addition of quinidine therapy in patients chronically anticoagulated with warfarin.[44] Such potentiation does not occur in the majority of patients treated with both drugs, however,[45] and the precise incidence of significant interaction is unknown.

**Procainamide.** Procainamide is a weak base, and approximately 50 to 60 percent of an administered dose is excreted unchanged by the kidneys.[46,47] Drugs that increase urinary pH, such as sodium bicarbonate and acetazolamide, interfere with procainamide excretion and can lead to elevated serum drug levels.[46] Acidification of the urine has opposite effects.

The major active metabolite of procainamide, N-acetylprocainamide (NAPA), is dependent almost entirely on renal excretion for its elimination.[48] The antidysrhythmic activity of this compound contributes considerably to the effectiveness of a given dose of procainamide,[49,50] and alterations in its rate of formation and elimination are likely to be of clinical importance. However, drug interactions affecting the generation and pharmacokinetics of N-acetylprocainamide have not been described. Similarly, although drugs that alter cardiac output and renal blood flow would be expected to appreciably influence the clearance of both procainamide and its metabolites, the clinical importance of these effects has not been determined.

As discussed previously, procainamide, quinidine, and disopyramide may cause additive cardiac toxicity. These drugs also have similar anticholinergic effects and may interact with other anticholinergic or cholinergic agents. However, clinically important interactions of this type are unusual with procainamide.

Finally, very high doses of procainamide may potentiate the effects of depolarizing and nondepolarizing muscle relaxants in experimental animals.[36,42] The clinical significance of these interactions is unknown.

**Phenytoin.** Phenytoin is metabolized by the liver and is affected by a variety of interactions which either potentiate or inhibit hepatic microsomal enzymes. Phenobarbital, diazoxide, and alcohol are all capable of enzyme induction, which accelerates phenytoin degradation.[51-53] Phenothiazines, phenylbutazone, isoniazid, dicumarol, chlordiazepoxide, diazepam, and several other drugs inhibit phenytoin biotransformation, thereby increasing serum drug levels and pharmacologic activity.[54-58] These effects are of clinical importance only during long-term antidysrhythmic therapy; under these circumstances, however, serum phenytoin concentrations must be followed carefully whenever any of these agents are added or withdrawn.

Conversely, phenytoin accelerates glucocorticoid degradation and may cause a loss of steroid effect.[59-61] Phenytoin also alters dicumarol pharmacokinetics due to accelerated metabolism as well as displacement from serum albumin.[62] The magnitude of these effects is difficult to predict, and any change in drug regimen should be followed closely with serial prothrombin time determinations.

Phenytoin is highly protein bound and may be partially displaced by a variety of other drugs. Since displacement only leads to a transient increase in free drug concentration, these interactions are generally not of clinical significance. However, phenytoin toxicity may be aggravated by such displacement, and drugs capable of this type of interaction (e.g., phenylbutazone and salicylates) should be avoided in patients with high serum phenytoin concentrations. In addition, phenytoin may itself displace other drugs from protein-binding sites and potentiate their pharmacologic effects. For example, phenytoin displaces thyroid hormone from its carrier protein and leads to increased free thyroxine levels.[63] Although normal individuals compensate for this effect by decreasing thyroxine synthesis, this homeostatic mechanism is lacking in athyrotic patients receiving replacement therapy. It has been suggested that phenytoin administration in such patients may precipitate signs of thyroxine excess, including cardiac dysrhythmias, although the clinical importance of this interaction remains unproven.[64]

**Propranolol.** Most of the beneficial and adverse effects of propranolol can be anticipated from a knowledge of its $\beta$-adrenergic blocking activity. For example, its pharmacologic effects are directly antagonistic to the actions of bronchodilating agents, and its ability to aggravate bronchospasm in patients with obstructive lung disease is well known.

Propranolol may also interact with insulin and the oral hypoglycemic agents by interfering with the usual sympathetic response to drug-induced hypoglycemia. $\beta$-adrenergic blockade reduces both glycogenolysis and the peripheral warning signs related to catecholamine excess.[65,66] Such effects may rarely lead to severe and unsuspected hypoglycemia in affected patients.

Chlorpromazine interferes with hepatic biotransformation of propranolol, and may lead to increased serum drug concentration and enhanced $\beta$-adrenergic blocking activity in some patients.[67] Orally administered propranolol, which is highly extracted by the liver, is particularly susceptible to this effect. Reported changes in propranolol clearance following intravenous administration have not been significant.[67]

Methyldopa therapy results in the accumulation of $\alpha$-methylnorepinephrine in sympathetic nerve endings. This compound has vasodilating effects in contrast to norepinephrine and is accordingly a less potent pressor agent. However, it has been suggested than propranolol may increase the pressor action of $\alpha$-methylnorepinephrine by inhibiting its $\beta$-adrenergic (vasodilating) effects and leading to unopposed $\alpha$-adrenergic stimulation. This interaction has been demonstrated experimentally in animals, although limited clinical studies have yielded conflicting results.[68] Since these drugs have been used successfully together in the treatment of hypertension, the clinical importance of this interaction would appear to be minor.

As with other antidysrhythmic agents mentioned previously, propranolol may potentiate the effects of both depolarizing and nondepolarizing muscle relaxants.[36,69] Although prolonged postoperative curarization has been reported in two thyrotoxic patients treated with this drug,[70] experimentally demonstrable interaction has generally required intravenous doses of propranolol greatly exceeding those used clinically.[36] The ultimate importance of this interaction remains to be determined.

**Atropine.** Potential drug interactions involving atropine can be anticipated from an appreciation of its potent anticholinergic effects. In practice, the usual brief duration of therapy with this agent makes such theoretical interactions clinically unimportant.

**Other Antidysrhythmic Agents.** The similar electrophysiologic effects and additive cardiac toxicity of disopyramide, quinidine, and procainamide have been referred to previously. Depression of myocardial contracility is particularly prominent with disopyramide, and caution is advisable when other negative inotropic agents, such as propranolol, are used concurrently. Anticholinergic effects are likewise prominent, and significant interaction with both anticholinergic and cholinergic drugs (similar to those described for quinidine and procainamide) are likely to occur. Clinical reports of such effects, however, have not yet appeared.

Bretylium, tocainide, mexiletine, aprindine, verapamil, and other new or experimental antidysrhythmic agents are likely to achieve more widespread use in the future. Although some cardiac interactions between these drugs are known (e.g., bretylium causes initial catecholamine release, which may aggravate digitalis-induced dysrhythmias),[71] or readily predictable (e.g., additive negative inotropic effects of verapamil and propranolol), clinical experience with these drugs in the United States is limited. Important interactions between these agents and noncardiac drugs are likely to be discovered, and multiple-drug therapy with any of these agents should be undertaken with appropriate caution.

Drug interactions involving antidysrhythmic agents are summarized in Table 40.2.

### Adrenergic Agents

Sympathomimetic drugs may act directly at adrenergic receptor sites located on the cell membrane (e.g., epinephrine, norepinephrine, isoproterenol, phenylephrine, dopamine, and dobutamine); indirectly by causing norepinephrine release from sympathetic nerve endings (e.g., amphetamine, tyramine); or have both direct and indirect actions (e.g., ephedrine, metaraminol). Direct-acting drugs further vary in the relative extent to which they stimulate $\alpha$- and $\beta$-adrenergic receptors. Isoproterenol is a pure $\beta$-agonist, while phenylephrine acts primarily on $\alpha$-adrenergic sites. Norepinephrine, epinephrine and dopamine all have $\alpha$- and $\beta$-adrenergic effects in differing ratios, while dopamine also acts on specific (dopaminergic) receptors. Recently, noncardiac ($\beta_2$) $\beta$-agonists have been developed (e.g., terbutaline, salbutamol, and metaproterenol), which stimulate $\beta$-recep-

**Table 40.2  Drug Interactions Involving Antidysrhythmic Agents**

| Drug Interaction | Effect | Mechanism | Clinical Significance | Comments |
|---|---|---|---|---|
| Bretylium with: | | | | |
| Digitalis | Aggravation of dysrhythmias due to digitalis toxicity | Initial catecholamine release by bretylium | Major | Alternative antidysrhythmic agents should be used in the treatment of digitalis toxicity |
| Disopyramide with: | | | | |
| Phenothiazines (and butyrophenones) | Additive cardiac toxicity | Similar electrophysiologic effects | Unestablished (probably major) | Dysrhythmias due to toxic doses of these agents should not be treated with disopyramide |
| Tricyclic Antidepressants | Additive cardiac toxicity | Similar electrophysiologic effects | Unestablished (probably major) | Dysrhythmias due to toxic doses of these agents should not be treated with disopyramide |
| Edrophonium (and other cholinergic agents) | Impaired cholinergic action | Intrinsic anticholinergic effect | Unestablished | Potentially important in patients with myasthenia gravis |
| Lidocaine with: | | | | |
| Barbiturates | Decreased serum lidocaine level | Accelerated hepatic biotransformation | Unestablished | Theoretically important during chronic barbiturate therapy; other enzyme-inducing drugs may have similar effects |
| Adrenergic agents | Altered serum lidocaine level | Altered lidocaine distribution and rate of biotransformation due to changes in cardiac output and hepatic blood flow | Unestablished | Theoretically important; clinical information is limited |
| Succinylcholine | More intense and prolonged muscle relaxation | Unknown | Minor | No problem with usual doses of lidocaine; other depolarizing muscle relaxants are similarly affected |
| d-Tubocurare | More intense and prolonged muscle relaxation | Unknown | Minor | No problem with usual doses of lidocaine; other nondepolarizing muscle relaxants are similarly affected |
| Vasodilating agents | Altered serum lidocaine level | Altered lidocaine distribution and rate of biotransformation due to changes in cardiac output and hepatic blood flow | Unestablished | Theoretically important; clinical information is limited |

**Table 40.2** (Continued)

| Drug Interaction | Effect | Mechanism | Clinical Significance | Comments |
|---|---|---|---|---|
| **Phenytoin with:** | | | | |
| Alcohol | Decreased serum phenytoin level | Accelerated hepatic biotransformation | Major | Important only during chronic phenytoin therapy |
| Barbiturates | Decreased serum phenytoin level | Accelerated hepatic biotransformation | Major | Important only during chronic phenytoin therapy |
| Chlordiazepoxide | Increased serum phenytoin level | Impaired hepatic biotransformation | Major | Important only during chronic phenytoin therapy |
| Diazepam | Increased serum phenytoin level | Impaired hepatic biotransformation | Major | Important only during chronic phenytoin therapy |
| Dicumarol | Increased serum phenytoin level | Impaired hepatic biotransformation | Major | Important only during chronic phenytoin therapy; phenytoin may also displace dicumarol from serum proteins and accelerate dicumarol biotransformation |
| Digitoxin | Decreased serum digitoxin level | Accelerated hepatic biotransformation of digitoxin | Moderate | Important only during chronic phenytoin therapy |
| Diazoxide | Decreased serum phenytoin level | Accelerated hepatic biotransformation | Major | Important only during chronic phenytoin therapy |
| Isoniazid | Increased serum phenytoin level | Impaired hepatic biotransformation | Major | Important only during chronic phenytoin therapy |
| Phenothiazines | Increased serum phenytoin level | Impaired hepatic biotransformation | Major | Important only during chronic phenytoin therapy |
| Phenylbutazone | Increased serum phenytoin level | Impaired hepatic biotransformation | Major | Important only during chronic phenytoin therapy |
| **Procainamide with:** | | | | |
| Acetazolamide (and sodium bicarbonate) | Increased serum procainamide level | Decreased renal excretion due to increased urinary pH | Major | N-acetylprocainamide (NAPA) similarly affected; urinary acidification has opposite effects |
| Phenothiazines (and butyrophenones) | Additive cardiac toxicity | Similar electrophysiologic effects | Major | Dysrhythmias due to toxic doses of these agents should not be treated with procainamide |
| Tricyclic antidepressants | Additive cardiac toxicity | Similar electrophysiologic effects | Major | Dysrhythmias due to toxic doses of these agents should not be treated with procainamide |

**Table 40.2 (Continued)**

| Drug Interaction | Effect | Mechanism | Clinical Significance | Comments |
|---|---|---|---|---|
| Propranolol with: | | | | |
| Chlorpromazine | Increased serum propranolol levels | Impaired hepatic biotransformation | Moderate | Important only with oral propranolol (no change in IV propranolol clearance); effects of other phenothiazines are unknown |
| Insulin | Impaired response to hypoglycemia | Reduced glycogenolysis and peripheral warning signs related to catecholamine excess | Major | |
| Methyldopa | Decreased hypotensive effect | Unknown; unopposed α-adrenergic stimulation by α-methylnorepinephrine postulated | Minor | Demonstrated in experimental animals; clinical reports are conflicting |
| Sulfonylureas (and other oral hypoglycemic agents) | Impaired response to hypoglycemia | Reduced glycogenolysis and peripheral warning signs related to catecholamine excess | Major | |
| d-Tubocurare | More intense and prolonged muscle relaxation | Unknown | Minor | Experimental demonstration requires very high doses of IV propranolol; other muscle relaxants may be similarly affected |
| Quinidine with: | | | | |
| Acetazolamide (and sodium bicarbonate) | Increased serum quinidine level | Decreased renal excretion due to increased urinary pH | Minor | Importance limited by relatively small amount of quinidine normally excreted in the urine |
| Digitalis | Increased serum digoxin level | Displacement from tissue binding sites; other mechanisms may also be involved | Probably major | Only recently described; effect on serum digitoxin concentration has not yet been established |
| Edrophonium (and other cholinergic agents) | Impaired cholinergic action | Intrinsic anticholinergic effect | Moderate | Potentially important in patients with myasthenia gravis |
| Phenothiazines (and butyrophenones) | Additive cardiac toxicity | Similar electrophysiologic effects | Major | Dysrhythmias due to toxic doses of these agents should not be treated with quinidine |
| Succinylcholine | More intense and prolonged muscle relaxation | Unknown | Moderate | More important than similar interactions involving other antidysrhythmic agents |
| Tricyclic antidepressants | Additive cardiac toxicity | Similar electrophysiologic effects | Major | Dysrhythmias due to toxic doses of these agents should not be treated with quinidine |
| Warfarin | Increased hypoprothrombinemia | Unknown | Moderate | Idiosyncratic; most patients are unaffected |

tors in bronchial and peripheral vascular smooth muscle in a relatively selective manner. Propranolol and several other agents competitively antagonize the effects of sympathomimetic amines on all $\beta$-receptors, while still others more selectively interfere with cardiac ($\beta_1$) or noncardiac ($\beta_2$) $\beta$-adrenergic stimulation. Metoprolol and butoxamine are examples of relatively selective $\beta_1$ and $\beta_2$ blocking agents, respectively. Finally, $\alpha$-adrenergic stimulation can also be antagonized nonselectively by the $\alpha$-receptor blocking agents phentolamine and phenoxybenzamine. The antihypertensive agent, prazosin, also acts as an $\alpha$-receptor blocking agent, exhibiting a much greater affinity for $\alpha_1$ (post-junctional) receptors than for $\alpha_2$ (pre-junctional) receptor sites.

The specific pharmacologic properties of these drugs can sometimes be exploited through the combined use of more than one sympathomimetic amine or the simultaneous administration of selective adrenergic stimulating and blocking agents. The use of adrenergic agents in conjunction with other drugs that exert independent effects on heart rate, myocardial contractility, or vasomotor tone likewise leads to predictable interactions based on the pharmacologic activity of the individual agents involved. These types of interactions will not be discussed further in this section.

Chronic therapy with either guanethidine or reserpine leads to a decrease in norepinephrine stores in sympathetic nerve endings.[72] Both drugs also increase the sensitivity of the neuroeffector cells to catecholamines,[72] an effect that resembles the hypersensitivity that develops following sympathetic denervation. The effects of indirect- or mixed-acting adrenergic agents are, therefore, highly variable in patients treated with these drugs.[73] In contrast, the activity of direct-acting sympathomimetic amines is uniformly increased.[73] If adrenergic stimulating agents are required in patients previously treated with guanethidine or reserpine, direct-acting drugs should be employed. However, such therapy must be undertaken cautiously, as smaller than usual doses may cause excessive hypertension or cardiac dysrhythmias.[72,74,75]

Methyldopa has been observed to decrease the mydriatic action of topically applied ephedrine.[76] The mechanism of this interaction is uncertain, although reduced norepinephrine stores due to the presence of $\alpha$-methylnorepinephrine as a "false" neurotransmitter have been postulated. Clinically significant interference with the systemic effects of indirect-acting adrenergic agents has not been reported, although such interactions might reasonably be anticipated. Methyldopa also enhances the pressor effects of exogenous norepinephrine by uncertain mechanisms.[74] Specific data concerning this interaction are limited, although caution is advisable when direct-acting adrenergic agents are given to patients previously treated with methyldopa.

Monamine oxidase (MAO) inhibitors (e.g., pargyline, phenelzine, tranylcypromine) increase the concentration of norepinephrine in sympathetic nerve endings by interfering with its degradation by oxidative deamination. Adrenergic-stimulating agents with indirect mechanisms of action, therefore, cause greater release of norepinephrine in the presence of these drugs.[77-81] Tyramine (an indirect-acting sympathomimetic amine) is present in many food products, and is normally degraded by intestinal and hepatic monamine oxidase. During treatment with MAO inhibitors, an increased proportion of ingested tyramine reaches the systemic circulation, an effect that further potentiates its adrenergic-stimulating action.[81] Indirect- or mixed-acting sympathomimetic drugs, tyramine-containing foods, and catecholamine precursors, such as levodopa, may cause severe hypertensive crises due to exaggerated norepinephrine release in patients treated with MAO inhibitors.[77-82] Such substances (including many over-the-counter "cold" remedies containing indirect-acting sympathomimetic amines)[83] should be avoided by these patients.

Amitriptyline, imipramine, and other tricyclic antidepressants interfere with norepinephrine reuptake by sympathetic neurons.[84] Variable activity of indirect-acting and hypersensitivity to direct-acting sympathomimetic agents would be predicted on this basis. Increased pressor effects and hypertensive crises have, in fact, been reported following amphetamine abuse by patients treated with these agents.[84] The incidence and clinical importance of such interactions have not been firmly established, however. Chlorpromazine and haloperidol act as inhibitors of central dopaminergic neurons.[85] These drugs are known to block certain peripheral as well as central actions of catecholamines and have been associated with a decreased pressor response to indirectly acting sympathomimetic agents.[86,87] Fortunately, clinically significant problems resulting from these interactions are unusual.

The combined use of $\beta$-adrenergic stimulating drugs and certain general anesthetic agents (e.g., cyclopropane, halothane, and other halogenated hydrocarbons) has been associated with an increased incidence of serious cardiac dysrhythmias.[88] The mechanism of these interactions has not been established, although increased myocardial sensitivity to the effects of adrenergic stimulation and concomitant hypoxemia or acid-base imbalance may both contribute. Nitrous oxide and ether are not known to be associated with such effects and are, therefore, preferable anesthetic agents in patients requiring the intraoperative administration of sympathomimetic drugs.

Theoretically, adrenergic agents may also interact with other drugs by altering their metabolism or excretion indirectly through changes in cardiac output or peripheral blood flow distribution. The extent to which the pharmacokinetics of concurrently administered drugs may be altered under these circumstances is difficult to predict, and serum drug levels are advisable to guide appropriate dosage adjustments.

Drug interactions involving adrenergic agents are summarized in Table 40.3.

## Vasodilators and Antihypertensive Agents

The combined use of more than one drug is often necessary in the treatment of hypertension. Such deliberate interactions make use of the varied mechanisms of action of different antihypertensive agents, and are generally predictable in their effects. However, interactions between antihypertensive agents and other types of drugs may occasionally cause unexpected clinical problems.

Specific drug interactions involving diuretics and propranolol are discussed in other sections (see Diuretics and Antiarrhythmic Agents, respectively). Metoprolol is a relatively selective $\beta$-adrenergic ($\beta_1$) blocking agent. However, in the dosages required for the treatment of hypertension, metoprolol also causes significant blockade of the $\beta$-adrenergic ($\beta_2$) receptors in bronchial and vascular smooth muscle. These effects competitively antagonize the action of bronchodilating agents and can cause bronchospasm in patients with asthma and chronic obstructive lung disease.[89] Metroprolol, like propranolol, can also interfere with catecholamine-dependent responses to hypoglycemia.[90] This agent should, therefore, be used with caution in diabetic patients treated with insulin or oral hypoglycemic agents.

Chronic therapy with guanethidine or reserpine variably alters the activity of indirect-acting sympathomimetic amines, while causing hypersensitivity to direct-acting adrenergic drugs.[73] Similar effects have been reported with methyldopa.[74,76] These interactions have been discussed in more detail in a previous section (see Adrenergic Agents).

Guanethidine is concentrated in sympathetic nerve endings by the same active transport system involved in norepinephrine reuptake.[72] Tricyclic antidepressants and phenothiazines inhibit this system, altering the action of adrenergic-stimulating agents as described previously. These drugs also interfere with neuronal uptake of guanethidine and diminish its hypotensive effect.[91] This interaction may require several days to become fully manifest, and may require up to a four-fold increase in guanethidine dosage. Residual effects often persist for prolonged periods after the responsible drugs are discontinued.[92] Inadequate blood pressure control can result from the combined use of these agents, whereas unexpected hypotension may develop when concomitantly administered tricyclic antidepressants or phenothiazines are discontinued.[92-94] Doxepin causes less antagonism than other tricyclic antidepressants[95] and is, therefore, a preferable drug in hypertensive patients requiring treatment with guanethidine.

The phenothiazines and tricyclic antidepressants may cause similar interference with the

**Table 40.3  Drug Interactions Involving Adrenergic Agents**

| Drug Interaction | Effect | Mechanism | Clinical Significance | Comments |
|---|---|---|---|---|
| Indirect-acting adrenergic stimulating agents (amphetamines, tyramine) with: | | | | |
| Guanethidine | Variably altered adrenergic stimulation | Decreased neuronal norepinephrine stores available for release; impaired norepinephrine reuptake by sympathetic nerve endings | Major | Few legitimate indications for amphetamines exist |
| Monamine oxidase inhibitors | Increased adrenergic stimulation | Increased neuronal norepinephrine stores available for release | Major | Tyramine-containing foods, nonprescription decongestants and other sources of indirect-acting sympathomimetic agents must be avoided |
| Phenothiazines (and butyrophenones) | Variably altered adrenergic stimulation | Decreased neuronal norepinephrine stores available for release; impaired norepinephrine reuptake by sympathetic nerve endings | Minor | Chlorpromazine has been used to reverse the adrenergic stimulation of amphetamine overdose |
| Reserpine | Decreased adrenergic stimulation | Decreased neuronal norepinephrine stores available for release | Unestablished | Well-documented experimentally; clinical evidence is inconclusive |
| Tricyclic antidepressants | Variably altered adrenergic stimulation | Decreased neuronal norepinephrine stores available for release; impaired norepinephrine reuptake by sympathetic nerve endings | Unestablished | Hypertensive crises have occurred with amphetamine abuse in patients treated with these agents |

**Table 40.3** (Continued)

| Drug Interaction | Effect | Mechanism | Clinical Significance | Comments |
|---|---|---|---|---|
| Mixed direct- and indirect-acting adrenergic agents (ephedrine, metaraminol) with:* | | | | |
| Anesthetic agents (cyclopropane, halothane, other halogenated hydrocarbons) | Serious cardiac dysrhythmias | Unknown; associated hypoxemia or acid-base imbalance may contribute | Major | Nitrous oxide and ether are safer anesthetic agents when intraoperative adrenergic drugs are required |
| Guanethidine | Variably altered adrenergic stimulation | Decreased neuronal norepinephrine available for release; impaired norepinephrine reuptake by sympathetic nerve endings | Major | Direct-acting agents should be used when adrenergic stimulation is necessary |
| Methyldopa | Decreased mydriatic action of topical ephedrine | Unknown; α-methyl norepinephrine may act as a "false" neurotransmitter | Minor | Interference with the systemic effects of ephedrine or other indirect- or mixed-acting adrenergic agents has not been demonstrated |
| Monoamine oxidase inhibitors | Increased adrenergic stimulation | Increased neuronal norepinephrine stores available for release | Major | Adrenergic agents with any indirect effects (including many nonprescription decongestants) must be avoided |
| Phenothiazines (and butyrophenones) | Variably altered adrenergic stimulation | Decreased neuronal norepinephrine stores available for release; impaired norepinephrine reuptake by sympathetic nerve endings | Minor | Direct-acting agents should be used when adrenergic stimulation is necessary |
| Reserpine | Decreased adrenergic stimulation | Decreased neuronal norepinephrine stores available for release | Unestablished | Well documented experimentally; clinical evidence is inconclusive |

**Table 40.3 (Continued)**

| Drug Interaction | Effect | Mechanism | Clinical Significance | Comments |
|---|---|---|---|---|
| Tricyclic antidepressants | Variably altered adrenergic stimulation | Decreased neuronal norepinephrine stores available for release; impaired norepinephrine reuptake by sympathetic nerve endings | Unestablished | Direct-acting agents should be used when adrenergic stimulation is necessary |
| Direct-acting adrenergic agents (dopamine, epinephrine, isoproterenol, norepinephrine, phenylephrine, dobutamine) with: * | | | | |
| Anesthetic agents (cyclopropane, halothane, other halogenated hydrocarbons) | Serious cardiac dysrhythmias | Unknown; associated hypoxemia or acid-base imbalance may contribute | Major | Nitrous oxide and ether are safer anesthetic agents when intraoperative adrenergic drugs are required |
| Guanethidine | Increased adrenergic stimulation | Probably related to inhibition of catecholamine membrane pump in sympathetic nerve endings | Major | Caution is necessary to avoid untoward hypertension or cardiac dysrhythmias |
| Methyldopa | Increased pressor response to norepinephrine | Unknown | Unestablished | Interactions with other direct-acting agents have not been established |
| Phenothiazines | Possible increased adrenergic stimulation | Inhibition of catecholamine membrane pump in sympathetic nerve endings | Unestablished | Theoretical consideration; clinical information lacking |
| Reserpine | Increased adrenergic stimulation | Unknown | Moderate | Smaller than usual doses may be effective |
| Tricyclic antidepressants | Possible increased adrenergic stimulation | Inhibition of catecholamine membrane pump in sympathetic nerve endings | Unestablished | Theoretical consideration; clinical information lacking |

* These agents may also theoretically alter the metabolism or excretion of a variety of other drugs indirectly through changes in cardiac output or peripheral blood flow distribution.

hypotensive effects of methyldopa.[96,97] It has been proposed that these agents block reuptake of α-methylnorepinephrine by sympathetic nerve endings, leading to a paradoxic hypertensive response. However, clinical evidence supporting this interaction is limited to single case reports involving either trifluoperazine [96] or amitriptyline,[97] and experimental studies have yielded conflicting results.[98,99] It is probable that the antihypertensive effects of methyldopa are unaffected in most patients treated with phenothiazines or tricyclic antidepressants, although individual exceptions may occur.

Methyldopa can interfere with the therapeutic effects of levodopa in some patients with parkinsonism.[100] The mechanism of this interaction is uncertain, although the extrapyramidal replacement of dopamine by a "false" neurotransmitter has been suggested.[101] Furthermore, the hypotensive effect of levodopa may be additive with that of methyldopa.[102] These drugs have sometimes been used together intentionally with beneficial results, particularly in patients with fluctuating responses to levodopa alone.[103] However, the possibility that this combination may worsen the clinical manifestations of parkinsonism, or lead to excessive hypotension, must be considered and alternative antihypertensive agents occasionally substituted.

Methyldopa has also been reported to increase the toxic effects of both lithium and haloperidol.[104] The mechanisms of these interactions are unknown, and their clinical importance remains to be established.

Clonidine is another hypotensive agent whose action is impaired by the tricyclic antidepressants.[105] The results of this interaction are typically gradual in onset and moderate in intensity, although more abrupt loss of blood pressure control may occur.[105] The mechanism by which these agents interact is unknown and may involve both central and peripheral effects. Clonidine has also been reported to inhibit the catecholamine response to hypoglycemia in diabetics treated with oral agents and to decrease the therapeutic effect of levodopa in patients with parkinsonism.[104] The mechanisms of these interactions and their clinical significance have not been established.

Monamine oxidase (MAO) inhibitors have occasionally been used as antihypertensive agents. Pargyline was, in fact, originally introduced for this purpose. These drugs interfere with the oxidative deamination of norepinephrine and potentiate the effects of indirect-acting sympathomimetic amines. The mechanism of their antihypertensive action is uncertain, although postural effects (without associated tachycardia) are prominent, indicating impaired sympathetic compensatory responses. Unfortunately, such agents also inhibit a variety of other drug-metabolizing enzymes, leading to frequent and often profound adverse effects. The activity of insulin, alcohol, and many sedatives and narcotics are potentiated by such interactions.[106-108] Severe toxicity has also resulted from the combined use of MAO inhibitors and tricyclic antidepressants, although the mechanism is uncertain and appears to be idiosyncratic.[109,110] The availability of a variety of alternative, safer, and more effective antihypertensive agents has eliminated any useful role of these drugs in the modern management of hypertension.

Hydralazine, nitroprusside, and other direct vasodilating agents (including nitroglycerin and the long-acting nitrates) are rarely involved in unexpected drug interactions. Each agent's relative effects on vascular resistance and capacitance combine predictably with the actions of other drugs that influence vasomotor tone (e.g., adrenergic stimulating or blocking agents), intravascular volume (e.g., diuretics), or myocardial performance (e.g., positive inotropic agents). These drugs may, however, indirectly influence the metabolism, distribution, or excretion of other agents by altering cardiac output or peripheral blood flow distribution. The clinical importance of these effects remains to be established.

Drug interactions involving vasodilators and antihypertensive agents are summarized in Table 40.4.

### Diuretics

Increased myocardial sensitivity to digitalis due to drug-induced hypokalemia is by far the most important drug interaction involving diuretics. Spironolactone (which can be used in

**Table 40.4  Drug Interactions Involving Vasodilators and Antihypertensive Agents**

| Drug Interaction | Effect | Mechanism | Clinical Significance | Comments |
|---|---|---|---|---|
| **Clonidine with:** | | | | |
| Levodopa | Decreased therapeutic effect of levodopa | Unknown | Unestablished | |
| Sulfonylureas (and other oral hypoglycemic agents) | Impaired response to hypoglycemia | Inhibition of normal catecholamine response | Unestablished | |
| Tricyclic antidepressants | Decreased hypotensive effect | Unknown | Moderate | Usually gradual onset |
| **Diazoxide with:** | | | | |
| Sulfonylureas (and other oral hypoglycemic agents) | Hyperglycemia | Decreased insulin release | Minor | Significance limited by usual brief duration of therapy with diazoxide |
| Warfarin | Transiently increased hypothrombinemic effect | Displacement of warfarin from serum proteins | Minor | Demonstrated experimentally; no clinical reports available |
| Diuretics (See Table 40.5) | | | | |
| **Guanethidine with:** | | | | |
| Adrenergic-stimulating agents | Variably altered effects of indirect- and mixed-acting agents; increased effects of direct-acting agents | Decreased neuronal norepinephrine stores available for release; impaired norepinephrine reuptake by sympathetic nerve endings | Major | Direct-acting agents should be used cautiously when adrenergic stimulation is necessary |
| Phenothiazines (and butyrophenones) | Decreased hypotensive effect | Impaired guanethidine uptake by sympathetic nerve endings | Major | Full interaction may take several days to develop; residual effects may last for weeks |
| Tricyclic antidepressants | Decreased hypotensive effect | Impaired guanethidine uptake by sympathetic nerve endings | Major | Full interaction may take several days to develop; residual effects may last for weeks; doxepin causes less antagonism than other tricyclic antidepressants |

969

**Table 40.4** (Continued)

| Drug Interaction | Effect | Mechanism | Clinical Significance | Comments |
|---|---|---|---|---|
| **Hydralazine \*** | | | | |
| **Methyldopa with:** | | | | |
| Adrenergic stimulating agents | Decreased mydriatic action of topical ephedrine; increased pressor response to norepinephrine | Unknown | Minor (ephedrine); unestablished (norepinephrine) | Interference with systemic effects of ephedrine or interactions involving other adrenergic agents have not been demonstrated |
| Levodopa | Decreased therapeutic effect of levodopa | Unknown; possible extrapyramidal replacement of dopamine with a "false" neurotransmitter | Moderate | Occasionally beneficial in patients with fluctuating response to levodopa |
| Lithium | Increased toxic effect of lithium | Unknown | Unestablished | Serum lithium levels should be followed serially when concurrent methyldopa therapy is started or stopped |
| Phenothiazines (and butyrophenones | Decreased hypotensive effect of methyldopa; increased haloperidol toxicity | Unknown | Minor | Clinical evidence is limited; experimental results are conflicting |
| Propranolol | Decreased hypotensive effect | Unknown; unopposed α-adrenergic stimulation by α-methylnorepinephrine postulated | Minor | Demonstrated in experimental animals; clinical reports are conflicting |
| Tricyclic antidepressants | Decreased hypotensive effect | Unknown | Minor | Clinical evidence is limited; experimental results are conflicting |
| **Metoprolol with:** | | | | |
| Insulin | Impaired response to hypoglycemia | Reduced glycogenolysis and peripheral warning signs related to catecholamine excess | Major | |

**Table 40.4** (Continued)

| Drug Interaction | Effect | Mechanism | Clinical Significance | Comments |
|---|---|---|---|---|
| Sulfonylureas and other oral hypoglycemic agents | Impaired response to hypoglycemia | Reduced glycogenolysis and peripheral warning signs related to catecholamine excess | Major | |
| Monamine Oxidase Inhibitors with: † | | | | |
| Adrenergic stimulating agents | Increased effects of indirect- and mixed-acting agents | Increased neuronal norepinephrine stores available for release | Major | Adrenergic agents with any indirect effects (including many nonprescription decongestants) must be avoided |
| Nitrates (isosorbide dinitrate, nitroglycerin, pentaerythritol tetranitrate) * | | | | |
| Nitroprusside * | | | | |
| Prazosin * | | | | |
| Propranolol (See Table 40.2) | | | | |
| Reserpine with: | | | | |
| Adrenergic stimulating agents | Decreased effects of indirect-acting agents; increased effects of direct-acting agents | Decreased neuronal norepinephrine stores available for release by indirect-acting agents; mechanism of hypersensitivity to direct-acting agents is unknown | Moderate | Direct-acting agents should be used when adrenergic stimulation is necessary although smaller than usual doses may be effective |
| Digitalis | Possible potentiation of digitalis toxicity | Unknown | Unestablished | Isolated case reports only |

\* These agents are rarely involved in unexpected drug interactions; however they may theoretically alter the metabolism or excretion of a variety of other drugs indirectly through changes in cardiac output or peripheral blood flow distribution.

† These agents also inhibit a variety of other drug-metabolizing enzymes leading to frequent and often severe adverse effects; they have no role in the modern management of hypertension.

combination with kaliuretic agents to maintain potassium balance) also induces enzymes that accelerate digitoxin degradation; and both spironolactone and triamterene interfere with renal digoxin secretion. These interactions were discussed previously in more detail (see Digitalis).

Thiazides and other kaliuretic diuretics can cause impaired glucose tolerance in some diabetic and nondiabetic patients.[111,112] The precise mechanism by which this occurs is uncertain, although impaired insulin release and diminished tissue responsiveness have both been implicated.[112,113] This effect is usually mild, and is often reversed by correcting associated potassium depletion,[114] although some patients may require increased doses of insulin or oral hypoglycemic agents. This interaction is not seen with potassium-sparing diuretics.

Thiazides and related drugs also interfere with uric acid excretion, and hyperuricemic patients treated with allopurinol or uricosuric agents may occasionally require increased doses of these medications. In addition, the pharmacologic effects of some diuretics may be influenced by concomitant antihyperuricemic therapy. Probenecid interferes with furosemide excretion, thereby increasing plasma furosemide levels and prolonging the time course of its diuretic effect.[115,116] The amount of furosemide and sodium ultimately excreted in response to a given dose is unchanged, however, restricting the importance of this interaction to situations in which a rapid diuretic response is required.

Of potentially greater significance is the observation that aspirin interferes with the natruretic effect of spironolactone.[117,118] The precise mechanism by which this occurs is uncertain, although competition for receptor sites on renal tubular cells has been suggested.[117] Regardless, in normal individuals given spironolactone chronically, the decrease in urinary sodium excretion induced by a single dose of aspirin is substantial.[118] Although the clinical importance of this interaction has not been fully established, aspirin alternatives should probably be used in patients taking spironolactone.

Another important interaction involves the potential effect of virtually all diuretics on lithium clearance. The role of sodium excretion in the production of lithium intoxication is well known.[119] Lithium is reabsorbed, along with sodium, in the proximal renal tubules, and diuretics that interfere with distal sodium reabsorption ultimately induce a compensatory increase in proximal reabsorption of both sodium and lithium.[120] Although single doses have little effect, chronic diuretic therapy in patients treated with lithium carbonate can significantly elevate serum lithium concentrations [120] and may lead to lithium toxicity.[121]

Finally, some caution must be used when ethacrynic acid and, to a lesser extent, furosemide are given to patients receiving aminoglycoside antibiotics. All of these drugs are capable of causing serious ototoxicity, particularly when given intravenously in high doses or to patients with abnormal renal function. Such effects may be additive, and combined therapy should be monitored closely or avoided if possible.

Drug interactions involving diuretics are summarized in Table 40.5.

## INTERACTIONS INVOLVING OTHER DRUGS COMMONLY USED IN CARDIOVASCULAR PATIENTS

### Anticoagulants

The oral anticoagulants have been involved in more therapeutically important drug interactions than any other class of drugs. The pharmacology and pharmacokinetics of these agents are complex and present multiple potential sites for interaction. In addition, their therapeutic index is relatively low so that small changes in drug activity readily lead to therapeutic failures or hemorrhagic complications. Two important clinical circumstances further contribute to the high incidence of recognized interactions involving these agents. First, oral anticoagulants are often prescribed for prolonged periods of time, and concurrent therapy with one or more additional drugs is almost invariable. Second, routine and reliable monitoring of anticoagulant effects provides a sensitive means of detecting adverse interactions unavailable with most other drugs. As a result, drug interactions

**Table 40.5  Drug Interactions Involving Diuretics**

| Drug Interaction | Effect | Mechanism | Clinical Significance | Comments |
|---|---|---|---|---|
| **Ethacrynic acid with:** | | | | |
| Allopurinol | Increased serum uric acid | Impaired uric acid excretion | Moderate | May require increased doses of allopurinol |
| Aminoglycoside antibiotics | Ototoxicity | Additive toxicity | Major | Combined therapy should be avoided if possible |
| Digitalis | Increased tissue sensitivity to digitalis | Potassium and magnesium depletion potentiates inhibition of Na-K-ATPase | Major | May have total body potassium deficit with normal serum potassium |
| Insulin | Impaired glucose tolerance | Decreased tissue responsiveness | Moderate | Often reversible with potassium replacement |
| Lithium | Increased serum lithium levels | Increased proximal tubular reabsorption of both sodium and lithium | Major | Serum lithium level must be followed when natriuretic diuretics are started or stopped |
| Probenecid | Increased serum uric acid | Impaired uric acid excretion | Moderate | May require increased doses of probenecid |
| Sulfonylureas (and other oral hypoglycemic agents) | Impaired glucose tolerance | Decreased insulin release; reduced tissue responsiveness | Moderate | Often reversible with potassium replacement |
| Warfarin | Transiently increased hypoprothrombinemic effect | Displacement of warfarin from serum proteins | Minor | Isolated case reports only |
| **Furosemide with:** | | | | |
| Allopurinol | Increased serum uric acid | Impaired uric acid excretion | Moderate | May require increased doses of allopurinol |
| Aminoglygoside antibiotics | Ototoxicity | Additive toxicity | Major | Combined therapy should be avoided if possible |
| Chloral hydrate | Vasomotor instability | Unknown | Unestablished | Isolated case reports only |

**Table 40.5  (Continued)**

| Drug Interaction | Effect | Mechanism | Clinical Significance | Comments |
|---|---|---|---|---|
| Digitalis | Increased tissue sensitivity to digitalis | Potassium and magnesium depletion potentiates inhibition of Na-K-ATPase | Major | May have total body potassium deficit with normal serum potassium |
| Insulin | Impaired glucose tolerance | Decreased tissue responsiveness | Moderate | Often reversible with potassium replacement |
| Lithium | Increased serum lithium levels | Increased proximal tubular reabsorption of both sodium and lithium | Major | Serum lithium level must be followed when natriuretic diuretics are started or stopped |
| Probenecid | Increased serum uric acid | Impaired uric acid excretion | Moderate | May require increased doses of probenecid |
| Sulfonylureas (and other oral hypoglycemic agents) | Impaired glucose tolerance | Decreased insulin release; reduced tissue responsiveness | Moderate | Often reversible with potassium replacement |
| Spironolactone with: Digitalis | Decreased serum digitoxin level; increased serum digoxin level | Accelerated hepatic biotransformation of digitoxin; impaired renal tubular secretion of digoxin | Moderate | May also interfere with digoxin radioimmunoassay |
| Salicylates | Decreased natriuretic effect | Probable competition for receptor sites on renal tubular cells | Unestablished | Substantial effect experimentally; aspirin alternatives are recommended |
| Thiazide diuretics with: Allopurinol | Increased serum uric acid | Impaired uric acid excretion | Moderate | May require increased doses of allopurinol |

974

**Table 40.5** (Continued)

| Drug Interaction | Effect | Mechanism | Clinical Significance | Comments |
|---|---|---|---|---|
| Cholestyramine (and colestipol) | Decreased diuretic effect | Decreased absorption due to intraluminal physicochemical binding | Moderate | Minimized by separating administration by several hours; effects on absorption of other diuretic agents are unknown |
| Digitalis | Increased tissue sensitivity to digitalis | Potassium and magnesium depletion potentiates inhibition of Na-K-ATPase | Major | May have total body potassium deficit with normal serum potassium |
| Insulin | Impaired glucose tolerance | Decreased tissue responsiveness | Moderate | Often reversible with potassium replacement |
| Lithium | Increased serum lithium levels | Increased proximal tubular reabsorption of both sodium and lithium | Major | Serum lithium level must be followed when natriuretic diuretics are started or stopped |
| Probenecid | Increased serum uric acid | Impaired uric acid excretion | Moderate | May require increased doses of allopurinol |
| Sulfonylureas (and other oral hypoglycemic agents) | Impaired glucose tolerance | Decreased insulin release; reduced tissue responsiveness | Moderate | Often reversible with potassium replacement |
| Triamterene with: Digitalis | Increased serum digoxin level | Impaired renal tubular secretion | Unestablished | Similar to spironolactone experimentally; no known effects on digitoxin metabolism |

have been reported to occur in from 34 to 53 percent of patients treated with these agents.[122,123] Although the oral anticoagulants can alter the pharmacologic action of several drugs, interference with anticoagulant effects by other agents is clinically much more important.

The two major types of oral anticoagulants have the same principal pharmacologic effect—inhibition of hepatic synthesis of vitamin K-dependent clotting factors. Theoretically, drugs that interfere with the bacterial synthesis of vitamin K or its subsequent absorption could potentiate the hypoprothrombinemic effects of these agents, but such interactions rarely cause problems in the absence of preexisting vitamin K deficiency.[124] Therapeutically important interactions result instead from drug-induced alterations in anticoagulant absorption or, more commonly, from changes in serum protein binding or hepatic biotransformation. Independent effects on prothrombin synthesis or unrelated hemostatic mechanisms are other important sources of interaction. The indandione anticoagulants (e.g., diphenadione, anisindione) are less frequently used than the coumarin derivatives (e.g., warfarin, dicumarol), with warfarin accounting for 95 percent of all anticoagulants prescribed.[123] Further discussion will focus on coumarin (and particularly warfarin) drug interactions.

Warfarin is completely and rapidly absorbed in the upper gastrointestinal tract and is rarely subject to drug interactions that decrease its bioavailability. Cholestyramine has been shown to bind warfarin, decreasing its absorption and subsequent hypoprothrombinemic effect in single-dose studies in normal volunteers.[125] The clinical importance of this interaction appears minor, however, and any potential problem can be minimized by administering these two drugs 3 to 6 hours apart. Dicumarol is less completely absorbed than other coumarin derivatives and is, therefore, more susceptible to drug-induced changes in bioavailability. Aluminum and magnesium-containing antacids may decrease dicumarol absorption, although warfarin absorption is unaffected.[125,126]

Warfarin is extensively (97 to 99 percent) bound to serum albumin, so that relatively small amounts of protein displacement may effectively double the concentration of active free drug. The effects of displacement are generally transient, with maximal hypoprothrombinemia developing in 3 to 5 days; the prothrombin time then returns, over several weeks, to near previous levels as enhanced metabolism and excretion reduce the concentration of unbound warfarin.

Phenylbutazone has about 2½ times greater affinity than warfarin for common albumin-binding sites, and uniformly causes an increase in free warfarin and an enhanced hypoprothrombinemic effect.[127-129] Oxyphenbutazone behaves similarly.[130] Indomethacin can also displace warfarin from serum albumin, although in vitro displacement is only about one-third that of phenylbutazone.[131] It does not, by itself, potentiate the anticoagulant effects of warfarin,[132] although increased hypoprothrombinemia has occurred following the combined use of both indomethacin and allopurinol.[133] All three of these drugs also inhibit platelet function, are ulcerogenic, and should probably be avoided in anticoagulated patients.

Other agents capable of displacing warfarin from albumin to varying degrees include iopanoic, ethacrynic, and naladixic acids; trichloracetic acid (a metabolite of choral hydrate); sulfinpyrazone; and diazoxide.[131,134-136] Although ethacrynic acid appears to have caused a substantial prolongation of the prothrombin time in a single patient,[137] significant clinical problems have not otherwise been reported with these drugs. The possibility of transiently increased hypoprothrombinemia should be anticipated, however, during the first 2 weeks of therapy with any drug capable of warfarin displacement interactions.

The coumarin anticoagulants are inactivated primarily by hepatic microsomal enzyme systems. Several drugs increase the hypoprothrombinemic effects of warfarin and other coumarin derivatives by inducing enzymes that accelerate this process of biotransformation. Such effects are fairly reproducible in a given individual, although interpatient variation is considerable. Phenobarbital, secobarbital, alcohol, glutethimide, carbamazepine, primidone, and rifampin all markedly accelerate warfarin metabolism.[138-142] Similar, although less important changes, occur with methaqualone, ethchlorvynol, and griseofulvin.[129,138] Rifampin is particularly potent in this regard, and may reduce plasma warfarin concentrations as much as sixfold.[141,142] The onset and duration of these effects are variable, but are generally apparent within 1 week after therapy with an interacting drug has been started.[124,141,142] Return to normal warfarin sensitivity may require several weeks to several months after enzyme-inducing agents are discontinued, although anticoagulant dosage will eventually have to be reduced.

A number of other drugs increase the hypoprothrombinemic effects of warfarin by inhibiting its hepatic biotransformation to inactive metabolites. Disulfiram, metronidazole, and isoniazid inhibit warfarin metabolism, while chloramphenicol, allopurinol, and certain tricyclic antidepressants interfere with dicumarol metabolism.[143-148] The effects of these latter drugs on warfarin metabolism have not been established, although caution is advisable in using these agents in combination with any oral anticoagulant.

Cotrimoxazole (trimethoprim-sulfamethoxazole) and other sulfonamides significantly increase the hypoprothrombinemic effects of warfarin.[149-153] Furthermore, both sulfamethizole and cotrimoxazole have been shown to inhibit warfarin metabolism experimentally.[149,152] This interaction necessitates either a reduction in warfarin dosage or use of alternative antimicrobial agents.

Clofibrate also potentiates the action of warfarin and other oral anticoagulants.[154,155] Increased hepatic receptor site affinity for these agents has been proposed, although other mechanisms may be involved as well.[154,156] Furthermore, this interaction may be less likely to develop in patients who either do not have elevated serum lipids or whose hyperlipidemia fails to respond to clofibrate.[129,156] Vitamin E has been reported to enhance the effect of warfarin in a clofibrate-treated patient, but has not been shown to increase the anticoagulant effects of warfarin when given alone.[157]

A number of drugs enhance the hypoprothrombinemic effects of anticoagulants without altering coumarin metabolism. Anabolic steroids (e.g., methandrostenolone, norethandrolone, oxymetholone) significantly increase the hypoprothrombinemic effects of warfarin and may lead to clinical bleeding.[158-161] Other C-17 alkylated androgens (e.g., methyltestosterone, fluoxymesterone) may have similar effects. The mechanism of this interaction is uncertain, although an increase in the affinity of hepatic receptor sites for coumarin derivatives has been postulated.[155] Dextrothyroxine more than doubles warfarin receptor site affinity, and usually decreases anticoagulant requirements after 1 to 4 weeks of therapy.[155,162] Increased catabolism of vitamin K-dependent clotting factors may also contribute to the enhanced hypoprothrombinemia caused by this drug, as has also been described in hyperthyroidism.

Salicylates in doses greater than 3.0 g daily may, by themselves, inhibit the synthesis of vitamin K-dependent clotting factors in some patients.[163,164] Aspirin also inhibits platelet aggregation and has direct effects on the gastric mucosa, both of which further increase the risk of bleeding in patients treated with warfarin. Acetaminophen and other alternative agents are generally preferable in these patients.

Quinidine has been reported to have an independent hypoprothrombinemic effect, which is additive to that of warfarin.[44] Most anticoagulated patients treated with quinidine experience no adverse effects,[45] although warfarin dosages may rarely have to be reduced.

The list of drugs known to interfere with the oral anticoagulants is extensive, and continues to expand as more experience is gained with newer therapeutic agents. Cimetidine has recently been shown to enhance the anticoagulant effects of warfarin by as much as 20 percent in a limited number of cases.[165,166] Similar effects have been observed with disopyramide in a single case report.[167] The continued emergence of newly recognized drug interactions serves to emphasize the caution that must be exerted in the use of multiple-drug therapy in patients treated with oral anticoagulants. Additional drugs can often be used safely and effectively in these patients if potential interactions are anticipated and serial prothrombin times utilized to monitor the effects of any change in drug regimen. Unnecessary drugs should be

**Table 40.6  Drug Interactions Involving Anticoagulants**

| Drug Interaction | Effect | Mechanism | Clinical Significance | Comments |
|---|---|---|---|---|
| **Dicumarol with:** | | | | |
| Allopurinol | Decreased hypoprothrombinemic effect | Impaired hepatic biotransformation | Minor | |
| Antiplatelet agents (dipyridamole, salicylates, sulfinpyrazone) | Increased risk of hemorrhagic complications | Additive interference with hemostatic mechanisms; gastric erosions (aspirin) | Major | Combination therapy occasionally used in thromboembolic disorders |
| Chloramphenicol | Increased hypoprothrombinemic effect | Impaired hepatic biotransformation | Minor | |
| Chlorpropamide | Increased hypoglycemic effect | Impaired hepatic biotransformation | Unestablished | |
| Nortriptyline | Increased hypoprothrombinemic effect | Impaired hepatic biotransformation | Minor | Effects of other tricyclic antidepressants unestablished |
| Phenytoin | Variably altered hypoprothrombinemic effect | Displacement of dicumarol from serum proteins; accelerated hepatic biotransformation of dicumarol | Moderate | Dicumarol may also inhibit phenytoin metabolism resulting in increased serum phenytoin levels |
| Tolbutamide | Increased hypoglycemic effect | Impaired hepatic biotransformation of tolbutamide | Unestablished | |
| **Heparin with:** | | | | |
| Antiplatelet agents (dipyridamole, salicylates, sulfinpyrazone) | Increased risk of hemorrhagic complications | Additive interference with hemostatic mechanisms; gastric erosions (aspirin) | Major | |
| **Warfarin with:** | | | | |
| Alcohol | Increased hypoprothrombinemic effect (acute); decreased hypoprothrombinemic effect (chronic) | Acute mechanism unknown; accelerated hepatic biotransformation with chronic alcohol abuse | Major | Excessive alcohol use should be avoided; prothrombin time must be followed closely when chronic alcohol consumption patterns are altered |
| Anabolic steroids (methandrostenolone, oxymetholone and other C-17 alkylated androgens) | Increased hypoprothrombinemic effect | Postulated increased affinity of hepatic receptor sites for warfarin | Major | Most patients will require a reduction in warfarin dosage |
| Antiplatelet agents (dipyridamole, salicylates, sulfinpyrazone) | Increased risk of hemorrhagic complications | Additive interference with hemostatic mechanisms; gastric erosions (aspirin) | Major | Combination therapy occasionally used in thromboembolic disorders |

**Table 40.6** (Continued)

| Drug Interaction | Effect | Mechanism | Clinical Significance | Comments |
|---|---|---|---|---|
| Barbiturates | Decreased hypoprothrombinemic effect | Accelerated hepatic biotransformation | Major | Most important with phenobarbital; short-term use of more rapidly-acting preparations is less clinically significant |
| Carbamazepine | Decreased hypoprothrombinemic effect | Accelerated hepatic biotransformation | Major | May double warfarin dosage requirements |
| Chloral hydrate | Transiently increased hypoprothrombinemic effect | Displacement of warfarin from serum proteins by trichloroacetic acid (a chloral hydrate metabolite) | Minor | Alternative agents (e.g., flurazepam) are recommended |
| Cimetidine | Increased hypoprothrombinemic effect | Unknown | Unestablished | Clinical information is limited; significant prolongation of the prothrombin time may occur in some patients |
| Cholestyramine | Decreased hypoprothrombinemic effect | Decreased absorption due to intraluminal physicochemical binding | Moderate | Minimized by separating administration by several hours |
| Clofibrate | Increased hypoprothrombinemic effect | Displacement of warfarin from serum proteins; increased affinity of hepatic receptor sites for warfarin; impaired hepatic biotransformation | Major | Less important in patients with normal serum lipids or hyperlipidemia unresponsive to clofibrate |
| Cotrimoxazole (trimethoprim-sulfamethoxazole) | Increased hypoprothrombinemic effect | Impaired hepatic biotransformation | Major | Alternative antimicrobial drugs are recommended |
| Dextrothyroxine | Increased hypoprothrombinemic effect | Increased affinity of hepatic receptor sites for warfarin; possible increased catabolism of vitamin K-dependent coagulation factors | Major | Most patients will require a reduction in warfarin dosage |
| Diazoxide | Transiently increased hypoprothrombinemic effect | Displacement of warfarin from serum proteins | Minor | Demonstrated experimentally; no clinical reports available |
| Disulfiram | Increased hypoprothrombinemic effect | Impaired hepatic biotransformation; possible increased affinity of hepatic receptor sites for warfarin | Moderate | |
| Ethacrynic acid | Transiently increased hypoprothrombinemic effect | Displacement of warfarin from serum proteins | Minor | Furosemide does not interact with warfarin |

979

**Table 40.6 (Continued)**

| Drug Interaction | Effect | Mechanism | Clinical Significance | Comments |
|---|---|---|---|---|
| Griseofulvin | Decreased hypoprothrombinemic effect | Accelerated hepatic biotransformation | Moderate | Alternative drugs are recommended |
| Indomethacin | Increased risk of hemorrhagic complications; possible increased hypoprothrombinemic effect in some patients | Inhibition of platelet function; ulcerogenic effects; displacement of warfarin from serum proteins | Moderate | Alternative drugs are recommended |
| Iopanoic acid | Transiently increased hypoprothrombinemic effect | Displacement of warfarin from serum proteins | Unestablished | Used for oral cholecystograms |
| Isoniazid | Increased hypoprothrombinemic effect | Impaired hepatic biotransformation | Minor | High doses of isoniazid should be used cautiously |
| Metronidazole | Increased hypoprothrombinemic effect | Impaired hepatic biotransformation | Unestablished | Single case report of prolonged prothrombin time and bleeding |
| Phenylbutazone (and oxyphenbutazone) | Transiently increased hypoprothrombinemic effect; increased risk of hemorrhagic complications | Displacement of warfarin from serum proteins; inhibition of platelet function; ulcerogenic effects | Major | Combined therapy should be avoided |
| Primidone | Decreased hypoprothrombinemic effect | Accelerated hepatic biotransformation | Major | |
| Quinidine | Increased hypoprothrombinemia | Unknown | Moderate | Idiosyncratic; most patients are unaffected |
| Rifampin | Decreased hypoprothrombinemic effect | Accelerated hepatic biotransformation | Major | |
| Sulfonamides | Increased hypoprothrombinemic effect | Impaired hepatic biotransformation; possible displacement of warfarin from serum proteins | Major | Alternative antimicrobial drugs are recommended |

avoided, however, and alterations in therapy minimized.

Heparin is much less susceptible than the oral anticoagulants to significant adverse drug interactions. Although drugs that independently alter coagulation parameters or platelet function must be given cautiously in heparinized patients, most cardiovascular agents can be used concurrently without difficulty.

Drug interactions involving anticoagulants are summarized in Table 40.6.

## Antiplatelet Agents

Aspirin, sulfinpyrazone, dipyridamole, and other agents that inhibit platelet function may directly increase the risk of bleeding in patients treated with systemic anticoagulants. In addition, sulfinpyrazone displaces warfarin from serum protein-binding sites,[131] and high doses of salicylates have an independent hypoprothrombinemic action.[163,164] Some of these agents (e.g., aspirin, indomethacin) also have direct effects on the gastric mucosa, which further predispose to gastrointestinal hemorrhage. Although platelet antagonists are sometimes given intentionally to anticoagulated patients with thromboembolic disorders, such therapy must be undertaken cautiously. Alternative analgesic, antipyretic, and uricosuric agents are available when the added effects of platelet inhibition are undesirable.

Drugs that increase urinary pH (including "nonsystemic" aluminum-and magnesium-containing antacids) facilitate renal clearance of salicylic acid, and result in a decrease in serum salicylate concentration.[168] Drugs that lower urinary pH have opposite effects. Salicylates also compete with several drugs for renal tubular receptor sites, and may consequently interfere with their excretion or pharmacologic activity. The uricosuric action of probenecid and sulfinpyrazone, and the natriuretic effect of spironolactone are inhibited in this manner.[117,118,169,170] Conversely, sulfinpyrazone may prevent the usual uricosuric effect of large doses of aspirin.[170]

Salicylates predispose to methotrexate toxicity by causing both reduced methotrexate excretion and displacement from serum proteins.[171]

Similar competition for protein-binding sites may cause excessive hypoglycemia in patients treated with sulfonylurea oral hypoglycemic agents.[172-174] Other mechanisms are involved in this interaction as well (see Antidiabetic Agents).

Sulfinpyrazone may also potentiate the sulfonylureas by interfering with both hepatic inactivation and serum protein binding.[175,176] However, these effects have been more clearly demonstrated with a structurally similar compound, phenylbutazone.[177,178] Additional interactions involving sulfinpyrazone and other antiplatelet agents are less well documented.

Drug interactions involving antiplatelet agents are summarized in Table 40.7.

## Antidiabetic Agents

The most important interactions involving insulin and the oral hypoglycemic agents have been referred to previously. Propranolol blocks both glycogenolysis and the peripheral manifestations of catecholamine excess induced by hypoglycemia;[65,66] thiazide and other diuretics may lead to worsening hyperglycermia in some diabetic patients.[111-114] The antidiabetic agents also interact with a variety of other drugs, however, the results of which may occasionally be of clinical significance.

Salicylates potentiate the hypoglycemic effects of chlorpropamide, tolbutamide, and probably other sulfonylureas. This is due partially to an intrinsic effect on carbohydrate metabolism, which lessens the hyperglycemia in diabetic patients,[172] although the mechanism involved is uncertain. In addition, salicylates displace tolbutamide and chlorpropamide from serum protein-binding sites[173] and may also interfere with renal tubular secretion of chlorpropamide.[174] Although these interactions rarely cause serious problems, clinically significant hypoglycemia has resulted from the addition of moderate doses of aspirin (serum levels of 10 mg/100 ml or less) to chronic sulfonylurea therapy.[174]

Phenylbutazone potentiates the hypoglycemic effect of tolbutamide, probably by interfering with both hepatic inactivation and serum protein binding.[177] This drug also increases the

**Table 40.7  Drug Interactions Involving Antiplatelet Agents**

| Drug Interaction | Effect | Mechanism | Clinical Significance | Comments |
|---|---|---|---|---|
| **Dipyridamole with:** | | | | |
| Anticoagulants (heparin, dicumarol, warfarin) | Increased risk of hemorrhagic complications | Additive interference with hemostatic mechanisms | Major | Combination therapy occasionally used in thromboembolic disorders |
| **Salicylates with:** | | | | |
| Acetazolamide (and sodium bicarbonate) | Decreased serum salicylate level | Enhanced renal excretion due to increased urinary pH | Major | |
| Antacids (magnesium hydroxide, aluminum hydroxide) | Decreased serum salicylate level | Enhanced renal excretion due to increased urinary pH | Major | Magnitude of effect varies among different antacids |
| Anticoagulants (heparin, dicumarol, warfarin) | Increased risk of hemorrhagic complications | Additive interference with hemostatic mechanisms; gastric erosions (aspirin) | Major | Alternative antiinflammatory and analgesic agents are recommended; combination therapy occasionally used in thromboembolic disorders |
| Methotrexate | Increased risk of methotrexate toxicity | Impaired methotrexate excretion; displacement of methotrexate from serum proteins | Unestablished | Probably a major interaction although little clinical information is available; salicylate alternatives are recommended |
| Probenecid | Decreased uricosuric effect of probenecid | Probable competition for renal tubular receptor sites | Moderate | |
| Spironolactone | Decreased natriuretic effect of spironolactone | Probable competition for renal tubular receptor sites | Unestablished | Substantial effect experimentally; aspirin alternatives are recommended |

**Table 40.7** (Continued)

| Drug Interaction | Effect | Mechanism | Clinical Significance | Comments |
|---|---|---|---|---|
| Sulfinpyrazone | Decreased uricosuric effect of sulfinopyrazone; decreased uricosuric effect of high doses of aspirin | Probable competition for renal tubular receptor sites | Moderate | |
| Sulfonylureas | Transiently increased hypoglycemic activity | Displacement from serum proteins | Minor | |
| Sulfinpyrazone with:<br>Anticoagulants (heparin, dicumarol, warfarin) | Increased risk of hemorrhagic complications | Additive interference with hemostatic mechanisms | Major | Combination therapy occasionally used in thromboembolic disorders |
| Salicylates | Decreased uricosuric effect of sulfinpyrazone; decreased uricosuric effect of high doses of aspirin | Probable competition for renal tubular receptor sites | Moderate | |
| Sulfonylureas | Increased hypoglycemic effect | Impaired hepatic biotransformation (tolbutamide); displacement from serum proteins (tolbutamide); impaired renal excretion of active metabolites (acetohexamide) | Unestablished | Theoretically postulated interaction due to structural similarity to phenylbutazone |

activity of acetohexamide by interfering with the renal excretion of its active metabolite, hydroxyhexamide.[178] Sulfinpyrazone is structurally similar to phenylbutazone and may be capable of similar interactions.[175,176] Such potential effects should be anticipated when either of these drugs are given to diabetic patients taking tolbutamide or acetohexamide. The effects of these agents on other sulfonylureas, phenformin, and insulin are uncertain.

Dicumarol may increase the serum half-life of chlorpropamide and tolbutamide, although the incidence of clinically important hypoglycemia resulting from this interaction is unknown.[179,180] Insulin is not affected by dicumarol, and indandione anticoagulants are not known to interact with oral hypoglycemic agents.

Clofibrate, allopurinol, and probenecid have all been shown to increase the serum half-life of chlorpropamide, presumably by interfering with its renal tubular secretion.[181] Guanethidine has been observed to exert an intrinsic hypoglycemic effect in small numbers of diabetic patients,[182] and clonidine has been reported to decrease the warning signs of hypoglycemia.[104] The mechanisms and clinical importance of these latter interactions have not been established.

Finally, a variety of other drugs in less common use among cardiac patients (including alcohol, monamine oxidase inhibitors, chloramphenicol, and sulfonamides) can also influence the hypoglycemic effects of some or all of the antidiabetic agents. These interactions are summarized in Table 40.8.

## Antihyperlipidemic Agents

The anion exchange resins, cholestyramine and cholestipol, may bind a variety of drugs as well as cholesterol. Such physiochemical interactions have been shown to significantly decrease the absorption of digoxin, digitoxin, thyroxine, warfarin and, to a lesser extent, the thiazide diuretics.[6,8,125,183,184] These interactions are dose and time dependent, and can be minimized by administering the resin several hours after other drugs.[6]

Other antihyperlipidemics, clofibrate and dextrothyroxine, can increase the hypoprothrombinemic effect of warfarin (see Anticoagulants).[154-156,162] In addition, clofibrate is competitively displaced from serum albumin by furosemide. This interaction has resulted in increased effects from both drugs in patients with hypoalbuminemia.[185]

Drug interactions involving antihyperlipidemic agents are summarized in Table 40.9.

## Sedatives and Narcotics

Drug interactions involving the narcotic analgesics are most often due to directly additive depressant effects on the central or autonomic nervous system. Such interactions commonly result in increased sedation, hypotension, respiratory depression, or enhanced anticholinergic activity. Antihistamines, phenothiazines, antidepressants, and sedative-hypnotics are all capable of potentiating the effects of these agents and should be used in combination cautiously.

Barbiturates are capable of acclerating the metabolism of a wide variety of other drugs by inducing hepatic microsomal enzyme systems. Among cardiac patients, digitoxin and the oral anticoagulants are the drugs most susceptible to these effects.[8,139] Phenobarbital is a particularly potent enzyme-inducing agent, although shorter-acting preparations may have similar actions when used chronically. Less important changes in warfarin metabolism have been observed with methaqualone and ethchlorvinol.[129,138]

Monamine oxidase inhibitors interfere with meperidine metabolism and may result in excessive central nervous system depression.[186] Paradoxic excitatory effects have also been described, apparently related to increases in cerebral serotonin concentrations.[187,188] Concurrent use of these drugs has resulted in coma and death in a small number of patients and is therefore contraindicated.[189] Morphine is a suitable alternative if narcotic analgesics are required in patients treated with monamine oxidase inhibitors, although such combinations should be used with caution.

Chloral hydrate potentiates the action of the oral anticoagulants through displacement from

**Table 40.8  Drug Interactions Involving Antidiabetic Agents**

| Drug Interaction | Effect | Mechanism | Clinical Significance | Comments |
|---|---|---|---|---|
| **Acetohexamide with:** | | | | |
| Alcohol | Increased hypoglycemic effect | Impaired gluconeogenesis | Moderate | Minor disulfiram-like reaction may also occur |
| Clonidine | Impaired response to hypoglycemia | Inhibition of normal catecholamine response | Unestablished | |
| Metoprolol | Impaired response to hypoglycemia | Reduced glycogenolysis and peripheral warning signs related to catecholamine excess | Major | |
| Phenylbutazone | Increased hypoglycemic effect | Impaired renal excretion of hydroxyhexamide (an active metabolite) | Unestablished | Severe hypoglycemia apparently due to this combination has been reported |
| Propranolol | Impaired response to hypoglycemia | Reduced glycogenolysis and peripheral warning signs related to catecholamine excess | Major | |
| Sulfinpyrazone | Increased hypoglycemic effect | Impaired renal excretion of hydroxyhexamide (an active metabolite) | Unestablished | Theoretically postulated interaction due to structural similarity to phenylbutazone |
| Thiazide diuretics | Impaired glucose tolerance | Decreased insulin release; reduced tissue responsiveness | Moderate | Often reversible with potassium replacement |
| **Chlorpropamide with:** | | | | |
| Alcohol | Disulfiram-like reaction; increased hypoglycemia | Inhibition of intermediary metabolism of alcohol; impaired gluconeogenesis | Moderate | Alcohol causes lesser disulfiram-like interactions with other sulfonylureas |
| Allopurinol | Increased hypoglycemic effect | Postulated competition for renal tubular secretion | Unestablished | Preliminary evidence suggests this interaction may be important in some patients |
| Chloramphenicol | Increased hypoglycemic effect | Impaired hepatic biotransformation | Moderate | |
| Clofibrate | Increased hypoglycemic effect | Postulated competition for renal tubular secretion | Probably minor | Clinical information is limited |
| Clonidine | Impaired response to hypoglycemia | Inhibition of catecholamine response | Unestablished | |
| Dicumarol | Increased hypoglycemic effect | Impaired hepatic biotransformation | Unestablished | |
| Metoprolol | Impaired response to hypoglycemia | Reduced glycogenolysis and peripheral warning signs related to catecholamine excess | Major | |

**Table 40.8 (Continued)**

| Drug Interaction | Effect | Mechanism | Clinical Significance | Comments |
|---|---|---|---|---|
| Probenecid | Increased hypoglycemic effect | Impaired renal tubular excretion of chlorpropamide | Moderate | Clinical information is limited |
| Propranolol | Impaired response to hypoglycemia | Reduced glycogenolysis and peripheral warning signs related to catecholamine excess | Major | |
| Salicylates | Increased hypoglycemic effect | Intrinsic hypoglycemic effect in some diabetic patients; displacement of chlorpropamide from serum proteins; impaired renal tubular secretion of chlorpropamide | Minor | Significant hypoglycemia has occasionally resulted |
| Thiazide diuretics | Impaired glucose tolerance | Decreased insulin release; reduced tissue responsiveness | Moderate | Often reversible with potassium replacement |
| Insulin with: | | | | |
| Alcohol | Increased hypoglycemic effect | Impaired gluconeogenesis | Moderate | Alcohol abusers may also be incapable of regular and accurate insulin self-administration |
| Clonidine | Impaired response to hypoglycemia | Inhibition of normal catecholamine response | Unestablished | Extrapolated from reported interactions involving the oral hypoglycemic agents |
| Metoprolol | Impaired response to hypoglycemia | Reduced glycogenolysis and peripheral warning signs related to catecholamine excess | Major | |
| Propranolol | Impaired response to hypoglycemia | Reduced glycogenolysis and peripheral warning signs related to catecholamine excess | Major | |
| Thiazide diuretics | Impaired glucose tolerance | Reduced tissue responsiveness | Moderate | Often reversible with potassium replacement |
| Tolbutamide with: | | | | |
| Alcohol | Increased hypoglycemic effect (acute); decreased hypoglycemic effect (chronic) | Decreased gluconeogenesis; accelerated hepatic biotransformation of tolbutamide (chronic) | Moderate | Minor disulfiram-like reaction may also occur |
| Anabolic steroids | Increased hypoglycemic effect | Inhibition of hepatic biotransformation by methandrostenolone (but not other agents); possible intrinsic hypoglycemic effect in some diabetic patients | Minor | Possible interactions with other oral hypoglycemic agents have not been tested |

**Table 40.8** (Continued)

| Drug Interaction | Effect | Mechanism | Clinical Significance | Comments |
|---|---|---|---|---|
| Chloramphenicol | Increased hypoglycemic effect | Impaired hepatic biotransformation | Moderate | |
| Clonidine | Impaired response to hypoglycemia | Inhibition of normal catecholamine response | Unestablished | |
| Dicumarol | Increased hypoglycemic effect | Impaired hepatic biotransformation | Unestablished | |
| Metoprolol | Impaired response to hypoglycemia | Reduced glycogenolysis and peripheral warning signs related to catecholamine excess | Major | |
| Phenylbutazone | Increased hypoglycemic effect | Displacement of tolbutamide from serum proteins; impaired hepatic biotransformation | Major | Severe hypoglycemia has been reported in a small number of patients; however the incidence of significant interaction is unknown |
| Propranolol | Impaired response to hypoglycemia | Reduced glycogenolysis and peripheral warning signs related to catecholamine excess | Major | |
| Rifampin | Possible decreased hypoglycemic effect | Accelerated hepatic biotransformation | Minor | |
| Salicylates | Increased hypoglycemic effect | Intrinsic hypoglycemic effect in some diabetic patients; displacement of tolbutamide from serum proteins | Minor | Significant hypoglycemia has occasionally resulted |
| Sulfinpyrazone | Increased hypoglycemic effect | Displacement of tolbutamide from serum proteins; impaired hepatic biotransformation | Unestablished | Theoretically postulated interaction due to structural similarity to phenylbutazone |
| Sulfonamides | Increased hypoglycemic effect | Impaired hepatic biotransformation; displacement of tolbutamide from serum proteins (sulfaphenazole) | Moderate | Significant interaction only with sulfaphenazole and sulfamethizole |
| Thiazide diuretics | Impaired glucose tolerance | Decreased insulin release; reduced tissue responsiveness | Moderate | Often reversible with potassium replacement |

987

**Table 40.9  Drug Interactions Involving Antihyperlipidemic Agents**

| Drug Interaction | Effect | Mechanism | Clinical Significance | Comments |
|---|---|---|---|---|
| Cholestyramine (and colestipol) with: | | | | |
| Digitalis | Decreased serum digoxin and digitoxin levels | Decreased absorption due to intraluminal physicochemical binding | Moderate | Minimized by separating administration by several hours |
| Levothyroxine | Decreased serum thyroxine level | Decreased absorption due to intraluminal physicochemical binding | Moderate | Minimized by separating administration by several hours |
| Thiazide diuretics | Decreased diuretic effect | Decreased absorption due to intraluminal physicochemical binding | Unestablished | Minimized by separating administration by several hours |
| Warfarin | Decreased hypoprothrombinemic effect | Decreased absorption due to intraluminal physicochemical binding | Moderate | Minimized by separating administration by several hours |
| Clofibrate with: | | | | |
| Furosemide | Increased effects of both clofibrate and furosemide | Mutual displacement from serum proteins | Minor | Significant effects reported only in patients with hypoalbuminemia |
| Warfarin | Increased hypoprothrombinemic effect | Displacement of warfarin from serum proteins; increased affinity of hepatic receptor sites for warfarin; impaired hepatic biotransformation | Major | Less important in patients with normal serum lipids or hyperlipidemia unresponsive to clofibrate |
| Dextrothyroxine with: | | | | |
| Warfarin | Increased hypoprothrombinemic effect | Increased affinity of hepatic receptor sites for warfarin; possible increased catabolism of vitamin K-dependent coagulation factors | Major | |

**Table 40.10  Drug Interactions Involving Sedatives and Narcotics ***

| Drug Interaction | Effect | Mechanism | Clinical Significance | Comments |
|---|---|---|---|---|
| **Barbiturates with: *†** | | | | |
| Corticosteroids | Decreased corticosteroid effects | Accelerated hepatic biotransformation | Moderate | |
| Digitoxin | Decreased serum digitoxin level | Accelerated hepatic biotransformation | Moderate | Important only during chronic barbiturate therapy; no effect on digoxin elimination |
| Phenothiazines | Increased sedative effects (acute); decreased phenothiazine effects (chronic) | Additive sedative effects (acute); accelerated hepatic biotransformation (chronic) | Moderate | |
| Rifampin | Decreased barbiturate effects | Accelerated hepatic biotransformation | Moderate | |
| Tricyclic antidepressants | Decreased antidepressant effects | Accelerated hepatic biotransformation | Moderate | |
| **Chloral Hydrate with: *** | | | | |
| Furosemide | Vasomotor instability | Unknown | Unestablished | |
| Warfarin | Transiently increased hypoprothrombinemic effect | Displacement of warfarin from serum proteins by trichloracetic acid (a chloral hydrate metabolite) | Minor | Alternative agents (e.g., flurazepam) are recommended |
| **Chlordiazepoxide with: *** | | | | |
| Phenytoin | Increased serum phenytoin level | Impaired hepatic biotransformation | Major | Important only during chronic phenytoin therapy |

**Table 40.10** (Continued)

| Drug Interaction | Effect | Mechanism | Clinical Significance | Comments |
|---|---|---|---|---|
| Diazepam with: Phenytoin | Increased serum phenytoin level | Impaired hepatic biotransformation | Major | Important only during chronic phenytoin therapy |
| Ethchlorvynol *,† | | | | |
| Flurazepam * | | | | |
| Glutethimide *,† | | | | |
| Meprobamate *,† | | | | |
| Methaqualone *,† | | | | |
| Meperidine with: * Monamine oxidase inhibitors | Variable central nervous system excitation and depression | Impaired hepatic biotransformation of meperidine; altered cerebral serotonin concentrations | Major | Coma and death may rarely occur; MAO inhibitor effects may persist for 14 days; alternative analgesics (e.g., morphine) are recommended |
| Methyprylon *,† | | | | |
| Morphine * | | | | |

* Combined therapy with other central nervous system depressants may cause excessive sedation, hypotension or respiratory depression. Directly additive depressant effects may occur with antihistamines, alcohol, antidepressants, phenothiazines, sedative-hypnotics, minor tranquilizers and narcotic analgesics.
† Barbiturates (especially phenobarbital) and related drugs may potentially alter the pharmacokinetics of any drug dependent on hepatic microsomal enzymes for biotransformation.

serum proteins, but significant complications due to this effect have not been reported.[135] This agent has also been associated with apparent vasomotor instability in patients treated with furosemide, although the mechanism of this interaction has not been established.[104]

Diazepam and chlordiazepoxide are among the many drugs capable of inhibiting phenytoin metabolism.[54] Limited use of these agents in the Coronary Care Unit is unlikely to appreciably alter phenytoin pharmacokinetics, although more chronic use may lead to increased serum drug levels. Except for effects that are additive with other central nervous system depressants, the benzodiazepines are not known to be involved in any other clinically important drug interactions.

Drug interactions involving commonly used sedatives and narcotic analgesics are summarized in Table 40.10.

## ACKNOWLEDGMENT

The authors wish to express their appreciation to Bruce Cromer for his assistance in the preparation of this chapter.

## REFERENCES

1. Koch-Weser J: Drug interactions in cardiovascular therapy. Am Heart J 90:93, 1975.
2. Smith JW, Seidl LG, Cluff LE: Studies on the epidemiology of adverse drug reactions V. clinical factors influencing susceptibility. Ann Intern Med 65:629, 1966.
3. Manninen V, Melin J, Apajalahti A, Karesoja M: Altered absorption of digoxin in patients given propantheline and metoclopramide. Lancet 1:398, 1973.
4. Manninen V, Apajalahti A, Simonen H, Reissell P: Effect of propantheline and metoclopramide on absorption of digoxin. Lancet 1:1118, 1973.
5. Brown DD, Juhl RP: Decreased bioavailability of digoxin due to antacids and kaolin-pectin. N Engl J Med 295:1034, 1976.
6. Brown DD, Juhl RP, Warner SL: Decreased bioavailability of digoxin due to hypocholesterolemic interventions. Circulation 58:164, 1978.
7. Bazzano G, Bazzano GS: Digitalis intoxication. Treatment with a new steroid-binding resin. JAMA 220:828, 1972.
8. Solomon HM, Abrams WB: Interactions between digitoxin and other drugs in man. Am Heart J 83:277, 1972.
9. Lindenbaum J, Maulity RM, Butler VP: Inhibition of digoxin absorption by neomycin. Gastroenterology 71:399, 1976.
10. Juhl RP, Summers RW, Guillory JK, Claug SM, Cheng FH, Brown DD: Effect of sulfasalazine on digoxin bioavailability. Clin Pharmacol Ther 20:387, 1976.
11. Lahari K, Ertel N: Mechanism of diphenylhydantoin induced decrease in serum digoxin levels (abstr). Clin Res 22:321A, 1974.
12. Storstein L, Janssen H: Studies on digitalis. VI. The effect of heparin on serum protein binding of digitoxin and digoxin. Clin Pharmacol Ther 20:15, 1976.
13. Leahey EB Jr, Reiffel JA, Drusin RE, Heissenbuttel RH, Lovejoy WP, Bigger JT Jr: Interaction between quinidine and digoxin. JAMA 240:533, 1978.
14. Ejvinsson G: Effect of quinidine on plasma concentrations of digoxin. Br Med J 1:279, 1978.
15. Leahey EB Jr, Giardina E-GV, Reiffel JA, Bigger JT Jr: Serum digoxin concentrations during quinidine and procainamide administration (abstr). Circulation (suppl II) 57,58:101, 1978.
16. Straub KD, Kane JJ, Bissett JK, Doherty JE: Alteration of digitalis binding by quinidine: A mechanism of digitalis-quinidine interaction (abstr). Circulation (suppl II) 57,58:58, 1978.
17. Solymoss B, Toth S, Varga S, Selye H: Protection by spironolactone and oxandrolone against chronic digitoxin or indomethacin intoxication. Toxicol Appl Pharmacol 18:586, 1971.
18. Steiness E: Renal tubular secretion of digoxin. Circulation 50:103, 1974.
19. Phillips AP: The improvement of specificity of radioimmunoassays. Clin Chim Acta 44:333, 1973.
20. Weintraub M: Interpretation of the serum digoxin concentration. Clin Pharmacokinet 2:205, 1977.
21. Steiness E: Suppression of renal excretion of digoxin in hypokalemic patients. Clin Pharmacol Ther 23:511, 1978.
22. Semple P, Tilstone WJ, Lawson DH: Furosemide and urinary digoxin clearance (letter). N Engl J Med 293:612, 1975.
23. Brown DD, Dormois JC, Abraham GN, Lewis K, Dixon K: Effect of furosemide on the renal

excretion of digoxin. Clin Pharmacol Ther 20:395, 1976.

24. Tilstone WJ, Semple PF, Lawson DH, Boyle JA: Effects of furosemide on glomerular filtration rate and clearance of practolol, digoxin, cephaloridine, and gentamycin. Clin Pharmacol Ther 22:389, 1977.

25. Malcolm AD, Leung FY, Tuchs JCA, Duarte JE: Digoxin kinetics during furosemide administration. Clin Pharmacol Ther 21:567, 1977.

26. Edmonds CJ, Jasani B: Total-body potassium in hypertensive patients during prolonged diuretic therapy. Lancet 2:8, 1972.

27. Brater DC, Morrelli HF: Digoxin toxicity in patients with normokalemic potassium depletion. Clin Pharmacol Ther 22:21, 1977.

28. Szekely P, Wynne NA: Effects of calcium chelation on digitalis-induced cardiac arrhythmias. Br Heart J 25:589, 1963.

29. Dowdy EG, Fabian LW: Ventricular arrhythmias induced by succinylcholine in digitalized patients: A preliminary report. Anesth Analg 42:501, 1963.

30. Dowdy EG, Duggar PN, Fabian LW: Effect of neuromuscular blocking agents on isolated digitalized mammalian hearts. Anesth Analg 44:608, 1965.

31. Lown B, Ehrlich L, Lipschultz B, Blake J: Effect of digitalis in patients receiving reserpine. Circulation 24:1185, 1961.

32. Soffer A: Digitalis intoxication, reserpine, and double tachycardia. JAMA 191:173, 1965.

33. Heinonen J, Takki, S, Jarho L: Plasma lidocaine levels in patients treated with potential inducers of microsomal enzymes. Acta Anaesthesiol Scand 14:89, 1970.

34. Benowitz N, Forsyth RP, Melmon KL, Rowland M: Lidocaine disposition kinetics in monkey and man. II. Effects of hemorrhage and sympathomimetic drug administration. Clin Pharmacol Ther 16:99, 1974.

35. Branch RA, Shand DG, Wilkinson GR, Nies AS: The reduction of lidocaine clearance by dl-propranolol: An example of hemodynamic drug interaction. J Pharmacol Exp Ther 184:515, 1973.

36. Harrah MD, Way WL, Katzung BG: The interaction of d-tubocurare with antiarrhythmic drugs. Anesthesiology 33:406, 1970.

37. Usubiaga JE, Wikinski JA, Morales RL, Usubiaga LEJ: Interaction of intravenously administered procaine, lidocaine, and succinylcholine in anesthetized subjects. Anesth Analg 46:39, 1967.

38. Kessler KM, Lowenthal DT, Warner H, Gibson T, Briggs W, Reidenberg MM: Quinidine elimination in patients with congestive heart failure or poor renal function. N Engl J Med 290:706, 1974.

39. Gerhardt RE, Knouss RF, Thyrum PT, Luchi RJ, Morris JJ Jr: Quinidine excretion in aciduria and alkaliuria. Ann Intern Med 71:927, 1969.

40. Gibaldi M, Grundhofer B, Levy G: Effects of antacids on pH of urine. Clin Pharmacol Ther 16:520, 1974.

41. Dreifus LS, deAzevedo IM, Watanabe Y: Electrolyte and antiarrhythmic drug interaction. Am Heart J 88:95, 1974.

42. Cuthbert MF: The effect of quinidine and procaine amide on neuromuscular blocking action of suxamethonium. Br J Anaesthesiol 38:775, 1966.

43. Miller RD, Way WL, Katzing BG: The potentiation of neuromuscular blocking agents by quinidine. Anesthesiology 28:1036, 1967.

44. Koch-Weser J: Quinidine-induced hypoprothrombinemic hemorrhage in patients on chronic warfarin therapy. Ann Intern Med 68:511, 1968.

45. Udall JA: Quinidine and hypoprothrombinemia (letter). Ann Intern Med 69:403, 1968.

46. Weily HS, Genton E: Pharmacokinetics of procainamide. Arch Intern Med 130:366, 1972.

47. Mark LC, Kayden HJ, Steele JM, Cooper JR, Berlin I, Rovenstine EA, Brodie BB: The physiological disposition and cardiac effects of procainamide. J Pharmacol Exp Ther 102:5, 1951.

48. Drayer DE, Lowenthal DT, Woosley RL, Nies AS, Schwartz A, Reidenberg MM: Cumulation of N-acetylprocainamide, an active metabolite of procainamide, in patients with impaired renal function. Clin Pharmacol Ther 22:63, 1977.

49. Elson J, Strong JM, Lee W-K, Atkinson AJ Jr: Antiarrhythmic potency of N-acetylprocainamide. Clin Pharmacol Ther 17:134, 1975.

50. Dreyfuss J, Bigger JT, Cohen AI, Schreiber EC: Metabolism of procainamide in rhesus monkey and man. Clin Pharm Ther 13:366, 1972.

51. Roe RF, Podosin RL, Blaskovics ME: Drug interaction: Diazoxide and diphenylhydantoin. Pediatrics 87:480, 1975.

52. Petro DJ, Vannucci RC, Kulin HE: Diazoxide-diphenylhydantoin interaction (letter). Pediatrics 89:331, 1976.

53. Kristensen M, Hansen JM, Skovsted L: The influence of phenobarbital on the half-life of

diphenylhydantoin in man. Acta Med Scand 185:347, 1969.

54. Vajda FJE, Prineas RJ, Lovell RRH: Interaction between phenytoin and the benzodiazepines (letter). Br Med J 1:346, 1971.

55. Andreasen PB, Frøland A, Skovsted L, Andersen SA, Hauge M: Diphenylhydantoin half-life in man and its inhibition by phenylbutazone: The role of genetic factors. Acta Med Scand 193:561, 1973.

56. Kutt H, Winters W, McDowell FH: Depression of parahydroxylation of diphenylhydantoin by antituberculosis chemotherapy. Neurology 16:594, 1966.

57. Hansen JM, Kristensen M, Skovsted L, Christensen LK: Dicoumarol-induced diphenylhydantoin intoxication. Lancet 2:265, 1966.

58. Kutt H, McDowell F: Management of epilepsy with diphenylhydantoin sodium. Dosage regulation for problem patients. JAMA 203:969, 1968.

59. Jubiz W, Merkle AW, Levinson RA, Mizutani S, West CD, Tyler FH: Effect of diphenylhydantoin on the metabolism of dexamethasone. N Engl J Med 283:11, 1970.

60. Petereit LB, Merkle AW: Effectiveness of prednisolone during phenytoin therapy. Clin Pharmacol Ther 22:912, 1977.

61. Wassner SJ, Pennisi AJ, Malekzadeh MH, Fine RN: The adverse effects of anticonvulsant therapy on renal allograft survival. J Pediatr 88:134, 1976.

62. Hansen JM, Siersback-Nielsen K, Kristensen M, Skovsted L, Christensen LK: Effect of diphenylhydantoin on the metabolism of dicoumarol in man. Acta Med Scand 189:15, 1971.

63. Oppenheimer JH, Tavernetti RR: Studies on the thyroxine-diphenylhydantoin interaction: Effects of 5,5'-diphenylhydantoin on the displacement of L-thyroxine from thyroxine-binding globulin (TBG). Endocrinology 71:496, 1962.

64. Fulop M, Widrow DR, Colmers RA, Epstein EJ: Possible diphenylhydantoin-induced arrhythmia in hypothyroidism. JAMA 196:454, 1966.

65. Kotler MN, Berman L, Rubenstein AH: Hypoglycemia precipitated by propranolol. Lancet 2:1389, 1966.

66. Abramson EA, Arley RA, Woeber KA: Effects of propranolol on the hormonal and metabolic responses to insulin-induced hypoglycemia. Lancet 2:1386, 1966.

67. Vestal RE, Kornhauser DM, Hollifield JW, Shand DG: Inhibition of propranolol metabolism by chlorpromazine. Clin Pharmacol Ther 1:19, 1979.

68. Nies AS, Shand DG: Hypertensive response to propranolol in a patient treated with methyldopa: A proposed mechanism. Clin Pharmacol Ther 14:823, 1973.

69. Norris FH Jr, Colella J, McFarlin D: Effects of diphenylhydantoin on neuromuscular synapse. Neurology 14:869, 1964.

70. Rozen MS, Whan FMcK: Prolonged curarization associated with propranolol. Med J Aust 1:467, 1972.

71. Anon: Bretylium (Bretylol) for ventricular arrhythmias. Med Lett Drugs Ther 20:105, 1978.

72. Nickerson M, Collier B: Drugs inhibiting adrenergic nerves and structures innervated by them. In: The Pharmacologic Basis of Therapeutics. 5th ed. Goodman LS, Gilman A, editors. MacMillan, New York, 1975, pp 553–559.

73. Mitchell JR, Oates JA: Guanethidine and related agents. I. Mechanism of selective blockade of adrenergic neurons and its antagonism by drugs. J Pharmacol Exp Ther 172:100, 1970.

74. Dollery CT: Physiological and pharmacological interactions of hypertensive drugs. Proc Roy Soc Med 58:983, 1965.

75. Mulheims GH, Entrup RW, Paiewonsky D, Mierzwiak DS: Increased sensitivity of the heart to catecholamine-induced arrhythmias following guanethidine. Clin Pharmacol Ther 6:757, 1965.

76. Sneddon JM, Turner P: Ephedrine mydriasis in hypertension and the response to treatment. Clin Pharmacol Ther 10:64, 1969.

77. Dorrell W: Tranylcyromine and intracranial bleeding. Lancet 2:414, 1963.

78. Hirsch MS, Walter RM, Hasterlik RJ: Subarachnoid hemorrhage following ephedrine and MAO inhibitors. JAMA 194:1259, 1965.

79. Horler AR, Wynne NA: Hypertensive crisis due to pargyline and metaraminol. Br Med J 2:460, 1965.

80. Elis J, Laurence DR, Mattie H, Prichard BNC: Modification by monamine oxidase inhibitors of the effect of some sympathomimetics on blood pressure. Br Med J 2:75, 1967.

81. Marley E, Blackwell B: Interactions of monamine oxidase inhibitors, amines, and food stuffs. Adv Pharmacol Chemother 8:226, 1970.

82. Hunter KR, Boakes AJ, Laurence DR, Stern GM: Monamine oxidase inhibitors and l-dopa. Br Med J 3:388, 1970.

83. Cuthbert MF, Greenberg MP, Moreley SW:

Cough and cold remedies: A potential danger to patients on monamine oxidase inhibitors. Br Med J 1:404, 1969.

84. Raisfeld IH: Cardiovascular complications of antidepressant therapy. Interactions at the adrenergic neuron. Am Heart J 83:129, 1972.

85. Cooper JR, Bloom FE, Roth RH: The Biochemical Basis of Neuropharmacology. 3rd ed. Oxford University Press, New York 1978. p. 177.

86. Eggers GWN, Corssen G, Allen CR: Comparison of vasopressor responses in the presence of phenothiazine derivatives. Anesthesiology 20:261, 1959.

87. Espelin DE, Done AK: Amphetamine poisoning: Effectiveness of chlorpromazine. N Engl J Med 278:1361, 1968.

88. Katz RL, Epstein RA: The interaction of anesthetic agents and adrenergic drugs to produce cardiac arrhythmias. Anesthesiology 29:763, 1968.

89. Formgren H: The effect of metoprolol and practolol on lung function and blood pressure in hypertensive patients. Br J Clin Pharmacol 3:1007, 1976.

90. Anon: Metoprolol (Lopressor). Med Lett Drugs Ther 20:97, 1978.

91. Ober KF, Wang RIH: Drug interactions with guanethidine. Clin Pharmacol Ther 14:190, 1973.

92. Meyer JF, McAllister CK, Goldberg LI: Insidious and prolonged antagonism of guanethidine by amitriptyline. JAMA 213:1487, 1970.

93. Janowsky DS, El-Yousef MK, Davis JM, Fann WE: Antagonism of guanethidine by chlorpromazine. Am J Psych 130:808, 1973.

94. Fann WE, Janowsky DS, Davis JM, Oates JA: Chlorpromazine reversal of the hypertensive action of guanethidine. Lancet 2:436, 1971.

95. Oates JA, Fann WE, Cavanaugh JH: Effect of doxepin on the norepinephrine pump. Psychosomatics 10:12, 1969.

96. Westervelt FB Jr, Atuk NO: Methyldopa-induced hypertension (letter). JAMA 227:557, 1974.

97. White AG: Methyldopa and amitriptyline. Lancet 2:441, 1965.

98. Kale AK, Satoskar RS: Modification of the central hypotensive effect of alpha-methyldopa by reserpine, imipramine and tranylcypromine. Eur J Pharmacol 9:120, 1970.

99. Mitchell JR, Cavanaugh JH, Arias L, Oates JA: Guanethidine and related agents. III. Antagonism by drugs which inhibit the norepinephrine pump in man. J Clin Invest 49:1596, 1970.

100. Kofman O: Treatment of Parkinson's disease with l-dopa: A current appraisal. Can Med Assoc J 104:483, 1971.

101. Hansten PD: Drug Interactions. 3rd ed. Lea and Febiger, Philadelphia, 1975, p 79.

102. Gibberd FB, Small E: Interaction between levodopa and methyldopa. Br Med J 2:90, 1973.

103. Sweet RD, Lee JE, McDowell FH: Methyldopa as an adjunct to levodopa treatment of Parkinson's disease. Clin Pharmacol Ther 13:23, 1972.

104. Anon: Adverse interactions of drugs. Med Lett Drugs Ther 21:5, 1979.

105. Briant RH, Reid JL, Dollery CT: Interaction between clonidine and desipramine in man. Br Med J 1:522, 1973.

106. Sjoqvist F: Interaction between monamine oxidase (MAO) inhibitors and other substances. Proc Roy Soc Med 58:967, 1965.

107. Markee S: The effects of monamine oxidase inhibitors on the hypotensive action of meperidine and the pressor action of norepinephrine. Anesthesiology 28:261, 1967.

108. Adnitt PI: Hypoglycemic action of monamine oxidase inhibitors (MAOI). Diabetes 17:628, 1968.

109. McCurdy RL, Kane FJ: Transient brain syndrome as a non-fatal reaction to combined pargyline imipramine therapy. Am J Psychiatry 121:397, 1964.

110. Schuckit M, Robins E, Feighner J: Tricyclic antidepressants and monamine oxidase inhibitors. Arch Gen Psychiatry 24:509, 1971.

111. Kanzal PC, Buse J, Buse MG: Thiazide diuretics and control of diabetes mellitus. South Med J 62:1374, 1969.

112. Fajans SS, Floyd JC Jr, Knopf RF, Rull J, Guntsche EM, Conn JW: Benzothiadiazine suppression of insulin release from normal and abnormal islet tissue in man. J Clin Invest 45:481, 1966.

113. Field JB, Mandell S: Effects of thiazides on glucose uptake and oxidation of rat muscle and adipose tissue. Metabolism 13:959, 1964.

114. Rapoport MI, Hurd HF: Thiazide-induced glucose intolerance treated with potassium. Arch Intern Med 113:405, 1964.

115. Honari J, Blair AD, Cutler RE: Effects of probenecid on furosemide kinetics and natriuresis in man. Clin Pharmacol Ther 22:395, 1977.

116. Homeida M, Roberto C, Branch RA: Influence

of probenecid and spironolactone on furosemide kinetics and dynamics in man. Clin Pharmacol Ther 22:402, 1977.

117. Elliott HC: Reduced adrenocortical steroid excretion rates in man following aspirin administration. Metabolism 11:1015, 1962.

118. Tweeddale MG, Ogilire RI: Antagonism of spironolactone-induced natriuresis by aspirin in man. N Engl J Med 289:198, 1973.

119. Singer I, Rotenberg D: Mechanisms of lithium action. N Engl J Med 289:254, 1973.

120. Petersen V, Hvidt S, Thomsen K, Schou M: Effect of prolonged thiazide treatment on renal lithium clearance. Br Med J 3:143, 1974.

121. Hurtig HI, Dyson WL: Lithium toxicity enhanced by diuresis (letter). N Engl J Med 290:748, 1974.

122. Laventurier MF, Talley RB: The incidence of drug-drug interactions in a Medi-Cal population. Calif Pharm 11:18, 1972.

123. Hull JH, Murray WJ, Brown HJ, Williams BO, Chi SL, Koch GG: Potential anticoagulant drug interactions in ambulatory patients. Clin Pharmacol Ther 24:644, 1978.

124. Koch-Weser J, Sellers EM: Drug interactions with coumarin anticoagulants. N Engl J Med 285:487,547, 1971.

125. Robinson DS, Benjamin DM, McCormack JJ: Interaction of warfarin and nonsystemic gastrointestinal drugs. Clin Pharmacol Ther 12:491, 1971.

126. Ambre JJ, Fisher LJ: Effect of coadministration of aluminum and magnesium hydroxides on absorption of anticoagulants in man. Clin Pharmacol Ther 14:231, 1973.

127. Aggeler PM, O'Reilly RA, Leong L, Kowitz PE: Potentiation of anticoagulant effect of warfarin by phenylbutazone. N Engl J Med 276:496, 1967.

128. Bull J, MacKinnon J: Phenylbutazone and anticoagulant control. Practitioner 215:767, 1975.

129. Udall JA: Drug interference with warfarin therapy. Clin Med 77:20, 1970.

130. Fox S: Potentiation of anticoagulants caused by pyrozole compounds. JAMA 188:320, 1964.

131. Henry RA, Wosilait WD: Drug displacement of warfarin from human serum albumin: A fluorometric analysis. Toxicol and Applied Pharmacol 33:267, 1975.

132. Vesell ES, Passananti GT, Johnson AO: Failure of indomethacin and warfarin to interact in normal human volunteers. J Clin Pharmacol 15:486, 1975.

133. Self TH, Evans WE, Ferguson T: Drug enhancement of warfarin activity. Lancet 2:557, 1975.

134. Sellers EM, Koch-Weser J: Kinetics and clinical importance of displacement of warfarin from albumin by acidic drugs. Ann NY Acad Sci 179:213, 1971.

135. Sellers EM, Koch-Weser J: Potentiation of warfarin-induced hypoprothrombinemia by chloral hydrate. N Engl J Med 283:827, 1970.

136. Sellers EM, Koch-Weser J: Displacement of warfarin from human albumin by diazoxide, and ethacrynic, mefenamic and nalidixic acids. Clin Pharmacol Ther 11:524, 1970.

137. Petrick RJ, Kronacher N, Alcena V: Interaction between warfarin and ethacrynic acid. JAMA 231:843, 1975.

138. Udall JA: Clinical implications of warfarin interactions with five sedatives. Am J Cardiol 35:67, 1975.

139. MacDonald MG, Robinson DS, Slywester D, Jaffe JJ: The effects of phenobarbital, chloral betaine and glutethimide administration on warfarin plasma levels and hypoprothrombinemic responses in man. Clin Pharmacol Ther 10:80, 1969.

140. Hansen JM, Siersbaek-Nielsen K, Skovsted L: Carbamazepine-induced acceleration of diphenylhydantoin and warfarin metabolism in man. Clin Pharmacol Ther 12:539, 1971.

141. O'Reilly RA: Interaction of chronic daily warfarin therapy and rifampin. Ann Intern Med 83:506, 1975.

142. Romankiewicz JA, Ehrman M: Rifampin and warfarin: A drug interaction. Ann Intern Med 82:224, 1975.

143. O'Reilly RA: Interaction of sodium warfarin and disulfiram (Antabuse) in man. Ann Intern Med 78:73, 1973.

144. Kazmier FJ: A significant interaction between metronidazole and warfarin. Mayo Clin Proc 51:782, 1976.

145. Rosenthal AR, Self TH, Baber ED, Linden RA: Interaction of isoniazid and warfarin. JAMA 238:2177, 1977.

146. Vesell ES, Passananti GT, Greene FE: Impairment of drug metabolism in man by allopurinol and nortriptyline. N Engl J Med 283:1484, 1970.

147. Christensen LK, Skovsted L: Inhibition of drug metabolism by chloramphenicol. Lancet 2:1397, 1969.

148. Koch-Weser J: Hemorrhagic reactions and

drug interactions in 500 warfarin-treated patients (abstr). Clin Pharmacol Ther 14:139, 1973.

149. Lumholtz B, Siersbaek-Nielsen K, Skovsted L, Kampmann J, Mølholm-Hansen J: Sulfamethizole-induced inhibition of diphenylhydantoin, tolbutamide and warfarin metabolism. Clin Pharmacol Ther 17:731, 1975.

150. Hassall CM, Feetam CL, Leach RH, Meynell MJ: Potentiation of warfarin by co-trimoxazole. Lancet 2:1155, 1975.

151. Errick JK, Keys PW: Co-trimoxazole and warfarin: Case report of an interaction. Am J Hosp Pharm 35:1399, 1978.

152. O'Reilly RA, Motley CH: Racemic warfarin and trimethoprim-sulfamethoxazole interaction in humans. Ann Intern Med 91:34, 1979.

153. Sioris LJ, Weibert RT, Pentel PR: Potentiation of warfarin anticoagulation by sulfisoxazole. Arch Intern Med (in press).

154. Oliver MF, Roberts SD, Hayes D, Pantridge JF, Suzman MM, Bersohn L: Effect of atromid and ethyl chlorophenoxyisobutyrate on anticoagulant requirements. Lancet 1:143, 1963.

155. Schrogie JJ, Solomon HM: The anticoagulant response to bishydroxy-coumarin. II. The effect of D-thyroxine, clofibrate and norethandrolone. Clin Pharmacol Ther 8:70, 1967.

156. Furman RH, Howard RP, Alaupovic P: Serum-lipid reducing agents and anticoagulant requirements (letter). Lancet 1:893, 1963.

157. Corrigan JJ Jr, Marcus FI: Coagulopathy associated with vitamin E ingestion. JAMA 230:1300, 1975.

158. McLaughlin GE, McCarty DJ, Segal DL: Hemarthrosis complicating anticoagulant therapy. JAMA 196:202, 1966.

159. Robinson BHB, Hawkins JB, Ellis JE, Moore-Robinson M: Decreased anticoagulant tolerance with oxymetholone. Lancet 1:1356, 1971.

160. Longridge RGM, Gillam PMS, Barton GMG: Decreased anticoagulant tolerance with oxymetholone. Lancet 2:90, 1971.

161. Edwards MS, Curtis JR: Decreased anticoagulant tolerance with oxymetholone. Lancet 2:221, 1971.

162. Solomon HM, Schrogie JJ: Change in receptor site affinity: A proposed explanation for the potentiating effect of d-thyroxine on the anticoagulant response to warfarin. Clin Pharmacol Ther 8:797, 1967.

163. O'Reilly RA, Aggler PM: Determinants of the response to the oral anticoagulant drugs in man. Pharmacol Rev 22:35, 1970.

164. O'Reilly RA: Impact of aspirin and chlorthalidone on the pharmacokinetics of oral anticoagulants in man. Ann NY Acad Sci 179:123, 1971.

165. Flind AC: Cimetidine and oral anticoagulants (letter). Lancet 2:1054, 1978.

166. Silver BA, Bell WR: Cimetidine potentiation of the hypoprothrombinemic effect of warfarin. Ann Intern Med 90:348, 1979.

167. Haworth E, Burroughs AK: Disopyramide and warfarin interaction. Br Med J 2:866, 1977.

168. Levy G, Lampam T, Kamath B, Garrettson LK: Decreased serum salicylate concentrations in children with rheumatic fever treated with antacids. N Engl J Med 293:323, 1975.

169. Pascale LR, Dubin A, Bronski D, Hoffman WS: Inhibition of the uricosuric action of benemid by salicylate. J Lab Clin Med 45:771, 1955.

170. Yu TF, Dayton PG, Gutman AB: Mutual suppression of the uricosuric effects of sulfinpyrazone and salicylate: A study in interactions between drugs. J Clin Invest 42:1330, 1963.

171. Liegler DG, Henderson ES, Hahn MA, Oliverio VT: The effect of organic acids on renal clearance of methotrexate in man. Clin Pharmacol Ther 10:849, 1969.

172. Seltzer HS: Drug-induced hypoglycemia: A review based on 473 cases. Diabetes 21:955, 1972.

173. Wishinsky H, Glasser EJ, Perkal S: Protein interactions of sulfonylurea compounds. Diabetes (suppl) 11:18, 1962.

174. Stowers JM, Constable LW, Hunter RB: Clinical and pharmacological comparison of chlorpropamide and other sulfonylureas. Ann NY Acad Sci 74:689, 1959.

175. Kaegi A, Pineo GF, Shimizu A, Trivedi H, Hirsh J, Gent M: Arterio-venous-shunt thrombosis. Prevention by sulfinpyrazone. N Engl J Med 290:304, 1974.

176. Anturane. Product information. Geigy Pharmaceuticals, 1978.

177. Christensen LK, Hansen JM, Kristensen M: Sulfaphenazole-induced hyperglycaemic attacks in tolbutamide-treated patients. Lancet 2:1298, 1963.

178. Field JB, Ohta M, Boyle C, Remer A: Potentiation of acetohexamide hypoglycemia by phenylbutazone. N Engl J Med 277:889, 1967.

179. Kirstensen M, Hansen JM: Accumulation of chlorpropamide caused by dicoumarol. Acta Med Scand 183:83, 1968.

180. Kristensen M, Hansen JM: Potentiation of the tolbutamide effect by dicoumarol. Diabetes 16:211, 1967.

181. Petitpierre B, Perin L, Rudhardt M: Behavior

of chlorpropamide in renal insufficiency and under the effect of associated drug therapy. Int J Clin Pharmacol 6:120, 1972.

182. Gupta KK: The anti-diabetic action of guanethidine. Postgrad Med J 45:455, 1969.

183. Kauffman RE, Azarnoff DL: Effect of colestipol on gastrointestinal absorption of chlorothiazide in man. Clin Pharmacol Ther 14:886, 1973.

184. Northcutt RC, Stiel JN, Hollifield JW, Stant EG Jr: The influence of cholestyramine on thyroxin absorption. JAMA 208:1857, 1969.

185. Bridgeman BF, Rosen SM, Thorp JM: Complications during clofibrate treatment of nephrotic-syndrome hyperlipoproteinemia. Lancet 2:506, 1972.

186. Eade NR, Renton KW: Effect of monamine oxidase inhibitors on N-demethylation and hydrolysis of meperidine. Biochem Pharmacol 19:2243, 1970.

187. Carlsson A, Lindquist M: Central and peripheral monaminergic membrane pump blockade by some addictive analgesics and antihistamines. J Pharm Pharmacol 21:460, 1969.

188. Rogers KJ: Role of brain monamines in the interaction between pethidine and tranylcypromine. Eur J Pharmacol 14:86, 1971.

189. London DR, Milne MD: Dangers of monamine oxidase inhibitors (letter). Br Med J 2:1752, 1962.

# 41 | Medical–Legal Problems in the Coronary Care Unit

## Douglas R. Reynolds, J.D.

In the beginning of a discussion of laws and legal principles as they apply to health care professionals in the Coronary Care Unit (CCU), it is important to include an explanation of the sources of these laws and legal principles. In addition, some insight into the practical application of these concepts is vital to understanding them. Members of the legal and health care professions are notoriously poor at communicating with each other. This frequently stems from the failure of one group to understand the practicalities of the other group's profession.

For example, the nonmedical person with little exposure to the diagnostic process frequently fails to understand the significance of the history and the role of clinical judgment in arriving at a diagnosis. Often, a patient (or an attorney making a legal evaluation of the quality of his client's medical care) will want black and white answers based on tests, x-ray studies, and other objective criteria, ignoring the importance of the other less objective but vitally important foundations of the diagnosis.

Similarly, physicians are often impatient with attorneys who do not give definite answers to questions or who are reluctant to attempt to predict (with any assurance) the outcome of a particular legal situation.

Once it is explained to the nonmedical person that in many cases the history may be the most important part of a diagnosis and the reasons for this importance explained, the person will usually approach the medical profession with a better understanding and more confidence. So, too, when the practical workings of the legal system, as it applies to health care professionals, are explained, it is hoped that greater confidence in the legal system, or at least more patience, will be the result.

Law, in the general sense, does not stem from any single source, but is a set of principles that creates rights and obligations in regard to various subjects. With regard to the medical profession, as is generally the case, the "law" is derived from three basic sources.

The three sources are: statutes, which are written laws enacted by legislative bodies; case law or decisional law, which is based on written opinions or decisions of appellate courts interpreting either written laws or historic principles of law known as precedents; and, administrative regulations, which are rules promulgated by administrative bodies, such as the Social Security Administration or the Internal Revenue Service.

On a practical level, the three basic sources intermingle. A statute written by a legislature attempts to set out a legal principle as a guide for regulating the relationships of individuals or organizations. When a dispute as to the effect or applicability of a written statute occurs, the matter is taken to court. Many statutes are subject to varying interpretations, and the interpretation placed on a written statute by an appellate court has the effect of establishing which interpretation will be accepted and thereafter have the force and effect of "law." Therefore, in order to understand the "official" meaning of a written statute, the person seeking to interpret it must be aware of any court decisions that have defined terms in the statute or otherwise interpreted its meaning.

Appellate court decisions are also made in areas where no written statute applies. Long lines of appellate court decisions on certain subjects have value as precedent and establish the "law" in the absence of legislative pronouncement. The legal definition of the "standard of care" applicable to health care providers is an example of this type of law in most states.

Administrative regulations are subject to interpretation by agencies that administer the regulations and also, under certain circumstances, to interpretation by the appellate court system. Thus, to properly interpret an administrative regulation one must read it, attempt to understand it, be aware of any interpretations placed upon it by the appropriate regulatory body, and, finally, know of any court decisions that have dealt with the particular regulation.

Another feature of the legal system that should be kept in mind is the variance among jurisdictions. Each state in our country operates according to an independent set of laws and regulations. Obviously, the legislatures of each of the states are independent of one another and, subject only to the constraint of the Constitution of the United States, are free to pass laws that are at variance with those of their sister states. The appellate court systems of each state are likewise independent and, again subject to constitutional restraints, need not follow the appellate court opinions from any other state.

Even within the Federal court system, the various "Circuit" Courts of Appeal may have differing decisional rules on the same subject. Until the Supreme Court has decided an issue in a certain way, a citizen in Texas operating out of the Fifth Circuit Court of Appeal may be subject to one rule, and a citizen of California, in the Ninth Circuit, to an opposite rule.

It is important to keep jurisdictional variations in mind when considering any statement as to what the "law is." Although the proposition may be a true statement in 45 states, other rules may apply in the remaining five.

Another extremely important concept to keep in mind with respect to the law is the concept of change. As in medicine, where new learning may lead to the rejection of a widely accepted doctrine, an accepted rule of law may change drastically with substantial impact.

Obviously, legislatures may pass new laws or repeal old ones. When this happens, important changes usually receive publicity and the effect is usually prospective.

Decisional changes, where appellate courts "reverse themselves," may have great impact, since these decisions by their very nature are usually retroactive.

A good example of the operation of this type of change in the law is afforded by the California experience with the doctrine of law that concerns the right of a husband or wife to recover money damages for the loss of services of an injured spouse.

Between 1958 and 1960, the California Supreme Court was faced with claims concerning the spouses of injured persons for damages in their own right, based on their loss of services, including companionship, sexual enjoyment, and related matters. After evaluating the claims, the California Supreme Court ruled that there should be no legal right to recovery on the part of the noninjured spouse, no matter how they might be affected by the injury.[1]

Thereafter, for a period of 14 years, no matter how severely injured a person's husband or wife was, the uninjured spouse was unable to make a valid claim for the loss. During that period, claims for money damages in personal injury and professional liability cases were evaluated with this law in mind by attorneys and insurance companies alike.

In 1974, however, the California Supreme Court in the case of *Rodriguez v. Bethlehem Steel*[2] reversed its field and ruled that the right to recover for such a loss would be recognized. The Court ruled that the decision would apply to any case that had not gone to trial before the effective date of the decision and overnight created thousands of substantial claims for money damages that had been nonexistent at the time the injuries were actually suffered.

In the *Rodriguez* case itself, which was tried a second time after the Supreme Court decision, the wife of a severely injured steel worker was awarded $500,000.00 for loss of services of her husband after having been correctly turned down under the law that existed at the first trial.[3]

Attorneys are aware of this type of change and must always realize, when advising a client, that no matter how correct the advice is when given, the law may change by the time the client comes to court or when the advice otherwise must take effect.

The effect of this type of far-reaching court decision can be compared to a referee in a football game declaring at half-time that forward passes are subject to a 15-yard penalty and then applying it to all the plays that have occurred during the first half.

This discussion of some of the uncertainties and difficulties in ascertaining what law governs a particular transaction is not to suggest that the system is a poor one or does not work. The system can and does work, but any discussion of legal problems must be considered in the light of the way in which the system functions.

## SELECTED MEDICAL-LEGAL PROBLEMS

Medical-legal problems arise in a wide array of subject areas with no particular interrelationship between the problems. The source of most medical-legal problems is, of course, the relationship between the patient and the health care professionals and institutions involved in patient care.

Professional negligence, or malpractice, is the medical-legal problem that probably first comes to any health care professional's mind. Simply stated, professional negligence involves a failure to measure up to the "standard of care"—the legal duty required of a professional in caring for a patient.

Another frequent medical-legal problem revolves around the right of the patient to control his care through consent to or refusal of a particular treatment. Problems in this area involve consent to treatment in the first instance, the question of informed consent to a particular treatment or procedure, and problems revolving around a patient's refusal of certain treatment,

including the refusal of lifesaving efforts or extraordinary means to prolong life. Physicians and personnel in the CCU are also faced with the question of termination of care in "hopeless" cases.

Underlying the entire range of problems relating to the patient's consent and intertwined with the patient's right to refuse to accept certain treatment is a progressively deepening concern for certain rights of the patient, such as freedom of choice and the right to privacy.

The interrelationship between health care professionals, such as physicians, surgeons, nurses, and technicians, as well as the institution in which health care is provided gives rise to a range of legal problems, including problems in malpractice cases as well as other aspects of medicine.

The personnel in a CCU see a large number of emergency situations and critically ill patients. Greater numbers of health care professionals become involved in patient care than is the rule in other areas of most hospitals. These characteristics of the CCU place emphasis on certain problems. With seriously ill patients, the result of faulty care, whether through the administration of improper treatment or the failure to institute proper or timely treatment, can result in significant detriment to the patient.

The nature of the CCU lends itself to frequent problems involving treatment of patients by nonphysicians in emergency settings, such as defibrillation or administration of medication to a patient without a specific order from a physician.

Some of the special procedures performed in the CCU again highlight the problem of "informed consent."

### Negligence

The medical-legal problem of most concern to health care professionals is probably professional negligence or "malpractice." In all jurisdictions in this country, patients may sue physicians, hospitals, and other medical personnel if they feel that they have been injured by negligent treatment. Every physician or health care professional is held by the law to a certain "standard of care" or standard of practice in the care of patients. Failure to meet this standard resulting in harm or injury to a patient may give rise to liability for money damages.[4] Persons working in areas where the chances of an unhappy result are high are particularly subject to claims of malpractice.

It is safe to say that many claims of "malpractice" are based on a poor result rather than improper treatment. Also, claims are frequently seen where there is admittedly some defect in the treatment without any real effect on the outcome of the patient's course. In neither of the above classes of case is legal liability on the part of the health care professional involved. Neither a bad result nor improper treatment that does not result in harm to the patient is properly the basis for a valid claim of malpractice. In any discussion of medical negligence, the concomitant requirements—negligence and resulting harm—must be kept in mind.

The first step in understanding the concept of medical negligence is a definition of the "standard of care." In almost every jurisdiction, the standard of care legally required by a physician or other health care professional consists of three basic concepts. First, the health care professional must have the level of skill and training ordinarily possessed by a similar individual performing the same basic type of care.[5] Many jurisdictions also impose a "locality rule;" that is, the health care professional must possess the level of skill and learning ordinarily possessed in the particular locality involved. The more enlightened jurisdictions have discarded strict adherence to the locality rule.[6]

The second concept is that the physician or health care professional must exercise the same level of skill and care ordinarily exercised by reputable members of the profession under the same or similar circumstances.[7]

The third concept incorporates the recognition that medicine promises neither perfection nor uniformity in its practice. Poor results or errors in judgment do not necessarily constitute negligence.[8] Similarly, failure to use a particular method of diagnosis or treatment, where more than one is accepted, is not negligence.

As a practical matter, litigation challenging the level of the knowledge or training of physicians is rarely encountered and the overwhelming number of claims focus upon the application of the physician's care and skill to a particular case. The level of care and training of nonphysician health care providers is, however, a frequent issue in litigation.

Defining the standard of care as that level of care ordinarily provided under the same or similar circumstances can easily lead to the conclusion that the standard of care can be determined by simply establishing the "majority rule." Many physicians employed by attorneys as expert witnesses in professional negligence cases will defend their opinion that some particular course of treatment fell below the standard of care by stating that they are sure the large majority of physicians in the community would have proceeded differently.

The legal definition of the standard of care, however, recognizes that there may be more than one course of treatment, method of diagnosis, or diagnosis in any particular case.

In California, in addition to the basic definition, jurors in medical negligence cases are instructed as follows:

> Where there is more than one recognized method of diagnosis or treatment, and no one of them is used exclusively and uniformly by all practitioners of good standing, a physician and surgeon is not negligent if, in exercising his best judgment, he selects one of the approved methods, which later turns out to be a wrong selection, or one not favored by certain other practitioners.[9]

Also included within the third component of the standard of care required of a health care professional is the concept that perfection is not required. In addition to the above-quoted statement, if it is appropriate to the particular case being tried, California juries are instructed as follows:

> A physician and surgeon is not negligent merely because his efforts were unsuccessful, he makes a mistake, or he errs in judgment in the matter for which he is engaged.
> However, if the physician and surgeon was negligent as defined in these instructions, it is not a defense that he did the best he could.[10]

Basically, then, the concept of standard of care requires that the physician or other health care professional proceed in a manner that is acceptable medical practice even though some others would have proceeded in a different fashion, used a different procedure, or arrived at a different diagnosis.

By way of illustration, with particular reference to the Cardiac Care Unit, a particular case history should be useful.

The case involved a 50-year-old male patient who complained to his wife of unspecified but rather severe chest pains. Becoming alarmed, his wife took him to the local emergency room where he gave the emergency room physician a history of having split some wood the previous day and described the chest pains as being in the area of his right back and shoulder. The physician examined the patient, ordered an ECG, which he interpreted as normal, and concluded that the patient had musculoskeletal pain. The patient was discharged home. The following day, the ECG was read by the hospital's cardiologist as a routine matter. The interpretation was as follows: "Record shows rather prominent junctional type depression in V3–4 and more suspicious type depression and straightening in V5. These changes are nondiagnostic."

This information was not specifically communicated to the emergency room physician. The patient, who had returned home, died of an acute myocardial infarction at approximately the time the cardiologist was interpreting the ECG. A lawsuit was filed against the emergency room physician, the hospital, and the cardiologist.

The claims against the cardiologist were twofold. It was claimed that he misreported the ECG and that, given his interpretation, he should have taken steps to ascertain the disposition of the patient and communicated the information to a treating physician.

The case was sent to several outside cardiologists for review, several of whom concluded that the reported interpretation of the ECG was below the required standard of care. Among the interpretations by the consulting cardiologists were:

1. "ST and T wave abnormalities compatible with inferior apical myocardial ischemia and/ or digitalis effect."

2. "Abnormal record with ST and T wave changes of subendocardial ischemia, possibly active. These changes could also be associated with the administration of digitalis and electrolyte imbalance."

From a legal standpoint, the interpretations of the various cardiologists, including the defendant, were considered virtually identical. However, the language of the interpretations led to disagreement among the physicians. The physicians who were critical of the defendant cardiologist were adamant that he should have listed the possible causes of the changes noted in the ECG in his report and that a failure to do so was a violation of the standard of care. However, other consulting cardiologists felt that the description by the defendant cardiologist was acceptable and was, in their opinion, within the standard of care. Interestingly, when the case finally went to trial, the cardiologist who testified against the defendant was not critical of the interpretation of the electrocardiogram or the description of it on the report.

The significance of this case from the standpoint of the interpretation and reporting of the electrocardiogram is that there is room for reasonable variance within the legal standard of care. Those physicians who felt that the report failed to meet the standard of care probably did not fully comprehend the flexibility within the legal definition of that term and were probably applying a more restrictive standard than the law imposes.

The second contention against the physician in this case serves to illustrate another area of the law of medical negligence that is frequently overlooked.

The claim that the physician should have communicated his findings to some treating physician instantly upon reading the electrocardiogram may or may not have some validity in the abstract. However, in the case under discussion, the fact that the patient died either before the ECG was read or so close to that time that there was no chance to be of benefit to the patient renders the failure to communicate the findings legally insignificant. Since there was no opportunity to help the patient, the failure to communicate the findings could in no way have harmed the patient and there could be no liability on the part of the physician.

A medical malpractice case is not a penalty for poor medical practice. There must be harm as a direct result of the failure to meet the standard of care or there is no civil liability.

A simple analogy may serve to illustrate this point. A physician who fails to meet the standard of care without harming a patient may be vulnerable to some administrative or staff remedies designed to improve future patient care. Similarly, a driver who fails to stop at a stop sign or red light may be cited by a police officer. In neither instance, however, is the person liable to any third party for money damages unless personal injury is a result of the transgression.

## Informed Consent

In any setting where seriously ill patients are seen, or where potentially hazardous procedures are performed, the issue of informed consent is particularly important. The law of informed consent varies from jurisdiction to jurisdiction, but in every area there is at least a basic requirement that the patient consent to treatment.

Historically, any treatment by health care providers that involved touching a patient without first obtaining the patient's consent was regarded as a technical "battery." [11] In English common law a battery was defined as any intentional offensive contact with the person of another without his consent. While medical treatment hardly fits the popular conception of a battery, there was for years no other legal rubric under which unauthorized medical care could be placed.

Most jurisdictions still use the "technical battery" theory for totally unauthorized treatment. [12] Since consent to treatment in the first instance can be express or implied, and since most patients are aware of treatment, it is quite unusual to find a claim being made merely because the patient was treated at all. The most common type of claim in this area is found in a situation where a patient consents to one type of treatment or operation and the physician or surgeon performs a totally different type. For example, in a case where a female patient consented to surgery solely for the repair of a hernia, she was granted recovery on a theory of a "technical battery" when the surgeon removed both ovaries. [13]

In situations where a patient consented to treatment but had not been informed by the physician of significant risks associated with the procedure, courts initially allowed recovery on the same battery theory. However, courts in various states became uncomfortable with the artificiality of the theory and began to consider other rationales for the requirement that a patient be informed not only of the fact of treatment itself, but also the risks that might be associated with it.

Today, the majority of jurisdictions impose upon the health care professional the duty to advise a patient of the significant risks of proposed treatments and view a failure to meet this duty as a breach of the basic standard of care to be applied. Thus, a failure to properly inform a patient is, in most areas, a form of professional negligence. [14]

There are enormous difficulties in applying this concept. The primary one is in determining with some degree of precision how far a physician must go in informing a patient. The basic rule is simple and cannot be quarreled with: the patient should be told enough to enable him to make an intelligent decision as to whether or not to undergo the proposed therapy. However, in the case of a patient about to undergo coronary angiography, is it legally sufficient for the physician to advise the patient that he or she may die or must the physician go through a long list of the other possible adverse consequences?

Some jurisdictions compound the difficulty by decreeing that if a common procedure involves relatively minor risks, which are commonly understood to be remote, there is no duty to inform the patient of them nor of the remote possibility of death or serious bodily injury. However, if the procedure is more complicated, the physician must discuss with the patient any risks of serious injury or death. [15]

No attempt has been made by the courts in California to draw the dividing line between common procedures or more complicated ones, nor has there been any quantification by way of percentages or otherwise as to what constitutes a remote risk of death or serious injury. The best that can be said is to repeat that the patient must be given enough information about the risks inherent in any particular procedure to make an intelligent decision as to whether to consent.

The saving grace in connection with informed consent is that, as with any other form of negligence, there must be a causal connection between the failure to inform and any resulting harm. Thus, if one of the risks inherent in a procedure materializes, the patient cannot recover against the physician unless the patient proves that had he or she been informed of that particular risk, the procedure would have been refused. Actually, the test is not whether the patient, having experienced the complication, would have consented to the treatment, but whether the average, reasonable, hypothetical patient, having been informed of the significant risks, under all the circumstances, would have agreed to the treatment.[16]

An interesting reverse twist in the area of informed consent was recently presented in a California Appellate Court decision. In a case entitled *Truman v. Thomas,*[17] a patient was advised by her physician to undergo a cervical smear. The patient refused to undergo the procedure even though the physician recommended it repeatedly. Later the patient was diagnosed as having advanced uterine cancer and died shortly thereafter. The patient's family sued, and among the theories presented as a basis for liability of the physician involved was that the physician had a duty to inform his patient of the risks involved and the consequences that could be envisioned if the patient refused the recommendation. The Court ruled that the physician did not have a duty to go into this kind of detail and that the patient's family did not have a valid claim against the physician under these circumstances.

The Court drew a distinction between the duty of a physician who has recommended some form of treatment to the patient, to disclose to the patient information sufficient for an intelligent choice, and the situation presented in the case. On this matter the Court said:

> To require a doctor, under pain of malpractice at the hands of a lay jury, routinely to deliver a dissertation regarding the potential adverse consequences of failure to take a recommended test, would degrade and demean both doctor and patient, treating both as dolts who lack even the most elementary respect for one-another's intelligence and judgment. We therefore hold that ordinarily there is no duty on the part of a physician to advise of the dangers of failure to submit to a test or course of treatment he recommends.[18]

Under the circumstances presented in the above case, the outcome and denial of the patient's right to successfully pursue a claim against the physician seems reasonable. However, in many cases the "standard of care" probably does require that a physician make a recommendation, with enough emphasis, so that the patient may be aware of the consequences of refusing treatment (see Addendum).

For example, there would seem to be a fundamental difference between the recommendation of a cervical smear and the recommendation of more complex and technical treatment, such as the use of a pacemaker or complicated drug therapy. If a patient with a severe rhythm disturbance were to refuse a physician's recommendation that a pacemaker be implanted and drug therapy instituted, it would surely behoove the physician to explain the risk the patient was undertaking by refusing this therapy. The "standard of care" among physicians faced with these circumstances would undoubtedly require, at the very least, an explanation that the procedures and therapy recommended were much less hazardous than the possible outcome if the arrhythmia were left untreated.

In the case referred to above, the Court recognized that there were definite exceptions to the rule regarding "informed refusal" and stated: "Everything, of course, is not as simple as a Pap smear, and there are doubtless occasions . . . where a doctor, along with recommended treatment, should undertake affirmatively to warn against the dangers of failing to take it. But that requirement is limited to situations dictated by the standard of practice in the medical community, according to expert testimony." [19]

Still another area where patient freedom of choice comes into play and one that will undoubtedly play a greater and greater role in CCUs throughout the country is the patient's right to refuse to accept the use of extraordinary means to prolong life. Although some of the underlying questions are common to the discussion below relating to termination of life-support systems, the physician and other health care providers are faced with a different conceptual approach when it is the patient who has requested or directed that no extraordinary means to prolong life be used or that life-support systems in use be withdrawn.

Physicians, particularly those in a CCU, face critical dilemmas in situations involving this freedom of choice by the patient.

A lucid patient who is terminally or gravely ill may direct his physician not to use artificial means to prolong life in the event of a potentially fatal crisis. Similarly, a lucid patient who is being maintained on such systems may direct that the physician discontinue them.

Still another situation presents even more troubling problems to the physician. A patient with severe, irreparable, and advancing coronary artery disease may be neither acutely ill nor "terminal" in the popular sense, but may wish to direct his physician that in the event of a life-threatening crisis no artificial means to prolong life or heroic measures be taken.

A physician in one of the above situations is faced with the threat of civil liability if his decision, under the circumstances, fails to meet the "standard of care" of other physicians in his specialty or in his community. In certain traditional and conservative geographic regions, a physician who acceded to a patient's request would run a grave risk of liability or perhaps even criminal prosecution, while in other areas of the country the decision would be accepted more easily.

California, in attempting to deal with this situation, has enacted the so-called Natural Death Act.[20] That act is based on a legislative finding that adult persons have a fundamental right to control the decisions relating to their own medical care, including decisions concerning life-sustaining procedures in the case of a terminal condition. The act has prescribed a procedure whereby a patient may issue a directive to withhold or withdraw a life-sustaining procedure.

The legislation, which is quite technical and designed to protect the patient as well as the physician, basically provides that an adult person may execute a document directing the withholding or withdrawal of life-sustaining procedures in the event a condition is terminal. A terminal condition under the act is basically defined as an "incurable condition caused by injury, disease, or illness," which regardless of treatment will produce death, and where life-sustaining procedures "serve only to postpone the moment of death of the patient." [21] The directive must be signed by the patient in the presence of two witnesses who are not heirs nor blood nor marital relatives and neither the patient's physician, employees of the physician, or the health facility in which the patient is being treated, nor any creditor, may be a witness.[22] A particular form is prescribed by the legislature on which a person may either sign the directive in advance of being diagnosed as terminal or may execute it after 14 days have passed since the terminal diagnosis.[23]

Directives may be revoked by any number of acts on the part of the patient and are good for a period of 5 years. A physician or health care facility giving effect to such a directive is insulated from civil and criminal liability and charges of unprofessional conduct.[24]

The burden is placed on the attending physician to determine that the directive complies with the appropriate code sections and is in full force and effect.

The California act, although subject to criticism on philosophic, moral, or ethical bases, and perhaps in some of its administrative procedures, is at least a step in attempting to assist physicians and other health care providers in determining when they may give effect to a patient's desires in the above-mentioned situations. Certainly this act will be of great interest to the personnel working on a daily basis in a CCU. It may be expected that other states will enact legislation dealing with the same issues.

## Cessation or Withholding of Life-Support Systems in a Comatose Patient

Related conceptually to the above discussion is the question frequently faced in a CCU as to when it would be permissible to remove life-support systems from a patient with extensive, irreversible brain injury or to fail to use such methods on a patient who has, in the judgment of the physician, suffered such an injury.

Where a patient has made such a choice, either in advance of need or following a diagnosis of a terminal illness, the physician giving effect to the choice may be comforted in that the will of the patient is being carried out. At least some of the moral questions surrounding decisions of this nature have been solved by the patient. However, a different problem is presented following an acute episode, such as a myocardial infarction or cerebrovascular accident, which leaves an incompetent or comatose patient.

A physician who undertakes to care for a patient has the duty to continue to use his or her best efforts to sustain the patient's life or health during the period of employment. When a patient becomes irreversibly comatose and requires life-sustaining equipment to survive, the question of the physician's duty is a difficult one. It has been debated in legal circles whether the withdrawal of life-support systems can actually constitute homicide on the part of the physician. Some legal authorities have proposed that a homicide can only be committed by an affirmative action on the part of a person, and therefore failure to provide life-support equipment to maintain life would not be homicide.[25] Logically, however, removal of existing equipment might be considered an affirmative act and could be homicide under this analysis. In order to avoid the difficulties of this approach, some commentators have advocated a solution that physicians only be required to provide "ordinary" care for patients with severe conditions incompatible with life without mechanical aids.[26]

The famous case of Karen Quinlan, which was eventually decided by the New Jersey Superior Court, involved many of the problems alluded to in this section. Faced with a diagnosis of severe brain damage and with medical testimony to the effect that Miss Quinlan was a victim of "brain death," viable only through the means of her life-support systems, her parents, as her legal guardians, requested that the life-support systems be withdrawn and that she be allowed to die. Over much opposition, the New Jersey Superior Court ruled that the patient, through her guardians, could enforce the request to have the systems withdrawn.[27]

It is interesting to note that the underlying rationale of this decision is remarkably similar to the rationale of the California Natural Death Act, that is, the "choice" of the patient. Since the daughter was unable to make a choice, the New Jersey court ruled that the parents were making the choice for her.

The case is also a good example of the difficulty faced in situations of this kind, since upon the removal of the life-support systems Miss Quinlan's circulatory and respiratory systems remain functional to this time.

A great many of the problems faced by physicians in connection with the brain-damaged patient as an end result of complications of cardiac disease (as well as other forms of pathology) have been lessened by the gradual change in the legal definition of death by a great number of states. Traditionally, the legal definition of death related to the circulatory system and basically stated that a patient with an intact circulatory system and functioning heart was "alive."[28] With the advent of organ transplants and more sophisticated monitoring and measuring devices, this standard was challenged and serious legal questions arose. For example, an individual in one case suffered a severe injury from a bullet wound that virtually destroyed the brain. He was utilized as an organ donor but because of intact circulation at the time the heart was removed, the person who shot him attempted to blame the physicians for his death.[29]

Because of cases such as this, legal authorities came to question whether the "circulatory" definition of "life" was a satisfactory one, and a search for an alternative ensued. This search lead to the adoption by a number of states of the so-called "brain death" standard to augment the more traditional and customary procedures for determining death. One such standard, contained in California's Health and Safety Code §7180, provides:

> A person shall be pronounced dead if it is determined by a physician that the person has suffered a total and irreversible cessation of brain function. There shall be independent confirmation of the death by another physician.
>
> Nothing in this chapter shall prohibit a physician from using other usual and customary procedures for determining death as the exclusive basis for pronouncing a person dead.

Other states have enacted similar laws. Among them are Alaska, Kansas, Maryland, New Mexico, Virginia, and West Virginia.[30] Thus, in those states where the appropriate diagnosis is made, the patient can be pronounced dead and life-support systems withdrawn, even when the heart is beating or the circulation is intact.

## LEGAL RELATIONSHIPS BETWEEN THE MEMBERS OF THE CCU TEAM

In a CCU, which may involve participation in patient care by a wide range of physicians, nurses, technicians, and auxillary personnel, the relationships between the personnel give rise to a number of important legal questions. These may relate to legal responsibility for the acts of others on the CCU team, such as the liability of a physician for the acts of a nurse or technician, or the hospital for the acts of a staff or outside physician. Also, they may involve the division of legal liability among members of the CCU team in a malpractice situation.

### Legal Responsibility for the Acts of Another

The law imposes responsibility on an individual for the consequences of his or her own acts. In the medical setting, a physician, nurse, vocational nurse, technician, orderly, or other person involved in patient care who negligently injures a patient is responsible for that injury. In certain circumstances, however, the acts of one individual may become the legal responsibility of another individual or an organization.

A simple example is a hospital's responsibility for the acts of its employees. A hospital can only act through the individuals it employs or has the power to direct. Thus, where an employee of a hospital acts in the course and scope of his employment, that act is said to be the act of the hospital.[31] A nurse, employed by a hospital, who turns off or detaches a cardiac monitor on a patient critically ill with an acute myocardial infarction clearly falls below the required standard of care. If the patient is harmed, the hospital is subject to liability for the nurse's acts. The same is true for any other regular employee of the hospital, including house staff.

The problems in determining liability among persons working in the hospital setting occur when there is not a clear cut employer-employee relationship or where, although the relationship is clearly not that of employer-employee, the right of one person to control another is involved.

An example of the first such ambiguous situation involves the so-called "independent contractors," such as radiologists or anesthesiologists who, although not employed by the hospital, perform virtually all of their work on the hospital premises and may even maintain their offices and billing facilities on hospital premises.

In many instances when independent contractors, such as these physicians, are alleged to have negligently injured a patient, an attempt is made to hold the hospital responsible for their acts. Such attempts have not usually been successful across the country, although there are a few instances in which courts have imposed liability on hospitals based on the acts of an individual who normally would have been an independent contractor.[32]

Under traditional legal analysis, the key difference between an employer-employee relationship and one where the person is acting as an independent contractor is the control exercised by the employer over the method by which the work is done. Hospitals do not normally control the methods used by an anesthesiologist or radiologist in performing their professional duties, and this is usually the basis for classifying them as independent contractors. However, professionals, whether they be nurses, therapists, or technicians, must perform the most important parts of their work in accordance with professional standards rather than minute-to-minute or day-to-day supervision by hospital administrative personnel. Even outside physicians performing in a hospital are subject to some rules and regulations.

This area of the law includes a gray area that may see future changes. In an era where many physicians are going without insurance coverage, it would not be surprising to find that in the future courts will consider them to be employees of the hospital for purposes of imposing liability. This would be especially likely for physicians who maintain their offices at a hospital.

Another gray area in the law of the relationships between physicians and auxillary personnel, such as in a CCU setting, involves problems engendered by the doctrine popularly known as the "Captain of the Ship." [33]

The Captain of the Ship doctrine, which goes by several other names, such as the "Borrowed Servant Rule" [34] or the "Special Employee Rule," [35] is basically a product of the operating room. Because the surgeon was historically said to be in "absolute" control during surgery, many jurisdictions held the surgeon responsible for the acts or omissions of any of the operating room personnel during the course of surgery. This did not necessarily free the individual from responsibility from his or her negligence, but imposed liability for the negligence of nurses and other operating room personnel on the physician, who was usually more financially responsible.

One of the major historic reasons for the development of this rule may have been that until approximately 20 years ago, a large majority of the hospitals in this country were immune from liability for the acts of their employees under the doctrines of governmental or charitable immunity. The doctrine of governmental immunity stated that some governmental institutions, such as hospitals, could not be held liable for most of the wrongful acts of their employees.[36] A similar rule applied to charitable institutions.[37] With the abolition of these immunities and imposition of liability on both charitable institutions and governmental entities, the need for a rule imposing liability on a physician for the acts of a nurse seems to have run its course.

A distinction must be made between the above cases and cases where a nurse follows a physician's order, which results in harm to the patient. In this type of case, the physician's responsibility is primary, and a nurse substantially following the order would usually not be found to be negligent. However, under the classic application of the "Captain of the Ship" doctrine, a surgeon could incur liability where a nurse improperly and negligently attempts to carry out an order in the operating room, even when the physician did not know of the impropriety and had no reasonable means of discovering it before the patient was harmed.

The Captain of the Ship rule has been eroded away in some jurisdictions, first by freeing the surgeon from liability for the acts of independent physicians in the room, such as the anesthesiologist.[38] Recently, a more realistic approach has been taken with courts ruling that a physician should only be responsible for the acts of an assistant where he directs the harmful act himself or where he is aware of the pending harmful act and does not use his authority to prevent it.

The application of the Captain of the Ship rule to the CCU in a nonsurgical setting is not merely of academic interest. The Captain of the Ship rule has been struck down in at least one jurisdiction [39] and has been infrequently applied in many others. The rule may also be questioned on sound intellectual grounds. Nevertheless, some jurisdictions still apply it and more give lip service to the rule. As more and more sophisticated techniques and procedures involving the services of a number of persons come into use in the CCU, it can be expected that there will be serious attempts to analogize the situation to the operating room and attempts made to impose liability on the head of the team for the acts of other members.

As an example of this, cases have occurred, during catheterization of a patient, involving malfunctions of the radiology equipment due to alleged negligence of the technical personnel. The procedures have been aborted, to be repeated at a later date. When complications occurred during the second procedure, the claim was made that the physician in charge of the catheterization was responsible for the alleged negligence of the technicians operating the equipment. This attempt at imposition of liability has not been officially approved by any lawmaking body as an extension of the Captain of the Ship doctrine, but the possibility that it could be extended is a real one.

In fact, the present status of the Captain of the Ship doctrine is a good example of the role change plays in the legal system. At this point, the law may well follow the direction chosen by some courts and abolish the unwarranted imposition of liability by the rule. However, other courts could extend the rule beyond the traditional confines of the operating room. As nonsurgeons become more and more involved in performing "team" procedures on critically ill patients with one physician in basic overall charge of the members of the group, the cardiologist may join the cardiac surgeon and incur legal responsibility for others on the team.

## DIVISION OR APPORTIONMENT OF LIABILITY

A subject related to the discussion just completed concerns situations where a number of health care professionals are charged with negligence in the same action. The typical malpractice complaint contains allegations of negligence against several physicians, a hospital, and perhaps other defendants. The other defendants may include nurses, technicians, manufacturers of equipment, drug companies, and perhaps even independent contracting firms performing such services as respiratory or physical therapy. When a number of defendants are sued and more than one of the defendants is ultimately found to be responsible for injury to a patient, the question of how to apportion the damages or fault arises. It is a rare case where numerous defendants are sued and the patient is successful against all of them. However, it is not uncommon at all for several defendants in the health care profession to be held responsible for a single injury to a patient.

There are three basic approaches toward resolving the situation where two or more defendants are held liable to a patient. The oldest solution and one that has all but been discarded in this country is that a patient entitled to a judgment against two or more defendants may collect the money from whichever defendant or defendants he or she desires without further recourse by the defendant who pays. As an example of this, if a doctor and hospital were held jointly liable to a patient for damages in the sum of $20,000.00, the patient would have the choice of collecting the entire sum from the physician, from the hospital, or in any combination from both. Under the traditional rule, neither the hospital nor the physician would have any choice in the matter and neither defendant could seek reimbursement of any amount from the other.[40]

A more modern approach, which is by far the majority rule today, utilizes a pro-rata split where two or more defendants are held liable to the same patient.

Using this approach, if a hospital, a surgeon, and an anesthesiologist were held liable to the same patient in the sum of $30,000.00, the pro-rata share of each would be $10,000.00, regardless of the fault involved or the degree to which any one of the three defendants contributed to the patient's injury. The patient would still have the option of collecting the entire judgment from any one of the defendants. However, with this approach a defendant paying more than his pro-rata share may seek reimbursement for the excess from the other defendants, under the doctrine known as "contribution."[41] For example, if the above judgment were all collected from the hospital, the hospital would then be entitled to seek $10,000.00 from the surgeon and the remaining $10,000.00 from the anesthesiologist. In the event that one of the defendants was unable to come up with the funds to pay his share the remaining defendants, rather than the patient, would bear the loss.

The third approach, which has only recently been developed, takes into consideration the degree of fault of the various defendants and attempts to apportion the dollar award accordingly.

In California in 1978, the Supreme Court

created what is known as "equitable partial indemnification" among codefendants in personal injury actions.[42] Simply stated, this means that in personal injury actions, including actions for medical malpractice, damages awarded against two or more defendants are apportioned according to fault.

The basic premise of the doctrine is just, but the practical application can become complicated.

An injured patient in a malpractice case may choose to sue any number of defendants he or she feels is responsible for injuries. The patient, likewise, may choose not to sue certain individuals who might arguably be partially responsible. Under the California rule, a defendant who has been sued may in turn file a lawsuit bringing additional persons before the Court for the purpose of "sharing the blame."

Once all the parties who are claimed to be at fault are before the Court, the first step is to determine how many, if any, of the defendants are liable. Once that preliminary question is decided, the question of apportionment among the defendants held responsible is reached.

To take a hypothetical case, if a jury were to find that a hospital, a cardiologist, and a radiologist were each partly responsible for injuries to a patient, the judge or jury trying the case would then determine the amount of damages to which the plaintiff was entitled. If, for example, that figure were $100,000.00, the judge or jury would then have to determine the proportional fault of each of the defendants found liable.

If the jury ruled that the hospital were 20 percent at fault, the cardiologist 60 percent at fault and the radiologist 20 percent at fault, the $100,000.00 figure would be apportioned by applying those percentages. As with the older rule of "contribution," the patient would still have the option to collect the entire $100,000.00 from any single defendant. If the hospital were to pay the entire $100,000.00, it would then be up to the hospital to seek $60,000.00 from the cardiologist and $20,000.00 from the radiologist in accordance with the percentages fixed at trial.

While the rule of apportioning damages appears more equitable than the older forms, which gave no consideration to the degree of fault involved, there are still problems that can result in substantial financial injustice with this system.

Because the plaintiff-patient has the choice of collecting the entire judgment from any particular defendant, as described above, it is obvious that the more financially responsible defendants are likely to be asked to pay the judgment in the first instance. In a situation where a physician is without insurance or substantial assets, or a hospital is insolvent, the apportionment according to fault may be meaningless, since the financially responsible defendant will be forced to pay and will have little or no recourse against the codefendants.

An example of this inequity can be seen in a situation where two physicians are sued by a patient with a resulting judgment against both of them in the sum of $100,000.00. The jury may assess the fault at 95 percent against the first physician and 5 percent against the second. However, if only the second physician is insured, the entire judgment would undoubtedly be collected from that physician's insurance carrier and unless the uninsured physician had substantial assets, the likelihood of the "fair share" being paid is slight. Thus, a physician who, according to the law, should have paid only $5,000.00 will be faced with the spectre of a $100,000.00 judgment on his record.

The significance of the various rules of apportionment of liability has impact in medical negligence litigation far beyond financial considerations. Where a number of health care professionals are sued in the same lawsuit, depending upon the rule in effect in the jurisdiction where the lawsuit is filed, there are many motivations to assist the patient in the lawsuit against codefendants or to "point the finger" at or attempt to increase the proportional share of fault of another health care provider.

A case history can serve here to illustrate the complexities of a multidefendant case.

The case involved a 36-year-old male with a history of several serious myocardial infarctions. The patient was evaluated by his family physician and a consulting cardiologist who referred him to a cardiac care center to be considered for bypass surgery. Upon evaluation by the cardiac surgeons and the center's cardiologists, and following angiograms and cineangiography, triple coronary bypass surgery was recommended.

The patient agreed and the surgery was performed by a well-trained surgical team with a cardiologist present in the operating room.

Immediately following surgery, chest radiographs were taken and revealed coiled linear densities in the area of the right pericardium, which were felt by the radiologist and the cardiac surgeon to be "pacing wires."

During the postoperative period, a series of chest radiographs were taken and reviewed by the surgeon, the cardiologist, and at least three radiologists. On each review, the coiled linear densities were seen and, when comments were made, the densities were described as "pacing wires."

The patient recovered from the surgery, but experienced a recurrence of symptoms, which lead to repeat cineangiography. These cineangiograms revealed that two of the three grafts were not patent and again showed the coiled linear densities in the area of the right pericardium.

The patient was referred to another cardiac center as a possible transplant candidate. Following a workup at that institution, a repeat triple bypass was performed at which time a surgical sponge was found on the surface of the patient's heart. On a subsequent review of all radiographs, including the repeat cineangiograms, the linear densities were clearly identified as radiopaque markers in the sponge.

The plaintiff-patient filed a lawsuit against the surgeon, the two assistant surgeons, the hospital, the three radiologists who had seen the films postoperatively, the cardiologist and the referring general practitioner.

In this case, it is easy to see how the defendants would have conflicting interests.

The hospital was responsible for the acts of the nurses in counting and in certifying the sponge count as correct. However, they could have argued that, had the physicians who reviewed the postoperative films appreciated the presence of the sponge, it could have been removed with little harm or inconvenience to the patient. Thus, the argument goes, even if the nurses are responsible for the sponge remaining in the patient, the damage should have been slight if the other physicians had correctly interpreted the films.

The surgeon and the assistant surgeon would, of course, argue that the nurses reported the sponge count as correct on two occasions and that surgeons are forced to rely on the nurses to perform their job and count sponges correctly.

The Captain of the Ship doctrine was invoked by the plaintiff, claiming that if the nurses erroneously counted the sponges, the surgeon would be responsible for the miscount. This puts additional pressure on the surgeon.

The surgeon also had a strong motive to blame the radiologists and he could have argued that as specialists, the radiologists have responsibility for the misinterpretation.

The radiologists, obviously, could turn this around and indicate that it would be the surgeon's function, together with the operating room nurses, to see that no sponges were left in the first place. The cardiologist could reasonably take the same position.

Given the conflicting interests and the different positions that can be taken, a case such as this one presents a strategic nightmare for the defendants. In the actual case, each of the defendants acknowledged his or her area of responsibility, making it largely unnecessary for the other defendants to attempt to shift responsibility away from themselves.

The hospital and the nurses accepted the responsibility for properly counting the sponges and acknowledged that if the sponges were miscounted it was the nurses who did it. The nurses testified that they followed accepted procedures, counted the sponges twice and informed the surgeon the count was correct. The surgeon indicated that he was in overall charge of the operating room and that it was his responsibility to see that all materials placed in the patient were removed before closing.

In defense of their failure to recognize the "coiled wires" as a sponge marker, the radiologists, the cardiologist, and the surgeon readily admitted that once it was pointed out to them that the density was a sponge marker, they could see it clearly. However, none of them had ever had occasion to see a sponge on an x-ray film before. This, combined with the presence of pacing wires that provided an explanation for the object on the film, caused each of them to fail to appreciate that what they were seeing was the sponge marker.

Since the patient suffered no demonstrable harm as a result of the sponge, and since there was no contention that the original grafts had closed off because of the presence of the sponge, and, probably, because of the lack of infighting among the various defendants, the jury in this case returned a verdict in favor of all defendants and no damages were awarded.

## CONCLUSION

The foregoing discussion of some selected medical-legal problems is obviously not intended as an exhaustive exposition of the law that relates to the medical profession or the CCU in particular. The discussion of several of the problems that can face physicians and auxillary personnel should serve to illustrate one basic feature of the medical-legal system that is not always appreciated by nonlawyers.

That feature is simply this: although the rules and regulations commonly called the law are extremely important, they act only as basic guidelines for governing any individual situation. The role of judgment and common sense is almost always the critical factor in determining what the proper course of action is in a situation or what the proper solution should be to a medical-legal problem.

When a complex and far-reaching legal system interacts with an equally complex and far-reaching medical system, conflicts and problems are bound to occur. Since perfection in either profession is beyond us, perfection in the interaction of the two professions is obviously impossible. However, if members of the medical profession understand the basic legal rules that apply, and approach these rules in a positive fashion with reasonable judgment, the end result will be a proper one in the overwhelming majority of situations.

## REFERENCES

1. Deshotel v. Atchison, Topeka & S.F. Ry. Co., (1958) 50 Cal.2d 664; West v. San Diego (1960) 54 Cal.2d 469.
2. (1974) 12 Cal.3d 382.
3. Rodriguez v. McDonnell Douglas Corp., (1979) 87 Cal.App.3d 626.
4. Landeros v. Flood (1976) 17 Cal.3d 399.
5. Wallach, *California Tort Guide* (2d ed.) p. 139.
6. Annos, 37 ALR 3d 420 (1971); 36 ALR 3d 440 (1971).
7. Sinz v. Owens (1949) 33 Cal.2d 749.
8. Huffman v. Lindquist (1951) 37 Cal.2d 465; Lawless v. Calaway (1944) 24 Cal.2d 81.
9. BAJI (6th ed.) No. 6.03.
10. BAJI (6th ed.) No. 6.02 (1977 Revision).
11. Berkey v. Anderson (1969) 1 Cal.App.3d 790; Corn v. French (1955) 71 Nev. 280; Gray v. Gunnagle (1966) 423 Pa. 144.
12. Comment, *Informed Consent in Medical Malpractice,* (1967) 55 Cal. L. Rev. 1396.
13. Zotorell v. Repp (1915) 187 Mich. 319.
14. Cobbs v. Grant (1972) 9 Cal.3d 229.
15. Cobbs v. Grant, *supra,* 244.
16. Canterbury v. Spence (D.C. Cir. 1972) 454 F.2d 772.
17. Truman v. Thomas (1979) 155 Cal.Rptr. 752.
18. Truman v. Thomas, *supra,* 759.
19. Truman v. Thomas, *supra,* 760.
20. California Health & Safety Code §7185, *et seq.*
21. California Health & Safety Code §7187(f).
22. California Health & Safety Code §7188.
23. California Health & Safety Code §7188.
24. California Health & Safety Code §7190.
25. Fletcher, *Prolonging Life,* 42 Wash. L. Rev. 999 (1967).
26. Kennedy, *The Karen Quinlan Case: Problems and Proposals,* (Mar. 1976) 2 J. Med. Ethics 3.
27. In re Karen Quinlan (1975) 137 N.J. Super. 227.
28. Black's Law Dictionary 481 (4th ed. 1968).
29. No. 56072 (Cal.Sup. Ct., Oakland, CA, 1974).
30. Alaska Stat. §09.65.120 (Supp. 1975); Cal. Health & Safety Code §7180 (West Supp. 1977); Kan. Stat. §77–202 (Supp. 1976); Md. Ann. Code art. 43, §54F (Supp. 1972); N.M. Stat. Ann. §1–2–2.2 (Supp. 1973); Va. Code §32–364.3:1 (Supp. 1976); W. Va. Code §16–19–1(c) (Supp. 1976).
31. Rice v. California Lutheran Hosp., (1945) 27 Cal.2d 296.
32. Quintal v. Laurel Grove Hosp., (1964) 62 Cal.2d 154.
33. Young, *Separation of Responsibility in the Oper-*

*ating Room: The Borrowed Servant, the Captain of the Ship and the Scope of Surgeons' Vicarious Liability,* 49 Notre Dame Lawyer 922 (1974).

34. Ault v. Hall, 119 Ohio St. 422.

35. Ybarra v. Spanguard (1944) 25 Cal.2d 486.

36. Talley v. Northern San Diego Hosp. Dist., (1953) 41 Cal.2d 33; 4 Witkin, *Torts,* §59.

37. Prosser, *Torts* (4th ed.) 992, *et seq.*

38. Marvulli v. Elshire (1972) 27 Cal.App.3d 180.

39. Sparger v. Worley Hospital, Inc. (1977) 547 S.W.3d 582.

40. 4 Witkin, *Torts,* §43.

41. Calif. Code of Civ. Proc. §875 *et seq.;* 9 Hastings L.J. 180.

42. American Motorcycle Assn. v. Superior Ct. (1978) 20 Cal.3d 578.

---

Addendum: Since this chapter was written, the California Supreme Court has overruled the lower court in *Truman v. Thomas,* providing an additional example of the changeability of the law as discussed above. The law in California as a result of the new decision is now that a physician must warn a patient of risks of not undergoing treatment. The California Supreme Court stated: "If a patient indicates that he or she is going to decline the treatment, then the doctor has the additional duty of advising of all material risks of which a reasonable person would want to be informed before deciding not to undergo the procedure." *Truman v. Thomas,* 165 Cal. Rptr. 308,312 (1980).

# 42 | *Statistical Interpretation: A Common-sense Approach*

*Elizabeth A. Gilpin, M.S.*

An understanding of statistical methodology is essential to evaluate properly the importance and impact of published medical research. Yet, the clinician who is attempting to keep up with the latest findings in his field is often ill-equipped to handle this task. Worse, the researchers whose work he reads are often equally handicapped.

We are all, in some sense, statistical beings who learn empirically from the events we encounter in our own personal universe. Some people jump to conclusions based on a single event and others are reluctant to make any judgment at all until they have had a chance to observe many similar events. These cautious types understand that although nature tends to act consistently, there may be a great deal of variability in response. Statistics is essentially the science (art?) of dealing with this variation so that an investigator can make inferences with some degree of confidence. Statistics do not prove anything. Realizing this fact is the first step toward understanding statistical methodology.

What statistics can accomplish depends on the soundness of the study or experimental design. Vague objectives, unreproducible methods, voluminous irrelevant data, and inappropriate statistical tests can produce "statistically significant results." In this case, statistics have only made a bad situation worse, since it has been sanctified by the aura of "statistical significance."

When statistical methodology is employed properly, it can give the investigator an idea of what chance he had of obtaining his results, assuming nature to be nothing but a colossal crap game. There is no magic to statistical methodology. The principles underlying it have been employed by good scientists long before it became a science in its own right.

In the discussion to follow, statistical terminology has inevitably been introduced. Where such terms are not defined in the text, refer to the Glossary for the definition.

## BACKGROUND

The father of applied statistics is generally considered to be R. A. Fisher, whose book, Statistical Methods for Research Workers [1] appeared in 1925. Ten years later he published The Design of Experiments.[2] The latter book actually sets the foundation for the earlier one by presenting the fundamental principles behind the significance tests with which the former is largely concerned. In order to take maximum advantage of the "methods," it is necessary to "design" the experiment properly. By the time Fisher and other early pioneers managed to sort out the implications of their methodology, statistical arithmetic had outdistanced statistical design and, unfortunately, statistical design has never caught up.[3]

Fisher [1] and many of the early statistical innovators worked in the agricultural sciences. They were able randomly to assign representative, homogeneous, experimental units (i.e., plots of land) to the treatments they wished to test in an unrestricted, randomized, and balanced fashion. Contrast this ideal situation with the plight of the medical research clinician. His experimental units, people, are each unique, and if he attempts to reduce heterogeneity by stratifying, for instance, according to sex or age, he may have difficulty achieving balance. In addition, the very availability of his subjects (those that reach him through the medical referral system and are willing to participate) might preclude generalizations from his results. Yet, the effective utilization of statistical methods is possible. It is essential that the researcher be familiar with the requisite underlying principles so that he can take all steps necessary to enhance the chances for a meaningful outcome.

## QUALITY OF STATISTICAL ANALYSES REPORTED IN THE MEDICAL LITERATURE

Various lamentations [3-10] have appeared concerning the state of statistics in medical research. One survey [8] examined 295 articles from 10 of the most frequently read and highly regarded medical journals. Experienced biostatisticians classified each article as either an analytical or a case study and then evaluated whether, "the conclusions drawn were valid in terms of the design of the experiment, the type of analysis performed, and the applicability of the statistical tests used or not used." Almost 50 percent (146) of the articles were classified as case studies, even though the authors (or editors) did not explicitly identify them as such. Among the 149 analytical studies, only 27.5 percent were considered acceptable. The most prevalent errors were those of omission rather than commission. Conclusions were drawn about very small differences without benefit of any statistical test, or no conclusions were drawn at all even though the study design and data collected would have allowed a statistical test. These two errors accounted for 43 percent of the total. Other errors, such as use of an improper statistical test, no identification of the

statistical test used, misleading data manipulation, misleading tables or charts, too much confidence in negative results with small sample sizes, absence of a control group, and improper design to answer the stated questions, accounted for the bulk of the remainder.

Another survey [9] involved the rigorous statistical scrutiny of 514 papers submitted to a leading medical journal for publication during 1964. Only 133 (26 percent) were considered acceptable when first reviewed. Of the original 514 papers submitted, 161 were finally published, and a post-hoc review by the original reviewers showed that 119 (74 percent) used acceptable statistical methodology. In order to judge the effectiveness of this program, random samples of studies published before the program and 1 year later were reviewed. The percentage of acceptable studies went from 35, before the program, to 70 a year later. The investigators concluded that the imposition of strict standards for statistical acceptability did improve the quality of published works.

As this study suggests, most investigators do receive a large part of their statistical education via the review process, and by reading quality journals. Unfortunately, when sloppy statistical methods get through the reviewing process, they are perpetuated. If the illustrious Dr. X of the prestigious institution Y analyzed his data in a particular way, then it must be correct (and I'll treat my data in the same manner). The program described above demonstrates that correct statistical methodology can be perpetuated as well.

Another factor that will undoubtedly have positive impact in the future is that more and more young researchers have had formal courses in experimental design and statistics. Also, they have had the opportunity to consult, during their training, with biostatisticians. The availability of such expertise is beginning to be a very important factor in obtaining research grants.

## IMPACT OF COMPUTERS

It is interesting that the bulk of the reported blunders still involve the absence of any statistical treatment at all. In this day and age of electronic computers and preprogrammed statistical packages, the effort required to do the analysis is minimal. Many analyses that would have been prohibitively tedious and prone to error by hand can be carried out correctly and rapidly, using a computer. Of course, the investigator has to recognize the need for statistical hypothesis testing before drawing conclusions and then have enough knowledge of statistical methods to choose the correct program and interpret the results—often a bewildering task even for the statistically cognizant worker.

In fact, it is debatable whether the computer has contributed to the quality of statistical methodology at all. The worker with a hand-held, preprogrammed calculator is especially vulnerable to three pitfalls. Very frequently he uses the wrong program; were he forced to look up the computational procedure in a textbook, he might realize its inappropriateness from the surrounding context. Even if he uses the right program, he might not understand or correctly interpret the displayed results. Of course, this might happen even if the computations were done by hand, but many programs give results based on certain assumptions concerning the worker's hypothesis that the directions for program use (documentation) might not sufficiently explain. Some examples will be given later in the section on evaluating the appropriateness of the statistical test used. Thirdly, when data can be so easily processed by computers, it is tempting to analyze everything in sight, whether or not it is relevant to the question at issue. A computer can be a useful tool for the investigator who knows what he is doing. If he doesn't, his ignorance is not the barrier it might have been had he to do the calculations by hand.

## OVERVIEW

In the limited space of one chapter, it is impossible to provide a comprehensive treatment of how one should go about the practice of statistics. Instead, the emphasis will be on the common errors that result from insufficient understanding of some of the underlying principles. What follows is a series of questions to guide the clinician in evaluating the publications he reads. The same set of questions can also guide the researcher to self-review his work. The most important tools for this undertaking are a large measure of common sense and a critical questioning attitude.

## EVALUATION OF THE PRODUCT

The first several questions pertain to the basic soundness of the study in terms of the objectives and methodologies employed. Next, is discussed the choice of a proper statistical test. The last two sets of questions address data presentation and the appropriateness of the conclusions drawn, based on the results obtained.

### Are the Objectives and Motivation Behind Them Clearly Stated?

It is unfortunately all too common to encounter journal articles that generally read as follows: From date one to two, we studied P patients selected by C criteria by M methods. We observed R ($p < .05$), which is (is not) in agreement with I investigators. We conclude Z. The description of P, C, M, R, I, and Z may be very straightforward and well written, but the reader is left asking, "so what?"

In order to evaluate any work, we must know the immediate purpose of the investigation as well as the more general or ultimate goals and why it is important that the problem be addressed at all. Also, it is important to understand the therapeutic implications in such cases where the issue is truly resolved. Within this framework, it is then possible to begin a careful scrutiny of the methods and procedures employed and of the stated results and conclusions.

Very often we see statements such as "our objective was to study the response of the heart to various conditions of stress," or "our goal was to determine whether exercise training improves left ventricular performance in patients with coronary artery disease." With a little imagination, the reader might be able to deduce both the ultimate goals and the implications of such work, but it is the investigator's responsibility to elaborate sufficiently so that the reader doesn't have to resort to speculation.

What specifically are the implications of understanding gained by the first investigation or by exercise-induced improvement in the second? What potential changes in therapy are implied for patients with coronary artery disease? If these changes are radical, we might insist on a more extreme significance level for the results than is usual, or that was used in that particular paper. Carefully formulated objectives are the foundation for the entire study.

## Are the Variables Measured Real Indices of the Phenomenon of Interest?

In the above examples, a potential association between two variables is of interest. The heart responds to stress, and exercise improves left ventricular performance. Even though there may or may not be a direct causal relationship, stress and exercise training are considered independent variables, and certain other variables are chosen to measure cardiac response or left ventricular performance. Are the variables chosen for observation really the relevant ones, or are they substitutions for the real variables of interest, which are impossible to measure directly? The most obvious example of this substitution is the use of an animal model and the inevitable leap from animal to human physiology. A more subtle example is the use of external blood pressure as a measure of intraarterial pressure, which has proved valid because a direct connection between the two has been established. The question to ask, therefore, is "has the variable measured actually been demonstrated to relate (mechanistically *not* statistically) to the real response variable of interest?"

## What are the Specific Hypotheses?

Assuming that the variables measured are valid indices of the phenomenon of interest, are specific hypotheses formulated in terms of the changes expected in the measured variables? Studying the response of the heart to various conditions of stress implies that the investigator expects some change in measured variable(s) as a result of the stressful conditions, perhaps

a greater response to some than to others. Given the expense and possible risk involved in exercise training, what level of improvement (change in the measured variables) should be realized before such a program is worthwhile? Such specific goals or hypotheses are the key to judge the adequacy of the design specifically in terms of the number of subjects studied.

## Are the Experimental Procedures (Methods) Designed Appropriately to Answer the Questions Posed by the Objective?

With the specific hypotheses in mind, do the study methods allow them to be tested appropriately? The study might involve an experiment in the strict sense; the investigator performs some maneuver on a subject and measures the result. For example, ejection fraction as an index of the left ventricular performance is measured before and after a fixed program of exercise training. Alternatively, the investigator may choose to conduct a survey of well-trained individuals and compare their ejection fractions to those of sedentary individuals. In this case, circumstances beyond the control of the investigator have assigned the level of the independent variable (active or sedentary) to the subject.

**Survey or Experiment?** When would an investigator choose one approach over the other? It is generally agreed, among scientists, that the experimental approach is best, since it allows a much greater degree of control of the degree of manipulation of the independent variable.[5] However, it is sometimes not possible, perhaps for ethical reasons, to conduct such monitored experiments on human subjects. The investigator may then resort to an animal model for his experiments or, if feasible, choose to survey the experiments already performed by the whims of Mother Nature. The question to ask, when judging whether a survey was the appropriate study method, therefore, is: "how could one design an actual experiment to test this same hypothesis?" If all efforts along this line prove inadequate, unethical, or completely impractical, then the survey approach is appropriate.

**Is the Type of Survey Method Optimal for the Situation?** There are several types of surveys and one type may be more appropriate for testing a given hypothesis than another. Surveys can be "longitudinal," implying that they look either backward from the present, retrospective surveys, or they look forward from the present, prospective surveys. Alternatively, they can simply be a snap shot or "cross-sectional" look at the current state of affairs.

A survey is retrospective if it starts with a group of subjects having some characteristic, for instance, an acute myocardial infarction, and then compares the incidence of certain risk factors hypothesized to contribute to the likelihood of this event compared to a group of similar subjects who did not experience an infarction.

Alternatively, the survey could identify two groups, one with and one without a suspicious factor, and observe the number of myocardial infarctions experienced by both groups in the future. Surveys deemed cross-sectional often resemble retrospective surveys in that the events tabulated have already occurred by the time the survey takes place. The most appropriate use of a cross-sectional survey is to answer a simple question such as: Has the incidence of a certain communicable disease reached X? If the survey results confirm this hypothesis, then the disease can be declared an epidemic and measures instituted to attempt to stop it. Another appropriate question for a cross-sectional survey is, "What is the normal creatine kinase level in healthy individuals?"

Prospective surveys have the advantage that the subjects are selected with full information available and the follow-up period is supervised by the investigators so that all pertinent information is gathered. Retrospective studies usually involve combing through old records that may be incomplete or unreliable; the full story is never known. However, prospective studies usually require large numbers of subjects in order that the number of events of interest, i.e., myocardial infarctions in the two groups with and without the suspicious factor, be large enough for meaningful comparisons. The cost of following these large numbers of patients may or may not be worth the effort.

### What Bias Might Exist in the Sample (Either Selected for Survey or As Experimental Subjects)?

In the description of the population selected, regardless of the type of survey or experiment, every possible reason for bias in the sampling procedures should be discussed by the researcher. What subjects are excluded? Why? How might this affect the answer to the question the survey or experiment was designed to answer? Were the subjects selected because they were readily at hand, i.e., had they been admitted to the hospital with which the investigator is affiliated? If the results of the study are to be applied only to these patients or patients admitted to similar hospitals, the sample is probably adequate. However, if wider application is anticipated, it is necessary to identify the characteristics of this institution, which might create a biased sample. Is the institution a private hospital for the well-to-do, a military hospital, or a public facility serving welfare recipients? Ideally, the sample should be selected by a randomization procedure that guarantees that every individual in the population about which inferences are to be made has an equal chance of being included.

### Compared to What?

In both surveys and experiments, the hypothesis to be tested nearly always implies that some comparison be made. Sometimes the comparison involves different states in the same subject, one of which is usually a "before" condition and the other an "after" state. There may be several "during" conditions of interest, too. In this situation, the subject is serving as his own control. In other cases, perhaps even in the same study, comparisons are made among groups of subjects, implying that these groups are in all ways identical except for some maneuver or state of the independent variable. Even in surveys, one group of subjects with a given characteristic is compared to a group without that characteristic. How comparable are these groups otherwise? Does the investigator provide sufficient information to allow the reader to judge that the groups are initially alike, as well as being representative of the inference population?

Why not compare the group undergoing a new therapy to patients who received conventional therapy in the past? Use of such historic controls has been the source of considerable controversy. Proponents of new therapies that seem to be vastly superior to conventional ones think that a randomized clinical trial (where patients are randomly assigned to the conventional and new therapy groups) is unethical; all patients should be given the new therapy and the results compared to data gathered in the past concerning the conventional therapy.[11]

However, the time factor may introduce biases that are subtle and impossible to detect and which could radically affect the results of trials utilizing historic data. Pocock [12] reviewed 19 large randomized clinical trials of drugs for treating lung cancer. The concurrent control group in each of the trials was given the same standard therapy. The differences in mortality rates between consecutive trials' control groups (*not* the drug groups) ranged from −46 to +24 percent! Of course, there is no guarantee that a randomized concurrent control group will be identical to the group receiving the new therapy, but at least the time factor is eliminated. Changes in patient management (i.e., initial period of hospitalization or extent of diagnostic procedures) over a period of time can introduce bias. If an investigator has elected to use historic controls, it is crucial that he examine any possible influence the time factor might introduce, as well as establish that his treatment and control groups can be considered identical otherwise.

**Appropriate Use of Controls?** One technique sometimes used in an attempt to obtain comparable groups is case matching. Especially in surveys, each patient in the group with a characteristic under scrutiny, say X, is matched with a patient in the group without this feature, not X, according to sex, age, occupation, and any other attributes that may be relevant. The more factors chosen as criteria, the more difficult it is to find a mate for each subject. Also, there is the danger of not covering the entire range of population with respect to each matching factor and, thus, limiting possible generaliza-

tions or even hiding the relationship the investigator wishes to demonstrate. If too many of the subjects end up having a certain attribute, say Z, and it is associated (unknown to the investigator) with the dependent variable Y, then he may fail to detect a real association of X with Y. For example, assume that most of the subjects available for study were male (Z = sex) and that only a few female-female pairs were used. The independent variable might have been a drug (X) suspected of altering cholesterol level (Y). The results of the pairwise analysis might show no effect, even when the few female-female pairs showed a marked difference due to an hormonal augmentation factor.

What factors might have influenced the controls during the course of an experiment or a longitudinal survey? In order to assure that the controls are handled, in all respects, identically, except for the independent variable, researchers often use double-blind trials, implying that neither the subject nor the investigator (or anyone who has contact with the subjects or investigator) knows whether the subject is in the control or experimental group. The coded list resulting from the randomization procedure is kept sealed and not opened by the investigator until the experiment is concluded. The subjects in the control group receive a placebo dispensed by a central pharmacy, which has no contact with the investigator, in the same manner as the drug being tested. Whenever such precautions are possible, it is advisable that they be taken; when the experiment is not conducted in this manner, it is a good idea to ask "why not?"

There may be some very good reasons. The most obvious is that the independent variable cannot be mimicked by a placebo. In our earlier example, the patients assigned to the control group, rather than the exercise-trained group, cannot be given a sham exercise course. However, what is to prevent them from being swept up by the jogging fad and training on their own? If this is discovered by the investigator, he can drop the subject from the investigation. He should not switch the patient to the experimental group because his training modality undoubtedly differed from the program experienced by the real experimental group. The investigator should report on precautions he took to make sure such an event does not go undetected.

If the research described is an experiment, the use of a matched subject as a control has the advantage in that it decreases intersubject variation and thereby requires fewer subjects in each group to demonstrate a given level of difference. One disadvantage of this approach is that if one subject in a pair is lost during the experiment or an equipment failure makes it impossible to make a second measurement on a subject acting as his own control, the data already collected are of little use because the conclusions depend on interpair differences.

Sometimes the investigator makes the mistake of thinking that because he uses "the subject as his own control" that no "control group" is necessary. The researcher interested in exercise training may have reasoned that if a group of subjects had an average initial ejection fraction of .41 and if, after the period of training, nearly all showed improvement and the group average was .48, that the training program was responsible for the improvement. It might be that these patients would have improved spontaneously over this period of time since they were all in the early stages of recovery after myocardial infarction. Following a control group consisting of such patients would eliminate this confusion, or, as the statisticians say, would eliminate the confounding of time and treatment.

Another example of confounding is when a new therapy is to be compared to an old one by giving Drug A to the patients for a certain length of time followed by an equal length period on Drug B. If the patients appear to respond differently to the drugs, how do we know that it is not due to the same type of spontaneous change as in the exercise training study? To account for this possibility, the investigator could assign patients at random to two sequences, half receiving Drug A followed by Drug B and the others the reverse sequence. This procedure is called a cross-over design. When treatments are administered sequentially, it is important that there be a rest period to allow the subject to return to the baseline state.

There may be carry-over effects from the first drug, a heightened period of symptoms due to drug withdrawal or even a benefit from withdrawal from the first drug. A placebo therapy can be given in the interim so that the patient still thinks he is on therapy.

It should be pointed out that the use of the subject as his own control, as just described, is *not* a more valid approach than randomly assigning subjects to two groups, one receiving Drug A and the other Drug B. Both designs, if implemented properly, can lead to a valid test of the hypothesis of interest. In some instances, one approach may be more efficient than the other, but both can lead to valid conclusions. The efficiencies of the paired approach in the drug-trial example are gained at the cost of more than doubling the duration of the experiment. In fact, if some of the potential disadvantages are objectionable enough, the investigator might have been better off using two groups at a relatively modest increase in the number of subjects required (often only about 25 percent).

**False Replication.** Are the experimental units or subjects truly independent? Suppose that a clinical trial extends over a period of time long enough for a patient to present twice for treatment. Some of the patients who entered the study early were treated but later suffered a recurrence. How was the second episode handled? Perhaps the end point for the first admission had already been attained (i.e., survival beyond 6 months). Is it valid for the investigator to use such patients twice? The answer to this question is an emphatic NO. The patient is likely to respond to treatment in the same manner both times so that the observations are not mutually independent.

This mistake is made more frequently in studies of organs. For instance, if measurements are taken from both lungs, and some patients are affected by some disease only in one and others in both, should patients or lungs be the observational units? Again, the answer is patients; lungs cannot be considered independent if they belong to the same patient. Such errors have been called false replication and occur with unfortunate frequency due, perhaps, to the pain it gives researchers to throw away data. For statistical tests to be meaningful, independent sample elements are required (see section on the appropriateness of a statistical test).

**More Than One Independent Variable?** In the examples discussed above, only one independent variable was involved at two or more states. In one case, a drug intervention (independent variable) was examined at two states (with and without). In another the response of the heart to stress (independent variable) was to be examined for several different conditions of stress (states). Many of the statistical designs advanced by Fisher [2] enable the investigator to examine the response to more than one independent variable at a time, using the same experimental units. The design is such that the *factors* (independent variables) are expected to produce significant *effects* (dependent variable). The terminology of "factors" and "effects" is used in the description of these designs, which go by such names as "factorial designs," "randomized block designs," and "Latin squares." All of these designs are collectively analyzed using multifactor analysis of variance.

In agriculture an investigator can assign the factor levels to his experimental units randomly with impunity. Furthermore, he can usually be certain that the experimental units (i.e., plots of land) are initially very uniform. He could, for instance, examine the yield for 10 different varieties of wheat using five types of fertilizer, three different row-spacing strategies, and four irrigation protocols. This would be a four-factor experiment (variety, fertilization, spacing and irrigation) having 10, 5, 3, and 4 levels, respectively. Such experiments are very efficient and can answer all his questions concerning which varieties are best, which fertilizers are best, etc., and what, if any, combinations of these factors produce synergistically the greatest yield. These analyses require balanced designs (same number of experimental units assigned to each factorial combination) for maximum efficiency. In the above example, the investigator would normally only use one plot for each of the $10 \times 5 \times 3 \times 4 = 600$ factorial combinations.

An example of a factorial design in medicine might involve different modalities of therapy, such as surgery or drug treatment, for coronary artery disease. Patients are assigned at random

**FACTOR 1**

| FACTOR 2 | No Surgery | Surgery |
|----------|-----------|---------|
| No Drugs | neither | only surgery |
| Drugs | only drugs | both |

Fig. 42.1  Design of factorial experiment to evaluate simultaneously the efficacy of medical and surgical treatment of coronary artery disease.

to each of the four categories shown in Figure 42.1. Thus, some patients receive only drug therapy, another group only has surgery, and a third group has both surgery and drug treatment, while a fourth group has neither. The dependent variable is presumably some measure of cardiac performance. The statistical analysis would allow the investigator to test the null hypotheses that surgery has no effect on cardiac performance, that drug treatment has no effect, or that there is no synergistic effect (bad or good) from both together. Such an experiment would not be feasible using human subjects because of the ethical considerations involved in allowing a group of patients to go untreated. (Who cares if a plot of wheat dies?)

These designs are occasionally utilized, usually in the following context. An investigator has measured the cholesterol level in the blood of a number of subjects. He makes himself a table, such as the one in Figure 42.2, and proceeds with a multifactor analysis of variance.

**FACTOR 2 - RACE**

| FACTOR 1 - SEX | Caucasian | Negroid | Mongoloid |
|----------------|-----------|---------|-----------|
| Male | 18 | 9 | 4 |
| Female | 16 | 11 | 8 |

Fig. 42.2  Subjects are not randomly assigned to the levels of the factors under consideration.

The fallacy here is that he did not randomly assign the experimental units to the various combinations of factor levels: Mother Nature did. Very likely there are other factors associated with sex or race that influence the dependent variable. The investigator might conclude that race makes a difference when the real factor is diet, due to socioeconomic factors. The results of such analyses may provide clues for further investigations, but drawing conclusions from such an analysis is a risky business.

## Is the Statistical Test Used Appropriate?

Before outlining a procedure for evaluating the appropriateness of a given statistical test, a few concepts need to be briefly reviewed. First of all, it should be remembered, once again, that a statistical test merely tells you how often a certain event could be expected to occur by chance. From the observed (dependent) variable values obtained during the experiment, a calculation is made according to some (usually complicated) formula that produces a "statistic" having its own underlying sampling probability distribution (see glossary). The event alluded to above then corresponds to obtaining a value for this statistic, which can be looked up in a table for its probability distribution to determine how likely such a value occurs by chance alone. The mathematicians who derive the various formulas used to calculate the test statistics usually were forced to make some assumptions regarding the nature and various characteristics of the probability distribution of the observed random variable.* More will be said about this later.

Evaluating whether the statistical test used is appropriate involves answering a number of questions. At the risk of oversimplifying this

complex task, a list of questions is offered as a guide. The remainder of this section will explore the implications of each of these questions, which are summarized in Figure 42.3.

**Is Using Any Statistical Test at All Justified?** All tests for statistical significance are based on the premise that the experimental units (subjects) are assigned to the levels of the independent variables under consideration (i.e., drug or control groups) by a strictly random method and that nothing happens during the course of the experiment to interfere with the effects of the randomization except the independent variable under study. If, from the description of the methods for selecting the sample and of the experimental or survey procedures, there is any evidence that bias has been introduced, the investigator has no business applying a statistical test at all. However, it is often the case that the description of the methods is not adequate to judge whether the randomization was done properly.

In an experiment involving dogs, the maneuver under investigation had to be applied to

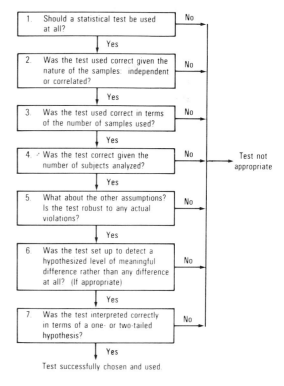

Fig. 42.3 Evaluation of the appropriateness of a statistical test.

---

* The distributions most frequently discussed in textbooks [13,14] include the normal, binomial, and Poisson distributions. IQ, as measured by standard intelligence test, is assumed to have a normal distribution. The number of heads observed in 25 coin tosses has a binomial distribution. The number of counts emitted within a given time interval from radioactive material has a Poisson distribution. Many other distributions are also possible. Procedures exist that allow the researcher to test whether his data fit any hypothesized distribution. [15,16]

one animal at a time. The animals in the control group were sham-operated. The description of the methods did not include any information on how it was determined what animal was chosen from the pool available, and how it was decided whether a sham or real maneuver was to be performed that day. What actually happened was that the friendliest animals were chosen first (they trotted to the door of the pen wagging their tails) and, to make matters worse, all the sham procedures were performed before the actual experimental operations (delivery of a special piece of equipment needed for the real procedure was delayed). Fate would have it that an equipment failure occurred just as the shams were completed. No statistical test exists that could guarantee that any differences seen between the control and experimental groups were not due to differences between friendly and nervous animals or to a difference in the piece of equipment before and after it has been repaired.

The critical reader should be suspicious if the description of the methods does not include any acknowledgment of the necessity to randomize. Very likely the investigator simply does not appreciate this point, and his work, even though meticulous in every other aspect, is not amenable to statistical tests of hypotheses.

**Does the Test Utilize Data for All the Samples?** When there is only one sample, this question is superfluous. For instance, in a cross-sectional survey, the objective was to estimate the incidence of a certain infectious disease and to test the hypothesis that this incidence is equal to some threshold value indicative of a potential epidemic. The square root of the sample variance (standard deviation) is used to compute the usual test statistic.[17]

If the hypothesis involves the comparison of observations on a control group to those on an experimental group, two samples of data (observations on the dependent variable) are obviously collected. Typically the investigator computes a test statistic,[18] which incorporates estimates of variation from both samples. For example, the unpaired $t$-test uses a pooled estimate of variance (see Glossary).

Where the researcher often gets into trouble is when there are more than two samples of data. Both in the two-sample and many-sample case, the investigator wants to see if the intersample variability is greater than the intrasample variability. Is the variability of response within each group so great that it overwhelms any differences that might exist among the groups? Just as in the two-sample cases, this intergroup variability should be based on *all* the samples. The many-sample tests, such as one-factor analysis of variance, do just that. These procedures first test the hypothesis that there are no differences among the samples. Then if this hypothesis can be rejected, the investigator proceeds with the two-sample tests he is interested in, but the intersample variability used in these tests is based on all the samples in the experiment.[19] The samples may be independent or correlated, and the method of analysis will be different depending on which is the case (see below).

**Are the Samples Independent or Correlated?** When subjects are paired or a subject acts as his own control, the data collected are not considered to come from two independent samples. Actually it is the difference (before-after value in the self control case) that is of interest, and these differences can be treated as one sample of data. Testing whether the means before and after treatment are the same is equivalent to testing whether the mean difference is zero.[20]

In the case where several observations of the same dependent variables are made on the same subjects, a repeated measures analysis of variance is appropriate.[21] This procedure averages all two-way differences between means (six for four observations) to obtain an estimate of the "treatment effect." It then compares this variability to the within-treatment variability after removing the source of variation due to intersubject differences.

Investigators frequently perform the wrong test due to the blind use of preprogrammed calculators or canned computer programs. Most programs available for the many-sample case are for independent samples, but the investigator fails to notice this fact and uses the program anyway. The paired $t$-test is usually part of most of the statistical packages, but data entry usually involves entering the raw sample data rather than subject differences and it's easy to wrongly use the procedure for independent samples. To guard against this pitfall, a quick phone call to the resident biostatistician is advisable.

**Small-Sample or Large-Sample Tests?** Of the many assumptions made by mathematicians when deriving a statistical test, sample size requirements are the easiest to verify. This question usually arises when the mathematician makes a statement such as, "the distribution of a given statistic can be approximated by the normal probability distribution for large samples." For the one- and two-sample test statistics described above, the general rule of thumb is to use the normal probability distribution approximation if the sample sizes involved are greater than 30. For smaller samples, the binomial (for proportions) or $t$-distributions should be used instead.[22]

The most frequent violation of this principle involves the chi-square statistic to test hypotheses involving differences in sample proportions when the samples are small. As an example, suppose that an investigator wants to test the hypotheses that the improvement rate of three out of 20 in a control group is no different from the rate of seven out of 10 in the group given an experimental drug. For two samples, the chi-square statistic has exactly the same probability distribution as the square of a normally distributed statistic. But using the normal distribution to test for differences in proportions requires "large" samples. Even for large samples, if the incidence in both groups is either very high or very low (the usual rule of thumb is five), the approximation may not be good. If only one group shows this characteristic, the discrepancy is probably minimal. In the example above, methods based on the computations of exact probabilities should be used.[23] Also, tables exist which allow the researcher to evaluate statistical significance directly.[24]

**Are Other Assumptions for the Test Satisfied?** Each statistical test is based on its own set of assumptions. The first assumptions in any statistical test is that the sample(s) are randomly selected and that the conditions of the experiment are such that it can be repeated. These assumptions have already been discussed above. Tests that involve estimates of population parameters such as means, standard deviations or proportions are called "parametric" tests. Examples are the $t$-tests, and the analysis of variance for many-sample experiments mentioned earlier. When no such estimates are required for the computation of the test statistic, the test is usually called a "nonparametric" test. Other assumptions for a given test usually involve the type and/or shape of the probability distribution governing the dependent variable. For instance, the $t$-test (independent samples) assumes that the dependent variable is continuous, is approximately normally distributed if the sample size is small, and that the two groups being compared have equal variances. The questions naturally arises as to how many of those assumptions may be relaxed and to what extent. Some tests are very robust (they remain valid) to violations of their assumptions and others are not.

If an investigator is worried about his data satisfying the underlying assumptions, he can either transform the data in an apprpropriate fashion, if possible, so that the new scale more nearly conforms to the assumptions,[25] or choose a test with different or fewer assumptions. For example, an investigator may choose to use a square-root transformation to make two group variances more nearly equal (assuming they are correlated with the group means which differ by an order of magnitude) before he applies a $t$-test. Or instead, he might choose to use the Wilcoxon rank sum test.

The transformation route, although traditional, implies that the hypotheses be reformulated on the new scale, which may or may not have any biologic meaning. It frequently happens that in his quest for statistical significance, a worker applies transforms in every conceivable fashion, regardless of the nature of his data, hoping that eventually a $p$-value $< .05$ will turn up. When a transform is used, a justification of the one chosen in terms of the peculiarities of the data should be presented.

The choice of the statistical test to be used should be made before the experiment is performed or the data gathered. If the literature is scanty and pilot studies too few to adequately explore the underlying distribution of the measured data, the choice of a nonparametric statistical test is appropriate. Nonparametric techniques are often very easy to understand and usually (although not always) easier to apply than their normal distribution theory counterparts. For example, many of the procedures require analysis, not of the actual magnitudes of the observations but only of their relative ranking. This might seem as if too much information is sacrificed, but some theoretical investigations have shown that the nonparametric procedures are only slightly less powerful (see Glossary) than their parametric counterparts when the underlying populations are truly normal and otherwise well behaved. That is, to achieve the same confidence of detecting a difference when it really exists, more (but not very many more) experimental units or subjects are required. However, when the underlying populations are *not* normally distributed, the nonparametric procedures can be vastly *more* efficient.

The number of nonparametric tests is growing rapidly, since this area of research has proven to be a fruitful one for mathematical statisticians. Several texts, such as Spiegel,[26] Tate,[27] Hollander,[28] and Bradley [29] give a comprehensive treatment of the topic. For a given problem, there may exist no single "best" procedure. However, some have prevailed since they are easy to understand and to apply and are efficient in a variety of situations. Table 42.1 gives the names of some of these nonparametric analogues in terms of the nature of the data and the hypotheses to be tested.

**Was the Hypothesized Level of Difference Incorporated into the Statistical Test?** From the stated objectives and the description of the methods, some indication of the magnitude of the difference to be expected in the dependent variable should be apparent. Gertrude Stein is reputed to have said, "A difference to be a difference must make a difference." Suppose that in a large, controlled study of hypertensives, a new drug showed an average decrease in systolic blood pressure of 22 mmHg. The control group of hypertensives, given the usual treatment, showed an average decrease (before-after treatment) of 18 mmHg. These means may be statistically different, but for all practical purposes the new drug did not perform sufficiently

better than the standard therapy to make it worth the trouble to market. The null hypothesis should include a meaningful threshold stated in terms of the dependent variable and the nature of the statistical test used. In the above example, the null hypothesis might be: Drug X is less than 50 percent more effective than the standard drug. Previous work would have established the standard drug's effectiveness as perhaps an average 20 mmHg reduction. This translates into a target reduction of 30 mmHg for the new drug compared to the standard one, and this value would be incorporated into the computation of the test statistic.[30] Unfortunately some canned programs do not allow the researcher to specify his threshold for a meaningful difference, and he usually forgets to recompute the statistic by hand. This is simple to do since the various other quantities used in the statistic's computation are generally program outputs.

In some cases, any difference at all may be worth detecting, but this should be stated explicitly. Often, especially in retrospective surveys, tables of findings are studded with asterisks, indicating statistically significant differences more for the purposes of description than as the result of rejecting stated null hypotheses. Although the asterisks do manage to draw the readers attention to statistically significant results, it is the author's responsibility to discuss these results by pointing out agreement with other studies, and if a result is completely unexpected, suggesting that further work is needed for confirmation (more will be said regarding this practice in the section on evaluating conclusions).

**Was the Test Interpreted Correctly in Terms of a One-Tailed or Two-Tailed Hypothesis?** This question is closely related to the last. The example described above shows the "one-tailed" case. The investigator has reason to believe that the new drug might be *more* effective than the standard one. If he had any reason to expect that it might, indeed, be less effective, he would not have gone to the expense and trouble to carry out the clinical trial in the first place. One possible null hypothesis, inferred from an earlier example, shows how this point is frequently confused: the incidence of a certain

**Table 42.1   Nonparametric Analogues to the Usual Statistical Testing Procedures**

| Type of Data | Usual Parametric Procedure | Nonparametric Procedure | Remarks |
|---|---|---|---|
| *One Sample* Central tendency | mean = c t-test | median = m signed rank procedures | Note that if $Z = X_1 - X_2$, procedures for paired data apply here. |
| Proportion | p = c normal approximation | p = c binomial test | |
| *Two Samples* | $\overline{X}_1 = \overline{X}_2$ (means equal) | medians equal | |
| Unpaired (independent) | unpaired t-test | Wilcoxon rank sum test | The alternative hypothesis is that one sample is shifted relative to the other. |
| Paired (correlated) | $Z = \overline{X}_1 - \overline{X}_2 = 0$ | treatment had no effect | |
| | paired t-test | Wilcoxon signed rank test or Fisher's sign test | |
| Proportions (independent) | $p_1 = p_2$ Chi-square test | Fisher's exact test | Use when total sample size small |
| *Many Samples* Independent | all means equal | all samples from same population | |
| | one-way analysis of variance | Kruskall-Wallis test | |
| Dependent | repeated measures analysis of variance | chi-square rank test | data in form of ranks |
| | | Q statistic[21] | data dichotomous |
| Multiple comparisons | Duncan's range test or Scheffe's multiple comparisons | Freidman rank sum procedures[28] | finds pairs of treatments that differ |
| *Independence* (correlation) | Pearson's correlation coefficient r = 0 t-test | Kendall test $\tau = 0$ | $\tau$ is a measure of association |
| *Regression* One line | t-test | Theil test | slope = 0: also can estimate slope |
| Two lines | t-test | Hollander test | slopes equal: also can estimate difference in slopes |

communicable disease is equal to a given threshold. This is stated as a "two-tailed" hypothesis and is rejected if the actual sample value is sufficiently larger *or* smaller than the given threshold value. The null hypothesis the investigator really wants to test is: The incidence of the disease is *less than* a given threshold value.

Rejecting this hypothesis means that the estimated incidence of the disease indicates that the true incidence is *greater than* or equal to the threshold value. Figure 42.4 illustrates this concept. In part A, the shaded area at *both* tails indicates the frequency of obtaining values of the statistic more extreme in absolute magni-

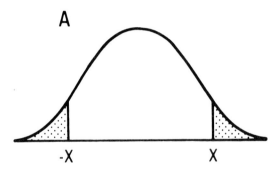

**A**

-X        X

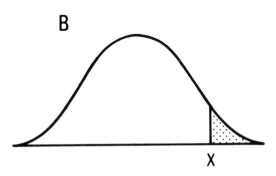

**B**

X

Fig. 42.4 The shaded area in the top panel corresponds to the probability of obtaining a more extreme value (greater than X or less than − X) than the value obtained, X. In the lower panel the shaded area corresponds to the probability of obtaining greater values than X.

tude than the value obtained. Part B shows the frequency of obtaining only greater values.

Interpreting the test as a two-tailed test when the hypothesis is really one-tailed, errs on the conservative side. The probability of obtaining a value for the test statistic more extreme rather than merely larger is twice as great. Again, many canned computer programs lead the investigator down a primrose path by displaying two-tailed *p*-values that he fails to convert before evaluating his one-tailed hypothesis. Looking up the statistic and the *p*-value in the appropriate statistical table can avoid this problem.

**An Example.** At this point, it might be helpful to use Figure 42.3 to evaluate a hypothetic study.

The objectives of the study were to test a new drug, which might alleviate angina pectoris via a mechanism different from the usual thera-

pies. This drug would be potentially useful in patients whose angina is unrelieved by the usual medications and may eventually prove more effective than conventional therapies in other patients as well. Another goal of the study was to develop and to test a method to quantitate the severity of angina.

Fifteen patients with coronary artery disease, suffering from stable angina pectoris, were referred to the study center by eight cardiologists practicing within a 35-mile radius of the study clinic. The maximum number of referrals by one physician was three. Ages ranged from 46 to 74 years, and there were 11 men and four women. The severity of the disease, as evaluated by angiography, varied considerably.

Each patient was to serve as his own control in a double-blind, crossover trial. The order of the medications, the new drug and a common standard one that had proved unsuccessful for each of the patients previously, was randomly determined. Each drug period lasted 4 weeks, with a 2-week placebo period in between. Each week the patients visited the clinic where they received the next week's medication and reviewed their angina "log" with a physician.

The patients were requested to log each angina attack with the date, time, duration of pain, what they had been doing, and the severity of the pain (mild, moderate, or severe). While at the clinic, together with the physician, they determined a score for each episode. The activity level that precipitated the attack was scored as: rest = 3, normal = 2, active = 1, and the pain graded as 1 = mild, 2 = moderate, and 3 = severe. The product of these two scores was further multiplied by the duration of pain in minutes. If the patient distinctly remembered that the pain, for instance, started at a mild but persisted at a moderate level, the pain score could be adjusted by using a value between 1 and 2, perhaps 1.3. Thus, severe pain at rest for 5 minutes would result in an episode score of $3 \times 3 \times 5 = 45$, while mild pain after exertion, persisting for 8 minutes would be scored as $1 \times 1 \times 8 = 8$. Before the randomization code was broken, an "angina index" was computed for the last 3 weeks of each drug period by summing the scores for all episodes within the period.

For any given patient, a reduction in the angina index on the new drug to less than half of what it was on the conventional drug was to be considered a successful outcome. The 50 percent reduction was chosen to assure meaningful relief beyond any impreciseness in the angina index itself. A sign test was used to test the hypothesis that the proportion of successful outcomes was not greater than what could be expected to occur by chance alone (i.e., half). The angina indices for each patient are shown in Table 42.2 for the two drug periods. The investigators rejected the above hypothesis, since the probability of obtaining 13 or more successes is $< .05$ under the null hypothesis.[31]

They concluded that the new drug was effective in reducing angina, as measured by the angina index for patients refractory to the conventional drug. They also reported that angina indices computed on a weekly basis had a range that was at most 20 percent of the median value for any 3-week period on the same drug in the same patient. Based on this evidence, they suggested that future studies, in possibly different populations, can be designed, using the angina index as a quantitative measure of anginal discomfort.

Even this rather long description of the study is barely adequate to evaluate the statistical methodology. The objectives seem reasonable. Whether the 15 patients entered into the trial can be considered a random sample of patients refractory to conventional antianginal therapy is difficult to determine, based on the information provided. However, no bias is apparent. The double-blind, randomized design guards against bias during the trial so a statistical test is appropriate (Question 1).

Each patient acted as his own control so the two sets of data collected are not independent (Questions 2,3). Due to lack of experience with the angina index, the investigators appropriately refrained from making any assumptions regarding the nature of its distribution (Questions 4,5). In the choice and application of the sign test, they assumed that a 50 percent reduction reflected a real relief beyond any lack of reproducibility in the angina index (Question 6). The interpretation of the test results was based on a one-tailed hypothesis. A two-tailed test would have looked at both extremes—the probability of obtaining either 13 or more successes or 13 or more failures (Question 7). Thus, an appropriate statistical test was successfully chosen and used. Also the investigators have qualified their conclusions to reflect the population of patients their study was designed to address.

Table 42.2 Angina Indices During Therapy with New and Conventional Drugs

| Patient | Angina Index | | Ratio New/conv | Success = + Failure = − |
| | New Drug | Conventional Drug | | |
|---|---|---|---|---|
| 1 | 72 | 825 | 0.09 | + |
| 2 | 194 | 462 | 0.42 | + |
| 3 | 201 | 1196 | 0.17 | + |
| 4 | 28 | 122 | 0.23 | + |
| 5 | 114 | 283 | 0.40 | + |
| 6 | 0 | 186 | 0.00 | + |
| 7 | 24 | 84 | 0.29 | + |
| 8 | 282 | 351 | 0.80 | − |
| 9 | 48 | 216 | 0.22 | + |
| 10 | 54 | 46 | 1.17 | − |
| 11 | 62 | 149 | 0.42 | + |
| 12 | 37 | 228 | 0.16 | + |
| 13 | 94 | 612 | 0.15 | + |
| 14 | 62 | 110 | 0.56 | − |
| 15 | 161 | 536 | 0.30 | + |
| Median | 62 | 228 | 0.23 | |
| Range | 282 | 1150 | 1.17 | |

Note that the formulation of the hypothesis tested and the choice of the statistical test used was done prior to any examination of the data. Given that the investigators now have some experience with the use of the angina index, future studies can be more precisely designed, perhaps using parametric procedures.

### Are the Data Presented Intelligently?

Were the data presented at all? Sometimes conclusions are stated without even sufficient summary information for the reader to judge their reasonableness. Just to determine whether the statistical test used was appropriate, much needs to be known about the data.

**Raw vs. Summary.** If the study involves a modest number of cases, nothing is clearer than a table of raw data. In fact, if such a table is not present, one begins to wonder what anomaly in the data the investigator is trying to hide. With the raw data at hand, the reader can reanalyze it as he feels appropriate, or recheck the computations if the results seem inconsistent for any reason. In addition, summary tables or graphs are useful to highlight the important results, but there is no substitute for seeing the raw data. Due to space limitations, some journals do not permit publication of lengthy tables of raw data. To overcome this problem, some journals ask that such information be deposited with documentary services and interested readers can obtain the data at a nominal cost.

There is one instance in which a plot of the raw data, no matter how voluminous, is absolutely essential. A correlation coefficient (see Glossary) without a plot can be misleading. Figure 42.5 shows four sets of data each having the same correlation coefficient. In plot A the correlation coefficient is a decent summary statistic. In the frames B and C the relation between the two variables can best be described by other means (such as a higher degree polynomial or periodic function) and in plot D, it is doubtful whether there is any relationship at all.

When the data are too voluminous to be presented in raw form, a clear organization of summary information is essential. Tables and graphs can work well provided they are kept

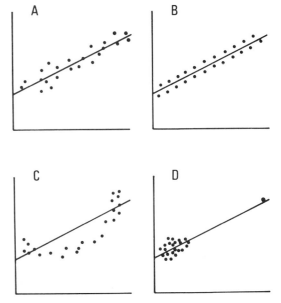

Fig. 42.5   In each case the correlation is 0.90!

simple. If the reader cannot interpret the table or graph *without* reading the legend, it is performing its function (i.e., communicating) poorly. Are scales on graphs obviously intended to be compared consistent? Are breaks in scale that might distort the data clearly indicated? Figure 42.6 gives examples where misinterpretation due to these blunders (?) might occur. The data depicted in Panel A were plotted on two scales, giving different impressions. In Panel B, the value the height represents for the bar on the right is actually only twice the value represented by the height of the left-most bar.

**The Ubiquitous Standard Error.** How does one interpret a plot of mean values as points with little bars sprouting vertically up and down? The author usually does indicate somewhere whether these brackets represent standard errors or standard deviations (see Glossary). But why use one rather than the other? The usual answer is that the data look "tighter" when the standard error is used. However, if the purpose is to present some indication of sample dispersion, the standard deviation is the appropriate statistic. On the other hand, if the purpose is to allow the reader to make inferences about a collection of means, 95 percent confidence intervals (see Glossary), rather than standard errors, would be more helpful. By

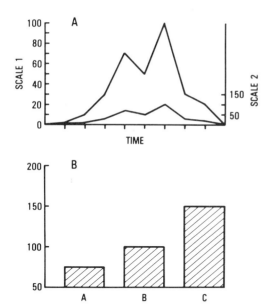

Fig. 42.6 The top panel illustrates how the choice of scale can influence interpretation. In the lower panel, the relative heights of the bars are misleading unless the scale begins at zero.

themselves, standard errors convey little useful information. Sometimes the author even has the misguided idea that the standard errors will help the reader judge whether two or more means are significantly different by some statistical test. Tests, such as the $t$-test or the analysis of variance, use a pooled estimate of the standard error, which implies that the intervals shown for the plotted means should all have the *same* width. If the purpose is to allow the reader to make such inferences, the author should use 95 percent confidence intervals computed using a pooled estimate of the standard error. If two intervals do not overlap, the corresponding means are significantly different ($p < .05$).

**The Typical Case.** Frequently, authors present a graph or table illustrating a "typical" case. Such data are difficult to interpret. If the case is truly typical, why isn't summary information given instead? If there are a modest number of cases, why aren't all the data presented? If one case is shown to demonstrate a problem with the data, how many of the other cases also exhibit this difficulty? In spite of these objections, there may be a good reason for presentation of a typical case, but this reason should

be explicitly justified. The presentation of an example can help clarify the experimental protocol.

**Obscure Manipulation of the Data.** Plots or summary tables should always show results in the same form in which they were analyzed. This, of course, is the actual dependent variable in terms of which the researcher has stated his hypotheses. If the researcher chooses to show some function of the dependent variable, such as percent change, this presentation should be in addition to, rather than instead of, the actual scale.

Very often investigators get into trouble when they start thinking in terms of percents. Thinking in this vein is a very natural tendency and can facilitate evaluation, if done properly. Whenever a percent is given, it should be indicated what and how many it is a percent of. If 50 percent of women in the 1968 freshman class at MIT became pregnant, this might be considered shocking, unless we knew that it represents only one out of the two women enrolled. Also, a percent without any comparison has little meaning. Maybe 50 percent of 1968 Radcliffe freshmen became pregnant, too. Misinterpretation can occur when an investigator attempts to combine such percentages. If the pregnancy rate at MIT in 1968 was 50 percent, at Radcliffe 20 percent, and at Bryn Mawr 15 percent, what is the overall rate at these three schools? It's not $(50 + 20 + 15)/3 = 28$ percent but rather $\frac{1 + 12 + 12}{2 + 60 + 80}$ or $25/142 = 18$ percent. In this context, the average percent is fallacious. Another pitfall involves deducing changes in absolute numbers from changes in percents. If the pregnancy rate at Radcliffe increased to 30 percent in 1978, this still might only mean 12 women became pregnant because enrollment in the 1978 freshman class was down to 40. The above examples all involve percentages of totals.

The use of a percent to indicate relative changes of status is also subject to misinterpretation. A decrease from 10 to 5 is probably a lot more meaningful than a change from 1 to 0.5 on the same scale, yet both "after" measurements are 50 percent of the "before" measurements. In the study investigating the effectiveness of a new drug for hypertensive patients, one patient's systolic blood pressure decreased from 190 mmHg before treatment to 140 mmHg after treatment, whereas a second patient actually became worse, increasing from 140 mmHg to 190 mmHg. Both represent an absolute change of 50 mmHg. Figure 42.7*A* shows these changes, using the before values as the basis for expressing the relative percent (see Glossary). Since one patient decreased 78 percent (140/190 = .78) and the other increased 136 percent (190/140 = 1.36), and the average of 78 and 136 is 107, blood pressure went up 7 percent. In Figure 42.7*B*, we can conclude exactly the opposite, overall blood pressure being 7 percent higher before relative to after the drug. Which is correct? Neither is. A different kind of average must be used, the geometric mean. Use either the before or after as the basis, multiply the numbers together, and take the square root of the result. (To get the geometric average of *n* numbers, multiply them all to-

gether and take the nth root.) For the above example $\sqrt{78 \times 136} = \sqrt{136 \times 78} = 100$, or overall blood pressure neither increased nor decreased.

Such manipulations of the data, unless analyzed carefully, can produce misleading results. Unless there are good physiologic reasons for using a relative percent scale (or percent differences—see Glossary), it is best to look at absolute changes. In the above example, the average absolute change is $(-50 + 50)/2 = 0$.

### Are the Conclusions Valid Based on the Design, the Data, and the Analysis?

First of all, can the conclusions even be identified? More is needed than the statement that Group X is significantly different from Group Y ($p < .05$). At the risk of being repetitive, it is necessary to refer back to the stated objectives. Have the specific objectives been achieved so that science is advanced toward achievement of the ultimate objectives? Has the investigator achieved meaningful results as well as statistically significant results? Does he go too far in generalizing the results to the inference population? Has he fully discussed any characteristics of his study group that might have biased his results and qualified his conclusions accordingly? These questions must all be carefully considered before the conclusions can be accepted.

**Negative Results.** If a given null hypothesis cannot be rejected at the chosen level of significance, do we conclude that the null hypotheses is true? A finding that is physiologically reasonable, which approaches a meaningful magnitude, and is consistent with the work of others should not be ignored. It is likely that the sample size was simply too small to allow statistical significance to be achieved.

Blunders along this line are all too common. Suppose seven out of 10 (70 percent) patients showed improvement on a given therapy when only two in the placebo group showed improvement (20 percent), a difference of 50 percent. Using samples of size 10, the probability of detecting a real treatment difference of 50 percent is fairly small. This probability is called "the power of the test." Researchers often fail to appreciate that they can control the power of

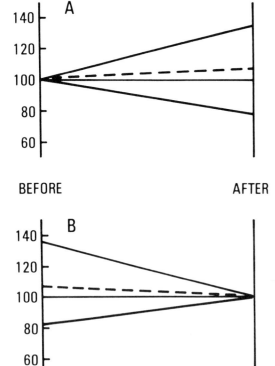

Fig. 42.7  In the top panel the basis is the before treatment value and blood pressure appears to increase. In the lower panel the basis is the after treatment value and blood pressure appears to decrease.

the test by choosing large enough sample sizes. A recent survey [32] of 71 "negative trials" reexamined the basis for the conclusion that a potential therapy was "no different from control," and found that the power of these tests was less than 90 percent for detecting a 25 percent therapeutic response for 67 of these studies. In 50 of these trials, the power was less than 90 percent for detecting a 50 percent therapeutic response. Rather than accepting the null hypothesis, the researcher can only conclude that his results are inconclusive. What a waste of scientific effort! Careful attention to power during the design of the experiment can avoid this unfortunate outcome (Type II error).[33]

One word of caution should be interjected at this point. It is often tempting for an investigator to keep entering subjects in a trial until significance is reached. The investigator rationalizes this practice by convincing himself that he misestimated the required sample size. Or, he wants to terminate a randomized clinical trial for ethical reasons as soon as the efficacy of the new drug is demonstrated so that all patients can then benefit from the new therapy. Special experimental designs called sequential analyses have been devised to handle this "multiple look" problem.[34,35] These are very useful methodologies when one specific hypothesis is to be tested and the time to gather an individual datum (conduct the intervention on a single subject) is small relative to that available for the entire study.

Multiple looks not part of a sequential design beg fate much in the same manner as multiple comparisons to be discussed in the next section. In fact, McPherson [36] reports that even when the null hypothesis is true, the possibility of rejecting it increases with the number of looks taken. Indeed, if an investigator keeps looking long enough, a true null hypothesis will be rejected.[29] At some stage the sample will be extreme enough for this to occur. Investigators are fooling themselves, as well as the readers of their publications, if they report the final sample size, obtained after more than one look (when significance at last is reached), as if they had planned it that way from the beginning. Often, much to the chagrin of such investigators, an early promising trend even disappears.

Careful design of the experiment, either on a one look or a sequential look basis, can eliminate this problem.

**Multiple Comparisons and Conclusions.** There are actually two types of comparisons: those made to test specific hypotheses decided upon as part of the original study design and those suggested by the data. It is important to identify which are which. Consider the following "experiment." Take a pack of index cards and have them represent a group of treated patients. Mark a card S for a successful outcome and F for failure depending upon the actual result. Now shuffle the deck and cut it in half. Mark the top half male and the bottom half female. Shuffle and cut the cards again, this time marking the top half old and the bottom half young. Repeat this procedure again and again adding such characteristics as treated early or late, sedentary or active, brown eyes or blue. During this procedure, you may have observed that sometimes many of the F's ended up in one half of the deck and very few in the other. If you had applied a statistical test in those instances, many would have resulted in $p$-values $< .05$. This same mechanism (the colossal crap game) is at work in any real set of data. Even when there is no actual association, some comparisons will be significant. If *only* those that appear different are analyzed and then conclusions are drawn based on these tests, the likelihood of being in error is enhanced. The only use such "a posteriori tests" have is to discover new hypotheses to be tested by a new, carefully designed investigation. Of course, the results of the new investigation must be analyzed separately. If they were combined with the original data, the sample is not random but selected because of its contents, at least with regard to the part contributed by the first investigation.

Even when the investigator has specified a priori exactly which hypotheses he wants to test, probability considerations can act to lead him astray. Before elaborating on how this can happen, it should be pointed out that probability theory is often not in accordance with one's intuition. (The next time you find yourself in a group of 30 or more people, assert that there are probably two persons in the room born on the same day of the year. Your chance of being correct is 50 percent!)

Back to the problem at hand, an example based on drawing cards from a deck is analogous to conducting multiple tests of significance. The probability of drawing an ace from a shuffled deck of playing cards is 4/52 or $1/13 = .08$, and the probability of *not* getting an ace is 12/13. The probability of two independent random events occurring together is the product of the probabilities that each occurs separately. The probability of not getting an ace twice in a row (replacing the card drawn first) is $(12/13)^2$ and the probability of drawing at least one ace * is thus $1-(12/13)^2 = .15$. Now let the event of drawing an ace be analogous to the event of obtaining an extreme value of a test statistic, a value corresponding to .05 probability. Also assume five tests are to be made as a result of one experiment. The probability of achieving at least one extreme event by chance alone (obtaining at least one significant result) is then $1-(.95)^5 = .23$ not .05! To maintain an overall specified level of significance, mathematicians have suggested that researchers divide the significance level by the number of tests made ($P' = P/K$, K = number of tests) and insist that any individual test, to be considered significant, achieve a significance less than or equal to $P'$.[37] In the above example, maintaining an overall significance level of .05 would require all tests to individually be significant at the $0.5/5 = .01$ level: $1-(.99)^5 = .05$. This seems a fairly drastic measure to take, and in some cases other "protection" methods are appropriate.[38] Unless some effort has been made to control this statistical phenomenon, publications peppered with P's should be taken with a grain of salt.

**Casuality and Association.** When an analysis shows that there is a relationship or correlation between two factors, drawing conclusions must

---

* For two draws there are four possible outcomes for which the probabilities sum to one.

$$P(A) \cdot P(A) + P(N) \cdot P(A) +$$
$$P(A) \cdot P(N) + P(N) \cdot P(N) = 1$$

Where P(A) = probability of drawing an ace and P(N) = probability of not drawing an ace

still be done with care. In fact, if there is not a well thought-out biologic hypothesis that led to the test in the first place, no conclusion should be drawn at all. This statements harks back to the *a posteriori* tests discussed above. Given that a biologic hypothesis does exist, there still might exist another hypothesis, which can exaplain the results just as well. Or, since biologic systems are exceedingly complex, a third factor might be associated with one of the factors under investigation, which is the actual causal agent.

## SUMMARY

The tone given this chapter risks imparting a negative attitude to the reader. Instead, it is hoped that this treatment, by pointing out errors common in statistical practice, and the principles they violate, will foster genuine understanding and give the reader of medical literature a certain degree of confidence in his evaluation of what he reads. Even people who have had formal courses in statistical methods sometimes fail to achieve this degree of understanding. Perhaps this is due to the cookbook format of most texts. Many potential students think that a cookbook is precisely what they need. They are wrong. They need a bit more—an appreciation of the foundations underlying statistical methodology.

The researcher, at this point, might feel that the "thou shalt nots" chronicled above leave little room for positive endeavor. However, once a background sufficient to appreciate what constitutes good statistical methodology is gained, life should actually be easier for researchers. A good experimental design means fewer false starts, even in the pilot study phase. Bias can best be kept at bay when vigilance is constant. A well-conceived study with clear objectives, translated into testable hypotheses and appropriate conclusions, avoids reviewer rejection. Correct analysis of the data and careful presentation of results minimizes manuscript revisions.

The hallmarks of a statistically well-crafted study are: clearly stated objectives, correct choice of independent and dependent variables, formulation of hypotheses to be tested in terms of those variables, use of random samples, proper use of controls, use of the appropriate statistical tests, clear presentation of the data, and carefully drawn conclusions. Each of these topics has been discussed above, but a few additional remarks seems appropriate at this point. These involve the use of samples which, though apparently without bias, are nevertheless not truly random.

The medical literature abounds with conflicting results. Other investigators do not observe the same trends in their work or cannot reproduce the results, even when they set out to do so by following exactly the methodology of the researcher whose work is in question. Was the researcher simply a victim of chance? He had a 5 percent chance of obtaining his results (maybe even greater if multiple tests were made), even when the relationship in question did not exist. And it happened! Or was some other demon at work besides fate? As long as the sample selected was not truly random, it is probably just as likely that the demon was bias rather than fate.

In medical research, the samples used are rarely ever selected randomly. Researchers use whatever experimental subjects present themselves, and it is folly to assume that this happens in a random fashion. Incorrectly, investigators often assume that attaining a $p$-value of .05 means that 95 times out of every 100, a study like theirs will yield the same result, and instead of testing the repeatability of their results by actually doing the experiment again or having others do it, they sit back and smugly draw their conclusions.

What did reputable scientists do to justify the conclusions indicated by their results before statistical methodologies became widespread? They actually demonstrated that their results were repeatable by doing the experiment or sampling again, and again, and again. Reputable scientists still follow these paths. In fact, this procedure is the only way to determine whether the results were a fluke due to some hidden sample bias. It is unlikely that the demon will rear its ugly head repeatedly.

One last comment: *Simple is better.* Often

researchers attempt to wring too much from one experiment. Realizing that it's tempting economically to use the same subjects to answer a number of questions, the potential problems outweigh the potential benefits on several grounds. First, what if fate had, indeed, dealt a bad sample? Not just one conclusion but possibly many would be erroneous. Also, the various measurements may perturb the subject in ways that bias observations on other dependent variables. Finally, we have discussed how multiple tests of significance degrade overall confidence for separate tests. Such a strategy is possibly useful in pilot studies, but to answer the various individual questions suggested, separate experiments should be conducted.

**Need Help?** Throughout this chapter various texts have been referenced, which elucidate a given point particularly well. It is difficult to recommend any one text as a basic reference to someone involved in doing or trying to interpret medical research. Instead, a small library might be more appropriate, although there will be considerable overlap in content. Elementary Medical Statistics by Mainland [39] emphasizes the importance of sound experimental design. It is a good companion text to some that are more oriented toward statistical computation. Statistics, Science and Sense by Shindell [10] also has this same orientation.

Several comprehensive texts stand out from among the hoards published. Statistical Methods in Medical Research by Armitage [14] focuses on medial applications, whereas Introduction to Statistical Analysis by Dixon and Massey [40] and Statistical Methods by Snedecor and Cochran [15] are more general in scope.

Less comprehensive and more elementary are Biostatistics, An Introductory Text by Goldstein [13] and Understanding Statistical Reasoning by Willemsen.[41]

For an intuitive and straightforward treatment of analysis of variance, Biometrical Interpretation by Gilbert [25] is superb. The text, Statistical Principles in Experimental Design, By Winer [27] emphasizes analysis of variance and is one of the only texts that treats repeated measures analysis of variance (several observations on the same subjects under different conditions) at all. It is mathematical in presentation but gives clear descriptions of computational procedures and underlying assumptions.

Finally, it would be useful to have within reach one of the texts on nonparametric methods. Any of those mentioned earlier is adequate but Nonparametric Statistical Methods by Hollander and Wolfe [28] tends toward medical applications and gives very clear descriptions and examples of computational procedures as well as guidance in selecting the appropriate test.

When a biostatistician is available for consultation, make use of such services. If the results of a published study could influence a clinical decision and there are potential problems with the study design which could have an impact on the validity of the conclusions, discuss it with a statistician.

Researchers, before you record a single datum, discuss your study design with a biostatistician. Don't expect miracles once the study is completed and the data are ready for analysis. Salvage operations after the fact are seldom completely satisfactory.

**A Plea for Common Sense.** The phrase "statistical significance" has intoxicated the reviewer or reader all too often. It has served to divert the audience from a careful consideration of whether the result has clinical or biologic significance, whether the logic of the objectives and hypotheses to be tested are sound, and from simply asking, "What else could this mean?" Don't let the arithmetic of statistical significance overshadow careful, critical evaluation of the validity of the underlying science.

# GLOSSARY

**Alternative Hypothesis.** An alternative hypothesis specifies the class of underlying distributions which do not satisfy the null hypothesis (i.e., [see null hypothesis] the proportion of red marbles is not .50 or the mean of the normal population is not 0.)

**Balanced Design.** An experiment is balanced if each treatment combination is assigned the same number of experimental units.

**Confidence Interval.** A confidence interval $(P_L, P_U)$ for some population parameter P is an interval derived from a random sample hav-

ing the property that the true, unknown population parameter is contained within this interval with a specified level of probability (i.e., .95).

**Correlation Coefficient.** The correlation coefficient of two random variables X and Y from the same sample is defined as:

$$r = \frac{\text{covariance of X and Y}}{\sqrt{(\text{variance of X})(\text{variance of Y})}}$$

**Covariance.** The covariance of two random variables from the same sample of size n is defined as:

$$\sum_{i=1}^{n}(X_i - \overline{X})(Y_i - \overline{Y})$$

where $\overline{X}$, $\overline{Y}$ are the sample means for the random variables X and Y respectively.

**Dependent Variable.** See page 1018.

**Distribution.** The distribution of a finite, discrete population is simply an enumeration of the various items in it and the frequency that they occur (i.e., 20 red marbles and 80 blue marbles in a jar. The chance of drawing a red marble is .20). When the population is continuous, the distribution can be represented by a curve on a graph above the horizontal axis. The total area under the curve and above the horizontal axis is one. The probability that a measurement in a given interval is obtained is the area under the curve above the horizontal axis and between the values defining the interval.

**Efficiency.** The relative efficiency of Test A to Test B for the same significance level is the ratio of $N_a/N_b$ where $N_a$ is the sample size of Test A required to achieve the same power as for Test B with a required sample size of $N_b$.

**Geometric Mean.** See page 1032.

**Independent Variable.** See page 1018.

**Independent Random Variables.** Two random variables are independent if the probability the first takes on a value in a given range *and* the second takes on a value in another range (possibly the same) is equal to the product of the probabilities each takes on a value in its own specified range. When this is not true, the variables are sometimes referred to as correlated (e.g., heart rates for two unrelated, isolated people are independent but the heart rates measured at two points in time for the same individual are not independent).

**Mean of a Sample.** The mean of a sample of size n is equal to

$$\overline{X} = \sum_{i=1}^{n} X_i/n$$

**Multiple Comparison Procedure.** A multiple comparison procedure based on sample observations evaluates simultaneously for a specified significance level a number of null hypotheses concerning various parameters of interest.

**Nonparametric Statistical Procedure.** A statistical procedure which has properties that hold under relatively mild assumptions regarding the underlying population is called a nonparametric statistical procedure.

**Null Hypothesis.** A null hypothesis specifies that the underlying population distribution (from which a sample came) is a member of a certain class and has a specified value for a population parameter (e.g. the proportion of red marbles in a jar is .50, or the mean of the population is 0).

**One-tailed Hypothesis.** The null hypothesis specifies that the underlying class of distributions has a parameter $<$, $\leq$, $>$, or $\geq$ a given value (e.g., the mean of a certain population is $< 0.$).

**Percent Difference.** The percent difference is 100 minus the relative percent of two numbers:

$$100 - 100\frac{a}{b} = 100\left(1 - \frac{a}{b}\right) = 100\left(\frac{b-a}{b}\right)$$

where b is the basis.

**Population.** A population is any set of individuals or objects having some common observable characteristic. The term population can refer to either the individuals measured or the measurements themselves. A population can be finite or infinite. When referring to measurements themselves, the values can be discrete or continuous.

**Population Parameter.** Any measurable characteristic of a population is a population parameter (e.g., the mean and variance).

**Pooled Variance Estimate.** If $S_1^2$, $S_2^2$, . . . , $S_k^2$ are sample variances for k samples of size $n_1$, $n_2$, . . . , $n_k$ the pooled variance estimate (sometimes referred to as "within sample variance" in analysis of variance) is

$$S^2 = \frac{(n_1 - 1)S_1^2 + (n_2 - 1)S_2^2 + . . . + (n_k - 1)S_k^2}{n_1 + n_2 + \cdots n_k - k}$$

**Power.** The power of a test is the probability of rejecting the null hypothesis when in fact the null hypothesis is true.

**Random Sample.** A sample is a random sample if each member of the population has the same chance of being included in the sample.

**Random Variable.** A characteristic or measurement whose possible values follow a probability distribution is called a random variable (e.g., the marbles in the jar are red or blue and have the distribution described above [see Distribution] or the random variable, basal temperature, has a normal distribution).

**Relative Percent.** The relative percent is 100 times the ratio of one value to another. The value used in the denominator is the basis.

**Sample.** A sample is any subset of a population.

**Sampling Distribution.** The value of a given statistic obtained from a random sample will vary depending on the sample selected. Thus, the statistic itself has a distribution of its own. This distribution is called the sampling distribution.

**Significance Level.** The significance level of a test is the probability of rejecting the null hypothesis when it is in fact true.

**Standard Deviation of a Sample.** The standard deviation for a random variable X from a sample of size n is the square root of its variance.

$$\text{S.D.} = \sqrt{\sum_{i=1}^{n} \frac{(X_i - \overline{X})^2}{n-1}}$$

where $\overline{X}$ is the sample mean.

**Standard Error.** The standard deviation of the sampling distribution is its standard error (i.e., the standard error of the mean is the standard deviation of the sample means for all possible samples which can be selected from a population).

**Statistic.** A statistic is any number computed from a sample (i.e., its mean, range, maximum value, etc.).

**Statistical test.** A statistical test is a procedure which, on the basis of random sample, either rejects or fails to reject a null hypothesis.

**Stratification.** A population can sometimes be divided into several groups or strata based on a specific characteristic. Subjects within such a strata are thus more homogeneous than for the population as a whole.

**Two-tailed Hypothesis.** The null hypothesis specifies that a parameter of the underlying distribution has a certain value. The alternative hypothesis then has values for the parameter either less than or greater than this value (i.e., the mean is 0).

**Type I Error.** A Type I error occurs when the null hypothesis is rejected when in fact it is true.

**Type II Error.** A Type II error occurs when the null hypothesis is *not* rejected when in fact the alternative hypothesis is true.

# REFERENCES

1. Fisher RA: Statistical Methods for Research Workers. Oliver and Boyd, Ltd., Edinburgh and New York, 1925.
2. Fisher RA: The Design of Experiments. Oliver and Boyd, Ltd., Edinburgh and London, 1935.
3. Mainland D: The use and misuse of statistics in medical publications. Clin Pharmacol Ther 1:411, 1960.
4. Feinstein AR: Clinical Biostatistics. The CV Mosby Company, St Louis, MO, 1977. p 6.
5. Hill AB: Principles of Medical Statistics. 9th ed. Oxford University Press, New York, 1971, p 274–308.
6. Mainland D: Statistical ward rounds—16. Clin Pharmacol Ther 10:576, 1969.
7. Saiger GL: Errors of medical studies. JAMA 173:678, 1960.
8. Schor S, Karten I: Statistical evaluation of journal manuscripts. JAMA 195:1123, 1966.
9. Schor S: Statistical reviewing program for medical manuscripts. Am Stat 21:28, 1967.
10. Shindell S: Statistics, Science and Sense. University of Pittsburgh Press, Pittsburgh, 1964, p 41–49.
11. Feinstein AR, Wells CK: Randomized trials vs historical controls: the scientific plagues of both houses. Trans Assoc Am Physicians 90:238, 1977.
12. Pocock S: Randomized clinical trials. Br Med J 1:1661, 1977.
13. Goldstein A: Biostatistics an Introductory Text. MacMillan, New York, 1964, p 34, 93, 117.
14. Armitage P: Statistical Methods in Medical Research. Blackwell Scientific Publications, Oxford, 1971, p 72, 59, 66.
15. Snedecor GW, Cochran WG: Statistical Methods. The Iowa State University Press, Ames, Iowa, 1956, p 25.
16. Hollander M, Wolfe D: Nonparametric Statistical Methods. John Wiley and Sons, New York, 1973, p 226.
17. Goldstein A: Biostatistics, An Introductory Text. MacMillan, New York, 1964, p 100.
18. Goldstein A: Biostatistics, An Introductory Text. MacMillan, New York, 1964, p 51–55.
19. Goldstein A: Biostatistics, An Introductory Text. MacMillan, New York, 1964, p 71–73.
20. Goldstein A: Biostatistics, An Introductory Text. MacMillan, New York, 1964, p 59–60.
21. Winer BJ: Statistical Principles in Experimental Design. McGraw-Hill, New York, 1971, p 261–308.
22. Goldstein A: Biostatistics, An Introductory Text. MacMillan, New York, 1964, p 93–101.
23. Goldstein A: Biostatistics, An Introductory Text. MacMillan, New York, 1964, p 110–111.
24. Pearson ES, Hartley HO: Biometrika Tables for Statisticians, Vol 1. Cambridge University Press, London, 1954, Table 38.
25. Gilbert N: Biometrical Interpretation. Clarendon Press, Oxford, 1973, p 56–62
26. Siegel S: Nonparametric Statistics for the Behavioral Sciences. McGraw-Hill, New York, 1956.
27. Tate MW, Clelland RC: Nonparametric and Shortcut Statistics in the Social, Biological and Medical Sciences. Interstate Printers and Publishers, Danville, Ill., 1957.
28. Hollander M, Wolfe D: Nonparametric Statistical Methods. John Wiley, New York, 1973.
29. Bradley, JV: Distribution-Free Statistical Tests. Prentice-Hall, Englewood Cliffs, NJ, 1968.
30. Snedecor GW, Cochran WG: Statistical Methods. The Iowa State University Press, Ames, Iowa, 1956, p 98.

31. Goldstein A: Biostatistics, An Introductory Text. MacMillan, New York, 1964, p 251.
32. Freiman JA, Chalmers TC, Smith H Jr, Kuebler RR: The importance of beta, the type II error and sample size in the design and interpretation of the randomized control trial. N Engl J Med 299:690, 1978.
33. Feinstein AR: Clinical Biostatistics. CV Mosby, St Louis, 1977, p 320.
34. Armitage P: Sequential Medical Trials. Blackwell Scientific Publications, Oxford, 1960.
35. McPherson CK, Armitage P: Repeated significance tests on accumulating data when the null hypothesis is not true. JR Stat Soc 134:15, 1971.
36. McPherson K: The problem of examining accumulating data more than once. N Engl J Med 290:501, 1974.
37. Dunn OJ: Multiple comparisons among means. J Am Stat Assoc 56:52, 1961.
38. Winer BJ: Statistical Principles in Experimental Design. McGraw-Hill, New York, 1971, p 185–204.
39. Mainland D: Elementary Medical Statistics. WB Saunders, Philadelphia, 1963.
40. Dixon WJ, Massey FJ: Introduction to Statistical Analysis. McGraw-Hill, New York, 1957.
41. Willemsen EW: Understanding Statistical Reasoning. WH Freeman and Company, San Francisco, 1974.

## ACKNOWLEDGMENT

This study supported by Specialized Center of Research on Ischemic Heart Disease NIH Research Grant HL-17682 from the National Heart, Lung and Blood Institute.

# 43 | Risk Assessment After Acute Myocardial Infarction

*Elizabeth A. Gilpin, M.S.*
*Joel S. Karliner, M.D.*
*John Ross, Jr., M.D.*

## SOME PURPOSES OF RISK ASSESSMENT

There are several advantages to be gained from accurate risk assessment of the individual patient. An obvious one is that clinical management of each patient could be optimized. As an example of one type of risk assessment, Swan et al.[1] have proposed that if by the fifth day after the acute event a patient is free from any of the complications listed below, he should respond favorably to short periods of bedrest (4 days) and hospitalization (9 to 14 days). These criteria include absence of evidence for:

1. Continued cardiac ischemia (pain, late enzyme increase)
2. Left ventricular failure (congestive heart failure, new murmurs, x-ray changes)
3. Shock (blood pressure drop, pallor, oliguria)
4. Important cardiac arrhythmias (premature ventricular contractions > 6/min, atrial fibrillation)
5. Conduction disturbances (bundle branch block, A-V block, hemiblock)
6. Complicating illness

Management of this type of patient by mobilization with progressive activity over the next week should reduce the average duration of hospital stay. Alternatively, patients identified as being at greater-than-average risk might be kept in the Coronary Care Unit (CCU) and monitored carefully for longer than the usual period or be candidates for more aggressive therapeutic measures. A variety of criteria for risk assessment based on such clinical criteria have been proposed by various investigators and are discussed in detail below.

Another advantage of accurate risk assessment concerns the research environment. In the design of clinical trials for new therapies, focusing on that portion of the patient population likely to benefit most from the proposed treatment will produce much more efficient designs regarding the number of patients required than if all patients were utilized. For instance, including patients at very low or very high risk may not provide any information. In the first case, virtually all patients will survive (assuming death to be the endpoint), whether or not they receive the therapy. In the second case, it might be unlikely that any therapy could help at all.

As an example, consider a drug trial in a group of patients from whom the 2-year mortality rate is 36 percent. Suppose it is hypothesized that the drug should reduce this rate by half (i.e. to 18 percent). With the standard two-tailed significance level of .05 and 90 percent power, the sample size required is 300 patients (150 in the control group and 150 in the treated group). Suppose that the patient population can be stratified into three groups, as shown in Table 43.1. Ignoring the low- and high-risk groups for which the therapy potentially will have no effect, the goal is to reduce the mortality of the middle group from 40 percent to 20 percent,

Table 43.1  Risk Stratification and Experimental Design

| Risk | Observed Untreated Mortality* | Design 1 Hypothesized Rates | Design 2 Hypothesized Rates |
|---|---|---|---|
| Low | $\frac{3}{10}$ (10)† | $\frac{3}{30}$ (10) | $\frac{3}{30}$ (10) |
| Medium | $\frac{24}{60}$ (40) | $\frac{6}{60}$ (10) | $\frac{12}{60}$ (20) |
| High | $\frac{9}{10}$ (90) | $\frac{9}{10}$ (90) | $\frac{9}{10}$ (90) |
| Overall | $\frac{36}{100}$ (36) | $\frac{18}{100}$ (18) | $\frac{24}{100}$ (24) |
| Sample size required | — | 300 | 260 |

\* The denominator indicates the incidence of low, medium, and high risk patients per 100 patients and the numerator the number dying in each group.
† Figures in parentheses are percentages.

which requires a total of 260 patients in the trial, a reduction in initial population of about 15 percent. However, the real danger in the first design is that the trial might turn out to be inconclusive. If the low- and high-risk patients are indeed unaffected by the drug, in order for overall mortality to be reduced by half, the middle group would have to show a reduction in mortality of 75 percent (See Table 43.1). In fact, the results of many negative clinical trials could possibly be altered if a group or groups of patients could be identified (by objective stratification criteria), which did indeed benefit from the therapy. Such retrospective data analysis, though very explanatory, often only points the way to a new experiment to confirm the apparent results. If appropriate criteria for patient entry based on risk assessment methodologies had been performed beforehand, the design would be optimally efficient and the results indisputable.

Another important implication of prognostic identification in clinical trials involves tests of extremely radical or controversial therapy. It would be unethical to subject patients to such treatment when it is known that other less extreme or more widely accepted measures are likely to be efficacious. If a very high-risk group can be identified for which the usual approach is ineffective, any improvement at all would be

noteworthy. For example, if the usual 6-month mortality rate for a group of patients is 97 percent, the upper 95 percent confidence limit on the survival rate would be about 10 percent. For 30 such people, at the most, three could be expected to survive by chance alone. Without even using a control group, if more than three people out of 30 survived 6 months, it is likely that the therapy deserves more attention. Plans can then be made to conduct a full-blown, controlled, clinical trial that included patients who are at less risk. If no more than three people survive the 6-month period, the therapy is probably not worth investigating further.

Finally, the process of constructing a risk assessment scheme can itself be enlightening. Often insight is gained concerning the relative importance of various factors in determining risk. Also patterns may emerge that actually might provide some insight into underlying mechanisms. For instance, clusters of patients with roughly the same profile might follow the same natural historic course.

## MORTALITY AFTER ACUTE MYOCARDIAL INFARCTION

A large proportion of patients who die following an acute myocardial infarction succumb before they even reach the hospital. Prehospital mortality is estimated to be between 40 and 60 percent of total deaths. The incidence of acute myocardial infarction in the United States is approximately 1,300,000 per year and an estimated 52 percent or about 650,000 fail to survive the acute episode. How long after the acute episode it can be considered the principal cause of death is not precisely defined. At some point, recovery should be sufficient that death after that time is no more likely than for persons with coronary heart disease who have not had an acute myocardial infarction.

Figure 43.1 shows a survival curve after acute myocardial infarction for a group of 256 patients studied at the University of California, San Diego Specialized Center of Research in Ischemic Heart Disease (UCSD SCOR) [2] and curves for a normal population,[3] and one with ischemic heart disease or angina pectoris.[4] In the first 30 days, 48 patients or 21 percent of the population with acute myocardial infarction died. Seventy-five percent of these deaths occurred in the CCU within 12 days of admission. The slope of the curve is clearly greater than the normal population or the population with angina pectoris until 7 or 8 months after the acute event, although the numbers of patients involved are too few for sweeping generalizations. However, these figures suggest that other

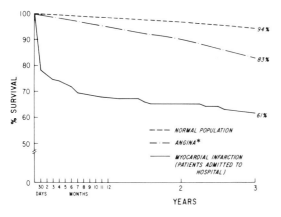

Fig. 43.1 Actuarial survival curve for UCSD-SCOR patients [2] with myocardial infarction *(solid line)*. The survival rates of an age- and sex-matched normal population *(dashed line)* computed from mortality rates published by the U.S. Public Health Service [3] and in patients with angina pectoris *(dashed and dotted line)* from Richards et al.[4] are shown for comparison.

than prehospital mortality, there are several potential target times for prognostication: early after admission (first day); in the hospital (from 2 days to 20 to 30 days); after discharge (1 to 12 months); and late mortality (after 1 year).

These divisions are somewhat arbitrary, as indicated by the ranges, and are conditioned by other factors as well. When a patient is admitted, it is customary to obtain a history, perform a physical examination, and order certain laboratory investigations, including an ECG, chest x-ray, and blood samples for serum enzyme determinations and hematology. A good deal of information is thus generated within a few hours after admission, which, if an accurate prognostic scheme were available, could be used to gauge immediate prognosis. Within the next few days, more information becomes available concerning arrhythmias, laboratory results, and serial changes in various factors such as arterial and possibly intracardiac pressures, enzyme levels, white blood cell count, and changes in heart size. Added to the admission findings, such data are potentially useful for determining prognosis during the hospital stay or, since this period varies from patient to patient, a fixed early point in time, such as 30 days. Assuming that a patient survives to be discharged from the hospital, all the data gathered during the hospital stay are available for risk assessment after discharge. It seems reasonable to focus on the postdischarge period, during which the patient's status is still, in part, determined by the acute event and his response to it as recorded during the hospital stay.

It is very likely that different factors will influence prognosis at each of the various stages. This phenomenon may, in part, be responsible for the lack of accord among the many studies of factors influencing prognosis after acute myocardial infarction. There are undoubtedly other reasons as well, including differences in study populations, factor definition or measurement, inadequate sample sizes, and different data-analysis methodologies.

## PROGNOSTIC VARIABLES

The search for a single factor that will accurately predict mortality and survival after acute myocardial infarction has occupied a number of investigators.[5-13] But even these reports qualify their results and either speculate or attempt to investigate other factors as well. The variables investigated can be classified broadly as those that provide some indication of the extent of cardiac damage and the resulting depression of cardiac performance, and those that are indicative of the patient's state, independent of the new acute event. This second set includes such factors as age, sex, presence of complicating illnesses such as chronic obstructive lung disease, hypertension or diabetes, and whether or not this is the first myocardial infarction. There is generally little that can be done to alter the patient's state with respect to this type of factor. Most therapeutic measures are aimed at improving the level of the variables associated with cardiac function.

With the possible exception of some hemodynamic indices obtained by invasive means, these variables are necessarily indirect measures of the variable of interest: the actual degree of pump dysfunction. As such, they are inevitably imprecise and, though they have proved useful for assessment of prognosis, perfect prediction is an unattainable goal. In fact, it is well-recognized that even when overt clinical manifestations of pump failure are absent, hemodynamic indices can be abnormal.[2,14] Conversely, severe congestive heart failure does not inevitably presage a poor prognosis, and occasionally such patients manage to survive for years beyond the acute event.

Table 43.2 lists, as comprehensively as possible, the factors that have been related to mortality at various times (prediction windows) after the acute event. The entries in the table are reference numbers, and the reader is urged to refer to these works for details concerning methods, definitions, and results. Although it rarely happens that two studies aimed at the same prediction window conclude that the same set of factors have predictive value, enough concordance does exist to warrant their inclusion in this list. If a reference number is not included for a certain factor, it could mean that factor was not investigated at all or it was investigated but not found to be significantly related to prognosis for that prediction window. Some of the possible reasons for the discrepancies apparent in Table 43.2 were mentioned above. The discussion below will attempt to go beyond the empirical evidence relating these factors to mortality and focus on the manner, often only hypothesized, in which they relate to either cardiac function or complicate a patient's condition and, thus, affect survival.

Factors Related to Function.

The class of factors indicative of function will be grouped under the following categories of findings: physical examination, chest radiograph, electrocardiogram (ECG), laboratory results, and hemodynamic observations.

**Physical Examination.** Assuming the patient has been calmed from the anxiety surrounding the initial onset of the event, admission heart rate and systolic blood pressure relate to immediate function and early mortality. In the absence of hypovolemia, an increased heart rate is indicative of a decreased stroke volume, and an elevated systolic blood pressure can be related to increased myocardial oxygen demands and raised vascular resistance, both of which may exacerbate left ventricular dysfunction.

A low systolic blood pressure in the presence of an adequate left ventricular filling pressure is one manifestation of cardiogenic shock. It is well known that this condition carries a very high early mortality (as high as 80 to 90 percent), regardless of exactly how it is defined (See Ch. 20).

Helmers [15-17] used respiratory rate as an index of the degree of cardiac failure. He stated that "congestive heart failure has long been recognized as one of the most important prognostic factors in acute myocardial infarction and that respiratory rate has been described as a reliable and easily measured indicator of the degree of heart failure." In his population, an increased respiratory rate was related to death within 24 hours of admission, in-hospital death, and 3-year mortality. (The exact levels of increase are mentioned in the section on multivariate studies.) Also, an elevated respiratory rate in the CCU was closely associated with a finding of pulmonary rales. Even though pain, anxiety,

Table 43.2   Variables Related to Prognosis Following Acute Myocardial Infarction*

| | | Mortality Time Window | | | |
|---|---|---|---|---|---|
| Factor | Very Early (first 48 hr) | In-hospital (20 days) | Early (1 mo) | Early Post Discharge (12 mo) | Late (over 1 yr) |
| **Function** | | | | | |
| Physical Examination | | | | | |
| Heart rate | | 44 | 2,55,49 | | 50,36 |
| Systolic blood pressure | | 26,21,43 | 2,55,51 | | 36 |
| Respiration rate | 15 | 15 | 49 | | 15 |
| Temperature | | 26 | 55,49 | | 36 |
| Hypertension | | | | 23 | 19 |
| Hypotension | | | | 37,51 | |
| Peripheral hyperprofusion | | 18 | | | |
| Shock | 15,23 | 26 | 49,51 | 49,51,52 | |
| Gallop rhythm | | 53 | 49 | 22,52 | 52,51 |
| Rales | | 8 | 2,49,51 | 22,23,51 | |
| Peripheral edema | | | 49 | | |
| X-ray | | | | | |
| Cardiomegaly | | 21 | 6,2 | 22,6,23 | 50,20,19 |
| Pulmonary congestion | | 18,26,44,21 | 6,51 | 22,6,23,37, 51–2 | 27,20,48,52 |
| **Laboratory** | | | | | |
| Leukocyte count | | 26 | 49 | 52,51 | 52 |
| Blood urea nitrogen level | | | 51 | 22,51,52 | 36 |
| Uric acid | | | | 22 | |
| Serum creatine | | | | 22 | |
| Enzymes | 15 | 15,41,40 | 2,11,51 | 22,11,51 | |
| Hemodynamics | | | | | |
| LV filling pressure | | 42 | 2 | | 42 |
| LV stroke work index | | 42 | | | 42 |
| Stroke volume index | | 43 | 2 | | |
| Cardiac output | | 43 | | | |
| Cardiac index | | 43 | 2 | | |
| AV-O$_2$ difference | | | 2 | | |
| Ejection fraction | | | 5 | 5,31,46,47 | |
| ECG | | | | | |
| Site of infarct | | 7,25,26,24 21,12,41 | 2,51 | 52,51 | 7,27,36 |
| QRS duration | 39 | 12 | 51 | | |
| QT interval | | | | | 13 |
| ST depression | | 41 | 49 | 51 | 50,9 |
| Q-wave | | 41 | | 51 | 50 |
| Conduction defects | 39 | 10 | 2,49,51 | 51,52 | 50,15,48,52 |
| Atrial dysrhythmias | | 29 | 2 | | 50,36 |
| Sinus tachycardia | | | 2 | | |
| Ventricular dysrhythmias | | | 2 | 6,32,31 | 50,33,36,27, 38,30,52 |
| **State** | | | | | |
| Age | | 15,23,26,21 | 2,55,49,51 | 52,51 | 15,38,20,52 |
| Sex | | 26 | 49 | 52,51 | 52 |
| Hx Previous MI | | 21 | 2,55 | | 50,36,27,20,48 |
| Hx Angina | | | 49 | 37,51 | 50,36,52 |
| Hx Congestive heart failure | | | 2 | | 19 |
| Hx Chronic obstructive pulmonary disease | | | 2 | | |
| Hx Diabetes | | 53 | | 23,51 | 52 |
| Cigarette smoking | | | | | 19,52 |
| Hx Hypertension | | | 49 | | |

* Numbers refer to references.

acidosis, and pulmonary infections affect respiratory rate, it still is a useful prognostic variable.

Other physical findings that can be incorporated into a prognostic scheme include an elevated temperature, which is hypothesized to be the result of the release of intracellular substances from the damaged myocardium. It is also partly due to inflammation resulting from the necrotic process. Jugular venous distention may indicate an elevated pulmonary arterial pressure or right ventricular dysfunction associated with right ventricular infarction. Gallop rhythm is common and is indicative of an elevated left ventricular filling pressure (see below), and often also of decreased diastolic compliance.

The clinical classification scheme developed by Killip et al.[8] seeks to use the presence and extent of pulmonary rales as an indication of left ventricular pump failure. Class I consists of patients without rales; the hospital mortality in this group is less than 10 percent. Patients with rales less than half-way up the lung fields are classified as Class II, and hospital mortality for this group is 10 to 15 percent. Class III patients have rales extending over half the lung fields or exhibit overt pulmonary edema. The mortality for this group is about 30 percent. Class IV consists of patients in shock and carries a high mortality ($\geq$ 80 percent). This classification scheme depends on adequate clinical determinations and is subject to error, even when correctly applied. Rales may result from noncardiac causes, or persist even when cardiac output is adequate, presumably due to decreased diastolic compliance, and may remain despite reduction of pulmonary venous pressure by diuretic therapy.

**Chest Radiograph.** A classification scheme developed by Forrester et al.[18] was based on the presence of pulmonary congestion (rales or an abnormal chest radiograph), and peripheral hypoperfusion (hypotension, tachycardia, confusion, cyanosis, and oliguria). The authors reasoned that pulmonary venous congestion often results from an elevated left ventricular end-diastolic pressure transmitted to the pulmonary venous system. Peripheral hypoperfusion is one of the consequences of reduced cardiac output. The mortality in 200 patients without either

of these clinical findings was only 1 percent. Patients with pulmonary congestion but without peripheral hypoperfusion had an 11 percent mortality. Those without pulmonary congestion but with peripheral hypoperfusion had an 18 percent mortality, and patients having both signs had a 60 percent mortality.

However, the degree of elevation of pulmonary venous pressure and the depression of cardiac output can only be approximated by these clinical manifestations. Also, these signs might be due to other causes. For instance, hypoperfusion might result from hypovolemia rather than pump failure and some patients with preexisting left ventricular failure might have very high left ventricular end-diastolic pressures, even though signs of pulmonary venous congestion are minimal.

Increased heart size is suggestive of left ventricular failure. Higher late mortality in patients with this finding [19,20] is likely related to more severe depression of cardiac function due to more extensive myocardial damage during the acute phase of myocardial infarction. Studies have related increased heart size to short-term survival as well.[2,21-23] It has also been hypothesized that there is some compensatory hypertrophy of residual normal myocardium following extensive myocardial infarction.

Recent work at the UCSD SCOR has examined both pulmonary venous congestion and heart size, as determined from the chest x-ray film taken with the patient in a half-upright, half-supine position.[6] The long-term survival curve for patients without congestion and with normal-sized hearts was different from the curve for patients without congestion but with enlarged hearts. The survival curve for patients with congestion but normal heart size was further depressed. Patients with both congestion and enlarged hearts fared worst of all.

**Electrocardiogram.** Infarct location, certain measurements from the ECG tracing, and the occurence of certain arrhythmias have all been related to prognosis.

The site of infarction and associated prognosis was investigated by Rigo and Murray.[12] Among 111 patients, those with transmural infarction had an in-hospital mortality rate of 22 percent, as compared to those with nontransmural infarction in whom the hospital mortality was 13 percent. However, when the group with nontransmural infarction was further subdivided into those with ST segment or T-wave changes alone, as opposed to those who also exhibited QRS abnormalities, the in-hospital mortality was zero for the former group and 27 percent in the latter. It is interesting to note that late mortality among survivors was the same for all groups.

Other studies concerning the site of infarction have produced conflicting results. Patients with transmural anterior infarction by ECG generally fared worse than those with transmural inferior infarcts,[24] or with infarcts not classified as anterior in location.[2,25-27] Another study of transmural versus nontransmural (subendocardial) infarctions[7] showed little difference in mortality, but patients with extensive subendocardial infarction, manifested by persistent ST depression in most leads, fared worse than patients with limited subendocardial infarction. These discordant results are likey due to small samples of differing populations, but the implication of these studies is that prognosis is likely to be worse if a large area of the left ventricle is involved, regardless of exact location or whether the infarct is transmural or nontransmural.

It has been hypothesized that an imbalance in cardiac sympathetic innervation prolongs the QT interval, increases the tendency to arrhythmias associated with coronary artery occlusion, and lowers the ventricular fibrillation threshold. Swartz and Wolf[13] found that a QT interval > 440 msec (corrected for heart rate) was associated with sudden death during the 10 years following the acute event. The QT intervals for 55 postmyocardial infarction patients and 55 controls were measured every 2 months during the first 4 years. Sixteen of the 28 patients who died suddenly had a prolonged QT interval, as compared to only five of the 27 survivors in this group. Interestingly, the one control subject with a prolonged QT interval also died suddenly.

The incidence of various arrhythmias in patients after acute myocardial infarction will depend, to a certain extent, on the methods used for arrhythmia detection. Conventional techniques use rate-triggered alarm systems and visual screening. However, earlier studies depended only on ECG recordings and very recently on-line computers have been utilized. It is understandable, therefore, that the findings with respect to mortality are plagued with inconsistencies. Arrhythmia frequency also depends on the elapsed time from the onset of symptoms and the monitoring period. The incidence of dysrhythmias is highest within the first hour and, for survivors, declines with time.[28]

Graboys[25] examined various types of arrhythmias in relation to sudden death in the hospital after discharge from the CCU. From a total of 1,378 patients over a 4-year period, 48 died, and 9 of those died suddenly. Those 9 patients were compared to 300 other patients who survived after CCU discharge. They exhibited a higher incidence of sinus tachycardia beyond 2 days without other evidence of pump failure, and an increased incidence of ventricular tachycardia, acute atrial fibrillation or flutter, acute intraventricular and/or atrioventricular conduction disturbances or anterior wall infarction. Also, the sudden-death group had a significantly prolonged CCU stay. Seven of the nine (78 percent) sudden-death patients had three or four of the above factors as compared to only 3 percent of the control group.

Atrial arrhythmias occur in about 10 percent of patients with acute myocardial infarction and the most common of these is atrial fibrillation, which has been associated with increased mortality. Atrial arrhythmias are generally associated with ischemic damage to the sinoatrial node due to occlusion of the artery supplying the area, either the proximal right coronary artery or proximal left circumflex coronary artery.[29] Yet, atrial arrhythmias occur more commonly in patients with anterior rather than inferior or lateral myocardial infarctions. Thus, in addition to injury to the sinoatrial node, other factors must play a significant role in producing atrial arrhythmias. The most obvious is the associated left ventricular failure and its severity, which, of course, relates to the extent of myocardial damage.

A number of investigators[9,30-33] have proposed that the incidence of premature ventricular contractions (PVCs) late in the hospital course might predispose a patient to episodes of ventricular fibrillation leading to sudden death. These studies classified the nature and severity of such ventricular arrhythmias (i.e. Wolf and Lown scheme [36a]) from an extended period of Holter monitoring (up to 12 hours) and assessed the mortality from sudden death in the late period following an acute myocardial infarction. The details of the classification scheme, time and duration of monitoring, length of follow-up, and number of patients studied differed. However, all theses studies demonstrated a difference in mortality from sudden death for patients without ventricular arrhythmia as opposed to those with complicated ventricular extrasystoles. Vismara et al.[30] studied 64 patients, of whom 20 died (average follow-up 25 months). Twelve of these were sudden deaths. None of the patients who died suddenly were free from ventricular arrhythmias. Four had uncomplicated PVCs and eight had complicated PVCs (> 5/min, paired or multifocal PVCs, R on T phenonenon, or ventricular tachycardia). Schulz et al.[31] studied 81 patients from 2 to 16 months following infarction. Eight patients died, all of them suddenly. Each were in Wolf and Lown Class III or greater, which corresponds roughly to the complicated group in Vismara's study. Schulze also noted that all eight patients who died suddenly had an ejection fraction < 0.40. Both studies also related arrhythmia class to ST segment findings. The complicated classes had more ST segment elevation in more leads than the uncomplicated classes. In another study of 160 male survivors of myocardial infarction under 65 years of age, the mortality from sudden death was 3 percent in patients without ventricular arrhythmias or less than 10 PVCs/hr and 14 percent for the more complicated classes.[32] These studies, with the exception of the small one by Schulze, failed to report the incidence of ectopic beats in patients who died from causes not classified as sudden death.

The Coronary Drug Project Research Group [33] examined data on 2,760 men who survived an acute myocardial infarction, in order to ascertain if the differential of frequent PVCs and associated ectopic characteristics (runs, multiform, interpolated, bigeminy, fusion) was greater for sudden death than for all deaths. The sudden death rate was 8.9 percent for patients with more than 10 PVCs per minute or complicated ectopic arrhythmias, and 5.3 percent for those without these findings. The corresponding total mortality rates were 27.7 percent and 11.7 percent, respectively. Thus, these data do not support the hypothesis that PVCs predispose a patient to sudden death. The Group concluded that PVCs are rather simply more frequent according to increasing severity of the clinical state and that PVCs and general mortality have a common base—a greater degree of myocardial disease. Note that the overall incidence of these arrhythmias is less than in the other studies. This is due to the fact that detection of PVCs was carried out using a 12-lead resting ECG with an average sample of 49.4 heart beats per record, rather than extended Holter monitoring. How this factor might affect the results and conclusions of this study is unclear, but recent evidence indicates that an accurate assessment of the frequency of PVCs requires two or more periods of extended ambulatory tape monitoring.[34,35] Nevertheless, complicated ventricular ectopic beats are apparently associated with prognosis after hospital discharge. Thus, a number of researchers have included such data in multivariate analyses for late mortality.[5,27,36,36a,37,38]

A prolonged QRS interval indicates slowing of conduction in the neighborhood of an infarcted or ischemic area. Depending on the site of the infarct, a bundle branch block or other conduction disturbance might also result. In-hospital death of patients with ventricular conduction abnormalities was investigated by Mullins and Atkins.[10] They compiled material from many published reports on the incidence of such disturbances (18 to 21 percent of acute myocardial infarctions); the associated mortality, depending on the type of block, ranged from 27 percent for a left anterior hemiblock to 57 percent for patients with a right bundle branch block and a left posterior hemiblock. Mortality for a left posterior hemiblock alone was 42 percent, for a right bundle branch block alone 46 percent, and for a left bundle branch block 44 percent. Together, a right bundle branch block and a left anterior hemiblock carried a 45 percent mortality. The mortality in patients without such disturbances was 15 percent. They also assessed the therapeutic value of both temporary and permanent pacemakers. The overall mortality of unpaced patients was 65 percent. Temporary pacing did not appear to alter this rate; however, permanent pacemakers reduced the mortality to only 9 percent. Sutton et al.[39] examined the utility of fixed versus demand pacing in 55 patients with second- or third-degree block, slow A-V junctional rhythm, or asystole. Although the small number of patients did not permit statistical analysis, mortality was 56 percent in the group of 18 patients with fixed pacing, compared to 38 percent in the group with demand pacing. Most studies have concluded that the poor prognosis in patients with conduction disturbances probably is not due to the disturbances themselves but rather to the extensive myocardial damage producing the disturbances *and* pump failure.

**Laboratory Data.** Blood urea nitrogen and uric acid elevation may be a consequence of diminished cardiac output, which results in diminished renal blood flow.[22] For similar reasons the serum creatinine may be elevated. The white cell count and erythrocyte sedimentation rate both reflect the presence of inflammation, as does a raised body temperature (see above).

In a number of studies it has been reported that either the maximum creatine kinase (CK) level [2,11,13] or maximum serum glutamic oxaloacetic transaminase (SGOT) level [15,17] relates to mortality. The level of enzyme release is believed to reflect the extent of myocardial damage. Enzymatic determination of "infarct size" was related to prognosis by Sobel et al.[40] In 33 patients, early death occurred in 8 of 12 patients with large infarcts compared to 1 of 21 patients with smaller infarcts. All 8 patients with large infarcts died as a result of pump failure. The one death in the small infarct group was sudden and unrelated to pump failure.

Recent work at the UCSD SCOR has shown that the peak CK value correlates well (r = .93) with CK area infarct-size estimates and relates to 30-day mortality.[11] Serial samples can be taken 6 hours apart and still yield a maximum CK value averaging 93 percent of the peak determined by sampling at 2-hour inter-

vals. A value greater than 85 percent of peak was obtained for 90 percent of all patients using 6-hour sampling.

Scheinman and Abbott [41] examined both the site of ECG changes and the level of enzyme rise in 230 patients with probable or definite myocardial infarctions. In 33 patients with ST segment or T wave changes, but only minimal enzyme rises, the Coronary Care Unit mortality was only 3 percent. For 45 patients with the same type of ECG findings, but having greater enzyme rises, the mortality was 37 percent. Among patients who developed Q waves in association with evolutionary changes in the ST segment and T wave, mortality was 19 percent. The authors concluded that the incidence of severe pump failure and mortality is closely reflected by the magnitude of the enzyme rise but not by the electrocardiographic changes.

**Hemodynamic Indices.** Chatterjee and Swan [42] constructed a classification based on left ventricular filling pressure (LVFP) and left ventricular stroke work index (LVSWI). For Group I patients with normal values (LVFP $<$ 15 mmHg and LVSWI 30 to 60 g-m/m²), mortality was 5.8 percent. Group II patients had an elevated LVFP ($>$ 16 mmHg) and a LVSWI $\geq$ 21 g-m/m², and a mortality of 26 percent. For Group III patients with an elevated LVFP and a depressed LVSWI ($<$21 g-m/m²), mortality was 80 percent. All patients received conventional therapy. Shubin et al.[43] used the technique of discriminant function analysis to construct an index based on cardiac output and blood flow velocity to correctly classify an estimated 95 percent of shock patients, but the study was based on only 20 patients.

Henning et al.[2] studied a representative group of patients from all Killip class strata and found that when LVFP, stroke volume index, and arteriovenous oxygen difference were included in a discriminant function analysis along with clinical and historic factors, 91 percent of early deaths (within 30 days) and 97 percent of survivors were correctly identified. This compares to 73 percent of early deaths and 97 percent of survivors when only noninvasive factors were used.

McHugh and Swan [44] also investigated various hemodynamic factors including LVFP, cardiac output, stroke volume, and the serial change in arterial $PO_2$ during $O_2$ breathing. The first three factors did not separate survivors and nonsurvivors well for their study group, and the authors concluded that a variety of compensatory mechanisms, such as catecholamine release, may result in increases in peripheral vascular resistance, heart rate, or the contractile state of the remaining myocardium so as to obscure the actual depressed state of myocardial function. Only when damage is so great that compensatory mechanisms fail are significant hemodynamic changes observed. They proposed that a temporary and reversible unmasking could be produced by a norepinehrine infusion. Serial arterial $PO_2$ measurements during $O_2$ breathing was another such challenge, and both did separate survivors from nonsurvivors better than hemodynamic variables. However, it should be emphasized that pressor challenge during acute myocardial infarction remains an experimental approach.

Several investigations have suggested that ejection fraction also might be a more sensitive indicator of function than the standard hemodynamic indices.[31,45,46] As an index of ventricular function, Nelson et al.[45] concluded that ejection fraction is more reliable than left ventricular end-diastolic pressure or cardiac index, since both of these indicators may be influenced by ventricular volume and compliance, while cardiac output is a function of numerous unrelated variables (venous return, aortic impedance, heart rate, stroke volume).

Until recently, this factor has not been routinely measured during the acute phase of myocardial infarction, but with the advent of radionuclide determinations of ejection fraction it is now feasible to obtain this measurement at the bedside (see Ch. 28). In the group of patients studied by Schulze,[27] all sudden deaths had an ejection fraction $< 40$ percent, together with Lown Class II to IV PVCs. Left ventricular ejection fraction by radionuclide angiography was assessed serially by Schelbert et al.[46] in 63 patients following acute myocardial infarction. The ejection fraction was reduced in 24 patients with mild to moderate left ventricular failure, and further reduced in 12 patients with overt pulmonary edema compared to the

24 patients with an uncomplicated infarct. Patients with an initially low or decreasing ejection fraction had a significantly greater incidence of early mortality (death within 60 days) than patients with initially normal ejection fractions or whose ejection fractions improved to normal (6/32 vs 0/18). The authors also found serial measurement of left ventricular ejection fraction a better measure of the functional state of the left ventricle than serial measurements of pulmonary artery wedge pressure or stroke volume.

Gated scintigraphy was used in a study by Rigo et al.[47] to compare left ventricular ejection fraction in a group of normal subjects to a group of patients with acute myocardial infarction. Twenty myocardial infarction patients were followed at 1 week and 3 months following the acute event, and the 14 who improved clinically also significantly increased their ejection fractions. Six patients who did not improve clinically showed no increase in ejection fraction. Also the ejection fraction was lower and the extent of akinesis higher in the patients who died compared to the survivors. Left ventricular filling pressure and cardiac index did not appear as sensitive as ejection fraction.

Recent work at the UCSD SCOR has shown that ejection fraction measured in early systole is more sensitive in detecting left ventricular dysfunction than is the total ejection fraction.[5] Accordingly, mortality at 1 year after myocardial infarction was examined for patients with a depressed first-third ejection fraction $(< .17)$ compared to those with a first-third ejection fraction $> .17$. Nine of the 23 patients in the second group died in the first year. It was concluded that a single determination of first-third ejection fraction early after infarction is just as good a predictor of prognosis as the serial approaches in earlier studies.

### Factors Related to the Patient's State.

Many of these factors are more likely to be related to long-term survival for the same reasons (sometimes only hypothesized) they are thought to be risk factors for coronary heart disease. Others probably have a direct complicating effect during the acute event.

**Age and Sex.** The incidence of myocardial infarction is much higher in men than in women, and women suffer their attacks at a more advanced age than men. In addition, compared to men in the same age group, the mortality for women is somewhat lower than for men. These two factors tend to cancel out each other. Women include a greater proportion of elderly patients more likely to die, but in each age group, women have a better chance of survival. The net result is that the overall mortality rate for women and men is equal.[23]

When patients were divided into "good-risk" and "bad-risk" groups according to whether or not they exhibited clinical shock or hypotension on admission, a history of congestive heart failure, dysrhythmias, gross cardiac enlargement, or diabetes mellitus, it was noted that good-risk patients had an increased mortality rate with advanced age. For bad-risk patients, however, this association was not apparent.[23] A similar observation based on high risk, defined by congestive heart failure, previous infarction, ventricular tachycardia, or conduction disturbances, was made by Weinberg.[48]

**Complicating Cardiac-Related Conditions.** Approximately 50 to 65 percent of patients with acute myocardial infarction give a history of ischemic heart disease, including angina pectoris, prior to infarction. Although this symptom usually indicates the presence of significant coronary artery obstructive lesions, the extent of the myocardium involved is extremely variable and, therefore, so is prognosis.[28] Patients with a previous myocardial infarction seem to have a poor prognosis after a second infarct, especially when reinfarction involves new areas of the left ventricle resulting in severe pump failure.[28]

Many studies have examined the relation of previous angina pectoris to short-term mortality (up to 1 month). However, not one has reported that the incidence of angina was significantly greater among those dying early. In one early study,[49] the incidence of angina among survivors (38 percent) was greater than for deaths (29 percent). The authors refer to the usual clinical impression that those patients without antecedent pain are caught unprepared, with less adequate collateral circulation, and suc-

cumb more easily. Several studies have, however, related the presence of angina to longer term mortality.[36,37,50-52] These studies indicate that a history of angina does have some bearing on the severity of the disease.

**Other Complicating Conditions.** Many of the factors commonly considered risk factors for the development of coronary artery disease have also been examined with respect to their influence on prognosis. These include such factors as hypertension,[49] diabetes,[23,51,52] obesity, lipid abnormalities, and cigarette smoking.[19,52] These factors are probably related more to the long-term progression of the disease than to prognosis immediately following the acute event. Only diabetes and hypertension have been related to early mortality (less than 1 month).[23,49]

Both a history of congestive heart failure and a history of chronic obstructive lung disease have been related to 30-day mortality.[2] A preliminary report by Oxman et al.[19] related a history of congestive heart failure to long-term mortality.

## MULTIVARIATE STUDIES

Many of the studies already cited related mortality not just to the primary factor of interest but also to the concomitant presence or absence of one or more other factors. The secondary factors in such studies were, in general, introduced because of specific mechanistic hypotheses, which might either worsen or ameliorate the primary condition.[7,9,30,32] Some investigators constructed classification schemes based on several specific factors, which then related directly to diminished cardiac performance due to myocardial damage.[12,18,31,41] A different philosophic direction from these approaches was taken by investigators who sought to utilize simultaneously a wide spectrum of factors that individually had previously been significantly related to prognosis.

This section describes the results of the application of these methodologies to mortality prediction or prognostic stratification following acute myocardial infarction. There are a few studies that manage to combine features of both major methodologies (see below), and these will be discussed where most appropriate. Following this review, the next section focuses on the advantages, disadvantages, features, and problems associated with the various methodologies and their clinical application. Finally, the last section emphasizes the importance of adequate validation.

Early approaches relied on trial and error directed by clinical judgment to select factors from those that were individually significant to use in the prognostic scheme. Some investigators used a computer to tabulate sample data, but the selection process was based on clinical judgment. Other investigators used the computer to exhaustively examine all possible combinations of two, three, and so on, factors and then, after examining the piles of generated output, selected the combinations that performed best. And, the computer itself has been called upon to select factors based on some programmed criteria.

## Approaches

There are basically two approaches to multivariate risk assessment. One approach seeks to determine a prognostic score for an individual patient based on a combination or weighted combination of various observed factors. It is unlikely that two patients will have identical prognostic scores, but presumably the range of scores can be broken into strata having increasing mortality. The second approach uses the factors themselves to define groups or strata with possibly differing mortality. For instance, patients with admission heart rates over 100/min and with systolic blood pressures less than 100 mmHg might be expected to have a higher mortality rate than patients without these findings, or with only one factor at risk.

**Prognostic Score Methodologies.** One of the first efforts toward multivariate prognostic assessment was made by Schnur in 1953.[53] He devised a "pathologic index" rating system that summed weights assigned to various factors, according to their relative importance in causing death. He acknowledged that these weights were derived from his own clinical experience and his review of other studies, and that others

might disagree with him concerning the significance of the factors selected. A total of 19 individual factors were included under the general headings of shock, congestive failure, serious arrhythmias, gallop rhythm, associated serious diseases, and a history of heart or vascular disease. Some factors such as shock, various arrhythmias, and gallop rhythm received fixed ratings. Others, such as congestive failure and associated diseases, both cardiovascular and otherwise, were given a range from which the user could select a rating according to his assessment of the severity of the findings. He applied his pathologic index rating to 230 patients surviving the first 24 hours after hospital admission, categorized them based on 20-point score increments into five groups, and then determined the 10-year mortality for each group. The mild group (with the lowest scores) experienced an 8 percent mortality and the critically-ill group (with the highest scores) a 95 percent mortality.

Peel et al. in 1962[54] improved upon this approach to develop their well-known "prognostic index." They limited the number of factors so that only six numbers had to be summed to obtain a patient's score. These numbers characterized: age and sex, previous history, shock, failure, the electrocardiogram, and rhythm disturbances. A great deal of effort went into carefully defining each rating within the categories to limit observer latitude and minimize differences of opinion. The derived prognostic index was applied to 628 patients and, again, patients were classified into five categories based on ranges of these index scores. The 30-day mortality for each class ranged from 2.5 percent for the lowest to 88.5 percent for the highest. Results for several sequential series of patients showed the same overall mortality trend with class, but mortality differed, sometimes very markedly (almost a factor of two), for a given class in the various series. The series were different in composition with respect to the proportion of cases falling within each class. Peel's prognostic index has been applied by other investigators and even used as a single "composite" variable in other multivariate schemes.[38,44]

Instead of defining the relative importance or weighting of various factors based on clinical judgment, statistical techniques have been used to derive them. Whether this is a step in the right direction remains to be seen.

These approaches—which include multiple regression, discriminant function analysis, and logistic discriminant function analysis—all derive weights, $W_i$, which are used to multiply the value of each factor, $X_i$, before the summation is made to obtain a score.

Score
$$= W_1X_1 + W_2X_2 + W_3X_3 + \cdots + W_kX_k$$

A discussion of the underlying assumptions and procedures for each of these methods will be given in the next section. Either the score, or some function of the score, is used as a basis for prognostic stratification or categorizing a patient as a death or a survivor.

Lemlich et al.[55] in 1963 applied stepwise linear regression to 371 patients in an attempt to determine which of nine factors first screened univariately were most important for predicting death or survival at 30 days. The goal of this project was more to explore the methodology applied to this problem than to develop a prognostic index. Attention was focused on the relative magnitude of the weights after all the factors had been scaled to standardized units. Blood pressure, a history of previous myocardial infarction, age, temperature, and duration of elevated temperature were identified, in the order listed, to be the most important factors.

Use of discriminant function analysis was reported by Hughes et al.[26] also in 1963 to predict in-hospital mortality in a group of 445 patients. Over 20 variables were included in the multivariate analysis. Variables with statistically significant weights were: age, white blood cell count, temperature, systolic blood pressure, presence of a conduction defect, pulmonary infarction, congestive heart failure, shock, hypertension along with congestive heart failure, and previous infarction together with diabetes. Variables included in the analysis, but not significant, were sex, previous infarction alone, angina, rhythm disturbance, hypertensive cardiovascular disease, diabetes alone, and selected combinations of two of the many factors. The resulting correct classification of the 445 patients was 97 percent for survivors and 80 percent for deaths. Only 37 patients were incorrectly classified, yielding an overall accuracy of 92 percent. Data on 38 of these patients were selected at random and given to 73 clinicians, who were asked to predict outcome. The average overall accuracy for the physicians was 68 percent, with the highest rate being 80 percent. The discriminant function correctly classified 35 of the 38 for an accuracy of 92 percent.

A report by Shubin et al.[43] in 1968 described discriminant function analysis applied to survival determination for 20 shock patients. Selected pairs and triplets from among 12 variables, not all of which were univariately significant, were submitted to discriminant function analysis. The pair that best discriminated deaths from survivors was stroke index and diastolic blood pressure. A discriminant score was computed for each of the 20 patients and compared to a cut-off point corresponding to a 50 percent chance of dying. The triplets, which rivaled the performance for this pair, included these factors and were not superior. Estimated prediction accuracy was 95 percent.

Norris and others[20,21] applied discriminant function methodology to both in-hospital mortality and 3-year mortality. Instead of using raw data (i.e, age in years or blood pressure in millimeters of mercury), all univariately significant variables were given values in the range of 0 to 1 based on the relative mortality observed for various intervals or categories. Scores were derived for patients using the discriminant function weights, applied to the scaled values, and then grouped into five categories that exhibited increasing mortality rates. These studies did not aim to predict survival in the individual patient but to define prognostic strata.

In 1968 McHugh and Swan[44] reported a prognostic index derived by linear regression analysis using hemodynamic, radiologic, and clinical factors. The study was based on only 42 patients but managed to classify these with 85 percent overall accuracy. The clinical criteria were synthesized into one number, the Peel index; also used were mixed venous $O_2$ saturation, and the product of heart rate and whether an x-ray film showed evidence of left ventricular failure (0 = no, 1 = yes). The authors did not mention how they selected the factors for analysis.

The Coronary Drug Project [33,50] submitted their extensive data on premature ventricular complexes and ECG findings to regression analysis along with other clinical data to investigate mortality in the late postinfarction period. The regression analysis was mainly used to examine the importance of various factors, but "clinical risk scores" were derived based on ECG data alone and the on the 10 best univariately significant clinical factors other than ECG data. Again, patients were grouped according to the level of their clinical risk score. Also the clinical score based on the non-ECG data was compared for the group of patients with normal baseline ECGs and those with abnormal findings. Baseline was taken about 1 month after the acute event. The mean clinical risk score was significantly higher for patients with abnormal ECGs compared to those with normal ECGs.

Sudden death up to 5 years following acute myocardial infarction was studied in 579 patients by Oxman et al.[19] and reported in 1973. Stepwise discriminant function analysis (see next section) was used and established cardiomegaly, diastolic hypertension, congestive heart failure, and cigarette smoking as the most important factors. The study classified 95 percent of survivors and 80 percent of sudden deaths correctly. Sex, angina postmyocardial infarction, and ventricular premature beats at 1 year were also univariately significant but were not selected by the stepwise discriminant function procedure.

A prognostic index for 2-year survival was reported by Luria et al.[36] in 1976 and was based on 143 patients surviving the hospital stay. From among 12 variables, which were significantly different for survivors, and the 27 patients who suffered cardiac death, the stepwise discriminant function analysis selected five factors. These were: admission systolic blood pressure, highest blood urea nitrogen level in the CCU, atrial arrhythmias in the CCU, angina pectoris for more than 3 months or a previous myocardial infarction, and more than one ventricular ectopic beat per hour recorded on a dynamic electrocardiogram during day 17 to 28 of hospitalization. Of the survivors, 93.6 percent were correctly classified, and of the deaths, 40.7 percent. These rates are based on a jackknife procedure (see Validation section).

A study from Europe, reported in 1978,[51] utilized linear regression applied to 42 factors established to be univariately significant in the population studied. The 312 myocardial infarction patients included were admitted to the study only if the onset of symptoms was within the previous 48 hours and the patient survived at least 48 hours after admission. Survival both at 1 and 6 months was predicted using different cut-off points on the scale of the prognostic score derived from the multivariate regression analysis. This scheme correctly classified 90.2 percent of the patients at 1 month and 85.7 percent at 6 months.

Henning et al.[2] recently reported the use of stepwise discriminant function analysis to predict 30-day mortality. First, only factors from the admission history were submitted to stepwise analysis. Next, factors from the physical examination, ECG, x-ray studies, and laboratory tests were added to the candidate set of factors. Finally, hemodynamic indices were also incorporated. The improvement in discrimination achieved by the addition of hemodynamic factors has already been discussed in the section on single factors. Factors selected by the discriminant function analysis for the set, including historic and noninvasive factors (based on 177 patients with complete data), included: age, history of a previous myocardial infarction, history of chronic obstructive lung disease, admission heart rate, whether rales could be detected above the scapula, the left heart dimension, the peak CK level in the first 24 hours, whether the ECG-determined infarct location was anterior, sinus tachycardia, and third-degree atrioventricular conduction block in the first 24 hours after admission. When hemodynamic factors were included in the analysis (94 patients with complete data), the set of variables selected differed. A history of congestive heart failure entered instead of chronic obstructive lung disease, rales and peak CK failed to enter, and ventricular fibrillation entered rather than sinus tachycardia. The hemodynamic variables that entered were: left ventricular filling pressure, atrioventricular oxygen difference, and stroke volume index. The different patient groups used in the analyses most likely account for these differences. Even though the patients studied hemodynamically came from all clinical strata, this group as a whole was probably more ill.

**Direct Factor Stratification.** This approach grew directly from the straightforward division of a patient population according to the level or the presence or absence of one or two factors. In some studies, the list of factors considered was limited to a specific type of factor, such as severity of rales or electrocardiographic findings, and these results have already been discussed.[8,30,32,42] In the work described below, the goal was to partition the postmyocardial infarction population into prognostic stata based on a wide spectrum of historic and clinical findings. Among the investigators involved in such studies have been Moss et al.[36-38] and Helmers.[15-17] Each has studied both the period immediately following hospitalization (4 to 6 months) and the long-term prediction window (2 to 3 years).

An early study by Moss et al.[38] used a combined regression and stratification approach. Patients (96 surviving beyond hospital discharge) were divided into two groups based on whether or not premature ventricular beats were present on a 6-hour, predischarge Holter monitor. Stepwise discriminant function analysis was then applied within each group to a variety of factors (univariately significant for that group), including the Peel and Norris indices. For the group without PVCs, age and the Peel index were selected. In the group with PVCs, age and whether or not the PVCs were frequent, in bigemial runs or pairs, and their degree of prematurity were selected. In the first group, 91 percent of both deaths and survivors were correctly classified. In the second group, 100 percent of deaths and 75 percent of survivors were classified correctly.

In 1976 these investigators reported a somewhat different approach.[27] The period studied was the 4 months immediately after hospital discharge, since most cardiac mortality following the acute myocardial infarction occurs during this time. Several schemes were constructed using 272 patients, and these were tested in 246 patients admitted later. A large number of variables were screened univariately and significant, clinically meaningful ones analyzed bivariately by looking at mortality in the groups with neither factor at risk, either factor at risk, and both factors at risk. All possible combinations of two and three factors were analyzed in this fashion.

The authors report on two such three-factor combinations, which best defined a high-risk group having a mortality significantly different from a low-risk group. The two schemes both included PVCs $\geq$ 20/hr on a 6-hour Holter recording prior to discharge, and a history of angina at ordinary levels of activity or rest. One scheme added a history of hypertensive cardiovascular disease and the other utilized CCU hypotension and/or congestive heart failure during hospitalization.

High-risk groups were defined as those patients having two or more of the three factors at risk. Note that this procedure is somewhat equivalent to assigning a prognostic score (0,1,2, or 3) and dividing the score range into two strata. The scheme utilizing CCU hypotension, congestive heart failure, or both, performed best. Mortality in the low-risk group was 3 percent as compared to 14 percent in the high-risk group. The authors mentioned a comparison of these results with those obtained using discriminant function analysis and logistic discriminant function analysis. Results were not presented but were said to be similar.

A recent preliminary report from this group[27] describes mortality in 940 patients based on a scheme utilizing the following factors: a previous myocardial infarction, pulmonary congestion in the CCU, and any PVC on a predischarge, 6-hour Holter monitor. The low-risk group had none of these factors, an intermediate group had either one or two, and the high-risk group all three. Mortality at 6 months was 2, 7, and 14 percent and at 24 months, 4, 12, and 23 percent for the low, intermediate, and high-risk groups, respectively.

The Helmers study[15] involved 606 patients and various periods of mortality: one day after admission, the second through the last day in the hospital, and up to 3 years following the acute event. A myriad of historic, symptomatic, physical, and ECG findings were examined with respect to each time interval. The Automatic Interaction Detector (AID) computer program was used in a stepwise fashion to select the most significant sets of variables for each time interval. The author noted that stepwise discriminant function analysis was also used and selected essentially the same sets. Rather than reproduce the resulting decision trees, which define the groups, only those groups having the largest and the smallest mortality rates will be described. For the first day, shock patients exhibited a 50 percent mortality compared to 1 percent in patients without shock who had, on admission, a respiration rate $< 26$/min and who were under age 70. For the duration of the hospital stay, the low mortality (5 percent) group was characterized by a respiration rate $< 20$/min and a maximum SGOT level $< 250$ IU. The high mortality (59 percent) group had a respiration rate $> 28$/min and a maximum SGOT $> 250$ IU. Low mortality (9 percent) for the long-term occurred in patients without a left bundle branch block (LBBB), who were under 70 years of age, or if older, who had a respiration rate $< 28$/min. High mortality (42 percent) was characterized by the presence of LBBB.

Identification of patients at high risk of in-hospital sudden death after discharge from the CCU was the goal of the study by Graboys.[25] In the study population of 759 definite myocardial infarctions, 144 in-hospital deaths occurred. Only 48 of these occurred after discharge from the CCU, and only nine of these patients died suddenly. One hundred patients who survived their hospital stay served as a comparison group. Compared to this group the sudden death group had a higher incidence of persistent sinus tachycardia, ventricular tachycardia, acute atrial fibrillation or flutter, conduction disturbances, and anterior wall infarction. Seven of the sudden death patients had at least three of these factors present compared to only 3 patients in the comparison group.

Weinberg[48] studied 154 patients who survived hospitalization and could be followed for 6 years. Many factors from the history, and especially the ECG during the hospital stay, were analyzed. Five factors were selected, which individually carried a higher risk of death

during this period, and a high-risk group was defined consisting of patients having one or more of these factors: congestive heart failure during hospitalization, major intraventricular conduction disturbances, history of a previous myocardial infarction, ventricular arrhythmias, and second- and third-degree atrioventricular block. One further modification was made to this scheme: both the low- and high-risk groups were subdivided according to age under and over 60 years. Mortality in the high-risk group was nearly the same for those under and over 60 years of age (48 and 51 percent, respectively). Those in the low-risk group under the age of 60, at the time of their myocardial infarction, had a 6-year death rate of 24 percent. In the over 60 category, mortality was 32 percent. Only the low-risk patients over 60 had a 6-year mortality comparable to actuarial projections for a normal age-matched population. In the other three groups, mortality was considerably higher than the actuarial projections.

Bigger et al.[22] recently reported a study of 6-month mortality in 100 patients who survived 10 days after the acute event. Eight variables from the history, physical examination, and hospital course were found to have prognostic value. All possible bivariate and trivariate combinations of these variables were examined in order to identify the best set for distinguishing deaths from survivors. For the bivariate combinations, patients with both factors present were compared to those with none or one. For the trivariate combinations, the comparison was between patients with all three and those having none, one, or two. The best combination was trivariate and included a peak CK level $> 585$ IU, a BUN level $> 20$ mg/dl at 2 weeks, and the presence of left ventricular failure (not defined) in the CCU. The mortality in the high-risk group was 55 percent compared to 5 percent for the low-risk group. The authors also observed that considering all eight factors, patients with two or three factors had 20 times the odds of dying in 6 months compared to those with none or one.

## Features and Limitations

The relative advantages and disadvantages of the various approaches to multivariate risk assessment can be summarized in a fashion to suit the prejudices of any individual investigator. An attempt will be made here to be as objective as possible.

**Prognostic Score Methods.** Techniques that count the number of factors present from a given list assign all an equal weight. Also, they assume that the presence of two factors is twice as bad as the presence of either one alone. In the realm of mathematics, this assumption is called "additivity." It may or may not be true, depending on the nature of the factors and how carefully they were selected. If some of the factors are simply different manifestations of the same underlying condition, the total score could be out of proportion to the importance of the underlying condition. On the other hand, the presence of two factors together might reflect a more severe state than indicated by the total contribution of the two separately. Many of the factor stratification studies are quests for this last eventuality. They seek to find a combination of factors that define a group having a mortality many-fold higher than the group with only one or neither of the factors present.

Straightforward, multiple, linear regression techniques, as applied to the problem at hand, predict death or survival as a linear function of a number of independent factors. Additivity for the independent factors is also assumed. However, these restrictions are not absolute and will be discussed in more detail below. The multiple regression procedure computes weights that minimize the sum of the squared difference between the actual and predicted state, using the weights over all patients in the sample analyzed. Once computed, these weights can be tested to see if they differ statistically from zero. Some of the studies described above report the set of weights for all variables, whether or not the weights are significant. Others point out that factors do have significant regression coefficients or weights. Just because a factor fails to have a significant weight does not mean that it is not related to prognosis. Indeed, most studies only analyze multivariately factors, which they have demonstrated to be univariately significant. What has happened is that one or more of the other predictive factors correlates with this factor and at the same time correlates slightly better with prognosis, so that the amount of additional variation in prognosis it accounts for is statistically insignificant.

The best possible prognostic score equation utilizes all of the predictive factors analyzed. The usual criterion for judging the "goodness of fit" is the square of the multiple correlation coefficient ($R^2$, where R is just a simple correlation coefficient between the predicted and actual outcomes), which gives the proportion of variation in the dependent variable explained by the set of independent variables used. Eliminating nonsignificant factors simplifies the application of the prognostic formula and usually only reduces the value of $R^2$ slightly. In fact, eliminating one of the significant factors might not reduce $R^2$ much at all, provided that one or more of the formally nonsignificant factors accounts for nearly the same amount of variance. Finding the smallest best possible set of factors from among all those to be analyzed would require repeated analyses of all possible combinations of two, three, four, and so on, of those considered—a tedious and expensive undertaking.

Fortunately, stepwise procedures exist that will seek out such a set of factors automatically. The factor that explains the greatest amount of variance in the dependent variable (death or survival) will enter first; the factor that explains the greatest amount of variance in conjunction with the first will enter second, and so on. Also, at any step factors previously entered may be removed if they do not explain a significant amount of variance given the others now included. The procedure terminates when all factors included do contribute significantly and those not included would not add appreciably to the amount of variance explained.

While most investigators employing regression techniques assume that the weighted factors are additive, the technique can be expanded to include combinations the investigator suspects may not be additive.

$$\text{Score} = W_1X_1 + W_2X_2 + W_3X_1X_2$$

The last term in the expression for the prognostic score would account for the additional severity above and beyond the sum of the contribution of each individually. The investigation by Hughes et al.[26] included such terms in its analysis.

Also, if the investigator has reason to suspect that the relationship between the dependent variable and an independent factor is not linear, he can introduce additional terms to account for this.

$$\text{Score} = W_1X_1 + W_2X_1^2 + W_3X_2$$

In this case the investigator suspects that the relation between death or survival and the factor $X_1$ is quadratic.

In the linear regression analysis technique just described, the dependent variable is assumed to be continuous; for predicting death or survival, this is clearly not the case. The researcher must arbitrarily divide the range of predicted scores into two regions, corresponding to death or survival. The technique of discriminant function analysis operates somewhat differently and does not make this assumption. Stepwise procedures seek, at each step, to select the variable that will increase the distance (in the space defined by the variables already selected plus the new one) between the group centroids. The centroids are simply the points in space corresponding to the mean value of each of the predictive factors considered. Also, at each step, factors already selected may be removed if they are found to reduce the distance between group centroids when combined with more recently selected factors.

Once the best set of predictors has been established, weights are determined for the discriminant function. Basically, these weights are computed by finding a hyperplane perpendicular to the direction determined by the group centroids. Figure 43.2 shows this geometry for two predictive factors $X_1$ and $X_2$. For two dimensions, the hyperplane is really a line. Where this line intersects the line determined by the centroids is a decision best made by the investigator. If a patient has values for $X_1$ and $X_2$ such that Score $= W_1X_1 + W_2X_2 \geq C$, he is classified into Group I, otherwise into Group II. The value of C determines where the intersection occurs.

Both the above methodologies use statistical tests to determine whether or not a factor contributes significantly. Strictly speaking, in order for these tests to be valid, the predictive factors

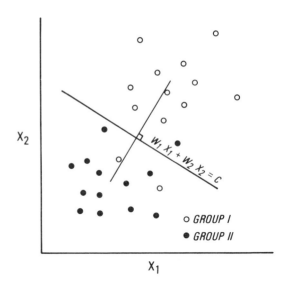

Fig. 43.2 A linear discriminant function based on two variables $X_1$ and $X_2$. A patient with data values such that $W_1X_1 + W_2X_2 \geq C$ would be classified into Group I. If instead, the values for $X_1$ and $X_2$ were such that $W_1X_1 + W_2X_2 < C$, the patient would be classified into Group II.

should have a joint multivariate normal probability distribution. In the context of mortality prediction after acute myocardial infarction, many of the factors, such as the presence or absence of pulmonary congestion, are not continuous, let alone normally distributed. In discriminant function analysis, the multivariate-normality theory allows a relationship to be derived which relates the discriminant score to the relative probability that a given patient belongs to one $P(G_1)$ of the two groups: typically, this relationship looks like the curve in Figure 43.3. The probability that he belongs to the other group is simply $P(G_2) = 1 - P(G_1)$. This interpretation is a useful tool for risk assessment in the individual patient.

Another assumption introduced by discriminant function analysis is that groups to be distinguished have equal variance-covariance matrices. This implies that the two distributions, though not centered at the same point in space defined by the predictive variables, have the same shape dispersion or scatter around that point.

Given that discriminant function analysis is such an appealing solution to the classification

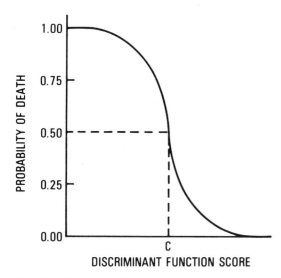

Fig. 43.3 The probability of early death as a function of the discriminant function score. The value C has been chosen to correspond to a probability of dying of 50 percent.

problem, statisticians have spent considerable effort trying to determine how robust the methodology is to the effects of violating the underlying assumptions. The chief consequence of differing covariance matrices is that cases are more likely to be classified into the group with the greatest overall dispersion. Many computer programs pool the covariance matrices to minimize this effect.[56] In cases where the best dividing partition is not a hyperplane but a curved hypersurface, the linear discriminant function method may only degrade classification performance slightly.[57] The use of existential or categorical predictive factors has also been investigated. It has been suggested [58] that transforming all predictive factors to the same scale or range might improve covariance homogeneity and classification performance. This possibility probably provided the motivation to Norris et al.[20,21] to give their factors values all in the zero-one range. Henning et al.[2] applied discriminant function analysis both to raw data, whether it be existential, categorical, or continuous, and to the same set of factors all converted to an existential scale. The results for each analysis were so similar that no advantage of one approach over the other was apparent.

Logistic discriminant function analysis avoids the normality assumption; factors need not even be continuous. Various approaches to this complex problem have been proposed.[59,60] All are conceptually complex. Only one report even mentions the use of this type of approach to the problem of risk assessment after acute myocardial infarction.[37] Results were not reported; it was reported only that they were similar to results obtained using discriminant function analysis and a direct factor stratification procedure. Packaged computer programs except for BMDP–79 do not as a rule include logistic discriminant techniques.[60a] The computational procedures that compute the weights are iterative and could be expensive in terms of computer time before convergence is reached. Additional experience with this technique relative to discriminant function analysis is necessary to see if the added complexity is worth any potential improvement in results. Although standard methodologies for both discriminant function analysis and logistic discriminant function analysis both assume linearity and additivity, both techniques can be modified, at the cost of added complexity and computational expense, to handle the more general case.

The regression approaches can produce, due to statistical artifact, weights that violate common sense. When this occurs, it is generally for a factor with relatively little prognostic value, given the other factors used and the sample of data analyzed. Eliminating the offending factor from the analysis usually improves overall classification slightly. Also, it is easy to see how the results of discriminant function analysis depend on the mean values (and less obviously, the dispersion) of the factors analyzed. If the sample used to construct the discriminant function is too small or aberrant to give good estimates of these population parameters, the resulting scheme may not perform well at all on a second set of data (see below).

These approaches have also been criticized because they do not demarcate discrete characteristics or groups but rather depend on a somewhat arbitrary division of the score scale to establish prognostic groups. Without such demarcation, the critics hold that little analytic or explicative insights are possible. For instance, subgroups with similar prognoses are disguised. These critics put more faith in schemes that seek out specific combinations of factors indicative of certain levels of mortality.

**Direct Factor Stratification Methodologies.** Many factors associated with prognosis are existential; either the finding is present or it is not present. A patient either has diabetes or he does not. Others are categorical, either discriptively or ordinally. Sex is descriptive and cardiac failure could be categorized as none, mild, moderate, or severe. Dividing the population using such factors is straightforward. However, other factors, such as heart rate and blood pressure, are measured more or less on a continuous scale. The factor stratification techniques reduce continuous data to a categorical and often to an existential scale. A patient's heart rate at hospital admission is greater than 100/min or it is not. Such data reduction can be looked upon as a loss of information or as a reduction in noise. Nevertheless, these techniques are free from any assumptions concerning the nature and shape of the underlying statistical distributions of the factors analyzed.

Finding combinations of factors that demark groups of patients having common prognoses is not a trivial task. Exhaustively examining all possible combinations of factors taken two at a time, three at a time, and so on, is no more appealing in this context than for the regression approaches, so analogous "stepwise" procedures have been developed. The various approaches explained in brief below all operate similarly. The main distinctions concern the specific criterion for factor selection. Basically, they select the factor that optimizes this criterion and partition the data sample into two subgroups based on the factor selected. For example, the first partition might be all patients under the age of 57 and all those older. Then for each subgroup so determined, a new search is made and the subgroup is further partitioned. Criteria for terminating the procedure usually involve some minimal subsample size or homogeneity consideration. Obviously, if all patients in a partition survived, there is no need to further subdivide it.

One approach uses as its factor selection criterion a variance reduction score.[61] Basically, an unpartitioned sample consisting of N cases, with mortality rate P and survival rate Q, has variance NPQ. After partitioning, the variance in each subsample is $n_i p_i q_i$. The proportionate reduction in overall variance is thus (NPQ − $\Sigma n_i p_i q_i$)/NPQ, which is called the variance reduction score. If the factor is not dichotomous, a cut-off point is first established for the factor, which maximizes the variance reduction score just for that factor. Partitioning continues until variance reduction is less than some arbitrary percent or the subsample is too small to partition further. The OSIRIS-AID computer program is based on this strategy.

Another approach maximizes the ratio of true-positives to false-positives (actual deaths/incorrectly predicted deaths) for each possible partition of a subgroup.[62] Again, it first establishes the best cut-off point for nondichotomous factors before selecting the best one. The effect of this criterion is to strip off extreme, homogeneous subgroups and then go to work on the residual group. The resulting scheme is called a diagnostic decision tree. A similar approach is described by Koss et al.[63] It simply selects the factor at each step, which cuts off the group having the highest mortality.

Recently the Kolmogorov-Smirnov criterion has been employed.[64,65] The technique, called recursive partitioning, selects the factor (first optimally dichotomized itself) that minimizes the overall misclassification rate within the subgroup being partitioned. Features have been incorporated into this methodology that will allow partitioning within a subgroup based on a discriminant function or some other weighted combination of the individual factors if it performs better than any single factor. Another potentially useful feature is that patients may be included, even if they have missing data for some factors. They simply are omitted in the analysis of that particular factor. If a partition is made using a factor for which a case has missing data, this case is classified during scheme construction according to the results of how the majority of a random sample from the parent subgroup were classified. When using such a scheme clinically, median values for the parent subgroup can be substituted for missing data. Other strategies are also possible.

The only reports so far of such schemes applied to the problem of prognosis after acute myocardial infarction are by Helmers.[15-17] The OSIRIS-AID computer program based on variance reduction was used. The diagnostic decision-tree was applied to the diagnosis of schizophrenic or excited versus nonschizophrenic and nonexcited patients.[62] The results in the second study were compared to those obtained by stepwise discriminant function analysis and were very similar. Some experience with the scheme, based on the Kolmogorov-Smirnov criteria, has been gained at the UCSD SCOR, using an expanded patient group from that described by Henning et al.[2] Preliminary results indicate that it is performing as well as discriminant function analysis, but included in the analyses are patients with incomplete data.

The classification problem has intrigued mathematicians for decades and their journals abound with schemes and theorems proving the optimal nature of various of their properties. No doubt some applications of these schemes exist, but experience with these methods in the relm of risk assessment after myocardial infarction is limited. However, these techniques hold much promise in that they do not make any assumptions concerning the nature of the factors' statistical distributions, additivity, or linearity. Conceivably, they might prove capable of isolating subgroups of patients with different characteristics, which, nonetheless, suffer the same mortality.

**Prognostic Stratification and Risk Prediction in the Individual Patient.** In many of the studies described above, categories were created either based on divisions along the scale of a prognostic score or by specific combinations of several factors. The mortality within each category was observed, thereby defining an associated level of risk. If the ultimate goal is to balance a clinical trial with respect to risk by including identical proportions from each risk category, this approach is adequate. But what about risk assessment in the individual patient? A patient's mortality is not 30 percent; it is either zero percent or 100 percent.

For patient management, it is not likely that a patient belonging to a group with a 20 percent risk of dying will be treated differently from one belonging to a 30 percent category. However, a patient in a group with a 20 percent risk of dying will almost surely be managed differently from one in a group having an 80 percent risk. Deciding on the cut-off point that will demarcate the low-risk from the high-risk group is tantamount to classifying patients as predicted survivors or predicted deaths. The threshold chosen will determine the error rate for such predictions.

Luria et al.[36] reported classification rates (93.6 percent for survivors and 40.7 percent for deaths) based on a 50 percent cut-off point and then noted that if the threshold for surviving was raised to 80 percent, the classification rates (72.7 percent for survivors and 77.8 percent for deaths) for both groups were nearly equal. The authors concluded that this second rule may be of greater usefulness for clinicians who are more interested in identifying deaths than concerned with incorrectly classifying survivors as deaths. This trade-off is a clinical decision and depends on the purpose of the risk assessment endeavor and the cost of misclassification and relative group sizes within that context.

**Sampling Considerations.** The results of the analysis will depend heavily on the actual sample of data collected. This fact explains, in part, the lack of concordance among the studies reviewed above. A previous history of myocardial infarction may well influence short- or long-term prognosis. If indeed it does, such influence is physiologic and should not be the product of sampling artifact. In one study, the incidence of previous infarction might be so nearly the same for both deaths and survivors that the factor has no prognostic value. In another study, the differential is pronounced and a history of previous infarction turns out to be very significant. Ideally, this shouldn't happen. In some sense, the early approaches by Schnur[53] and Peel[54] did not have to contend with the sampling problem. The weights were determined by clinical judgment rather than statistically from one sample of data.

For any prognostic scheme to be widely applicable, it should be based on a large, representative sample from the population of patients it is ultimately supposed to classify. It might be necessary to include patients from a broad spectrum of hospitals. Alone, none of the following types of hospitals could be expected to yield a representative sample: county hospital (largely treating an indigent patient population); Veterans Administration or military hospital; prepaid medical plan hospital; or exclusive private clinic.

The design of a risk-assessment scheme is necessarily retrospective. Data must be available that describe the initial state of a group of patients and the final target event—death or survival at some point in time after the initial state. Data are complete only after the target event has occurred so that the analysis can only be performed after the fact or retrospectively. The data can be obtained from routine medical records or from a preplanned research study, but the analysis required to develop the risk assessment scheme is nevertheless retrospective.

**Practical Considerations.** The investigator decides which factors to analyze initially, based on clinical judgment and the cost of obtaining certain data relative to its potential usefulness. If the scheme is to be widely applicable, factors not available to most clinicians, even if important, probably should not be used. Another investigator might argue with the choice of factors, the definitions of these factors and, if used, the weights applied to them. After screening the initial set univariately, some, probably not all, are included in the prognostic scheme. Whether the investigator makes this determination himself or relies on a computer to do it for him, the resulting scheme must make sense clinically.

Also, if the scheme is to be used in a clinical setting it must be logistically feasible. If any computations are required, it is essential that a computer programmed to do them be readily available. Hand-held, programmed calculators are probably adequate for most schemes. A doctor or nurse simply keys in a patient's data and either a prognostic score or a prognostic stratum identification is displayed.

Enough time must be allowed for data to be collected and verified prior to the time the actual risk assessment is to be made. This is a very real problem when predictions are made at admission regarding prognosis in the next several days. If factors such as an elevated BUN or leukocyte count are included, procedures must be specified for determining whether the elevated value is due to the patient's myocardial infarction or to some other chronic condition. Finally, how are patients with missing data to be handled? Using population mean values is not a very satisfactory solution. A possible solution might be to define a range of risk assuming the missing factor is at its worst or best possible state.

## Validation

Once a prognostic scheme is constructed, how can its expected accuracy be determined? One indication is how well it classifies the patients in the sample used to construct it. This procedure is called "resubstitution," and is what most reports cite. Obviously, such results depend on the sample used to construct the scheme and to give a biased view of how well the scheme might perform on a new, independent sample.

Ideally, the scheme should indeed be applied to new, independent samples and these "external" results compared ·‡ the ·internal" results obtained by resubstitution. A number of studies have reported results based on at least one validation sample with various degrees of success.[2,33,36,37,43,54,66]

There are, however, methods that can establish expected classification rates based on the original data sample, which are nearly unbiased. Two suggested procedures are called the Jackknife method [67] and the Bootstrap [68] method. Conceptually, these methods are easy to understand but tedious to apply, unless handled by a computer.

The Jackknife procedure omits, in turn, each patient from scheme construction and classifies the patient omitted based on the scheme derived from the other patients in the sample. The estimated correct classification rates are based on how each patient is classified using this procedure. Assuming that the original sample is representative, the Jackknife classification rates take into account the variability expected in the population and bias is reduced. Confidence limits can be constructed for the Jackknife classification rates. Henning et al.,[2] Luria,[36] and

Moss[38] reported their classification results based on the procedure.

The Bootstrap procedure selects subsamples with replacement (i.e., after a patient is drawn, he is put back in the hopper and can be drawn again), then it constructs a classification scheme based on the subsample and computes the difference (called the bias) for the classification rate determined by applying the scheme to all patients in the original sample and the resubstitution rates for the original scheme. After many repetitions, the average bias is computed and is used to adjust the resubstitution classification rate. Confidence limits can also be constructed for the adjusted or bootstrapped classification rates.

When discriminant function analysis is used and the predictive factors are truly multivariate normal (see above), a theoretical classification rate may be derived based on the degree of group overlap. Shubin et al.[43] computed this "reliability" for their discriminant function, using hemodynamic variables to predict death or survival for shock patients.

If an investigator is reasonably confident that his original sample is representative of the population to which his scheme will ultimately be applied, these classification-rate estimation procedures can help him evaluate whether it is worth validating his scheme using independent samples. Typically, resubstitution classification rates are too inflated to provide such guidance. If he proceeds with a validation in a new sample, and the results are not in agreement with the original resubstitution rates, he might feel he has failed. In reality, the scheme may have worked adequately and produced classification rates within the expected confidence limits.

## SUMMARY

Many researchers have devoted a great deal of effort to the search for accurate risk assessment following acute myocardial infarction. Yet the goals discussed in the introduction remain largely unrealized. The authors are unaware of a single reported instance where any prognostic scheme, using any of the methodologies described above, has actually been used either for patient management or in the design of clinical trials involving patients in a particular risk group. There have been some applications to the analysis of study results.[69,70] In these reports, multivariate regression techniques were applied to the study group to define risk strata within which the therapy of interest was evaluated.

Perhaps the very multitude of studies, each with its own unique set of factors, tends to discourage the actual use of such risk-assessment schemes. For patient management, clinicians prefer to rely on their own judgment and experience with the patient group they see. Indeed, there are undoubtedly factors that influence prognosis greatly that will never be objectively determined. These factors are intuitively apparent to the attending physician but can never be quantitated into a risk-assessment scheme. One wonders how the physicians in the study reported by Hughes et al.[26] would have performed if they had actually seen the patients rather than just their data. No doubt there would have been differences of opinion among the physicians due to their varied experience, skills, and sensitivity, but each would probably be willing to bet that his batting average would be better than that of any prognostic scheme. There is certainly a need for just such a (blinded) study.

In the design of randomized clinical trials, however, a prognostic index is clearly superior to the judgment of individual physicians. As long as the scheme has been properly validated on patient groups similar to those to be used in the trial, it can be used *reproducibly* and *without bias* to determine a patient's risk level. Patients in the risk group of interest can then be randomly assigned to either therapy or a control group. The concurrent, randomized, control group will then serve to establish that the population has not changed over time so that the assumptions incorporated into the design of the trial remain valid.

By far the biggest obstacle to the application of risk assessment methodologies is the necessity for accurate and timely data collection. Appropriate data collection forms and procedures are difficult enough to devise and implement in a research setting. In a clinical setting, the lack of time and personnel compound the problem. Only physicians dedicated to the goals and ideas behind risk assessment can successfully put it into practice.

# REFERENCES

1. Swan HJC, Blackburn HW, De Sanctis R, Frommer PL, Hurst JW, Paul O, Rapaport E, Wallace A, Weinberg S: Duration of hospitalization in "uncomplicated" completed acute myocardial infarction. Am J Cardiol 37:413, 1976.

1a. Schroeder JS, Lamb IH, and Hu M: Do patients in whom myocardial infarction has been ruled out have a better prognosis after hospitalization than those surviving infarction? N Engl J Med 303:1, 1980.

2. Henning H, Gilpin EA, Covell JW, Swan EA, O'Rourke RA, Ross J Jr: Prognosis after acute myocardial infarction: A multivariate analysis of mortality and survival. Circulation 59:1124, 1979.

3. California State Life Tables: 1959–1961. US Department of Health, Education and Welfare. Public Health Service, Washington, DC, 1966, pp 64.

4. Richards DW, Bland EF, White PD: A completed twenty-five year follow-up study of 456 patients with angina pectoris. J Chron Dis 4:423, 1956.

5. Battler A, Slutsky R, Karliner J, Froelicher V, Ashburn W, Ross J Jr: Left ventricular ejection fraction and first-third ejection fraction early after acute myocardial infarction: Predictive value for mortality and survival. Am J Cardiol 45:797, 1980.

6. Battler A, Karliner JS, Higgins CD, Slutsky R, Gilpin EA, Froelicher VF, Ross J Jr: The initial chest x-ray in acute myocardial infarction: prediction of early and late mortality and survival. Circulation 61:1004, 1980.

7. Cannom DS, Levy W, Cohen LS: The short and long term prognosis of patients with transmural and nontransmural myocardial infarction. Am J Med 61:452, 1976.

8. Killip T, Kimball JT: A survey of the coronary care unit: Concepts and results. In: Acute Myocardial Infarction in the Coronary Care Unit. Friedberg CK, editior. Grune and Stratton, New York, NY, 1969, p 281.

9. Kotler MN, Tabatanik B, Mower MN, Tominaga S: Prognostic significance of ventricular ectopic beats with respect to sudden death in the late post infarction period. Circulation 47:959, 1973.

10. Mullins CB, Atkins JM: Prognosis and management of ventricular conduction blocks in acute myocardial infarction. Mod Concepts Cardiovasc Dis 45:129, 1976.

11. Ryan W, Karliner JS, Gilpin EA, Covell JW, Deluca M, Ross J Jr: The creatine kinase (CK) curve area and peak CK after acute myocardial infarction: usefulness and limitations. Submitted for publication.

12. Rigo P, Murray M, Taylor DR, Weisfeldt ML, Strauss HW, Pitt B: Hemodynamic and prognostic findings in patients with transmural and nontransmural infarction. Circulation 51:1064, 1975.

13. Scwartz PJ, Wolf S: QT interval prolongation as predictor of sudden death in patients with myocardial infarction. Circulation 57:1074, 1978.

14. Kostuk W, Barr JW, Simon AL, Ross J Jr: Correlations between the chest film and hemodynamics in acute myocardial infarction. Circulation 48:624, 1973.

15. Helmers C: Short and long term prognostic indices in acute myocardial infarction: A study of 606 patients initially treated in a CCU. Acta Med Scand (Suppl) 555, 1973.

16. Helmers C: Assessment of 3-year prognosis in survivors of acute myocardial infarction. Br Heart J 37:593, 1975.

17. Helmers C: Respiratory rate and its relationship to mortality and mode of death in and after acute myocardial infarction. Herz 2:459, 1977.

18. Forrester JS, Diamond GA, Swan HJC: Correlative classification of clinical and hemodynamic function after acute myocardial infarction. Am J Cardiol 39:137, 1977.

19. Oxman H, Connolly DC, Nobrega FT, Titus JL: Identification of patients at highest risk for sudden death within five years following their first myocardial infarction (abstr). Am J Cardiol 31:150, 1973.

20. Norris RM, Caughey DE, Mercer CJ, Deeming LW, Scott PJ: Coronary prognostic index for predicting survival after recovery from acute myocardial infarction. Lancet 2:485, 1970.

21. Norris RM, Brandt PWT, Caughey DE, Lee AJ, Scott PJ: A new coronary prognostic index. Lancet 1:224. 1969.

22. Bigger JT, Heller CA, Wenger TL, Weld FM: Risk stratification after acute myocardial infarction. Am J Cardiol 42:202, 1978.

23. Honey GE, Truelove SC: Prognostic factors in myocardial infarction. Lancet 1:1155, 1957.

24. Meltzer LE, Kitchell R: The development and current status of coronary care. In: Textbook of Coronary Care. Meltzer LE, Danning AJ, edi-

tors. The Charles Press, Philadelphia, 1972, p 3.

25. Graboys TB: In-hospital sudden death after coronary care unit discharge. A high-risk profile. Arch Intern Med 135:513, 1975.

26. Hughes WL, Kalbfleish JM, Brandt EN, Costiloe JP: Myocardial infarction prognosis by discriminant analysis. Arch Intern Med 111:120, 1963.

27. Moss AJ, Davis H, DeCamilla J: Survivorship patterns after myocardial infarction: Implications for intervention trials (abstr). Circulation 57, 58 (suppl II):152, 1978.

28. Chatterjee K, Brundage BH: Prognostic factors in acute myocardial infarction. Pract Cardiol March:23, 1978.

29. James TN: Myocardial infarction and atrial arrhythmias. Circulation 24:761, 1961.

30. Vismara LA, Amsterdam EA, Mason DT: Relation of ventricular arrhythmias in the late hospital phase of acute myocardial infarction to sudden death after hospital discharge. Am J Med 59:6, 1975.

31. Schulze RA, Strauss HW, Pitt B: Sudden death in the year following myocardial infarction. Am J Med 62:192, 1977.

32. Ruberman W, Weinblatt E, Frank CW, Goldberg JD, Shapiro S, Feldman CL: Ventricular premature beats and mortality of men with coronary heart disease. Circulation 51, 52 (suppl III):199, 1975.

33. The Coronary Drug Project Research Group: The prognostic importance of premature ventricular complexes in the late post-infarction period. Acta Cardiol (Suppl) 18:33, 1974.

34. Morganroth J, Michelson EL, Horowitz LN, Josephson ME, Pearlman AS, Dunkman WB: Limitations of routine long-term electrocardiographic monitoring to assess ventricular ectopic frequency. Circulation 58:408, 1978.

35. Engler R, Ryan W, LeWinter M, Bluestein H, Karliner JS: Assessment of long-term antiarrhythmic therapy: Studies on the long-term efficacy and toxicity of tocanide. Am J Cardiol 43:612, 1979.

36. Luria MH, Knoke JD, Margolis RM, Hendricks FH, Kuplic JB: Acute myocardial infarction: Prognosis after recovery. Ann Intern Med 85:561, 1976.

36a. Lown B, Wolf MA: Approaches to sudden death from Coronary heart disease. Circulation 44:130, 1971.

37. Moss AJ: The early posthospital phase of myocardial infarction. Prognostic stratification. Circulation 54:58, 1976.

38. Moss AJ, DeCamilla J, Engstrom F, Hoffman W, Odoroff C, Davis H: The post hospital phase of myocardial infarction: Identification of patients with increased mortality risk. Circulation 49:460, 1974.

39. Sutton R, Chatterjee K, Leatham A: Heart block following acute myocardial infarction. Lancet 2:648, 1968.

40. Sobel BE, Breshnahan GF, Shell WE, Yoder RD: Estimation of infarct size in man and its relation to prognosis. Circulation 46:640, 1972.

41. Scheinman MM, Abbott JA: Clinical significance of transmural versus nontransmural electrocardiographic changes in patients with acute myocardial infarction. Am J Med 55:602, 1973.

42. Chatterjee K, Swan HJC: Hemodynamic profile in acute myocardial infarction. In Myocardial Infarction. Corday E, Swan HJC, editors. Williams and Wilkins, Baltimore, 1975, p 51.

43. Shubin H, Afifi AA, Rand WM, Weil MH: Objective index of hemodynamic status for quanitation of severity and prognosis of shock complicating myocardial infarction. Cardiovasc Res 4:329, 1968.

44. McHugh TJ, Swan HJC: Prognostic indicators in acute myocardial infarction. Geriatrics 26:72, 1971.

45. Nelson GR, Cohn PF, Gorlin R: Prognosis in medically treated coronary artery disease: Influence of ejection fraction compared to other parameters. Circulation 52:408, 1975.

46. Schelbert HR, Henning H, Ashburn WL, Verba JW, Karliner JS, O'Rourke RA. Serial measurements of left ventricular ejection fraction by radionuclide angiography early and late after myocardial infarction. Am J Cardiol 38:407, 1976.

47. Rigo R, Murray M, Strauss NW, Taylor D, Kelly D, Weisfeldt M, Pitt B. Left ventricular function in acute myocardial infarction evaluated by gated scintiphotography. Circulation 50:678, 1974.

48. Weinberg SL: Natural history six years after acute myocardial infarction. Is there a low-risk group? Chest 69:23, 1976.

49. Rosenbaum FF, Levine FA: Prognostic value of various clinical and electrocardiographic features of acute myocardial infarction. Arch Intern Med 68:913, 1941.

50. The Coronary Drug Project Research Group: The prognostic importance of the electrocardiogram after myocardial infarction. Ann Intern Med 77:677, 1972.

51. Beaume J, Touboul P, Boissel JP, Delahaye JP: Quantitative assessment of myocardial infarction prognosis 1 and 6 months—from clinical data. Eur J Cardiol 8:629, 1978.

52. Cole DR, Singian EB, Katz LN: The long-term

prognosis following myocardial infarction and some factors which affect it. Circulation 9:321, 1954.

53. Schnur S: Mortality rates in acute myocardial infarction, II: A proposed method for measuring quantitatively severity of illness on admission to the hospital. Ann Intern Med 39:1018, 1953.

54. Peel AA, Semple T, Wang I: A coronary prognostic index for grading the severity of infarction. Br Heart J 26:745, 1962.

55. Lemlich A, Covo G, Ziffer H: Multivariate analysis of prognostic factors in myocardial infarction. In: Data Acquisition and Processing in Biology and Medicine. Proceedings. Vol 3. Rochester Conference on Data Acquisition and Processing in Biology and Medicine. Enslein K, editor. Macmillan, New York, 1963, pp 65–81.

56. Cornfield J: Discriminant functions. In Proceedings, Sixth IBM Medical Symposium. White Plains, NY, 1964, pp 567–589.

57. Michaels J: Simulation experiments with multiple group linear and quadratic discriminant analysis. In: Discriminant Analysis and Applications. Cacoullos T, editor. Academic Press, New York, 1973, pp 225–238.

58. Gilbert E: On discrimination using qualitative variables. J Am Stat Assoc 63:1399, 1968.

59. Anderson JA: Logistic Discrimination with Medical Applications. In: Discriminant Analysis and Applications. Cacoullos T, editor. Academic Press, New York, 1973, pp 1–16.

60. Walker SH, Duncan DB: Estimation of probability of an event as a function of several independent variables. Biometrika 54:167, 1967.

60a. Biomedical Computer Programs P-Series. Dixon WJ, Brown MB, editors. University of California Press, Los Angeles, 1979, p. 517.1–517.13.

61. Feinstein AR: The process of prognostic stratification, part I. Clin Pharmacol Ther 13:442, 1972.

62. Klein DF, Honigfeld G, Feldmen S: Prediction of drug effect by diagnostic decision tree. Dis Nerv Syst 29:159, 1968.

63. Koss N, Feinstein AR: Computer aided prognosis II: Development of a prognostic algorithm. Arch Intern Med 127:448, 1971.

64. Gordon L, Olshen RA: Asymptotically efficient solutions to the classification problem. Ann Stat 6–3:515, 1978.

65. Friedman JH: A recursive partioning decision rule for nonparametric classification. IEEE Trans on Comp C-26:104, 1977.

66. Luria MH, Knoke JD, Wachs JS, et al: Survival after recovery from acute myocardial infarction; two year and five year prognostic indices. Am J Med 67:9, 1979.

67. Lachenbruch PA: An almost unbiased method of obtaining confidence intervals for the probability of misclassification in discriminant analysis. Biometrics 23:639, 1967.

68. Efron B: Bootstrap methods: Another look at the Jackknife. Ann Stat 7–1:1, 1979.

69. Wilhelmsen L, Sann H, Elmfeldt D, et al: A controlled trial of physical training after myocardial infarction. Prev Med 4:491, 1975.

70. Miettines OS: Stratification by a multivariate confounder score. Am J of Epidemiol 104:609, 1976.

## ACKNOWLEDGMENT

Supported by Specialized Center of Research on Ischemic Heart Disease NIH Research Grant HL-17682 from the National Heart, Lung and Blood Institute.

# INDEX